Textbook of Neural Repair and Rehabilitation

In two freestanding volumes, Textbook of Neural Repair and Rehabilitation provides comprehensive coverage of the science and practice of neurological rehabilitation. This volume, Medical Neurorehabilitation, can stand alone as a clinical handbook for neurorehabilitation. It covers the practical applications of the basic science principles presented in Volume I, provides authoritative guidelines on the management of disabling symptoms, and describes comprehensive rehabilitation approaches for the major categories of disabling neurological disorders. Emphasizing the integration of basic and clinical knowledge, this book and its companion are edited and written by leading international authorities. Together they are an essential resource for neuroscientists and provide a foundation for the work of clinical neurorehabilitation professionals.

Michael E. Selzer is Professor of Neurology at the University of Pennsylvania and Research Director in the Department of Physical Medicine Rehabilitation. He is editor-in-chief of Neurorehabilitation and Neural Repair, the official Journal of the American Society of Neurorehabilitation and the World Federation of Neurorehabilitation.

Leonardo G. Cohen is Chief of the Human Cortical Physiology Section and the Stroke Rehabilitation Clinic at the National Institute of Neurologic Disorders and Stroke, National Institutes of Health, Bethesda.

Stephanie Clarke is Professor and Head of Neuropsychology at the University Hospital, Lausanne and President of the Swiss Society of Neurorehabilitation.

Pamela W. Duncan is Professor of Health Services Administration and Physical Therapy, and Director

of the Brooks Center for Rehabilitation Studies,
University of Florida.

Fred H. Gage is Professor in the Laboratory of
Genetics at the Salk Institute, and served as
President of the Society for Neuroscience,
2001–2002. He is a fellow of the American
Association for the Advancement of Science
and a member of the National Academy of
Sciences and the Institute of Medicine.

Textbook of
Neural Repair
and Rehabilitation

Volume II
Medical
Neurorehabilitation

EDITED BY

Michael E. Selzer
University of Pennsylvania

Stephanie Clarke
University of Lausanne

Leonardo G. Cohen
National Institutes of Health

Pamela W. Duncan
University of Florida

Fred H. Gage
The Salk Institute

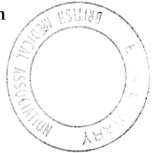

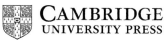

CAMBRIDGE
UNIVERSITY PRESS

CAMBRIDGE UNIVERSITY PRESS
Cambridge, New York, Melbourne, Madrid, Cape Town, Singapore, São Paulo

CAMBRIDGE UNIVERSITY PRESS
The Edinburgh Building, Cambridge CB2 2RU, UK

Published in the United States of America by Cambridge University Press, New York

www.cambridge.org
Information on this title: www.cambridge.org/9780521856416

First published 2006

Printed in the United Kingdom at the University Press, Cambridge

A catalog record for this book is available from the British Library

Library of Congress Cataloging in Publication data

Volume I:
ISBN-10 0-521-85641-8
ISBN-13 978-0-521-85641-6
Volume II:
ISBN-10 0-521-85642-6
ISBN-13 978-0-521-85642-3
2 Volume set:
ISBN-10 0-521-83639-5
ISBN-13 978-0-521-83639-5

Every effort has been made in preparing this book to provide accurate and up-to-date information which is in accord with accepted standards and practice at the time of publication. Although case histories are drawn from actual cases, every effort has been made to disguise the identities of the individuals involved. Nevertheless, the authors editors and publishers can make no warranties that the information contained herein is totally free from error, not least because clinical standards are constantly changing through research and regulation. The authors, editors and publishers therefore disclaim all liability for direct or consequential damages resulting from the use of material contained in this book. Readers are strongly advised to pay careful attention to information provided by the manufacturer of any drugs or equipment that they plan to use.

Contents (contents of Volume II)

Contents (contents of Volume I)

Preface

Neurorehabilitation is a medical specialty that is growing rapidly because medical advances have extended life expectancy and saved the lives of persons who previously would not have survived neurological injury. It is now urgent to develop a rigorous scientific basis for the field. The basic science relevant to functional recovery from neural injury is perhaps the most exciting and compelling of all the medical sciences. It encompasses areas of plasticity, regeneration and transplantation in the nervous system that individually have been the subjects of many monographs. With the *Textbook of Neural Repair and Rehabilitation*, these areas are integrated with each other and with the clinical topics to which they apply.

The *Textbook of Neural Repair and Rehabilitation* is organized into two volumes. *Volume I, Neural Repair and Plasticity* can stand alone as a textbook for graduate or advanced undergraduate level courses on recovery from neural injury. It is subdivided into two sections: *Section A, Neural Plasticity and Section B, Neural Repair.* Following an injury to the nervous system, most patients partially regain function. *Section A, Plasticity*, addresses the mechanisms that underlie spontaneous recovery as well as the added recovery induced by therapies based on use, retraining and pharmacological manipulations. The chapters cover the anatomical and physiological responses of neurons to injury, mechanisms of learning and memory, and plasticity in specific areas of the nervous system consequent to intense use, disuse and injury. Ultimately, interventions aimed at repairing the damaged neural circuitry will be required if full function is to be restored. Thus *Section B, Neural Repair*, covers topics on neuronal death, trophic factors, axonal regeneration and the molecules that inhibit it, stem cell biology, and cell transplantation. *Section B* builds on *Section A* because the mechanisms of plasticity will have to be invoked to translate restored neuronal connections into useful function.

Volume II, Medical Neurorehabilitation can stand alone as a clinical handbook for physicians, therapists, rehabilitation nurses and other neurorehabilitation professionals. It is organized into three sections. *Section A, The Technology of Neurorehabilitation*, is a direct transition from *Volume I*, emphasizing the applications of basic scientific principles to the practice of neurorehabilitation. This section includes material on functional imaging, motor control, gait and balance assessment, electrodiagnosis, virtual reality, and bioengineering and robotic applications to prosthetics and orthotics. *Section B, Symptom-Specific Neurorehabilitation*, provides guidelines to managing spasticity, gait disorders, autonomic and sexual dysfunction, cognitive deficits and other disabling neurological symptoms that are common to many disorders. *Section C, Disease-Specific Neurorehabilitation*, describes comprehensive approaches to the rehabilitation of persons suffering from the major categories of disabling neurological disorders, such as spinal cord injury, multiple sclerosis, stroke and neurodegenerative diseases.

Wherever possible, the chapters in this book refer the reader back to chapters that deal with relevant material at a different level. It is hoped that by stressing the integration of clinical and basic scientific knowledge, this book will help to advance the quality and scientific rigor of neurorehabilitation.

Contributors (contributors of Volume II)

Mindy L. Aisen, MD
United Cerebral Palsy Research and Education
Foundation
Department of Neurology and Neuroscience,
Georgetown University

Gad Alon, PT, PhD
Department of Physical Therapy and
Rehabilitation Science
University of Maryland School of Medicine
Baltimore, MD, USA

Frank Andrasik, PhD
Institute for Human and Machine Cognition
University of West Florida
Pensacola, FL, USA

Antoaneta Balabanov, MD
Department of Neurological Sciences
Rush Medical College
Chicago, IL, USA

Michael P. Barnes, MD, FRCP
Department of Neurological Rehabilitation
Hunters Moor Regional Neurological
Rehabilitation Centre
Newcastle upon Tyne, UK

Serafin Beer, MD
Department of Neurology and Neurorehabilitation
Rehabilitation Centre
Valens, Switzerland

Claire Bindschaedler, PhD
Division de Neuropsychologie
Centre Hospitalier Universitaire Vaudois
Lausanne, Switzerland

Sarah Blanton, DPT, NCS
Department of Rehabilitation Medicine
Emory University
Atlanta, GA, USA

Michael L. Boninger, MD
Department of Rehabilitation
Science & Technology
University of Pittsburgh School of
Health and Rehabilitation Sciences
Pittsburgh, PA, USA

Carole W. Brown, EdD
Department of Education
The Catholic University of America
Washington, DC, USA

Stefano F. Cappa, MD
Department of Neuroscience
Vita-Salute University and San Raffaele
Scientific Institute
Milano, Italy

Diana D. Cardenas, MD, MHA
Department of Rehabilitation Medicine
University of Washington
Seattle, WA, USA

Leeanne Carey, BAppSc(OT), PhD
School of Occupational Therapy
Faculty of Health Sciences
LaTrobe University
Bundoora, Victoria, Australia

Stephanie Clarke, MD
Division de Neuropsychologie
Centre Hospitalier Universitaire Vaudois
Lausanne, Switzerland

Rory A. Cooper, PhD
Department of Rehabilitation
Science & Technology
University of Pittsburgh School of
Health and Rehabilitation Sciences
Pittsburgh, PA, USA

Rosemarie Cooper, MPT, ATP
Department of Rehabilitation
Science & Technology
University of Pittsburgh School of
Health and Rehabilitation Sciences
Pittsburgh, PA, USA

Mark D'Esposito, MD
Departments of Neuroscience and Psychology
Helen Wills Neuroscience Institute
University of California, Berkeley
Berkeley, CA, USA

Volker Dietz, MD, FRCP
Spinal Cord Injury Center
University Hospital Balgrist
Forchstr, Zurich, Switzerland

Bruce H. Dobkin, MD, FRCP
Department of Neurology
David Geffen School of Medicine, UCLA
Los Angeles, CA, USA

Neila J. Donovan, MA
Department of Communicative Disorders
VA RR&D Brain Rehabilitation Research Center
University of Florida
Gainesville, FL, USA

William K. Durfee, PhD
Department of Mechanical Engineering
University of Minnesota
Minneapolis, MN, USA

Gammon M. Earhart, PT, PhD
Program in Physical Therapy
Washington University School of Medicine
St. Louis, MO, USA

Georg Ebersbach, MD
Neurologisches Fachkrankenhaus
für Bewegungsstörungen/Parkinson
Beelitz-Heilstätten, Germany

Jonathan Evans, PhD
Section of Psychological Medicine
Gartnavel Royal Hospital
Glasgow, UK

Uri Feintuch, PhD
School of Occupational Therapy
Hadassah-Hebrew University
Jerusalem, Israel
Caesarea-Rothschild Institute for Interdisciplinary
Applications of Computer Science, University of
Haifa
Haifa, Israel

Peter J. Flett, MD
Department of Child and Adolescent Development,
Neurology and Rehabilitation, Women's and
Children's Hospital
North Adelaide
Melbourne, Victoria, Australia
Present Address:
Paediatric Rehabilitation,
Calvary Rehabilitation Services,
Hobart, Tasmania

Herta Flor, PhD
Department of Clinical and Cognitive
Neuroscience
University of Heidelberg
Central Institute of Mental Health
Mannheim, Germany

Richard S.J. Frackowiak, MD, PhD
Wellcome Department of Imaging Neuroscience
Institute of Neurology
University College London
London, UK

Adam Gazzaley
Helen Wills Neuroscience Institute and
Department of Psychology

University of California, Berkeley
Berkeley, CA, USA

David A. Gelber, MD
Springfield Clinic Neuroscience Institute
Springfield, IL, USA

Peter H. Gorman, MD
Department of Neurology and Rehabilitation
The James Lawrence Kernan Hospital
Baltimore, MD, USA

H. Kerr Graham, MD
Department of Orthopaedics,
University of Melbourne
The Royal Children's Hospital
Parkville, Victoria, Australia

Murray Grossman, MD, EdD
Department of Neurology
University of Pennsylvania School of Medicine,
Philadelphia, PA, USA

Amparo Gutierrez, MD
Department of Neurology
Louisiana State University Medical Center
New Orleans, LA, USA

Courtney D. Hall, PT, PhD
Atlanta Veterans Administration
Rehabilitation Research and Development, Decatur
Department of Rehabilitation Medicine
Emory University
Atlanta, GA, USA

Hans-Peter Hartung, MD
Department of Neurology
Heinrich-Heine-University
Düsseldorf, Germany

Susan J. Herdman, PhD, PT FAPTA
Atlanta Veterans Administration
Rehabilitation Research and Development, Decatur

Departments of Rehabilitation Medicine and
Otolaryngology-Head and Neck Surgery
Emory University
Atlanta, GA, USA

Hugh M. Herr, PhD
The Media Laboratory and The Harvard/MIT
Division of Health Sciences and Technology
Cambridge, MA, USA

Neville Hogan, PhD
Departments of Mechanical Engineering,
and Brain and Cognitive Sciences
Massachusetts Institute of Technology
Cambridge, MA, USA

Fay B. Horak, PhD, PT
Neurological Sciences Institute
Oregon Health & Science University
Beaverton, OR, USA

Jessica Johnson, OTR
Department of Occupational Therapy
University of Florida
Gainesville, FL, USA

Andres M. Kanner, MD
Department of Neurological Sciences
Rush Medical College
Chicago, IL, USA

Noomi Katz, MD
School of Occupational Therapy
Hadassah-Hebrew University,
Jerusalem, Israel

Danielle M. Kerkovich, PhD
Rehabilitation Research and Development Service
Department of Veterans Affairs
Washington, DC, USA

Jürg Kesselring, MD
Department of Neurology and
Neurorehabilitation
Rehabilitation Centre
Valens, Switzerland

Rachel Kizony, MSc
School of Occupational Therapy
Hadassah-Hebrew University, Jerusalem, Israel
Department of Occupational Therapy
University of Haifa
Haifa, Israel

Hubertus Köller, MD
Department of Neurology
Heinrich-Heine-University
Düsseldorf, Germany

Hermano Igo Krebs, PhD
Department of Mechanical Engineering
Massachusetts Institute of Technology,
Cambridge, MA, USA
Department of Neuroscience
The Winifred Masterson Burke Medical
Research Institute
Weill Medical College of Cornell University
New York, NY, USA

Catherine E. Lang, PT, PhD
Program in Physical Therapy
Washington University School of Medicine
St. Louis, MO, USA

James S. Lieberman, MD
Department of Rehabilitation Medicine
Columbia University College of Physicians and
Surgeons
New York, NY, USA

Francesco Lombardi, MD
Riabilitazione Intensiva Neurologica
Ospedale di Correggio
Correggio, Reggio, Emilia, Italy

Marilyn MacKay-Lyons, PhD
School of Physiotherapy
Dalhousie University
Halifax, Nova Scotia, Canada

Brenda S. Mallory, MD
Department of Rehabilitation Medicine
Columbia University College of Physicians &
Surgeons
New York, NY, USA

Francine Malouin, PhD, PT
Department of Rehabilitation and Centre for
Interdisciplinary Research in Rehabilitation and
Social Integration
Laval University
Quebec City, Quebec, Canada

William C. Mann, OTR, PhD
Department of Occupational Therapy
University of Florida
Gainesville, FL, USA

Beth Mineo Mollica, PhD
Center for Applied Science & Engineering and
Department of Linguistics
University of Delaware
Wilimington, DE, USA

C. Warren Olanow, MD
Departments of Neurology
Mount Sinai School of Medicine
New York, NY, USA

P. Hunter Peckham, PhD
Department of Biomedical Engineering
Case Western Reserve University and FES Center of
Excellence
Cleveland VA Medical Center
Cleveland, OH, USA

Thomas Platz, MD
Department of Neurological Rehabilitation
Free University Berlin
Berlin, Germany

Werner Poewe, MD
Department of Neurology
Medical University Innsbruck
Innsbruck, Germany

Karen T. Reilly, PhD
Department of Neurobiology and Anatomy
University of Rochester School of Medicine &
Dentistry
Rochester, NY, USA

Carol L. Richards, PhD
Department of Rehabilitation and Centre for
Interdisciplinary Research in Rehabilitation and
Social Integration
Laval University
Quebec City, Quebec, Canada

Keith M. Robinson, MD
Department of Physical Medicine and
Rehabilitation
University of Pennsylvania School of Medicine
Philadelphia, PA, USA

John C. Rosenbek, PhD
Department of Communicative Disorders
VA RR&D Brain Rehabilitation Research Center
University of Florida
Gainesville, FL, USA

Marc H. Schieber, MD, PhD
Department of Neurology
University of Rochester School of Medicine &
Dentistry
Rochester, NY, USA

Brian J. Snyder, MD
Department of Neurosurgery
Mount Sinai School of Medicine
New York, NY, USA

Jill Campbell Stewart, MS, PT, NCS
Department of Biokinesiology and Physical
Therapy
University of Southern California
Los Angeles, CA, USA

Nancy E. Strauss, MD
Department of Rehabilitation Medicine
Columbia University College of Physicians and
Surgeons
New York, NY, USA

Sheela Stuart, PhD
Children's Hearing and Speech Center
Children's National Medical Center
Washington, DC, USA

Austin J. Sumner, MD
Department of Neurology
Louisiana State University Medical Center
New Orleans, LA, USA

Antonio De Tanti, MD
Responsabile U.O. Gravi Cerebrolesioni e Disturbi
Cognitivi
Centro Riabilitativo "Villa Beretta"
Costamasnaga, Lecco, Italy

Cheryl Y. Trepagnier, PhD
Department of Psychology
The Catholic University of America
Washington, DC, USA

Nick S. Ward, MD, MRCP
Wellcome Department of Imaging Neuroscience
Institute of Neurology
University College London
London, UK

Catherine Warms, PhD, RN, ARNP, CRRN
Department of Rehabilitation Medicine
University of Washington
Seattle, WA, USA

Patrice L. Weiss, PhD
Department of Occupational Therapy
University of Haifa
Haifa, Israel

Carolee J. Winstein, PhD, PT, FAPTA
Department of Biokinesiology and Physical
Therapy
University of Southern California
Los Angeles, CA, USA

Jörg Wissel, MD
Neurologische Rehabilitationsklinik
Kliniken Beelitz GmbH
Beelitz-Heilstätten, Germany

Steven L. Wolf, PhD, PT, FAPTA
Department of Rehabilitation Medicine
Emory University
Atlanta, GA, USA

Sharon Wood-Dauphinee, PhD, PT
School of Physical and Occupational Therapy
McGill University
Montreal, Quebec, Canada

Richard D. Zorowitz, MD
Department of Physical Medicine
and Rehabilitation
University of Pennsylvania School of
Medicine
Philadelphia, PA, USA

Contributors (contributors of Volume I)

Evangelos G. Antzoulatos
Department of Neurobiology and Anatomy
University of Texas Health Science Center at Houston
Houston, TX, USA

Zafar I. Bashir, PhD
Department of Anatomy
MRC Centre for Synaptic Plasticity
University of Bristol
Bristol, UK

Niels Birbaumer, PhD
Institute of Behavioural Neurosciences
Eberhard-Karls-University
Tubingen, Germany

Cesar E. Blanco, PhD
Department of Biomedical Engineering
A.E. Mann Institute for Biomedical Engineering
University of Southern California
Los Angeles, CA, USA

Mary Bartlett Bunge, PhD
The Miami Project to Cure Paralysis
University of Miami School of Medicine
Miami, FL, USA

John H. Byrne, PhD
Department of Neurobiology and Anatomy
University of Texas Health Science Center
at Houston
Houston, TX, USA

Huaibin Cai, PhD
Computational Biology Section
Laboratory of Neurogenetics, NIA
National Institutes of Health
Bethesda, MD, USA

Kimberly M. Christian
Neuroscience Program
University of Southern California
Los Angeles, CA, USA

Hollis T. Cline, PhD
Cold Spring Harbor Laboratory
Cold Spring Harbor, NY, USA

Leonardo G. Cohen, MD
Human Cortical Physiology Section
National Institute of Neurological Disorders and
Stroke
National Institutes of Health
Bethesda, MD, USA

Matthew B. Dalva, PhD
Department of Neuroscience
University of Pennsylvania School of Medicine
Philadelphia, PA, USA

Marco Domeniconi
Department of Biological Sciences
Hunter College
City University of New York
New York, NY, USA

John P. Donoghue, PhD
Department of Neuroscience
Brown University
Providence, RI, USA

V. Reggie Edgerton, PhD
Department of Physiological Science and
Neurobiology
University of California, Los Angeles
Los Angeles, CA, USA

Ines Eisner-Janowicz
Department of Molecular and
Integrative Physiology
University of Kansas Medical Center
Kansas City, KS, USA

Marie T. Filbin, PhD
Department of Biology
Hunter College
City University of New York
New York, NY, USA

Diasinou Fioravante
Department of Neurobiology and
Anatomy
University of Texas Health Science Center
at Houston
Houston, TX, USA

Itzhak Fischer, PhD
Department of Neurobiology and Anatomy
Drexel University College of Medicine
Philadelphia, PA, USA

Agnes Floel, MD
Human Cortical Physiology Section
National Institute of Neurological
Disorders and Stroke
National Institutes of Health
Bethesda, MD, USA

Thomas W. Gould
Department of Neurobiology and Anatomy and the
Neuroscience Program
Wake Forest University School of Medicine
Winston-Salem, NC, USA

John W. Griffin, MD
Departments of Neurology and Neuroscience
Johns Hopkins University School of Medicine
Baltimore, MD, USA

Kurt Haas, PhD
Department of Anatomy and Cell Biology
University of British Columbia
Vancouver, British Columbia, Canada

Peter Hagell, RN PhD
Department of Nursing
Faculty of Medicine
Lund University
Lund, Sweden

Steve Sang Woo Han, MD, PhD
Department of Neurobiology and Anatomy
Drexel University College of Medicine
Philadelphia, PA, USA

Ahmet Höke, MD, PhD
Department of Neurology
Johns Hopkins University School of Medicine
Baltimore, MD, USA

Ronaldo M. Ichiyama, PhD
Department of Physiological Science
University of California, Los Angeles
Los Angeles, CA, USA

Bharathi Jagadeesh, PhD
Department of Physiology and Biophysics
University of Washington
Seattle, WA, USA

Jon H. Kaas, PhD
Department of Psychology
Vanderbilt University
Nashville, TN, USA

Un Jung Kang, MD
Department of Neurology
University of Chicago
Chicago, IL, USA

Matthew S. Kayser
Department of Neuroscience
University of Pennsylvania School
of Medicine
Philadelphia, PA, USA

Gerd Kempermann, MD
Max Delbruck Center for Molecular
Medicine (MDC)
Berlin-Buch, Germany

Timothy E. Kennedy, PhD
Department of Neurology and Neurosurgery
Montreal Neurological Institute
McGill University
Montreal, Quebec, Canada

Angelo C. Lepore
Department of Neurobiology and Anatomy
Drexel University College of Medicine
Philadelphia, PA, USA

Joel M. Levine, PhD
Department of Neurobiology and Behavior
State University of New York at Stony Brook
Stony Brook, NY, USA

Tong Li
Department of Pathology
Johns Hopkins University School of Medicine
Baltimore, MD, USA

Olle F. Lindvall, MD, PhD
Section of Restorative Neurology
Wallenberg Neuroscience Center/BMC A11
Lund University Hospital
Lund, Sweden

Gerald E. Loeb, MD
Department of Biomedical Engineering
A.E. Mann Institute for Biomedical Engineering
University of Southern California
Los Angeles, CA, USA

Jeffrey D. Macklis, MD, DHST
Department of Neurology
MGH–HMS Center for Nervous System Repair
Harvard Medical School
Boston, MA, USA

Peter V. Massey, PhD
Department of Anatomy
MRC Centre for Synaptic Plasticity
University of Bristol
Bristol, UK

Lisa J. McKerracher, PhD
Départment de Pathologie et Biologie Cellulaire
Université de Montreal
Montreal, Quebec, Canada

Lorne M. Mendell, PhD
Department of Neurobiology and Behavior
State University of New York at Stony Brook
Stony Brook, NY, USA

Jared H. Miller
Department of Neurosciences
Case Western Reserve University
School of Medicine
Cleveland, OH, USA

Simon W. Moore
Department of Neurology and Neurosurgery
Center for Neuronal Survival
Montreal Neurological Institute
McGill University
Montreal, Quebec, Canada

Ken Nakamura, MD, PhD
Department of Neurology
University of California, San Francisco
San Francisco, CA, USA

Thien Nguyen, MD, PhD
Departments of Neurology and Neuroscience
Johns Hopkins University, School of Medicine
Baltimore, MD, USA

Randolph J. Nudo, PhD
Department of Molecular and Integrative Physiology
University of Kansas Medical Center
Kansas City, KS, USA

Catherine L. Ojakangas, PhD
Department of Neuroscience
Brown University
Providence, RI, USA

Ronald W. Oppenheim, MD, PhD
Department of Neurobiology and Anatomy
Wake Forest University
Winston-Salem, NC, USA

Tim P. Pons, PhD
Department of Neurosurgery
Wake Forest University School of Medicine
Winston-Salem, NC, USA

Andrew M. Poulos
Neuroscience Program
University of Southern California
Los Angeles, CA, USA

Donald L. Price, MD
Division of Neuropathology
Johns Hopkins University School of Medicine
Baltimore, MD, USA

Josef P. Rauschecker, PhD
Department of Physiology and Biophysics
Georgetown Institute for Cognitive and
Computational Sciences
Georgetown University Medical Center
Washington, DC, USA

Serge Rossignol, MD, PhD
du centre de rechercher en sciences
University de Montreal
Montreal, Quebec, Canada

Roland R. Roy, PhD
Brain Research Institute
University of California, Los Angeles
Los Angeles, CA, USA

Krishnankutty (Krish) Sathian, MD, PhD
Department of Neurology
Emory University
Atlanta, GA, USA

Ralf Schneggenburger, PhD
Abteilung Membranbiophysik and AG synaptische
Max-Planck Institut für Biophysikalische Chemie
Gottingen, Germany

Michael E. Selzer, MD, PhD
Department of Neurology
University of Pennsylvania School of Medicine
Philadelphia, PA, USA

Jerry Silver, PhD
Department of Neurosciences
School of Medicine
Case Western Reserve University
Cleveland, OH, USA

Tim Spencer
Department of Biological Sciences
Hunter College
City University of New York
New York, NY, USA

Oswald Steward, PhD
Departments of Anatomy and Neurobiology,
Neurobiology and Behavior, and Neurosurgery
Reeve-Irvine Research Center
College of Medicine
University of California, Irvine
Irvine, CA, USA

Ann M. Stowe
Department of Molecular and Integrative
Physiology
University of Kansas Medical Center
Kansas City, KS, USA

Alan R. Tessler, MD
Department of Neurobiology and Anatomy
Drexel University College of Medicine
Philadelphia, PA, USA

Richard F. Thompson, PhD
Department fo Psychology and Biological
Sciences
University of Southern California
Keck School of Medicine
Los Angeles, CA, USA

Wesley J. Thompson, PhD
Section of Neurobiology
University of Texas
Austin, TX, USA

Stephen G. Waxman, MD, PhD
Department of Neurology
Yale University School of Medicine
New Haven, CT, USA

Jonathan R. Wolpaw, MD
Laboratory of Nervous System Disorders
Wadsworth Center, NYS Department of Health
Department of Biomedical Sciences,
State University of New York at Albany
Albany, NY, USA

Philip C. Wong, PhD
Department of Pathology
Johns Hopkins University School of Medicine
Baltimore, MD, USA

Patrick M. Wood, PhD
The Miami Project to Cure Paralysis
Department of Neurological Surgery
University of Miami School of Medicine
Miami, FL, USA

Neural repair and rehabilitation: an introduction

Michael E. Selzer[1], Stephanie Clarke[2], Leonardo G. Cohen[3], Pamela W. Duncan[4] and Fred H. Gage[5]

[1]University of Pennsylvania, Philadelphia, PA, USA; [2]University of Lausanne, Lausanne, Switzerland;
[3]National Institutes of Health, Bethesda, MD, USA; [4]University of Florida, Gainesville, FL, USA; [5]The Salk Institute, La Jolla, CA, USA

Among medical specialties, rehabilitation has been one of the slowest to develop a basic science framework and to establish evidence-based practices as its norms. The reasons for this relate in part to the urgent need for clinical service and the dearth of experienced practitioners in the field during its formative years. It is imperative now, that the perceived lack of a scientific basis be reversed in order for rehabilitation medicine to achieve its full academic recognition and fulfill its great potential for relieving human suffering. This book represents an attempt to place the practice of neurorehabilitation in a rigorous scientific framework. Precisely because the need and the potential are so great, the editors have devoted equal space and emphasis to the clinical practice of neurorehabilitation and to its basic science underpinnings. In particular, two areas of basic science are highlighted – neuroplasticity and neural repair. In this respect, the book differs from most clinical textbooks. However, the professional neurorehabilitation community has been especially supportive of this direction and has taken very active steps to further the development of a basic scientific underpinning for its field. Similarly, the field of rehabilitation medicine, and in particular neurorehabilitation, has begun to put great emphasis on the development of evidence-based medical practices (DeLisa et al., 1999; Ottenbacher and Maas, 1999; Practice PPoE-B, 2001). The chapters in the clinical sections of this book stress those therapies for which evidence exists based on controlled clinical trials.

1 Definitions

Neurorehabilitation

Neurorehabilitation is the clinical subspecialty that is devoted to the restoration and maximization of functions that have been lost due to impairments caused by injury or disease of the nervous system. According to the social model of disability adopted by the World Health Organization (WHO), "' impairment' refers to an individual's biological condition …," whereas "… 'disability' denotes the collective economic, political, cultural, and social disadvantage encountered by people with impairments" (Barnes, 2001). These definitions have collapsed older distinctions of the WHOs 1980 International Classification of Impairments, Disabilities and Handicap (ICIDH) (Thuriaux, 1995). In that classification, "impairment" referred to a biological condition: for example, spinal cord injury; "disability" referred to the loss of a specific function: for example, loss of locomotor ability consequent to the impairment; and "handicap" referred to the loss of functioning in society: for example, inability to work as a postman, consequent to the disability. In order to improve healthcare data reporting by the nations of the world, the WHO replaced ICIDH with an International Classification of Functioning, Disability and Health (ICF) in 2001. ICF has two *parts*, each with two *components*:

- Part 1: Functioning and disability:
    - (a) body functions and structures,
    - (b) activities and participation.

- Part 2: Contextual factors:
    - (c) environmental factors,
    - (d) personal factors.

It is not possible to review the entire classification here, but because of its widespread use, including some of the chapters in this book, a brief summary is presented in Chapter 32 of volume II. The complete version can be found at http://www3.who.int/icf/icftemplate. cfm. By focusing on components of health, ICF can be used to describe both healthy and disabled populations, whereas the ICIDH focused on consequences of disease and thus had a narrower usefulness. However, the older classification is more useful in understanding the level of interventions and research performed by the rehabilitation community. Traditionally, rehabilitation medicine has concerned itself with disabilities and handicaps but very little with the level of impairment and even less with the molecular and cellular mechanisms that underlie impairments. In recent years, this state of affairs has begun to change as rehabilitation professionals have come to recognize the continuity that exists from molecular pathophysiology to impairments to disabilities and handicaps. Neurorehabilitation has come to represent the application of this continuum to neurologically impaired individuals.

Over the last 30 years, interest in understanding the mechanisms underlying recovery of function has increased. An expression of this interest has been the substantial increment in basic science and translational studies geared to characterize the extent to which the central nervous system (CNS) can reorganize to sustain clinical rehabilitation.

Neuroplasticity

The term "neuroplasticity" is used to describe the ability of neurons and neuron aggregates to adjust their activity and even their morphology to alterations in their environment or patterns of use. The term encompasses diverse processes, as from learning and memory in the execution of normal activities of life, to dendritic pruning and axonal sprouting in response to injury. Once considered overused and trite, the term "neuroplasticity" has regained currency in the neurorehabilitation community as a concise way to refer to hypothetical mechanisms that may underlie spontaneous or coaxed functional recovery after neural injury and can now be studied in humans through such techniques as functional imaging (including positron-emission tomography (PET) and functional magnetic resonance imaging (fMRI)), electrical and magnetic event-related potentials (including electroencephalogram (EEG), evoked potentials (Eps), and magneto-encephalography (MEG)) and non-invasive brain stimulation in the form of transcranial magnetic or electrical stimulation (TMS and trancranial direct current stimulation, tDCS).

Neural repair

The term "neural repair" has been introduced in the past several years to describe the range of interventions by which neuronal circuits lost to injury or disease can be restored. Included in this term are means to enhance axonal regeneration, the transplantation of a variety of tissues and cells to replace lost neurons, and the use of prosthetic neuronal circuits to bridge parts of the nervous system that have become functionally separated by injury or disease. Although there is overlap with aspects of "neuroplasticity," the term "neural repair" generally refers to processes that do not occur spontaneously in humans to a degree sufficient to result in functional recovery. Thus therapeutic intervention is necessary to promote repair. The term is useful as part of the basic science of neurorehabilitation because it encompasses more than "regeneration" or "transplantation" alone. In recent years, concepts of neural plasticity have been accepted as important elements in the scientific understanding of functional recovery. The rehabilitation community has been slower to embrace repair as a relevant therapeutic goal. "Neural repair" has been used in the title of this textbook in order to convey the breadth of subject matter that it covers and is now considered relevant to neurorehabilitation.

2 History of neurorehabilitation as a medical subspecialty

Origins of rehabilitation medicine

In late 19th century America, interest developed in the possibility that then exotic forms of energy, that is, electricity, could help to heal patients with diseases and disabilities. In particular, high-frequency electrical stimuli were applied to generate deep heat in tissues (diathermy) and some physicians adopted this treatment modality as a specialty. In the early days, X-ray treatments and radiology were closely linked to electrotherapy (Nelson, 1973) and in 1923, the American College of Radiology and Physiotherapy was formed, changing its name to the American Congress of Physical Therapy in 1925. This organization merged with the American Physical Therapy Association in 1933 and in 1945, it adopted the name American Congress of Physical Medicine, then American Congress of Physical Medicine and Rehabilitation, and finally in 1966, the American Congress of Rehabilitation Medicine (ACRM). This is a multidisciplinary organization with membership open to physicians from many specialties and to non-physician rehabilitation specialists. With the large number of injuries to soldiers in World War I, the need for therapists to attend to their retraining and reintroduction to productive life created a new specialty that was based on physical modalities of treatment, including physical and occupational therapy, diathermy, electro-stimulation, heat and massage. These modalities were expanded during World War II. Training programs for physical therapy technicians were started in the 1920s and an American Medical Association (AMA) Council on Physical Therapy (later the Council on Physical Medicine) was started in 1926. By 1938, a medical specialty organization, the American Academy of Physical Medicine and Rehabilitation (AAPM&R) was formed and in 1947, the Academy sponsored a specialty board with a residency requirement and qualifying examination (Krusen, 1969). Gradually, the focus of rehabilitation has broadened to include the social and psychological adjustment to disability, treatment of medical complications such as bedsores, autonomic instability and urinary tract infections, management of pain syndromes and other medical aspects of the treatment of chronically ill patients. As with the name of the ACRM, the term "Rehabilitation Medicine" has replaced "Physical Medicine and Rehabilitation" in the naming of some hospital and university departments, since the latter term is associated with limitations to specific therapeutic modalities, such as physical therapy, rather than to a target patient population or therapeutic goal, i.e., restoration of function. With variations, parallel developments have occurred in many countries throughout the world.

A concomitant of the broadening of the focus of rehabilitation has been a trend toward specialization, including organ system-specific specialization. Previously, the tendency was to approach disabilities generically, based on their symptoms (e.g., gait disorder) and signs (e.g., spasticity), regardless of the cause. But with a growing conviction that the rehabilitation of patients requires knowledge of the pathophysiological basis of their disorders, medical specialists outside of physical medicine and rehabilitation (PM&R) became more interested in the rehabilitation of patients whom they might have treated during the acute phase of their illness. This was especially true among neurologists. The American Academy of Neurology formed a section on rehabilitation and in 1990, members of that section formed the American Society for Neurorehabilitation. National societies of neurorehabilitation were also formed in Europe and more recently in other parts of the world. In 2003, these national societies confederated officially as the World Federation of Neurorehabilitation, designating *Neurorehabilitation and Neural Repair* as its official journal.

Epidemiology of neurological disabilities

For many years, and especially during the two world wars, the practice of rehabilitation medicine was dominated by orthopedic problems, such as bone fractures and limb amputations. More recently, progress in keeping severely neurologically injured

patients alive has shifted the emphasis toward rehabilitation of patients with developmental neurological disorders, stroke, traumatic injuries of the brain
and spinal cord, and other chronic disabling diseases. It is estimated that in the USA, chronic health
conditions cause activity limitations 61,047,000
times each year (Kraus et al., 1996). The five conditions causing the most limitations are: heart disease
(7,932,000); back problems (7,672,000); arthritis
(5,721,000); asthma (2,592,000); and diabetes
(2,569,000). However, the conditions causing people
to have major activity limitations most often are:
mental retardation (87.5% of people with the condition have a limitation); multiple sclerosis (69.4%);
malignant neoplasm of the stomach, intestine,
colon, and rectum (62.1%); complete and partial
paralysis of extremities (60.7%); malignant neoplasm of the lung, bronchus, and other respiratory
sites (60.6%); and blindness in both eyes (60.3%).
The WHO estimates that more than 300 million
people worldwide are physically disabled, of whom
over 70% live in the developing countries. In the USA,
approximately 300,000 people are admitted to inpatient rehabilitation facilities each year. In a recent
survey, orthopedic conditions (hip and limb fractures, amputations, hip replacements) accounted for
20% of rehabilitation admissions, while neurological
conditions (stroke, traumatic brain injury, spinal
cord injury, polyneuropathy, and other neurological
conditions) accounted for 80% (Deutsch et al., 2000).
The survey excluded Guillain–Barré syndrome, so
the prevalence of neurological disabilities may have
been underestimated. Thus disorders of the nervous
system are those most often requiring intensive
rehabilitation interventions.

3 Outcomes measurement in rehabilitation medicine

The complex medical, emotional, and social problems of the medically disabled patient population,
and the complexity of the treatment regimens, has
made assessing outcomes difficult. As practiced in
most countries, rehabilitation is a multidisciplinary
process, involving combinations of treatment
modalities administered by multiple therapists.
Moreover, the most important outcome of the rehabilitation process is the degree of reintegration of the
patient in society, in terms of roles in work, family,
and community. This also was difficult to assess with
the limited instruments available only one generation ago. In order to catch up to other fields in the
practice of evidence-based medicine, the rehabilitation field has been forced to become extremely
resourceful in designing outcomes measures to evaluate the efficacy of its treatments (Stineman, 2001).
The resulting sophistication of outcomes measurement has had an important impact on all of medicine, which now routinely considers quality of life in
the evaluation of effectiveness in clinical trials.

4 Impact of evidence-based medicine on neurorehabilitation

Ironically, while outcomes measurement has begun
to have an important impact on the evaluation of
systems of rehabilitation, and on complex aspects of
rehabilitation outcomes, the evaluation of outcomes
for specific physical therapy treatments has lagged. A
consensus conference was held in 2002, which
developed a structured and rigorous methodology to
improve formulation of evidence-based clinical
practice guidelines (EBCPGs; Practice PPoE-B, 2001).
This was used to develop EBCPGs based on the literature for selected rehabilitation interventions in the
management of low back, neck, knee, and shoulder
pain, and to make recommendations for randomized clinical trials. To date, only two large-scale,
prospective, multicenter, randomized clinical trials
have been carried out to test-specific physical therapy treatments. These are the trial of body weight-
supported treadmill training for spinal cord injury
(Dobkin et al., 2003; see Chapter 3 of volume II) and
the trial of constraint-induced movement therapy for
upper extremity dysfunction after stroke (Winstein
et al., 2003; see Chapter 18 Volume II). Evidence that
amphetamines combined with physical therapy can
enhance recovery in several animal models of stroke

and traumatic brain injury has led to several small-scale randomized clinical trials. These have suggested a tendency toward effect in human patients with ischemic stroke (Long and Young, 2003). A larger clinical trial is underway.

5 Impact of the revolution in the science of neuroplasticity and regeneration on neurorehabilitation

Between 1980 and 2003, there was a relatively constant 3.8-fold increase in annual publications in the field of rehabilitation medicine (best searched on Medline using the term "physical rehabilitation"). A Medline search using the terms "neuroplasticity" or "nerve regeneration" showed a steady or slightly accelerating 7.8-fold increase during the same time (Fig. 1). However, the combination of "rehabilitation" and either "neuroplasticity" or "regeneration" did not appear until after the term "neurorehabilitation" became current.

As indicated in Fig. 2, the term "neurorehabilitation" was used less than 10 times/year in Medline-indexed articles until 1994. From then until 2003, the annual number of articles on "neurorehabilitation" increased 9.4-fold. During that same period, the number of articles on ("neuroplasticity" or "regeneration") and "physical rehabilitation" increased 7.6-fold. Similarly, the terms "rehabilitation" and "evidence-based medicine" did not appear in the same article until 1994. From then until 2003, their coincidence increased 25.5-fold. Thus there is a correlation between the use of the term "neurorehabilitation" and acceleration in the application of basic science and evidence-based medicine to rehabilitation research. This can be ascribed to the accelerated interest in organ-specific rehabilitation, and in particular, to interest in the rehabilitation of patients disabled by neurological disorders. As in other fields of medicine, the trend toward specialization in the field of rehabilitation medicine carried with it recognition of the need to develop a basic science research underpinning and to become more rigorous in the evaluation of its therapies and clinical practices.

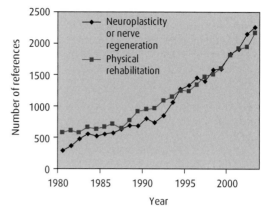

Figure 1. Parallel growth of research in medical rehabilitation and in neural plasticity and repair over the past 25 years. In order to estimate research in medical rehabilitation, a PubMed search was conducted using the term "physical rehabilitation," which yielded the highest combination of sensitivity and specificity among such terms as "medical rehabilitation," "rehabilitation," and "rehabilitation medicine." In order to estimate research on neuroplasticity, the term "neuroplasticity" was sufficient. In order to estimate research on regeneration in the nervous system, the best combination of specificity and sensitivity was achieved by searching for the term "nerve regeneration."

From the above, it can be seen that the maturation of neurorehabilitation as a clinical specialty has experienced two phases, which replicates the pattern seen in other specialties. In the first phase, the enormous need for clinical service was met by reliance on the experience and a priori reasoning of medical clinicians and therapists in devising methods to maximize function. In the second phase, scientific exploration in animal models was used to buttress the rationale for these therapies, while the rigors of prospective, controlled clinical trials were applied to test the effectiveness of those treatments in patients. This second phase is still very active, but we are already witnessing the beginning of a third phase, in which therapy is directed not only at maximizing function based on the post-injury residual anatomical substrate, but incorporates attempts at repairing that substrate. As with clinical trials of neuroprotective agents in human stroke and trauma, early results of cell and gene therapies for

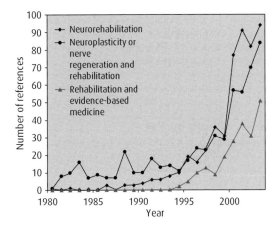

Figure 2. The subspecialization represented by the term "neurorehabilitation" has followed closely the application to rehabilitation medicine of basic research on neural plasticity and repair, and has closely led evidence-based clinical research. In order to estimate the frequency with which research on neuroplasticity and neural repair is applied to rehabilitation medicine, the best combination of sensitivity and specificity was obtained with the terms "rehabilitation," "neuroplasticity," and "nerve regeneration." Similarly the term "evidence-based medicine" was best paired with "rehabilitation" rather than other terms pairing "rehabilitation" with modifiers.

human injuries and diseases of the CNS have highlighted the need for caution in translating animal studies into human therapies. The most notable example is Parkinson's disease. Based on results in animal models, attempts to replace dopaminergic cells in human patients have been carried out for more than a decade. Yet despite promising results in small-scale studies on special populations (Lindvall, 1998; Chapter 34 of Volume I), larger double-blind, sham operated controlled clinical trials have not suggested major benefits in idiopathic Parkinson's disease (Olanow et al., 2003; Chapter 6 of Volume II). Despite favorable results in animals, intraventricular infusions of glial cell line-derived neurotrophic factor (GDNF) also failed to provide improvement in human Parkinson's disease. It turns out that because of the large size of the human brain, the GDNF failed to penetrate far enough into the brain parenchyma.

Thus a small-scale clinical trial of intraputamenal GDNF injections has been reported (Gill et al., 2003). A multicenter trial of *in vivo* gene therapy, using an adeno-associated virus vector containing the gene for neurturin, a GDNF-related peptide that has similar biological activity, is planned. A multicenter clinical trial of autologous macrophages activated by exposure to skin and injected into the spinal cord (Bomstein et al., 2003) is currently under way. The US Food and Drug Administration has approved small-scale clinical trials of intracerebral transplantation of tumor-derived neuronal progenitors for stroke, nerve growth factor-secreting fibroblasts for Alzheimer's disease, and epidural injection of a rho-A antagonist for spinal cord injury. In countries where clinical research is less stringently regulated, many patients have received transplants of stem cells and other highly invasive treatments for a variety of disabling neurological disorders, in the absence of evidence for effectiveness or experimental controls. The technical difficulties of carrying out controlled trials of these novel, highly invasive therapies are matched by ethical concerns. How do you convince patients to undergo a neurosurgical procedure that might be a sham operation? Should a clinical trial be performed on only the most severely disabled patients, who may have less to lose? Or should they be done on less disabled patients, who might have a better chance of responding favorably to an effective treatment, knowing that a failed trial might make it difficult to mount a subsequent one on a more favorable patient population? These and other questions are under intensive discussion and guidelines for the application of these advanced therapies to human patients are needed.

6 Rehabilitation of cognitive functions

Although rehabilitation is commonly thought of as relating primarily to motor retraining, the most disabling aspects of injury to the nervous system often relate to impairments in other domains, such as autonomic, sensory, and especially cognitive functions. Most major neuropsychological syndromes,

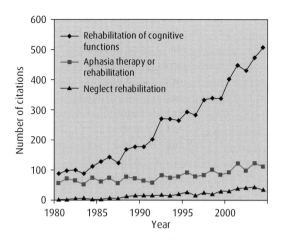

Figure 3. Increase in publications on neuropsychological rehabilitation. A PubMed search was conducted to identify articles published between 1980 and 2004 on rehabilitation of cognitive functions key words: (neuropsychological OR aphasia) AND (rehabilitation OR therapy); aphasia (therapy OR rehabilitation); and neglect rehabilitation. The titles of the included publications were then checked for appropriateness.

such as aphasia, apraxia, visual agnosia, or neglect, have been identified in the second half of the 19th and the first half of the 20th century. Many of the original reports described the course of spontaneous recovery and proposed specific rehabilitative measures. During the last 25 years the field of rehabilitation of cognitive functions has expanded rapidly. The annual number of publications concerning neuropsychological rehabilitation, including aphasia therapy, has increased from about 100 in 1980 to over 500 in 2004, with a steep increase beginning around 1987 (Fig. 3). A small but important part of this increase can be accounted for by studies of specific neuropsychological syndromes. Most of the studies published in the early 1980s concerned aphasia, which continued to be investigated and experienced a 2-fold increase between 1980 and 2004. In recent years, research in other cognitive syndromes has grown even faster. Unilateral neglect, very little investigated in the 1980s, witnessed a 10-fold increase by 2004. This current expansion of rehabilitation studies of specific syndromes is linked to the application of cognitive models to rehabilitation and

to a better understanding of post-lesional plasticity as apparent in functional imaging studies.

However, most of the impressive increase in studies of neuropsychological rehabilitation was due to studies of disease-specific rehabilitation. Thus, rehabilitation of traumatic brain injury, stroke, tumors, degenerative diseases such as Parkison's disease or progressive diseases such as multiple sclerosis are increasingly investigated in their own rights. This type of research requires more than ever a multidisciplinary approach to neuropsychological rehabilitation, with close interactions between physicians, neuropsychologists, speech therapists, and physiotherapists and occupational therapists.

The chapters on rehabilitation of cognitive functions and on disease-specific rehabilitation demonstrate the necessity and the putative strength of evidence-based approaches. Although we need to understand the mechanisms underlying recovery from cognitive deficits, we also must have proof of the efficacy of our interventions. Specific fields, such as aphasia and neglect rehabilitation, have started accumulating this type of evidence. However, many more studies, and in particular large-scale multicenter investigations, are needed and should be carried out during the next decade.

7 Purpose and organization of this book

If most severely disabling disorders are neurological, why write a separate textbook of neurorehabilitation rather than incorporating it with the rest of rehabilitation medicine into a general rehabilitation textbook? The editors believe that it is time for rehabilitation medicine to go beyond optimizing function based on what is left to the body after an injury or illness. Rather, the goal should be full restoration of function by any means necessary, including actual repair of the injured tissues and organs. By focusing on the nervous system, we can present a cogent and intellectually rigorous approach to restoration of function, based on principles and professional interactions that have a deep vertical penetration. This requires two additions to the traditional rehabilitation approach, which had considered disabilities and handicaps in the abstract, apart from the specific disease processes that underlay them. First, there is a need to understand the pathophysiological bases of disabling neurological disorders. Second, there is a need to apply basic scientific knowledge about the plastic properties of the nervous system in order to effect anatomical repair and physiological restoration of lost functions.

This book is presented in two volumes, designed to be used either separately or as an integrated whole. *Volume I, Neural Plasticity and Repair,* explores the basic science underpinnings of neurorehabilitation and can be used as a textbook for graduate level courses in recovery of function after neural injury. It is divided into two sections. *Section A, Neural plasticity*, includes chapters on the morphological and physiological plasticity of neurons that underlie the ability of the nervous system to learn, accommodate to altered patterns of use, and adapt to injury. *Section B, Neural repair*, includes chapters on the neuronal responses to injury, stem cells and neurogenesis in the adult CNS, the molecular mechanisms inhibiting and promoting axon regeneration in the CNS, and strategies to promote cell replacement and axon regeneration after injury, the design of prosthetic neural circuitry, and translational research, applying animal experimental results to human patients. *Volume II, Medical Neurorehabilitation*, will be of greatest interest to clinical rehabilitation specialists, but will be useful to basic scientists who need to understand the clinical implications of their work. The volume is divided into three sections. *Section A, Technology of neurorehabilitation*, contains chapters on outcomes measurement, diagnostic techniques such as functional imaging and clinical electrophysiology, rehabilitation engineering and prosthetics design, and special therapeutic techniques. *Section B, Symptom-specific rehabilitation*, considers rehabilitation approaches to neurological symptoms that are common to many types of neurological disorders; for example, spasticity and other motor dysfunctions, autonomic, and sexual dysfunctions, sensory disturbances including chronic pain, and cognitive dysfunctions. *Section C, Disease-specific neurorehabilitation systems*, considers the integrated approaches that have been developed to address the rehabilitation of patients with specific diseases and disease categories; multiple sclerosis, stroke, traumatic brain injury, neurodegenerative diseases, etc.

Throughout the two volumes, efforts have been made to relate the basic science to the clinical material, and to cross-reference relevant chapters where the integration is supported. In this way, we hope to stimulate basic scientists to broaden their understanding of the clinical relevance of their work. At the same time clinicians and clinical scientists in the various fields of rehabilitation medicine will be encouraged to enhance their curiosity and understanding of the mechanisms underlying their practice. Ultimately, we hope that encouraging communication between basic and clinical scientists in relevant areas of research will help to accelerate the translation of basic research into effective clinical treatments that will expand the degree of functional recovery of neurologically disabled persons.

REFERENCES

Barnes, C. (2001). World Health Organization – Disability and Rehabilitation Team Conference Report and Recommendations. In: *Rethinking Care from the Perspective of Disabled People*. WHO, Oslo, Norway.

Bomstein, Y., Marder, J.B., Vitner, K., Smirnov, I., Lisaey, G., Butovsky, O., Fulga, V. and Yoles, E. (2003). Features of skin-coincubated macrophages that promote recovery from spinal cord injury. *J Neuroimmunol*, **142**, 10–16.

DeLisa, J.A., Jain, S.S., Kirshblum, S. and Christodoulou, C. (1999). Evidence-based medicine in physiatry: the experience of one department's faculty and trainees. *Am J Phys Med Rehabil*, **78**, 228–232.

Deutsch, A., Fiedler, R.C., Granger, C.V. and Russell, C.F. (2000). The uniform data system for medical rehabilitation report of patients discharged from comprehensive medical rehabilitation programs in 1999. *Am J Phys Med Rehabil*, **81**, 133–142.

Dobkin, B.H., Apple, D., Barbeau, H., Basso, M., Behrman, A., Deforge, D., Ditunno, J., Dudley, G., Elashoff, R., Fugate, L., Harkema, S., Saulino, M. and Scott, M. (2003). Methods for a randomized trial of weight-supported treadmill training versus conventional training for walking during inpatient rehabilitation after incomplete traumatic spinal cord injury. *Neurorehabil Neural Repair*, **17**, 153–167.

Gill, S.S., Patel, N.K., Hotton, G.R., O'Sullivan, K., McCarter, R., Bunnage, M., Brooks, D.J., Svendsen, C.N. and Heywood, P. (2003). Direct brain infusion of glial cell line-derived neurotrophic factor in Parkinson disease. *Nat Med*, **9**, 589–595.

Kraus, L., Stoddard, S. and Gilmartin, D. (1996). Section 3: Causes of disabilities. In: *Chartbook on Disability in the United States. An InfoUse Report*. U.S. National Institute on Disability and Rehabilitation Research, Washington, DC.

Krusen, F.H. (1969). Historical development in physical medicine and rehabilitation during the last forty years. Walter J. Zeiter Lecture. *Arch Phys Med Rehabil*, **50**, 1–5.

Lindvall, O. (1998). Update on fetal transplantation: the Swedish experience. *Mov Disord*, **13**, 83–87.

Long, D. and Young. J. (2003). Dexamphetamine treatment in stroke. *Quart J Nuclear Med*, **96**, 673–685.

Nelson, P.A. (1973). History of the once close relationship between electrotherapeutics and radiology. *Arch Phys Med Rehabil*, **54**(**Suppl.**), 608–640.

Olanow, C.W., Goetz, C.G., Kordower, J.H., Stoessl, A.J., Sossi, V., Brin, M.F., Shannon, K.M., Nauert, G.M., Perl, D.P., Godbold, J. and Freeman, T.B. (2003). A double-blind controlled trial of bilateral fetal nigral transplantation in Parkinson's disease. *Ann Neurol*, **54**, 403–414.

Ottenbacher, K.J. and Maas, F. (1999). How to detect effects: statistical power and evidence-based practice in occupational therapy research. *Am J Occup Ther*, **53**, 181–188.

Practice PPoE-B (2001). Philadelphia panel evidence-based clinical practice guidelines on selected rehabilitation interventions: overview and methodology. *Phys Ther*, **81**, 1629–1640.

Stineman, M.G. (2001). Defining the population, treatments, and outcomes of interest: reconciling the rules of biology with meaningfulness. *Am J Phys Med Rehabil*, **80**, 147–159.

Thuriaux, M.C. (1995). The ICIDH: evolution, status, and prospects. *Disabil Rehabil*, **17**, 112–118.

Winstein, C.J., Miller, J.P., Blanton, S., Taub, E., Uswatte, G., Morris, D., Nichols, D. and Wolf, S. (2003). Methods for a multisite randomized trial to investigate the effect of constraint-induced movement therapy in improving upper extremity function among adults recovering from a cerebrovascular stroke. *Neurorehabil Neural Repair*, **17**, 137–152.

SECTION A

Technology of neurorehabilitation

CONTENTS

Outcomes measurement and diagnostic technology

CONTENTS

Outcomes measurement: basic principles and applications in stroke rehabilitation

Carol L. Richards[1], Sharon Wood-Dauphinee[2] and Francine Malouin[1]

[1]Department of Rehabilitation and Centre for Interdisciplinary Research in Rehabilitation and Social Integration, Laval University, Quebec City and [2]School of Physical and Occupational Therapy, McGill University, Montreal, Quebec, Canada

1.1 Summary

The objective of this chapter is to give an overview of basic principles guiding the development and application of outcome measures. This chapter starts by introducing basic concepts related to the development of outcome measures, and demonstrates their applications in stroke rehabilitation. Specifically, the first section includes a theoretical discussion of reliability, validity and responsiveness, and how to approach interpretation. This discussion is based on classical test theory. For each property the theory is applied to development of a measure of "participation". Future trends related to computer-adapted testing (CAT) are also briefly described. In the second section, the evaluation of "walking competency" after stroke is used to illustrate the selection of appropriate outcome measures for this population, as well as their relation to "participation". These measures include self-reported scales, performance-based ratings and laboratory assessments. This chapter concludes with examples of how laboratory-based gait assessments and measures of brain reorganization help explain changes in clinical scales and performance-based measures.

1.2 Introduction

"Outcomes are the end results of medical care: what happened to the patient in terms of palliation, control of illness, cure or rehabilitation" (Brook et al., 1976). Outcome measures used in stroke rehabilitation can be divided into three categories: scales that assess constructs such as function, mobility and quality of life, performance-based measures that evaluate such areas as gait speed and upper limb dexterity, and measures of brain plasticity. This chapter introduces basic concepts related to the development of outcome measures and demonstrates their applications in stroke rehabilitation. To avoid a redundant review of traditional scales (Wood-Dauphinee et al., 1994; Finch et al., 2002), a section on how to create an evaluative scale that measures "participation" is provided. This information will enable the reader to critique published scales when selecting them for clinical practice or research. In the second part, the evaluation of "walking competency" after stroke is used as an example to illustrate the selection of appropriate outcome measures for this population as well as their relation to participation. This chapter ends with discussions as to how laboratory-based gait assessments and measures of brain reorganization help explain changes in clinical scales and performance-based measures.

1.3 Developing and testing measures

Measures used to evaluate the outcomes of rehabilitation for individuals with stroke generally reflect physical, psychologic or social characteristics of people. Physical attributes or abilities are most easily assessed as they are observed directly. They can be evaluated using electromechanical devices or functional status scales. Psychologic and social characteristics are more difficult to evaluate because they are concepts and often cannot be observed directly. To assess a concept, we must make inferences from what we observe and decide if, for instance, an individual is independent, depressed, motivated, receiving sufficient support or coping with life's challenges. When one cannot directly observe these concepts or behaviors, they are termed constructs (Portney and Watkins, 2000). Other constructs we might want to assess include impairment, ability/disability, community mobility, health status, self-efficacy, fitness, participation or quality of life. Such constructs are evaluated using standardized scales.

Development and testing of evaluative scales

Generating the items

A series of well-defined steps is necessary for the development and testing of a standardized scale (Juniper et al., 1996; Streiner and Norman, 2003). First one must decide what the instrument is to measure and the type of measure to be developed. We are interested in creating an evaluative scale (Kirshner and Guyatt, 1985) to assess "participation" of an individual or a group at baseline, and again at one or more points later on, principally to determine if change has occurred. In optimal circumstances, one would begin with a conceptual framework such as the International Classification of Functioning, Disability and Health (ICF) (World Health Organization, 2001), which proposes multiple interactions between the health condition, body functions and structures, activities, participation in life, environmental and personal factors. Such a framework names broad categories, suggests relationships among categories and anchors a measure to an extensive body of knowledge. It also provides a guide to evaluating the validity of the measure, and adds to its interpretability.

In the absence of a theoretical framework, or even in addition to it, pertinent information is obtained from a review of literature to identify existing instruments assessing similar constructs that

may incorporate useful items. Ideas are also obtained from patients, significant others in their lives and involved health professionals. Individual un- or semi-structured interviews and/or focus groups are conducted with these persons to gather information that is sufficiently specific to provide the basis for scale items. For the "participation" example, one might solicit issues related to caring for oneself or one's home, moving around the home or the community, traveling, communicating and interacting with family, friends and colleagues, and engaging in work and leisure activities as well as about factors in the social or physical environments that impede or assist "participation". The overall goal of this step is to amass a large number of ideas that will form the basis for writing many items that represent the construct of interest.

Reducing the number of items

The goal of this step is to select the items that are the most suitable for the scale. Knowledgeable individuals who, preferably, have not been involved in their creation must carefully review all items. Each item is initially judged qualitatively to eliminate those that are unclear. Decisions are then made about the response options and the time frame of the questions. For example, the time frame may refer to today, the past week, etc. and the response options may be dichotomous (yes/no), may contain several ordinal categories or may be a visual analog scale (VAS). A categorical scale needs descriptors for each choice and a VAS needs descriptive anchors at each end.

The items are then administered to a convenience sample of approximately 100 people who reflect the characteristics of the individuals who will be using the scale (Juniper et al., 1996). If possible, a subset of this group (30–40 people) can be asked to complete the items a second time. These data provide information useful for further item reduction. Item frequency distributions tell us about the spread of responses across the sample, and provide the first hint as to whether or not the item will be responsive. Items that are highly correlated with another item may be redundant, and items with very low correlations to other items may not belong in the scale. Items with similar means and standard deviations (SD) can be summed to provide subscale or total scores (Likert, 1952). Items with missing data may indicate that the content was unclear or offensive to the respondent. Item reliabilities may also be estimated using data from the group that completed the items twice. Kappa statistics are often used for this purpose (Cohen, 1960). If criteria for excluding items are set a priori, these data allow a quantitative approach to reducing the number of items.

Pre-testing the scale

A pre-test on a small sample that reflects the characteristics of subjects in the target population (Juniper et al., 1996) is conducted to reduce problems related to understanding the content, or to the format of the measure. It should be completed by five to ten subjects using the same mode of administration as intended for routine use. Following completion of the scale, subjects should be debriefed. It is currently advocated that each item be examined using cognitive testing procedures (Collins, 2003). This process ensures that respondents really understand the item and that all respondents understand it in the same way. This process may need to be repeated until no further changes are necessary.

Testing the reliability, validity and responsiveness of the new scale

The measurement properties of the scale need to be examined on a new sample of subjects with stroke.

Reliability reflects the degree to which a measure is free from random error, or in other words, the degree to which the observed score is different from the true score (Scientific Advisory Committee, 2002). Traditionally, reliability has been categorized as either reflecting internal consistency or stability. Internal consistency denotes precision, how well the items are inter-correlated or measure the same characteristic. To examine internal consistency, one administration of the scale to an appropriate sample of subjects is needed. Coefficient alpha (Cronbach, 1951) is the test statistic most often used. It provides an estimate of the amount of error that is due to the sampling of items, by assessing the correlation between the scale and another hypothetical scale selected from the same group of items at the same time.

In general, stability of a scale is examined over time (test–retest and intra-rater (including the situation in which the subject self-completes the scale twice)) or between raters. Two administrations of the scale are required. The interval between administrations should be sufficiently short to minimize changes in the subjects but far enough apart to avoid the effects of learning memory or fatigue. For intra- and inter-rater reliability tests, rater training prior to testing is usually provided. Inter-rater reliability is most easily assessed if all raters can observe the subject simultaneously but independently, for example through the use of videotapes. Scales that require interactions between the subject and the rater may not lend themselves to this approach and multiple tests need to be conducted. In this situation issues related to the testing intervals are again important. The intra-class correlation coefficient (Cronbach, 1957) is the preferred test statistic as it assesses agreement, using estimates of variance obtained from an analysis of variance (ANOVA). Different versions, reflecting different test situations, are available (Portney and Watkins, 2000). For "participation" internal consistency and test–retest reliability would be assessed.

Reliability coefficients range between 0 and ± 1.00, and are interpreted by their closeness to ± 1.00. A coefficient of 0.85 tells us that the data contain 85% true variance and 15% error variance. Commonly accepted minimal standards for reliability coefficients are 0.70 for use with groups and 0.90 for use with individuals as in the clinical setting. Lower coefficients yield confidence intervals that are too wide for monitoring an individual over time (Scientific Advisory Committee, 2002).

Validity is defined as the extent to which a scale measures what it claims to measure, and it can be divided into three main types: content, criterion-related and construct (Portney and Watkins, 2000; Scientific Advisory Committee, 2002). *Content validity* signifies that the items contained in the measure provide a representative sample of the universe of content of the construct being measured. For instance, a measure of "participation" should contain items reflecting each of the domains listed earlier in this chapter. *Content validity* is usually judged by the thoroughness of the item generation and reduction processes previously described. A subjective judgment is required as there is no statistical test to assess this type of validity.

Criterion-related validity is based on the relationship between a new scale and a criterion measure, a "gold standard", which is examined at the same point in time or in the future. The most difficult aspect of this type of validation is finding a "gold standard" that reflects the same criterion and is measurable. A gold standard for "participation" is probably not available, but one might choose the reintegration to normal living index (Wood-Dauphinee et al., 1988) or the impact on participation and autonomy questionnaire (Cardol et al., 2002) as measures tapping a similar construct to evaluate *concurrent-criterion validity*. The new scale and one of the existing measures would be administered at the same time to an appropriate sample of community-dwelling individuals with stroke and the scores would be correlated to assess the strength of the association. *Predictive-criterion validity* attempts to demonstrate that a new measure can successfully predict a future criterion. For instance, a measure of "participation" could be tested in the stroke sample noted earlier to determine if it would predict institutionalization over time. This type of validation would use regression to determine if the "participation" scores obtained, for example, a month after discharge could predict the living situation over the next 2 years.

Construct validity examines evidence that a measure performs according to theoretical expectations by examining relationships to different constructs. One might hypothesize that "participation" among community-dwelling stroke survivors was positively and moderately correlated with the ability to drive a car. It might also be negatively correlated with the

absence of a significant other who was willing to plan and execute activities with the stroke survivor (*convergent construct validity*). One could also hypothesize that the extent of functional recovery following the stroke would be more highly correlated with "participation" than would the presence of shoulder pain (divergent construct validity). These hypotheses would be tested on appropriate samples of stroke survivors by evaluating both "participation" and the other constructs at the same point in time. *Known groups*, another form of construct validation, examines the performance of a new measure through the use of existing external reference groups. For example, one might expect that stroke survivors living (1) at home with a willing and able caregiver, (2) at home with paid assistance or (3) in an institution would demonstrate different levels of "participation". By collecting "participation" data on each of the groups and comparing mean scores across the groups via ANOVA one can determine if the measure can discriminate as hypothesized. Finally, because the "participation" measure is to be based on the ICF framework, validity could also be evaluated by testing hypotheses that support the conceptual framework. Environmental or personal factors that assist or limit the stroke survivor in terms of participating could be explored, as could the relationships between "activities" or "body structures and functions" and "participation".

To finish this brief section on validity it is important to note that validation is never completed. One must always ask if a measure is valid for a certain population or in a specific setting. When developing a new measure most investigators select a few tests of validity according to available time and resources.

While reliability and validity are traditional psychometric properties with a long history in the social sciences, *responsiveness* is a relative newcomer. In fact, there has been considerable discussion as to whether it is simply another aspect of validity (Hays and Hadorn, 1992; Stratford et al., 1996; Terwee et al., 2003). Nonetheless, a taxonomy for responsiveness, that incorporates three axes (who is to be studied; which scores are to be contrasted; and what type of change is to be assessed), has been proposed (Beaton et al., 2001). The different types of change being assessed have served to categorize various definitions of responsiveness. These have been grouped as the ability to detect change in general, clinically important change and real change in the concept being measured (Terwee et al., 2003). For this chapter we have selected a definition from the third group – "the accurate detection of change when it has occurred" (De Bruin et al., 1997) because it encompasses all types of change (Beaton et al., 2001).

In addition to many definitions there are also many approaches to measuring responsiveness. Most depend on assessing patients longitudinally over time during a period of anticipated change. For example, a person with mild stroke returning home would be expected to gradually resume participation in former activities and roles. A protocol to evaluate responsiveness is strengthened when one can collect data on both: a group that is expected to change as well as one not expected to change (Guyatt et al., 1987; Tuley et al., 1991; Scientific Advisory Committee, 2002). In addition, patients who perceive positive or negative changes need to be separated from those who report no change. The various statistical approaches to quantifying responsiveness, along with their strengths and weaknesses, have been extensively presented in recent literature (Husted et al., 2000; Crosby et al., 2003; Terwee et al., 2003). Examples include the use of a paired t-test to test the hypothesis that a measure has not changed over time, calculations of effect size, standardized response mean (SRM) or Guyatt's responsiveness statistic, as well as others that are based on sample variation, and those based on measurement precision such as the index of reliable change and the standard error of measurement. The developer needs to choose one or more approaches based on the data collection protocol.

Following a stroke we expect considerable recovery during the first 6 weeks (Richards et al., 1992; Skilbeck et al., 1983; Jorgensen et al., 1995), after which time the gradient flattens somewhat but there is considerable improvement until around 6 months from the index event. At that time recovery tends to plateau although further gains are clearly possible, particularly in the functional and social realms. For testing responsiveness of the measure of "participation" one could enroll subjects upon return to their home setting and monitor them for a defined number of months. At each evaluation point, in addition to completing the scale, patients and their caregivers should independently be asked if they are "better, the same or worse" since the previous evaluation. Given sufficient subjects this will allow like responders to be grouped for analysis. People saying they are better form a positive response group and those who report being worse make up a deteriorating group. As noted above, there are many statistical approaches from which to choose. To date, in addition to descriptive data, the different versions of the effect size based on sample variation are most commonly found in the literature. One should be aware, however, that because of the different methods of calculation they are not interchangeable for interpretative purposes.

Interpretability means the capacity to assign a qualitative meaning to a quantitative score (Ware and Keller, 1996). As clinicians and researchers have only a short history of trying to interpret the meaning of scale scores as compared to clinical tests, contextual relationships are required to facilitate understanding. Two basic approaches have been proposed to help interpret scalar data (Lydick and Epstein, 1993). The first, a distribution-based approach, relies on the statistical distributions of the results of a study, usually an effect size as calculated from the magnitude of change and the variability of the subjects at baseline or over time. The term effect size, coined by Cohen (1988), is a standardized, unitless measure of change in a group. Limitations of this approach include differing variability across groups being tested and the meaning of the values obtained. While Cohen suggested that 0.2, 0.5 and 0.8 represent small medium and large effects, respectively, these values are somewhat arbitrary (Guyatt et al., 2002).

The second approach, termed anchor based, examines the relationship between the change score on the instrument being tested, to that of an independent measure that is well known, associated with the measure being tested and clinically meaningful

(Guyatt et al., 2002). Population norms, severity classifications, symptom scores, global ratings of change by patients or physicians, and the minimum important difference (MID) have all been used. The MID is defined as "the smallest difference in score in the domain of interest which patients perceive as beneficial and which would mandate, in the absence of troublesome side effects and excessive costs, a change in the patient's management" (Jaeschke et al., 1989). Investigators have proposed several methods of calculating MIDs (Jaeschke et al., 1989; Redelmeier et al., 1996; Wyrwich et al., 2002), discussions of which are beyond the scope of this chapter. It is sufficient to say that the magnitude of MIDs tend to vary across measures. On a more positive note, there is some empirical evidence that in certain situations the distribution- and anchor-based approaches provide similar information (Norman et al., 2001; Guyatt et al., 2002). Neither of these approaches is without limitations but each provides a framework for investigation and contributes information important for understanding scale scores.

For the scale developer, a group of psychometric experts (Scientific Advisory Committee, 2002) has recommended that several types of information would be useful in interpreting scale scores. If the measure is to be used with stroke survivors, possibilities include data on the relationship of scores or change scores to ratings of the MID by those with stroke, their significant others or their clinicians, information on the relationship of scores on the new measure to other measures used with people who have had a stroke, comparative data on the distribution of scores from population groups, and eventually, results from multiple studies that have used the instrument and reported findings. This will increase familiarity with the measure and thus, assist interpretation.

Applications

During the past 25 years the authors of this chapter have used these steps, with modifications, to develop and test a number of measures for use with individuals who have sustained a stroke: the reintegration to normal living index (Wood-Dauphinee et al., 1988); the balance scale (Berg et al., 1989, 1992a, b, 1995; Wood-Dauphinee et al., 1997), the stroke rehabilitation assessment of movement (STREAM) (Daley et al., 1997, 1999; Ahmed et al., 2003); a fluidity scale for evaluating the motor strategy of the rise-to-walk test (Malouin et al., 2003) and the preference-based stroke index (Poissant et al., 2003).

Dynamic assessments

The prior paragraphs outlined the development of a scale based on classical test theory as advocated by many psychometricians during the last century. In the 1990s, several health researchers (Fisher, 1993; Bjorner and Ware, 1998; McCorney, 1997; Revicki and Cella, 1997) recognized the need for a new approach to creating health scales, primarily because a number of limitations to the psychometric approach were known. Foremost was the difficulty of any one scale covering the entire spectrum of a construct such as physical functioning (Revicki and Cella, 1997). Indeed, a scale with a very large number of items would be needed to encompass the entire continuum of activities for people with stroke, considering that they range from having extremely severe limitations to only minor limitations and a high level of functioning. This scale would be time consuming and perhaps distressing for persons to complete as they are faced with items far beyond or below their capabilities (Cleary, 1996; McHorney, 1997). In addition, traditional scaling techniques do not allow one to separate the properties of the items from the subject's abilities (Hambleton et al., 1991; Hays, 1998). In other words, scores of the test sample determine how much of the trait is present and this, in turn, is related to test norms (Streiner and Norman, 2003). Theoretically at least, the known psychometric properties of a test apply only to those in the testing sample. This means that if the measure is to be used with others who are different, the psychometric properties need to be reexamined. Finally, a statistical disadvantage is that only an overall reliability estimate is possible with a traditionally developed scale, but we know that measurement precision changes according to the level of the subject's ability (Hays, 1998).

To address these issues and others, statistical and technical methods, namely item response theory (IRT), computer adapted testing (CAT) and computer-assisted scale administration, have been combined to create a modern approach to scale construction and delivery. To start, all known items that assess the same underlying construct (i.e. mobility or self-care or physical activities outside the home) are collected, most often from existing measures. New items reflecting missing areas may also be written. All items undergo careful analyses to examine dimensionality and item fit, and then they are calibrated onto a common ruler to create a measure with one metric. Items are further analyzed to determine if the construct is adequately represented, both statistically and clinically (Cella et al., 2004). Additional validation, field testing and analyses lead to the creation of a "data bank" of items relating to one domain. Thus, a data bank is a group of items that is able to define and quantify one construct (Revicki and Cella, 1997). Information describing the inter-item relationships as well as the relationships of responses to the various items is available. A framework for developing an item bank has been described by Cella and colleagues (2004).

To use CAT with an individual patient, a computer algorithm is employed to select the items for the subject, according to his or her level of performance. At the beginning of the test, the subject responds to a series of items and an initial classification of performance is made. For example, a person with stroke may be classified as having a low level of functional performance. After confirming this classification in a second series of items of similar difficulty, the computer algorithm adapts the third series of items to reflect the subject's level of performance, and this process continues until his or her performance stabilizes. This means that the time to complete the test is usually shortened because after determining the general level of performance, subjects are presented only with items close to their level of ability. It also means that different subjects take different versions of the same test, but results can be compared across subjects using IRT. IRT is a statistical framework related to a subject's performance on individual items and on the test as a whole, and how this performance is associated with the abilities assessed by test items (Hambleton and Jones, 1993). It is based on two assumptions: that the items tap only one construct, and that the probability of answering in a manner that reflects an increasing amount of the trait (i.e. physical function) is unrelated to the probability of answering any other item positively for subjects with the same amount of the trait (Streiner and Norman, 2003). A subject's response to each item is described by a curve, called an item characteristic curve. This curve depicts the relationship between the actual response to the item and the underlying ability, and is thus, a measure of item effectiveness. IRT places each subject on the continuum underlying the construct of interest, allowing the comparison across subjects noted previously.

Before finishing this section of this chapter, it should be noted that the review criteria (Scientific Advisory Committee, 2002), referenced frequently in the paragraphs related to classical scale development, were expanded from a previous version to reflect modern test theory principles and methods. Given the current stage of development as well as the large numbers of subjects and technical support needed to create the new scales, it is predicted that scales developed according to the methods of classical test theory will be used well beyond the next decade. Nonetheless, dynamic testing is being developed in several areas and we can expect to read more and more about it in the near future. It is important that researchers in rehabilitation are involved with research teams creating dynamic measures so that constructs useful in rehabilitation are included. Already, the US National Institutes of Health has announced two initiatives related to IRT. One is from the National Institute of Neurological Disorders and Stroke, and it is expected to create item banks for use in clinical research for people with neurologic conditions. Stroke researchers should benefit from the new technology.

1.4 Principles guiding the selection of outcomes to measure walking competency after stroke

The term *walking competency* (Salbach et al., 2004) is used to describe an ensemble of abilities related to walking that enables the individual to navigate the community proficiently and safely. Elements of walking competency include being able to: walk fast enough to cross the street safely (Robinett and Vondran, 1988; Perry et al., 1995), walk far enough to accomplish activities of daily living (Lerner-Frankiel et al., 1986), negotiate sidewalk curbs independently, turn the head while walking without losing balance, react to unexpected perturbations while walking without loss of stability, and demonstrate anticipatory strategies to avoid or accommodate obstacles in the travel path (Shumway-Cook and Woollacott, 1995). Thus walking competency is linked to the accomplishment of basic every-day tasks, leisure activities and participation in life.

Reliability, validity and responsiveness of gait speed

Gait speed at a comfortable pace is likely the best-known measure of walking performance (Wade, 1992; see Volume II, chapter 3). Timed walking tests (over 5, 10 or 30 m) are easy to carry out and when standardized instructions are used, the *inter-rater* (Holden et al., 1984; Wade et al., 1987) and *test–retest reliability* (Holden et al., 1984; Evans et al., 1997) of measures of walking speed in persons with stroke are high. The *construct validity* of walking speed is also very good. In persons with stroke, comfortable walking speed has been shown to be positively correlated to strength ($r = 0.25$–0.67) of the lower extremity (Bohannon, 1986; Bohannon and Walsh, 1992), to balance ($r = 0.60$; Richards et al., 1995), to motor recovery ($r = 0.62$; Brandstater et al., 1983), to functional mobility ($r = 0.61$; Podsiadlo and Richardson, 1991), and negatively correlated to spasticity of the lower extremity (Norton et al., 1975; Lamontagne et al., 2001; Hsu et al., 2003). Moreover, subjects who walk faster tend to have a better walking pattern (Wade et al., 1987; Richards et al., 1995).

Thus, in terms of *reliability* and *validity*, the 10-min walk (10mW) test at natural or free pace is a very good measure, but is it always the most *responsive* measure? For example, should maximum gait speed also be tested to assess the capacity of persons with stroke to have a burst of speed to, for example cross a busy street (Nakamura et al., 1988; Suzuki et al., 1990; Bohannon and Walsh, 1992)? Others believe measuring gait speed over 5 m is enough. For the sake of argument, let us define "measure of choice" as the measure that is most responsive to change as determined by the SRM. Salbach et al. (2001) examined the responsiveness of four different timed gait tests in 50 persons, tested an average of 8 and 38 days after stroke. They found the 5-min walk (5mW) at comfortable pace test was most responsive followed by the 5mW maximum pace, the 10mW comfortable and the 10mW maximum pace. Responsiveness of a measure of physical performance cannot be generalized because it is related to stroke severity. Table 1.1 compares data from two studies, one with subjects in the early (Salbach et al., 2001) and the other in a sub-acute phase (Richards et al., 2004) post-stroke. It gives estimates of the magnitude of change that can be expected in clinical measures over 8 weeks.

As demonstrated by the Salbach et al. data, the 5mW was more responsive than the timed up and go (TUG) (Podsiadlo and Richardson, 1991) or the balance scale (Berg et al., 1989, 1992a, b, 1995). On the other hand, in the Richards et al. data, the Barthel index (Mahoney and Barthel, 1954) ambulation subscore was the most sensitive measure, followed by the balance scale and the TUG. In this group of subjects, walking speed was less sensitive, likely due to the more severe disability as indicated by the walking speed and TUG time. The balance scale scores, however, are comparable between groups at both evaluations and the SRMs indicate that it is the second most responsive measure for both groups.

To further examine the relation between stroke severity, as gauged by walking speed, and *responsiveness*, data from the sub-acute stroke subjects in the Richards et al. (2004) study were subdivided

Table 1.1. Magnitude of change over 8-week period in persons with acute and sub-acute stroke.

Measure (max. score)	Acute stroke ($n = 50$)			Sub-acute stroke ($n = 62$)				
	Baseline	Post-therapy	SRM	Baseline	Post-therapy	Change	Change (%)	SRM
STREAM (100)	77 ± 25	88 ± 18	0.89					
FM-L (34)				19.7 ± 6.8	22.5 ± 6.4	2.8 ± 3.7	20 ± 29	0.77
FM-A (66)				25.6 ± 19.8	30.6 ± 21.9	5.0 ± 6.8	25 ± 36	0.74
Barthel index (100)	75 ± 26	90 ± 17	0.99					
Barthel ambulation (47)				19.4 ± 8.6	37.7 ± 7.8	18.3 ± 8.5	120 ± 86	2.14
Balance scale (56)	37 ± 18	47 ± 11	1.04	36.1 ± 10.6	45.9 ± 7.6	9.8 ± 7.5	38 ± 46	1.31
TUG (time, s)	32.3 ± 29.1	19.6 ± 17.5	0.88	53.5 ± 24.2	31.3 ± 17.9	22.2 ± 18.3	40 ± 22	1.22
$5mW_{com}$ (cm/s)	59 ± 34	88 ± 38	1.22					
$5mW_{max}$ (cm/s)	83 ± 50	1.16 ± 55	1.00					
$10mW_{com}$ (cm/s)	59 ± 34	84 ± 36	0.92	26.3 ± 14.1*	57 ± 35.8	30.7 ± 29.0	127 ± 130	1.06
$10mW_{max}$ (cm/s)	79 ± 47	105 ± 47	0.83					

Data for subjects with acute stroke obtained from Salbach et al. (2001); subjects, undergoing regular rehabilitation were evaluated 1-week post-stroke and 8 weeks later. Data for subjects with sub-acute stroke taken from Richards et al. (2004); subjects who received task-oriented physical therapy, were evaluated on average 52-days post-stroke and 8 weeks later. SRM that represents the average change score over a set period of time divided by the SD of that change.
*Comfortable walking speed measured over 5, 10 or 30 m. Maximum (max.) score for each measure shown in first column; values give mean or mean ± 1 SD.

according to whether the subjects walked <0.3 or ⩾0.3 m/s at baseline. Figure 1.1 compares the SRM values of the different measures in the two groups. Although the Barthel ambulation subscore remains the most responsive, the SRM is closer to the TUG and gait speed values in the faster walking group and conversely, the balance scale is more responsive in the slower walking group. These results are similar to those reported by Salbach et al. (2001) and Richards et al. (1995), in persons with acute stroke. Such results illustrate how *floor* and *ceiling* effects relate to responsiveness. When selecting a locomotor-related outcome measure it is important to consider the locomotor abilities of the persons to be evaluated. The Fugl-Meyer leg (FM-L) (Fugl-Meyer et al., 1975) subscale and the balance scale which rate the achievement of movement tasks, have a ceiling effect when evaluating higher-performing subjects. Conversely, walking speed can have a floor effect when evaluating subjects who walk at very slow speeds and require assistance

(Richards et al., 1995). The TUG also has a floor effect because many subjects cannot complete the test 2 months after stroke (Richards et al., 1999).

We must now question the classical recovery curve that has been defined by plotting change over time in clinical measures that have a ceiling effect. Thus, it is generally accepted that most recovery occurs in the first 6-week post-stroke when the effects of rehabilitation augment natural recovery. Thereafter, recovery slows but continues up to about 6-month post-stroke (Skilbeck et al., 1983; Richards et al., 1992; Jorgensen et al., 1995). With a continuous measure such as gait speed, however, recovery has been documented up to 2-year post-stroke (Richards et al., 1995). Moreover, a number of intervention studies in persons with chronic stroke have confirmed that recovery of function (Dean et al., 2000; Tangeman et al., 1990; Teixeira-Salmela et al., 1999, 2001; Salbach et al., 2004) and changes in brain organization (Liepert et al., 2000) occur beyond 6 months post-stroke.

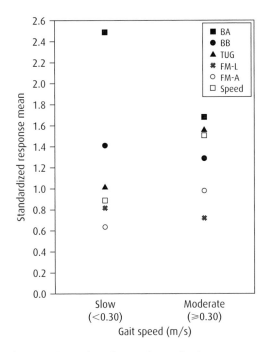

Figure 1.1. Comparison of responsiveness for six outcome measures as determined by the SRM (*y*-axis) in subjects (*n* = 62) with sub-acute stroke who walked at slow (<0.30 m/s) or moderate speeds (≥0.30 m/s) at baseline. BA: Barthel index ambulation subscale; BB: balance scale; FM-A: Fugl-Meyer arm subscale; speed: walking speed at comfortable pace. Data from Richards et al. (2004).

When examining change in outcome measures, it is important to question whether the amount of change is larger than the *measurement error*. For continuous measures, such as walking speed, systematic and random error in repeated measures (measurement error) can be mathematically derived (Evans et al., 1997). It is also possible to calculate the standard error of the mean of scale scores from published reliability studies (Stratford, 2004). Once it is established if the change is greater than the error estimation, it becomes important to decide the MID. For example, the MID of the balance scale is 6 points (Stevenson, 2001), for the 6-min walk (6 MINW) test it is 54 m (Redelmeier et al., 1997) and for the Stroke Impact Scale it is 10–15 points on a subscale (Duncan et al., 1999). One suggested MID

for scale scores is a change of about 11% (Iyer et al., 2003), another is the value one-half an SD of baseline scores (Norman et al., 2003).

Clearly, walking speed alone will not evaluate aspects of walking competency related to endurance, the ability to ascend or descend stairs, or navigate in different terrains under various environmental conditions (Malouin and Richards, 2005). In real life, one usually must rise from a bed or a chair before beginning to walk, not easy tasks for persons with stroke, in part because the affected leg supports less than 50% of the body weight (Engardt and Olsson, 1992; Malouin et al., 2003, 2004a, b). The physical demands of rising from a chair, as measured by the percent maximum muscle activation level (PMAL) of the vastus medialis, are more than triple the approximately 25% PMAL needed for walking, and larger than the 65% PMAL required for stair ascent in healthy subjects (Richards, 1985; Richards et al., 1989). A mobility test like the TUG thus also assesses the ability to perform the sub-tasks of rising and sitting, walking initiation and walking. Stair ascent and descent of a flight of 14 stairs can be added to the TUG to create the more difficult stair test (Perron et al., 2003). Although persons with a dynamic strength deficit of about 25% in the knee extensors (Moffet et al., 1993a, b) can walk without apparent disability, stair climbing will reveal the impairment. The recently developed rise-to-walk test (Dion et al., 2003; Malouin et al., 2003) combines the sit-to-rise test with walking initiation, thus combining two different motor programs while remaining an easier test than the TUG because it does not require the subject to walk 3 m. Subjects with more severe stroke are less able to smoothly transfer from one activity to another and tend to perform first one task and then the second (Dion et al., 2003). This decreased fluidity of task merging can be evaluated in the laboratory (Dion et al., 2003), or by a recently validated clinical method (Malouin et al., 2003).

Poor endurance (Potempa et al., 1995; Macko et al., 1997), largely ignored in clinical practice, has become the focus of much research and the 6 MINW test, that measures functional endurance, has been selected as an outcome measure in a number of stroke trials (Visintin et al., 1998; Dean et al., 2000; Nilsson et al., 2001; Duncan et al., 2003; Salbach et al., 2004). Moreover, the practice of calculating the distance walked in 6 min from the walking speed over 10 m overestimates the actual distance (Dean et al., 2001). Even persons with chronic stroke who walk at near-normal speed (122–142 cm/s) may require functional endurance training (Richards et al., 1999), highlighting the importance of using tests with increasing physical demands.

"Walking competency" as a goal of therapy is relatively new, particularly those aspects related to cognitive processes such as *anticipatory control* and *navigational skills*. Clinicians and researchers alike are grappling to develop new approaches for both therapy and evaluation. The *dynamic gait index* evaluates the ability to modify gait in response to changing task demands. It is able to predict falls in the elderly (Shumway-Cook et al., 1997) and in persons with vestibular problems (Whitney et al., 2000), although the reliability of certain items has been questioned in this population (Wrisley et al., 2003). Others have investigated the dimensions of the physical environment that might impact on mobility. Understanding the relationship of environment to mobility is crucial to both prevention and rehabilitation of mobility problems in older adults (Shumway-Cook et al., 2002). One can argue that the best test of walking competency is to be able to participate in daily routines such as evaluated by the fitness, personal care, housing and mobility categories of the assessment of life habits (Life-H) instrument, based on the handicap creation process model (Fougeyrollas et al., 1998). It has been validated to assess many aspects of life participation of people with disabilities, regardless of the type of underlying impairment (Fougeyrollas and Noreau, 2001). It is not surprising that Desrosiers et al. (2003) have reported high correlations between participation (handicap situations) measured by the Life-H, and impairment and disability measures of the leg, supporting the importance of mobility and gait speed (Perry et al., 1995) to promote social integration after stroke.

1.5 The use of laboratory-based gait assessments and measures of brain reorganization help explain changes in clinical scales and performance-based measures

Laboratory outcome measures

This section will briefly illustrate how *laboratory outcome measures* can be used to:

1 validate clinical measures,
2 explain the results of clinical outcomes,
3 develop new measures,
4 guide therapy.

In-depth gait studies (see Volume II, chapter 19) have elucidated the disturbed motor control during gait in persons after chronic stroke. Low muscle activations (paresis), hyperactive stretch reflexes, excessive coactivation of antagonist muscles and hypoextensibility of muscles and tendons (Knutsson and Richards, 1979; Dietz et al., 1981; Lamontagne et al., 2000a, b, 2001, 2002) may be present to a different extent across subjects. While analysis of gait movements and muscle activations recorded concomitantly during a laboratory gait study allow for the differentiation of the salient motor disturbance (Knutsson and Richards, 1979) to guide therapy, such analyses are not available to usual clinical practice. From studies of moments of force and mechanical power produced by the muscle activations during walking, we know that the main propulsive force comes from the "push-off" contraction of the ankle plantarflexors (generation of power) at the end of the stance phase aided by the "pull-off" contraction of the hip flexors (generation of power) at swing initiation and the contraction of the hip extensors in early stance (Olney et al., 1991; Winter, 1991; Olney and Richards, 1996). Moreover, in persons with chronic stroke, Olney et al. (1994) found the power generated by the hip flexors and ankle plantarflexors of the paretic lower extremity to be the best predictors of walking speed. These laboratory results point to the ankle plantarflexors and hip flexors as muscles to be targeted in therapy to promote better walking speed (Olney et al., 1997;

Richards et al., 1998; Dean et al., 2000; Teixeira-Salmela et al., 2001; Richards et al., 2004).

While gait speed can be used to discern a change in functional status, it does not explain why the person walks faster. An analysis of gait kinetics (muscle activations, moments, powers, work) is needed to pinpoint the source of the increased speed. For example, in a recent trial evaluating the effects of task-oriented physical therapy, Richards et al. (2004) were able to attribute 27% of the improvement in walking speed to a better plantarflexor power burst.

Many new therapeutic approaches and outcome measures are first developed in the laboratory. Much work, for example, has been done on obstacle avoidance in healthy persons (McFadyen and Winter, 1991; Gérin-Lajoie et al., 2002) and persons with stroke (Said et al., 1999, 2001). Virtual reality technology is now being applied to the development of training paradigms to enable persons with stroke to practice navigational skills safely in changing contextual environments (Comeau et al., 2003; McFadyen et al., 2004).

An example of the use of laboratory data to validate a clinical measure is recent work related to the rise-to-walk test. The clinical fluidity scale of the rise-to-walk test was validated by comparing clinical decisions to the smoothness of the momentum curve derived from a biomechanical analysis made in the laboratory (Dion et al., 2003) and led to the development of a fluidity scale (Malouin et al., 2003).

Neuroimaging techniques for studying changes in brain activation patterns and their relationship with functional recovery

With the rapid development of neuroimaging techniques (Volume II, chapter 5), such as positron-emitted tomography (PET), functional magnetic resonance imaging (fMRI) and transcranial magnetic stimulations (TMS; Volume I, Chapter 15), it has become possible to study neural organization associated with motor recovery after brain damage.

Numerous studies have looked at the *predictive value* of TMS (Hendricks et al., 2002; Liepert, 2003).

It provides important prognostic information in the early stage after stroke. For instance, the persistence of motor evoked potentials (MEPs) in paretic muscles has been correlated with good motor recovery, whereas the lack of TMS responses is predictive of poor motor recovery. Patterns of brain activation can also be used early after stroke for predicting functional outcomes. In a longitudinal fMRI study, where hand motor scores were compared to the whole sensorimotor network activation, the early recruitment and high activation of the supplementary motor area (SMA) was correlated with faster or better recovery (Loubinoux et al., 2003). Based on findings from a study combining fMRI and TMS, it has been proposed that the early bilateral activation of the motor networks seen in patients with rapid and good recovery may be a prerequisite to regain motor function rapidly, and thus, may be predictive of motor recovery (Foltys et al., 2003).

Functional imaging and electrophysiologic brain imaging techniques have provided substantial information about adaptive changes of cerebral networks associated with *recovery* from brain damage (Calautti and Baron, 2003). For example, in two rigorously controlled studies, the effects of task-oriented training for the upper limb on brain activation patterns were studied using fMRI (Carey et al., 2002) and PET (Nelles et al., 2002). Both studies found that, in contrast to patients in control groups whose brain activation patterns remained unchanged, patients in the treatment groups displayed enhanced activations in the lesioned sensorimotor cortex in parallel with improved motor function. Similar correlations between changes in brain activation patterns and motor recovery have also been reported after a single dose of fluoxetine (Pariente et al., 2001). TMS mapping studies (Liepert, 2003) provide further evidence of a relationship between training-induced cerebral changes and motor recovery. In these studies, TMS was used to map the motor output area (motor representation) of targeted muscles. Increased cortical excitability and a shift in the motor maps after active rehabilitation (Traversa et al., 1997) or constraint-induced therapy (Liepert et al.,

2000) are associated with improved motor function suggesting treatment-induced reorganization in the affected hemisphere (Liepert et al., 2000).

Recently, the laterality index (LI) has been proposed to quantify changes of brain activation patterns observed in functional neuroimaging studies of recovery post-stroke (Cramer et al., 1997). LI provides an estimate of the relative hemispheric activation in motor cortices. LI values range from +1 (activation exclusively ipsilesional or affected hemisphere) to −1 (activation exclusively contralesional or unaffected hemisphere). These LIs are generally lower in patients, especially in poorly recovered chronic patients, indicating a relatively greater activation of the unaffected hemisphere consistent with the aforementioned general patterns of changes (Calautti and Baron, 2003). Dynamic changes in LI values over time have also been reported in a longitudinal study (Marshall et al., 2000; Calautti et al., 2001). After specific finger-tracking training, Carey

et al. (2002) found increases in LI values corresponding to a switch of activation to the affected hemisphere to be related to improved hand function, suggesting that the LI is a good *marker of brain reorganization*.

Likewise, inter-hemispheric motor reorganization can be quantified using TMS input/output (i/o) curves. The i/o curves, provide a reliable measure (Carroll et al., 2001) of the increase of MEP amplitudes against incrementing levels of TMS intensity (Devanne et al., 1997). Comparisons of the excitability of the motor cortex of the two hemispheres (Fig. 1.2), indicate that in a patient with good motor recovery, the excitability of the motor cortex contralateral to the paretic tibialis anterior (TA) muscle (LI of motor threshold = 0.78) is greater (lower motor threshold, steeper slope and higher plateau of MEP amplitude) compared to the ipsilateral motor cortex and resembles the pattern seen in a healthy individual (LI of motor threshold = 1.0). In contrast,

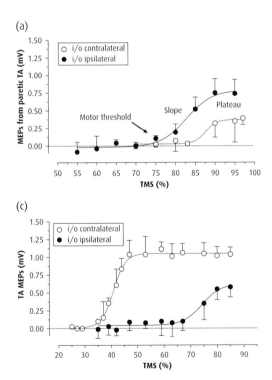

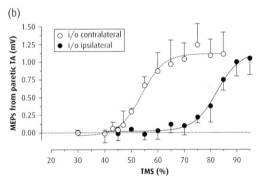

Figure 1.2. Examples of the contralateral and ipsilateral i/o curves of the paretic TA in a patient with (a) poor motor recovery (LI: −0.28) and (b) good recovery (LI = 0.78) compared to normal curves from a (c) healthy subject (LI = 1.0). Each symbol represents the mean of 4 MEPs (±1 SD). See text for more details (Schneider and Malouin, unpublished data).

in a person with poor recovery, a greater excitability is observed in the motor cortex ipsilateral to the paretic TA (LI of motor threshold = −0.28), corresponding to a relatively greater activation from the unaffected hemisphere (Schneider and Malouin, unpublished data). An LI can be calculated for each parameter (motor threshold, slope and MEP plateau) and for the ensemble (Fig. 1.2).

These examples show the potential of combining clinical, laboratory and brain imaging measures to better understand the recovery of locomotor function after stroke.

REFERENCES

Ahmed, S., Mayo, N.E., Higgins, J., Salbach, N.M., Finch, L. and Wood-Dauphinee, S. (2003). The stroke rehabilitation assessment of movement (STREAM): a comparison with other measures used to evaluate effects of stroke and rehabilitation. *Phys Ther*, **83**, 617–630.

Beaton, D.E., Bombardier, C., Katz, J.N. and Wright, J.G. (2001). A taxonomy for responsiveness. *J Clin Epidemiol*, **54**, 1207–1217.

Berg, K., Wood-Dauphinee, S., Williams, J.I. and Gayton, D. (1989). Measuring balance in the elderly: preliminary development of an instrument. *Physiother Can*, **41**, 304–311.

Berg, K., Maki, B., Williams, J.I., Holliday, P. and Wood-Dauphinee, S. (1992a). A comparison of clinical and laboratory measures of postural balance in an elderly population. *Arch Phys Med Rehabil*, **73**, 1073–1080.

Berg, K., Wood-Dauphinee, S., Williams, J.I. and Maki, B. (1992b). Measuring balance in the elderly: validation of an instrument. *Can J Public Health*, **83**(**Suppl. 2**), S7–S11.

Berg, K., Wood-Dauphinee, S. and Williams, J.I. (1995). The balance scale: reliability assessment with elderly residents and patients with acute stroke. *Scand J Rehabil Med*, **27**, 27–36.

Bjorner, J.B. and Ware, J.E. (1998). Using modern psychometric methods to measure health outcomes. *Med Outcome Trust Monit*, **3**, 12–16.

Bohannon, R.W. (1986). Strength of lower limb related to gait velocity and cadence in stroke patients. *Physiother Can*, **38**, 204–210.

Bohannon, R.W. and Walsh, S. (1992). Nature, reliability, and predictive value of muscle performance measures in patients with hemiparesis following stroke. *Arch Phys Med Rehabil*, **73**, 721–725.

Brandstater, M.E., de Bruin, H., Gowland, C. and Clark, B.M. (1983). Hemiplegic gait: analysis of temporal variables. *Arch Phys Med Rehabil*, **64**, 583–587.

Brook, R.H., Williams, K.N. and Avery, A.D. (1976). Quality assurance today and tomorrow: forecast for the future. *Ann Intern Med*, **85**, 809–817.

Calautti, C. and Baron, J.C. (2003). Functional neuroimaging studies of motor recovery after stroke in adults. *Stroke*, **34**, 1553–1566.

Calautti, C., Leroy, F., Guincestre, J.Y. and Baron, J.C. (2001). Dynamics of motor network overactivation after striatocapsular stroke: a longitudinal PET study using a fixed-performance paradigm. *Stroke*, **32**, 2534–2542.

Cardol, M., Beelen, A., van den Bos, G.A., de Jong, B.A., de Grout, I.J. and de Haan, R.J. (2002). Responsiveness of the impact on participation and autonomy questionnaire. *Arch Phys Med Rehabil*, **83**, 1524–1529.

Carey, J.R., Kimberly, T.J., Lewis, S.M., Auerbach, E.J., Dorsey, L., Runqist, P. and Ugurbil, K. (2002). Analysis of fMRI and finger tracking training in subjects with chronic stroke. *Brain*, **125**, 773–788.

Carroll, T.J., Riek, S. and Carson, R.G. (2001). Reliability of the input–output properties of the cortico-spinal pathway obtained from transcranial magnetic and electrical stimulation. *J Neurosci Method*, **112**, 193–202.

Cella, D., Lai, J. and Item Bank Investigators. (2004). Core item banking programs: past, present and future. *Qual Life News Lett*, Fall, Sage Publications, 5–8.

Cleary, P.D. (1996). Future directions of quality of life research. *Qual Life Med Rehabil*, **83**, 1524–1529.

Cohen, J. (1960). Coefficient of agreement for nominal scales. *Educ Psychol Measure*, **20**, 37–46.

Cohen, J. (1988). *Statistical Power Analysis for the Behavioral Sciences*, 2nd edn., Laurence Erlbaum, Hillsdale, NJ.

Collins, D. (2003). Pretesting survey instruments: an overview of cognitive methods. *Qual Life Res*, **12**, 229–238.

Comeau, F., Chapdelaine, S., McFadyen, B.J., Malouin, F., Lamontagne, A., Galiana, L., Laurendeau, D., Richards, C.L. and Fung, J. (2003). Development of increasingly complex virtual environment for locomotor training following stroke. *Second International Workshop on Virtual Rehabilitation*, Piscataway, NJ, September.

Cramer, S.C., Nelles, G., Benson, R.R., Kaplan, J.D., Parker, R.A., Kwong, K.K., Kennedy, D.N., Finklestein, S.P. and Rosen, B.R. (1997). A functional MRI study of subjects recovered from hemiparesis stroke. *Stroke*, **28**, 2518–2527.

Cronbach, L.J. (1951). Coefficient alpha and the internal structure of tests. *Psychometrika*, **16**, 297–334.

Cronbach, L.J. (1957). The two disciplines of scientific psychology. *Am Psychol*, **12**, 671–684.

Crosby, R.D., Kolotkin, R.L. and Williams, G.R. (2003). Defining clinically meaningful change in health-related quality of life. *J Clin Epidemiol*, **56**, 395–407.

Daley, K., Mayo, N., Danys, I., Cabot, R. and Wood-Dauphinee, S. (1997). The stroke rehabilitation assessment of movement (STREAM). *Physiother Can*, **49**, 269–276.

Daley, K., Mayo, N. and Wood-Dauphinee, S. (1999). Testing the reliability of the stroke rehabilitation assessment of movement (STREAM). *Phys Ther*, **79**, 9–23.

De Bruin, A.F., Diederiks, J.P.M., De Witte, L.P., Stevens, F.C.J. and Philipsen, H. (1997). Assessing the responsiveness of a functional status measure: the sickness impact profile versus the SIP68. *J Clin Epidemiol*, **50**, 529–540.

Dean, C.M., Richards, C.L. and Malouin, F. (2000). Task-related circuit training improves performance of locomotor tasks in chronic stroke: a randomized, controlled pilot trial. *Arch Phys Med Rehabil*, **81**, 409–417.

Dean, C.M., Richards, C.L. and Malouin, F. (2001). Walking speed over 10 metres overestimates locomotor capacity after stroke. *Clin Rehabil*, **15**, 415–421.

Desrosiers, J., Malouin, F., Bourbonnais, D., Richards, C.L., Rochette, A. and Bravo, G. (2003). Arm and leg impairments and disabilities after stroke rehabilitation: relation to handicap. *Clin Rehabil*, **17**, 666–673.

Devanne, H., Lavoie, B.A. and Capaday, C. (1997). Input–output properties and gain changes in the human corticospinal pathway. *Exp Brain Res*, **114**, 329–338.

Dietz, V., Quintern, J. and Berger, W. (1981). Electrophysiological studies of gait spasticity and rigidity: evidence that mechanical properties of muscles contribute to hypertonia. *Brain*, **104**, 431–439.

Dion, L., Malouin, F., Mcfadyen, B. and Richards, C.L. (2003). Assessing mobility and locomotor coordination after stroke with the rise-to-walk task. *Neurorehabil Neural Repair*, **17**, 83–92.

Duncan, P., Studenski, S., Richards, L., Gollub, S., Lai, S.M., Reker, D., Perera, S., Yates, J., Koch, V., Regler, S. and Johnson, D. (2003). Randomized clinical trial of therapeutic exercise in sub-acute stroke. *Stroke*, **34**, 2173–2180.

Duncan, P.W., Wallace, D., Lai, S.M., Johnson, D., Embretson, S. and Laster, L.J. (1999). The stroke impact scale version 2.0. Evaluation of reliability, validity and sensitivity to change. *Stroke*, **30**, 2131–2140.

Engardt, M. and Olsson, E. (1992). Body weight-bearing while rising and sitting down in patients with stroke. *Scand J Rehabil Med*, **24**, 67–74.

Evans, M.D., Goldie, P.A. and Hill, K.D. (1997). Systematic and random error in repeated measurements of temporal and distance parameters of gait after stroke. *Phys Ther*, **78**, 725–729.

Finch, E., Brooks, D., Stratford, P. and Mayo, N. (2002). *Physical Rehabilitation Outcome Measures. A Guide to Enhanced Clinical Decision Making*, 2nd edn., B.C. Decker Inc., Hamilton, Ontario.

Fisher, W.P. (1993). Measurement-related problems in functional assessment. *Am J Occup Ther*, **47**, 331–338.

Foltys, H., Krings, T., Meister, I.G., Sparing, R., Boroojerdi, B., Thron, A. and Topper, R. (2003). Motor representation in patients rapidly recovering after stroke: a functional magnetic resonance imaging and transcranial magnetic stimulation study. *Clin Neurophysiol*, **114**, 2404–2415.

Fougeyrollas, P. and Noreau, L. (2001). *Life Habits Measure – Shortened Version (LIFE-H 3.0)*. CQCIDIH, Lac St-Charles, Quebec, Canada.

Fougeyrollas, P., Noreau, L., Bergeron, H., Cloutier, R., Dion, S.A. and St-Michel, G. (1998). Social consequences of long term impairments and disabilities: conceptual approach and assessment of handicap. *Int J Rehabil Res*, **21**, 127–141.

Fugl-Meyer, A.R., Jaaskp, L., Leyman, I., Olsson, S. and Steglind, S. (1975). The post-stroke hemiplegia patient. I. A method for evaluation of physical performance. *Scand J Rehabil Med*, **7**, 13–31.

Gérin-Lajoie, M., McFadyen, B.J., Richards, C.L. and Vallis, L. (2002). Walking around static and mobile upright obstacles. *World Congress of Biomechanics*, Calgary, August.

Guyatt, G., Walter, S. and Norman, G. (1987). Measuring change over time: assessing the usefulness of evaluative instruments. *J Chron Dis*, **40**, 171–178.

Guyatt, G.H., Osoba, D., Wu, A., Wyrwich, K. and Norman, G.R. (2002). Methods to explain the clinical significance of health status measures. *Mayo Clinic Proc*, **77**, 371–383.

Hambleton, R.K. and Jones, R.W. (1993.) Comparison of classical test theory and item response theory and their applications to test development. *Educ Measure Issue Pract*, **12**, 38–47.

Hambleton, R.K., Swaminathan, H. and Rogers, H.J. (1991). *Fundamentals of Item Response Theory.*, Sage, Newbury Park, NJ.

Hays, R.D. (1998). Item response theory models. In: *Quality of Life Assessment in Clinical Trials* (eds Staquet, M.J., Hays, R.D. and Fayers, P.M.), Oxford University Press, Oxford., pp. 183–190.

Hays, R.D. and Hadorn, D. (1992). Responsiveness to change: an aspect of validity not a separate dimension. *Qual Life Res*, **1**, 73–75.

Hendricks, H.T., Zwarts, M.J., Plat, E.F. and van Limbeek, J. (2002). Systematic review for the early prediction of motor and functional outcome after stroke by using motor-evoked potentials. *Arch Phys Med Rehabil*, **83**, 1303–1308.

Holden, M.K., Gill, K.M., Magliozzi, M.R., Nathan, J. and Piehl-Baker, L. (1984). Clinical gait assessment in the neurologically impaired. Reliability and meaningfulness. *Phys Ther*, **64**, 35–40.

Hsu, A.-L., Tang, P.-F. and Jan, M.-H. (2003). Analysis of impairments influencing gait velocity and asymmetry of hemiplegic patients after mild to moderate stroke. *Arch Phys Med Rehabil*, **84**, 1185–1193.

Husted, J.A., Cook, R.J., Farewell, V.T. and Gladman, D.D. (2000). Methods for assessing responsiveness: a critical review and recommendations. *J Clin Epidemiol*, **53**, 459–468.

Iyer, L.V., Haley, S., Watkins, M.P. and Dumas, H.M. (2003). Establishing minimal clinically important difference scores on the pediatric evaluation of disability inventory for inpatient rehabilitation. *Phys Ther*, **83**, 888–898.

Jaeschke, R., Singer, J. and Guyatt, G.D. (1989). Measurement of health status: ascertaining the minimal clinically important difference. *Control Clin Trial*, **10**, 407–415.

Jorgensen, H.S., Nakayama, H., Raaschou, H.O. and Olsen, T.S. (1995). Recovery of walking function in stroke patients. The Copenhagen Stroke Study. *Arch Phys Med Rehabil*, **76**, 27–32.

Juniper, E.F., Guyatt, G.H. and Jaeschke, R. (1996). How to develop and validate a new health-related quality of life instrument. In: *Quality of Life and Pharmacoeconomics in Clinical Trials* (ed. Spilker, B.), Lippencott-Raven, Philadelphia, PA., pp. 49–56.

Kirshner, B. and Guyatt, G. (1985). A methodological framework for assessing health indices. *J Chron Dis*, **38**, 27–36.

Knutsson, E. and Richards, C.L. (1979). Different types of disturbed motor control in gait of hemiparetic patients. *Brain*, **102**, 405–430.

Lamontagne, A., Malouin, F. and Richards, C.L. (2000a). Contribution of passive stiffness to ankle plantarflexor moment during gait after stroke. *Arch Phys Med Rehabil*, **81**, 351–358.

Lamontagne, A., Richards, C.L. and Malouin, F. (2000b). Coactivation during gait as an adaptive behavior after stroke. *J Electromyogr Kinesiol*, **10**, 407–415.

Lamontagne, A., Malouin, F. and Richards, C.L. (2001). Locomotor task-specific measure of spasticity of plantarflexor muscles after stroke. *Arch Phys Med Rehabil*, **82**, 1696–1704.

Lamontagne, A., Malouin, F., Richards, C.L. and Dumas, F. (2002). Mechanisms of disturbed motor control in ankle weakness during gait after stroke. *Gait Posture*, **15**, 244–255.

Lerner-Frankiel, M.B., Vargus, S., Brown, M.B., et al. (1986). Functional community ambulation: What are your criteria? *Clin Manage*, **6**, 12–15.

Liepert, J. (2003). TMS in stroke. In: *Transcranial Magnetic Stimulation and Transcranial Direct Current Stimulation* (eds Paulus, W., Tergau, F., Rothwell, J.C., Ziemann, U. and Hallett, M.), Elsevier Science. *Clin Neurophysiol*, **56**(**Suppl.**), S368–S380.

Liepert, J., Bauder, H., Miltmer, H.R., Taub, E. and Weiller, C. (2000). Treatment-induced cortical reorganization after stroke in humans. *Stroke*, **31**, 1210–1216.

Likert, R.A. (1952). A technique for the development of attitudes. *Educ Psychol Measure*, **12**, 313–315.

Loubinoux, I., Carel, C., Pariente, J., deChaumont, S., Albucher, J.F., Marque, P., Manelfe, C. and Chollet, F. (2003). Correlation between cerebral reorganization and motor recovery after subcortical infarcts. *Neuroimage*, **20**, 2126–2180.

Lydick, E.G. and Epstein, R.S. (1993). Interpretation of quality of life changes. *Qual Life Res*, **2**, 221–226.

Macko, R.F., DeSouza, C.A., Tretter, L.D., Silver, K.H., Smith, G.V., Anderson, P.A., Tomoyasu, N., Gorman, P. and Dengel, D.R. (1997). Treadmill aerobic exercise training reduces the energy expenditure and cardiovascular demands of hemiparetic gait in chronic stroke patients. A preliminary report. *Stroke*, **28**, 326–330.

Mahoney, F.I. and Barthel, D.W. (1954). Rehabilitation of the hemiplegic patient: a clinical evaluation. *Arch Phys Med Rehabil*, **35**, 359–362.

Malouin, F. and Richards, C.L. (2005). Assessment and training of locomotor function after stroke: evolving concepts. In: *Science-Based Rehabilitation: Theory into Practice* (eds Refshauge, K., Ada, L. and Ellis, E.), Butterworth-Heinemann, Sydney, Australia, pp. 185–222.

Malouin, F., McFadyen, B., Dion, L. and Richards, C.L. (2003). A fluidity scale for evaluating the motor strategy of the rise-to-walk task after stroke. *Clin Rehabil*, **17**, 674–685.

Malouin, F., Belleville, S., Desrosiers, J., Doyon, J. and Richards, C.L. (2004a). Working memory and mental practice after stroke. *Arch Phys Med Rehabil*, **85**, 177–183.

Malouin, F., Richards, C.L., Belleville, S., Desrosiers, J. and Doyon, J. (2004b). Training mobility tasks after stroke with combined physical and mental practice: a feasibility study. *Neurorehabil Neural Repair*, **18**, 66–75.

Marshall, R.S., Perera, G.M., Lazar, R.M., Krakauer, J.W., Costantine, R.C. and DeLaPaz, R.L. (2000). Evolution of cortical activation during recovery from corticospinal tract infarction. *Stroke*, **31**, 656–661.

McFadyen, B.J. and Winter, D.A. (1991). Anticipatory locomotor adjustments during obstructed walking. *Neurosci Res Commun*, **9**, 37–44.

McFadyen, B.J., Malouin, F., Fung, J., Comeau, F., Chapdelaine, S., Beaudoin, C., Lamontagne, A., Laurendeau, D. and Richards, C.L. (2004). *Development of Complex Virtual*

Environments for Locomotor Training Following Stroke. International Society of Electrophysiology and Kinesiology, Boston, USA.

McHorney, C.A. (1997). Generic health measurement: past accomplishments and a measurement paradigm for the 21st century. *Ann Intern Med*, **15**, 743–750.

Moffet, H., Richards, C.L. and Malouin, F. (1993a). Load-carrying during stair ascent: a new functional test. *Gait Posture*, **1**, 35–44.

Moffet, H., Richards, C.L., Malouin, F. and Bravo, G. (1993b). Impact of knee extensor strength deficits on stair ascent performance in patients after medial meniscectomy. *Scand J Rehabil Med*, **25**, 63–71.

Nakamura, R.A., Handa, T., Watanabe, S. and Morohashi, I. (1988). Walking cycle after stroke. *Tohoku J Exp Med*, **154**, 241–244.

Nelles, G., Jentzen, W., Jueptner, M., Muller, S. and Diener, H.C. (2002). Arm training induced brain plasticity in stroke studied with serial positron emission tomography. *Neuroimage*, **13**, 1146–1154.

Nilsson, L., Carlsson, J., Danielsson, A., Fugl-Meyer, A., Hellstrom, K., Kristensen, L., Sjolund, B., Sunnerhagen, K.S. and Grimby, G. (2001). Walking training of patients with hemiparesis at an early stage after stroke: a comparison of walking training on a treadmill with body weight support and walking training on the ground. *Clin Rehabil*, **15**, 515.

Norman, G.R., Sridhar, F.G., Guyatt, G.H. and Walter, S.D. (2001). Relation of distribution- and anchor-based approaches in interpretation of changes in health-related quality of life. *Med Care*, **39**, 1039–1047.

Norman, G.R., Sloan, J.A. and Wyrwich, K.W. (2003). Interpretation of changes in health-related quality of life: the remarkable universality of half a standard deviation. *Med Care*, **41**, 582–592.

Norton, B.J., Bomze, H.A., Sahrmann, S.A., et al. (1975). Correlation between gait speed and spasticity at the knee. *Phys Ther*, **55**, 355–359.

Olney, S., Nymark, J., Zee, B., Martin, C. and McNamara, P. (1997). Effects of computer-assisted gait training (BioTRAC) on early stroke – a randomised clinical trial. *North American Stroke Meeting*, Montreal. *Neurol Rev*, **5**, 38.

Olney, S.J. and Richards, C.L. (1996). Hemiplegic gait following stroke. Part I. Characteristics. *Gait Posture*, **4**, 136–148.

Olney, S.J., Griffin, M.P., Monga, T.N. and McBride, I.D. (1991). Work and power in gait of stroke patients. *Arch Phys Med Rehabil*, **72**, 309–314.

Olney, S.J., Griffen, M.P. and McBride, I.D. (1994). Temporal, kinematic and kinetic variables related to gait speed in sub-jects with hemiplegia: a regression approach. *Phys Ther*, **74**, 872–885.

Pariente, J., Loubinoux, I., Carel, C., Albucher, J.F., Leger, A., Manelfe, C., Rascol, O. and Chollet, F. (2001). Fluoxetine modulates motor performance and cerebral activation of patients recovering from stroke. *Ann Neurol*, **50**, 718–729.

Perron, M., Malouin, F. and Moffet, H. (2003). Assessing loco-motor recovery after total hip arthroplasty with the timed stair test. *Clin Rehabil*, **17**, 780–786.

Perry, J., Garrett, M., Gronley, J.K. and Mulroy, S.J. (1995). Classification of walking handicap in the stroke population. *Stroke*, **26**, 982–989.

Podsiadlo, D. and Richardson, S. (1991). The timed "up an go". A test of basic functional mobility for frail elderly persons. *J Am Geriatr Soc*, **39**, 142–149.

Poissant, L., Mayo, N., Wood-Dauphinee, S. and Clarke, A. (2003). The development and preliminary validation of the preference-based stroke index (PBS). *Health Qual Life Outcome*, **1**, 43.

Portney, L.G. and Watkins, M.P. (2000). *Foundations of Clinical Research: Applications to Practice*, 2nd edn., Prentice Hall Health, Upper Saddle River, NJ.

Potempa, K., Lopez, M., Braun, L.T., Szidon, J.P., Fogg, L. and Tincknell, T. (1995). Physiological outcomes of aerobic exercise training in hemiparetic stroke patients. *Stroke*, **26**, 101–105.

Redelmeier, D.A., Guyatt, G.H. and Goldstein, R.S. (1996). Assessing the minimal important difference in symptoms: a comparison of two techniques. *J Clin Epidemiol*, **49**, 1215–1219.

Redelmeier, D.A., Bayoumi, A.M., Goldstein, R.S. and Guyatt, G.H. (1997). Interpreting small differences in functional status: the six minute walk test in chronic lung disease patients. *Am J Respir Crit Care Med*, **155**, 1278–1283.

Revicki, D.A. and Cella, D.F. (1997). Health status assessment for the twenty-first century: item response theory, item banking and computer testing. *Qual Life Res*, **6**, 595–600.

Richards, C.L. (1985). EMG activity level comparisons in quadriceps and hamstrings in five dynamic activities. In: *Biomechanics IX-A* (eds Winter, D., Wells, R., Norman, R., Hayes, K. and Patla, A.), Human Kinetics Publishers, Champaign, IL, pp. 313–317.

Richards, C.L., Malouin, F., Durand, A. and Moffet, H. (1989). Muscle activation level comparisons for determining func-tional demands of locomotor tasks. *Semin Orthoped*, **4**, 120–129.

Richards, C.L., Malouin, F., Dumas, F. and Wood-Dauphinee, S. (1992). The relationship of gait speed to clinical measures of function and muscle activations during recovery post-stroke.

In: *Proceedings of NACOBII: The Second North American Congress on Biomechanics* (eds Draganich, L., Wells, R. and Bechtold, J.), Chicago, pp. 299–302.

Richards, C.L., Malouin, F., Dumas, F. and Tardif, D. (1995). Gait velocity as an outcome measure of locomotor recovery after stroke. In: *Gait Analysis: Theory and Applications* (eds Craik, R.L. and Oatis, C.), Mosby, St-Louis, pp. 355–364.

Richards, C.L., Malouin, F., Dumas, F. and Lamontagne, A. (1998). Recovery of ankle and hip power during walking after stroke. *Can J Rehabil*, **11**, 271–272.

Richards, C.L., Malouin, F. and Dean, C. (1999). Assessment and rehabilitation. *Clin Geriatric Med*, **15**, 833–855.

Richards, C.L., Malouin, F., Bravo, G., Dumas, F. and Wood-Dauphinee, S. (2004). The role of technology in task-oriented training in persons with sub-acute stroke: a randomized controlled trail. *Neurorehabil Neural Repair*, **18**, 199–211.

Robinett, C.S. and Vondran, M.A. (1988). Functional ambulation velocity and distance requirements in rural and urban communities. A clinical report. *Phys Ther*, **68**, 1371–1373.

Said, C.M., Goldie, P.A., Patla, A.E., Sparrow, W.A. and Martin, K.E. (1999). Obstacle crossing in subjects with stroke. *Arch Phys Med Rehabil*, **80**, 1054–1059.

Said, C.M., Goldie, P.A., Patla, A.E. and Sparrow, W.A. (2001). Effect of stroke on step characteristics of obstacle crossing. *Arch Phys Med Rehabil*, **82**, 1712–1719.

Salbach, N.M., Mayo, N.E., Higgins, J., Ahmed, S., Finch, L.E. and Richards, C.L. (2001). Responsiveness and predictability of gait speed and other disability measures in acute stroke. *Arch Phys Med Rehabil*, **82**, 1204–1212.

Salbach, N.M., Mayo, N.E., Wood-Dauphinee, S., Hanley, J.A., Richards, C.L. and Côté R. (2004). A mobility intervention enhances walking competency in the first year post-stroke: a randomized controlled trial. *Clin Rehabil*, **5**, 509–519.

Scientific Advisory Committee of the Medical Outcomes Trust (2002). Assessing health status and quality of life instruments: attributes and review criteria. *Qual Life Res*, **11**, 193–205.

Shumway-Cook, A. and Woollacott, M. (1995). *Motor Control: Theory and Practical Applications.*, Williams & Wilkins, Baltimore, MD.

Shumway-Cook, A., Baldwin, M., Polissar, N.L. and Gruber, W. (1997). Predicting the probability for falls in community-dwelling older adults. *Phys Ther*, **77**, 812–819.

Shumway-Cook, A., Patla, A.A.E., Stewart, A., Ferrucci, L., Ciol, M.A. and Guralnik, J.M. (2002). Environmental demands associated with community mobility in older adults with and without mobility disabilities. *Phys Ther*, **82**, 670–681.

Skilbeck, C.E., Wade, D.T., Hewer, R.L. and Wood, V.A. (1983). Recovery after stroke. *J Neurol Neurosurg Psychiatr*, **46**, 5–8.

Stevenson, T. (2001). Detecting change in patients with stroke using the Berg balance scale. *Aust J Physiother*, **7**, 29–38.

Stratford, P. (2004). Getting more from the literature: estimating the standard error of measurement from reliability studies. *Physiother Can*, **56**, 27–30.

Stratford, P.W., Binkley, J.M. and Riddle, D.L. (1996). Health status measures: strategies and analytic methods for assessing change scores. *Phys Ther*, **76**, 1109–1123.

Streiner, D.L. and Norman, G.R. (2003). *Health Measurement Scales: A Practical Guide to Their Development and Use*, 3rd edn., Oxford University Press, Oxford.

Suzuki, K., Nakamura, R., Yamada, Y. and Handa, T. (1990). Determinants of maximum walking speed in hemiparetic stroke patients. *Tohoku J Exp Med*, **162**, 337–344.

Tangeman, P., Banaitis, D. and Williams, A. (1990). Rehabilitation for chronic stroke patients: changes in functional performance. *Arch Phys Med Rehabil*, **71**, 876–880.

Teixeira-Salmela, L.F., Olney, S.J., Nadeau, S. and Brouwer, B. (1999). Muscle strengthening and physical conditioning to reduce impairment and disability in chronic stroke survivors. *Arch Phys Med Rehabil*, **10**, 1211–1218.

Teixeira-Salmela, L.F., Nadeau, S., McBride, I. and Olney, S.J. (2001). Effects of muscle strengthening and physical conditioning training on temporal, kinematic and kinetic variables during gait in chronic stroke survivors. *J Rehabil Med*, **33**, 53–60.

Terwee, C.B., Dekker, F.W., Wiersinga, W.M., Prummel, M.F. and Bossuyt, P.M.M. (2003). On assessing responsiveness of health related quality of life instruments: guidelines for instrument evaluation. *Qual Life Res*, **12**, 349–362.

Traversa, R., Cicinelli, P., Bassi, A., Rossinin, P.M. and Bernardi, G. (1997). Mapping of motor cortical reorganization after stroke: a brain stimulation study with focal magnetic pulses. *Stroke*, **28**, 110–117.

Tuley, M.R., Mulrow, C. and McMahan, A. (1991). Estimating and testing an index of responsiveness and the relationship of the index to power. *J Clin Epidemiol*, **44**, 417–421.

Visintin, M., Barbeau, H., Korner-Bitensky, N. and Mayo, N.E. (1998). A new approach to retrain gait in stroke patients through body weight support and treadmill stimulation. *Stroke*, **29**, 1122–1128.

Wade, D.T. (1992). *Measurement in Neurological Rehabilitation.*, Oxford Medical Publications, Oxford University Press, Oxford.

Wade, D.T., Wood, V.A., Heller, A., Maggs, J. and Langton, H.R. (1987). Walking after stroke: measurement and recovery over the first 3 months. *Scand J Rehabil Med*, **19**, 25–30.

Ware, J.E. and Keller, S.D. (1996). Interpreting general health measures. In: *Quality of Life and Pharmacoeconomics in*

Clinical Trials (ed. Spilker, B.), Lippencott-Raven, Philadelphia, PA, pp. 445–460.

Whitney, S.L., Hudak, M.T. and Marchetti, G.F. (2000). The dynamic gait index relates to self-reported fall history in individuals with vestibular dysfunction. *J Vestib Res*, **10**, 99–105.

Winter, D.A. (1991). *The Biomechanics and Motor Control of Human Gait: Normal, Elderly and Pathological*, 2nd edn., University of Waterloo Press, Waterloo, ON.

Wood-Dauphinee, S., Williams, J.I., Opzoomer, A., Marchand, B. and Spitzer, W.O. (1988). Assessment of global function: the reintegration to normal living index. *Arch Phys Med Rehabil*, **69**, 583–590.

Wood-Dauphinee, S., Berg, K. and Daley, K. (1994). Monitoring status and evaluating outcomes: an overview of rating scales for use with patients who have sustained a stroke. *Top Geriat Rehabil*, **10**, 22–41.

Wood-Dauphinee, S., Berg, K., Bravo, G. and Williams, J.I. (1997). The balance scale: responsiveness to clinically meaningful changes. *Can J Rehabil*, **10**, 35–50.

World Health Organization (2001). *International Classification of Functioning, Disability and Health.*, World Health Organization, Geneva.

Wrisley, D.M., Walker, M., Echternach, J.L. and Strasnick, B. (2003). Reliability of the dynamic gait index in people with vestibular disorders. *Arch Phys Med Rehabil*, **84**, 1528–1533.

Wyrwich, K.W., Tierney, W.M. and Wolinsky, F.D. (2002). Using the standard error of measurement to identify important changes in the asthma quality of life questionnaire. *Qual Life Res*, **11**, 1–7.

Human voluntary motor control and dysfunction

Catherine E. Lang[1], Karen T. Reilly[2] and Marc H. Schieber[2,3]

[1]*Program in Physical Therapy, Washington University School of Medicine, St. Louis, MO, USA and*
[2]*Departments of Neurobiology and Anatomy and* [3]*Neurology, University of Rochester, Rochester, NY, USA*

The ability to promote functional recovery after nervous system injury depends in part on understanding how the normal brain works and how the damaged brain reorganizes itself. This chapter discusses the current understanding of how areas of the cerebral cortex and their descending pathways contribute to voluntary motor control in humans in the context of how these areas may provide compensatory control for each other in the damaged brain. Primary motor cortical (M1) areas and non-primary motor cortical areas (NPMAs) are presented as a flexible control system for voluntary movement, with an inherent capacity for reorganization. In part, this capacity for flexible reorganization arises from the intrinsic organization of cortical areas, in part from the network of connections among areas, and in part from the availability of more than one descending pathway. The concluding section of this chapter discusses how, in addition to lesion size and lesion location, territories and tracts that are spared after a lesion can affect the capacity for functional recovery of movement.

2.1 The M1

The current view of M1 organization

Our thinking about M1 has been shaped largely by the oversimplification of two related concepts. First, the concept of motor somatotopy, which was carried farthest by the work of Penfield and his memorable cartoon, the homunculus (Penfield and Boldrey, 1937; Penfield and Rasmussen, 1950), has been interpreted to mean that different segments of the body are controlled from spatially separate regions of M1, down to the level of a different region for each finger of the hand. Second, the concept of the upper motor neuron, which can be traced to Gowers (Phillips and Landau, 1990), has been interpreted to mean that cortical neurons are simply higher order neurons whose physiologic behavior is essentially like that of lower motoneurons. Following these two concepts, M1 has previously been viewed as a somatotopically organized sheet of separate groups of upper motor neurons, each of which controls a pool of spinal motoneurons, and thereby moves a particular body segment (illustrated schematically in Fig. 2.1(a)). The current view of M1 is quite different (Schieber, 2001) such that different spinal motoneuron pools receive input from broad, overlapping cortical territories, and many M1 neurons have projections that diverge to more than one motoneuron pool (Fig. 2.1(b)). In the current view, neurons distributed over a wide cortical region are active during the movement of a given body segment. This section reviews evidence that supports the current, more complex view of M1, and discusses how the current view indicates that M1 is a flexible control system with an inherent capacity for plastic reorganization after brain injury.

Three important points provide evidence for this current, more complex view of M1. First, whereas the prior view of M1 suggested that stimulation of different regions of M1 should elicit movement of different body segments, the current view indicates

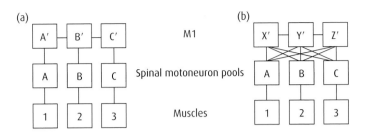

Figure 2.1. Classical view (a) and current view (b) of the manner in which M1 neurons connect to the spinal motoneuron pools and their muscles.

that focal stimulation can elicit movement of the same body part from multiple sites in a broad region. Thus, regions where stimulation elicits movements of different body segments must overlap extensively. Early studies of electrical stimulation of the cortical surface, including those of Penfield, show that within the face region, arm region, or leg region, the territories from which stimulation can elicit movement of different segments overlap considerably (Leyton and Sherrington, 1917; Penfield and Boldrey, 1937; Woolsey et al., 1952). Despite the development of more focal stimulation of the cortex over the past few decades, the spatial resolution of motor maps has not become finer. Intracortical microstimulation shows a broadly overlapping mosaic of points where stimulation elicits movements of different body segments (Sato and Tanji, 1989; Waters et al., 1990; Park et al., 2001). Moreover large cortical territories have projections that converge on single spinal motoneurons (Andersen et al., 1975). Taken together, these studies support the view that output from a broad cortical territory converges on the spinal motoneuron pool for a given muscle and that the cortical territories for different muscles overlap extensively.

Second, whereas the prior view of M1 suggested that each M1 neuron with corticospinal output influences just one muscle, the current view indicates that a given M1 neuron may influence the motoneuron pools of several muscles. Evidence that single M1 neurons provide output to multiple muscles has been obtained using spike-triggered averaging, an analysis technique that is used to detect and quantify

relatively direct relationships between a cortical neuron and a spinal motoneuron pool. Spike-triggered averaging studies in awake monkeys have shown that single M1 neurons usually connect to two or more muscles (Fetz and Cheney, 1980; Buys et al., 1986) and that some single M1 neurons connect to both proximal and distal muscles (McKiernan et al., 1998). Anatomically, horseradish peroxidase staining has shown that some single corticospinal axons have terminal arbors in multiple spinal motoneuron pools (Shinoda et al., 1981). Thus, although some corticospinal neurons may influence only one muscle, many others diverge to multiple muscles.

Third, whereas the prior view of M1 suggested that neurons in one region of M1 would be active during movement of one body segment and neurons in another region of M1 would be active during movement of another body segment, the current view indicates that neurons in overlapping M1 territories will be active during movements of different body segments. Evidence supporting the current view has been found in monkeys and in humans. Recording the activity of single M1 hand area neurons in monkeys trained to flex and extend each of their fingers revealed that (1) a given neuron could be active with movement of several different fingers and (2) the region of M1 where active neurons were found during movement of a given digit was co-extensive with the region where active neurons were found during the movement of any other digit (Schieber and Hibbard, 1993). Reversible inactivation studies in similarly trained monkeys show that small amounts of muscimol injected into the hand area disrupt some finger movements more than others, but the movements that are disrupted were unrelated to the mediolateral location of the inactivation along the central sulcus (Schieber and Poliakov, 1998). Similarly, other reports of small reversible (Brochier et al., 1999) and permanent (Friel and Nudo, 1998) lesions to the M1 hand area have documented impairment in movements of body segments proximal to the hand, as well as in the hand itself. In humans, regional cerebral blood flow studies have shown that, although a small somatotopic shift for the center of activation can be identified, extensively overlapping M1 regions are activated during movements of a single finger, several fingers, or of the more proximal arm segments (Grafton et al., 1993; Sanes et al., 1995; Kleinschmidt et al., 1997; Beisteiner et al., 2001; Hlustik et al., 2001; Indovina and Sanes, 2001). Likewise, cases of small lesions to the M1 hand territory suggest that although there is a general somatotopic gradient in human M1 (Lee et al., 1998; Schieber, 1999; Kim, 2001), a strict mediolateral somatotopy with discrete regions for each finger and for the wrist, elbow, and shoulder likely does not exist. Taken together, this evidence shows that natural movements of different body parts involve activation of M1 in broad, overlapping territories.

Implications of M1 organization for recovery after brain injury

What implications do these advances in our understanding of M1 have for functional recovery and neurorehabilitation after brain injury? First, note that the current view suggests that any region of M1 normally participates in the control of many body parts. Neurologists, physiatrists, and rehabilitation professionals witness this in clinical practice daily. One never sees a cortical lesion produce weakness of just the thumb, or just the little finger, or just the upper lip. Rather, any lesion affecting M1 that is large enough to produce clinical findings produces simultaneous weakness of multiple contiguous body segments. The entire face on one side, the entire hand, or the entire foot becomes weak from a cortical lesion. The weakness may be greater in the thumb and index

than in the ulnar fingers, or greater distally than proximally in an extremity, but weakness is not confined to one small body segment. This observation is customarily ascribed to the fact that disease processes do not respect physiologic boundaries. But if this were the reason, some patients should have a weak face and thumb, but strong fingers, or a weak leg and little finger, but a strong thumb. Instead, these patterns do not occur because the physiologic boundaries do not exist.

If any one region of M1 normally participates in the control of many body parts, then when part of M1 is injured, spared regions of M1 may be able to restore function, not because they have assumed entirely new functions, but because they were participating in those functions before the injury. This may explain, in part, why after small experimental lesions to the M1 hand territory in monkeys with subsequent forced use of the affected hand, intracortical microstimulation in the territory surrounding the lesion that had originally represented more proximal muscles, now produced contractions in hand muscles (Nudo et al., 1996a, see also Volume I, Chapter 8 on Plasticity in motor functions and Chapter 14, Plasticity after Brain Lesions). Similarly, in people with small lesions of the hand knob area of M1 (Yousry et al., 1997), recovery may be nearly complete, such that impairments in motor control can be detected only during kinematic testing of independent finger movements (Lang and Schieber, 2003). Thus, if some M1 territory is spared, part of the functional recovery seen after brain injury may arise from the inherent flexibility of the remaining M1 territory.

Redistribution of function within M1 may be capable of occurring over greater cortical distances and faster than previously thought. For example, the areas of M1 devoted to control of the fingers have been shown to enlarge when a normal subject practices a complex finger movement task (Karni et al., 1995). Enlargement of the M1 hand area over several weeks has been observed with intracortical microstimulation mapping in monkeys (Nudo et al., 1996b), and studies employing transcranial magnetic stimulation suggest that in humans, such enlargement can occur within minutes (Pascual-Leone et al., 1994). Simply repositioning the forelimb in rodents has been shown to shift the boundary between the forelimb and vibrissae (whisker) representations in M1 (Sanes et al., 1992). Permanent changes in the human M1's neural connections with the periphery, such as those occurring with spinal cord injury or amputation, have been shown to alter the M1 map (Levy et al., 1990; Giraux et al., 2001). Likewise, temporary ischemic anesthesia of the forearm for 30 min produces greater activation of proximal arm muscles by a constant transcranial magnetic stimulus compared to before the ischemic anesthetic (Brasil-Neto et al., 1993). M1 can thus reorganize extensively and promptly.

An important and rapidly developing topic in neurorehabilitation research is how this capacity for flexible reorganization of M1 might be exploited in humans with brain injury to enhance functional recovery. For example, Muellbacher and colleagues are exploring how afferent input from proximal versus distal upper extremity segments may be manipulated to increase the M1 representation of the hand, and potentially result in improved hand function in people with chronic stroke (Muellbacher et al., 2002; see Volume I, Chapter 15 on Influence of theories of plasticity on humans). While it could be many years until these novel approaches might be proven efficacious enough to be used routinely in clinical practice, we speculate that neurorehabilitation will eventually be able to make use of M1's ability to flexibly redistribute its function, by identifying the injured regions and then designing specific rehabilitative strategies that make maximal use of nearby uninjured regions.

2.2 NPMAs

The current view of NPMA organization

The classical view of voluntary motor control was that, when an action is willed, the frontal association areas pass a command to the "premotor" cortical areas, which in turn select a motor plan and pass it to M1. M1 executes the movement via direct and indirect commands to the spinal motoneurons. Evidence has emerged over the past few decades suggesting that this sequential, hierarchical model of voluntary motor control is inaccurate and should be replaced with a more parallel, distributed model. In a parallel, distributed model, NPMAs and M1 areas are engaged together in generating the motor plan and controlling spinal motoneurons. Whereas the sequential, hierarchical model suggested that destruction of any single area in the hierarchy would prevent voluntary movement, the parallel, distributed model implies that if one center is destroyed, other centers may be able to take over.

What evidence is there that voluntary motor control should be viewed as a parallel, distributed process? It is now known that there are many more frontal cortical motor areas than formerly thought, that these areas are extensively interconnected with M1 and with one another, and that many NPMAs have significant corticospinal projections themselves. Primate studies have identified multiple NPMAs in the frontal lobe (Fig. 2.2). Anterior to the M1 in area 4, area 6 contains a ventral premotor area (PMv), and a dorsal premotor area (PMd) on the lateral surface of the hemisphere, and the supplementary motor area (SMA) on the medial surface. PMv and PMd can be further subdivided into a ventrorostral premotor area (PMvr), ventrocaudal premotor area (PMvc), dorsorostral premotor area (PMdr), and dorsocaudal premotor area (PMdc). Rostral to the SMA, area 6 also contains the pre-supplementary motor area (pre-SMA). Area 24 in the superior and inferior banks of the cingulate sulcus contains at least dorsal (CMAd), rostral (CMAr), and caudal (CMAc) cingulate motor areas. These NPMAs can be distinguished from one another because they have: (1) different cytoarchitechtonic features; (2) separate microstimulation maps; (3) separate reciprocal interconnections with the thalamus, with M1 and/or with one another; and (4) different features of physiologic activity (for reviews see Rizzolatti et al., 1998; Dum and Strick, 2002). Figure 2.3 shows our current road map of the interconnections between these areas. Corticospinal projections arise not only from

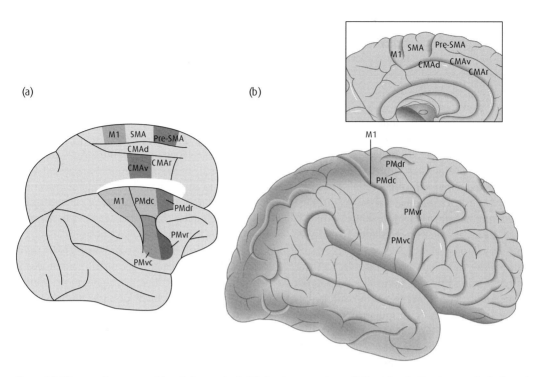

(a)

(b)

Figure 2.2. Diagram of a macaque (a) and a human brain (b) showing current parcellation of cortical motor areas in the frontal lobe. Note that the various NPMAs are defined based on research in the non-human primate and that the human parcellation is currently under investigation.

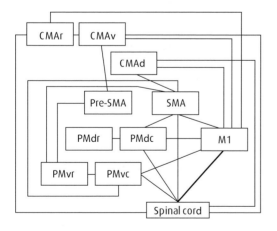

Figure 2.3. Connections of the cortical motor areas. See text for definitions of abbreviations. Most corticocortical connections are reciprocal. The thick line from M1 to the spinal cord indicates that this corticospinal projection is stronger than corticospinal projections from other areas.

M1, but also from PMv, PMd, SMA, CMAd, CMAr, and CMAc. Corticospinal axons from the NPMAs terminate in the intermediate zone and the ventral horn of the spinal cord, in a distribution that is quantitatively less but qualitatively similar to axonal projections from M1 (for review see Dum and Strick, 2002).

Further evidence supporting a parallel, distributed model of motor control and not a sequential, hierarchical model comes from reaction time and neuronal firing time data. Given that conduction times from M1 to spinal motoneurons and then to hand muscles require only 20–30 ms, human reaction times, approximately 200 ms for visual cues, and 100 ms for somatosensory cues (Cordo and Flanders, 1989), allow sufficient time for information sharing within and between multiple cortical and subcortical areas prior to a motor response.

Likewise in non-human primates, task-related M1 neurons and NPMA neurons increase their firing approximately 50–200 ms prior to the onset of movement (Tanji et al., 1988; Shima et al., 1991), allowing for the exchange of information between multiple cortical and subcortical areas related to the planning and execution of the intended movement. Although the average onset of increased task-related neuronal firing in the NPMAs slightly precedes the average onset of firing in M1, the distributions of onset times are broadly overlapping, making it unlikely that a motor command would progress in a sequential, hierarchical manner.

Understanding the roles played by these NPMAs in voluntary motor control is a focus of ongoing research. Though this work cannot be reviewed thoroughly here, current research suggests that different NPMAs may have overlapping but partially separate functions. A good example is the difference between the PMv and the SMA during visually-cued versus self-paced movements. Passingham and his coworkers have shown that bilateral lesions of the premotor cortex (which include PMv) produce profound deficits in a monkey's ability to choose which movement to make based on visual cues, but these same lesions do not impair the ability to generate self-paced, internally-cued movements (Passingham, 1987). Conversely, bilateral SMA lesions produce a deficit in internally-cued movements but not in visually-cued choices. Though one might conclude that visually-cued movements are controlled only by the PMv, and internally-cued movements only by the SMA, physiologic recordings show some overlap of function. Mushiake et al. (1991) trained monkeys to press three buttons in sequence. At first, a new sequence was cued to the monkey by illuminating the buttons one at a time on each trial. Once the monkey had practiced the sequence enough, he could continue performing it for several trials without having the buttons illuminated, guided by remembered internal cues. Though the PMv and SMA both contained neurons that were active during both visually-cued and internally-cued movements, PMv neurons on average were more active during visually-cued movements, whereas SMA neurons on average were more

active during internally-cued movements. So although the PMv may play a greater role in visually-cued movements, and the SMA in internally-cued movements, these are quantitative differences and there is some overlap of function between PMv and SMA.

Although the majority of studies investigating NPMAs have been done with animals, there is now a considerable amount of evidence indicating that humans have multiple NPMAs similar to those identified in monkeys (Fig. 2.2(b)). Cortical surface stimulation via implanted subdural electrode grids up to 30 mm anterior to the Rolandic fissure (i.e., 20 mm anterior to the precentral gyrus) produces motor effects in humans (Uematsu et al., 1992). Motor related cortical potentials derived from electroencephalography suggest that both the SMA and M1 are normally involved in self-paced movements (Tarkka and Hallett, 1991; Ikeda et al., 1992). Studies of regional cerebral blood flow showing activation of NPMAs – including SMA, PMv, PMd, CMAd, CMAr, CMAc – during various motor tasks suggests that the human brain contains NPMAs that are homologous to the NPMAs identified in non-human primates (see Picard and Strick, 2001 for review). And finally, resections of NPMAs such as the SMA, where the surgical resection leaves M1 intact, produces an initial hemiparesis that almost completely resolves (Laplane et al., 1977; Krainik et al., 2001). Though the correspondence between particular activated regions in humans and those more precisely defined in monkeys has yet to be fully understood, all the above evidence indicates that human voluntary movement control normally requires NPMAs along with M1 and that voluntary movement is controlled via a parallel, distributed process.

Implications of NPMA organization for recovery after brain injury

Compared with a hierarchical control process, a parallel, distributed control process would allow for better recovery after damage to one part of the system. The NPMAs are therefore well-suited to provide compensatory control of voluntary movement after damage to M1. With their individual loosely somatotopic representations and corticospinal projections, neurons in NPMAs could provide compensatory control of spinal motoneurons after damage to the M1. Although each NMPA has its own unique inputs and neural activation patterns in relation to various aspect of movement control, subsets of neurons in each area have activation patterns that are similar to M1 neurons (Tanji and Kurata, 1982; Shima et al., 1991; Cadoret and Smith, 1997; Boudreau et al., 2001). Furthermore, neurons in NPMAs are more frequently related to bilateral movements than neurons in M1 (Tanji et al., 1988), and thus may be able to exert control over spinal motor neurons via both corticospinal pathways. Electrical stimulation in patients with structural cortical lesions, and magnetic stimulation in patients with traumatic quadriplegia, both have been found to evoke muscle contractions from a much wider area of cortex than just M1, suggesting that NPMAs have developed more output to motoneurons (Levy et al., 1990; Uematsu et al., 1992). Imaging studies indicate that PM and SMA are more active during finger movements in hemiparetic subjects compared to control subjects (Weiller et al., 1992, 1993; Seitz et al., 1998), suggesting that these NPMAs are providing compensatory control of voluntary movements after damage to M1. Interestingly, many imaging studies after stroke show increased activity not only in the NPMAs described above, but also in parietal regions and in ipsilateral M1. Thus NPMAs, which play a role in generating normal voluntary movements, take on an increasingly important role after brain injury.

We speculate that as the particular situations that maximally engage each NPMA are better understood, rehabilitation professionals will be better able to promote functional recovery. For example, if a particular patient has a lesion that affects M1 and the human equivalent of PMv but spares the SMA, movements made in response to visual cues might be most severely impaired, whereas internally generated movements that are mediated in part by the SMA might be relatively spared. The most effective rehabilitative approach might then primarily employ internally generated movements, or teach the patient compensatory strategies to substitute internal cues

in situations where visual cues normally suffice. In this way, each patient's neurorehabilitation might be better tailored to their particular brain injury.

2.3 The corticospinal tract

Motor control signals from M1 and the NPMAs travel to the spinal cord via several descending tracts (Fig. 2.4). The corticospinal tract is the most

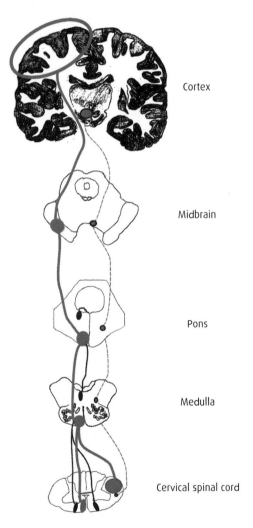

Figure 2.4. Pathway of the corticospinal tract (green, thick line), reticulospinal tract (blue, thinner line), and the rubrospinal tract (red, dashed line).

direct pathway from the cerebral cortex to the spinal motoneurons. The corticospinal tract originates from multiple areas in the frontal and parietal lobes. In the frontal lobe of primates, the greatest proportion of axons originates from M1 (approximately 30% of the total corticospinal tract), with the remaining frontal lobe axons (another 30% of the total corticospinal tract) originating from the SMA, the premotor areas, and the cingulate motor areas (Dum and Strick, 1991). In the parietal lobe, corticospinal axons originate from Brodmann's areas 1, 2, 3, 5, and 7 (approximately 40% of the total corticospinal tract) and project to the dorsal horn of the spinal cord to regulate sensory inflow.

Corticospinal axons arise from the large pyramid-shaped cell bodies in cortical layer V. The axons leave the cortex, pass through the corona radiata, and enter the internal capsule, along with many other corticofugal projections. In the internal capsule, the corticospinal axons are found in the posterior limb, where axons from the NPMAs pass through the genu and anterior third of the posterior limb, axons from M1 pass through the middle third of the posterior limb, and axons from parietal areas pass through just posterior to the primary motor axons (Fries et al., 1993; Axer and Keyserlingk, 2000; Morecraft et al., 2002). As the axons descend through the internal capsule, they shift posteriorly (Axer and Keyserlingk, 2000) and pass below the thalamus. The corticospinal tract then descends through the cerebral peduncle of the midbrain, concentrating in its middle third. In the pons, the corticospinal axons pass around the nuclei in the base of the pons (basis pontis). In the medulla, the corticospinal tract forms the medullary pyramid. At the spinomedullary junction, the majority of corticospinal axons cross the midline and form the lateral corticospinal tract on the opposite side of the spinal cord. The remaining corticospinal axons descend uncrossed as the ventral corticospinal tract near the ventral midline of the spinal cord. In the spinal cord, the corticospinal axons branch and enter the spinal gray matter, synapsing on interneurons in the intermediate zone and synapsing directly on motoneurons in the ventral horn. Axons traveling in the crossed lateral corticospinal tract tend to synapse

on motoneurons and interneurons involved in the control of more distal musculature, whereas axons traveling in the uncrossed ventral corticospinal tract tend to synapse on motoneurons and interneurons involved in the control of axial and more proximal limb muscles. A small number of corticospinal axons recross the midline in the spinal cord and terminate in the ventral horn ipsilateral to their origin.

In humans, strokes affecting the white matter in the territory of the middle cerebral artery frequently damage the corticospinal tract, as well as other structures, resulting in hemiparesis. Relatively isolated lesions of the corticospinal tract can occur in humans when a small ischemic lesion is located in the posterior limb of the internal capsule or in the basis pontis, resulting in the clinical syndrome of pure motor hemiparesis (Fisher and Curry, 1964; Fisher, 1979). After damage to the corticospinal tract, axons carried in the uncrossed ventral corticospinal tract from the opposite hemisphere may be able to exert compensatory control over muscles on the affected side of the body (Fisher, 1992; Cao et al., 1998). These uncrossed axons terminate in the ventromedial portion of the ventral horn and are likely to exert more control over proximal and axial rather than distal musculature (Kuypers and Brinkman, 1970). This spared ventromedial input to spinal motoneurons controlling the affected side of the body may therefore account for the relative preservation of axial and proximal motor control seen after stroke (Colebatch and Gandevia, 1989).

2.4 Other descending motor tracts

Descending motor tracts such as the reticulospinal tract and the rubrospinal tract may contribute to voluntary movement and may assist in recovery of function after damage to the motor cortex or to the corticospinal tract (Fig. 2.4). The reticulospinal tract arises from the pontine and medullary reticular formation and descends in the ventral and ventrolateral columns of the spinal cord. In man, the reticulospinal tract exists as scattered bundles of fibers that terminate primarily in the ventromedial portion of the spinal gray matter at or above the cervical enlargement (Nathan et al., 1996). Only a small proportion of the fibers continue into the thoracic, lumbar, and sacral levels of the spinal cord (Nathan et al., 1996). The origin of the reticulospinal tract, the reticular formation, receives input from a variety of sources, including bilateral motor cortical areas (Kuypers and Lawrence, 1967), and is heavily interconnected with other brainstem structures such as the vestibular nuclei (Kuypers, 1982). The reticular formation, via the reticulospinal tract, exerts control chiefly over axial and proximal limb musculature to assist with postural control and orientation (Lawrence and Kuypers, 1968b; Kuypers, 1982). In man, the reticulospinal tract has been cited as an anatomical substrate for the recovery of function, along with the ipsilateral corticospinal tract, after partial cordotomy (Nathan and Smith, 1973) and after capsular stroke (Fries et al., 1991). If the reticulospinal tract provides compensatory control over spinal motoneurons after damage to the motor cortex or the corticospinal tract, this compensatory control would be greatest over the axial and proximal upper limb muscles.

The rubrospinal tract arises from the magnocellular red nucleus, crosses directly to the opposite side in the anterior tegmental decussation, and descends in the lateral column of the spinal cord, just anterior to and somewhat intermingled with the corticospinal tract. Axons from the rubrospinal tract terminate in dorsal and lateral parts of the intermediate zone of the spinal cord. In contrast to the bilateral motor cortical input to the reticular formation, the red nucleus receives input from the ipsilateral cerebral cortex (Kuypers and Lawrence, 1967). In non-human primates, the rubrospinal tract exerts control over proximal and distal limb motoneurons and can provide some degree of compensatory control after damage to the corticospinal tract (Lawrence and Kuypers, 1968a, b; Kuypers, 1982; Cheney et al., 1991; Belhaj-Saif and Cheney, 2000). In man, the rubrospinal tract is considerably smaller and only a minimal number of axons likely extend down into the upper cervical cord (Nathan and Smith, 1982). Although the extent and relative importance of the

rubrospinal tract in man remains unclear, the possibility exists that the rubrospinal tract could provide some compensatory control of voluntary movement after damage to the motor cortex or corticospinal tract in humans. If the rubrospinal tract were to provide compensatory control of motoneurons in man, then this control would have to be exerted primarily through the most rostral cervical segments.

2.5 The importance of spared territory for reorganization and functional recovery

The previous sections in this chapter have discussed how various cortical areas and descending pathways contribute to voluntary movement in the context of how these areas might provide compensatory control for each other after brain injury. The M1 areas, NPMAs, and descending pathways appear to be a relatively flexible system, controlling movement through parallel, distributed processes. This final section discusses how, in addition to lesion size and location, spared territories and tracts might affect the capacity for functional recovery of movement.

With the development of imaging techniques such as computed tomography (CT) and magnetic resonance (MR), researchers have examined the relationships between lesion size, lesion location, and motor function. The degree of motor impairment and recovery of function cannot be predicted by just lesion size or just lesion location (Chen et al., 2000; Binkofski et al., 2001). Rather, motor impairments and potential for functional recovery can be better predicted by determining what percentage of the corticospinal system is affected (Pineiro et al., 2000). Although we intuitively think that larger lesions will produce more severe motor impairments with less potential for recovery, this relationship is confounded by lesion location and by what territory or tracts are spared. Two lesions of comparable size but in different locations can produce differing degrees of motor impairments and differing prognoses for functional recovery. For example, a small lesion relatively confined to the M1 hand knob results in initial paresis of only the hand and arm (Kim, 2001), yet within a few months, the patient typically can use the hand and arm well except for activities requiring fine independent finger movements, such as typing. In contrast, a lesion of comparable size on one side of the basis pontis, affecting the entire corticospinal tract, results in initial paresis affecting the face, hand, arm, and leg (Fisher, 1982), and although much of the initial deficit typically improves over time, the patient often is left with permanent residual deficits in the hand, arm, and leg. Differences in functional recovery reflect both the structures affected by the lesion and the structures that remain intact. The first lesion damages M1 territory controlling the hand and arm, but compensatory control for functional recovery can arise from both spared M1 territory and the NPMAs, reaching the spinal cord over an otherwise intact corticospinal tract. The latter lesion damages the entire corticospinal tract, so that compensatory control from the intact M1 and NPMAs can reach the spinal cord only through alternate descending pathways. Thus, lesion size, lesion location, and spared territories interact in a complex manner to affect not only motor impairments, but the capacity for plastic reorganization and the resulting recovery of function.

Lesion size and location may also influence which cortical motor areas undergo plastic reorganization after brain injury (Liu and Rouiller, 1999). In the case of very small experimental lesions that affect only a portion of monkey M1, reorganization was observed primarily in the spared territory within M1. In the case of small to moderate lesions that affected the entire M1 territory, reorganization occurred primarily in NPMAs in the same hemisphere. And in the case of large lesions that affected M1 and NPMAs, reorganization occurred in the contralateral M1 and NPMAs. Similarly in humans after stroke, better functional recovery is associated with less activation in the NPMAs of the same hemisphere and with less activation in the contralateral M1 and NPMAs (Ward et al., 2003). Patients with more complete recovery were likely to have near normal brain activation patterns, while patients with poor recovery were more likely to activate additional motor areas in the same and in the contralateral hemispheres. Furthermore,

the probability of recovery of upper extremity function is greatest after lesions relatively isolated to M1 and decreases progressively with descending lesions affecting the descending corticospinal axons (Shelton and Reding, 2001). Taken together, these data suggest that spared territories and tracts can control voluntary movement in humans after brain injury, but that the spared territories and tracts cannot fully compensate for the highly selective control provided by M1 and the crossed corticospinal system.

In summary, rehabilitation professionals should evaluate what areas and tracts remain intact after each patient's brain injury, as well as assessing lesion location, and size. A better understanding of the anatomy and physiology of the spared components of the nervous system and their capacity for reorganization may improve the ability to design and implement effective individualized rehabilitative strategies, and thus promote greater functional recovery.

REFERENCES

Andersen, P., Hagan, P.J., Phillips, C.G. and Powell, T.P. (1975). Mapping by microstimulation of overlapping projections from area 4 to motor units of the baboon's hand. *Proc R Soc Lond B Biol Sci*, **188**, 31–36.

Axer, H. and Keyserlingk, D.G. (2000). Mapping of fiber orientation in human internal capsule by means of polarized light and confocal scanning laser microscopy. *J Neurosci Methods*, **94**, 165–175.

Beisteiner, R., Windischberger, C., Lanzenberger, R., Edward, V., Cunnington, R., Erdler, M., Gartus, A., Streibl, B., Moser, E. and Deecke, L. (2001). Finger somatotopy in human motor cortex. *Neuroimage*, **13**, 1016–1026.

Belhaj-Saif, A. and Cheney, P.D. (2000). Plasticity in the distribution of the red nucleus output to forearm muscles after unilateral lesions of the pyramidal tract. *J Neurophysiol*, **83**, 3147–3153.

Binkofski, F., Seitz, R.J., Hacklander, T., Pawelec, D., Mau, J. and Freund, H.J. (2001). Recovery of motor functions following hemiparetic stroke: a clinical and magnetic resonance-morphometric study. *Cerebrovasc Dis*, **11**, 273–281.

Boudreau, M.J., Brochier, T., Pare, M. and Smith, A.M. (2001). Activity in ventral and dorsal premotor cortex in response to predictable force-pulse perturbations in a precision grip task. *J Neurophysiol*, **86**, 1067–1078.

Brasil-Neto, J.P., Valls-Sole, J., Pascual-Leone, A., Cammarota, A., Amassian, V.E., Cracco, R., Maccabee, P., Cracco, J., Hallett, M. and Cohen, L.G. (1993). Rapid modulation of human cortical motor outputs following ischaemic nerve block. *Brain*, **116(Pt 3)**, 511–525.

Brochier, T., Boudreau, M.J., Pare, M. and Smith, A.M. (1999). The effects of muscimol inactivation of small regions of motor and somatosensory cortex on independent finger movements and force control in the precision grip. *Exp Brain Res*, **128**, 31–40.

Buys, E.J., Lemon, R.N., Mantel, G.W. and Muir, R.B. (1986). Selective facilitation of different hand muscles by single corticospinal neurones in the conscious monkey. *J Physiol*, **381**, 529–549.

Cadoret, G. and Smith, A.M. (1997). Comparison of the neuronal activity in the SMA and the ventral cingulate cortex during prehension in the monkey. *J Neurophysiol*, **77**, 153–166.

Cao, Y., D'Olhaberriague, L., Vikingstad, E.M., Levine, S.R. and Welch, K.M. (1998). Pilot study of functional MRI to assess cerebral activation of motor function after poststroke hemiparesis. *Stroke*, **29**, 112–122.

Chen, C.L., Tang, F.T., Chen, H.C., Chung, C.Y. and Wong, M.K. (2000). Brain lesion size and location: effects on motor recovery and functional outcome in stroke patients. *Arch Phys Med Rehabil*, **81**, 447–452.

Cheney, P.D., Fetz, E.E. and Mewes, K. (1991) Neural mechanisms underlying corticospinal and rubrospinal control of limb movements. *Prog Brain Res*, **87**, 213–252.

Colebatch, J.G. and Gandevia, S.C. (1989). The distribution of muscular weakness in upper motor neuron lesions affecting the arm. *Brain*, **112(Pt 3)**, 749–763.

Cordo, P.J. and Flanders, M. (1989). Sensory control of target acquisition. *Trend Neurosci*, **12**, 110–117.

Dum, R.P. and Strick, P.L. (1991). The origin of corticospinal projections from the premotor areas in the frontal lobe. *J Neurosci*, **11**, 667–689.

Dum, R.P. and Strick, P.L. (2002). Motor areas in the frontal lobe of the primate. *Physiol Behav*, **77**, 677–682.

Fetz, E.E. and Cheney, P.D. (1980). Postspike facilitation of forelimb muscle activity by primate corticomotoneuronal cells. *J Neurophysiol*, **44**, 751–772.

Fisher, C.M. (1979). Capsular infarcts: the underlying vascular lesions. *Arch Neurol*, **36**, 65–73.

Fisher, C.M. (1982). Lacunar strokes and infarcts: a review. *Neurology*, **32**, 871–876.

Fisher, C.M. (1992). Concerning the mechanism of recovery in stroke hemiplegia. *Can J Neurol Sci*, **19**, 57–63.

Fisher, C.M. and Curry, H.B. (1964). Pure motor hemiplegia. *Trans Am Neurol Assoc*, **89**, 94–97.

Friel, K.M. and Nudo, R.J. (1998). Recovery of motor function after focal cortical injury in primates: compensatory movement patterns used during rehabilitative training. *Somatosens Mot Res*, **15**, 173–189.

Fries, W., Danek, A. and Witt, T.N. (1991). Motor responses after transcranial electrical stimulation of cerebral hemispheres with a degenerated pyramidal tract. *Ann Neurol*, **29**, 646–650.

Fries, W., Danek, A., Scheidtmann, K. and Hamburger, C. (1993). Motor recovery following capsular stroke. Role of descending pathways from multiple motor areas. *Brain*, **116(Pt 2)**, 369–382.

Giraux, P., Sirigu, A., Schneider, F. and Dubernard, J.M. (2001). Cortical reorganization in motor cortex after graft of both hands. *Nat Neurosci*, **4**, 691–692.

Grafton, S.T., Woods, R.P. and Mazziotta, J.C. (1993). Within-arm somatotopy in human motor areas determined by positron emission tomography imaging of cerebral blood flow. *Exp Brain Res*, **95**, 172–176.

Hlustik, P., Solodkin, A., Gullapalli, R.P., Noll, D.C. and Small, S.L. (2001). Somatotopy in human primary motor and somatosensory hand representations revisited. *Cereb Cortex*, **11**, 312–321.

Ikeda, A., Luders, H.O., Burgess, R.C. and Shibasaki, H. (1992). Movement-related potentials recorded from supplementary motor area and primary motor area. Role of supplementary motor area in voluntary movements. *Brain*, **115(Pt 4)**, 1017–1043.

Indovina, I. and Sanes, J.N. (2001). On somatotopic representation centers for finger movements in human primary motor cortex and supplementary motor area. *Neuroimage*, **13**, 1027–1034.

Karni, A., Meyer, G., Jezzard, P., Adams, M.M., Turner, R. and Ungerleider, L.G. (1995). Functional MRI evidence for adult motor cortex plasticity during motor skill learning. *Nature*, **377**, 155–158.

Kim, J.S. (2001). Predominant involvement of a particular group of fingers due to small, cortical infarction. *Neurology*, **56**, 1677–1682.

Kleinschmidt, A., Nitschke, M.F. and Frahm, J. (1997). Somatotopy in the human motor cortex hand area. A high-resolution functional MRI study. *Eur J Neurosci*, **9**, 2178–2186.

Krainik, A., Lehericy, S., Duffau, H., Vlaicu, M., Poupon, F., Capelle, L., Cornu, P., Clemenceau, S., Sahel, M., Valery, C.A., Boch, A.L., Mangin, J.F., Bihan, D.L. and Marsault, C. (2001). Role of the supplementary motor area in motor deficit following medial frontal lobe surgery. *Neurology*, **57**, 871–878.

Kuypers, H.G. (1982). A new look at the organization of the motor system. *Prog Brain Res*, **57**, 381–403.

Kuypers, H.G. and Brinkman, J. (1970). Precentral projections to different parts of the spinal intermediate zone in therhesus monkey. *Brain Res*, **24**, 29–48.

Kuypers, H.G. and Lawrence, D.G. (1967). Cortical projections to the red nucleus and the brain stem in the rhesus monkey. *Brain Res*, **4**, 151–188.

Lang, C.E. and Schieber, M.H. (2003). Differential impairment of individuated finger movements in humans after damage to the motor cortex or the corticospinal tract. *J Neurophysiol*, **90**, 1160–1170.

Laplane, D., Talairach, J., Meininger, V., Bancaud, J. and Orgogozo, J.M. (1977). Clinical consequences of corticectomies involving the supplementary motor area in man. *J Neurol Sci*, **34**, 301–314.

Lawrence, D.G. and Kuypers, H.G. (1968a). The functional organization of the motor system in the monkey. I. The effects of bilateral pyramidal lesions. *Brain*, **91**, 1–14.

Lawrence, D.G. and Kuypers, H.G. (1968b). The functional organization of the motor system in the monkey. II. The effects of lesions of the descending brain-stem pathways. *Brain*, **91**, 15–36.

Lee, P.H., Han, S.W. and Heo, J.H. (1998). Isolated weakness of the fingers in cortical infarction. *Neurology*, **50**, 823–824.

Levy Jr., W.J., Amassian, V.E., Traad, M. and Cadwell, J. (1990). Focal magnetic coil stimulation reveals motor cortical system reorganized in humans after traumatic quadriplegia. *Brain Res*, **510**, 130–134.

Leyton, A.S.F. and Sherrington, C.S. (1917). Observations on the excitable cortex of the chimpanzee, orangutan, and gorilla. *Q J Exp Physiol*, **11**, 137–222.

Liu, Y. and Rouiller, E.M. (1999). Mechanisms of recovery of dexterity following unilateral lesion of the sensorimotor cortex in adult monkeys. *Exp Brain Res*, **128**, 149–159.

McKiernan, B.J., Marcario, J.K., Karrer, J.H. and Cheney, P.D. (1998). Corticomotoneuronal postspike effects in shoulder, elbow, wrist, digit, and intrinsic hand muscles during a reach and prehension task. *J Neurophysiol*, **80**, 1961–1980.

Morecraft, R.J., Herrick, J.L., Stilwell-Morecraft, K.S., Louie, J.L., Schroeder, C.M., Ottenbacher, J.G. and Schoolfield, M.W. (2002). Localization of arm representation in the corona radiata and internal capsule in the non-human primate. *Brain*, **125**, 176–198.

Muellbacher, W., Richards, C., Ziemann, U., Wittenberg, G., Weltz, D., Boroojerdi, B., Cohen, L. and Hallett, M. (2002). Improving hand function in chronic stroke. *Arch Neurol*, **59**, 1278–1282.

Mushiake, H., Inase, M. and Tanji, J. (1991). Neuronal activity in the primate premotor, supplementary, and precentral motor cortex during visually guided and internally determined sequential movements. *J Neurophysiol*, **66**, 705–718.

Nathan, P.W. and Smith, M.C. (1973). Effects of two unilateral cordotomies on the motility of the lower limbs. *Brain*, **96**, 471–494.

Nathan, P.W. and Smith, M.C. (1982). The rubrospinal and central tegmental tracts in man. *Brain*, **105**, 223–269.

Nathan, P.W., Smith, M. and Deacon, P. (1996). Vestibulospinal, reticulospinal and descending propriospinal nerve fibres in man. *Brain*, **119**(Pt 6), 1809–1833.

Nudo, R.J., Milliken, G.W., Jenkins, W.M. and Merzenich, M.M. (1996a). Use-dependent alterations of movement representations in primary motor cortex of adult squirrel monkeys. *J Neurosci*, **16**, 785–807.

Nudo, R.J., Wise, B.M., SiFuentes, F. and Milliken, G.W. (1996b). Neural substrates for the effects of rehabilitative training on motor recovery after ischemic infarct. *Science*, **272**, 1791–1794.

Park, M.C., Belhaj-Saif, A., Gordon, M. and Cheney, P.D. (2001). Consistent features in the forelimb representation of primary motor cortex in rhesus macaques. *J Neurosci*, **21**, 2784–2792.

Pascual-Leone, A., Grefman, J. and Hallet, M. (1994). Modulation of cortical motor output maps during development of implicit and explicit knowledge. *Science*, **263**, 1289–1289.

Passingham, R.E. (1987). Two cortical systems for directing movement. In: *Motor Areas of the Cerebral Cortex*, Wiley, Chichester, pp. 151–164.

Penfield, W. and Boldrey, E. (1937). Somatic motor and sensory representation in the cerebral cortex of man as studied by electrical stimulation. *Brain*, **37**, 389–443.

Penfield, W. and Rasmussaen, T. (1950). *The Cerebral Cortex of Man*, MacMillan, New York.

Phillips, C.G. and Landau, W.M. (1990). Clinical neuromythology. VIII. Upper and lower motor neuron: the little old synecdoche that works. *Neurology*, **40**, 884–886.

Picard, N. and Strick, P.L. (2001). Imaging the premotor areas. *Curr Opin Neurobiol*, **11**, 663–672.

Pineiro, R., Pendlebury, S.T., Smith, S., Flitney, D., Blamire, A.M., Styles, P. and Matthews, P.M. (2000). Relating MRI changes to motor deficit after ischemic stroke by segmentation of functional motor pathways. *Stroke*, **31**, 672–679.

Rizzolatti, G., Luppino, G. and Matelli, M. (1998). The organization of the cortical motor system: new concepts. *Electroencephalogr Clin Neurophysiol*, **106**, 283–296.

Sanes, J.N., Wang, J. and Donoghue, J.P. (1992). Immediate and delayed changes of rat motor cortical output representation with new forelimb configurations. *Cereb Cortex*, **2**, 141–152.

Sanes, J.N., Donoghue, J.P., Thangaraj, V., Edelman, R.R. and Warach, S. (1995). Shared neural substrates controlling hand movements in human motor cortex. *Science*, **268**, 1775–1777.

Sato, K.C. and Tanji, J. (1989). Digit-muscle responses evoked from multiple intracortical foci in monkey precentral motor cortex. *J Neurophysiol*, **62**, 959–970.

Schieber, M.H. (1999). Somatotopic gradients in the distributed organization of the human primary motor cortex hand area: evidence from small infarcts. *Exp Brain Res*, **128**, 139–148.

Schieber, M.H. (2001). Constraints on somatotopic organization in the primary motor cortex. *J Neurophysiol*, **86**, 2125–2143.

Schieber, M.H. and Hibbard, L.S. (1993). How somatotopic is the motor cortex hand area? *Science*, **261**, 489–492.

Schieber, M.H. and Poliakov, A.V. (1998). Partial inactivation of the primary motor cortex hand area: effects on individuated finger movements. *J Neurosci*, **18**, 9038–9054.

Seitz, R.J., Hoflich, P., Binkofski, F., Tellmann, L., Herzog, H. and Freund, H.J. (1998). Role of the premotor cortex in recovery from middle cerebral artery infarction. *Arch Neurol*, **55**, 1081–1088.

Shelton, F.N. and Reding, M.J. (2001). Effect of lesion location on upper limb motor recovery after stroke. *Stroke*, **32**, 107–112.

Shima, K. and Tanji, J. (1998). Both supplementary and presupplementary motor areas are crucial for the temporal organization of multiple movements. *J Neurophysiol*, **80**, 3247–3260.

Shima, K., Aya, K., Mushiake, H., Inase, M., Aizawa, H. and Tanji, J. (1991). Two movement-related foci in the primate cingulate cortex observed in signal-triggered and self-paced forelimb movements. *J Neurophysiol*, **65**, 188–202.

Shinoda, Y., Yokota, J. and Futami, T. (1981). Divergent projection of individual corticospinal axons to motoneurons of multiple muscles in the monkey. *Neurosci Lett*, **23**, 7–12.

Tanji, J. and Kurata, K. (1982). Comparison of movement-related activity in two cortical motor areas of primates. *J Neurophysiol*, **48**, 633–653.

Tanji, J., Okano, K. and Sato, K.C. (1988). Neuronal activity in cortical motor areas related to ipsilateral, contralateral, and bilateral digit movements of the monkey. *J Neurophysiol*, **60**, 325–343.

Tarkka, I.M. and Hallett, M. (1991). Topography of scalp-recorded motor potentials in human finger movements. *J Clin Neurophysiol*, **8**, 331–341.

Uematsu, S., Lesser, R., Fisher, R.S., Gordon, B., Hara, K., Krauss, G.L., Vining, E.P. and Webber, R.W. (1992). Motor and sensory cortex in humans: topography studied with chronic subdural stimulation. *Neurosurgery*, **31**, 59–71; discussion, 71–72.

Ward, N.S., Brown, M.M., Thompson, A.J. and Frackowiak, R.S. (2003). Neural correlates of outcome after stroke: a cross-sectional fMRI study. *Brain*, **126**, 1430–1448.

Waters, R.S., Samulack, D.D., Dykes, R.W. and McKinley, P.A. (1990). Topographic organization of baboon primary motor cortex: face, hand, forelimb, and shoulder representation. *Somatosens Mot Res*, **7**, 485–514.

Weiller, C., Chollet, F., Friston, K.J., Wise, R.J. and Frackowiak, R.S. (1992). Functional reorganization of the brain in recovery from striatocapsular infarction in man. *Ann Neurol*, **31**, 463–472.

Weiller, C., Ramsay, S.C., Wise, R.J., Friston, K.J. and Frackowiak, R.S. (1993). Individual patterns of functional reorganization in the human cerebral cortex after capsular infarction. *Ann Neurol*, **33**, 181–189.

Woolsey, C.N., Settlage, P., Meyer, D.R., Sencer, W., Hamuy, T.P. and Travis, A.M. (1952). Patterns of localization in precentral and "supplementary" motor areas and their relation to the concept of a premotor area. *Res Pub Assoc Res Nerv Ment Dis*, **30**, 238–264.

Yousry, T.A., Schmid, U.D., Alkadhi, H., Schmidt, D., Peraud, A., Buettner, A. and Winkler, P. (1997). Localization of the motor hand area to a knob on the precentral gyrus. A new landmark. *Brain*, **120(Pt 1)**, 141–157.

Assessments, interventions, and outcome measures for walking

Bruce H. Dobkin

Professor of Neurology, University of California Los Angeles; Director, Neurologic Rehabilitation and Research Program, Reed Neurologic Research Center, Los Angeles, CA, USA

3.1 When walking fails

Difficulty walking is reported by 10% of Americans (Iezzoni, 2003). One-third report major difficulty. They are unable to walk or climb stairs or stand. The most rapid rates of increase occur after ages 54 and 74 years old. Musculoskeletal and joint diseases account for 24% of causes of major difficulty, back pain for 8%, stroke for 5%, and multiple sclerosis for 2%. Falls affect 41% of these people yearly. Eleven percent never leave their homes and only 32% get out of the home daily. By report, 25% receive some physical therapy during the year of major difficulty walking. At this level of difficulty, 48% with stroke use a cane, 28% use a walker, and 44% a wheelchair.

Six months after a traumatic spinal cord injury (SCI), 2% of subjects graded by the American Spinal Injury Association (ASIA) scale as ASIA A (sensorimotor complete) at 24 h after onset are able to walk at least 25 ft, 30% of those graded ASIA B (motor complete), and 94% graded ASIA C (Geisler et al., 2001). Six months after stroke, 85% of patients with a pure motor impairment, 75% with sensorimotor loss, and 35% with sensorimotor and hemianopsia deficits will recover the ability to walk at least 150 ft without physical assistance (Patel et al., 2000). These levels of gains do not necessarily lead to walking well enough to navigate outside of the home. In general, walking speeds greater than 80 cm/s make it more likely that a person can participate in the community (Perry et al., 1995; Lord et al., 2004). Only 40% of patients who recover walking ability after stroke achieve community-walking velocities. Indeed, half of those who are walking do so at less than 50 cm/s (about 1 mph). The push for faster, more functional walking speeds and longer distances walked is an underplayed goal in rehabilitation. Successful approaches to improve these walking outcomes would lead to greater participation. More functional walking may also reduce risk factors for cardiovascular disease, recurrent stroke, and frailty by permitting more opportunity for exercise and fitness (Chapter 21 of Volume II) (Macko et al., 2001; Greenlund et al., 2002; Gill et al., 2002; Kurl et al., 2003).

The rehabilitation of walking poses some common questions about the services provided by clinicians (Dobkin, 2003a). How do we know when our patients have received enough goal-directed therapy for their level of motor control? What measures should we use to rate progress? What do we really mean when we say that a patient has reached a plateau in recovery and will no longer benefit from therapy? Do outside-the-box therapies exist that might augment gains?

3.2 Rationales for gait retraining

Interneuron-linked oscillators within the lumbar cord for flexion and extension of the hindlimbs, called central pattern generators (CPGs), have become a target for both locomotor training interventions and for neural repair (Chapter 13 of Volume I). This circuitry may be driven by the timing of cutaneous and weight-bearing inputs from the soles and by proprioceptive and load information from joints, especially the hips, during the practice of stepping. Following a low thoracic spinal cord transection, cats and rats have been trained to step with their hindlimbs on a moving treadmill belt with support for the sagging trunk. Pulling down on their tails or a noxious input enhances hindlimb loading in extension. The animals are not as successful walking over ground. Training-induced adaptations within the cord in these animal models point to the potential of plasticity induced by rehabilitation to lead to behavioral gains. It seems likely that a network of locomotor spinal motoneurons and interneurons has been conserved in humans (Dimitrijevic et al., 1998), along with other forms of spinal organization (Lemay and Grill, 2004) that increase the flexibility of supraspinal regions to control hindlimb and lower extremity movements.

Studies in patients with clinically complete SCI reveal similar responses to limb loading and hip inputs as were found in spinal transected cats (Chapter 30 Volume II). However, plasticity within the cord may be no more important than plasticity induced within cortical and subcortical nodes of the sensorimotor network for walking in patients who have residual descending supraspinal input to the lumbosacral motor pools. Review articles may overstate the evidence for the case that spinal networks, in concert with specific sensory information, are responsible for locomotion in man. Rationales for gait retraining in patients can draw from animal models about specific sensory inputs that aid the timing and efficacy of the step cycle. These sensory inputs, however, act at many levels of the neuroaxis, beyond the CPGs.

Figure 3.1 shows the extent of cortical reorganization induced by a conus/cauda equina SCI followed by gait training. This 52-year-old subject suffered a burst fracture of the first lumbar vertebral body 8 years prior to the functional magnetic resonance imaging (fMRI) study. He had no movement or sensation below L3 on the left and L4 on the right. He dorsiflexed his right ankle a maximum of 5° and could not offer resistance. He was able to extend each knee against gravity and minimal resistance. The subject walked modest distances with a reciprocal gait at 1.5 mph wearing bilateral solid ankle–foot orthoses with a cane in each hand for balance. The fMRI study of voluntary right ankle dorsiflexion (Fig. 3.1(a)) reveals significantly greater recruitment compared to control subjects, involving the contralateral thoracolumbar representation in primary sensorimotor cortex (M1S1) and in bilateral M1S1 that represents the whole leg, the supplementary motor area, basal ganglia, and cerebellar hemispheres. Contralateral cingulate motor cortex and premotor area activation and bilateral parietal, insula, and dorsolateral prefrontal cortex (dlpf) activity also significantly

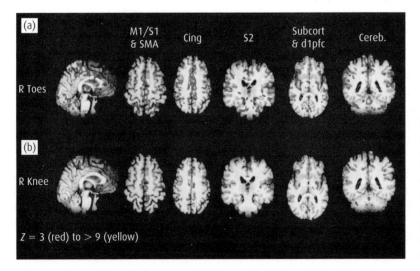

Figure 3.1. Right ankle dorsiflexion and right quadriceps contraction during fMRI of a subject with a SCI at the conus. R Toes: right toes; R Knee: right knee; SMA: supplementary motor area; Cing: cingulate motor cortex; Subcort: subcortical nodes; Cereb: cerebellum.

exceeded that of healthy subjects. The evoked activity for contraction of the quadriceps, however, was similar to that of control subjects (Fig. 3.1(b)), with the exception of recruitment of the bilateral secondary sensory (SII) area and the trunk representation within M1S1. In this subject, a portion of the CPG network is likely damaged, but residual cortical control and practice led to useful motor control for gait.

In human subjects who are healthy or have had a stroke or incomplete SCI, functional neuroimaging and other neurophysiological studies of walking reveal considerable contributions from supraspinal nodes of the distributed locomotor network for effective bipedal walking (Dobkin, 2000b; Miyai et al., 2001; Dobkin, 2003c; Nielsen, 2003; Grasso et al., 2004). By better defining supraspinal components and the means to engage them by voluntary action, visuoperception, planning, mechanisms for declarative and procedural learning, and through drugs and electrical stimulation procedures, a broad range of strategies for gait training suggest themselves for further evaluation.

3.3 Assessments

Analysis of gait

Figure 3.2 shows a quantitative gait analysis in a normal subject for the timing and amplitude of electromyographic (EMG) activation of muscle groups (3.2a), the ground reaction forces elicited (3.2b), and the joint angles at the hip, knee, and ankle (3.2c) during the step cycle (Dobkin, 2003a). Surface and wire electrodes are used for EMG data. Electrogoniometers, computerized video analysis with joint markers, and electromagnetic field motion analysis will reveal the kinematics in two or three dimensions. Kinetics are measured by a force plate in the ground or embedded in a treadmill, as well as by a load cell embedded in a shoe. Energy cost is also measurable by oxygen consumption studies. These procedures take considerable expertise, time, and equipment to perform and analyze. The numerous variables collected and their interactions demand special statistical and modeling approaches. Of clinical importance, walking velocity correlates with many of the measured temporal parameters of the gait cycle. Formal gait studies are best reserved for a research laboratory and for presurgical evaluations of orthopedic and neurosurgical procedures. Knowledge of the typical patterns revealed by analyses in normal, hemiparetic, and paraparetic subjects does help inform an observational analysis of a new patient.

Common gait deviations

The gait cycle can be assessed by educated observational skills and knowledge of the disease and its resulting symptoms and impairments. By combining a visual assessment of the stance (initial heel contact, foot flat, midstance, heel off) and swing phases (toe off, midswing, and end of swing heel contact), the clinician can look for temporal as well as kinematic asymmetries between the phase components for each leg. For example, a hemiparetic gait often reveals temporal differences – a shorter step length for the unaffected leg because the affected leg is impaired as it supports single-limb stance; greater double-limb support time compared to healthy persons, mostly from less time spent in single-limb stance on the affected leg; and shorter duration of swing for each leg. Kinematic differences include excessive flexion at the hip during midstance which, by moving the center of gravity forward, increases the knee extensor moment; decreased lateral shift to the paretic side during single-limb stance; less knee flexion and ankle dorsiflexion during swing, which may lead to circumduction of the affected leg or vaulting off the unaffected one to clear the affected foot; and initial contact with the whole foot or forefoot rather than heel contact followed by a rocker motion onto the forefoot that provides forward momentum. Using cluster analysis, formal gait studies characterized differences among patients based on walking velocity, knee extension in terminal stance, and peak dorsiflexion in swing during inpatient rehabilitation for stroke (Mulroy et al., 2003). At 6 months, explanatory variables of impairment were velocity, knee extension in terminal

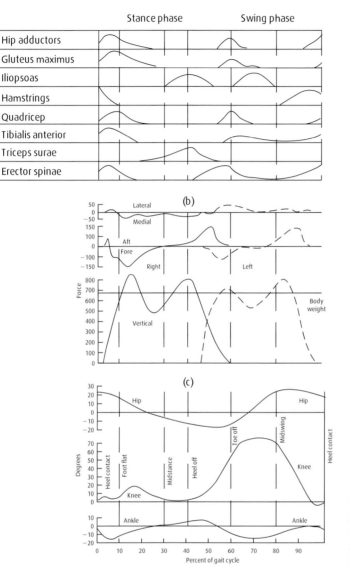

Figure 3.2. Normal gait cycle: EMG, ground reaction force, and kinematic data starting at heel strike (taken from Dobkin, 2003a), *courtesy* of Oxford University Press.

stance, and knee flexion in pre-swing. Treatment approaches could address each of these patterns.

Paraparetic gait (Chapter 30 of Volume II) during the stance phase may include absent heel strike, excessive hip and knee flexion and plantar flexion, pelvic drop with compensatory lateral shift of the trunk to the stance leg, and poor plantar flexor force for push off. During the swing phase, excessive plantar flexion and insufficient hip or knee flexion may impair foot clearance. The pelvis may drop on the swing side from weakness and overactive hip adductors may narrow the base of support. As in children with spastic diplegia from cerebral palsy, motor control of paraparetic gait is complicated by variations in residual selective strength, use of synergistic movements, loss of coordination of muscle firing patterns, hypertonicity that is state dependent, limitations in range of motion, tissue changes in muscles and across joints, and truncal and multi-joint interactions during stance and swing phases.

3.4 Interventions for retraining gait

Strategies for retraining gait start with interventions to improve control of the head and trunk when necessary, then proceed to sitting and standing balance (Chapter 8 of Volume II). Practice paradigms ought to include a clear schedule and form of reinforcement (Chapter 7 of Volume II). Rehabilitation approaches for walking are listed in Table 3.1. Locomotor interventions are limited only by the imagination of the rehabilitation team. An eclectic problem-solving approach is taken by most therapists. Walkers, canes, ankle–foot orthoses, and on occasion, knee–ankle–foot braces are used to improve balance, lessen the need for full lower extremity weight support, and aid foot clearance and knee control. A trial-and-error approach for fitting and employing these aids and a reassessment over the time of improved motor control is usually needed. For step-training *per se*, as well as confounders such as hemi-inattention, lateral pulsion (pusher syndrome), truncal ataxia, gait apraxia, and extrapyramidal features, no particular style of care has been shown to be better than another, but few comparisons have been made. Anti-spasticity agents and intramuscular botulinum toxin may improve aspects of the gait cycle, primarily in patients with excessive plantar flexion/inversion.

Several of the approaches in Table 3.1 are being tested in randomized clinical trials (RCTs).

Task-oriented training

Body weight-supported treadmill training (BWSTT) is partially derived from treadmill training experiments on spinal transected animals and CPGs (Barbeau, 2003). It also provides task-oriented, massed practice under more optimal conditions for managing weight bearing and walking speed (Dobkin, 1999; Sullivan

Table 3.1. General approaches for retraining walking.

- Bobath, NDT, et al. to improve head and trunk control, balance, stance
- Progression from parallel bars; correct qualitative gait deviations
- Massed practice of walking
- Braces and assistive devices
- Increase muscle strength (Moreland et al., 2003)
- Increase walking speed and distance
- Reverse deconditioning (Teixeira-Salmela et al., 1999; MacKay-Lyons and Makrides, 2002)
- Task-specific shaping of more selective movements (Taub et al., 2002)
- Treadmill training ± body weight support
- Circuit training (Dean et al., 2000)
- Functional electrical stimulation for reflexive flexion or to fire a critical muscle group during the step cycle (Daly and Ruff, 2000; Loeb and Richmond, 2001; Herman et al., 2002)
- Robotic and electromechanical assists for stepping (Hesse et al., 2003)
- Pharmacological adjuncts for learning or neuromodulation
- Biofeedback – kinematic or EMG ± induced muscle stimulation (Moreland et al., 1998; Sinkjaer et al., 2000)
- Practice in virtual environments
- Imagery (Lafleur et al., 2002; Malouin et al., 2004)
- Increase cortical excitation during practice (Dobkin, 2003b) – peripheral nerve, transcranial magnetic or direct motor cortex stimulation

et al., 2002). Forms of BWSTT have been employed after SCI, stroke, cerebral palsy (Schindl et al., 2000), multiple sclerosis (Lord et al., 1998), and Parkinson's disease (Miyai et al., 2002).

Reviews and some initial reports of BWSTT after SCI often suggest that the beneficial effect of locomotor training in incomplete SCI patients is "well established" and that "even chronic SCI patients who underwent locomotor training had greater mobility compared with a control group with conventional rehabilitation" (Dietz and Harkema, 2004). The studies that are usually quoted have not, however, included control subjects at all (Field-Fote, 2001; Barbeau, 2003) or they employed "historical" controls (Wernig et al., 1995). Only one trial with clinically meaningful outcome measures obtained by blinded

Table 3.2. Six-month outcomes for a clinical trial of BWSTT versus conventional mobility training for 60 ASIA C and D subjects randomized within 8 weeks of SCI, graded at time of admission for rehabilitation.

	BWSTT	CONV
FIM walking score (0–7)	5.8 ± 1.2	5.6 ± 1.9
LEMS (0–50)	43 ± 10	41 ± 12
Walking speed (ft/s)	1.9	2.5
Median	3.3	3.8
FIM total motor score	85 ± 15	86 ± 17
6-min walk (ft)	1125 ± 618	1197 ± 564
WISCI (0–20)	15 ± 5	14 ± 7
Median	18	18
Berg balance (0–58)	44 ± 19	43 ± 19
Median	52	55

CONV: conventional physical therapy; LEMS: lower extremity motor score.

observers has been reported, and that revealed no benefit of BWSTT over conventional care in incomplete subjects. The SCI Locomotor Trial (SCILT) randomized 145 subjects with incomplete SCI who could not walk on admission to six regional SCI facilities. Subjects received 12 weeks of BWSTT complemented by over ground training when feasible or an equal amount of conventional over ground training, in addition to usual inpatient and outpatient therapies (Dobkin et al., 2003). Table 3.2 is an overview of the results for ASIA C and D subjects with upper motor neuron impairments. No benefit of the intervention was found for ASIA B subjects, most of whom did not recover any ability to walk, or to ASIA C and D subjects, most of whom did walk at remarkably functional speeds and distances (Dobkin et al., 2004).

In patients who cannot stand and yet have some proximal motor control that may be brought out by an upright posture, BWSTT may enable some loading and foster rhythmic stepping. For example, the patient whose fMRI is shown in Fig. 3.1 was enabled to stand upright, bear some weight in the legs, and activate the iliopsoas and quadriceps muscles reciprocally 3 months after the SCI, when he could not stand or step after routine rehabilitation. The upright posture and leg assistance allowed him to concentrate on finding some motor control over residual descending pathways to surviving motoneurons that still innervated these muscles. Training and neuromuscular activity may then drive cerebral control for gait over various surfaces and speeds. Trophic substances produced by activity can increase peripheral axon regeneration to re-innervate muscle. (Dobkin and Havton, 2004). As interesting as this recovery seems, the same result may have been possible using more aggressive conventional therapies.

BWSTT when instituted a mean of 70 days after acute hemiparetic stroke revealed statistically significant gains in gait when compared to treadmill training without BWS (Visintin et al., 1998; Barbeau and Visintin, 2003). This comparison is of interest, but not a clinically useful distinction for evidence-based practices. Also, the outcomes were statistically significant for walking speed, but not clinically significant. Other RCTs of BWSTT during acute inpatient rehabilitation after stroke revealed no clinical benefits for walking independence or speed (Nilsson et al., 2002; Lennihan et al., 2003). RCTs are needed to determine if BWSTT ought to be offered to patients who cannot walk over ground with a reciprocal gait or to those who still walk too slowly to ambulate outside of the home (<50 cm/s) more than 6 months after onset of hemiplegic stroke or SCI in ASIA C subjects. Such trials will need to establish training scenarios for the manipulation of BWS and treadmill speeds, along with justifying the duration and intensity of treatment. Even greater attention will be necessary for the design of RCTs of BWSTT augmented by robotic assistive devices (Colombo et al., 2000; Werner et al., 2002), functional electrical stimulation (Hesse et al., 1995; Chaplin, 1996; Barbeau et al., 2002), and pharmacological interventions (Norman et al., 1998; Dobkin, 2003a). Dose–response studies for the amount of training, as is typically required for drug studies, and a demonstration of the reproducibility of training techniques will require considerable pilot data (Dobkin, 2004).

Pulse therapies

The efficacy of a pulse of various training strategies for walking has been demonstrated in well-designed trials from months to years after stroke (Hesse et al., 1994; Sullivan et al., 2002; Ada et al., 2003; Duncan et al., 2003b) and other chronically disabling neurological diseases. The duration of effect will be limited in progressive diseases. That should not dissuade the clinician from attempting to maintain functional walking through a home-based exercise program and a brief course of goal-directed therapy to improve the gait pattern, strengthen leg muscles, or recondition a patient to lessen disability. A home-based program might include sets of practice in sit-to-stand, supine and prone leg lifts, partial squats while braced against a wall, pool exercise, treadmill walking, specified goals for progressive gains in walking distance or walking speed, modest resistance exercises with weights or latex bands, and practice walking on uneven surfaces and stairs.

3.5 Outcome measures for clinical care

Whether an individual patient is in rehabilitation as an inpatient or outpatient or participating in a clinical trial, sensitive and reliable outcome measures help determine the success of an intervention for walking.

Physiological measures

Walking speed over 10 m or 50 ft, 2- or 6-min walking distance and heart rate change from rest, a timed stand up and walk task, and measures of impairment such as the Berg balance scale, Fugl-Meyer motor assessment, and ASIA motor score provide quick and reliable measures relevant to walking after stroke or SCI (Steffen et al., 2002; Duncan et al., 2003b). These measures may be more sensitive to changes during a subacute intervention compared to a treatment in chronically disabled subjects. The Multiple Sclerosis Functional Composite scale includes a 25-foot timed walk that, with its other two measures, has proven valuable for clinical trials (Kalkers et al., 2000). Serial monitoring of walking speed can serve as both

a measure and an incentive for progress during formal rehabilitation and for practice at home. Scales for spasticity, such as the Ashworth scale, are of no value as an outcome measure. Resistance to movement tested at a single joint while supine cannot be correlated with hypertonicity and impaired motor control during walking.

Time spent walking can be measured using an accelerometer that records activity (Coleman et al., 1999; Zhang et al., 2003). With well-designed software, accelerometers placed on the trunk, each thigh, and under each foot reveal both temporal aspects of the gait cycle and acceleration forces at key points in the step cycle, such as at toe off and initial swing. Figure 3.3 shows the step cycle from one foot accelerometer obtained using a commercial device, the Intelligent Device for Energy Expenditure and Physical Activity (IDEEA) system (MiniSun, Fresno, CA). Table 3.3 was calculated from gait cycle data recording from bilateral foot and thigh accelerometers.

Functional neuroimaging may serve to reveal the nodes of the supraspinal networks that are engaged over the course of a training intervention. For example, near-infrared spectroscopy has assessed changes in M1S1 and premotor cortex that contribute to improved motor control during walking on a treadmill (Miyai et al., 2003). Using an ankle dorsiflexion fMRI activation paradigm, changes over time of gait training can be shown after SCI, stroke, and in children after hemispherectomy for epilepsy (Dobkin, 2000b; Dobkin et al., 2004; de Bode et al., 2005). These techniques may provide insight into the optimal duration of an intervention and the effects of medications on cortical representational plasticity. Ankle dorsiflexion or other active and passive leg movements may also be of value in discerning the completeness of a SCI and in determining the functional effects of a subcortical or spinal neural repair strategy.

Functional measures

The locomotor score (0–7) of the Functional Independence Measure (FIM) and of the Barthel Index (dependent, need help, independent) offer insight into the need for assistance and thus the burden of

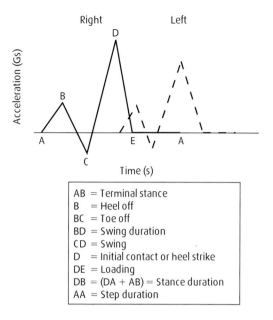

AB = Terminal stance
B   = Heel off
BC = Toe off
BD = Swing duration
CD = Swing
D   = Initial contact or heel strike
DE = Loading
DB = (DA + AB) = Stance duration
AA = Step duration

Figure 3.3. Gait cycle defined by accelerometry of each foot.

care related to walking. A measure such as the Walking Index for SCI (WISCI) takes into account the physical help, braces and assistive devices needed and reflects, in part, functional limitations (Ditunno and Ditunno, 2001). In the SCILT trial, the locomotor FIM and the WISCI correlated with lower extremity strength and walking speed. The Stroke Impact Scale and the physical activity portion of the SF-36 for any neurological disease may reveal how patients assess themselves for mobility tasks in everyday activities, which reflects health-related quality of life (Ware and Sherbourne, 1992; Vickrey et al., 1995, 2000; Duncan et al., 2003a).

3.6 Neural repair strategies and gait training

A well-defined approach for the retraining of walking will be needed to engage and incorporate new neurons, axons, synapses, and networks created by

Table 3.3. Healthy subject walking with IDEEA system foot accelerometers.

Statistics	Left leg		Right leg		Bilateral	
Steps	281		281		562	
Duration	2 min, 51 s		2 min, 54 s		5 min, 46 s	
Distance (km)	0.197		0.200		0.396	
	Mean	*SD*	*Mean*	*SD*	*Mean*	*SD*
Single support (ms)	450.9	19.1	445.4	16.4	448.2	18.0
Double support (ms)	170.1	17.7	167.3	17.9	168.7	17.8
SLS/DLS (%)	265.1	26.9	266.3	25.2	265.7	26.3
Swing duration (ms)	445.4	16.4	450.9	19.1	448.2	18.0
Step duration (ms)	618.1	27.4	615.4	25.2	616.8	26.3
Cycle duration (ms)	1.23	0.046	1.24	0.089	1.24	0.071
Pulling acceleration foot (Gs)	0.518	0.054	0.565	0.048	0.542	0.056
Pulling acceleration *thigh* (Gs)	0.297	0.057	0.326	0.047		
Swing power (Gs)	0.759	0.094	0.750	0.103	0.754	0.099
Ground impact (Gs)	1.45	0.345	1.55	0.376	1.50	0.364
Foot fall (G) deceleration	2.88	0.265	2.90	0.278	2.89	0.271
Push-off (°) angle at B	79.5	12.8	87.9	7.22	83.7	11.2
Speed (m/min)	68.6	4.51	68.7	4.40	68.7	4.46
Cadence (steps/min)	98.5	9.51	96.9	4.13	97.7	7.37
Step length (m)	0.7	0.041	0.710	0.032	0.705	0.037
Stride length (m)	1.41	0.056	1.41	0.051	1.41	0.054

SDL/DLS: single-limb support/double-limb support.

neural repair strategies (Dobkin, 2000a). Any trial of a repair intervention ought to include a physical therapy approach that is relevant to a potential treatment goal of the repair intervention. An RCT ought to assign the experimental and control arms to the same rehabilitation therapies, given the gains that can be made at any time after onset of walking disability in many patients. Finding a means to encourage and assist locomotor training may be a critical element for driving activity-dependent plasticity through intrinsic mechanisms such as long-term potentiation, release of neurotrophins, and dendritic sprouting (Chapters 4, 7, and 20 of Volume I) (Dobkin and Havton, 2004).

3.7 Summary

The ability to walk 150 ft without physical help, which is the definition of recovery of typical measurement tools for rehabilitation studies, is achieved by most patients after stroke, traumatic brain injury (TBI), and incomplete SCI by 3–6 months after onset. This artificial ceiling on walking gains in rehabilitation studies is set too low, however. Many studies suggest that rehabilitation approaches for those who can walk ought to seek independent community ambulation as the goal, which means walking at least 80 cm/s for at least 200 m. Few RCTs have set this goal for a well-defined intervention. In addition, creative rehabilitation efforts built upon an understanding of the biological adaptability of networks for motor control are needed to get non-walkers who have some residual lower extremity movement to become more independent. Future trials would make a meaningful contribution to evidence-based practices if subjects were entered based on level of independence and initial walking speed. Trial designs should employ a reproducible therapy that is defined by its intensity and duration of actual practice to maximize gains in ambulation.

REFERENCES

Ada, L., Dean, C.M., Hall, J.M., Bampton, J. and Crompton, S. (2003). A treadmill and overground walking program improves walking in persons residing in the community after stroke: a placebo-controlled, randomized trial. *Arch Phys Med Rehabil*, **84**, 1486–1491.

Barbeau, H. (2003). Locomotor training in neurorehabilitation: emerging rehabilitation concepts. *Neurorehabil Neural Repair*, **17**, 3–11.

Barbeau, H. and Visintin, M. (2003). Optimal outcomes obtained with body-weight support combined with treadmill training in stroke subjects. *Arch Phys Med Rehabil*, **84**, 1458–1465.

Barbeau, H., Ladouceur, M., Mirbagheri, M. and Kearney, R. (2002). The effect of locomotor training combined with functional electrical stimulation in chronic spinal cord injured subjects: walking and reflex studies. *Brain Res Rev*, **40**, 274–291.

Chaplin, E. (1996). Functional neuromuscular stimulation for mobility in people with spinal cord injuries. The parastep I system. *J Spinal Cord Med*, **19**, 99–105.

Coleman, K., Smith, D., Boone, D., Joseph, A. and del Aguila, M. (1999). Step activity monitor: long-term, continuous recording of ambulatory function. *J Rehabil Res Dev*, **36**, 8–18.

Colombo, G., Joerg, M., Schreier, R. and Dietz, V. (2000). Treadmill training of paraplegic patients using a robotic orthosis. *J Rehab Res Develop*, **37**, 693–700.

Daly, J. and Ruff, R. (2000). Electrically induced recovery of gait components for older patients with chronic stroke. *Am J Phys Med Rehabil*, **79**, 349–360.

de Bode, S., Firestine, A. and Dobkin, B. (2005). Residual motor control and cortical representations of function following hemispherectomy. *J Child Neurol*, **20**, 64–75.

Dean, C., Richards, C. and Malouin, F. (2000). Task-related circuit training improves performance of locomotor tasks in chronic stroke: a randomized, controlled pilot trial. *Arch Phys Med Rehabil*, **81**, 409–417.

Dietz, V. and Harkema, S. (2004). Locomotor activity in spinal cord-injured persons. *J Appl Physiol*, **96**, 1954–1960.

Dimitrijevic, M., Gerasimenko, Y. and Pinter, M. (1998). Evidence for a spinal central pattern generator in humans. *Ann NY Acad Sci*, **860**, 360–376.

Ditunno, P. and Ditunno J. (2001). Walking index for spinal cord injury scale revision (WISCI II). *Spinal Cord*, **39**, 654–656.

Dobkin, B. (1999). Overview of treadmill locomotor training with partial body weight support: a neurophysiologically sound approach whose time has come for randomized clinical trials. *Neurorehabil Neural Repair*, **13**, 157–165.

Dobkin, B. (2000a). Functional rewiring of brain and spinal cord after injury: the three R's of neural repair and neurological rehabilitation. *Curr Opin Neurol*, **13**, 655–659.

Dobkin, B. (2000b). Spinal and supraspinal plasticity after incomplete spinal cord injury: correlations between functional magnetic resonance imaging and engaged locomotor networks. In: *Progress in Brain Research* (ed. Seil, F.), Vol. 128, Elsevier, Amsterdam, pp. 99–111.

Dobkin, B. (2003a). *The Clinical Science of Neurologic Rehabilitation*, Oxford University Press, New York.

Dobkin, B. (2003b). Do electrically stimulated sensory inputs and movements lead to long-term plasticity and rehabilitation gains? *Curr Opin Neurol*, **16**, 685–691.

Dobkin, B. (2003c). Functional MRI: a potential physiologic indicator for stroke rehabilitation interventions. *Stroke*, **34**, e23–e24.

Dobkin, B. for the SCILT Group. (2004). Walking-related gains over the first 12 weeks of a RCT for incomplete traumatic spinal cord injury. *Neurol Rehabil*, **4**, S15.

Dobkin, B.H. (2004). Strategies for stroke rehabilitation. *Lancet Neurol*, **3**, 528–536.

Dobkin, B. and Havton, L. (2004). Basic advances and new avenues in therapy of spinal cord injury. *Annu Rev Med*, **55**, 255–282.

Dobkin, B., Apple, D., Barbeau, H., Basso, M., Behrman, A., Deforge, D., et al. (2003). Methods for a randomized trial of weight-supported treadmill training versus conventional training for walking during inpatient rehabilitation after incomplete traumatic spinal cord injury. *Neurorehabil Neural Repair*, **17**, 153–167.

Dobkin, B.H., Firestine, A., West, M., Saremi, K. and Woods, R. (2004). Ankle dorsiflexion as an fMRI paradigm to assay motor control for walking during rehabilitation. *Neuroimage*, **23**, 370–381.

Duncan, P., Lai, S., Bode, R., Perera, S. and DeRosa, J. (2003a). Stroke impact scale-16. *Neurology*, **60**, 291–296.

Duncan, P., Studenski, S., Richards, L., Golub, S., Lai, S., Reker, D., et al. (2003b). Randomized clinical trial of therapeutic exercise in subacute stroke. *Stroke*, **34**, 2173–2180.

Field-Fote, E. (2001). Combined use of body weight support, functional electrical stimulation, and treadmill training to improve walking ability in individuals with chronic incomplete spinal cord injury. *Arch Phys Med Rehabil*, **82**, 818–824.

Geisler, F., Coleman, W., Grieco, G., Poonian, D. and Group, S.S. (2001). Measurements and recovery patterns in a multicenter study of acute spinal cord injury. *Spine*, **26**, S68–S86.

Gill, T., Baker, D., Gottschalk, M., Peduzzi, P., Allore, H. and Byers, A. (2002). A program to prevent functional decline in physically frail, elderly persons who live at home. *New Engl J Med*, **347**, 1068–1074.

Grasso, R., Ivanenko, Y.P., Zago, M., Molinari, M., Scivoletto, G. and Castellano, V., et al. (2004). Distributed plasticity of locomotor pattern generators in spinal cord injured patients. *Brain*, **127**, 1019–1034.

Greenlund, K., Giles, W., Keenan, N., Croft, J. and Mensah, G. (2002). Physician advice, patient actions, and health-related quality of life in secondary prevention of stroke through diet and exercise. *Stroke*, **33**, 565–571.

Herman, R., He, J., D'Luzansky, S., Willis, W. and Dilli, S. (2002). Spinal cord stimulation facilitates functional walking in a chronic incomplete spinal cord injured. *Spinal Cord*, **40**, 65–68.

Hesse, S., Jahnke, M., Bertelt, C., Schreiner, C., Lucke, D. and Mauritz, K. (1994). Gait outcome in ambulatory hemiparetic patients after a 4-week comprehensive rehabilitation program and prognostic factors. *Stroke*, **25**, 1999–2004.

Hesse, S., Malezic, M., Schaffrin, A. and Mauritz, K-H. (1995). Restoration of gait by combined treadmill training and multichannel electrical stimulation in nonambulatory hemiparetic patients. *Scand J Rehab Med*, **27**, 199–203.

Hesse, S., Schmidt, H., Werner, C. and Bardeleben, A. (2003). Upper and lower extremity robotic devices for rehabilitation and for studying motor control. *Curr Opin Neurol*, **16**, 705–710.

Iezzoni, L. (2003). *When Walking Fails*, University of California Press, Berkeley.

Kalkers, N., de Groot, V., Lazeron, R., Killestein, J., Ader, H., Barkhof, F., et al. (2000). MS functional composite: relation to disease phenotype and disability strata. *Neurology*, **54**, 1233–1239.

Kurl, S., Laukkanen, J.A., Rauramaa, R., Lakka, T.A., Sivenius, J. and Salonen, J.T. (2003). Cardiorespiratory fitness and the risk for stroke in men. *Arch Intern Med*, **163**, 1682–1688.

Lafleur, M., Jackson, P., Malouin, F., Richards, C., Evans, A. and Doyon, J. (2002). Motor learning produces parallel dynamic functional changes during the execution and imagination of sequential foot movements. *Neuroimage*, **16**, 142–157.

Lemay, M. and Grill, W. (2004). Modularity of motor output evoked by intraspinal microstimulation in cats. *J Neurophysiol*, **91**, 502–514.

Lennihan, L., Wootten, M., Wainwright, M., Tenteromano, L., McMahon, D. and Cotier, J. (2003). Treadmill with partial body-weight support versus conventional gait training after stroke. *Arch Phys Med Rehabil*, **84**, E5 (abstract).

Loeb, G. and Richmond, F. (2001). BION implants for therapeutic and functional electrical stimulation. In: *Neural Prostheses for Restoration of Sensory and Motor Function* (eds Chapin, J. and Moxon, K.), CRC Press, Boca Raton, 75–99.

Lord, S., Wade, D. and Halligan, P. (1998). A comparison of two physiotherapy treatment approaches to improve walking in multiple sclerosis: a pilot randomized controlled study. *Clin Rehabil*, **12**, 477–486.

Lord, S., McPherson, K., McNaughton, H., Rochester, L. and Weatherall, M. (2004). Community ambulation after stroke: how important and obtainable is it and what measures appear predictive? *Arch Phys Med Rehabil*, **85**, 234–239.

MacKay-Lyons, M. and Makrides, L. (2002). Exercise capacity early after stroke. *Arch Phys Med Rehabil*, **83**, 1697–1702.

Macko, R., Smith, G., Dobrovolny, C., Sorkin, J., Goldberg, A. and Silver, K. (2001). Treadmill training improves fitness reserve in chronic stroke patients. *Arch Phys Med Rehabil*, **82**, 879–884.

Malouin, F., Belleville, S., Richards, C., Desrosiers, J. and Doyon, J. (2004). Working memory and mental practice outcomes after stroke. *Arch Phys Med Rehabil*, **85**, 177–183.

Miyai, I., Tanabe, H., Sase, I., Eda, H., Oda, I., Konishi, I., et al. (2001). Cortical mapping of gait in humans: a near-infrared spectroscopic topography study. *Neuroimage*, **14**, 1186–1192.

Miyai, I., Fujimoto, Y., Yamamoto, H., Ueda, Y., Saito, T., et al. (2002). Long-term effect of body weight-supported treadmill training in Parkinson's disease: a randomized controlled trial. *Arch Phys Med Rehabil*, **83**, 1370–1373.

Miyai, I., Yagura, H., Hatakenaka, M., Oda, I., Konishi, I. and Kubota, K. (2003). Longitudinal optical imaging study for locomotor recovery after stroke. *Stroke*, **34**, 2866–2870.

Moreland, J., Thomson, M. and Fuoco, A. (1998). Electromyographic biofeedback to improve lower extremity function after stroke: a meta-analysis. *Arch Phys Med Rehabil*, **79**, 134–140.

Moreland, J.D., Goldsmith, C.H., Huijbregts, M.P., Anderson, R.E., Prentice, D.M., Brunton, K.B., et al. (2003). Progressive resistance strengthening exercises after stroke: a single-blind randomized controlled trial. *Arch Phys Med Rehabil*, **84**, 1433–1440.

Mulroy, S., Gronley, J., Weiss, W., Newsam, C. and Perry, J. (2003). Use of cluster analysis for gait pattern classification of patients in the early and late recovery phases following stroke. *Gait Posture*, **18**, 114–125.

Nielsen, J. (2003). How we walk: central control of muscle activity during human walking. *Neuroscientist*, **9**, 195–204.

Nilsson, L., Carlsson, J., Danielsson, A., Fugl-Meyer, A., Sunnerhagen, K., Grimby, G., et al. (2002). Walking training of patients with hemiparesis at an early stage after stroke: a comparison of walking training on a treadmill with body weight support and walking training on the ground. *Clin Rehabil*, **15**, 515–527.

Norman, K., Pépin, A. and Barbeau, H. (1998). Effects of drugs on walking after spinal cord injury. *Spinal Cord*, **36**, 699–715.

Patel, A., Duncan, P., Lai, S. and Studenski, S. (2000). The relation between impairments and functional outcomes post-stroke. *Arch Phys Med Rehabil*, **81**, 1357–1363.

Perry, J., Garrett, M., Gromley, J. and Mulroy, S. (1995). Classification of walking handicap in the stroke population. *Stroke*, **26**, 982–989.

Schindl, M., Forstner, C., Kern, H. and Hesse, S. (2000). Treadmill training with partial body weight support in non-ambulatory patients with cerebral palsy. *Arch Phys Med Rehabil*, **81**, 301–306.

Sinkjaer, T., Andersen, J., Ladouceur, M., Christensen, L. and Nielsen, J. (2000). Major role for sensory feedback in soleus EMG activity in the stance phase of walking in man. *J Physiol*, **523(3)**, 817–827.

Steffen, T.M., Hacker, T.A. and Mollinger, L. (2002). Age- and gender-related test performance in community-dwelling elderly people: six-minute walk test, Berg balance scale, timed up & go test, and gait speeds. *Phys Ther*, **82**, 128–137.

Sullivan, K., Knowlton, B. and Dobkin, B. (2002). Step training with body weight support: effect of treadmill speed and practice paradigms on post-stroke locomotor recovery. *Arch Phys Med Rehabil*, **83**, 683–691.

Taub, E., Uswatte, G. and Elbert, T. (2002). New treatments in neurorehabilitation founded on basic research. *Nature Rev Neurosci*, **3**, 228–236.

Teixeira-Salmela, L., Olney, S. and Nadeau, S. (1999). Muscle strengthening and physical conditioning to reduce impairment and disability in chronic stroke survivors. *Arch Phys Med Rehabil*, **80**, 1211–1218.

Vickrey, B., Hays, R., Harooni, R., Myers, L. and Ellison, G. (1995). A health-related quality of life measure for multiple sclerosis. *Qual Life Res*, **4**, 187–206.

Vickrey, B., Hays, R. and Beckstrand, M. (2000). Development of a health-related quality of life measure for peripheral neuropathy. *Neurorehabil Neural Repair*, **14**, 93–104.

Visintin, M., Barbeau, H., Korner-Bitensky, N. and Mayo, N. (1998). A new approach to retrain gait in stroke patients through body weight support and treadmill stimulation. *Stroke*, **29**, 1122–1128.

Ware, J. and Sherbourne, C. (1992). The MOS 36-item short-form health survey (SF-36): conceptual framework and item selection. *Med Care*, **30**, 473–483.

Werner, C., von Frankenberg, S., Treig, T., Konrad, M. and Hesse, S. (2002). Treadmill training with partial body weight support and electromechanical gait trainer for restoration of gait in subacute stroke patients. *Stroke*, **33**, 2895–2901.

Wernig, A., Muller, S., Nanassy, A. and Cagol, E. (1995). Laufband therapy based on "Rules of Spinal Locomotion" is effective in spinal cord injured persons. *Europ J Neurosci*, **7**, 823–829.

Zhang, K., Werner, P., Sun, M., Pi-Sunyer, F.X. and Boozer, C.N. (2003). Measurement of human daily physical activity. *Obes Res*, **11**, 33–40.

Electromyography in neurorehabilitation

Amparo Gutierrez and Austin J. Sumner

Department of Neurology, Louisiana State University Medical Center, New Orleans, LA, USA

4.1 Introduction

One of the fundamental principles of electrodiagnostic medicine is the assessment of the peripheral nervous system's ability to conduct an electrical impulse (Dumitru et al., 2002). Nerve conduction studies (NCs) and needle electromyography (EMG), are commonly referred to as *electrodiagnostic* or *EMG* studies. Electrodiagnostic studies play a crucial role in identifying disorders that affect the peripheral nerve, the dorsal root ganglia, the nerve root, or the anterior horn cell. Electrodiagnostic studies can also identify disturbances at the level of the neuromuscular junction and in the muscle. Additionally, EMG studies can provide useful information in disorders involving the upper motor neurons or disorders of volition as well as evaluating gait.

Thus, electrodiagnostic testing serves as an important diagnostic and prognostic tool when applied within the context of the clinical neurologic examination. A detailed, focused history and neurologic examination should serve as the template upon which one designs and performs the EMG study. Data acquired during the EMG study must always be interpreted within the clinical context because the same data may have very different interpretations depending on the clinical situation. An EMG study performed in isolation of the clinical context may provide little useful information.

4.2 Basic principles in EMG

The primary goals of the EMG study are to localize the lesion, characterize the underlying nerve pathophysiology, quantitate the severity of the lesion, and assess the temporal course of the disorder (Preston et al., 1998).

Localizing a lesion within the peripheral nervous system is best determined with the use of an EMG study. The EMG study can be tailored in such a fashion as to specifically localize the lesion to the nerve roots, plexus, trunks, or individual peripheral nerves. The clinician designing the EMG study must have intimate knowledge of the anatomy of the peripheral nervous system for precise lesion localization.

EMG studies can often identify the underlying pathologic process involving a nerve lesion. The EMG study can determine whether the pathology leading to the clinical deficit is secondary to axonal loss, demyelination or if the underlying disorder is secondary to muscle disease or neuromuscular dysfunction. This differentiation between pathologic processes allows for a narrowing of the differential diagnosis.

The EMG study can also assess the degree or extent of axonal loss versus demyelination, which then allows the clinician to predict the extent of recovery from a particular lesion and the expected time frame in which this recovery should take place. A lesion that primarily involves axonal loss will carry a worse prognosis and therefore a less complete recovery would be expected. A lesion that is the result of demyelination can be expected to recover fully when given the required time for remyelination. Lesions with mixed pathology will recover in an intermediate time frame.

The EMG study can provide data on the temporal course and rate of recovery of a lesion. Abnormalities seen on the EMG can separate lesions into hyperacute (less than 1 week), acute (less than a few weeks), or chronic. The electromyographer must therefore be aware of the patient's clinical time course to accurately interpret the abnormalities observed during the study.

4.3 Assessment of weakness

A motor deficit can result as a consequence of a lesion that lies within various places in the neuraxis. Weakness can be secondary to a lesion in the upper motor neuron pool (corticospinal tracts) or within the lower motor neuron pool (anterior horn cell and its peripheral process). Weakness may also be secondary to neuromuscular junction dysfunction. Finally, weakness can be due to muscle disease. Differentiating between these various etiologic factors in the clinical setting can be quite challenging. The EMG study provides an excellent tool for determining the cause of weakness. In a study performed by Nardin et al. (2002), the diagnostic accuracy of electrodiagnostic testing in the evaluation of patient weakness had an overall accuracy of 91%.

Upper motor lesions

Clinically, patients with lesions of the brain and/or spinal cord present with weakness and most often also have numbness. These patients usually have increased deep tendon reflexes, extensor plantar responses, and increased muscle tone that marks the lesion site. Assessment of a lesion that involves the upper motor neuron pool is done during the EMG portion of the study. These patients have a delayed onset of EMG activity and a decreased ability to recruit motor unit potentials. Several studies have documented that there is a delay of initiation and prolonged termination of muscle contraction in paretic muscles from upper motor impairment (Chae et al., 2002). Following a stroke, changes in descending input may modify interneuronal excitability throughout the cord (Grimby, 1963). The loss of excitability at the level of the spinal interneurons may account for the delayed onset of EMG activity observed in paretic limbs in an upper motor neuron lesion

(Dewald et al., 1999). Additional discussion of upper motor lesions are found in several chapters of this volume (e.g., Volume II, Chapters 17, 18, 36, and 38).

Lower motor lesions

In a patient undergoing rehabilitation, there is the potential for the patient to be immobilized for protracted periods of time. These patients may consequently develop superimposed patterns of weakness, due to deconditioning, development of contractures and joint problems. Additionally, they may develop a lower motor neuron lesion secondary to either a compressive neuropathy or a polyneuropathy (see Volume II, Chapter 40). Being able to distinguish between these varying patterns of weakness is important. NCs are extremely useful in assessing these types of patients. Compressive and entrapment neuropathies usually lead to numbness and weakness in the area of the involved nerve. Although the terms compression and entrapment are often used interchangeably, it is important to recognize the distinction between a nerve entrapped in a fibroosseous tunnel where chronic low pressure and ischemia are the major mechanisms of nerve injury and external compression where, in acute situations, high mechanical pressures can result in a unique structural deformation of the nerve producing a focal demyelination (a neuropraxia). Certain forms of compression, with moderately high external pressure for limited time periods, result in a failure of action potential propagation (conduction block) but not in Wallerian degeneration (Fowler et al., 1972). If the compression is more prolonged, even with relatively low pressures there is a mixed lesion with both action potential blockade and Wallerian degeneration. These histologic findings can be anticipated from careful electrodiagnostic studies.

Electrodiagnostic studies performed on a nerve with a compressive lesion should reveal that the conduction velocity above and below the region of the segmental demyelination are normal (McDonald, 1962). However, across the demyelinated region of the nerve, the velocity of action potential propagation is significantly slowed. Conduction block is defined as

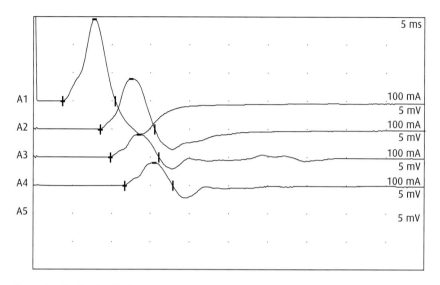

Figure 4.1. Conduction block.

a normal motor response when stimulating the affected nerve distal to the lesion, but either a reduced or absent response is elicited when stimulating proximal to the lesion. (Fig. 4.1) Neuropraxic lesions, (conduction block), may take up to 6 months to resolve, although typically block reverses over 2 weeks to 3 months. The presence of Wallerian degeneration can be especially observed during EMG. In this situation of axon loss, one can see fibrillation potentials of the involved muscles. These patients usually have an incomplete recovery. When a diagnosis of a compressive neuropathy is made, the patient's caretakers can then be given specific instructions for positioning of the patient or other equipment utilized in the care of the patient. Therefore, early recognition of this pattern of weakness is important.

Frequently distal weakness is secondary to a polyneuropathy. Patients commonly develop this neuropathy insidiously. The most common neuropathy is a generalized axonal sensorimotor polyneuropathy. Etiologic causes can be varied: metabolic, nutritional, secondary to a systemic disorder, infectious, or cryptogenic. The most common etiology of a generalized distal axonal sensorimotor polyneuropathy is diabetes mellitus (Melton and Dyck, 1987). The risk of developing a diabetic peripheral neuropathy

correlates with the duration of the diabetes, the control of hyperglycemia, and the presence of retinopathy and nephropathy (Dyck et al., 1993). Other causes of axonal polyneuropathy are shown in Table 4.1.

Patients with an axonal polyneuropathy first develop a distal pattern of sensory loss followed by distal weakness. The reflexes, when lost, are in a length-dependent fashion. Electrodiagnostic studies reveal reduced amplitudes of sensory and motor action potentials. Conduction velocities are minimally affected (Oh, 1993). EMG reveals a pattern compatible with denervation mostly affecting the distal muscles. Motor unit potentials are usually large with an increased recruitment and decreased interference pattern (Brown and Bolton, 1987). Spontaneous activity is usually sparse. Identifying the underlying etiology can lead to improvement or at least a stabilization of the polyneuropathy.

Occasionally, patients develop another pattern of weakness that involves both proximal and distal muscles. This pattern of weakness is most consistently seen in a demyelinating polyneuropathy. Demyelinating neuropathies may be divided into acute or chronic presentations. Guillain–Barre syndrome (GBS) or acute inflammatory demyelinating polyradiculoneuropathy (AIDP) has become the most

Table 4.1. Causes of axonal polyneuropathies.

Nutritional deficiencies
Thiamine
Pyridoxine (B$_6$)
Cobalamin (B$_{12}$)
Folate
Vitamin E
Strachan syndrome

Toxins
Alcohol
Drugs

Chloramphenicol	Hydralazine
Chloroquine	Aminodarone
Dapsone	Propafenone
Metronidazole	FK 506 (Prograf)
Nitrofurantoin	Colchicine
Zalcitabine and other	Vincristine
nucleoside analogs	Disulfiram
Cisplatinum	Glutethimide
Paclitaxel	Simivastin and other statins
Misonidazole	
Thalidomide	

Heavy metals
Hexacarbons
Acrylamide
Carbon disulfide
Ethylene glycol
Organophosphates

common cause of acute paralysis in Western countries since the virtual elimination of poliomyelitis with vaccination programs (Parry, 1993). GBS is clinically a predominant motor neuropathy affecting the patient in a symmetrical fashion. At the nadir of the illness there is approximately equal weakness of proximal and distal muscles in about 50% of cases (Ropper and Shahani, 1984). Roughly 60–70% of patients with AIDP note some form of acute illness (e.g., a viral syndrome) 1–3 weeks before the onset of neurologic symptoms. In a recent case control study of 154 patients with GBS, serologic evidence of recent infections with *Campylobacter jejuni* (32%), cytomegalovirus (13%), Epstein–Barr virus (10%), and *Mycoplasma pneumoniae* (5%) were more frequent than in the control population (Jacobs et al., 1998).

The early and accurate diagnosis of GBS depends primarily on NCs. Carefully performed NCs of multiple nerves, including cranial nerves and proximal segments of spinal nerves, if indicated, are almost always abnormal even when the cerebrospinal fluid protein is normal. The electrophysiologic diagnosis of GBS requires the demonstration of the characteristic changes associated with acute demyelination (Gilliatt, 1966). The most studied aspects in AIDP are motor nerves; distal latencies, compound action potentials, conduction velocities, waveform duration and morphology, and F-waves. The electrophysiologic hallmarks include prolongation of the distal latencies, slow conduction velocities, temporal dispersion, conduction block, and prolonged F-waves. Another electrodiagnostic finding often seen in GBS is superimposed axonal degeneration (Ensurd and Krivickas, 2001). The degree of axonal loss has been shown to correlate with both acute mortality and long-term disability in patients with GBS (Chio et al., 2003).

Nearly 40% of patients hospitalized with GBS will require inpatient rehabilitation (Meythaler et al., 1994). The electrodiagnostic study aids in identifying these patients.

Chronic inflammatory demyelinating polyneuropathy (CIDP) is an acquired demyelinating polyradiculoneuropathy that shares a similar pathology and presumed autoimmune etiology with AIDP but differs primarily in the time course of presentation and evolution of clinical signs. In typical CIDP, motor and sensory symptoms develop slowly over the course of weeks to months, or even years. The clinical course may be relapsing, with variable periods of remission, or stepwise and chronically progressive. The diagnosis of CIDP is based on a combination of clinical and electrophysiologic findings as well as evaluation of the cerebrospinal fluid. The patient with CIDP has variable weakness in proximal and distal muscles. Sensory impairment is common, and tendon reflexes are either reduced or absent (McCombe et al., 1987). Electrodiagnostic studies usually reveal absent sensory responses. Motor conduction velocities are very slow, usually below 80% of normal values, and distal latencies may be prolonged.

Table 4.2. Concurrent diseases with CIDP.

HIV infection
Diabetes mellitus
Chronic active hepatitis
Inflammatory bowel disease
Connective tissue disease
Nephrotic syndrome
Melanoma
Monoclonal gammopathy
Lyme disease
Lymphoma

Table 4.3. Drugs that may cause a myopathy.

Amiodarone	Gemfibrozil
Anesthetics	Interferon alpha
Cytarbine	Isoniazid
Cyclosporine	Neuroleptics
Cyclophosphamide	Penicillamine
Cholesterol-lowering agent	Steroids
Colchicine	Tacrolimus
Corticosteroids	Vasopressin
Diazepam	Zidovudine
Diuretics	

If the pathology is concentrated proximally, the F-wave latencies are markedly abnormal (Nicolas et al., 2002; Scarlato and Comi, 2002). Some patients with CIDP may have a concurrent illness (Table 4.2).

Muscle disease

Some patients may, in the course of their rehabilitation, develop a pattern of proximal weakness. This weakness usually begins in the lower extremities and then progresses to involve the proximal arms. There may or may not be associated muscle pain. In this setting, the most common etiology would be a toxic or iatrogenic myopathy. Certain drugs are known to cause an immunologic reaction directed against muscle (Scarlato and Comi, 2002) (Table 4.3). Electrolyte imbalances have also been associated with vacuolar muscle damage (Saleh and Seidman, 2003). Prompt recognition of this clinical picture is important because toxic or iatrogenic myopathies are potentially reversible, thus reducing their damaging effect.

Inflammatory myopathies are another cause of proximal weakness. The inflammatory myopathies are a diverse group, ranging from focal varieties to widespread skeletal involvement. Etiologic factors are mainly immune-mediated or infectious agents. The most common immune-related varieties in clinical practice are dermatomyositis and polymyositis, each of which have distinctive clinical and histopathological features, and may occur in isolation or associated with a systemic connective tissue disease (Amato and Barohn, 1997). Human immunodeficiency virus (HIV) causes a myopathy in almost a third of infected patients (Dalakas et al., 1986). Another infectious agent is human T-cell lymphotropic virus 1 (HTLV-1).

Electrodiagnostically, patients with a myopathy should have normal nerve conductions. EMG in these patients demonstrates short duration, small amplitude, polyphasic motor unit potentials with early recruitment (Mastaglia et al., 2003). For additional discussion of myopathies, see Volume II, Chapter 41.

Neuromuscular transmission defect

Infrequent causes of muscle weakness are the diseases of the neuromuscular junction (Volume II, Chapter 40). Neuromuscular transmission defect can be a result an autoimmune disease like Myasthenia gravis (MG) or Eaton–Lambert syndrome (LEMS), or toxins that block neuromuscular transmission. MG occurs with a prevalence of 20 per 100,000 (Phillips, 2003). Like other autoimmune disorders, it is characterized by periods of relapses and remissions (Richman and Agius, 2003). The target of the autoimmune attack in MG is the nicotinic acetylcholine receptor, which is located on the postsynaptic muscle endplate membrane (Tzartos and Lindstrom, 1980). Patients present with weakness of the ocular and or bulbar musculature that over time may generalize to involve proximal limb muscles. An important characteristic of patients with neuromuscular transmission defect is fatigability. Additionally, these patients can present with unexplained respiratory failure.

Repetitive nerve stimulation is a useful electro-physiologic test in the evaluation of patients with suspected neuromuscular junction disorders. In patients with MG, there is a decremental response seen on the compound motor action potential (CMAP) with slow rates of stimulation. In patients with LEMS, fast rates of repetitive stimulation produce a marked increase in the CMAP (Kimura, 1989).

4.4 EMG in movement

Surface EMG (SEMG) can provide a simple, non-invasive method to assess the activation of muscles involved in performing specific tasks. Likewise SEMG can aid in determining the timing and intensity of muscular activation and contraction during task specific performance. Thus, SEMG analysis has been widely employed in the field of ergonomics, biomechanics, sports science, and kinesiology (McGill, 2004).

SEMG can serve as a useful tool specifically in gait analysis, the origins of which date back to Europe in the 17th century. Vern Inman, and colleagues moved the science of gait analysis dramatically forward by adding kinesiologic EMG, 3-D force, and energy measurements in the study of walking in normal subjects and amputees (1944–1947) (Sutherland, 2001). Kinesiologic EMG is a technique which is used to determine the relationship of muscle activation to joint movement and to the gait (see Volume II, Chapter 19).

These techniques of dynamic EMG have been employed to evaluate varies disease states, such as children with cerebral palsy, stroke patients and in patients with prosthetic devices. The use of gait analysis in children with cerebral palsy has allowed for better surgical intervention to influence gait function. Finally, electromyographic biofeedback has been used to improve lower extremity function after stroke (Moreland et al., 1998).

4.5 Interpreting the EMG report

An electrodiagnostic consultation is best interpreted within the context of a specific clinical question.

Clear identification of the clinical question allows the electromyographer to design the appropriate electrical tests. Most EMG reports should include various sections: chief complaint, history, physical examination, nerve conductions, needle EMG, summary of findings, and impression.

Likewise it is important to understand the limitations of electrodiagnostic testing. NCs and EMG display a limited repertoire of abnormalities that include loss of myelinated motor or sensory nerve fibers, or both, abnormalities in myelin that affect conduction properties and membrane characteristics, compensatory changes associated with reinnervation of muscle fibers, and changes that are consistent with acute or chronic lesions (Krarup, 2003). Routine nerve conductions only assess the large myelinated fibers usually in their more distal distribution. Symptoms that are as a result of pathology of the small myelinated or unmyelinated fibers require alternative methods of evaluation.

The timing of the electrodiagnostic evaluation is important, as there is an orderly sequence of electrophysiologic changes that follow nerve injury. Knowledge of these changes is necessary for proper interpretation of results.

4.6 Use of the EMG as an outcome measure

The ability to predict a patient's eventual prognosis is an important part of the overall treatment plan. Unfortunately the current literature dealing with electrodiagnostic prognostication is meager. There are only a few areas that electrophysiologic testing provides important outcome data. One of these areas is the evaluation of traumatic peripheral nerve injury. Traumatic nerve injuries can result in different grades of injuries as outlined by Seddon; neuropraxic, axonotmesis, and neurotmesis. They are based on morphologic criteria and the presence of Wallerian degeneration. The electromyographer is frequently asked to participate in the clinical evaluation and therapeutic decision-making of patients with peripheral nerve injury. Careful EMG evaluation can identify a lesion that is a result of neuropraxia versus axonotmesis and neurotmesis. In the latter case there is varying degrees of Wallerian degeneration. The timing of the EMG study is important and is guided by experimental studies of sensory and motor nerve regeneration (Gilchrist and Sachs, 2004). Nerves have been shown to regenerate at an average rate of 1–2 mm/day (Seddon et al., 1943). Knowing when the lesion occurred allows the evaluator a time course in which one can predict the course of regeneration and likewise when a nerve is not regenerating as one would anticipate. For most nerve lesions in continuity, surgical exploration is generally recommended if there is no evidence of axonal regeneration by 3–6 months post injury. Prognostically, lesions with the least amount of Wallerian degeneration recover best (Cros, 2001).

NCs are useful in mapping the recovery from a compression neuropathy or a neuropraxic lesion. Neuropraxic lesions result from a disruption of myelin with intact axons and stroma. This type of lesion can also be seen in traumatic brachial plexus injuries. In this situation the large myelinated fibers are more susceptible. Thus motor fibers are usually more affected than sensory fibers, resulting in motor paralysis. Motor paralysis from, a neuropraxic lesion, is expected to last from 1 to 6 months, although most resolve by 3 months (Rudge, 1974). Nerve conductions serve to document and outline the recovery of this type of injury.

Electrodiagnostic testing is perhaps the most important predictor of outcome in patients with GBS (Katirji et al., 2002). Patients with severe axonal loss have poorer outcomes. The amplitude of the CMAP is the most reliable measure of axonal loss: low CMAP amplitude (less than 10–20% of normal) has been correlated with poor outcomes (McKhann et al., 1985).

NCs can be used in assessing the response of diabetic neuropathy to various therapeutic interventions. Early studies revealed improvement in conduction velocity following glycemic control in newly diagnosed diabetics (Fraser et al., 1977).

Lastly, electrophysiologic testing has played an important role in determining the extent of facial nerve injury when there is early, complete paralysis of the facial muscles. Testing is best performed on the 5th day after onset or within 2 weeks (Gutierrez and Sumner, 2003). The facial nerve conduction is the most useful. CMAP side-to-side comparisons seem to hold the best prognostic values. May demonstrated that a 25% or greater sparing of CMAP amplitude when compared to the unaffected side had a 98% chance of satisfactory recovery (May et al., 1983).

REFERENCES

Amato, A. and Barohn, R.J. (1997). Idiopathic inflammatory myopathies. *Neurol Clin N Amer*, **15**, 615–641.

Brown, W.F. and Bolton, C.F. (1987). *Clinical Electromyography*, Butterworth, Boston, pp. 379–381.

Chae, J., Yang, G., Park, B.K. and Labatia, I. (2002). Delay initiation and termination of muscle contraction, motor impairment, and physical disability in upper limb hemiparesis. *Muscle Nerve*, **25**, 568–575.

Chio, A., Cocito, D., Leone, M., et al. (2003). Guillain–Barre syndrome: a prospective, population-based incidence and outcome survey. *Neurology*, **60**, 1146–1150.

Cros, D. (2001). *Peripher Neuropath: A Practical Approach to Diagnosis and Management*, Lippincott Williams & Wilkins, Boston.

Dalakas, M.C., Pezeshkpour, G.H., Gravell, M., et al. (1986). Polymyositis associated with AIDS retrovirus. *J Am Med Assoc*, **256**, 2381.

Dewald, J.P.A., Beer, R.F., Given, J.D., et al. (1999). Reorganization of flexion reflexes in the upper extremity of hemiparetic subjects. *Muscle Nerve*, **22**, 1209–1221.

Dumitru, D., Amato, A.A. and Zwarts, M.J. (2002). *Electrodiagnostic Medicine*, 2nd edn., Hanley & Belfus Inc., Philadelphia.

Dyck, P.J., Kratz, K.M., Litchy, W.J., et al. (1993). The prevalence by staged severity of various types of diabetic neuropathy, retinopathy, and nephropathy in a population-based cohort: the Rochester diabetic neuropathy study. *Neurology*, **43**, 817–824.

Ensurd, E.R. and Krivickas, L.S. (2001). Acquired inflammatory demyelinating neuropathies. *Phys Med Rehabil Clin N Am*, **12**, 321–324.

Fowler, T.J., Danta, G. and Gilliatt, R.W. (1972). Recovery of nerve conduction after a pneumatic tourniquet: observations on the hind-limb of the baboon. *J Neurol Neurosurg Psychiatr*, **35**, 638–647.

Fraser, D.M., Campbell, I.W., Ewing, D.J., et al. (1977). Peripheral and autonomic nerve function in newly diagnosed diabetes mellitus. *Diabetes*, **26**, 546–550.

Gilchrist, J.M. and Sachs, G.M. (2004). Electrodiagnostic studies in the management and prognosis of neuromuscular disorders. *Muscle Nerve*, **29**, 165–190.

Gilliatt, R.W. (1966). Nerve conductions in human and experimental neuropathies. *Proc Roy Soc Med*, **59**, 989–993.

Grimby, L. (1963). Pathological plantar response: disturbances of the normal integration of flexor and extensor reflex components. *J Neurol Neurosurg Psychiatr*, **26**, 314–321.

Gutierrez, A. and Sumner, A.J. (2003). *Idiopathic (Bell's) Facial Palsy. Neurological Disorders Course and Treatment*, Academic Press, Boston (Chapter 14).

Jacobs, B.C., Rothbarth, P.H., Vander Meche, N., et al. (1998). The spectrum of antecedent infections in Guillain–Barre syndrome. A case control study. *Neurology*, **51**, 1110–1115.

Katirji, B., Kaminski, H.J., Preston, D., et al. (2002). *Neuromuscular Disorders in Clinical Practice*, Butterworth Heinemann, Boston (Chapter 41).

Kimura, J. (1989). *Electrodiagnosis in Diseases of Nerve and Muscle*, Davis, Philadelphia.

Krarup, C. (2003). An update on electrophysiological studies in neuropathy. *Curr Opin Neurol*, **16**, 603–612.

Mastaglia, F.L., Garlep, M.J., Philips, B.A., et al. (2003). Inflammatory myopathies: clinical, diagnostic, and therapeutic aspects. *Muscle Nerve*, **27**, 407–425.

May, M., Blumenthal, F. and Klein, S.R. (1983). Acute Bell's P5falsy: prognostic value of evoked electromyography, maximal stimulation and other electrical test. *Am J Otol*, **5**, 1–7.

McCombe, P.A., Pollard, J.D. and McLeod, J.G. (1987). Chronic inflammatory demyelinating polyradiculoneuropathy: a clinical and electrophysiological study of 92 case. *Brain*, **110**, 1617–1630.

McDonald, W.I. (1962). Conduction in muscle afferent fibres during experimental demyelination in cat nerve. *Acta Neuropath*, **1**, 425–432.

McGill, K.C. (2004). Surface electromyography signal modeling. *Med Biol Eng Comput*, **42**, 446–454.

McKhann, G.M., Griffin, J.W., Cornblath, D.R., et al. (1985). Prognosis in Guillain–Barre syndrome. *Lancet*, **1**, 1202–1203.

Melton, L.J. and Dyck, P.J. (1987). Clinical features of diabetic neuropathies. In: *Diabetic Neuropathy* (eds Dyck, P.J., Thomas, P.K. and Asbury, A.K.), W.B. Saunders, Philadelphia, pp. 27–35.

Meythaler, J., DeVivo, M., Clausen, G., et al. (1994). Prediction of outcome in Guillain–Barre syndrome patients admitted to rehabilitation. *Arch Phys Med Rehabil*, **75**, 1027.

Moreland, J.D., Thomson, M.A. and Fuoco, A.R. (1998). Electromyographic biofeedback to improve lower extremity function after stroke: a meta-analysis. *Arch Phys Med Rehabil*, **79**, 134–140.

Nardin, R.A., Rutkove, S.B. and Raynor, E.M. (2002). Diagnostic accuracy of electrodiagnostic testing. In: *Neuromuscular Disorders in Clinical Practice*, (eds Katirji, B., Kaminski, H.J., Preston, D., et al.), Butterworth Heinemann, Boston (Chapter 41).

Nicolas, G., Maisonobe, T., Le Forestier, N., et al. (2002). Proposed revised electrophysiological criteria for chronic inflammatory demyelinating polyradiculoneuropathy. *Muscle Nerve*, **25**, 26–30.

Oh, S.J. (1993). *Clinical Electromyography Nerve Conductions Studies*, 2nd edn., Williams & Wilkens, Baltimore, MD, pp. 482–485.

Parry, G.J. (1993). *Guillain–Barre Syndrome.*, Thieme Medical Publishers Inc., New York, p. 10.

Phillips, L.H. (2003). The epidemiology of myasthenia gravis. *Ann New York Acad Sci*, **998**, pp. 407–412.

Preston, D.C., Shapiro, B.E. and Katirji, B. (1998). *Electromyography and Neuromuscular Disorders: Clinical–Electrophysiologic Correlations*, Butterworth-Heinemann, Boston (Chapter 7).

Richman, D.P. and Agius, M.A. (2003). Treatment of autoimmune myasthenia gravis. *Neurology*, **61**, 1652–1661.

Ropper, A.H. and Shahani, B.T. (1984). Diagnosis and management of areflexic paralysis with emphasis on Guillain–Barre syndrome. In: *Peripheral Nerve Disorders* (eds Asbury, A.K. and Gilliatt, R.W.), Butterworth, London, pp. 21–45.

Rudge, P. (1974). Tourniquey paralysis with prolonged conduction block. An electrophysiological study. *J Bone Joint Surg*, **56B**, 716–720.

Saleh, F.G. and Seidman, R.J. (2003). Drug-induced myopathy and neuropathy. *J Clin Neuromusc Dis*, **5**, 81–92.

Scarlato, G. and Comi, G.P. (2002). Metabolic and drug-induced muscle disorders. *Curr Opin Neurol*, **15**, 533–538.

Seddon, H.J., Medawar, P.B. and Smith, H. (1943). Rate of regeneration of peripheral nerves in man. *J Physiol*, **102**, 191–215.

Sutherland, D.H. (2001). *Gait and Posture*, **14**, 61–70.

Tzartos, S.J. and Lindstrom, J.M. (1980). Monoclonal antibodies used to probe acetylcholine receptor structure: localization of the main immunogenic region and detection of similarities between subunits. *Proc Natl Acad Sci*, **77**, 755–759.

Functional neuroimaging

Nick S. Ward and Richard S.J. Frackowiak

Wellcome Department of Imaging Neuroscience, Institute of Neurology, University College London, London, UK

5.1 Introduction

Patients who survive focal brain injury for example stroke, undergo complete or more commonly partial recovery of function (Twitchell, 1951). The management of patients with incomplete recovery draws on specific rehabilitation interventions aimed at assisting adaptation to impairment. However there is a growing interest in designing therapeutic strategies to promote cerebral reorganisation as a way of reducing rather than compensating for impairment. This interest stems largely from experiments in animal models, which have unequivocally demonstrated post-lesional changes in cerebral organisation related to recovery. In addition, it is clear that focal cortical damage in adult brains renders widespread surviving cortical regions more able to change structure and function in response to afferent signals in a way normally only seen in the developing brain (Schallert et al., 2000; Bury and Jones, 2002) (see Chapter 14 of Volume I, pp. 21–28 for a more extensive discussion of these changes). Activity-driven changes in these regions may be enhanced by experiential (Nudo et al., 1996) or pharmacological (Feeney, 1997) context, and correlate with functional recovery. These findings are clearly very exciting for clinicians. It has been suggested that similar injury-induced changes occur in the human brain, and that their manipulation will provide a means of promoting functional recovery in patients with focal brain damage. One crucial aspect of developing such strategies involves building an empirical understanding of how the brain responds to injury and how such changes may be manipulated in a way that promotes functional

recovery. The investigation of cerebral reorganisation after focal brain injury in humans is less well advanced than similar work in animal models. There are clearly greater limitations in studying the human brain, but functional imaging, a technique that allows measurement of task-related brain activation, provides an opportunity to do so. Furthermore, one must consider that the findings from animals apply almost exclusively to cortical damage, whereas much of the work in humans to date has been performed in patients with deep subcortical infarcts. Nevertheless, both approaches have yielded important results from which a clearer picture of functional cerebral reorganisation is beginning to emerge.

5.2 Functional imaging techniques

The detailed theoretical background to the techniques positron emission tomography (PET) and functional magnetic resonance imaging (fMRI) are beyond the scope of this chapter. In brief however, both techniques rely on the assumption that neuronal activity is closely coupled to a local increase in cerebral blood flow (CBF) secondary to an increase in metabolism. PET relies on mapping the distribution of inert, freely diffusible radioactive tracers deposited in tissue as a function of regional perfusion (rCBF). Functional MRI comprises different methods, but the studies described below use blood oxygen level-dependent (BOLD) imaging techniques. During an increase in neuronal activation there is an increase in local CBF, but only a small proportion of the greater amount of oxygen delivered locally to the tissue is used. There is a resultant net increase in the tissue concentration of oxyhaemoglobin and a net reduction in paramagnetic deoxyhaemoglobin in the local capillary bed and draining venules. The magnetic properties of haemoglobin depend on its level of oxygenation so that this change results in an increase in local tissue derived signal intensity on T2*-weighted MR images.

5.3 Methodological considerations

The study of patients with motor impairment requires careful consideration. Many early studies were performed in fully recovered patients so that comparisons with healthy controls could be made. However, to address the issue of whether differences between stroke patients and controls are related to recovery, patients with a wide range of outcomes must be studied. In this way, correlations between task-related brain activation and outcome can be identified. There are two consequences of this consideration. Firstly, outcome must be characterised in a detailed and appropriate way. Secondly, patients must perform the *same task* during the acquisition of fMRI data so that a meaningful comparison can be made across subjects or scanning sessions. Equality of task may be interpreted in a number of ways. In patients with different abilities a task may be the same in terms of *absolute* or *relative* parameters. For example a simple motor paradigm can be equated in terms of absolute parameters of force and rate of task performance across subjects, or in terms of how effortful the task is. The experimenter is interested in different states of cerebral reorganisation. However depending on paradigm selection, changes in brain activation patterns across subjects may also be attributable to differences in absolute performance parameters (if effort is equated) or differences in effort (if absolute task parameters are equated).

Most studies have used finger tapping as the motor task. This task is problematic as many stroke patients with poor outcome are unable to perform fractionated finger movements adequately. As a result neither effort nor absolute task parameters can be controlled

for. The return of fractionated finger movements represents an excellent outcome and is therefore of clinical interest but this does not mean that it is the best paradigm to use, for the reasons described above. An important concept in experimental design is that it is not possible to scan patients in order to determine the neural correlates of something they cannot do (Price and Friston, 1999). An experimenter must find alternative ways to probe the system of interest. An alternative task is dynamic hand grip which is used in several studies described in this chapter (Ward and Frackowiak, 2003; Ward et al., 2003a,b). Hand grip can be performed by patients with even minimal recovery and its performance correlates well with other measures of upper limb recovery (Heller et al., 1987; Sunderland et al., 1989). In order to control as much as possible for the effort involved in performing a hand grip task subjects (controls and patients) can be set target forces that are a fixed percentage of their own maximum hand grip. This is therefore a task that all can perform. In our series of experiments all patients were able to perform repetitive hand grips at 10%, 20%, 40%, etc. of their own maximum exertable force. The results of these studies pertain to how a damaged motor system is able to perform *this* task. Thus by using a motor task (hand grip) that reflects intrinsic motor recovery more than adaptation (Sunderland et al., 1989) and by controlling for motor effort as much as possible, the results within known motor-related regions are then more likely to reflect cerebral reorganisation rather than change of strategy after focal brain damage. The interpretation of results from all functional imaging studies involving patients with differing abilities needs to take these factors into consideration (Poldrack, 2001).

5.4 Cerebral reorganisation in chronic stroke

Early functional imaging studies were performed in recovered chronic subcortical stroke patients. These patients demonstrated relative overactivations in a number of motor-related brain regions when performing a motor task compared to control subjects.

In particular, overactivations were seen in dorsolateral premotor cortex (PMd), ventrolateral premotor cortex (PMv), supplementary motor area (SMA), cingulate motor areas (CMA), parietal cortex, and insula cortex (Chollet et al., 1991; Weiller et al., 1992, 1993; Cramer et al., 1997; Seitz et al., 1998). Such findings contributed to the notion that recruitment of these brain regions, particularly those in the unaffected hemisphere, might be responsible for recovery. However, in order to make inferences about the mechanisms underlying functional recovery it is necessary to study patients with different degrees of recovery. If one studies patients with a range of late post-stroke outcomes, it appears that those patients with the best outcome have a "normal" activation pattern when compared to normal controls, whereas

those with poorer outcome show excessive activation of the primary and non-primary motor areas in both hemispheres (Ward et al., 2003a). These relative overactivations are often bilateral, involving sensorimotor, premotor, posterior parietal, prefrontal and insular cortices, SMA, CMA, and cerebellum.

When this relationship is explored formally, a significant negative linear correlation is found between the size of brain activation and outcome in a number of brain regions (Fig. 5.1). This result does not initially seem to support the notion that recruitment of these regions facilitates recovery. A key determinant of motor recovery is the integrity of fast direct motor output pathways from primary motor cortex (M1) to spinal cord motor neurons (Heald et al., 1993; Cruz et al., 1999; Pennisi et al., 1999).

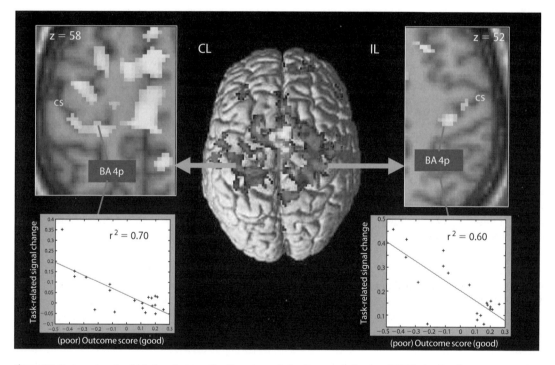

Figure 5.1. Brain regions in which there is a negative (linear) correlation between task-related BOLD signal and outcome score in a group of 20 chronic stroke patients. Results are surface rendered onto a canonical brain shown from above (left hemisphere on the left). The panels represent the same result displayed on axial slices through a canonical T_1-weighted image. The plots represent task-related signal change versus outcome score for the peak voxel in BA 4p, contralesional (CL) on the left and ipsilesional (IL) on the right. Each "+" represents one patient. All voxels are significant at $P < 0.05$, corrected for multiple comparisons across whole brain. cs: central sulcus.

Thus it is likely that those patients with poorer outcome have greater disruption to this cortico-motoneuronal (CMN) pathway. The work of Strick (1988) and others suggests that in primates at least, the non-primary motor system is organised as a number of neural networks or loops involving pre-motor (both lateral and medial wall), parietal and subcortical regions (see also Chapter 14 of Volume I, p. 12). These motor loops are independent of those involving M1 but crucially they are interconnected at the level of the cortex (Strick, 1988; Dum and Strick, 1991). Furthermore, each has its own direct projection to spinal cord motor neurons. In the face of disruption to the CMN pathway the generation of an output to the musculature requires an increase in signals to spinal cord motor neurons via alternative pathways. The non-primary motor loops described by Strick provide an ideal substrate. The implication is that damage in one of these networks could be compensated for by activity in another, thus explaining the recruitment of regions seen in recovered stroke patients. These projections are unlikely to completely substitute for projections from M1 as they are less numerous and less efficient at exciting spinal cord motor neurons (Maier et al., 2002). Thus patients who rely on these alternative pathways to augment or substitute for CMN pathways are unlikely to fully regain dextrous finger movements. In attempting to reconcile these results with those from early studies it seems likely that patients in many previous studies may not have been fully recovered. Some patients found the finger tapping task more effortful to perform (Chollet et al., 1991) and results in those patients were similar to results in patients with residual motor deficit in a later study (Ward et al., 2003a).

The question of the functional relevance of these additionally recruited regions remains. If one could explain differential recovery in a group of patients with identical anatomical damage by the degree to which certain areas are recruited, that would constitute direct evidence of their functional significance in relation to recovery. Due to the heterogeneous nature of infarcts such a result is very difficult to achieve. An alternative approach is to study the same chronic stroke patients before and after a therapeutical intervention. In chronic stroke patients there should be no change in anatomical connections as a result of treatment, but differences in brain activation seen in relation to improved functional status might suggest that certain regions were causally involved. Increased activity in ipsilesional (IL) PMd has been associated with therapy-induced improvement in both upper limb function (Johansen-Berg et al., 2002a) and gait (Miyai et al., 2003). There is also evidence to suggest that disruption of IL PMd (Fridman et al., 2004) and contralesional (CL) PMd (Johansen-Berg et al., 2002b) by transcranial magnetic stimulation (TMS) impairs performance of a simple motor task in chronic stroke patients but not controls. Fridman et al. (2004) however failed to find any behavioural effect from disruption of CL PMd. It is possible that the patients studied by Johansen-Berg et al. (2002b) had greater impairment, and thus were more reliant on CL PMd, but outcomes were not well characterised in either study so it is difficult to make a comparison.

Thus "alternative" brain regions appear to be recruited after focal damage in those patients with greatest need. In addition, there is evidence that IL PMd takes on an executive motor role, such that task-related BOLD signal increases linearly as a function of hand grip force in chronic stroke patients with significant impairment, but not in good recoverers or in controls. Thus it is unlikely that the response to focal injury involves the simple substitution of one cortical region for another, as nodes within a remaining motor network may take on new roles, that is there is true lesion-induced reprogramming in the human central nervous system.

The studies discussed so far have been on chronic stroke patients. It appears that the relationship between size of brain activation and outcome in the late post-stroke phase holds true for patients in the early post-stroke phase also, at least when considering the primary and non-primary motor regions discussed above (Ward et al., 2004). Thus patients with greater initial deficit recruited more of the primary and non-primary motor network during hand grip. This result suggests that rather than slowly being recruited over time, brain regions in non-primary motor loops can participate in motor action very early after stroke in those patients that have the greatest need. Such rapid cerebral reorganisation can also be seen in normal people after repetitive TMS (rTMS) to the hand area of M1, which reduces M1 cortical excitability without altering task performance. Lee et al. (2003) demonstrated an immediate increase in recruitment of ipsilateral PMd following rTMS to M1 suggesting that this compensation allowed maintenance of task performance.

In other brain regions there is an interaction between outcome and time after stroke. In CL middle intraparietal sulcus, CL cerebellum, and IL rostral premotor cortex there is a negative correlation between size of activation and outcome in the early but not late post-stroke phase (Fig. 5.2) (Ward et al., 2004). In other words patients with poorer outcome scores recruit these areas only in the early and not in the late post-stroke phase suggesting that those with greater deficit engage attentional networks more in the early compared to late post-stroke phase. Attention may no longer be a useful tool for optimising motor performance in the late post-stroke phase. Alternatively, increasing the degree to which a motor task is attended to by chronic stroke patients might facilitate performance by enhancing detection of discrepancies between predicted and actual consequences of any action. These findings need to be explored further, but in those patients with most to gain from rehabilitation, different therapeutical approaches may be required at different stages after stroke.

The role of CL (ipsilateral to the affected hand) M1 in recovery of motor function after stroke remains controversial. Anatomical studies suggest that both direct (corticospinal) and indirect (corticoreticulospinal) pathways from ipsilateral M1 end in projections to axial and proximal stabilising muscles rather than hand muscles (Brinkman and Kuypers, 1973; Carr et al., 1994). However, repetitive TMS to

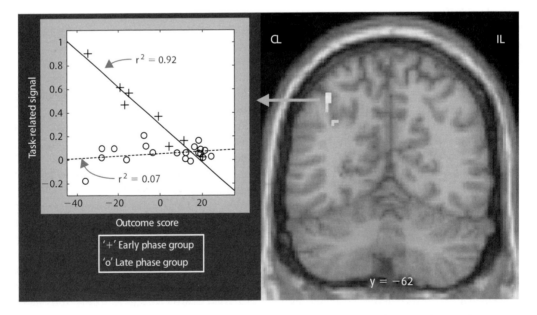

Figure 5.2. A plot of task-related signal change in posterior contralesional (CL) intraparietal sulcus versus outcome/recovery score for a group of early phase patients (10–14 days post stroke) and a group of late phase stroke patients (over 3 months post stroke). The peak voxel in intraparietal sulcus is shown on canonical coronal T_1-weighted brain slice ($P < 0.05$, corrected for multiple comparisons across whole brain).

M1 results in errors in both complex and simple motor tasks with the ipsilateral hand (Chen et al., 1997) suggesting that ipsilateral M1 may play a role in planning and organisation of normal hand movement. CL M1 recruitment not present in normal controls has been described in some chronic stroke patients (see Calautti and Baron, 2003, for review), but its contribution to functional recovery remains controversial. A negative correlation between size of activation and outcome, similar to that described in non-primary motor regions, has been demonstrated for CL posterior M1 (Brodmann area, BA 4p) but not anterior M1 (BA 4a) (Ward et al., 2003a). Studies using TMS to disrupt local cortical function have failed to find any functional significance of increased CL M1 activation after stroke (Johansen-Berg et al., 2002b; Werhahn et al., 2003). TMS to the motor hot spot for hand muscles (corresponding to M1) may affect predominantly BA 4a, rather than BA 4p, and so it remains plausible that parts of CL M1 can generate a motor output to an affected hand in patients with a significant deficit, in whom a dependency on alternative motor projections has developed.

For chronic stroke patients with preserved IL M1 shifts in the peak IL sensorimotor activations have been found by comparison to control subjects (Weiller et al., 1993; Pineiro et al., 2001). As with other motor regions, this recruitment depends on the final outcome of the patient. A negative correlation between size of brain activation and outcome is seen in IL BA 4p and in BA 4a, ventral to the peak hand region of M1 (Ward et al., 2003a). Overall, these data suggest that there is a certain amount of remapping of hand representation in M1, even though undamaged, which may result from functionally relevant changes in both its afferent and efferent connections. Changes in somatotopical representation in non-primary motor regions might result in stronger connections with different (e.g. more ventral or caudal) regions of M1 in order to facilitate access to intact portions of the direct corticospinal pathway. Shifts in somatotopic representation in non-primary motor regions might also facilitate recruitment of surviving ischaemia-resistant small diameter myelinated

corticospinal fibres, such as those arising from premotor cortex, to compensate for loss of large diameter fibres. In our studies, parts of SMA, CMA, and PMd that were outside regions normally activated by the task in the control group, were recruited by chronic patients with poorer outcome (Ward et al., 2003a). Thus shifts in the hand representation in M1 as well as in non-primary motor regions occurred primarily in patients with greatest deficit and presumably with the most significant damage to CMN pathways. Support for lesion-induced changes in connectivity comes from the observation that rTMS to M1 leads to the stimulated part of M1 becoming less responsive to input from PMd and SMA, as well as increased coupling between an inferomedial portion of M1 and anterior motor areas (Lee et al., 2003).

5.5 The evolution of cerebral reorganisation after stroke

It appears that in the chronic setting a damaged brain will utilise those remaining structures and networks that can generate some form of motor signal to spinal cord motor neurons, and that in addition some areas such as PMd take on a new role in motor performance. What such studies do not tell us is how this reorganised state evolved from the time of infarction. Two early longitudinal studies with early and late time points demonstrated initial task-related overactivations in motor-related brain regions followed by a reduction over time in patients said to recover fully (Marshall et al., 2000; Calautti et al., 2001). Feydy and co-workers (2002), found no relationship between longitudinal changes and recovery scores and another study found no correlates of functional improvement outside the ipsilateral (CL) cerebellum, in which increases in task-related activation were seen with recovery (Small et al., 2002). A more detailed longitudinal fMRI study of patients with infarcts not involving M1 indicated an initial overactivation in many primary and non-primary motor regions that was more extensive in those with greatest clinical deficit (Ward et al., 2003b). The subsequent longitudinal changes were predictably different in each patient but there were changes common to all. After early overactivation, a negative correlation between size of activation and recovery scores was observed in all patients throughout IL M1, and in inferior CL M1, as well as in anterior and posterior PMd, bilaterally (BA 6 and BA 8), CL PMv, and IL SMA-proper, pre-SMA, prefrontal cortex (superior frontal sulcus), and caudal cingulate sulcus (Fig. 5.3). A positive correlation between size of activation and recovery across sessions was seen in some brain regions in four patients (including IL M1 in one patient), but there were no consistent increases in a group analysis (Ward et al., 2003b).

These longitudinal recovery-related changes are reminiscent of those seen during motor learning experiments in normal people. One model of motor learning suggests that during early motor learning movements are encoded in terms of spatial coordinates, a process requiring high levels of attention (Hikosaka et al., 2002). Encoding is performed within a frontoparietal network and in parts of the basal ganglia and cerebellum. Once learning has occurred and a task has become automatic, movement is encoded in terms of a kinematic system of joints, muscles, limb trajectories, etc., by a network involving primary motor cortex, and parts of the basal ganglia and cerebellum that are different from those involved in early learning (Hikosaka et al., 2002). Interaction between these parallel systems and the transfer of reliance from one to the other, occurs not only in cerebellum and basal ganglia but also via intracortical connections involving particularly premotor cortex and pre-SMA (Hikosaka et al., 1999, 2002). An important aspect of any motor learning model is the generation of an error signal. Attempted movements by hemiparetic patients will result in significant discrepancies between predicted and actual performance. The error signals thus generated in normal subjects are used by the cerebellum to optimise subsequent sensorimotor accuracy (Blakemore et al., 2001). Thus the longitudinal recovery-related changes described above are in part similar to those seen when normal subjects learn a motor sequence. The need to re-learn simple motor

tasks after stroke is likely to engage such a mechanism, but the degree to which this is successful will depend on the degree of overall damage to the motor network. The role of error signal generation in a damaged motor system is clearly of interest, particularly as it may diminish with chronicity of impairment (Ward et al., in press Ward et al 2004). These important issues remain to be explored, and may have significant implications for rehabilitative interventions.

In summary, the goal of cerebral reorganisation after focal damage to the motor system appears to be to re-establish a connection between IL M1 and spinal cord motor neurons via fast direct CMN pathways if possible. This allows recovery of fractionated finger movements. In the face of partial CMN damage, one potential strategy is to re-map the somatotopic representations in M1 and in those parts of the motor system that project to M1. If CMN pathways are completely lost then parallel motor loops become useful only for their projections to spinal cord, not by virtue of their projections to M1. Studies in adults with damage to the entire middle cerebral artery territory are scarce. However, data from young adults who suffer unilateral brain damage in the perinatal period suggest that the ipsilateral hemisphere becomes the main source of motor output in these circumstances (Cao et al., 1998).

A process such as cerebral reorganisation during motor learning occurs in the normal brain and is a reflection of changes occurring at synaptic and systems levels. The degree to which such "normal processes" are successfully employed in the recovery process will depend on a number of variables, not least the precise amount and site of anatomical damage caused by an infarct and the amount of retraining available to the patient. However, the evidence from animal models suggests that the lesioned brain has an increased capacity for plastic change, at least early after damage. For example, widespread areas of cortical hyperexcitability appear immediately after cerebral infarction in animal brains, changes which subside over subsequent months (Buchkremer-Ratzmann et al., 1996). These changes occur in regions structurally connected to the lesion in both hemispheres as a consequence of

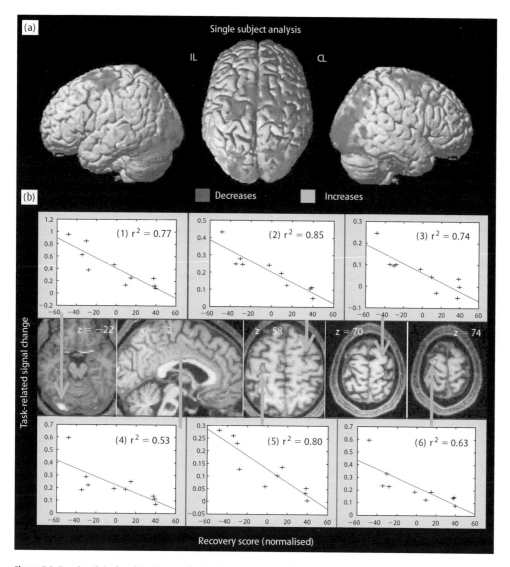

Figure 5.3. Results of single subject longitudinal analysis examining for linear changes in task-related brain activations over sessions as a function of recovery. The patient suffered from a left sided pontine infarct resulting in right hemiparesis. (a) Results are surface rendered onto a canonical brain; red areas represent recovery-related decreases in task-related activation across sessions, and green areas represent the equivalent recovery related increases. All voxels are significant at $P < 0.001$ (uncorrected for multiple comparisons) for display purposes. The brain is shown (from left to right) from the left ipsilesional (IL) side, from above (left hemisphere on the left), and from the right contralesional (CL). (b) Results are displayed on patients own normalised T_1-weighted anatomical images (voxels significant at $P < 0.05$, corrected for multiple comparisons across the whole brain), with corresponding plots of size of effect against overall recovery score (normalised), for selected brain regions. Coordinates of peak voxel in each region are followed by the correlation coefficient and the associated P value: (1) ipsilesional (IL) cerebellum ($x = -26, y = -84, z = -22$) ($r^2 = 0.77, P < 0.01$), (2) contralesional (CL) PMd ($x = 38, y = 0, z = 58$) ($r^2 = 0.85, P < 0.01$), (3) contralesional (CL) M1 ($x = 28$, $y = -14, z = 70$) ($r^2 = 0.74, P < 0.01$), (4) ipsilesional (IL) SMA ($x = -2, y = -2, z = 60$) ($r^2 = 0.53, P = 0.02$), (5) ipsilesional (IL) M1 ($x = -30, y = -14, z = 58$) ($r^2 = 0.80, P < 0.01$), (6) contralesional (CL) PMd ($x = -18, y = -10, z = 74$) ($r^2 = 0.63, P = 0.01$) (from Ward et al. *Brain*, 2003; **126**: 2476–2496, by permission of Oxford University Press).

downregulation of the α1-gamma-aminobutyric acid (GABA) receptor subunit and a decrease in GABAergic inhibition (Neumann-Haefelin et al., 1998) (see Chapter 14 of Volume I, pp. 18–21 for further discussion of these phenomena). This would be of particular interest to clinicians as it is easier to induce long-term potentiation (LTP) in hyperexcitable cortex, that is the cortex is more responsive to afferent input. In humans, acute limb deafferentation leads to reduced levels of GABA within minutes (Levy et al., 2002). It is tempting to think that the same thing may happen in areas of partially disconnected cortex after stroke. There is evidence of hyperexcitability in the CL motor cortex after both cortical and subcortical stroke in humans with at least moderate recovery (Bütefisch et al., 2003). Such hyperexcitability decreases with time after infarction, in keeping with data from animals (Buchkremer-Ratzmann et al., 1996; Witte, 1998; Shimizu et al., 2002). This window of opportunity, if therapeutically useful, may last only for a limited time.

One final caveat should be mentioned. After injury-induced reorganisation of the brain the capacity for subsequent adaptive change is reduced (Kolb et al., 1998). Adaptive changes in older brains have been described (Ward and Frackowiak, 2003) and these may themselves limit the capacity for further reorganisation after injury in older patients. This may have implications for what can be expected from therapy designed to promote cerebral reorganisation after stroke in older subjects.

Cerebral reorganisation undoubtedly contributes to functional recovery after stroke, but it is clear that a more detailed understanding of the natural history of these processes is required, together with the factors that influence them, before they can be utilised to rationalise therapeutical strategies in individual patients or groups.

5.6 Therapeutic interventions

A number of studies have appeared recently that have attempted to evaluate therapeutically driven change with functional imaging techniques (Pariente et al., 2001; Carey et al., 2002; Schaechter et al., 2002; Johansen-Berg et al., 2002a; Jang et al., 2003; Miyai et al., 2003). Each study uses functional imaging before and after a particular therapeutical intervention. In general these studies have shown increased task-related activation in affected hemispheres (e.g. in PMd) and reduced activation in unaffected hemispheres after a period of treatment. Although of interest as discussed earlier in this chapter, these are likely to represent the consequences of functional improvement rather than the mechanism. However, this approach has limitations. Functional imaging is unlikely to be useful purely as a marker of clinical improvement, something that is measurable with simple outcome scores. Functional imaging will become a useful marker of the *potential* for change in damaged brain. Furthermore, it is to be hoped that the potential of different therapeutical interventions can be assessed, both in groups and individuals. Functional imaging, in conjunction with other techniques such as TMS, electro-encephalography (EEG), and magneto-EEG, has the potential to achieve these aims.

5.7 Other imaging modalities

The interpretation of functional imaging data from patients with brain lesions will be influenced by the site and extent of lesions. Two separate imaging techniques can provide accurate objective anatomical data that can be used to address hypotheses about the structure–function relationships of surviving brain regions. Voxel-based morphometry (VBM) and diffusion tensor imaging (DTI) are both MRI-dependent techniques.

VBM is used to characterise grey and white matter differences in structural MRI scans (Ashburner and Friston, 2000) thus providing objective anatomical data about which regions of the brain have been damaged. A number of studies have validated VBM techniques against more traditional region of interest volumetric approaches (Good et al., 2002; Maguire et al., 2003). In stroke patients VBM has been used to identify structural changes in peri-lesional tissue and at distant sites compared to controls (Schormann and Kraemer, 2003). It is this ability to search for structural differences across the whole brain in an objective, automated and therefore in a reproducible manner that makes VBM such a valuable technique.

DTI is a technique that provides quantitative information about the integrity and orientation of white matter fibre tracts in the brain. It is based on the principle that water diffuses preferentially along nerve axons rather than across nerve bundles and that the direction of water diffusion within a brain voxel (typically $2–3 \, mm^3$) can be assessed and quantified. This parameter is used to test the direction of most coherent diffusion in all voxels and therefore the likelihood of connection to a specified starting point (a technique termed tractography) (Parker et al., 2002). Construction of statistical maps of the likelihood of connections between cortical areas, deep nuclei, and motor output pathways is then possible (Behrens et al., 2003; Ciccarelli et al., 2003; Guye et al., 2003). The technique is ideal for examination of the structural integrity of the corticospinal tract in health and disease (Kunimatsu et al., 2003; Toosy et al., 2003; Sach et al., 2004).

These precise and objective measurements of anatomical damage will become invaluable for the interpretation of functional imaging data.

ACKNOWLEDGEMENTS

N.S.W. and R.S.J.F. are supported by The Wellcome Trust. We would like to thank Peter Aston and Eric Featherstone (Wellcome Department of Imaging Neuroscience) for the design and programming involved in creating the hand grip manipulandum and the staff of the Acute Brain Injury Unit and Neurorehabilitation Unit at the National Hospital for Neurology and Neurosurgery, Queen Square, London, for their assistance.

REFERENCES

Ashburner, J. and Friston, K.J. (2000). Voxel-based morphometry – the methods. *Neuroimage*, **11**, 805–821.

Behrens, T.E., Johansen-Berg, H., Woolrich, M.W., Smith, S.M., Wheeler-Kingshott, C.A., Boulby, P.A., Barker, G.J., Sillery, E.L., Sheehan, K., Ciccarelli, O., Thompson, A.J., Brady, J.M. and Matthews, P.M. (2003). Non-invasive mapping of connections between human thalamus and cortex using diffusion imaging. *Nat Neurosci*, **6**, 750–757.

Blakemore, S.J., Frith, C.D. and Wolpert, D.M. (2001). The cerebellum is involved in predicting the sensory consequences of action. *NeuroReport*, **12**, 1879–1884.

Brinkman, J. and Kuypers, H.G. (1973). Cerebral control of contralateral and ipsilateral arm, hand and finger movements in the split-brain rhesus monkey. *Brain*, **96**, 653–674.

Buchkremer-Ratzmann, I., August, M., Hagemann, G. and Witte, O.W. (1996). Electrophysiological transcortical diaschisis after cortical photothrombosis in rat brain. *Stroke*, **27**, 1105–1109.

Bury, S.D. and Jones, T.A. (2002). Unilateral sensorimotor cortex lesions in adult rats facilitate motor skill learning with the unaffected forelimb and training-induced dendritic structural plasticity in the motor cortex. *J Neurosci*, **22**, 8597–8606.

Bütefisch, C.M., Netz, J., Wessling, M., Seitz, R.J. and Homberg, V. (2003). Remote changes in cortical excitability after stroke. *Brain*, **126**, 470–481.

Calautti, C. and Baron, J.C. (2003). Functional neuroimaging studies of motor recovery after stroke in adults: a review. *Stroke*, **34**, 1553–1566.

Calautti, C., Leroy, F., Guincestre, J.Y. and Baron, J.C. (2001). Dynamics of motor network overactivation after striato capsular stroke: a longitudinal PET study using a fixed-performance paradigm. *Stroke*, **32**, 2534–2542.

Cao, Y., D'Olhaberriague, L., Vikingstad, E.M., Levine, S.R. and Welch, K.M. (1998). Pilot study of functional MRI to assess cerebral activation of motor function after poststroke hemiparesis. *Stroke*, **29**, 112–122.

Carey, J.R., Kimberley, T.J., Lewis, S.M., Auerbach, E.J., Dorsey, L., Rundquist, P. and Ugurbil, K. (2002). Analysis of fMRI and finger tracking training in subjects with chronic stroke. *Brain*, **125**, 773–788.

Carr, L.J., Harrison, L.M. and Stephens, J.A. (1994). Evidence for bilateral innervation of certain homologous motoneurone pools in man. *J Physiol*, **475**, 217–227.

Chen, R., Gerloff, C., Hallett, M. and Cohen, L.G. (1997). Involvement of the ipsilateral motor cortex in finger movements of different complexities. *Ann Neurol*, **41**, 247–254.

Chollet, F., DiPiero, V., Wise, R.J., Brooks, D.J., Dolan, R.J. and Frackowiak, R.S. (1991). The functional anatomy of motor recovery after stroke in humans: a study with positron emission tomography. *Ann Neurol*, **29**, 63–71.

Ciccarelli, O., Toosy, A.T., Parker, G.J., Wheeler-Kingshott, C.A., Barker, G.J., Miller, D.H. and Thompson, A.J. (2003). Diffusion tractography based group mapping of major white-matter pathways in the human brain, *Neuroimage*, **19**, 1545–1555.

Cramer, S.C., Nelles, G., Benson, R.R., Kaplan, J.D., Parker, R.A., Kwong, K.K., Kennedy, D.N., Finklestein, S.P. and Rosen, B.R. (1997). A functional MRI study of subjects recovered from hemiparetic stroke. *Stroke*, **28**, 2518–2527.

Cruz, M.A., Tejada, J. and Diez, T.E. (1999). Motor hand recovery after stroke. Prognostic yield of early transcranial magnetic stimulation. *Electromyogr Clin Neurophysiol*, **39**, 405–410.

Dum, R.P. and Strick, P.L. (1991). The origin of corticospinal projections from the premotor areas in the frontal lobe. *J Neurosci*, **11**, 667–689.

Feeney, D.M. (1997). From laboratory to clinic: noradrenergic enhancement of physical therapy for stroke or trauma patients. *Adv Neurol*, **73**, 383–394.

Feydy, A., Carlier, R., Roby-Brami, A., Bussel, B., Cazalis, F., Pierot, L., Burnod, Y. and Maier, M.A. (2002). Longitudinal study of motor recovery after stroke: recruitment and focusing of brain activation. *Stroke*, **33**, 1610–1617.

Fridman, E.A., Hanakawa, T., Chung, M., Hummel, F., Leiguarda, R.C. and Cohen, L.G. (2004). Reorganization of the human ipsilesional premotor cortex after stroke. *Brain*, Brain Advanced Access Published January 28, 2004: 0.1093/brain/awh 082.

Good, C.D., Scahill, R.I., Fox, N.C., Ashburner, J., Friston, K.J., Chan, D., Crum, W.R., Rossor, M.N. and Frackowiak, R.S. (2002). Automatic differentiation of anatomical patterns in the human brain: validation with studies of degenerative dementias. *Neuroimage*, **17**, 29–46.

Guye, M., Parker, G.J., Symms, M., Boulby, P., Wheeler-Kingshott, C.A., Salek-Haddadi, A., Barker, G.J. and Duncan, J.S. (2003). Combined functional MRI and tractography to demonstrate the connectivity of the human primary motor cortex in vivo. *Neuroimage*, **19**, 1349–1360.

Heald, A., Bates, D., Cartlidge, N.E., French, J.M. and Miller, S. (1993). Longitudinal study of central motor conduction time following stroke. 2. Central motor conduction measured within 72 h after stroke as a predictor of functional outcome at 12 months. *Brain*, **116**, 1371–1385.

Heller, A., Wade, D.T., Wood, V.A., Sunderland, A., Hewer, R.L. and Ward, E. (1987). Arm function after stroke: measurement and recovery over the first three months. *J Neurol Neurosurg Psychiatr*, **50**, 714–719.

Hikosaka, O., Nakahara, H., Rand, M.K., Sakai, K., Lu, X., Nakamura, K., Miyachi, S. and Doya, K. (1999). Parallel neural networks for learning sequential procedures. *Trend Neurosci*, **22**, 464–471.

Hikosaka, O., Nakamura, K., Sakai, K. and Nakahara, H. (2002). Central mechanisms of motor skill learning. *Curr Opin Neurobiol*, **12**, 217–222.

Jang, S.H., Kim, Y.H., Cho, S.H., Lee, J.H., Park, J.W. and Kwon, Y.H. (2003). Cortical reorganization induced by task-oriented training in chronic hemiplegic stroke patients. *NeuroReport*, **14**, 137–141.

Johansen-Berg, H., Dawes, H., Guy, C., Smith, S.M., Wade, D.T. and Matthews, P.M. (2002a). Correlation between motor improvements and altered fMRI activity after rehabilitative therapy. *Brain*, **125**, 2731–2742.

Johansen-Berg, H., Rushworth, M.F., Bogdanovic, M.D., Kischka, U., Wimalaratna, S. and Matthews, P.M. (2002b). The role of ipsilateral premotor cortex in hand movement after stroke. *Proc Natl Acad Sci USA*, **99**, 14518–14523.

Kolb, B., Forgie, M., Gibb, R., Gorny, G. and Rowntree, S. (1998). Age, experience and the changing brain. *Neurosci Biobehav Rev*, **22**, 143–159.

Kunimatsu, A., Aoki, S., Masutani, Y., Abe, O., Mori, H. and Ohtomo, K. (2003). Three-dimensional white matter tractography by diffusion tensor imaging in ischaemic stroke involving the corticospinal tract. *Neuroradiology*, **45**, 532–535.

Lee, L., Siebner, H.R., Rowe, J.B., Rizzo, V., Rothwell, J.C., Frackowiak, R.S. and Friston, K.J. (2003). Acute remapping within the motor system induced by low-frequency repetitive transcranial magnetic stimulation. *J Neurosci*, **23**, 5308–5318.

Levy, L.M., Ziemann, U., Chen, R. and Cohen, L.G. (2002). Rapid modulation of GABA in sensorimotor cortex induced by acute deafferentation. *Ann Neurol*, **52**, 755–761.

Maguire, E.A., Spiers, H.J., Good, C.D., Hartley, T., Frackowiak, R.S. and Burgess, N. (2003). Navigation expertise and the human hippocampus: a structural brain imaging analysis. *Hippocampus*, **13**, 250–259.

Maier, M.A., Armand, J., Kirkwood, P.A., Yang, H.W., Davis, J.N. and Lemon, R.N. (2002). Differences in the corticospinal projection from primary motor cortex and supplementary motor area to macaque upper limb motoneurons: an anatomical and electrophysiological study. *Cereb Cortex*, **12**, 281–296.

Marshall, R.S., Perera, G.M., Lazar, R.M., Krakauer, J.W., Constantine, R.C. and DeLaPaz, R.L. (2000). Evolution of cortical activation during recovery from corticospinal tract infarction. *Stroke*, **31**, 656–661.

Miyai, I., Yagura, H., Hatakenaka, M., Oda, I., Konishi, I. and Kubota, K. (2003). Longitudinal optical imaging study for locomotor recovery after stroke. *Stroke*, **34**, 2866–2870.

Neumann-Haefelin, T., Staiger, J.F., Redecker, C., Zilles, K., Fritschy, J.M., Mohler, H. and Witte, O.W. (1998).

Immunohistochemical evidence for dysregulation of the GABAergic system ipsilateral to photochemically induced cortical infarcts in rats. *Neuroscience*, **87**, 871–879.

Nudo, R.J., Wise, B.M., SiFuentes, F. and Milliken, G.W. (1996). Neural substrates for the effects of rehabilitative training on motor recovery after ischemic infarct. *Science*, **272**, 1791–1794.

Pariente, J., Loubinoux, I., Carel, C., Albucher, J.F., Leger, A., Manelfe, C., Rascol, O. and Chollet, F. (2001). Fluoxetine modulates motor performance and cerebral activation of patients recovering from stroke. *Ann Neurol*, **50**, 718–729.

Parker, G.J., Wheeler-Kingshott, C.A. and Barker, G.J. (2002). Estimating distributed anatomical connectivity using fast marching methods and diffusion tensor imaging. *IEEE T Med Imaging*, **21**, 505–512.

Pennisi, G., Rapisarda, G., Bella, R., Calabrese, V., Maertens, D.N. and Delwaide, P.J. (1999). Absence of response to early transcranial magnetic stimulation in ischemic stroke patients: prognostic value for hand motor recovery. *Stroke*, **30**, 2666–2670.

Pineiro, R., Pendlebury, S., Johansen-Berg, H. and Matthews, P.M. (2001). Functional MRI detects posterior shifts in primary sensorimotor cortex activation after stroke: evidence of local adaptive reorganization? *Stroke*, **32**, 1134–1139.

Poldrack, R.A. (2001). Imaging brain plasticity: conceptual and methodological issues – a theoretical review. *Neuroimage*, **12**, 1–13.

Price, C.J. and Friston, K.J. (1999). Scanning patients with tasks they can perform. *Hum Brain Mapp*, **8**, 102–108.

Sach, M., Winkler, G., Glauche, V., Liepert, J., Heimbach, B., Koch, M.A., Buchel, C. and Weiller, C. (2004). Diffusion tensor MRI of early upper motor neuron involvement in amyotrophic lateral sclerosis. *Brain*, **127**, 340–350.

Schaechter, J.D., Kraft, E., Hilliard, T.S., Dijkhuizen, R.M., Benner, T., Finklestein, S.P., Rosen, B.R. and Cramer, S.C. (2002). Motor recovery and cortical reorganization after constraint-induced movement therapy in stroke patients: a preliminary study. *Neurorehabil Neural Repair*, **16**, 326–338.

Schallert, T., Leasure, J.L. and Kolb, B. (2000). Experience-associated structural events, subependymal cellular proliferative activity, and functional recovery after injury to the central nervous system. *J Cereb Blood Flow Metab*, **20**, 1513–1528.

Schormann, T. and Kraemer, M. (2003). Voxel-guided morphometry (VGM) and application to stroke. *IEEE T Med Imaging*, **22**, 62–74.

Seitz, R.J., Hoflich, P., Binkofski, F., Tellmann, L., Herzog, H. and Freund, H.J. (1998). Role of the premotor cortex in recovery from middle cerebral artery infarction. *Arch Neurol*, **55**, 1081–1088.

Shimizu, T., Hosaki, A., Hino, T., Sato, M., Komori, T., Hirai, S. and Rossini, P.M. (2002). Motor cortical disinhibition in the unaffected hemisphere after unilateral cortical stroke. *Brain*, **125**, 1896–1907.

Small, S.L., Hlustik, P., Noll, D.C., Genovese, C. and Solodkin, A. (2002). Cerebellar hemispheric activation ipsilateral to the paretic hand correlates with functional recovery after stroke. *Brain*, **125**, 1544–1557.

Strick, P.L. (1988). Anatomical organization of multiple motor areas in the frontal lobe: implications for recovery of function. *Adv Neurol*, **47**, 293–312.

Sunderland, A., Tinson, D., Bradley, L. and Hewer, R.L. (1989). Arm function after stroke. An evaluation of grip strength as a measure of recovery and a prognostic indicator. *J Neurol Neurosurg Psychiatr*, **52**, 1267–1272.

Toosy, A.T., Werring, D.J., Orrell, R.W., Howard, R.S., King, M.D., Barker, G.J., Miller, D.H. and Thompson, A.J. (2003). Diffusion tensor imaging detects corticospinal tract involvement at multiple levels in amyotrophic lateral sclerosis. *J Neurol Neurosurg Psychiatr*, **74**, 1250–1257.

Twitchell, T.E. (1951). The restoration of motor function following hemiplegia in man. *Brain*, **74**, 443–480.

Ward, N.S. and Frackowiak, R.S.J. (2003). Age-related changes in the neural correlates of motor performance. *Brain*, **126**, 873–888.

Ward, N.S., Brown, M.M., Thompson, A.J. and Frackowiak, R.S.J. (2003a). Neural correlates of outcome after stroke: a cross-sectional fMRI study. *Brain*, **126**, 1430–1448.

Ward, N.S., Brown, M.M., Thompson, A.J. and Frackowiak, R.S.J. (2003b). Neural correlates of motor recovery after stroke: a longitudinal fMRI study. *Brain*, **126**, 2476–2496.

Ward N.S., Brown, M.M., Thompson, A.J. and Frackowiak, R.S.J. (2004). The influence of time after stroke on brain activations during a motor task. *Ann Neurol*, **55**, 829–834.

Weiller, C., Chollet, F., Friston, K.J., Wise, R.J. and Frackowiak, R.S. (1992). Functional reorganization of the brain in recovery from striatocapsular infarction in man. *Ann Neurol*, **31**, 463–472.

Weiller, C., Ramsay, S.C., Wise, R.J., Friston, K.J. and Frackowiak, R.S. (1993). Individual patterns of functional reorganization in the human cerebral cortex after capsular infarction. *Ann Neurol*, **33**, 181–189.

Werhahn, K.J., Conforto, A.B., Kadom, N., Hallett, M. and Cohen, L.G. (2003). Contribution of the ipsilateral motor cortex to recovery after chronic stroke. *Ann Neurol*, **54**, 464–472.

Witte, O.W. (1998). Lesion-induced plasticity as a potential mechanism for recovery and rehabilitative training. *Curr Opin Neurol*, **11**, 655–662.

Therapeutic technology

CONTENTS

Cell transplantation therapy for Parkinson's disease

Brian J. Snyder[1] and C. Warren Olanow[2]

Departments of [1]Neurosurgery and [2]Neurology, Mount Sinai School of Medicine, New York, NY, USA

6.1 Introduction

Parkinson's disease (PD) is an age-related progressive neurodegenerative disorder that affects approximately 1–2% of the population (see Volume II, Chapter 35). It is characterized by bradykinesia, rigidity, postural instability and tremor (Lang and Lozano, 1998; Olanow et al., 2001). Pathologically the hallmark of PD is degeneration of the substantia nigra pars compacta (SNc) with the loss of midbrain dopaminergic neurons combined with the presence of intraneuronal inclusion (Lewy) bodies. Importantly, degeneration also occurs in non-dopaminergic regions including epinephrine neurons of the locus coeruleus, serotonin neurons of the dorsal raphe, cholinergic neurons of the nucleus basalis of Meynert, and nerve cells in the dorsal motor nucleus of the vagus, the pedunculopontine nucleus, and peripheral autonomic system. Despite the involvement of multiple brain regions and multiple transmitter systems, treatment of PD is primarily based on a dopamine replacement strategy. Levodopa is the most widely employed and most effective symptomatic agent. It is converted to dopamine within the brain by an aromatic acid decarboxylase (AADC). Treatment with levodopa is extremely effective in the early stages of the disease, however, chronic levodopa treatment is associated with the development of motor complications (motor fluctuations and dyskinesias) which affect as many as 80% of patients after 5–10 years of treatment (Marsden and Parkes, 1976; Ahlskog and Muenter, 2001; Olanow,

2004). Motor complications can be an important source of disability for many patients who cycle between "on" periods in which they respond to levodopa but have complicating dyskinesia, and "off" periods in which they do not respond to the drug and suffer features of parkinsonism. Dopamine agonists are associated with reduced motor complications, but patients eventually require levodopa treatment with the risk of motor complications (Olanow, 2003). Deep brain stimulation (DBS) of the subthalamic nucleus (STN) or globus pallidus pars interna (GPi) is now widely used to reduce the incidence and severity of levodopa-induced dyskinesias, but this treatment is associated with side-effects related to the surgery, the implantation system and stimulation (2001). PD is also associated with features that do not respond to levodopa or other available treatments. These include freezing of gait, postural instability, dysphagia, speech difficulties, sleep disturbances, autonomic impairment (orthostatic hypotension and gastrointestinal, urinary and sexual dysfunction), depression, and dementia, which likely reflect degeneration of non-dopaminergic neurons (Lang and Lozano, 1998; Olanow et al., 2001). Finally, the disease continues to progress despite levodopa treatment. Indeed, there is a theoretical concern that exogenous administration of levodopa may be toxic to dopamine neurons based on its oxidative metabolism and its capacity to damage dopamine neurons in tissue culture. While the drug has not been shown to be toxic in the *in vivo* experiments (Olanow et al., 2004), the imaging component of the recently completed

ELLDOPA study noted a faster rate of decline in an imaging biomarker of the nigrostriatal system in levodopa compared to placebo-treated patients consistent with a toxic effect of levodopa (Fahn et al., 2004).

It is thus clear that PD patients can suffer intolerable disability despite currently available therapies, and a treatment that slows disease progression and/or restores function is an urgent priority. At present, no treatment intervention has been demonstrated to provide such an effect in PD. Much attention has focused on transplantation strategies as a treatment option because of the potential of transplanted dopamine nerve cells to replace degenerating dopamine neurons. While transplantation of dopaminergic cells may not address all of the problems in PD, dopamine cell loss is primarily responsible for the motor features of the disease. Restoration of dopamine in a more physiologic manner might provide the benefits of levodopa with a reduced risk of motor complications. Further, successful transplantation could obviate the need for levodopa therapy and protect against the potentially toxic effects of exogenously administered levodopa. It is also theoretically possible that early and physiologic replacement of dopamine might prevent degeneration in non-dopaminergic regions that occurs secondary to dopamine loss (Rodriguez et al., 1998).

6.2 Early transplant studies

Studies in the late 1970s first reported that transplantation of fetal ventral mesencephalic tissue into the striatum could improve motor function in the 6-hydroxy dopamine (6-OHDA) lesioned rat model of PD (Bjorklund and Stenevi, 1971; Perlow et al., 1979). Autopsy studies in these animals showed that transplantation was associated with significant increases in striatal tyrosine hydroxylase (TH) immunoreactive staining and dopamine levels (Nikkhah et al., 1994). Motor improvement in this model was proportional to the number of transplanted fetal ventral mesencephalic cells (Brundin et al., 1986). Transplantation of dopamine neurons into the SNc failed to produce similar benefits unless axons extended to the

striatum, illustrating the importance of striatal dopamine innervation for motor function (Dunnett et al., 1983; Collier et al., 2002). Implanted cells have been shown to manufacture and release dopamine, to form normal appearing synapses, to have normal electrical firing patterns, and to be capable of autoregulation (Wuerthele et al., 1981; Schmidt et al., 1982; Brundin et al., 1988). The specificity of the transplant procedure is illustrated by the observation that benefits are not detected if the right tissue (fetal mesencephalon) is implanted into the wrong part of the brain (cerebellum), or if the wrong tissue (non-dopaminergic cells) is implanted into the right place (striatum) (Dunnett et al., 1988). Importantly, numerous studies have demonstrated motor benefits following transplantation of fetal nigral dopamine cells into the striatum of both the 6-OHDA lesioned rodent and the MPTP-lesioned primate (Dunnett and Annett, 1991; Olanow et al., 1996).

6.3 Open label human trials

The first studies of transplantation in humans utilized autologous adrenomedullary cells implanted into the caudate nucleus. Dramatic benefits were reported in a small group of patients (Madrazo et al., 1987), but these were not confirmed in subsequent studies (Lindvall et al., 1987; Goetz et al., 1989; Olanow et al., 1990) and few if any surviving cells were detected at autopsy (Peterson et al., 1989). The procedure was associated with substantial morbidity and this treatment approach has been abandoned.

Transplantation using fetal nigral dopamine cells derived from human ventral mesencephalon provides superior results in the laboratory (Dunnett and Annett, 1991; Olanow et al., 1996). In the clinic, several open label studies reported benefit following fetal nigral transplantation (Lindvall et al., 1990; 1992; Freed et al., 1992; Peschanski et al., 1994; Freeman et al., 1995; Bjorklund et al., 2003). Improvement was observed in a variety of measures of motor function including motor score on the unified Parkinson's disease rating scale (UPDRS) performed in the practically defined off state (approximately 12 h after the last evening dose of levodopa) and in percent on time without dyskinesia based on home diary assessments. Benefits have been reported to be long-lasting (Lindvall et al., 1994; Hauser et al., 1999), and some transplanted patients no longer required levodopa. On the other hand, some patients did not improve following transplant, possibly reflecting differences in patient selection and the transplant variables employed (reviewed in Olanow et al., 1996). Variables that must be considered in developing a transplant protocol include method of tissue storage prior to surgery, donor age (ontogeny studies suggest age 6.5–9 weeks post conception is the optimal time), number of donors implanted (most studies have chosen 1–4 donors per side), site of transplantation (putamen, caudate, or both), type of transplant (cell suspension or solid graft), and the use of immunosuppression. The rationale for considering these various transplant variables is discussed in detail in reference (Olanow et al., 1996).

Clinical improvement in PD features following fetal nigral transplantation has been associated with a significant and progressive increase in striatal fluorodopa (FD) uptake on positron emission tomography (PET) in some studies (Lindvall et al., 1994; Kordower et al., 1995; Remy et al., 1995). FD–PET is a surrogate biomarker of dopamine terminal function, and increased striatal FD uptake has been interpreted to represent an index of the survival of transplanted dopamine neurons (Lindvall et al., 1994). Post-mortem studies on transplanted patients have shown healthy appearing graft deposit with survival of more than 100,000 transplanted cells per side (Kordower et al., 1995; 1996; Mendez et al., 2005). In these studies, individual implanted cells express a normal dopamine phenotype; TH positive processes extended from the graft into the striatum providing continuous dopamine innervation between graft deposits with a patch-matrix pattern; grafted regions stained positively for cytochrome oxidase indicating increased metabolism, and expressed TH mRNA consistent with functional activity; no host-derived sprouting was observed; electron microscopy demonstrated normal appearing synaptic connections; and no overt graft rejection was detected, although there was increased expression of immune markers in grafted regions (Kordower et al., 1997).

6.4 Double-blind controlled studies to assess fetal nigral transplantation in PD

To better define the safety and efficacy of fetal nigral transplantation as a treatment for PD, the National Institutes of Health in the USA supported two double-blind, placebo-controlled trials. These studies were not without controversy. Some felt it was premature to carry out a double-blind clinical trial, others argued against the use of sham controls for a surgical procedure, and the use of embryonic tissue as a source of dopamine cells remains a controversial topic (Cohen, 1994; Freeman et al., 1999; Macklin, 1999).

The first of these studies was a 1 year trial in which 40 advanced PD patients were randomized to receive bilateral transplantation or a sham placebo operation (Freed et al., 2001). Ventral mesencephalic tissue was stored for up to 4 weeks, and solid grafts derived from two donors per side were implanted longitudinally into the putamen using two deposits or "noodles". The sham procedure consisted of a burr hole without needle penetration of the brain. Immunosuppression was not employed. The primary endpoint of the study was the change from baseline to final visit in a measure of quality of life. The study failed to meet its primary endpoint, as transplanted patients were not improved in comparison to those in the placebo group (0.0 ± 2.1 on UPDRS in the transplant group and −0.4 ± 1.7 in the sham surgery group). A pre-specified analysis demonstrated a significant benefit of transplantation in younger patients (<60 years) in UPDRS motor score performed in the practically defined off state (P < 0.1), but not in older patients. The authors noted further improvement during the course of follow-up (38% at 3 years), although it should be noted that these later evaluations were performed by unblinded investigators. A subsequent analysis by the authors suggested that baseline response to levodopa rather than patient's age best predicted a good response to transplantation (Bjorklund et al., 2003; Freed et al., 2004). FD–PET studies showed improvement in striatal FD uptake, and the authors considered the findings indicative of graft survival in 17/20 transplanted patients. Autopsy in two patients confirmed survival of TH+ neurons in each of the transplant tracks with fibers extending approximately 2–3 mms into the striatum. Cell counting noted survival of approximately 7000–40,000 cells per side. Some evidence of inflammation was observed in transplanted regions based on immunostaining for CD3 and HLA class II antigen. Neurophysiologic assessments of reaction time (RT) and movement time (MT) noted significant improvement in transplanted patients in comparison to patients in the sham group, who in contrast demonstrated significant worsening over time (Gordon et al., 2004). The procedure itself was well tolerated, however, 5 transplanted patients developed severe and disabling dyskinesias that were not alleviated by a reduction or cessation in the dose of levodopa (see discussion below).

In the second double-blind, placebo-controlled study, 34 patients were randomized to one of three treatment groups; bilateral transplantation of fetal mesencephalic tissue derived from one donor per side (11 patients), bilateral transplantation of fetal mesencephalic tissue derived from four donors per side (12 patients) or sham surgery (11 patients) (Olanow et al., 2003). Fetal mesencephalic tissue was stored for no more than 48 h in cool hibernation media and was not cultured. Solid grafts were implanted exclusively into the post-commissural putamen with deposits placed no more than 5 mm apart in an attempt to achieve continuous reinnervation of the striatum. Patients in the placebo-control group received bilateral partial burr holes which did not penetrate the inner table of the skull. All patients received cyclosporine beginning 2 weeks prior to surgery and continuing for 6 months following the operation. The primary endpoint was the change in UPDRS motor score during the practically defined off state. Transplanted patients had a significant increase in striatal FD uptake on PET ($P < 0.01$ compared to controls) (Fig. 6.1).

Post-mortem studies demonstrated robust graft survival with more than 100,000 TH+ cells in each striatum and extensive reinnervation of the striatum, similar to what we have seen in open label studies (Fig. 6.2). However, this study also failed to meet its primary endpoint ($P = 0.244$), although a paired comparison of the four donor versus placebo group just failed to meet significance ($P = 0.096$). It is noteworthy that transplanted patients in both the one and four donor groups did show improvement at 6 and 9 months ($P < 0.05$) and deteriorated afterwards (Fig. 6.3). Interestingly, this time period corresponds with the discontinuation of cyclosporine, raising the possibility that immune rejection might have compromised continued benefit. In support of this concept, post-mortem studies did show increased CD45 immunostaining in the region of graft deposits.

Post hoc analysis of the data in this study demonstrated that transplanted patients with milder disease in both the one and four donor groups were significantly improved in comparison to the placebo group despite the small sample size ($P < 0.01$). No difference between younger and older patients or in baseline response to levodopa was observed in patients who did or did not respond to transplantation. The surgical procedure was also well tolerated in this study, but a blinded and randomized review of videotapes obtained during visits conducted in the practically defined off state noted that 13/23 transplanted patients developed off-medication dyskinesia. This problem was not observed in any patient in the control group. Off-medication dyskinesias in this study were characterized by stereotypic, rhythmic, involuntary movements that predominantly affected the lower extremities and were associated with parkinsonism in other body regions. Off-medication dyskinesias thus resembled diphasic dyskinesias, and differed from classical on period levodopa-related dyskinesias which typically are more choreiform in nature and affect the head, neck, torso, and upper extremities to an equal or greater degree than the lower extremities. In this study, off-medication dyskinesias were generally mild, but were sufficiently severe in three to warrant surgical intervention.

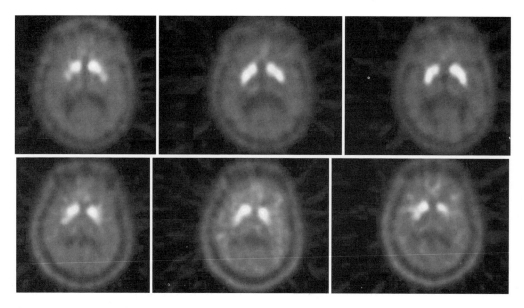

Figure 6.1. FD–PET studies in a representative patient receiving bilateral transplantation with four donors per side (top panels) and a patient receiving a sham procedure (lower panels). Scans were obtained at baseline (left panels), 1 year (middle panels) and 2 years (right panels). Note the progressive increase in striatal FD uptake in the transplanted patient in comparison to the progressive loss of striatal FD uptake consistent with continued disease progression in the placebo treated patient (Olanow et al., 2003).

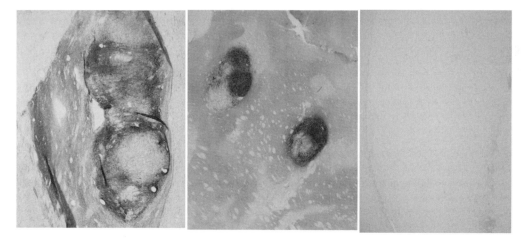

Figure 6.2. TH immunostaining of striatum in patients receiving treatment with bilateral grafts using four donors per side (left panel), one donor per side (middle panel), and a sham placebo procedure (right panel). Note healthy appearing graft deposits and extensive striatal TH innervation with both four and one donors per side. Note also that grafts in the four donor group are larger and have a cylindric appearance whereas in the one donor group they are smaller, more concentric, and more densely packed (Olanow et al., 2003).

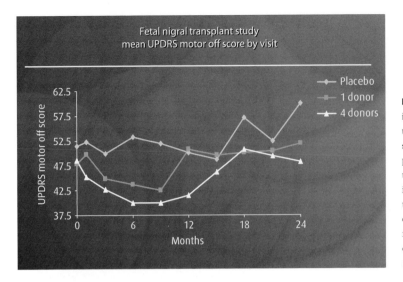

Figure 6.3. Mean UPDRS scores in patients receiving bilateral transplantation with one donor per side, four donors per side, or a sham placebo procedure. Note that transplantation is associated with improvement for 6–9 months, and that transplant-related benefit disappears after approximately 9 months coincident with the cessation of cyclosporine treatment (Olanow et al., 2003).

6.5 Commentary

It is clear that fetal nigral transplantation remains an experimental procedure and cannot be presently recommended as a therapy for PD. It is not certain why benefits were observed in open label studies but not in two double-blind studies, despite using similar protocols and evidence of graft survival on both PET studies and post-mortem examination. It is certainly possible that benefits observed in open label studies were exaggerated by placebo effect or bias. It is also not certain why transplanted patients developed off-medication dyskinesias. Insight into the cause of this complication and the development of methods to prevent this complication from occurring are required before further trials of fetal nigral transplantation or other forms of cell-based therapy can be resumed. While these results are disappointing, these studies provide some clues that might permit better results to be obtained with a variety of protocol modifications (Winkler et al., 2005). These are discussed below.

6.6 Patient selection

Patient selection is an important factor in the design of transplantation studies. It is obviously important to ensure the correct diagnosis, and most groups utilize the UK brain bank criteria in order to minimize the risk of an atypical Parkinsonism. There is no evidence to suggest that fetal nigral transplantation will benefit patients with atypical Parkinsonism where degeneration occurs in the striatum and pallidum and likely precludes any benefit from restoration of the nigrostriatal system. Freed et al. suggest that transplantation is more effective in younger patients who respond well to levodopa, possibly because there is less degeneration of non-dopaminergic systems and transplant has a better chance of improving patient disability (Freed et al., 2001). Olanow et al. did not find an age effect, but observed significant benefits with transplantation in the subset of patients with milder disease, possibly reflecting the same phenomenon (Olanow et al., 2003). Interestingly, several studies have reported that patients who do best following transplantation are receiving relatively lower doses of levodopa than those who do poorly (Wenning et al., 1997; Hagell et al., 1999; Brundin et al., 2000a). This observation is consistent with the notion that the patients who do best with transplantation have relatively mild disease. More advanced patients who require higher levodopa doses may benefit less, possibly because of involvement of non-dopaminergic regions (Lang and Obeso, 2004a). To this point, studies in the 6-OHDA model in the rat similarly note greater benefits with intrastriatal transplantation in animals that have lesions confined to the striatum in comparison to those with lesions involving both striatal and non-striatal forebrain dopaminergic projections (Kirik et al., 2001). Longer periods of follow-up may also be required to see the full benefits of transplantation. Freed et al. noted continued improvement over 3 years, although observations during the last 2 years were unblinded. Additionally, late improvement in physiologic measures of motor performance and a delay in recovery in movement-related cortical function have been reported (Brundin et al., 2000a; Gordon et al., 2004). Collectively, these observations suggest that the best candidates for fetal nigral transplantation and other cell-based therapies might be younger PD patients with relatively mild disease who respond well to levodopa and have minimal or no evidence of non-dopaminergic lesions.

6.7 Immunosuppression

A fundamental question in transplantation is whether immunosuppression is necessary in order to permit host tolerance of the graft. The brain has been considered to be an immunologically privileged site, but immune rejection can still occur even following transplantation of autografts (Fisher and Gage, 1993; Drucker-Colin and Verdugo-Diaz, 2004). While intracerebral grafts can survive in the absence of immunosuppression, differences in the expression of major and minor histocompatability antigens between graft and host can result in a long-term inflammatory response with macrophage and microglial activation and upregulation of immunological markers (Duan et al., 1993; Shinoda et al., 1995; 1996; Baker-Cairns et al., 1996). Such immune reactions could be detrimental to graft survival and function, and are likely relevant to human transplantation. Indeed, evidence of some degree of an immune response was seen in post-mortem studies of patients in each of the double-blind trials. In addition, we have previously demonstrated dense HLA-DR immunostaining and numerous pan macrophages, T-cells, and B-cells

in otherwise normal appearing graft deposits, 18 months following fetal nigral transplantation (Kordower et al., 1997). Further, Freed et al. did not use immunosuppression and had much less survival of transplanted cells than did Olanow et al. who employed cyclosporine for 6 months (Kordower et al., 1995; 1996; Freed et al., 2001; Olanow et al., 2003). Indeed, in the latter group it was suggested that an immune response may have limited the clinical benefit of fetal nigral transplantation, as benefits deteriorated following withdrawal of cyclosporine and there was evidence of increased CD45 staining in grafter regions at post-mortem (Olanow et al., 2003). These studies each used solid tissue grafts, and it has been suggested that solid grafts are more likely to generate an immune response as the blood vessels within the graft are of donor origin and likely to express major histocompatability type 1 antigens which are intensely immunogenic (Baker-Cairns et al., 1996). In this regard, the Lund group used suspension grafts and a "cocktail" of three immunosuppressive agents, and reported long-lasting benefits with the ability to stop levodopa in some patients (Wenning et al., 1997; Piccini et al., 2000). Thus, current evidence suggests that long-term immunosuppression might be desirable in future transplant regimens.

6.8 Off-medication dyskinesia

Off-medication dyskinesia is an important and potentially disabling side-effect of transplantation that currently represents a major obstacle to future studies of fetal nigral transplantation and other cell-based therapies in PD. The precise cause of off-medication dyskinesia is not known. Current evidence indicates that levodopa-induced on-medication dyskinesias are related to abnormal intermittent or pulsatile stimulation of denervated dopamine receptors (Obeso et al., 2000). Transplantation of functioning dopamine neurons and terminals might thus be expected to provide dopamine to the striatum in a more continuous and physiologic manner than regular oral formulations of levodopa and so reduce rather than increase the risk of dyskinesia. Indeed,

Lee et al. found a reduction in levodopa-induced dyskinesia following transplantation of dopamine neurons in a rodent model of PD (Lee et al., 2000). However, patchy reinnervation of the striatum or abnormal synaptic connectivity such as could occur with an immune reaction, could lead to regional pulsatility and consequent dyskinesia. Indeed, regional areas of increased FD uptake on PET were observed in one study (Ma et al., 2002). The authors suggested that dopamine released from innervated regions of the striatum or "hot spots" could stimulate upregulated, hypersensitive receptors in denervated neighboring areas leading to dyskinesia. In contrast to these findings, PET scans in other transplant studies have not shown inhomogeneities (Olanow et al., 2003), although this does not exclude this possibility.

A variety of other hypotheses have been put forward. Freed et al. proposed that off-medication dyskinesia might be due to excessive dopamine release from grafts (Freed et al., 2001), but there is no evidence of excess dopaminergic activity on PET or post-mortem examination in any of the studies performed to date. Further, we have reported reduced dyskinesia with survival of larger numbers of implanted dopaminergic neurons (Kordower et al., 1995), and found no correlation between off-medication dyskinesia and the number of implanted donor cells (Olanow et al., 2003). Hagell et al. suggested that off-medication dyskinesia might relate to long-term storage of cells in tissue culture prior to transplantation, and noted a correlation in their studies with the severity of on-medication dyskinesia at baseline (Hagell et al., 2002). However, in a larger double-blind study, off-medication dyskinesia were observed with freshly transplanted cells that were not cultured and there was no correlation with on-medication dyskinesia scores at baseline or at any other time point during the trial (Olanow et al., 2003). Finally, it has been observed that off-medication dyskinesia resemble diphasic dyskinesia, a form of dyskinesia that is seen with suboptimal dopaminergic levels, and that striatal FD uptake, while increased in comparison to baseline, did not return to the lower limits of normal in any patient (Olanow et al., 2003). These observations suggest that off-medication may be due to partial, but incomplete, reinnervation of the striatum. This hypothesis raises the intriguing possibility that transplantation of increased numbers of functioning dopamine neurons might both enhance efficacy and eliminate off-medication dyskinesia.

Further insight into the cause of off-medication dyskinesia and the development of methods that prevent their occurrence are crucial before studies of fetal nigral transplantation can be resumed in PD patients. It remains uncertain whether this side-effect will prove to be a problem with other cell-based therapies such as stem cells and laboratory studies to assess grafts in animals who have been exposed to levodopa and who experience levodopa-related dyskinesia must be performed prior to commencing clinical trials.

6.9 Attempts to enhance survival of transplanted dopamine neurons

Only about 5% of neurons in the SNc are dopaminergic, and only about 5–20% of grafted dopamine neurons survive transplantation (Kordower et al., 1998; Sortwell et al., 2004). Approximately 20–30% of mesencephalic cells die during preparation of the tissue for transplantation probably due to ischemia or trauma associated with dissection and dissociation of the cells (Fawcett et al., 1995; Brundin et al., 2000a) and another 60–70% of cells die during the first week post-transplantation (Barker et al., 1996; Sortwell et al., 2000). Enhanced survival of transplanted cells would facilitate the logistics of performing a fetal nigral transplant procedure and could potentially yield enhanced clinical results. Considerable research has focused on ways of trying to improve this yield. Mesencephalic cell graft aggregates can be maintained in culture and exposed to agents such as antioxidants and trophic factors that promote their survival that promote their survival following transplantation (Meyer et al., 1998).

Neurotrophic factors promote the survival of dopaminergic neurons *in vitro* and *in vivo* (Lin et al., 1993; Nikkhah et al., 1993; Altar et al., 1994; Studer et al., 1995) and might therefore be expected to enhance survival and functional effects of dopamine cell transplants. Trophic factors can be administered by direct infusion into the striatum, through co-transplantation of cells that manufacture and secrete neurotrophic factors, and by gene therapy approaches. Approximately 94% of melanized neurons within the SNc normally contain fibroblast growth factor 2 (FGF-2) receptors suggesting this might be an important trophic factor for dopamine neurons (Tooyama et al., 1994). Indeed, co-transplantation of Schwann cells that express FGF-2 enhances the survival of intrastriatal dopamine grafts and promotes striatal reinnervation and functional recovery in the rat model of PD (Timmer et al., 2004). Glial derived neurotrophic factor (GDNF) is a member of the transforming growth factor β family and appears to have the greatest capacity amongst trophic factors to protect dopaminergic neurons both in culture and *in vivo*. GDNF infusion in MPTP lesioned primates enhances survival of nigral neurons, increases TH staining in the striatum, and improves behavioral features even when delivered weeks after the insult (Gash et al., 1995; 1996; Winkler et al., 1996). Lentivirus delivery of GDNF similarly is associated with marked behavioral and anatomic benefits in both the 6-OHDA rodent and the MPTP monkey (Bensadoun et al., 2000; Kordower et al., 2000). GDNF has been shown to improve survival of grafted dopamine neurons and to increase striatal reinnervation in the 6-OHDA rat (Granholm et al., 1997; Zawada et al., 1998), suggesting that co-administration of GDNF might be a way to enhance the clinical effects associated with fetal nigral grafts. The carotid body contains DA rich chromaffin cells which release neurotrophic factors such as GDNF, as well as brain derived neurotrophic factor (BDNF) and neurotrophin-3 (NT3). Co-transplantation of carotid body cells has been shown to enhance the survival of grafted fetal ventral mesencephalic dopaminergic cells, striatal TH immunoreactivity and dopamine levels, and functional recovery in 6-OHDA lesioned rats (Shukla et al., 2004). Encapsulated cells that constitutively express high levels of VEGF have also been reported to improve behavior and decrease TH cell loss in a rat model of PD, but have not been tested

in conjunction with transplanted dopamine cells (Yasuhara et al., 2004).

Increased expression or co-administration of anti-apoptotic and antioxidant agents is another approach that has been tried in an attempt to increase the survival of transplanted dopamine neurons. The Jun-N-terminal kinase (JNK) stress pathway is central to apoptotic neuronal death in several model systems (Chun et al., 2001; Gearan et al., 2001) and mixed lineage kinase (MLK) activation is a critical event in this sequence of events (Xu et al., 2001). MLK inhibitors have been shown to protect against dopaminergic cell death in culture systems (Harris et al., 2002; Murakata et al., 2002), and to improve long-term survival, graft size and fiber outgrowth following transplantation of rat ventral mesenecephalic cells (Boll et al., 2004). Caspase inhibitors also reduce apoptosis in many model systems and increase the survival of dopaminergic grafts in the 6-OHDA rat model (Schierle et al., 1999). Antioxidants also improve graft survival, striatal TH-immunoreactivity and behavioral function when co-administered with ventral mesencephalic grafts (Agrawal et al., 2004). Co-administration of lazaroids with fetal nigral transplantation has now been attempted in PD patients with good clinical results (Brundin et al., 2000b), but it is not possible to say with any certainty how much the lazaroids contributed to the observed benefit based on this anecdotal report.

6.10 Combined striatal and SNc grafts

Combined striatal and SNc grafts are reported to provide enhanced behavioral benefits in complex tasks in animal models of PD in comparison to intrastriatal grafts alone (Baker et al., 2000). This approach theoretically provides for dopamine reinnervation of the striatum as well as regions of the basal ganglia and the cerebral cortex that receive dopaminergic inputs from the SNc. Mendez and colleagues transplanted fetal ventral mesencephalic tissue into both the striatum and the SNc in a small numbers of PD patients and reported clinical benefits along with increased striatal FD uptake on

PET in an open label study (Mendez et al., 2002). At autopsy, surviving transplanted cells were detected in both the striatum and the SNc and stained positively for TH, G-protein-coupled inward rectifying current potassium channel type 2 (Girk2), and calbindin. The procedure was well tolerated with no side-effects related to implantation into the midbrain. Off-medication dyskinesias were not recorded. The magnitude of clinical improvement and degree of survival of implanted neurons was similar to that reported in previously reported studies. Double-blind trials are required to confirm these results.

6.11 Other cell-based approaches to transplantation in PD

The limited clinical benefits obtained with fetal nigral transplantation to date coupled with the societal and logistic issues involved in the use of human embryonic tissue, has led to a search for alternate sources of dopaminergic cell types for transplantation in PD. As previously discussed, adrenomedullary tissue has been abandoned as patients did not maintain long-term benefit and the procedure was associated with considerable morbidity. Extra-adrenal chromaffin tissue has attracted some attention. The organ of Zuckerkandl is a paired organ located adjacent to the abdominal aorta which represents a source of GDNF (Bohn et al., 1982). Transplant of this tissue has been reported to induce functional improvement in Parkinsonian rats (Espejo et al., 2001). Autologous sympathetic ganglia cells have been tested in small groups of patients with advanced PD. In one study, patients were reported to have a decrease in "off" time (Nakao et al., 2001), while another found amelioration of bradykinesia and gait dysfunction in half of transplanted patients (Itakura et al., 1997). Transplantation of autologous carotid body cells improved motor function in Parkinsonian rodents and (Luquin et al., 1999; Toledo-Aral et al., 2003) were reported to provide some benefits to a small number of PD patients (Arjona et al., 2003). However, post-mortem studies demonstrated no evidence of graft integration into the brain nor evidence that they secreted dopamine. Carotid body

tissue undergoes atrophy with increasing age and it has been suggested that any improvement seen in these experiments was due to the release of trophic factors and not from restoration of the nigrostriatal system (Toledo-Aral et al., 2003). None of these procedures has been studied in double-blind placebo-controlled trials.

Transplantation of porcine fetal nigral cells has been reported to provide some benefit in open label studies in PD patients (Schumacher et al., 2000). However, there were only a few surviving transplanted dopaminergic cells at post-mortem (Deacon et al., 1997), and no benefit was detected in double-blind studies (unpublished studies). Human retinal epithelial cells secrete levodopa, are relatively resistant to immune rejection and survive following transplantation when implanted attached to gelatin microcarriers (Spheramine®) (Subramanian et al., 2002). Spheramine transplantation has been reported to provide anti-Parkinson effects when transplanted into the striatum of the MPTP monkey and in open label trials in PD patients (Watts et al., 2003). No serious adverse events related to the microcarrier system have been noted and no patient has yet been reported with off-medication dyskinesia. A double-blind placebo-controlled study to test this approach in PD patients is currently under way.

Most optimism for the treatment of PD with a cell-based therapy rests on stem cells as a source of dopamine neurons for transplantation, although there are still many hurdles that must be overcome. Stem cells are pluripotent cells that have the potential to differentiate into all of the different cell types of the body. Several types of stem cells have been studied: embryonic stem cells (ES cells), neural stem cells (NSCs) that are found within the fetal and adult brain, and primitive cells that are found in the bone marrow and umbilical cord. In the laboratory, ES cells are the most promising as approximately 50% spontaneously differentiate into a neuronal phenotype. ES cells are harvested from the inner cell membrane of the blastocyst and offer the potential of being expanded to provide a renewable source of dopamine neurons. Mouse ES cells have been shown to spontaneously differentiate into neurons following transplantation, with a few showing phenotypic features of dopamine neurons

(Bjorklund et al., 2002). The yield can be increased by inducing ES cells to differentiate into dopamine neurons while in culture using agents such as Nurr-1, trophic factors, sonic hedgehog, Bcl-XL, and ascorbate (Kim et al., 2003; Park et al., 2005). A higher yield of TH+ cells for transplantation can be accomplished by using a cell sorter to identify dopaminergic cells that have been transfected with a green fluorescent protein reporter (Yoshizaki et al., 2004). More recently, studies have demonstrated that human ES cells can also be induced to differentiate into dopamine neurons (Perrier et al., 2004). Transplanted dopamine neurons derived from ES cells have now been shown to be able to survive and to provide behavioral improvement in the 6-OHDA rat model (Bjorklund et al., 2002). Importantly, ES cells have also been reported to improve motor features and to increase striatal FD uptake on PET in MPTP-lesioned monkeys (Takagi et al., 2005).

Neural stem cells initially generated considerable enthusiasm because they already have a neuronal lineage, but results have been disappointing as they primarily differentiate into astroglia (Gage, 2000; Magavi and Macklis, 2001; Storch et al., 2004). A few cells spontaneously differentiate into dopamine phenotypes following transplantation (Yang et al., 2002), and they can be induced to differentiate into midbrain dopaminergic neurons by exposure to agents such as cytokines and trophic factors (Carvey et al., 2001; Burnstein et al., 2004; Wang et al., 2004). Behavioral effects can be observed following transplantation into the rat model of PD, but only a few TH+ positive cells are found at post-mortem. Autologous stem cells derived from the umbilical cord or bone marrow are also of great interest because they can avoid the immunological and societal issues associated with embryonic stem cells. However, they also default to glial cells and to date it has proven difficult to generate large numbers of dopamine neurons suitable for transplantation. *In vitro* treatment with GDNF increase TH positivity in bone marrow stromal cells, and following transplantation they have been shown to produce behavioral improvement in the 6-OHDA rat (Dezawa et al., 2004).

Stem cells offer the theoretical advantage of providing a source of virtually unlimited and optimized dopamine neurons for transplantation in PD. There are however many issues that remain to be resolved. It has not yet proven easy to routinely generate large numbers of dopamine neurons for transplantation, and the optimal type of stem cell and method of inducing them to differentiate into dopamine neurons remain to be determined. Studies in models of PD show limited cell survival and do not provide benefits superior to fetal nigral transplants, which to date have not been confirmed to yield significant results in PD patients in double-blind trials. The adverse event profile must be defined. Transplantation of pluripotential stem cells carries with it the risk of unregulated growth and tumor formation. Indeed, 5 of 17 rats transplanted with stem cells had teratomas at post-mortem examination (Bjorklund et al., 2002). Studies will also have to be conducted to determine if stem cells are associated with off-medication dyskinesia, and if so how to prevent them. In addition, extensive laboratory testing will have to be performed to exclude unanticipated side-effects, to the extent possible, prior to entering into clinical trial. Stem cells will also need to be proven to be more effective than just pharmacologic replacement of lost dopamine. Finally, it is by no means assured that even complete and physiologic restoration of the nigrostriatal dopamine system will eliminate disability in PD patients caused by degeneration of non-dopaminergic neurons (see below).

6.12 Need for double-blind controlled trials and sham surgery

While there has been some resistance to the use of double-blind placebo-controlled trials to assess new surgical therapies, we believe that it is essential to employ this study design in evaluating the safety and efficacy of cell-based therapies for PD (Freeman et al., 1999). Placebo and bias effects can be powerful and seriously distort the results of a trial (McRae et al., 2004). Placebo therapy can also be associated with dopamine release with possible clinical consequences (de la Fuente-Fernandez et al., 2001). There are numerous examples of surgical procedures that were adopted into general practice based on anecdotal observations that were discarded after negative results in more formal clinical trials (Freeman et al., 1999). In PD, we have recently seen that positive results in open label trials of human fetal nigral transplantation, porcine fetal nigral transplantation, and GDNF infusion were not confirmed in double-blind trials. Transplantation therapies in PD are particularly appropriate for evaluation in double-blind trials as the intervention is relatively standardized and the treatment has much in common with drug therapies; issues such as dose, distribution, metabolism/degeneration, delayed response, and immune reactivity must all be considered (Olanow, 2005). Indeed, a recent survey showed that 97% of PD investigators would insist on a double-blind placebo-controlled trial before accepting that a cell-based or gene therapy procedure was efficacious, despite the need for a sham control (Kim et al., 2005). While a sham procedure is not fully without risk, the alternative is to expose patients to a procedure that might not work, and whose safety and efficacy profile has not been fully defined.

6.13 Conclusion

The future of mesencephalic cell transplantation for PD is uncertain at this time. Laboratory studies have demonstrated that transplanted dopamine cells can survive, release dopamine, reinnervate the striatum and provide benefit in animal models of PD. Open label studies of fetal nigral transplantation showed positive clinical benefits associated with increased striatal FD uptake on PET. Post-mortem studies reveal histologic evidence of robust graft survival with extensive and organotypic striatal reinnervation. However, two double-blind studies failed to demonstrate that transplanted patients were superior to placebo with respect to their primary endpoints. Further, transplantation of fetal mesencephalic dopamine neurons was associated with a potentially disabling off-medication dyskinesia. Thus, fetal nigral transplantation can not be currently recommended as a treatment for PD. It is still possible that transplantation using different transplant

protocols or different dopaminergic cells will prove helpful for PD patients. Post hoc analyses in the double-blind transplant studies suggest that improved clinical results might be obtained with protocols that employ younger patients with milder disease and long-term use of immunosuppression. It remains to be determined if transplantation of larger numbers of cells or co-administration of agents that enhance cell survival will influence outcome. It is also possible that enhanced benefit can be derived by transplantation of other dopaminergic cell types such as stem cells.

It is also important to question whether transplantation of dopaminergic cells can provide benefits any greater than can be achieved with levodopa (Lang and Obeso, 2004b). Levodopa does not improve potentially disabling features of PD such as sleep disturbances, autonomic dysfunction, freezing of gait, postural instability, and dementia presumably because they result from degeneration of non-dopaminergic neurons. It is not clear that transplanted dopamine cells will provide better results. Indeed, Lindvall et al. report the best results in patients whose clinical features can be best controlled with levodopa, and suggest that these are the optimal candidates for a transplant procedure. It is possible that early replacement of dopaminergic tone will have downstream effects that prevent damage to non-dopaminergic regions. For example, it has been postulated that dopamine depletion-induced increased firing of glutamatergic neurons in the STN could cause excitotoxic damage in target neurons such as the globus pallidus, substantia nigra pars reticulata, the pedunculopontine nucleus, as well as the SNc (Rodriguez et al., 1998). Early restoration of dopamine might prevent these non-dopaminergic consequences. It is also possible that degeneration of dopaminergic pathways to cerebral cortex and other brain regions might contribute to the gait, autonomic, and cognitive dysfunction that occurs in PD. It is by no means clear, however, that transplantation of dopamine neurons into the striatum will have any effect on these non-dopaminergic systems and that these types of disability that occur in PD will persist despite complete restoration of the nigrostriatal dopamine system. For additional discussion of transplantation therapies in Parkinson's and other neurodegenerative disease, see Volume I, Chapter 34.

REFERENCES

Deep Brain stimulation study group. (2001). Deep-brain stimulation of the subthalamic nucleus or the pars interna of the globus pallidus in Parkinson's disease. *New Engl J Med*, **345**, 956–963.

Agrawal, A.K., Chaturvedi, R.K., Shukla, S., Seth, K., Chauhan, S., Ahmad, A. and Seth, P.K. (2004). Restorative potential of dopaminergic grafts in presence of antioxidants in rat model of Parkinson's disease. *J Chem Neuroanat*, **28**, 253–264.

Ahlskog, J.E. and Muenter, M.D. (2001). Frequency of levodopa-related dyskinesias and motor fluctuations as estimated from the cumulative literature. *Mov Disord*, **16**, 448–458.

Altar, C.A., Boylan, C.B., Fritsche, M., Jones, B.E., Jackson, C., Wiegand, S.J., Lindsay, R.M. and Hyman, C. (1994). Efficacy of brain-derived neurotrophic factor and neurotrophin-3 on neurochemical and behavioral deficits associated with partial nigrostriatal dopamine lesions. *J Neurochem*, **63**, 1021–1032.

Arjona, V., Minguez-Castellanos, A., Montoro, R.J., Ortega, A., Escamilla, F., Toledo-Aral, J.J., Pardal, R., Mendez-Ferrer, S., Martin, J.M., Perez, M., Katati, M.J., Valencia, E., Garcia, T. and Lopez-Barneo, J. (2003). Autotransplantation of human carotid body cell aggregates for treatment of Parkinson's disease. *Neurosurgery*, **53**, 321–328, discussion 328–330.

Baker, K.A., Sadi, D., Hong, M. and Mendez, I. (2000). Simultaneous intrastriatal and intranigral dopaminergic grafts in the Parkinsonian rat model: role of the intranigral graft. *J Comp Neurol*, **426**, 106–116.

Baker-Cairns, B.J., Sloan, D.J., Broadwell, R.D., Puklavec, M. and Charlton, H.M. (1996). Contributions of donor and host blood vessels in CNS allografts. *Exp Neurol*, **142**, 36–46.

Barker, R.A., Dunnett, S.B., Faissner, A. and Fawcett, J.W. (1996). The time course of loss of dopaminergic neurons and the gliotic reaction surrounding grafts of embryonic mesencephalon to the striatum. *Exp Neurol*, **141**, 79–93.

Bensadoun, J.C., Deglon, N., Tseng, J.L., Ridet, J.L., Zurn, A.D. and Aebischer, P. (2000). Lentiviral vectors as a gene delivery system in the mouse midbrain: cellular and behavioral improvements in a 6-OHDA model of Parkinson's disease using GDNF. *Exp Neurol*, **164**, 15–24.

Bjorklund, A. and Stenevi, U. (1971). Growth of central catecholamine neurones into smooth muscle grafts in the rat mesencephalon. *Brain Res*, **31**, 1–20.

Bjorklund, A., Dunnett, S.B., Brundin, P., Stoessl, A.J., Freed, C.R., Breeze, R.E., Levivier, M., Peschanski, M., Studer, L. and

Barker, R. (2003). Neural transplantation for the treatment of Parkinson's disease. *Lancet Neurol*, **2**, 437–445.

Bjorklund, L.M., Sanchez-Pernaute, R., Chung, S., Andersson, T., Chen, I.Y., McNaught, K.S., Brownell, A.L., Jenkins, B.G., Wahlestedt, C., Kim, K.S. and Isacson, O. (2002). Embryonic stem cells develop into functional dopaminergic neurons after transplantation in a Parkinson rat model. *Proc Natl Acad Sci USA*, **99**, 2344–2349.

Bohn, M.C., Goldstein, M. and Black, I.B. (1982). Expression of phenylethanolamine *N*-methyltransferase in rat sympathetic ganglia and extra-adrenal chromaffin tissue. *Dev Biol*, **89**, 299–308.

Boll, J.B., Geist, M.A., Kaminski Schierle, G.S., Petersen, K., Leist, M. and Vaudano, E. (2004). Improvement of embryonic dopaminergic neurone survival in culture and after grafting into the striatum of hemiparkinsonian rats by CEP-1347. *J Neurochem*, **88**, 698–707.

Brundin, P., Nilsson, O.G., Strecker, R.E., Lindvall, O., Astedt, B. and Bjorklund, A. (1986). Behavioural effects of human fetal dopamine neurons grafted in a rat model of Parkinson's disease. *Exp Brain Res*, **65**, 235–240.

Brundin, P., Strecker, R.E., Widner, H., Clarke, D.J., Nilsson, O.G., Astedt, B., Lindvall, O. and Bjorklund, A. (1988). Human fetal dopamine neurons grafted in a rat model of Parkinson's disease: immunological aspects, spontaneous and drug-induced behaviour, and dopamine release. *Exp Brain Res*, **70**, 192–208.

Brundin, P., Karlsson, J., Emgard, M., Schierle, G.S., Hansson, O., Petersen, A. and Castilho, R.F. (2000a). Improving the survival of grafted dopaminergic neurons: a review over current approaches. *Cell Transplant*, **9**, 179–195.

Brundin, P., Pogarell, O., Hagell, P., Piccini, P., Widner, H., Schrag, A., Kupsch, A., Crabb, L., Odin, P., Gustavii, B., Bjorklund, A., Brooks, D.J., Marsden, C.D., Oertel, W.H., Quinn, N.P., Rehncrona, S. and Lindvall, O. (2000b). Bilateral caudate and putamen grafts of embryonic mesencephalic tissue treated with lazaroids in Parkinson's disease. *Brain*, **123**(**Part 7**), 1380–1390.

Burnstein, R.M., Foltynie, T., He, X., Menon, D.K., Svendsen, C.N. and Caldwell, M.A. (2004). Differentiation and migration of long term expanded human neural progenitors in a partial lesion model of Parkinson's disease. *Int J Biochem Cell Biol*, **36**, 702–713.

Carvey, P.M., Ling, Z.D., Sortwell, C.E., Pitzer, M.R., McGuire, S.O., Storch, A. and Collier, T.J. (2001). A clonal line of mesencephalic progenitor cells converted to dopamine neurons by hematopoietic cytokines: a source of cells for transplantation in Parkinson's disease. *Exp Neurol*, **171**, 98–108.

Chun, H.S., Gibson, G.E., Degiorgio, L.A., Zhang, H., Kidd, V.J. and Son, J.H. (2001). Dopaminergic cell death induced by

MPP(+), oxidant and specific neurotoxicants shares the common molecular mechanism. *J Neurochem*, **76**, 1010–1021.

Cohen, J. (1994). New fight over fetal tissue grafts. *Science*, **263**, 600–601.

Collier, T.J., Sortwell, C.E., Elsworth, J.D., Taylor, J.R., Roth, R.H., Sladek Jr., J.R. and Redmond Jr., D.E. (2002). Embryonic ventral mesencephalic grafts to the substantia nigra of MPTP-treated monkeys: feasibility relevant to multiple-target grafting as a therapy for Parkinson's disease. *J Comp Neurol*, **442**, 320–330.

de la Fuente-Fernandez, R., Ruth, T.J., Sossi, V., Schulzer, M., Calne, D.B. and Stoessl, A.J. (2001). Expectation and dopamine release: mechanism of the placebo effect in Parkinson's disease. *Science*, **293**, 1164–1166.

Deacon, T., Schumacher, J., Dinsmore, J., Thomas, C., Palmer, P., Kott, S., Edge, A., Penney, D., Kassissieh, S., Dempsey, P. and Isacson, O. (1997). Histological evidence of fetal pig neural cell survival after transplantation into a patient with Parkinson's disease. *Nat Med*, **3**, 350–353.

Dezawa, M., Kanno, H., Hoshino, M., Cho, H., Matsumoto, N., Itokazu, Y., Tajima, N., Yamada, H., Sawada, H., Ishikawa, H., Mimura, T., Kitada, M., Suzuki, Y. and Ide, C. (2004). Specific induction of neuronal cells from bone marrow stromal cells and application for autologous transplantation. *J Clin Invest*, **113**, 1701–1710.

Drucker-Colin, R. and Verdugo-Diaz, L. (2004). Cell transplantation for Parkinson's disease: present status. *Cell Mol Neurobiol*, **24**, 301–316.

Duan, W.M., Widner, H., Bjorklund, A. and Brundin, P. (1993). Sequential intrastriatal grafting of allogeneic embryonic dopamine-rich neuronal tissue in adult rats: will the second graft be rejected? *Neuroscience*, **57**, 261–274.

Dunnett, S.B. and Annett, L.E. (1991). Nigral transplants in primate models of parkinsonism. In: *Intracerebral Trans-plantation in Movement Disorders* (eds Lindvall, O., Bjorklund, A. and Widermer, H.R.), Elsevier Science Publishers, New York.

Dunnett, S.B., Bjorklund, A., Schmidt, R.H., Stenevi, U. and Iversen, S.D. (1983). Intracerebral grafting of neuronal cell suspensions. IV. Behavioural recovery in rats with unilateral 6-OHDA lesions following implantation of nigral cell suspensions in different forebrain sites. *Acta Physiol Scand Suppl*, **522**, 29–37.

Dunnett, S.B., Hernandez, T.D., Summerfield, A., Jones, G.H. and Arbuthnott, G. (1988). Graft-derived recovery from 6-OHDA lesions: specificity of ventral mesencephalic graft tissues. *Exp Brain Res*, **71**, 411–424.

Espejo, E.F., Gonzalez-Albo, M.C., Moraes, J.P., El Banoua, F., Flores, J.A. and Caraballo, I. (2001). Functional regeneration in a rat Parkinson's model after intrastriatal grafts of glial cell line-derived neurotrophic factor and transforming growth factor beta1-expressing extra-adrenal chromaffin cells of the Zuckerkandl's organ. *J Neurosci*, **21**, 9888–9895.

Fahn, S., Oakes, D., Shoulson, I., Kieburtz, K., Rudolph, A., Lang, A., Olanow, C.W., Tanner, C. and Marek, K. (2004). Levodopa and the progression of Parkinson's disease. *New Engl J Med*, **351**, 2498–2508.

Fawcett, J.W., Barker, R.A. and Dunnett, S.B. (1995). Dopaminergic neuronal survival and the effects of bFGF in explant, three dimensional and monolayer cultures of embryonic rat ventral mesencephalon. *Exp Brain Res*, **106**, 275–282.

Fisher, L.J. and Gage, F.H. (1993). Grafting in the mammalian central nervous system. *Physiol Rev*, **73**, 583–616.

Freed, C.R., Breeze, R.E., Rosenberg, N.L., Schneck, S.A., Kriek, E., Qi, J.X., Lone, T., Zhang, Y.B., Snyder, J.A., Wells, T.H., et al. (1992). Survival of implanted fetal dopamine cells and neurologic improvement 12 to 46 months after transplantation for Parkinson's disease. *New Engl J Med*, **327**, 1549–1555.

Freed, C.R., Greene, P.E., Breeze, R.E., Tsai, W.Y., Dumouchel, W., Kao, R., Dillon, S., Winfield, H., Culver, S., Trojanowski, J.Q., Eidelberg, D. and Fahn, S. (2001). Transplantation of embryonic dopamine neurons for severe Parkinson's disease. *New Engl J Med*, **344**, 710–719.

Freed, C.R., Breeze, R.E., Fahn, S. and Eidelberg, D. (2004). Preoperative response to levodopa is the best predictor of transplant outcome. *Ann Neurol*, **55**, 896, author reply 896–897.

Freeman, T.B., Olanow, C.W., Hauser, R.A., Nauert, G.M., Smith, D.A., Borlongan, C.V., Sanberg, P.R., Holt, D.A., Kordower, J.H., Vingerhoets, F.J., et al. (1995). Bilateral fetal nigral transplantation into the postcommissural putamen in Parkinson's disease. *Ann Neurol*, **38**, 379–388.

Freeman, T.B., Vawter, D.E., Leaverton, P.E., Godbold, J.H., Hauser, R.A., Goetz, C.G. and Olanow, C.W. (1999). Use of placebo surgery in controlled trials of a cellular-based therapy for Parkinson's disease. *N Engl J Med*, **341**, 988–992.

Gage, F.H. (2000). Mammalian neural stem cells. *Science*, **287**, 1433–1438.

Gash, D.M., Zhang, Z., Cass, W.A., Ovadia, A., Simmerman, L., Martin, D., Russell, D., Collins, F., Hoffer, B.J. and Gerhardt, G.A. (1995). Morphological and functional effects of intranigrally administered GDNF in normal rhesus monkeys. *J Comp Neurol*, **363**, 345–358.

Gash, D.M., Zhang, Z., Ovadia, A., Cass, W.A., Yi, A., Simmerman, L., Russell, D., Martin, D., Lapchak, P.A., Collins, F., Hoffer, B.J. and Gerhardt, G.A. (1996). Functional recovery in parkinsonian monkeys treated with GDNF. *Nature*, **380**, 252–255.

Gearan, T., Castillo, O.A. and Schwarzschild, M.A. (2001). The parkinsonian neurotoxin, MPP+ induces phosphorylated c-Jun in dopaminergic neurons of mesencephalic cultures. *Parkinsonism Relat Disord*, **8**, 19–22.

Goetz, C.G., Olanow, C.W., Koller, W.C., Penn, R.D., Cahill, D., Morantz, R., Stebbins, G., Tanner, C.M., Klawans, H.L. and Shannon, K.M. (1989). Multicenter study of autologous adrenal medullary transplantation to the corpus striatum in patients with advanced Parkinson's disease. *New Engl J Med*, **320**, 337–341.

Gordon, P.H., Yu, Q., Qualls, C., Winfield, H., Dillon, S., Greene, P.E., Fahn, S., Breeze, R.E., Freed, C.R. and Pullman, S.L. (2004). Reaction time and movement time after embryonic cell implantation in Parkinson disease. *Arch Neurol*, **61**, 858–861.

Granholm, A.C., Mott, J.L., Bowenkamp, K., Eken, S., Henry, S., Hoffer, B.J., Lapchak, P.A., Palmer, M.R., Van Horne, C. and Gerhardt, G.A. (1997). Glial cell line-derived neurotrophic factor improves survival of ventral mesencephalic grafts to the 6-hydroxydopamine lesioned striatum. *Exp Brain Res*, **116**, 29–38.

Hagell, P., Schrag, A., Piccini, P., Jahanshahi, M., Brown, R., Rehncrona, S., Widner, H., Brundin, P., Rothwell, J.C., Odin, P., Wenning, G.K., Morrish, P., Gustavii, B., Bjorklund, A., Brooks, D.J., Marsden, C.D., Quinn, N.P. and Lindvall, O. (1999). Sequential bilateral transplantation in Parkinson's disease: effects of the second graft. *Brain*, **122**(Pt 6), 1121–1132.

Hagell, P., Piccini, P., Bjorklund, A., Brundin, P., Rehncrona, S., Widner, H., Crabb, L., Pavese, N., Oertel, W.H., Quinn, N., Brooks, D.J. and Lindvall, O. (2002). Dyskinesias following neural transplantation in Parkinson's disease. *Nat Neurosci*, **5**, 627–628.

Harris, C.A., Deshmukh, M., Tsui-Pierchala, B., Maroney, A.C. and Johnson Jr., E.M. (2002). Inhibition of the c-Jun N-terminal kinase signaling pathway by the mixed lineage kinase inhibitor CEP-1347 (KT7515) preserves metabolism and growth of trophic factor-deprived neurons. *J Neurosci*, **22**, 103–113.

Hauser, R.A., Freeman, T.B., Snow, B.J., Nauert, M., Gauger, L., Kordower, J.H. and Olanow, C.W. (1999). Long-term evaluation of bilateral fetal nigral transplantation in Parkinson disease. *Arch Neurol*, **56**, 179–187.

Itakura, T., Uematsu, Y., Nakao, N., Nakai, E. and Nakai, K. (1997). Transplantation of autologous sympathetic ganglion into the brain with Parkinson's disease. Long-term follow-up of 35 cases. *Stereotact Funct Neurosurg*, **69**, 112–115.

Kim, S.Y.H., Frank, S., Holloway, R., Zimmerman, C., Wilson, R. and Kierburtz, K. (2005). Science and ethics of sham surgery: a survey of Parkinson's disease clinical researchers. *Arch Neurol*, **62**, 1357–1360.

Kim, T.E., Lee, H.S., Lee, Y.B., Hong, S.H., Lee, Y.S., Ichinose, H., Kim, S.U. and Lee, M.A. (2003). Sonic hedgehog and FGF8 collaborate to induce dopaminergic phenotypes in the Nurr1-overexpressing neural stem cell. *Biochem Biophys Res Commun*, **305**, 1040–1048.

Kirik, D., Winkler, C. and Bjorklund, A. (2001). Growth and functional efficacy of intrastriatal nigral transplants depend on the extent of nigrostriatal degeneration. *J Neurosci*, **21**, 2889–2896.

Kordower, J.H., Freeman, T.B., Snow, B.J., Vingerhoets, F.J., Mufson, E.J., Sanberg, P.R., Hauser, R.A., Smith, D.A., Nauert, G.M., Perl, D.P., et al. (1995). Neuropathological evidence of graft survival and striatal reinnervation after the transplantation of fetal mesencephalic tissue in a patient with Parkinson's disease. *New Engl J Med*, **332**, 1118–1124.

Kordower, J.H., Rosenstein, J.M., Collier, T.J., Burke, M.A., Chen, E.Y., Li, J.M., Martel, L., Levey, A.E., Mufson, E.J., Freeman, T.B. and Olanow, C.W. (1996). Functional fetal nigral grafts in a patient with Parkinson's disease: chemoanatomic, ultrastructural, and metabolic studies. *J Comp Neurol*, **370**, 203–230.

Kordower, J.H., Styren, S., Clarke, M., Dekosky, S.T., Olanow, C.W. and Freeman, T.B. (1997). Fetal grafting for Parkinson's disease: expression of immune markers in two patients with functional fetal nigral implants. *Cell Transplant*, **6**, 213–219.

Kordower, J.H., Freeman, T.B., Chen, E.Y., Mufson, E.J., Sanberg, P.R., Hauser, R.A., Snow, B. and Olanow, C.W. (1998). Fetal nigral grafts survive and mediate clinical benefit in a patient with Parkinson's disease. *Mov Disord*, **13**, 383–393.

Kordower, J.H., Emborg, M.E., Bloch, J., Ma, S.Y., Chu, Y., Leventhal, L., McBride, J., Chen, E.Y., Palfi, S., Roitberg, B.Z., Brown, W.D., Holden, J.E., Pyzalski, R., Taylor, M.D., Carvey, P., Ling, Z., Trono, D., Hantraye, P., Deglon, N. and Aebischer, P. (2000). Neurodegeneration prevented by lentiviral vector delivery of GDNF in primate models of Parkinson's disease. *Science*, **290**, 767–773.

Lang, A.E. and Lozano, A.M. (1998). Parkinson's disease. First of two parts. *New Engl J Med*, **339**, 1044–1053.

Lang, A.E. and Obeso, J.A. (2004a). Challenges in Parkinson's disease: restoration of the nigrostriatal dopamine system is not enough. *Lancet Neurol*, **3**, 309–316.

Lang, A.E. and Obeso, J.A. (2004b). Time to move beyond nigrostriatal dopamine deficiency in Parkinson's disease. *Ann Neurol*, **55**, 761–765.

Lee, C.S., Cenci, M.A., Schulzer, M. and Bjorklund, A. (2000). Embryonic ventral mesencephalic grafts improve levodopa-induced dyskinesia in a rat model of Parkinson's disease. *Brain*, **123**(Pt 7), 1365–1379.

Lin, L.F., Doherty, D.H., Lile, J.D., Bektesh, S. and Collins, F. (1993). GDNF: a glial cell line-derived neurotrophic factor for midbrain dopaminergic neurons. *Science*, **260**, 1130–1132.

Lindvall, O., Backlund, E.O., Farde, L., Sedvall, G., Freedman, R., Hoffer, B., Nobin, A., Seiger, A. and Olson, L. (1987). Transplantation in Parkinson's disease: two cases of adrenal medullary grafts to the putamen. *Ann Neurol*, **22**, 457–468.

Lindvall, O., Brundin, P., Widner, H., Rehncrona, S., Gustavii, B., Frackowiak, R., Leenders, K.L., Sawle, G., Rothwell, J.C., Marsden, C.D., et al. (1990). Grafts of fetal dopamine neurons survive and improve motor function in Parkinson's disease. *Science*, **247**, 574–577.

Lindvall, O., Widner, H., Rehncrona, S., Brundin, P., Odin, P., Gustavii, B., Frackowiak, R., Leenders, K.L., Sawle, G., Rothwell, J.C., et al. (1992). Transplantation of fetal dopamine neurons in Parkinson's disease: one-year clinical and neurophysiological observations in two patients with putaminal implants. *Ann Neurol*, **31**, 155–165.

Lindvall, O., Sawle, G., Widner, H., Rothwell, J.C., Bjorklund, A., Brooks, D., Brundin, P., Frackowiak, R., Marsden, C.D., Odin, P., et al. (1994). Evidence for long-term survival and function of dopaminergic grafts in progressive Parkinson's disease. *Ann Neurol*, **35**, 172–180.

Luquin, M.R., Montoro, R.J., Guillen, J., Saldise, L., Insausti, R., Del Rio, J. and Lopez-Barneo, J. (1999). Recovery of chronic parkinsonian monkeys by autotransplants of carotid body cell aggregates into putamen. *Neuron*, **22**, 743–750.

Ma, Y., Feigin, A., Dhawan, V., Fukuda, M., Shi, Q., Greene, P., Breeze, R., Fahn, S., Freed, C. and Eidelberg, D. (2002). Dyskinesia after fetal cell transplantation for parkinsonism: a PET study. *Ann Neurol*, **52**, 628–634.

Macklin, R. (1999). The ethical problems with sham surgery in clinical research. *New Engl J Med*, **341**, 992–996.

Madrazo, I., Drucker-Colin, R., Diaz, V., Martinez-Mata, J., Torres, C. and Becerril, J.J. (1987). Open microsurgical autograft of adrenal medulla to the right caudate nucleus in two patients with intractable Parkinson's disease. *New Engl J Med*, **316**, 831–834.

Magavi, S.S. and Macklis, J.D. (2001). Manipulation of neural precursors in situ: induction of neurogenesis in the neocortex of adult mice. *Neuropsychopharmacology*, **25**, 816–835.

Marsden, C.D. and Parkes, J.D. (1976). "On-off" effects in patients with Parkinson's disease on chronic levodopa therapy. *Lancet*, **1**, 292–296.

McRae, C., Cherin, E., YAmazaki, T.G., Diem, G., Vo, A.H., Russell, D., Ellgring, J.H., Fahn, S., Greene, P., Dillon, S., Winfield, H., Bjugstad, K.B. and Freed, C.R. (2004). Effects of perceived treatment on quality of life and medical outcomes in a double-blind placebo surgery trial. *Arch Gen Psychiatry*, **61**, 412–420.

Mendez, I., Dagher, A., Hong, M., Gaudet, P., Weerasinghe, S., McAlister, V., King, D., Desrosiers, J., Darvesh, S., Acorn, T. and Robertson, H. (2002). Simultaneous intrastriatal and intranigral fetal dopaminergic grafts in patients with Parkinson disease: a pilot study. Report of three cases. *J Neurosurg*, **96**, 589–596.

Mendez, I., Sanchez-Pernaute, R., Cooper, O., Vinuela, A., Ferrari, D., Bjorklund, L., Dagher, A. and Isacson, O. (2005). Cell type analysis of functional fetal dopamine cell suspension transplants in the striatum and substantia nigra of patients with Parkinson's disease. *Brain*, **128**, 1498–1510.

Meyer, M., Widmer, H.R., Wagner, B., Guzman, R., Evtouchenko, L., Seiler, R.W. and Spenger, C. (1998). Comparison of mesencephalic free-floating tissue culture grafts and cell suspension grafts in the 6-hydroxydopamine-lesioned rat. *Exp Brain Res*, **119**, 345–355.

Murakata, C., Kaneko, M., Gessner, G., Angeles, T.S., Ator, M.A., O'Kane, T.M., McKenna, B.A., Thomas, B.A., Mathiasen, J.R., Saporito, M.S., Bozyczko-Coyne, D. and Hudkins, R.L. (2002). Mixed lineage kinase activity of indolocarbazole analogues. *Bioorg Med Chem Lett*, **12**, 147–150.

Nakao, N., Kakishita, K., Uematsu, Y., Yoshimasu, T., Bessho, T., Nakai, K., Naito, Y. and Itakura, T. (2001). Enhancement of the response to levodopa therapy after intrastriatal transplantation of autologous sympathetic neurons in patients with Parkinson disease. *J Neurosurg*, **95**, 275–284.

Nikkhah, G., Odin, P., Smits, A., Tingstrom, A., Othberg, A., Brundin, P., Funa, K. and Lindvall, O. (1993). Platelet-derived growth factor promotes survival of rat and human mesencephalic dopaminergic neurons in culture. *Exp Brain Res*, **92**, 516–523.

Nikkhah, G., Cunningham, M.G., Jodicke, A., Knappe, U. and Bjorklund, A. (1994). Improved graft survival and striatal reinnervation by microtransplantation of fetal nigral cell suspensions in the rat Parkinson model. *Brain Res*, **633**, 133–143.

Obeso, J.A., Rodriguez-Oroz, M.C., Rodriguez, M., Lanciego, J.L., Artieda, J., Gonzalo, N. and Olanow, C.W. (2000). Pathophysiology of the basal ganglia in Parkinson's disease. *Trends Neurosci*, **23**, S8–S19.

Olanow, C.W. (2003). Present and future directions in the management of motor complications in patients with advanced PD. *Neurology*, **61**, S24–S33.

Olanow, C.W. (2004). The scientific basis for the current treatment of Parkinson's disease. *Annu Rev Med*, **55**, 41–60.

Olanow, C.W. (2005). Double-blind, placebo-controlled trials for surgical interventions in Parkinson's disease. *Arch Neurol*, **62**, 1343–1344.

Olanow, C.W., Koller, W., Goetz, C.G., Stebbins, G.T., Cahill, D.W., Gauger, L.L., Morantz, R., Penn, R.D., Tanner, C.M., Klawans, H.L., et al. (1990). Autologous transplantation of adrenal medulla in Parkinson's disease. 18-month results. *Arch Neurol*, **47**, 1286–1289.

Olanow, C.W., Kordower, J.H. and Freeman, T.B. (1996). Fetal nigral transplantation as a therapy for Parkinson's disease. *Trends Neurosci*, **19**, 102–109.

Olanow, C.W., Watts, R.L. and Koller, W.C. (2001). An algorithm (decision tree) for the management of Parkinson's disease (2001): treatment guidelines. *Neurology*, **56**, S1–S88.

Olanow, C.W., Goetz, C.G., Kordower, J.H., Stoessl, A.J., Sossi, V., Brin, M.F., Shannon, K.M., Nauert, G.M., Perl, D.P., Godbold, J. and Freeman, T.B. (2003). A double-blind controlled trial of bilateral fetal nigral transplantation in Parkinson's disease. *Ann Neurol*, **54**, 403–414.

Olanow, C.W., Agid, Y., Mizuno, Y., Albanese, A., Bonucelli, U., Damier, P., de Yebenes, J., Gershanik, O., Guttman, M., Grandas, F., Hallett, M., Hornykiewicz, O., Jenner, P., Katzenschlager, R., Langston, W.J., Lewitt, P., Melamed, E., Mena, M.A., Michel, P.P., Mytilineou, C., Obeso, J.A., Poewe, W., Quinn, N., Raisman-Vozari, R., Rajput, A.H., Rascol, O., Sampaio, C. and Stocchi, F. (2004). Levodopa in the treatment of Parkinson's disease: current controversies. *Mov Disord*, **19**, 997–1005.

Park, C.H., Minn, Y.K., Lee, J.Y., Choi, D.H., Chang, M.Y., Shim, J.W., Ko, J.Y., Koh, H.C., Kang, M.J., Kang, J.S., Rhie, D.J., Lee, Y.S., Son, H., Moon, S.Y., Kim, K.S. and LEE, S.H. (2005). In vitro and in vivo analyses of human embryonic stem cell-derived dopamine neurons. *J Neurochem*, **92**, 1265–1276.

Perlow, M.J., Freed, W.J., Hoffer, B.J., Seiger, A., Olson, L. and Wyatt, R.J. (1979). Brain grafts reduce motor abnormalities produced by destruction of nigrostriatal dopamine system. *Science*, **204**, 643–647.

Perrier, A.L., Tabar, V., Barberi, T., Rubio, M.E., Bruses, J., Topf, N., Harrison, N.L. and Studer, L. (2004). Derivation of midbrain dopamine neurons from human embryonic stem cells. *Proc Natl Acad Sci USA*, **101**, 12543–12548.

Peschanski, M., Defer, G., N'Guyen, J.P., Ricolfi, F., Monfort, J.C., Remy, P., Geny, C., Samson, Y., Hantraye, P., Jeny, R., et al. (1994). Bilateral motor improvement and alteration of L-dopa effect in two patients with Parkinson's disease following intrastriatal transplantation of foetal ventral mesencephalon. *Brain*, **117**(Pt 3), 487–499.

Peterson, D.I., Price, M.L. and Small, C.S. (1989). Autopsy findings in a patient who had an adrenal-to-brain transplant for Parkinson's disease. *Neurology*, **39**, 235–238.

Piccini, P., Lindvall, O., Bjorklund, A., Brundin, P., Hagell, P., Ceravolo, R., Oertel, W., Quinn, N., Samuel, M., Rehncrona, S., Widner, H. and Brooks, D.J. (2000). Delayed recovery of movement-related cortical function in Parkinson's disease after striatal dopaminergic grafts. *Ann Neurol*, **48**, 689–695.

Remy, P., Samson, Y., Hantraye, P., Fontaine, A., Defer, G., Mangin, J.F., Fenelon, G., Geny, C., Ricolfi, F., Frouin, V., et al. (1995). Clinical correlates of [18F]fluorodopa uptake in five grafted parkinsonian patients. *Ann Neurol*, **38**, 580–588.

Rodriguez, M.C., Obeso, J.A. and Olanow, C.W. (1998). Subthalamic nucleus-mediated excitotoxicity in Parkinson's disease: a target for neuroprotection. *Ann Neurol*, **44**, S175–S188.

Schierle, G.S., Hansson, O., Leist, M., Nicotera, P., Widner, H. and Brundin, P. (1999). Caspase inhibition reduces apoptosis and increases survival of nigral transplants. *Nat Med*, **5**, 97–100.

Schmidt, R.H., Ingvar, M., Lindvall, O., Stenevi, U. and Bjorklund, A. (1982). Functional activity of substantia nigra grafts reinnervating the striatum: neurotransmitter metabolism and [14C]2-deoxy-d-glucose autoradiography. *J Neurochem*, **38**, 737–748.

Schumacher, J.M., Ellias, S.A., Palmer, E.P., Kott, H.S., Dinsmore, J., Dempsey, P.K., Fischman, A.J., Thomas, C., Feldman, R.G., Kassissieh, S., Raineri, R., Manhart, C., Penney, D., Fink, J.S. and Isacson, O. (2000). Transplantation of embryonic porcine mesencephalic tissue in patients with PD. *Neurology*, **54**, 1042–1050.

Shinoda, M., Hudson, J.L., Stromberg, I., Hoffer, B.J., Moorhead, J.W. and Olson, L. (1995). Allogeneic grafts of fetal dopamine neurons: immunological reactions following active and adoptive immunizations. *Brain Res*, **680**, 180–195.

Shinoda, M., Hudson, J.L., Stromberg, I., Hoffer, B.J., Moorhead, J.W. and Olson, L. (1996). Microglial cell responses to fetal ventral mesencephalic tissue grafting and to active and adoptive immunizations. *Exp Neurol*, **141**, 173–180.

Shukla, S., Agrawal, A.K., Chaturvedi, R.K., Seth, K., Srivastava, N., Sinha, C., Shukla, Y., Khanna, V.K. and Seth, P.K. (2004). Co-transplantation of carotid body and ventral mesencephalic cells as an alternative approach towards functional restoration in 6-hydroxydopamine-lesioned rats: implications for Parkinson's disease. *J Neurochem*, **91**, 274–284.

Sortwell, C.E., Pitzer, M.R. and Collier, T.J. (2000). Time course of apoptotic cell death within mesencephalic cell suspension grafts: implications for improving grafted dopamine neuron survival. *Exp Neurol*, **165**, 268–277.

Sortwell, C.E., Collier, T.J., Camargo, M.D. and Pitzer, M.R. (2004). An in vitro interval before transplantation of mesencephalic reaggregates does not compromise survival or functionality. *Exp Neurol*, **187**, 58–64.

Storch, A., Sabolek, M., Milosevic, J., Schwarz, S.C. and Schwarz, J. (2004). Midbrain-derived neural stem cells: from basic science to therapeutic approaches. *Cell Tissue Res*, **318**, 15–22.

Studer, L., Spenger, C., Seiler, R.W., Altar, C.A., Lindsay, R.M. and Hyman, C. (1995). Comparison of the effects of the neurotrophins on the morphological structure of dopaminergic neurons in cultures of rat substantia nigra. *Eur J Neurosci*, **7**, 223–233.

Subramanian, T., Marchionini, D., Potter, E.M. and Cornfeldt, M.L. (2002). Striatal xenotransplantation of human retinal pigment epithelial cells attached to microcarriers in hemiparkinsonian rats ameliorates behavioral deficits without provoking a host immune response. *Cell Transplant*, **11**, 207–214.

Takagi, Y., Takahashi, J., Saiki, H., Morizane, A., Hayashi, T., Kishi, Y., Fukuda, H., Okamoto, Y., Koyanagi, M., Ideguchi, M., Hayashi, H., Imazato, T., Kawasaki, H., Suemori, H., Omachi, S., Iida, H., Itoh, N., Nakatsuji, N., Sasai, Y. and Hashimoto, N. (2005). Dopaminergic neurons generated from monkey embryonic stem cells function in a Parkinson primate model. *J Clin Invest*, **115**, 102–109.

Timmer, M., Muller-Ostermeyer, F., Kloth, V., Winkler, C., Grothe, C. and Nikkhah, G. (2004). Enhanced survival, reinnervation, and functional recovery of intrastriatal dopamine grafts co-transplanted with Schwann cells overexpressing high molecular weight FGF-2 isoforms. *Exp Neurol*, **187**, 118–136.

Toledo-Aral, J.J., Mendez-Ferrer, S., Pardal, R., Echevarria, M. and Lopez-Barneo, J. (2003). Trophic restoration of the nigrostriatal dopaminergic pathway in long-term carotid body-grafted parkinsonian rats. *J Neurosci*, **23**, 141–148.

Tooyama, I., McGeer, E.G., Kawamata, T., Kimura, H. and McGeer, P.L. (1994). Retention of basic fibroblast growth factor immunoreactivity in dopaminergic neurons of the substantia nigra during normal aging in humans contrasts with loss in Parkinson's disease. *Brain Res*, **656**, 165–168.

Wang, X., Lu, Y., Zhang, H., Wang, K., He, Q., Wang, Y., Liu, X., Li, L. and Wang, X. (2004). Distinct efficacy of pre-differentiated versus intact fetal mesencephalon-derived human neural progenitor cells in alleviating rat model of Parkinson's disease. *Int J Dev Neurosci*, **22**, 175–183.

Watts, R.L., Raiser, C.D., Stover, N.P., Cornfeldt, M.L., Schweikert, A.W., Allen, R.C., Subramanian, T., Doudet, D., Honey, C.R. and Bakay, R.A. (2003). Stereotaxic intrastriatal implantation of human retinal pigment epithelial (hRPE) cells attached to gelatin microcarriers: a potential new cell therapy for Parkinson's disease. *J Neural Transm Suppl*, 215–227.

Wenning, G.K., Odin, P., Morrish, P., Rehncrona, S., Widner, H., Brundin, P., Rothwell, J.C., Brown, R., Gustavii, B., Hagell, P., Jahanshahi, M., Sawle, G., Bjorklund, A., Brooks, D.J., Marsden, C.D., Quinn, N.P. and Lindvall, O. (1997). Short- and long-term survival and function of unilateral intrastriatal dopaminergic grafts in Parkinson's disease. *Ann Neurol*, **42**, 95–107.

Winkler, C., Sauer, H., Lee, C.S. and Bjorklund, A. (1996). Short-term GDNF treatment provides long-term rescue of lesioned nigral dopaminergic neurons in a rat model of Parkinson's disease. *J Neurosci*, **16**, 7206–7215.

Winkler, C., Kirik, D. and Bjorklund, A. (2005). Cell transplantation in Parkinson's disease: how can we make it work? *Trends Neurosci*, **28**, 86–92.

Wuerthele, S.M., Freed, W.J., Olson, L., Morihisa, J., Spoor, L., Wyatt, R.J. and Hoffer, B.J. (1981). Effect of dopamine agonists and antagonists on the electrical activity of substantia nigra neurons transplanted into the lateral ventricle of the rat. *Exp Brain Res*, **44**, 1–10.

Xu, Z., Maroney, A.C., Dobrzanski, P., Kukekov, N.V. and Greene, L.A. (2001). The MLK family mediates c-Jun N-terminal kinase activation in neuronal apoptosis. *Mol Cell Biol*, **21**, 4713–4724.

Yang, M., Stull, N.D., Berk, M.A., Snyder, E.Y. and Iacovitti, L. (2002). Neural stem cells spontaneously express dopaminergic traits after transplantation into the intact or 6-hydroxydopamine-lesioned rat. *Exp Neurol*, **177**, 50–60.

Yasuhara, T., Shingo, T., Kobayashi, K., Takeuchi, A., Yano, A., Muraoka, K., Matsui, T., Miyoshi, Y., Hamada, H. and Date, I. (2004). Neuroprotective effects of vascular endothelial growth factor (VEGF) upon dopaminergic neurons in a rat model of Parkinson's disease. *Eur J Neurosci*, **19**, 1494–1504.

Yoshizaki, T., Inaji, M., Kouike, H., Shimazaki, T., Sawamoto, K., Ando, K., Date, I., Kobayashi, K., Suhara, T., Uchiyama, Y. and Okano, H. (2004). Isolation and transplantation of dopaminergic neurons generated from mouse embryonic stem cells. *Neurosci Lett*, **363**, 33–37.

Zawada, W.M., Zastrow, D.J., Clarkson, E.D., Adams, F.S., Bell, K.P. and Freed, C. R. (1998). Growth factors improve immediate survival of embryonic dopamine neurons after transplantation into rats. *Brain Res*, **786**, 96–103.

List of abbreviations

6-OHDA	6-hydroxyl dopamine
AADC	Aromatic acid decarboxylase
BDNF	Brain derived neurotrophic factor
DBS	Deep brain stimulation
ES	Embryonic stem cell
FD	Flourodopa
FGF2	Fibroblast growth factor 2
GDNF	Glial derived neurotrophic factor
GPi	Globus pallidus pars interna
NSC	Neural stem cell
PD	Parkinson's disease
PET	Positron emission tomography
SNc	Substantia nigra pars compacta
STN	Subthalamic nucleus
TH	Tyrosine hydroxylase
UPDRS	Unified Parkinson's disease rating scale
VEGF	Vascular endothelial growth factor

Conditions of task practice for individuals with neurologic impairments

Carolee J. Winstein and Jill Campbell Stewart

Department of Biokinesiology and Physical Therapy, University of Southern California, LOS Angeles, CA

7.1 Introduction

Significant growth and interest in the field of rehabilitation medicine has been fueled in part by advances in rehabilitation science within an interdisciplinary research model (DeLisa, 2004). More importantly, research in rehabilitation has witnessed the application of the scientific method to specific functional problems such as the recovery of walking in neurologic populations (Barbeau and Fung, 2001) and the recovery of upper extremity (UE) use after stroke-hemiparesis (Taub and Uswatte, 2003). Recently, this translational research has spawned various protocol-based treatments, for example, to enhance walking in individuals with spinal cord injury (Field-Fote, 2001) and chronic stroke (Sullivan et al., 2002), and to enable use of the hemiparetic UE in adults with sub-acute stroke (Winstein et al., 2003). However, if rehabilitation medicine is to join the ranks of other evidence-based medical and pharmaceutical practices, objective treatment protocols will become a necessary component of valid efficacy and effectiveness research (Whyte and Hart, 2003). The development of specific and objective rehabilitation treatment protocols will be a clear signal of progress in the field of rehabilitation medicine. At present, the majority of published protocols in neurologic rehabilitation lack an explicit scientific rationale for the intensity, duration, and content (e.g., task-specific versus muscle-specific) of training used within the rehabilitation treatments. Without an explicit rationale (or even hypothesis), the precise parameters of training for a given rehabilitation treatment can take

on a mythical quality with hidden meaning at worst, and lead to "blind" following at best (Dromerick, 2003). This process undermines scientific enquiry and in some cases tends to hinder the development of alternative and innovative approaches. For example, Why is the signature constraint-induced therapy (CIT) protocol of 6 h/day (60 h total) with one-on-one supervised training for no less than a 2-week period (10 days) "optimal" for achieving an effect (Taub and Uswatte, 2003)?[1] How important is the "constraint" within a CIT training protocol? Why is a typical bout of step training with body weight support during treadmill walking 20 min in duration, 3 times/week for 4 weeks (Sullivan et al., 2002)? These rhetorical questions suggest that the field of rehabilitation medicine is at a critical cross-road in its development. On one hand, defining rehabilitation treatments is necessary for this field to advance, but on the other hand, its practitioners must heed the temptation to simply adopt these protocols without questioning their rationale, refining patient selection criteria, revising the parameters of training to fit patient characteristics and rehabilitation goals, and developing reliable prognostic indicators of outcome (Dobkin, 2004; Whitall, 2004).

Stroke is the leading cause of disability among American adults. Nearly 3 million of Americans are stroke affected; each year, approximately 700,000 people suffer a stroke and the estimated economic

[1] It is perhaps no accident that most behavior modification programs that are based on traditional operant-conditioning methods are 2 weeks in duration.

burden from stroke-related disability is 35 billion dollars annually in direct costs (American Heart Association, 2005). More effective acute management of stroke has resulted in declining mortality while the number of stroke survivors who need long-term care or rehabilitation is expected to greatly increase, imposing an enormous economic burden on individuals and society (Rundek et al., 2000; Chapter 36 of Volume II). Residual burden of care is significant with 44% of community-based individuals post-stroke in a National Survey reporting difficulty with at least five to six activities of daily life (Chan et al., 2002). Surprisingly, despite these impressive statistics, there has been little principled and systematic research to determine the most effective and efficient parameters of training or conditions of task practice for the rehabilitation of the motor skills that constitute a significant portion of daily life.

In cases where movement deficits result from a stroke, intense task practice, defined as repeated attempts to produce motor behaviors beyond present capabilities, is considered the most crucial component for recovery (Butefisch et al., 1995; Kwakkel et al., 1999; Wolf et al., 2002). Previous work that has invoked performance improvements and/or experience-dependent neuroplasticity shows that large amounts of practice (consisting of 1000s sometimes 10,000s of trials) are needed (Pavlides et al., 1993; Karni, 1995; Nudo et al., 1996; Doyon et al., 1997). See Chapters 8 and 14 in Volume I for details about cortical re-organization and learning-dependent changes associated with task practice. These large amounts of practice are a dramatic contrast to the limited time that patients post-stroke spend in therapeutic activities: on average between 30 and 40 min/day (Keith and Cowell, 1987; Lincoln et al., 1996). Further, patients typically spend 70% of the day in activities largely unrelated to physical outcome and less than 20% of the day in activities that could *potentially* contribute to their recovery (Mackey et al., 1996). In sum, current medical "practice" models in stroke rehabilitation are not designed to enhance recovery and maximize functional outcomes. Thus, a critical goal of rehabilitation science is to understand the parameters of training and conditions of task practice that will optimize functional outcomes from rehabilitation programs (Whitall, 2004; Weinrich et al., 2005).

7.2 Parameters of exercise training depend on the goal

Would you choose different parameters of exercise training, including frequency (number of training sessions in a given period), intensity (within session attributes for training goal and progression), and duration (total number of sessions or hours), if the goals were specific for: (1) muscle strengthening; (2) cardiovascular endurance; (3) reversal of "learned-non-use"; or (4) motor skill acquisition? We ask this rhetorical question to emphasize the point that without explicit discussion of the goals of exercise training for individuals with neurologic impairments, the selection of precise parameters will have undefined rationale. Perhaps, more importantly, without a sound theoretical framework for exercise parameter selection, future clinical trials in this field will be limited to a purely empirical approach, an approach that will not survive the rigors of scientific review (Verville and DeLisa, 2003). Future advances in rehabilitation science will depend on the development of hypothesis-driven clinical trials that are designed to test relevant and innovative ideas about exercise training (Dobkin, 2004).

For these reasons, we distinguish between exercise and task-specific training in neurorehabilitation. The term "exercise training" in the classical sense refers to cardiovascular fitness training (aerobic and anaerobic) or muscle strength training. The goal for these exercise training protocols is either cardiovascular conditioning as evidenced by various performance-based tests including VO_2 peak in the former or targeted levels of voluntary muscle force (e.g., maximum torque) or muscle endurance (e.g., sub-maximal torque levels for a given duration) in the latter. There is an extensive literature in both of these areas that can be used to develop appropriate exercise parameters for the desired goal, including in individuals with neurologic impairments. The reader is referred to Chapter 21 by MacKay-Lyons in this volume for an excellent discussion of cardiovascular fitness and training in neurorehabilitation and Chapter 18 by Blanton and Wolf for a review of UE muscle weakness following stroke.

Task-specific training, in contrast to a generic exercise program, focuses on improving the performance of functional tasks through repetition and goal-oriented practice. A task-specific training program and a generic exercise program, therefore, have fundamentally different goals. Further, task-specific training can be quite limited without a foundation grounded in the rubric of skill learning. For purposes of this chapter, we define a motor skill as one in which the task is performed effectively, efficiently, and within a variety of environmental contexts (Gordon, 2000). When the goal of rehabilitation is to enhance skilled task performance, the appropriate resources such as strength, endurance, motor control, and coordination provide the foundation that supports task practice. Given this specific therapeutic goal, the purpose of this chapter is to provide a scientific rationale for choosing the conditions of practice that best promote skill learning in the context of task-specific training for diminished functional ability in the neurologically impaired patient. First, we define skill and motor learning within the context of neurorehabilitation. Next, we discuss the differences between "use" and "skill" as these terms apply to UE and manual actions. We argue that this distinction becomes important for choosing the appropriate conditions of practice for individuals post-stroke. Next, we review the literature pertaining to two important conditions of practice known to be critical for motor skill learning: (1) augmented feedback and explicit information and (2) task scheduling. For each we outline how these conditions might be manipulated to promote recovery of functional skills in the neurologically impaired patient.

7.3 Motor learning, skills and the disablement model

A 1997 research agenda that emanated from a workshop focused on facilitating patient learning during medical rehabilitation proposed that "the effectiveness and efficiency of learning-oriented practices will likely be enhanced by well-formulated investigations grounded in available learning theory and research" (Fuhrer and Keith, 1998, p. 560). More recently others have argued for the need to investigate and better explain the specific ingredients of rehabilitation protocols including the conditions of practice that optimize learning and recovery (Whyte and Hart, 2003). A program that focuses on the learning of motor skills can take a "top-down approach" whereby the inability to perform a personal or societal role is identified first. Then, further evaluation and analysis determines the functional skills required to meet those roles and the impairments (strength, coordination, endurance, etc.) that are interfering with an individual's ability to perform these skills (Gordon, 2000). Such a model takes into account the levels of Nagi's model of disablement, including: pathology, impairment, functional limitation, and disability. For neurologic disorders in which motor control deficits are marked (e.g., stroke-hemiparesis), the underlying impairments require attention if functional ability is to improve (Sunderland and Tuke, 2005; Wolf et al., 2005). Emphasis on the underlying impairments, termed resources, in the top-down model allows the development of more efficient and flexible movement strategies that can be used in a variety of task and environmental contexts.

Task-specific training focused on improving the skill with which an individual performs motor tasks draws heavily upon the principles of learning derived from the cognitive neuroscience and movement science literature. Motor learning is a set of processes associated with "practice" or experience leading to relatively permanent changes in the capability for responding (Schmidt and Lee, 2005). Three key terms/phrases that are critical for determining optimal parameters and conditions of training are "practice", "relatively permanent", and "capability". Amount of practice is the most important variable for motor skill learning (Schmidt and Lee, 2005). Equally important, however, is that the learner be actively involved in solving the motor problem during practice (Lee and Maraj, 1994; Gordon, 2000). Simple repetition of a task is not sufficient to increase skill or promote the associated cortical re-organization (Plautz et al., 2000). The learner must perform the task under conditions that require variations in speed, timing, and environmental conditions that require him/her to generate successful motor solutions. If the learner is challenged to assess task conditions and to prepare and generate an appropriate response over practice trials, the probability is greater that an ability is acquired to adapt those responses to the ever-changing circumstances of daily life. It is this ability to adapt that provides the individual with the capability to perform a task over time (relatively permanent change).

7.4 Spontaneous use versus skilled performance in arm and hand rehabilitation training

Programs that employ task-specific training can do so for a variety of reasons. In the context of CIT, practice is designed to reverse the sub-acute conditioning that leads to decreased spontaneous use of an extremity, referred to as "learned-non-use" (Taub et al., 1994, 2003). By contrast, a training program for patients with diminished motor control and impaired functional ability is designed to promote skilled performance (Dean and Shepherd, 1997; Sunderland and Tuke, 2005; Winstein and Prettyman, 2005).

CIT protocols grew out of the behavioral model put forth by Taub and colleagues (1994) in which it is proposed that during the early post-injury phase (e.g., deafferentation), use of the limb is suppressed when spontaneous attempts to move it are unsuccessful (negative reinforcement). This conditioned response is "learned" and ultimately results in diminished spontaneous use. The design of CIT protocols is therefore directed towards the reversal of learned-non-use

and the increase of spontaneous use of the hemiparetic limb in individuals post-stroke. Since the goal of CIT is to promote spontaneous hand use and not necessarily to develop skilled use, the conditions of practice are designed directly from operant-conditioning principles and include the "shaping" procedure. With shaping, a behavior is progressively modified towards the goal through successive approximation and positive reinforcement. In contrast to a motor-learning-based approach, the "shaping" procedure as described within the context of CIT (Morris et al., 1997; Taub et al., 2003), does not address the known resource impairments of motor control, strength and coordination (Sunderland and Tuke, 2005).

Skinner (1968) taught us that shaping was a form of operant conditioning in which the probability of experimenter determined behaviors are "elicited" through reinforcement (reward or punishment). Using this procedure he shaped pigeons to peck a ping-pong ball over a net. Obviously, the pigeon is not aware that this is a game-like, goal-oriented behavior. In fact, the learner (i.e., pigeon in this case) is relatively passive in this process while performance is progressively "shaped" towards the behavioral objective (task goal) in small steps through reinforcement or reward (positive feedback).

The shaping procedure is designed around the elicitation of behavior and not the acquisition of a voluntary skill. In fact, the pigeon, or any animal, can be shaped without knowing or ever understanding the goal behavior. The shaping procedure stands in sharp contrast to the procedures employed when designing task practice to optimize motor skill learning in the context of neurorehabilitation. For skill acquisition, the learner practices under a set of active learning principles that are derived from more modern theories of learning and memory (Cahill et al., 2001) such as those reviewed in Chapter 2 of Volume I. For example, an operant-conditioning model treats "augmented feedback" as a form of "reinforcement" or reward, while a skill-learning model treats "augmented feedback" as information about performance for cognitive processing (e.g., problem-solving) relevant to the preparation for the next practice trial.

If augmented feedback operates like positive rein-forcement, designing practice with frequent rewards should enhance learning within an operant-conditioning-based approach. In contrast, if aug-mented feedback operates like post-response information that elicits cognitive processing and problem-solving, designing practice with a faded feedback schedule, where feedback is provided on progressively fewer trials, should enhance learning within a motor-learning-based approach. Table 7.1 compares and contrasts training principles derived from each of these two learning models (operant con-ditioning and voluntary skill) as they apply to the choice of task practice variables to enhance recovery. In the remaining sections of this chapter, we review the literature and expand the discussion of two of

Table 7.1. Comparison of training principles between operant-conditioning and motor-learning-based interventions.

Practice variable	Operant-conditioning training principles	Motor-learning training principles
	Lifting of learned suppression explains the increased use of the affected limb in real-world activities: • Learned-non-use develops from negative reinforcement during the acute stage where non-reinforced behavior becomes suppressed. • Successful performance and positive reinforcement are necessary to lift the suppression allowing the behavior to be expressed in a real-world environment.	Skill acquisition, motor program, or schema formation and the development of internal representations for action explain the increased functional use of the affected limb for purposeful, volitional activities: • Automatic and implicit procedural knowledge develops with practice of motor tasks. • Tasks are controlled more automatically and with less cognitive effort; this manifests as skill develops.
Amount and scheduling of practice	Massed practice is essential for cortical re-organization and reversal of learned-non-use: • "Massed" practice in CIT is the term used to mean intense or extensive practice that is necessary to reverse learned-non-use and leads to cortical re-organization. • The optimal duration, intensity, or challenge (level of difficulty) of practice for enhancing functional recovery has not been determined.	Physical practice is the most important variable for motor learning: • Practice that challenges the learner is motivating and optimal for learning-dependent cortical re-organization. • The term "massed" practice is contrasted with "distributed" practice where within a bout of practice the distribution of practice-rest is manipulated. In "massed" practice, there is little to no rest and performance decrements due to fatigue are generally not considered detrimental to learning.
Task progression	Shaping of motor behavior is essential especially for patients with limited ability: • Shaping is based on the idea of successive approximations. • Guidelines for progression are performance based and not learning based.	Task progression is learning based and depends on an analysis of underlying motor control deficits (strength, coordination, etc.): • Progression can be accomplished by manipulating a variety of variables depending on individual needs (e.g., speed, ROM, adding or freeing degrees of freedom, part-whole task practice). • These progression techniques are recommended especially for the lower or beginning levels of skill acquisition. • Task complexity and parameterization within a class of actions are important components of task progression.

(Cont.)

Table 7.1. (*Cont.*)

	Operant-conditioning training principles	Motor-learning training principles
Practice variability	Diversity of tasks leads to a more generalized benefit of practice: • During shaping, no more than two sets of 10 trials of a given task should be practiced in a single day.	Contextual variety enhances problem-solving and retention of skills: • The task practice schedule is designed to challenge the cognitive operations important for future capability in variable contexts.
Augmented feedback	Constant and frequent feedback is necessary for optimal lifting of learned suppression: • The informational content of feedback is de-emphasized while reinforcement and encouragement are emphasized.	Reduced augmented feedback (KR, KP) frequency and faded schedules that promote problem-solving and the development of internal error-detection capabilities are more beneficial for learning than constant and frequent feedback: • The informational content of feedback is emphasized and is distinct from the encouragement provided during practice.
Role of errors	Errors during performance are ignored: • Error feedback serves as negative reinforcement and is detrimental to the reversal of learned suppression of behavior. • Errors are viewed as punishment that leads to avoidance of the behavior.	Errors during performance are beneficial to learning and therefore should be provided as information feedback to the performer: • Errors are viewed as information that can be useful for planning the next trial. • Movement problems are effectively solved partially through the provision of error information (feedback).
Social-cognitive factors	Behaviors are "elicited" in this model. These behaviors can be shaped through successive approximations during practice with positive reinforcement: • Collaboration with the patient for task selection or engagement for self-management and development of self-efficacy are not directly addressed in this model.	The development of skill through practice is by nature embedded into a meaningful and social context: • The choice of tasks to practice and the development of self-efficacy as performance improves are intertwined with this approach and are recognized mediators for self-management and maintenance after training ends.

KP: knowledge of performance; ROM: range of motion.

these practice variables, augmented feedback and task scheduling, as they relate to motor skill acquisition in neurorehabilitation.

7.5 Conditions of practice to promote functional recovery of motor skills

Augmented feedback and explicit information

It is well known that augmented feedback provided during or after trial completion can be manipulated to enhance motor learning. Following a movement, the learner is able to evaluate performance based on internally generated, intrinsic feedback provided through the perceptual and sensory systems. Augmented feedback, in contrast, is provided by an external source, such as a trainer or therapist, and provides error information that can be used in addition to the learner's own intrinsic error signals. Knowledge of results (KR) is one form of augmented feedback and is defined as "verbal (or verbalizable), terminal (i.e., post-movement) feedback about the outcome of the movement in terms of the environmental goal"

(Schmidt and Lee, 1999, p. 325). KR can be provided after every practice trial, after only a portion of trials, termed reduced relative frequency of KR, or when performance falls outside a pre-determined acceptable range, called bandwidth KR. Here we review the effect of reducing the relative frequency of KR as an example of how manipulating augmented feedback can impact motor skill learning.

Relative frequency of KR refers to the percentage of total practice trials for which KR is provided, such as 50% (half of the trials) or 25% (one-quarter of the trials). The prescribed relative frequency or scheduling can be accomplished in different ways. For example, a 50% relative frequency schedule may be achieved by providing KR on every other trial. It may also be achieved by use of a faded schedule whereby an average relative frequency of 50% is obtained by providing more frequent KR during early practice (say 100%) and progressively reducing the frequency over trials (e.g., to 25%) (Winstein and Schmidt, 1990; Schmidt and Lee, 2005).

While several studies found no benefit of a decreased KR frequency on learning a linear positioning task (Sparrow and Summers, 1992; Sparrow, 1995), multiple studies have found a beneficial effect on the learning of other motor tasks in healthy young adults (Ho and Shea, 1978; Wulf and Schmidt, 1989; Lee et al., 1990; Winstein and Schmidt, 1990; Vander Linden et al., 1993; Wulf et al., 1993, 1994; Winstein et al., 1994; Lai and Shea, 1998; Goodwin et al., 2001). This benefit seen when KR is provided only after a percentage of practice trials has also been demonstrated in older, healthy adults (Behrman et al., 1992; Swanson and Lee, 1992) except in one study where a reduced frequency KR schedule did not benefit either younger or older subjects (Wishart and Lee, 1997). Why might reducing the frequency of augmented feedback benefit learning? KR is beneficial in that it provides useful information that leads to improved performance on the next trial and, therefore, facilitates learning of the motor task. If feedback is provided after every trial or at high relative frequencies though, the learner may become dependent on the KR such that it can be detrimental to performance on trials without KR (i.e., retention test) and actually

degrade learning. In essence, an optimal schedule of KR provides an opportunity for practice that attenuates dependence on the extrinsic KR, promotes the development of intrinsic error-detection capabilities, and allows active engagement in information processing activities required for future skillful action (Salmoni et al., 1984; Schmidt, 1991). Additionally, it is imperative for the learner to be able to perform a given task without augmented feedback as this is how tasks are performed in the "real world". This is an important point when discussing feedback in rehabilitation; patients must be able to perform tasks once they leave the sheltered rehabilitation setting. Conditions of practice that promote the development of intrinsic error-detection capabilities are important for self-maintenance and persistence of skilled performance in the future.

While a reduced KR frequency may benefit learning of relatively simple laboratory tasks, it is yet unclear if such a KR schedule also benefits learning more complex real-world skills that may require several days to learn and involve multiple degrees of freedom (Wulf and Shea, 2002; Guadagnoli and Lee, 2004). Research that used summary KR, where a summary of performance is provided after a specified number of trials, suggested that more frequent feedback may be needed when practicing a complex motor skill (Wulf and Shea, 2002). Additionally, Wulf et al. (1998) found that reducing KR frequency did not benefit the learning of a complex ski simulation task. In fact, the group that practiced the task while receiving continuous, 100% KR performed better on a retention test than did the 50% KR group. Therefore, it seems that there is something different about learning a complex task compared with a simple task. One hypothesis is that the cognitive processing demands may be inherently greater for the learning of a complex task (Wulf and Shea, 2002). If a reduced KR frequency schedule requires more processing by the learner compared to one with feedback after every trial, then we might imagine that the aggregate processing demands could be quite large for the learning of a complex task under conditions of reduced KR frequency. In this case, the processing demands may be too high resulting in diminished learning. There is a great deal yet to be learned about the interaction of task complexity and augmented feedback scheduling to enhance motor learning.

Several studies have demonstrated that individuals post-stroke have the ability to learn a new motor task (Platz et al., 1994; Hanlon, 1996; Pohl and Winstein, 1999; Winstein et al., 1999). Only one study to date has directly investigated the effect of reducing the relative frequency of KR on learning in individuals post-stroke. Winstein et al. (1999) used a lever task that required subjects to learn a series of elbow flexion–extension movements with specific amplitude and timing requirements using the less-involved UE. While their performance was not as accurate as age-matched controls, the subjects with stroke were able to demonstrate learning of the task as measured by a delayed retention test. Both control and stroke Participants that practiced the task under a faded feedback schedule (67% average KR frequency) condition demonstrated similar learning when compared to their peers who received KR after every trial (100% KR frequency). While the faded schedule of KR did not enhance learning, it was not detrimental either. Additionally, the subjects with stroke demonstrated very similar performance curves to control subjects when compared across feedback conditions. Therefore, the results of this study suggest that the literature on relative frequency of KR with healthy control subjects may be applicable to individuals with stroke (Winstein et al., 1999).

Further work is needed to better understand the benefits of augmented feedback for motor learning in individuals with central nervous system pathology. While the Winstein et al. (1999) study suggests that individuals with stroke benefit from feedback similarly to controls, this research needs to be replicated and expanded to include other tasks. Recent work that manipulated explicit instructions (Boyd and Winstein, 2004) found that when individuals post-stroke were provided with explicit information during practice of an implicit lever task, performance and learning was disrupted. This was not the case for age-matched control subjects who actually demonstrated better learning across days when explicit information was provided than when it was not. Although explicit prescriptive information about the movement strategy is distinctly different from post-response augmented feedback, this work in general suggests that there may be differences in the way in which motor skills are learned between individuals post-stroke and age-matched controls. The information provided, including augmented feedback or explicit task information, may be processed in different ways after brain damage. It is hoped that these ideas will invoke new approaches and hypotheses for rehabilitation science as researchers from multiple disciplines including psychologic and physiologic science collaborate to gain a better understanding of the neural correlates of motor learning (Miller and Keller, 2000).

Task scheduling

Individuals post-stroke generally need to learn or re-learn numerous tasks during rehabilitation. Optimal scheduling of to-be-learned items has been the subject of considerable behavioral research since early in the 20th century. The literature emphasizes two key principles of task scheduling: (1) spacing of trials is better than massing trials (for reviews see Lee and Genovese, 1988; Druckman and Bjork, 1991; Dempster, 1996; Donovan and Radosevich, 1999) and (2) a random task practice schedule is better than a blocked task practice schedule (for reviews see Magill and Hall, 1990; Brady, 2004) for the learning of motor skills in healthy adults. While there is limited research about how these principles apply to individuals post-stroke, the findings from these lines of research can be used to provide some guidance for clinicians and researchers as to the best way to structure practice for motor learning (Marley et al., 2000).

One of the most robust finding in this domain of study is the so-called "spacing effect" according to which distributed presentation of an item strongly increases the retention of learned material compared to massed presentations. In a massed practice schedule, there is typically little to no time between presentations of the same task (Fig. 7.1(a)). In a distributed practice schedule, the inter-trial interval between task presentations is longer than in a massed schedule, an arrangement that can persist for

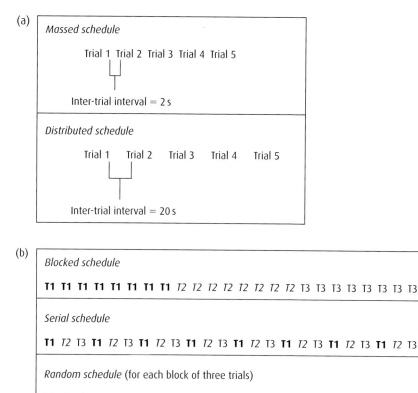

Figure 7.1. Examples of the micro-scheduling of practice for motor-learning studies. (a) Practice of five trials of a single task in a massed and distributed schedule. (b) Practice of three different tasks for eight trials each in schedules with varying levels of contextual variety. **T1**: Task 1; *T2*: Task 2; and T3: Task 3.

dozens of seconds to weeks in duration. A benefit for distributed practice has been shown in a variety of motor tasks from pursuit rotor (Bourne and Archer, 1956) to typing (Baddeley and Longman, 1978). Lee and Genovese (1989), however, found that a distributed practice schedule did not benefit learning of a discrete tapping task compared to a massed schedule. In addition, others have suggested that a distributed practice schedule may not always be optimal and that boundary conditions likely exist related to task type, overall task complexity, and the length of the inter-trial interval (Donovan and Radosevich, 1999).

Distributing practice of several items during a rehabilitation session, however, would be extremely time consuming if the inter-trial interval contained only empty time. An alternative would be to insert other tasks within the vacant "space" so that multiple tasks could be practiced simultaneously. Contextual interference (CI) is "the interference effects in performance and learning that arise from practicing one task in the context of other tasks" (Schmidt and Lee, 1999, p. 412). It is well accepted that a random practice schedule (Fig. 7.1(b)) provides greater CI than a blocked schedule and is generally thought to be better for learning motor skills in healthy adults (Shea and Morgan, 1979; Lee and Magill, 1983; Shea et al., 1990; Sekiya et al., 1994, 1996; Wright and Shea, 2001). It is important to note that a random practice schedule also provides space between repeated trials of the same task. For example, a blocked schedule for the practice of three tasks would provide 0 intervening items between presentations of the same task.

A random schedule, in comparison, would provide a range from 0 to 4 intervening items between presentations of a single item. Therefore, a random practice schedule provides greater spacing, or number of intervening items, than a blocked schedule.

Why might a random practice schedule be better for learning than a blocked practice schedule? One hypothesis is that the processing demands for learning are different for these two practice schedules. In a blocked schedule, the learner knows which item will be presented on the next trial. In a random schedule, the learner does not know which item will be presented next. Therefore, a random schedule is thought to require greater attention and deeper processing (Shea and Zimny, 1983; Lee and Magill, 1985; Lee and Maraj, 1994). However, Lee and Magill (1983) showed that a serial schedule, where the task schedule was predictable but not blocked, was equivalent in effect to that of a random schedule. The predictability of the next task was not the critical factor in this study, but rather the process of determining the movement requirements, and preparing and generating a new solution with each trial. This process required the learner to be more actively engaged in the practice session under random or serial task schedules compared with the blocked task schedule. This analysis suggests that it is the engagement in information processing surrounding task performance and not just the task performance itself that is critical for effective motor learning. In this case, what is learned enables the individual to perform the task with skill effectively with differing speeds and directions and under a variety of environmental contexts.

Recently, though, some authors have questioned whether the CI effect generalizes to all tasks and conditions. It is not clear if random practice is always better for learning more difficult, real-world tasks (Wulf and Shea, 2002; Brady, 2004). Albaret and Thon (1998) found such an effect when studying the learning of a drawing task. Random practice was better for learning the easy version but not the more difficult version of the task. Applying a more difficult practice schedule to an already difficult task may make the processing demands too high for adequate learning (Wulf

and Shea, 2002). The skill level of the learner is another variable that may play a role in designing optimal practice schedules for learning. It has been suggested that novices may benefit from a blocked schedule while those who have more experience may benefit from a random schedule (Guadagnoli and Lee, 2004). Some have supported this idea (Shea et al., 1990) while others have not (Ollis et al., 2005).

Only two studies have examined the effect of practice schedules on neural recovery from stroke. Hanlon (1996) investigated the effect of practice schedules on learning a functional reaching task with the hemiparetic UE in individuals post-stroke. Subjects were assigned to either a blocked practice, random practice, or no practice control group. While there was no significant difference between the two practice groups for the number of trials to reach criterion (three consecutive successful trials), the random group had a significantly greater number of successful trials on the 2- and 7-day retention tests compared to the blocked group. Thus, this study provides some evidence that random practice may be more beneficial than blocked practice to improve function of the paretic limb in patients with stroke. However, because the functional task used was a complex five-step sequential task that involved grasping and moving a cup, success of the task was only measured by the cup not being dropped, and no kinematics or force measures were taken, it is hard to know which motor control parameters benefited from the random schedule. Furthermore, the random practice group practiced additional movements with the hemiparetic UE between presentations of the criterion task giving subjects in that group overall more practice in moving the arm, thus confounding a precise interpretation of the results.

In a study by Cauraugh and Kim (2003), subjects post-stroke performed three different movements (wrist/finger extension, elbow extension, and shoulder abduction) with the hemiparetic UE. In the blocked and random practice groups, movements were completed with a combination of active muscle activity and neuromuscular stimulation. A control group performed the same movements without stimulation. After four sessions lasting 90 min each over a

2-week period, subjects in both experimental groups performed better than controls on several behavioral measures but there was no difference in performance between the blocked and random groups. The lack of difference between groups practicing under different schedules is partially explained by the nature of the task, which was more a force production task than a functional task (see Winstein et al., 2004) and did not require the demands of skill acquisition.

Stroke severity and lesion location are important factors to consider when discussing motor learning in this population. Some work has suggested that individuals with more severe motor impairments may not demonstrate the same degree of short-term performance change (Dancause et al., 2002; Cirstea et al., 2003) or learning (Pohl et al., 2001) as individuals with less severe symptoms. This is a relatively open area for additional research to better understand the relationship between stroke severity, concomitant motor control deficits, and motor learning. The effect of lesion location on motor skill learning is not well understood either. Recent work has shown that if the primary locus of the stroke-affected area is the basal ganglia, there is more difficulty using explicit information to benefit implicit motor learning than age-matched controls (Boyd and Winstein, 2004). However, this is only a beginning. More research is needed to determine if differences in motor learning exist for individuals with specific stroke locations and levels of severity. For example, the optimal practice schedule may need to be tailored differently to accommodate individuals with more severe motor impairments compared with those with less severe deficits. More importantly, in order to effectively incorporate motor-learning principles into rehabilitation treatments and to design effective protocols, the interaction of stroke severity, lesion location, and conditions of practice will need a concentrated and focused research program.

7.6 Conclusions

Over the past decade, tremendous advances have been made in developing effective programs to enhance neurorecovery and rehabilitation. For the purposes of this chapter, we distinguish between exercise training and task-specific training designed for skill acquisition. The 1997 call for "well-formulated investigations grounded in available learning theory and research" (Fuhrer and Keith, 1998, p. 560) has only just begun to be addressed. We discussed the top-down model of rehabilitation that focuses on the skills necessary for rehabilitation. We have reviewed the literature relevant to a motor-learning-theory-based design of training that emphasizes the acquisition of skilled functional behaviors and contrasted this with an operant-conditioning approach that focuses on elicited behaviors and spontaneous use. The emergent principles of training from these two learning theories have tremendous implications for future developments in the area of neurorehabilitation. Further research is needed to better determine the optimal conditions of practice for motor skill learning in individuals with neurologic impairments. We are at an exciting time in rehabilitation medicine, but one that warrants a careful, theory-based analysis as we proceed to develop a scientific rationale for our interventions to promote recovery and rehabilitation.

ACKNOWLEDGEMENT

The authors wish to thank Nicolas Schweighofer for valuable discussions of scientifically derived and optimal task practice schedules and funding support to CJW from the NIH, NS 45485 and the Foundation for Physical Therapy.

REFERENCES

Albaret, J.M. and Thon, B. (1998). Differential effects of task complexity on contextual interference in a drawing task. *Acta Psychol*, **100**, 9–24.

American Heart Association (2005). *Heart Disease and Stroke Statistics – 2005 Update*, American Heart Association, Dallas, Texas.

Baddeley, A.H. and Longman, D.J.A. (1978). The influence of length and frequency on training sessions on the rate of learning to type. *Ergonomics*, **21**, 627–635.

Barbeau, H. and Fung, J. (2001). The role of rehabilitation of walking in the neurological population. *Curr Opin Neurol*, **12**(**6**), 735–740.

Behrman, A.L., Vander Linden, D.W. and Cauraugh, J.H. (1992). Relative frequency knowledge of results: older adults learning a force–time modulation task. *J Hum Mov Stud*, **23**, 233–250.

Bourne, L.E. and Archer, E.J. (1956). Time continuously on target as a function of distribution of practice. *J Exp Psychol*, **51**, 25–33.

Boyd, L.A. and Winstein, C.J. (2004). Providing explicit information disrupts implicit motor learning after basal ganglia stroke. *Learn Memory*, **11**, 388–396.

Brady, F. (2004). Contextual interference: a meta-analytic study. *Percept Motor Skill*, **99**, 116–126.

Butefisch, C., Hummelsheim, H., Denzler, P. and Mauritz, K.H. (1995). Repetitive training of isolated movements improves the outcome of motor rehabilitation of the centrally paretic hand. *J Neurol Sci*, **130**, 59–68.

Cahill, L., McGaugh, J.L. and Weinberger, N.M. (2001). The neurobiology of learning and memory: some reminders to remember. *Trend Neurosci*, **24**, 578–581.

Cauraugh, J.H. and Kim, S.B. (2003). Stroke motor recovery: active neuromuscular stimulation and repetitive practice schedules. *J Neurol Neurosurg Psychiatr*, **74**, 1562–1566.

Chan, L., Beaver, S., MacLehose, R.F., Jha, A., Maciejewski, M. and Doctor, J.N. (2002). Disability and health care costs in the medicare population. *Arch Phys Med Rehabil*, **83**, 1196–1201.

Cirstea, M.C., Ptito, A. and Levin, M.F. (2003). Arm reaching improvements with short-term practice depend on the severity of the motor deficit in stroke. *Exp Brain Res*, **152**(**4**), 476–488.

Dancause, N., Ptito, A. and Levin, M.F. (2002). Error correction strategies for motor behavior after unilateral brain damage: short-term motor learning processes. *Neuropsychologia*, **40**, 1313–1323.

Dean, C.M. and Shepherd, R.B. (1997). Task-related training improves performance of seated reaching tasks after stroke. A randomized controlled trial. *Stroke*, **28**(**4**), 722–728.

DeLisa, J.A. (2004). Shaping the future of medical rehabilitation research: using the interdisciplinary research model. *Arch Phys Med Rehabil*, **85**, 531–537.

Dempster, F.N. (1996). Distributing and managing the conditions of encoding and practice. In: *Memory* (eds Bjork, E.L. and Bjork, R.A.), Academic Press, San Diego, CA, pp. 317–344.

Dobkin, B.H. (2004). Strategies for stroke rehabilitation. *Lancet Neurol*, **3**(**9**), 528–536.

Donovan, J.J. and Radosevich, D.J. (1999). A meta-analytic review of the distribution of practice effect: now you see it, now you don't. *J Appl Psychol*, **84**(**5**), 795–805.

Doyon, J., Gaudreau, D., Laforce, R., Castonguay, M., Bedard, P.J., Bedard, F. and Bouchard, J.P. (1997). Role of the striatum, cerebellum, and frontal lobes in the learning of a visuomotor sequence. *Brain Cognit*, **34**(**2**), 218–245.

Dromerick, A. (2003). Evidence-based rehabilitation: the case for and against constraint-induced movement therapy. *J Rehabil Res Dev*, **40**(**6**), vii–ix.

Druckman, D. and Bjork, R.A. (1991). Optimizing long-term retention and transfer. In: *In the Mind's Eye: Enhancing Human Performance* (eds Druckman, D. and Bjork, R.A.), National Academy Press, Washington, DC, pp. 23–56.

Field-Fote, E.C. (2001). Combined use of body weight support, functional electric stimulation, and treadmill training to improve walking ability in individuals with chronic incomplete spinal cord injury. *Arch Phys Med Rehabil*, **82**(**6**), 818–824.

Fuhrer, M.J. and Keith, R.A. (1998). Facilitating patient learning during medical rehabilitation: a research agenda. *Am J Phys Med Rehabil*, **77**(**6**), 557–561.

Goodwin, J.E., Eckerson, J.M. and Voll, C.A. (2001). Testing specificity and guidance hypotheses by manipulating relative frequency of KR scheduling in motor skill acquisition. *Percept Motor Skill*, **93**(**3**), 819–824.

Gordon, J.G. (2000). Assumptions underlying physical therapy intervention: theoretical and historical perspectives. In: *Movement Science. Foundations for Physical Therapy in Rehabilitation* (eds Carr, J. and Shepard, R.), 2nd edn., Aspen Publishers, Gaithersburg, MD, pp. 1–30.

Guadagnoli, M.A. and Lee, T.D. (2004). Challenge point: a framework for conceptualizing the effects of various practice conditions in motor learning. *J Motor Behav*, **36**(**2**), 212–224.

Hanlon, R.E. (1996). Motor learning following unilateral stroke. *Arch Phys Med Rehabil*, **77**, 811–815.

Ho, L. and Shea, J.B. (1978). Effects of relative frequency of knowledge of results on retention of a motor skill. *Percept Motor Skill*, **46**(**3 Pt 1**), 859–866.

Karni, A. (1995). When practice makes perfect. *Lancet*, **345**(**8946**), 395.

Keith, R.A. and Cowell, K.S. (1987). Time use of stroke patients in three rehabilitation hospitals. *Soc Sci Med*, **24**(**6**), 529–533.

Kwakkel, G., Wagenaar, R.C., Twisk, J.W., Lankhorst, G.J. and Koetsier, J.C. (1999). Intensity of leg and arm training after primary middle-cerebral artery stroke: a randomized trial. *Lancet*, **354**, 191–196.

Lai, Q. and Shea, C.H. (1998). Generalized motor program learning: effects of reduced frequency of knowledge of results and practice variability. *J Motor Behav*, **30**(**1**), 51–59.

Lee, T.D. and Genovese, E.D. (1988). Distribution of practice in motor skill acquisition: learning and performance effects reconsidered. *Res Quart Exercise Sport*, **59**(**4**), 277–287.

Lee, T.D. and Genovese, E.D. (1989). Distribution of practice in motor skill acquisition: different effects for discrete and continuous tasks. *Res Quart Exercise Sport*, **60**(**1**), 59–65.

Lee, T.D. and Magill, R.A. (1983). The locus of contextual interference in motor-skill acquisition. *J Exp Psychol Learn Memory Cognit*, **9**(**4**), 730–746.

Lee, T.D. and Magill, R.A. (1985). Can forgetting facilitate skill acquisition? In: *Differing Perspectives in Motor Learning, Memory, and Control* (eds Goodman, D., Wilberg, R.B. and Franks, I.M.), Elsevier Science Publishing B.V., North-Holland, pp. 3–22.

Lee, T.D. and Maraj, B.K. (1994). Effects of bandwidth goals and bandwidth knowledge of results on motor learning. *Res Quart Exercise Sport*, **65**(**3**), 244–249.

Lee, T.D., White, M.A. and Carnahan, H. (1990). On the role of knowledge of results in motor learning: exploring guidance hypothesis. *J Motor Behav*, **22**(**2**), 191–208.

Lincoln, N.B., Willis, D., Philips, S.A., Juby, L.C. and Berman, P. (1996). Comparison of rehabilitation practice on hospital wards for stroke patients. *Stroke*, **27**(**1**), 18–23.

Mackey, F., Ada, L., Heard, R. and Adams, R. (1996). Stroke rehabilitation: are highly structured units more conducive to physical activity than less structured units? *Arch Phys Med Rehabil*, **77**(**10**), 1066–1070.

Magill, R.A. and Hall, K.G. (1990). A review of the contextual interference effect in motor skill acquisition. *Hum Mov Sci*, **9**, 241–289.

Marley, T.L., Exekiel, H.J., Lehto, N.K., Wishart, L.R. and Lee, T.D. (2000). Application of motor learning principles: the physiotherapy client as a problem-solver. II. Scheduling practice. *Physiother Can*, **52**, 311–316.

Miller, G.A. and Keller, J. (2000). Psychology and neuroscience: making peace. *Psychol Sci*, **9**, 212–215.

Morris, D., Crago, J., Deluca, S., Pidikiti, R. and Taub, E. (1997). Constraint-induced (CI) movement therapy for motor recovery after stroke. *Neurorehabilitation*, **9**, 29–43.

Nudo, R.J., Wise, B.M., SiFuentes, F. and Milliken, G.W. (1996). Neural substrates for the effects of rehabilitative training on motor recovery after ischemic infarct. *Science*, **272**(**5269**), 1791–1794.

Ollis, S., Button, C. and Fairweather, M. (2005). The influence of professional expertise and task complexity upon the potency of the contextual interference effect. *Acta Psychol*, **118**, 229–244.

Pavlides, C., Miyashita, E. and Asanuma, H. (1993). Projection from the sensory to the motor cortex is important in learning motor skills in the monkey. *J Neurophysiol*, **70**(**2**), 733–741.

Platz, T., Denzler, P., Kaden, B. and Mauritz, K.H. (1994). Motor learning after recovery from hemiparesis. *Neuropsychologia*, **32**(**10**), 1209–1223.

Plautz, E., Milliken, G.W. and Nudo, R.J. (2000). Effects of repetitive motor training on movement representations in adult squirrel monkeys: role of use versus learning. *Neurobiol Learn Memory*, **74**, 27–55.

Pohl, P.S. and Winstein, C.J. (1999). Practice effects on the less-affected upper extremity after stroke. *Arch Phys Med Rehabil*, **80**, 668–675.

Pohl, P.S., McDowd, J.M., Filion, D.L., Richards, L.G. and Stiers, W. (2001). Implicit learning of a perceptual-motor skill after stroke. *Phys Ther*, **81**(**11**), 1780–1789.

Rundek, T., Mast, H., Hartmann, A., Boden-Albala, B., Lennihan, L., Lin, I.F., Paik, M.C. and Sacco, R.L. (2000). Predictors of resources use after acute hospitalization. The Northern Manhattan Stroke Study. *Neurology*, **55**, 1180–1187.

Salmoni, A.W., Schmidt, R.A. and Walter, C.B. (1984). Knowledge of results and motor learning: a review and critical reappraisal. *Psychol Bull*, **95**(**3**), 355–386.

Schmidt, R.A. (1991). Frequent augmented feedback can degrade learning: evidence and interpretations. In: *Tutorials in Motor Neuroscience* (eds Stelmach, G.E. and Requin, J.), Kluwer, Dordrecht, pp. 59–75.

Schmidt, R.A. and Lee, T.D. (1999). *Motor Control and Learning: A Behavioral Emphasis*, 3rd edn., Human Kinetics, Champaign, Ill.

Schmidt, R.A. and Lee, T.D. (2005) *Motor Control and Learning: A Behavioural Emphasis*, 4th edn., Human Kinetics, Champaign, Ill.

Sekiya, H., Magill, R.A., Sidaway, B. and Anderson, D.I. (1994). The contextual interference effect for skill variations from the same and different generalized motor programs. *Res Quart Exercise Sport*, **65**(**4**), 330–338.

Sekiya, H., Magill, R.A. and Anderson, D.I. (1996). The contextual interference effect in parameter modifications of the same generalized motor program. *Res Quart Exercise Sport*, **67**(**1**), 59–68.

Shea, J.B. and Morgan, R.L. (1979). Contextual interference effects on the acquisition, retention, and transfer of a motor skill. *J Exp Psychol Hum Learn Memory*, **5**(**2**), 179–187.

Shea, J.B. and Zimny, S.T. (1983). Context effects in memory and learning movement information. In: *Memory and Control of Action* (ed. Magill, R.A.), North Holland Publishing Company, Amsterdam, pp. 345–366.

Shea, C.H., Kohl, R. and Indermill, C. (1990). Contextual interference: contributions of practice. *Acta Psychol*, **73**, 145–157.

Skinner, B.F. (1968). *The Technology of Teaching*, Appleton-Century-Crofts, East Norwalk, CT.

Sparrow, W.A. (1995). Acquisition and retention effects of reduced relative frequency of knowledge of results. *Aust J Psychol*, **47**(**2**), 97–104.

Sparrow, W.A. and Summers, J.J. (1992). Performance on trials without knowledge of results (KR) in reduced frequency presentations of KR. *J Motor Behav*, **24**(**2**), 197–209.

Sullivan, K., Knowlton, B.J. and Dobkin, B.H. (2002). Step training with body weight support: effect of treadmill speed and practice paradigms on poststroke locomotor recovery. *Arch Phys Med Rehabil*, **83**, 683–691.

Sunderland, A. and Tuke, A. (2005). Neuroplasticity, learning and recovery after stroke: a critical evaluation of constraint-induced therapy. *Neuropsychol Rehabil*, **15**(**2**), 81–96.

Swanson, L.R. and Lee, T.D. (1992). Effects of aging and schedules of knowledge of results on motor learning. *J Gerontol Psychol Sci*, **47**(**6**), P406–P411.

Taub, E. and Uswatte, G. (2003). Constraint-induced movement therapy: bridging from primate laboratory to the stroke rehabilitation laboratory. *J Rehabil Med*, **419**(**Suppl.**), 34–40.

Taub, E., Crago, J.E., Burgio, L.D., Groomes, T.E. and Cook, E.W. (1994). An operant approach to overcoming learned nonuse after CNS damage in monkeys and man: the role of shaping. *J Exp Anal Behav*, **61**, 281–293.

Taub, E., Uswatte, G. and Morris, D.M. (2003). Improved motor recovery after stroke and massive cortical reorganization following constraint-induced movement therapy. *Phys Med Rehabil Clin North Am*, **14**(**Suppl. 1**), S77–S91, ix.

Vander Linden, D.W., Cauraugh, J.H. and Greene, T.A. (1993). The effect of frequency of kinetic feedback on learning an isometric force production task in nondisabled subjects. *Phys Ther*, **73**, 79–87.

Verville, R. and DeLisa, J. (2003). Evolution of National Institutes of Health options for rehabilitation research. *Am J Phys Med Rehabil*, **82**(**8**), 565–579.

Weinrich, M., Stuart, M. and Hoyer, T. (2005). Rule for rehabilitation: an agenda for research. *Neurorehabil Neural Repair*, **19**, 72–83.

Whitall, J. (2004). Stroke rehabilitation research: time to answer more specific questions? *Neurorehabil Neural Repair*, **18**, 3–8.

Whyte, J. and Hart, T. (2003). It's more than a black box; it's a Russian doll: defining rehabilitation treatments. *Am J Phys Med Rehabil*, **82**(**8**), 639–652.

Winstein, C.J. and Schmidt, R.A. (1990). Reduced frequency of knowledge of results enhances motor skill learning. *J Exp Psychol Learn Memory Cognit*, **16**(**4**), 677–691.

Winstein, C.J. and Prettyman, M.G. (2005) Constraint-induced therapy for functional recovery after brain injury: unraveling the key ingredients and mechanisms. In: *Synaptic Plasticity* (eds Baudry, M., Bi, X. and Schreiber, S.), Marcel Dekker, Inc., New York.

Winstein, C.J., Pohl, P.S. and Lewthwaite, R. (1994). Effects of physical guidance and knowledge of results on motor learning: support for the guidance hypothesis. *Res Quart Exercise Sport*, **65**(**4**), 316–323.

Winstein, C.J., Merians, A. and Sullivan, K. (1999). Motor learning after unilateral brain damage. *Neuropsychologia*, **37**, 975–987.

Winstein, C.J., Miller, J.P., Blanton, S., Morris, D., Uswatte, G., Taub, E., Nichols, D. and Wolf, S. (2003). Methods for a multi-site randomized trial to investigate the effect of constraint-induced movement therapy in improving upper extremity function among adults recovering from a cerebrovascular stroke. *Neurorehabil Neural Repair*, **17**, 137–152.

Winstein, C.J., Rose, D.K., Tan, S.M., Lewthwaite, R., Chui, H.C. and Azen, S.P. (2004). A randomized controlled comparison of upper-extremity rehabilitation strategies in acute stroke: a pilot study of immediate and long-term outcomes. *Arch Phys Med Rehabil*, **85**, 620–628.

Wishart, L.R. and Lee, T.D. (1997). Effects of aging and reduced relative frequency of knowledge of results on learning a motor skill. *Percept Motor Skill*, **84**(**3 Pt 1**), 1107–1122.

Wolf, S., Blanton, S., Baer, H., Breshears, J. and Butler, A.J. (2002). Repetitive task practice: a critical review of constraint induced therapy in stroke. *Neurologist*, **8**, 325–338.

Wolf, S.L., Butler, A.J., Alberts, J.L. and Kim, M.W. (2005). Contemporary linkages between EMG, kinetics and stroke rehabilitation. *J Electromyogr Kinesiol*, **15**, 229–239.

Wright, D.L. and Shea, C.H. (2001). Manipulating generalized motor program difficulty during blocked and random practice does not affect parameter learning. *Res Quart Exercise Sport*, **72**(**1**), 32–38.

Wulf, G. and Schmidt, R.A. (1989). The learning of generalized motor programs: reducing the relative frequency of knowledge of results enhances memory. *J Exp Psychol Learn Memory Cognit*, **15**(**4**), 748–757.

Wulf, G. and Shea, C.H. (2002). Principles derived from the study of simple skills do not generalize to complex skill learning. *Psychonom Bull Rev*, **9**(**2**), 185–211.

Wulf, G., Schmidt, R.A. and Deubel, H. (1993). Reduced feedback frequency enhances generalized motor program learning but not parameterization learning. *J Exp Psychol Learn Memory Cognit*, **19**(**5**), 1134–1150.

Wulf, G., Lee, T.D. and Schmidt, R.A. (1994). Reducing knowledge of results about relative versus absolute timing: differential effects on learning. *J Motor Behav*, **16**(**4**), 362–369.

Wulf, G., Shea, C.H. and Matschiner, S. (1998). Frequent feedback enhances complex motor skill learning. *J Motor Behav*, **30**(**2**), 180–192.

Balance training

Gammon M. Earhart[1] and Fay B. Horak[2]

[1]*Washington University School of Medicine, Program in Physical Therapy and* [2]*Oregon Health and Science University, Neurological Sciences Institute*

8.1 Why balance matters

Introduction

Consider riding a bicycle, standing on one leg, or walking along a narrow beam. All of these tasks require active control of balance. In order to successfully complete these tasks one may have to make a conscious effort to keep from falling and practice may be necessary to improve performance. Next consider sitting on a stool, standing quietly, or walking across the floor. It may not be immediately obvious that these tasks also require active balance control and practice, as these tasks can often be performed without devoting attention specifically to the maintenance of an upright posture. However, all of the tasks mentioned above and most other tasks that we perform on a daily basis require the ability to maintain balance. Whether consciously or more automatically controlled, balance is a key, complex skill for successful movement within our changing environments. Although balance is generally viewed as a function of the cerebellum and the vestibular system, balance skills can be compromised by a variety of central neurologic pathologies, such as stroke and Parkinson disease (PD), and by peripheral pathologies such as sensory loss or musculoskeletal injuries. In fact, damage or pathology to almost any part of the body may affect balance because it is a complex skill requiring many resources. Balance performance is a very sensitive measure of health, although it is often not a very specific diagnostic indicator of particular diseases.

Statistics on the incidence and cost of falls

Loss of balance, and the falls that result, are serious problems. Although all age groups are subject to falls, the risk of falling increases exponentially with age (Samelson et al., 2002). In fact, more than one-third of community-dwelling elderly and 60% of nursing home residents fall each year (Hornbrook et al., 1994; Fuller, 2000; Hausdorff et al., 2001). In addition, the incidence of falls in people with neurologic pathology such as PD may be more than double that of age-matched healthy subjects. Falls are often the precursor to immobility, lack of independence, and even death. In fact, falls are the leading cause of death in people over 85 years and the leading cause of injuries in people over 65 years (Alexander et al., 1992; Murphy, 2000). The total cost of all fall injuries in people age 65 or older in the USA was over $20.2 billion in 1994 (Englander et al., 1996). This cost is expected to increase to $32.4 billion by 2020, as the elderly population grows. Given the high personal and economic cost of falls and the high incidence of balance problems in patients seen for rehabilitation, a basic understanding of balance control, assessment, and rehabilitation is essential for effective treatment.

8.2 Balance control

Basic terminology

Balance, a skill required to maintain upright posture, has both orientation and stability components.

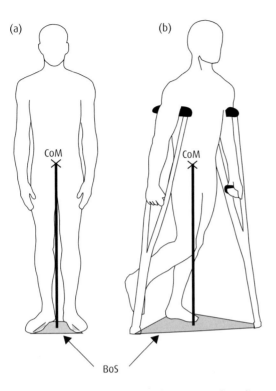

Figure 8.1. Illustration of the CoM and BoS in normal standing (a) and when using an assistive device (b).

Orientation involves interpreting sensory information and using it to maintain the appropriate alignment of the body with respect to the environment and the task. The body may be aligned using several references, including gravity, the support surface, the visual environment, and internal representations. Postural stability, or equilibrium, involves controlling the center of body mass (CoM) relative to the base of support (BoS) to resist perturbations or allow functional movement. CoM refers to the point at which the entire mass of the body may be considered to be concentrated (Winter, 1990). BoS is the region bounded by the points of contact between body segments and the support surface. For example, during unsupported stance, the BoS consists of an area under the base of foot support and when the subject is using an assistive device, the BoS includes the combined area under both the assistive device and the feet (Fig. 8.1). For static equilibrium, the

CoM must be kept over the BoS. The boundaries of the region in which the CoM can be moved safely without changing the BoS are referred to as the limits of stability. For dynamic equilibrium, such as during walking, the CoM must be controlled both within and outside a changing BoS (Winter, 1990). During dynamic tasks such as locomotion or arising from a chair, the limits of stability depend on the momentum, as well as the position, of the body CoM (Pai et al., 1994).

Systems model of balance control

Control of body orientation and stability results from complex interactions among the individual, the environment, and the task being performed. Successful accomplishment of the desired task depends on processing and integrating multiple sensory inputs to determine the relative orientation among body segments and body position relative to the environment. This information is used to plan and execute movements that allow maintenance of balance during task performance. Older models of postural control as parallel sensory reflexes (such as visual, vestibular, and proprioceptive righting responses) are no longer considered useful (Horak et al., 1997; Mergner et al., 2003).

Figure 8.2 shows a contemporary model of postural control (adapted from Merfeld et al., 1993) that outlines how the process of selection and adaptation of balance responses may occur. In this model, the central nervous system uses sensory inputs in combination with knowledge of biomechanical constraints to form internal models of body and sensory dynamics. A postural control strategy is selected to achieve the desired body orientation and a copy of the control strategy is fed to the internal models to yield estimated orientation and expected sensory afferent signals. These expected afferent signals are then compared to actual sensory afferent signals that result from the postural movement performed. A sensory conflict, or difference between expected and actual afferent signals, is relayed to the internal model of body dynamics, the model is changed, and the next postural strategy modified

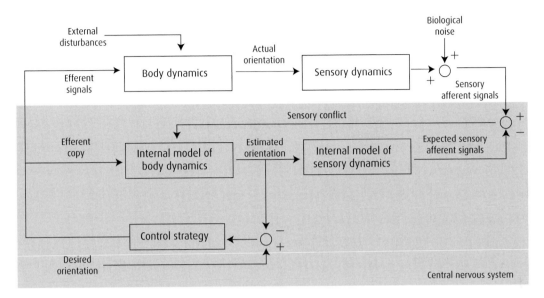

Figure 8.2. Contemporary model of postural control that outlines how balance responses may be selected and adapted. See text for details (adapted from Merfeld et al., 1993).

such that estimated orientation more closely approaches actual orientation. External, as well as self-initiated postural disturbances cause changes in afferent signals and these, too, drive change in the internal model of body dynamics, resulting in implementation of a more efficient and effective postural control strategy to regain the desired orientation. This type of model explains how postural strategies can be rapid, and somewhat stereotyped, although they are constantly being improved based on prior experience and knowledge of results. This model also assumes that sensory information is integrated by the nervous system to form an internal representation of the body and world that is used for both perception of postural orientation as well as for automatic control of posture (Mergner et al., 2003).

Multiple resources required for postural stability and orientation

Multiple resources are required for postural stability and orientation (Fig. 8.3), and a basic understanding of these functional systems is necessary in order to diagnose balance disorders and design treatments

that focus specifically on the affected systems. Biomechanical constraints, such as muscle strength and range of motion, play an important role in balance control, as they can limit the strategies available for use. Dynamic control is essential for challenges to balance that occur during gait, such as proactive modifications in order to avoid or accommodate obstacles. Disruptions of cognitive control may make balance difficult in dual-task situations where attention is divided, and/or make it difficult to improve postural control based on prior experience. Abnormal perception of spatial orientation relative to the environment can skew the internal model of the body. Two additional resources that are crucial for balance control are sensory strategies and movement strategies, both of which are covered in more detail in the following sections.

Sensory integration and weighting

Multiple sources of sensory information are required for postural stability and orientation (Fig. 8.3). Sensory contributions to balance control come from three major sensory systems: visual, vestibular, and

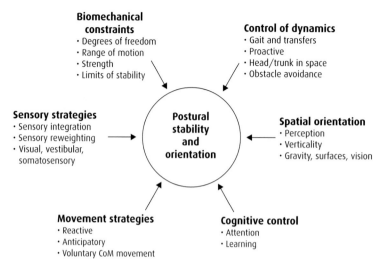

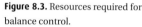

Figure 8.3. Resources required for balance control.

somatosensory. The visual system allows recognition of, and detection of orientation and movement of, objects in the environment. This information can be used to determine the orientation of the body with respect to the environment and to adapt movements to meet environmental conditions, for example, avoiding an obstacle in one's path during locomotion. The visual system also detects relative motion of the self with respect to the environment, such as postural sway during standing or progression during locomotion. Objects at about arm's length away allow for more effective balance control than objects at a great distance, as the nearer an object the greater angular displacement of its image on the retina with body movement. Objects greater than 2.5 m away cannot be used to effectively control sway during quiet stance (Paulus et al., 1984) and sway increases for many subjects in the absence of vision (Romberg, 1851; Chiari et al., 2001). As the visual system cannot differentiate self-motion from environmental motion, vision can induce illusions of movement when the visual scene moves slowly with respect to a stationary individual. An example of this phenomenon that many of us have experienced is the sensation of movement that is briefly felt when sitting in a parked car as the neighboring car starts to move. Forward motion of the neighboring car results

in an illusion of self-motion backwards. The influence that vision has on postural control varies with changes in lighting conditions, visual acuity, and the location and size of a visual stimulus within the visual field (Leibowitz et al., 1972).

The vestibular system is specialized for the control of postural orientation and balance (see Chapter 20 of Volume II). The system can detect both linear and rotational accelerations of the head in space. The otoliths sense all of the linear accelerations acting on the head, including the constant acceleration due to gravity. As such, the otoliths are sensitive to changes in orientation (e.g. tilt) with respect to gravity and provide an important source of information for the perception of verticality. In contrast, the semicircular canals sense angular head accelerations. Pitch (sagittal) and roll (frontal) movements of the head are detected by the anterior and posterior canals, whereas yaw movements are detected by the horizontal canals. Since pitch and roll movements move the body CoM toward its limits of stability, the anterior and posterior semicircular canals are particularly important for control of postural sway. The semicircular canals are most sensitive to high-frequency head movements, such as during locomotion, in contrast to the low-frequency sensitive otoliths that are suited to control static postural alignment (Nashner, 1972; Nashner et al., 1989; Mittelstaedt, 1999).

Both the visual and the vestibular systems are located in the head, which moves independently from the body. Thus, these two systems do not provide direct information about body orientation in space. This important information comes from somatosensors, such as muscle spindles, Golgi tendon organs, cutaneous mechanoreceptors, pressure receptors, and joint receptors, that are distributed throughout the body. In fact, without important somatosensory information from the neck and trunk, visual and vestibular information alone cannot help the nervous system distinguish between: (1) head movements on a stable body and head movements accompanied by movement of the body CoM that may result in postural instability and (2) forward head movements when the body CoM moves backward via hip flexion and forward head movements when the body CoM moves forward via ankle dorsiflexion. In addition to relaying information about body configuration, the somatosensory system also provides information about the support surface and the forces exerted by the body against those surfaces. For example, cutaneous and deep mechanoreceptors on the soles of the feet are activated in relation to forces under the feet.

It has been clear for some time that the visual, vestibular, and somatosensory systems all contribute to balance control, as evidenced by the fact that stimulation of each of the three systems can induce body sway (Coats and Stoltz, 1969; Lestienne et al., 1977; Hlavacka and Nijiokiktjien, 1985). But information from each of these sources alone would not be sufficient to allow selection of an appropriate postural response. For example, if an image moves across the retina this could be interpreted as body movement with respect to the object being viewed or as movement of the object relative to a stationary body. Without vestibular and/or proprioceptive information to use in addition to the visual input, the retinal slip signal cannot be successfully interpreted.

The processing and integration of information from the three systems, obviously an essential component of successful balance, relies on sensory integration and sensory channel reweighting (Peterka, 2002). Sensory channel reweighting refers to the ability of the nervous system to modify the relative contributions of the three sensory systems to balance control based on the context in which balance is to be maintained. For example, movement of a visual surround has a stronger influence when the support surface is also moving, which provides evidence of an increased weighting of visual information in conditions where the support surface is unstable or compliant (Soechting and Berthoz, 1979; Peterka and Benolken, 1992). Recent studies have established that a healthy subject standing on a stable surface in a well-lit room relies primarily upon somatosensory information for postural orientation (Peterka and Benolken, 1992). However, that same person will gradually increase dependence on vestibular information (and vision, if available) in proportion to the amplitude of random surface orientations (Peterka, 2002). Light haptic touch from a single finger on a stable support can also provide a powerful sensory reference, even more powerful than the effects of vision (Jeka and Lackner, 1994). This may explain why the use of a cane as a sensory substitution device, rather than as a mechanical support, is so effective in improving balance and reducing falls in patients with sensory deficits (Jeka, 1997; Dickstein et al., 2001; Horak et al., 2002). Thus, sensory reweighting occurs not only in response to the context in which a task in being performed, but also in response to injury to one of the sensory systems. When one of the sensory systems is damaged, the nervous system can increase the weight placed on the intact sensory systems to compensate for the damage (Nashner et al., 1982; Marchand and Amblard, 1984; Horak and Hlavacka, 2001). Studies have shown that patients with loss of somatosensory or vestibular information can increase the sensitivity of their other senses for balance control and particularly benefit from substituting light touch for their missing sensory information for postural stability.

Balance strategies

Postural movement strategies take advantage of body biomechanics to allow for effective and efficient control of body CoM. Although postural strategies are rather stereotyped, they are constantly being shaped, or adapted, based on prior experience and knowledge of results. Anticipatory postural adjustments are those that occur prior to a voluntary movement. For example, prior to pulling on a handle to open a door, calf muscles are activated to stabilize the body and prevent a forward fall during the pull (Cordo and Nashner, 1982). These anticipatory postural adjustments are specific to each particular voluntary movement pattern and do not consist of simple stiffening of the body (Horak and Anderson, 1980). Anticipatory postural adjustments are dependent on predictive, feedforward control, as the postural muscles are activated prior to, or at the same time as, the muscles that are the prime movers

for the voluntary movement (Crenna et al., 1987; Oddsson and Thorstensson, 1987). Thus, sensory feedback is not available to trigger anticipatory postural adjustments. However, sensory feedback control is important for postural responses to unexpected external perturbations. Patients with injuries affecting the cerebellum or parts of frontal cortex may have poor control of anticipatory postural adjustments.

Responses to external perturbations, which can be elicited by movement of the support surface or of the body, consist of a continuum of strategies that may or may not involve changes in the BoS (Horak et al., 1997). Fixed support strategies are those where the BoS is not altered (Fig. 8.4). One fixed support strategy, the ankle strategy, is generated in response to small perturbations experienced when standing

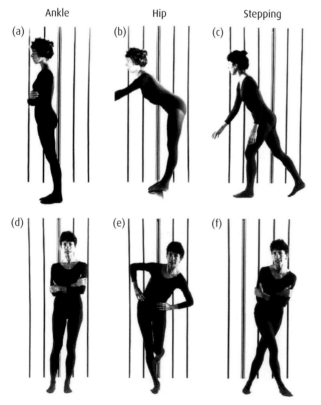

Figure 8.4. Illustration of ankle, hip, and stepping strategies used in response to backward (a–c) and lateral (d–f) perturbations (reprinted with permission from Horak and Shumway-Cook, 1990).

on a firm, wide surface (Horak and Nashner, 1986). Use of the ankle strategy in response to forward or backward perturbations is characterized by distal-to-proximal activation of muscles on the side of the body opposite the direction of sway with torque generated primarily around the ankles. Use of a similar strategy in response to lateral perturbations involves hip abduction/adduction and loading/unloading of the limbs, allowing upright orientation of the body during motion of the body CoM (Henry et al., 1998). Another fixed support strategy, the hip strategy, is generated in response to larger perturbations or perturbations experienced on support surfaces that do not allow use of ankle torque. The hip strategy in response to forward or backward perturbations is characterized by proximal-to-distal activation of muscles, resulting in hip torque that rotates the trunk opposite the legs to more rapidly move the body CoM (Runge et al., 1999). Use of a similar strategy that involves lateral flexion of the trunk in response to lateral perturbations involves activation of trunk paraspinal muscles (Henry et al., 1998). The ankle and hip strategies both have muscle activation latencies of 75–100 ms and represent the two extremes of the continuum of fixed support strategies. Different combinations of the ankle and hip strategies can be used depending on the characteristics of the perturbation, expectations based on prior experience, and the environmental context in which the perturbation is experienced.

Change in support strategies are those that involve an alteration in the BoS (Maki and McIlroy, 1997). Stepping is one example of a change in support strategy that is used for very large or fast perturbations. A second change in support strategy is to grasp a nearby object, increasing the size of the BoS. These strategies are more complex than the hip and ankle strategies in that they involve anticipatory unloading of the stepping leg and longer latencies than the ankle and hip strategies, but they are not simply used as a last resort when fixed support strategies are unsuccessful (Maki and McIlroy, 1997). For example, elderly subjects who are prone to falls or who fear falling are more likely to use a stepping or arm reaching strategy than a fixed support strategy.

8.3 Assessment and treatment of balance disorders

Framework/goal of assessment and treatment

Nagi's (1965) disablement scheme (Fig. 8.5) is a helpful model to use in approaching balance assessment, the first step in balance rehabilitation. Assessment may identify the underlying pathology causing the balance problem (such as PD, vestibular loss, etc.),

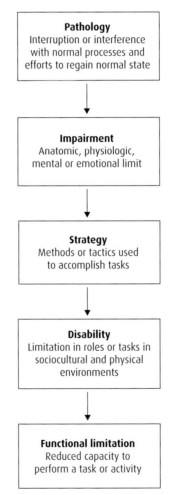

Figure 8.5. Nagi's disablement model (adapted from Nagi, 1965).

but the clinician should be aware that diagnosis of pathology itself is not sufficient. The same pathology may affect individuals quite differently, so an assessment must also identify specific impairments and functional limitations that stem from the pathology. The ultimate goal of assessment is to make a differential diagnosis of a postural disorder that allows for development of an intervention that is patient-specific and targets the particular impairments and functional limitations identified. Nagi's disablement scheme does not include another level that therapists should consider in their assessment and treatment of balance and movement disorders, the *strategies* by which individuals accomplish a functional task given their impairments. The strategy level is located between the impairment and functional levels and represents the tactics or methods by which a subject accomplishes a task. A therapist must decide if the individual is using the most effective and efficient strategy possible given their particular impairments and pathology.

Balance assessment

A complete assessment includes evaluation of both intrinsic and extrinsic factors that may influence balance. Intrinsic factors that could limit balance ability include biomechanical factors, motor coordination for static and dynamic tasks, sensory orientation, and cognitive limitations (Fig. 8.3). Biomechanical factors include range of motion, strength, flexibility, and postural alignment during standing and sitting. Biomechanical constraints at the feet, which provide the BoS for standing and walking, are particularly important. Motor coordination is also central to balance control. Assessment of a person's ability to select and coordinate appropriate postural movement strategies in response to external perturbations, in anticipation of voluntary movements, and during voluntary movements of the whole body is also essential (Horak, 1997). Responses to external perturbations may be evaluated by examining responses to a tug at the shoulders or hips, or by the push and release test (Horak et al., 2004). Anticipatory postural adjustments may be examined

by asking a patient to rapidly raise both arms to shoulder level or to place one foot on a step. In addition, one should consider the adaptation of these strategies to different environmental contexts. For example, how long does it take for a patient to use a hip strategy to balance with a narrow BoS or to take an effective compensatory step in response to a large perturbation? The effects of cognitive processing on postural control may be evaluated by asking subjects to perform a secondary cognitive task while they are also doing a balance task. For example, therapists may ask a subject to count backwards from 100 in increments of 3 while they are walking or trying to stand on one foot. If either the cognitive task or the balancing task, or both deteriorate significantly, this may suggest either that the balancing task has not become automatic or that the patient lacks sufficient attentional resources to safely and accurately perform both a cognitive and a balancing task (Woollacott and Shumway-Cook, 2002).

One means of quantifying postural control is through dynamic posturography, the use of an instrumented movable platform, motion analysis, and/or electromyography (EMG) to quantify sway, body kinematics, and muscle activation patterns (see Horak et al., 1997 or Monsell et al., 1997 review). Posturography can be used to evaluate stance, reactions to movements of the support surface, voluntary movements, gait, and sensory organization. Sensory organization is quantified by measuring increases in postural sway when visual and/or surface information is no longer providing adequate postural feedback (Nashner et al., 1982). Measures of sway during quiet stance are not necessarily good predictors of instability or fall risk for some neurologic conditions. For example, in PD sway is markedly reduced during stance in people who are actually quite unstable (Horak et al., 1992). Reactions to movements of the support surface can discriminate among problems with force scaling, strategy selection, response latency, sense of vertical, and difficulties with sensorimotor integration (Horak et al., 1997). Dynamic posturography is more effective than vestibulo-ocular reflex testing in identifying dizziness (Stewart et al., 1999), correlates with fall history of elderly persons (Topp et al., 1998), and differentiates between diabetics with and without neuropathy (Simmons et al., 1997). However, despite the usefulness of dynamic posturography, it is expensive and requires sophisticated equipment. As such, it is not always feasible to include dynamic posturography in a balance assessment.

One inexpensive alternative for clinical assessment of sensory organization is the clinical test for sensory integration in balance (CTSIB) (Shumway-Cook and Horak, 1986). This test, modeled after a dynamic posturography sensory organization protocol (Nashner et al., 1982), requires only a piece of foam, a paper lantern, and a stopwatch. The CTSIB has six different conditions in which the accuracy or availability of visual and somatosensory information is altered. For each condition, subjects are asked to stand quietly for 30 s. Visual information is eliminated by closing the eyes or is rendered inaccurate by having the person wear a paper lantern over his head such that as the head moves the visual surround moves with it. Somatosensory information is altered by having the person stand on 4-in. thick Temper foam (Kees Goebel Medical Specialties, Hamilton, OH) of medium density. Figure 8.6 shows the six CTSIB conditions. All three senses (visual, vestibular, and somatosensory) are available and accurate in condition one. The eyes are closed in condition two, leaving only vestibular and somatosensory information. People with somatosensory loss as a result of spinal cord injury, peripheral neuropathy, or other conditions have difficulty on condition two (Allison, 1995). In condition four, the subject stands on foam to reduce the accuracy of somatosensory information from the feet and ankles. People with visual deficits may have difficulty with condition four. In condition five, the eyes are closed and the person stands on the foam. In this case only vestibular information is accurate. Not surprisingly, people with vestibular loss have difficulty in condition five. In the remaining conditions, three and six, the person wears the lantern on his head. These conditions test the ability to suppress inaccurate visual information and rely on other sources for balance control. Those with central nervous system

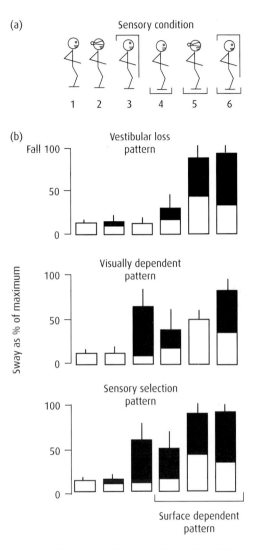

Figure 8.6. Illustration of the six conditions of the CTSIB (a). Patterns of sway in healthy subjects (open bars) and subjects with vestibular loss, visual dependence, and sensory selection problems (black bars) are shown in (b) (adapted from Black et al., 1988).

lesions such as multiple sclerosis (MS), head injury, and stroke, and some patients with vestibular pathology leading to increased visual dependence may have difficulty with these conditions. Figure 8.6 (adapted from Black et al., 1988) shows the patterns of sway in control subjects and patients with various sensory organization problems.

Clinical assessment of sensory organization should also include evaluation of the person's perceived limits of stability (by asking them to lean in all directions without moving their feet) and postural vertical (by assessing their standing and sitting postural alignment with respect to gravity with and without vision and on an unstable surface). Postural stability and strategies may be affected similarly whether a patient's perceived or actual limits of stability are small or distorted. Patients with somatosensory loss in the feet show reduced limits of stability in standing whereas patients after some strokes or unilateral vestibular loss may show asymmetrical limits of stability (as well as a tilted postural verticality).

One should also consider the role of extrinsic factors in balance control. It is important to recognize that people must balance in a variety of environments in the community and the home. Extrinsic factors that may contribute to balance problems include slippery, wet, uneven, and cluttered surfaces and stairs. Lighting can also greatly influence balance, as improper or inadequate lighting can reduce the usefulness of visual inputs (Birge, 1993).

Balance assessment is complex because balance control is multifactorial. In addition to the factors mentioned above, there are many others. For example, elderly individuals who are taking psychoactive medications, or more than four medications, are twice as likely to fall when compared to those not taking these medications (Cumming, 1998). Current clinical instruments have been developed to predict whether patients are at risk for falls rather than to determine the underlying reason for the balance problems. Review of these balance instruments is beyond the scope of this chapter (see Allison, 1995; Whitney et al., 1998, for more information).

Balance rehabilitation: approaches and efficacy

Just as assessment of balance is multifactorial, so too is treatment of balance disorders. Many different approaches have been used to treat balance disorders, including generalized exercise programs, balance-specific exercises, training of postural strategies, sensory organization training, biofeedback, and environmental modifications paired with education. The most effective balance retraining programs are customized for the particular constraints on balance control in each individual patient (Tinetti et al., 1994; Shumway-Cook et al., 1997).

Tai Chi, a Chinese conditioning exercise known for its slow, controlled movements, has a beneficial effect on balance. Several studies have shown that Tai Chi training can improve balance (see Lan et al., 2002 for review). Tai Chi reduces the risk of falls in the elderly (Li et al., 2001). Although Tai Chi improves balance and functional mobility, it does not reduce, but appears to increase, postural sway in stance (Wolf et al., 1997; Zwick et al., 2000; Taggart, 2002). Increase of postural sway may indicate larger limits of stability, which improves postural stability. Other generalized exercise programs, such as aerobics and strength training, do not improve balance or postural stability, likely because subjects differ in their underlying balance problems (Lichtenstein et al., 1989).

Treatment of the musculoskeletal system is imperative to address balance constraints including weakness, reduced range of motion, reduced flexibility, and improper postural alignment. Strength training of the leg muscles, for example, can improve dynamic balance and walking speed (Fiatarone et al., 1990; Nelson et al., 1994).

In conjunction with treatment of musculoskeletal constraints, neuromuscular constraints must also be addressed. Customized, multidimensional exercise programs are more effective than generic exercises for improving balance (Shepard and Telian, 1995; Shumway-Cook et al., 1997). These treatments should address problems with response latency, scaling, relative timing of muscle activity, and appropriate selection and adaptation of motor strategies.

There are several ways that one can train motor strategies for balance. For example, to promote the ankle strategy, postural responses should be practiced on a broad, stable surface and movement at the ankles without movement at the hips or knees should be facilitated. To promote the hip strategy, postural responses should be practiced on narrow surfaces where the ability to generate ankle torque is reduced. The stepping strategy can be encouraged by practicing unweighting of the stepping leg during gait initiation and moving the CoM outside the BoS. Balance during dynamic gait exercise should also be practiced in a variety of environments. Use of a dual-task paradigm may also help to make balance a more automatic process, as attention must be diverted to the secondary task rather than being focused on keeping balance (Woollacott and Shumway-Cook, 2002).

Recent work has also focused on promoting sensory substitution. For example, people with vestibular loss tend to rely heavily on visual inputs for balance control and as a result are unstable in situations where visual information is not accurate or is not available. Visual over-dependence can be discouraged by provision of accurate and secure somatosensory inputs, gradual reduction of availability and complexity of visual inputs, and introduction of movement of the visual surround to create sensory conflict situations where the appropriate sense must be relied upon in order to maintain balance. If, on the other hand, a person is overly dependent on somatosensory inputs for balance control, this can be discouraged by practicing standing and walking on a variety of surfaces such as carpet, gravel, sand, and grass. Sensory organization training based on the six conditions of the CTSIB is an effective means of rehabilitation (Hu and Woollacott, 1994). They key to successful sensory organization training is to first identify which senses are being used effectively and which are not, and then have the person practice balance tasks in contexts where sensory information is reduced or eliminated. Progressive reduction of information from the overused sense will promote increased utilization of the underused source(s) of information.

Several tools are available to assist with sensory retraining for balance control. Optokinetic stimulation, the use of moving visual stimuli to create sensory conflict, is one such tool. Following optokinetic stimulation, patients with vestibular loss and presbyastasia demonstrate less postural sway (Sémont et al., 1992; Vitte et al., 1994). Optokinetic stimulation is particularly useful because nervous system adaptation to deficits is more efficient when the person must actively deal with complex and natural sensory conflicts. Another means of inducing sensory conflicts is through the use of virtual reality. Virtual reality can be used to induce movement of the visual environment relative to a stationary subject, thus challenging the subject to rely on somatosensory and vestibular information to remain upright and stable. Preliminary studies of virtual reality for balance training in subjects with traumatic brain injury and vestibular loss are promising (McComas and Sveistrup, 2002; Whitney et al., 2002). Virtual reality allows a person to interact with a complex and realistic environment in a manner that is safe and can be adapted to suit individual needs. Although some subjects experience motion sickness as a result of virtual environment immersion, the after-effects on postural stability are mild and short lived (Cobb and Nichols, 1998; Cobb, 1999).

For those with complete loss of a sense, another approach has been the use of prosthetic devices to provide information that would normally be provided by the impaired sensory system. For example, sensory prostheses are being developed that can reduce postural sway in subjects with vestibulopathy (Dozza et al., 2003; in press; Wall and Weinberg, 2003). The devices consist of an accelerometer that provide signals used to estimate the fore/aft tilt angle of the subject. This tilt estimate is fed into a digital controller which activates either a series of vibrotactile devices, called tactors, that are in contact with the subject's skin or a set of earphones that provides audio biofeedback. As the subject leans forward, tactors on different parts of the torso vibrate or the subject hears tone changes correlated with body sway and direction.

EMG biofeedback can also be used in balance rehabilitation. For subjects with excessive or unwanted postural muscle activity, visual biofeedback of muscle activity can be used to assist healthy people and people with neurologic injuries to relax overactive muscles (Poppen et al., 1988; Duckett and Kramer, 1994). Muscles important for control of posture (such as the ankle strategy muscles) can also be activated with surface electrodes based on feedback from force sensors under the feet. Force platform biofeedback training is another methodology used to treat balance disorders. Force platform biofeedback systems consist of two force platforms, a computer, and a monitor that provides visual feedback about weight distribution during standing. Force platform biofeedback is an effective means of reducing the number of falls in patients with peripheral neuropathy (Wu, 1997), and can be used to train a more symmetrical weight distribution and reduce postural sway during quiet stance following stroke (Lee et al., 1996; Nichols, 1997; Sackley and Lincoln, 1997; Simmons et al., 1998). There is controversy, however, about the use of force platform biofeedback. When used in conjunction with conventional balance rehabilitation, force platform biofeedback may not confer an added benefit (Walker et al., 2000). Furthermore, evidence suggests that improvements in quiet stance stability following biofeedback training do not translate to improvements in dynamic balance during gait (Winstein et al., 1989).

Environment and education

Just as assessment of balance must consider both intrinsic and extrinsic factors, so, too, must treatment of balance. Modification of the home environment to reduce or eliminate fall hazards is advisable. Measures to be taken include: removing throw rugs or securing them to the floor with double-sided tape, wearing supportive shoes with non-skid soles, using adequate lighting, using a rubber mat or a shower seat when bathing, and installing handrails on stairways. Another treatment option is to prescribe an assistive device, such as a cane or a walker. Both standard and quad canes reduce postural sway in people with hemiparesis (Milczarek et al., 1993; Laufer, 2003), and people with peripheral neuropathy are less likely to fall while standing on an unstable surface when using a cane (Ashton-Miller et al., 1996). In fact, even light fingertip touch on a stable

surface substantially stabilizes postural sway in healthy people and people with peripheral neuropathy or vestibular loss (Jeka, 1997; Dickstein et al., 2001). Despite their usefulness, however, assistive devices can increase the attentional demands associated with walking (Wright and Kemp, 1992) and prevent patients from effectively grabbing onto a stable support in response to external perturbation (Maki and McIlroy, 1997). As such, those using assistive devices need to practice allocating attention during walking with the device and may need to refrain from performing other tasks while walking. Patients must be educated regarding the nature of their particular balance deficits, the situations they should avoid or use caution in given their particular problems, and the measures they can take to make their environment safer.

Synthesis of principles: balance in PD

Postural instability is one of the hallmark features of PD and often does not respond well to medications or surgical treatments that ameliorate other symptoms (McAuley, 2003). Postural instability in PD frequently leads to gait difficulties and falls. People with PD often have disordered postural alignment characterized by thoracic kyphosis and reduced lumbar lordosis accompanied by a narrow base of support, all of which contribute to reduced limits of stability. Postural responses to perturbations as well as anticipatory postural adjustments prior to a voluntary movement in patients with PD are normal in latency, but reduced in amplitude with excessive muscle co-contraction (Horak et al., 1992, 1996; Chong et al., 1999). People with PD show inflexibility of postural set as evidenced by difficulty modifying postural strategies based on environmental context (Bloem, 1992; Chong et al., 2001). For example, patients with PD have difficulty suppressing unnecessary leg muscle activity in response to postural perturbations when sitting or when holding onto a stable support (Chong et al., 2001). Most research indicates that postural instability in PD stems from insufficient and slow force production such that responses are not adequate to counteract perturbations (Romero and Stelmach, 2003). There is also evidence that people with PD show more dramatic deficits than control subjects in postural control when tested in dual-task conditions (Morris et al., 2000; Woollacott and Shumway-Cook, 2002).

When assessing balance in an individual with PD, it is important to consider the direct effects of PD, such as bradykinesia and rigidity, but also indirect effects such as reduced flexibility secondary to altered postural alignment (Schenkman et al., 1998; Schenkman, 2001). Treatment of balance deficits in PD can and should be aimed at a number of different goals. These include: reducing biomechanical impairments such as weakness and poor axial range of motion, improving force control (perhaps with biofeedback), improving self-awareness of body somatosensory information regarding postural alignment, improving dual-task abilities through practice or learning to avoid dual-task situation, and improving initiation and sequencing of movement via use of external cues, mental imagery, explicit directions, etc. (Morris, 2000). Patients with PD should also be taught how to fall more gracefully to avoid injuries, and how to arise from the floor safely. Through careful assessment and treatment, it is possible to significantly improve balance and reduce fall injuries in individuals with PD (Hirsch et al., 2003; Stankovic, 2004). PD is but one example of many conditions that affect balance at multiple levels and must be assessed and treated at each of these levels. Only through a combination of approaches ranging from strengthening to home modification is it possible to maximally improve postural stability in individuals with PD and other balance disorders, and thereby reduce the risk of falls.

REFERENCES

Alexander, B.H., Rivara, F.P. and Wolf, M.E. (1992). The cost and frequency of hospitalization for fall-related injuries in older adults. *Am J Public Health*, **82**(**Suppl. 7**), 1020–1023.

Allison, L. (1995). Balance disorders. In: *Neurological Rehabilitation* (ed. Umphred, D.A.), Mosby-YearBook, Inc. St. Louis, MO, pp. 802–837.

Ashton-Miller, J.A., Yeh, M.W., Richardson, J.K. and Galloway, T. (1996). A cane reduces loss of balance in patients with peripheral neuropathy: results from a challenging unipedal balance test. *Arch Phys Med Rehabil*, **77**, 446–452.

Birge, S.J. (1993). Osteoporosis and hip fracture. *Clin Geriatr Med*, **9**, 69–86.

Black, F.O., Shupert, C.L., Horak, F.B. and Nashner, L.M. (1988). Abnormal postural control associated with peripheral vestibular disorders. *Prog Brain Res*, **76**, 263–275.

Bloem, B.R. (1992). Postural instability in Parkinson's disease. *Clin Neurol Neurosurg*, **94**(**Suppl.**), S41–S45.

Chiari, L., Kluzik, J., Lenzi, D., Horak, F.B. and Cappello, A. (2001). Different postural behaviors in normal subjects: sensory strategy or control strategy? *ESMAC-SIAMOC Joint Congress*, Rome.

Chong, R.K., Jones, C.L. and Horak, F.B. (1999). Postural set for balance control is normal in Alzheimer's but not in Parkinson's disease. *J Gerontol A Biol Sci Med Sci*, **54**, M129–M135.

Chong, R.K., Barbas, J., Garrison, K., Herzog, A., Teheng, R. and Sethi, K. (2001). Does balance control deficit account for walking difficulty in Parkinson's disease? *Int J Clin Pract*, **44**, 411–412.

Coats, A.C. and Stoltz, M.S. (1969). The recorded body-sway response to galvanic stimulation of the labyrinth: a preliminary study. *Laryngoscope*, **79**, 85–103.

Cobb, S.V.C. (1999). Measurement of postural stability before and after immersion in a virtual environment. *Appl Ergn*, **30**, 47–57.

Cobb, S.V.C. and Nichols, C. (1988). Static posture tests for the assessment of postural instability after virtual environment use. *Brain Res Bull*, **47**, 459–464.

Cordo, P.J. and Nashner, L.M. (1982). Properties of postural adjustments associated with rapid arm movements. *J Neurophysiol*, **47**, 287–302.

Crenna, P., Frigo, C., Massion, J. and Pedotti, A. (1987). Forward and backward axial synergies in man. *Exp Brain Res*, **65**, 538–548.

Cumming, R.F. (1998). Epidemiology of medication-related falls in the elderly. *Drug Aging*, **12**, 43–53.

Dickstein, R., Shupert, C.L. and Horak, F.B. (2001). Fingertip touch improves postural stability in patients with peripheral neuropathy. *Gait Posture*, **14**, 238–247.

Dozza, M., Chiari, L., Peterka, R., Horak, F.B. and Hlavacka, F. (2003). Controlling posture using an audio biofeedback system. *Human Posture Control Meeting*, Bratislava, Slovakia.

Dozza, M., Chiari, L. and Horak, F.B. (2005) Audio-biofeedback improves balance in patients with bilateral vestibular loss. *Arch Phys Med Rehabil*, **86**, 1401–1403.

Duckett, S. and Kramer, T. (1994). Managing myoclonus secondary to anoxic encephalopathy through EMG biofeedback. *Brain Injury*, **8**, 185–188.

Englander, F., Hodson, T.J. and Terregrossa, R.A. (1996). Economic dimensions of slip and fall injuries. *J Foren Sci*, **41**(**Suppl. 5**), 733–746.

Fiatarone, M.A., Marks, E.C., Ryan, N.D., Meredith, C.N., Lipsitz, L.A. and Evans, W.J. (1990). High-intensity strength training in nonagenarians. Effects on skeletal muscle. *J Am Med Assoc*, **263**, 3029–3034.

Fuller, G.F. (2000). Falls in the elderly. *Am Family Physician*, **61**(**Suppl. 7**), 2159–2168.

Hausdorff J.M., Rios, D.A. and Edelber, H.K. (2001). Gait variability and fall risk in community-living older adults: a 1-year prospective study. *Arch Phys Med Rehabil*, **82**(**Suppl. 8**), 1050–1056.

Henry, S., Fung, J. and Horak, F.B. (1998). Control of stance during lateral and anterior/posterior surface translations. *IEEE Trans Rehabil Eng*, **6**(**Suppl. 1**), 32–42.

Hlavacka, F. and Nijiokiktjien, C. (1985). Postural responses evoked by sinusoidal galvanic stimulation of the labyrinth. *Acta Otolaryngol*, **99**, 107–112.

Hirsch, M.A., Toole, T., Maitaland, C.G. and Rider, R.A. (2003). The effects of balance training and high-intensity resistance training on persons with idiopathic Parkinson's disease. *Arch Phys Med Rehabil*, **84**, 1109–1117.

Horak, F.B. (1997). Clinical assessment of balance disorders. *Gait Posture*, **6**, 76–84.

Horak, F.B. and Anderson, M.A. (1980). Preparatory postural activity associated with movement. *Phys Ther*, **60**(**Suppl. 5**), 580.

Horak, F.B. and Nashner, L.M. (1986). Central programming of postural movements: adaptation to altered support-surface configurations. *J Neurophysiol*, **55**, 1369–1381.

Horak, F.B. and Hlavacka, F. (2001). Somatosensory loss increases vestibulospinal sensitivity. *J Neurophysiol*, **86**(**Suppl. 2**), 575–585.

Horak, F.B., Nutt, J. and Nashner, L.M. (1992). Postural inflexibility in parkinsonian subjects. *J Neurol Sci*, **111**, 46–58.

Horak, F.B., Frank, J. and Nutt, J. (1996). Effects of dopamine on postural control in parkinsonian subjects: scaling, set, and tone. *J Neurophysiol*, **75**, 2380–2396.

Horak, F.B., Henry, S.M. and Shumway-Cook, A. (1997). Postural perturbations: new insights for treatment of balance disorders. *Phys Ther*, **77**(**Suppl. 5**), 517–533.

Horak, F.B., Buchanan, J., Creath, R. and Jeka, J. (2002). Vestibulospinal control of posture. *Adv Exp Med Biol*, **508**, 139–145.

Horak, F.B., Jacobs, J.V., Tran, V.K. and Nutt, J.G. (2004). The push and release test: an improved clinical postural stability test

for patients with Parkinson's disease. *Mov Disord*, **19**(**Suppl. 9**), S170.

Hornbrook, M.C., Stevens, V.J., Wingfield, D.J., Hollis, J.F., Greenlick, M.R. and Ory, M.G. (1994). Preventing falls among community-dwelling older persons: results from a randomized trial. *Gerontologist*, **34**(**Suppl. 1**), 16–23.

Hu, M.H. and Woollacott, M.H. (1994). Multisensory training of standing balance in older adults. I. Postural stability and one-leg stance balance. *J Gerontol*, **49**, M52–M61.

Jeka, J.J. (1997). Light touch contact as a balance aid. *Phys Ther*, **77**(**Suppl. 5**), 476–487.

Jeka, J.J. and Lackner, J.R. (1994). Fingertip contact influences human postural control. *Exp Brain Res*, **100**(**Suppl. 3**), 495–502.

Lan, C., Lai, J.S. and Chen, S.Y. (2002). Tai Chi Chuan: an ancient wisdom on exercise in health promotion. *Sport Med*, **32**, 217–224.

Laufer, Y. (2003). The effect of walking aids on balance and weight-bearing patterns of patients with hemiparesis in various stance positions. *Phys Ther*, **83**, 112–122.

Lee, M.Y., Wong, M.K. and Tang, F.T. (1996). Clinical evaluation of a new biofeedback standing balance training device. *J Med Eng Technol*, **20**, 60–66.

Leibowitz, H.W., Johnson, C.A. and Isabelle, E. (1972). Peripheral motion detection and refractive error. *Science*, **177**, 1207–1208.

Lestienne, F., Soechting, J. and Berthoz, A. (1977). Postural readjustments induced by linear motion of visual scenes. *Exp Brain Res*, **28**, 363–384.

Li, J.X., Hong, Y. and Chan, K.M. (2001). Tai Chi: physiological characteristics and beneficial effects on health. *Br J Sport Med*, **35**, 148–156.

Lichtenstein, M.J., Shields, S.L., Shiavi, R.G. and Burger, C. (1989). Exercise and balance in aged women: a pilot controlled clinical trial. *Arch Phys Med Rehabil*, **70**, 138–143.

Maki, B.E. and McIlroy, W.E. (1997). The role of limb movements in maintaining upright stance: the "change-in-support" strategy. *Phys Ther*, **77**, 488–507.

Marchand, A.R. and Amblard, B. (1984). Locomotion in adult cats with early vestibular deprivation: visual cue substitution. *Exp Brain Res*, **54**, 395–405.

McAuley, J.H. (2003). The physiological basis of clinical deficits in Parkinson's disease. *Prog Neurobiol*, **69**, 27–48.

McComas, J. and Sveistrup, H. (2002). Virtual reality applications for prevention, disability awareness, and physical therapy rehabilitation in neurology: our recent work. *Neurol Report*, **l**(**26**), 55–61.

Merfeld, D.M., Young, L.R., Oman, C.M. and Shelhamer, M.J. (1993). A multidimensional model of the effect of gravity on the spatial orientation of the monkey. *J Vestibul Res*, **3**, 141–161.

Mergner, T., Maurer, C. and Peterka, R.J. (2003). A multisensory posture control model for human upright stance. *Prog Brain Res*, **142**, 189–201.

Milczarek, J.J., Kirby, R.L., Harrision, E.R. and MacLeod, D.A. (1993). Standard and four-footed canes: their effect on the standing balance of patients with hemiparesis. *Arch Phys Med Rehabil*, **74**, 281–285.

Mittelstaedt, H. (1999). The role of the otoliths in perception of the vertical and in path integration. *Ann NY Acad Sci*, **871**, 334–355.

Monsell, E.M., Furman, J.M., Herdman, S.J., Konrad, H.R. and Shepard, N.T. (1997). Computerized dynamic platform posturography. *Otolaryngol Head Neck surg*, **117**, 394–398.

Morris, M., Iansek, R., Smithson, F. and Huxham, F. (2000). Postural instability in Parkinson's disease: a comparison with and without a concurrent task. *Gait Posture*, **12**, 205–216.

Morris, M.E. (2000). Movement disorders in people with Parkinson's disease: a model for physical therapy. *Phys Ther*, **80**, 578–597.

Murphy, S.L. (2000). Deaths: final data for 1998. *National Vital Statistics Reports*, **48**(11). National Center for Health Statistics, Hyattsville, MD.

Nagi, S. (1965). Some conceptual issues in disability and rehabilitation. In: *Sociology and Rehabilitation* (ed. Sussman, M.), American Sociological Association, Washington, DC, pp. 100–113.

Nashner, L.M. (1972). A vestibular posture control model. *Kybernetik*, **10**, 106–110.

Nashner, L.M., Black, F.O. and Wall III, C. (1982). Adaptation to altered support and visual conditions during stance: patients with vestibular deficits. *J Neurosci*, **2**, 536–544.

Nashner, L.M., Shupert, C.L., Horak, F.B. and Black, F.O. (1989). Organization of posture control: an analysis of sensory and mechanical constraints. *Prog Brain Res*, **80**, 411–418.

Nelson, M.E., Fiatarone, M.A., Morganti, C.M., Trice, I., Greenberg, R.A. and Evans, W.J. (1994) Effects of high-intensity strength training on multiple risk factors for osteoporotic fractures. A randomized controlled trial. *J Am Med Assoc*, **272**(Suppl. 24), 1909–1914.

Nichols, D. (1997). Balance retraining after stroke using force platform biofeedback. *Phys Ther*, **77**, 553–558.

Oddsson, L. and Thorstensson, A. (1987). Fast voluntary trunk movements in standing: motor patterns. *Acta Physiol Scand*, **129**, 93–106.

Pai, Y.-C., Naughton, B.J. and Chang, R.W. (1994). Control of body center of mass momentum during sit-to-stand among young and elderly adults. *Gait Posture*, **2**, 109–116.

Paulus, W.M., Straube, A. and Brandt, T. (1984). Visual stabilization of posture: physiological stimulus characteristics and clinical aspects. *Brain*, **107**, 1143–1164.

Peterka, R.J. (2002). Sensorimotor integration in human postural control. *J Neurophysiol*, **88**, 1097–1118.

Peterka, R.J. and Benolken, M.S. (1992). Role of somatosensory and vestibular cues in attenuating visually-induced human postural sway. In: *Posture and Gait: Control Mechanisms* (eds Woollacott, M. and Horak, F.), University of Oregon Books, Eugene, OR, pp. 272–275.

Poppen, R., Hanson, H.B. and Ip, S.M. (1988). Generalization of EMG biofeedback training. *Biofeedback Self Regul*, **13**, 235–243.

Romberg, M.H. (1851). *Lehrbuch der Mercenkrankheiten des Menschen.*, Duncker, Berlin.

Romero, D.H. and Stelmach, G.E. (2003). Changes in postural control with aging and Parkinson's disease. *IEEE Eng Biol Med Mag*, **22**, 27–31.

Runge, C.F., Shupert, C.L., Horak, F.B. and Zajac, F.E. (1999). Ankle and hip postural strategies defined by joint torques. *Gait Posture*, **10**, 161–170.

Sackley, C.M. and Lincoln, N.B. (1997). Single blind randomized controlled trail of visual feedback after stroke: effects on stance symmetry and function. *Disabil Rehabil*, **19**, 536–546.

Samelson, E.J., Zhang, Y., Kiel, D.P., Hannan, M.T. and Felson, D.T. (2002). Effect of birth cohort on risk of hip fracture: age-specific incidence rates in the Framingham study. *Am J Public Health*, **92**(Suppl. 5), 858–862.

Schenkman, M. (2001). *Topics in Neurology: Parkinson's Disease: Update on Clinical Features, Physiology and Treatment.* University of Colorado Health Science Center, Denver, CO, pp. 1–74.

Schenkman, M., Custon, T.M., Kuchibhatla, M., Chandler, J., Pieper, C.F., Ray, L. and Laub, K.C. (1998). Exercise to improve spinal flexibility and function for people with Parkinson's disease: a randomized controlled trail. *J Am Geriatr Soc*, **46**, 1207–1216.

Sémont, A., Vitte, E. and Freyss, G. (1992). Falls in the elderly: a therapeutic approach by optokinetic reflex stimulations. In: *Falls, Balance and Gait Disorders in the Elderly* (eds Vellas, B., Toupet, M., Rubenstein, L., Albarede, J.I. and Christen, Y.), Elsevier, Paris, pp. 153–159.

Shepard, N.T. and Telian, S.A. (1995). Programmatic vestibular rehabilitation. *Otolaryngol Head Neck Surg*, **112**, 173–182.

Shumway-Cook, A. and Horak, F.B. (1986). Assessing the influence of sensory interaction on balance: suggestions from the field. *Phys Ther*, **66**, 1548–1550.

Shumway-Cook, A., Gruber, W., Baldwin, M. and Liao, S. (1997). The effect of multidimensional exercises on balance, mobility, and fall risk in community-dwelling older adults. *Phys Ther*, **77**, 46–57.

Simmons, R.W., Richardson, C. and Pozos, R. (1997). Postural stability of diabetic patients with and without cutaneous sensory deficit in the foot. *Diabetes Res Clin Pract*, **36**, 153–160.

Simmons, R.W., Smith, K., Erez, E., Burke, J.P. and Pozos, R.E. (1998). Balance retraining in a hemiparetic patient using center of gravity biofeedback: a single-case study. *Percept Motor Skill*, **87**, 603–609.

Soechting, J.F. and Berthoz, A. (1979). Dynamic role of vision in the control of posture in man. *Exp Brain Res*, **36**, 551–561.

Stankovic, I. (2004). The effect of physical therapy on balance of patients with Parkinson's disease. *Int J Rehabil Res*, **27**, 53–57.

Stewart, M.G., Chen, A.Y., Wyatt, J.R., Favrot, S., Beinart, S., Coker, N.J. and Jenkins, H.A. (1999). Cost-effectiveness of the diagnostic evaluation of vertigo. *Laryngoscope*, **109**, 600–605.

Taggart, H.M. (2002). Effects of Tai Chi exercise on balance, functional mobility, and fear of falling among older women. *Appl Nurs Res*, **15**, 235–242.

Tinetti, M.E., Baker, D.I., McAvay, G., Claus, E.B., Garrett, P., Gottischalk, M.G., Koch, M.L., Trainor, K. and Horwitz, R.I. (1994). A multifactorial intervention to reduce the risk of falling among elderly people living in the community. *New Eng J Med*, **331**, 821–827.

Topp, R., Mikesky, A. and Thompson, K. (1998). Determinants of four functional tasks among older adults: an exploratory regression analysis. *J Orthop Sport Phys Ther*, **27**, 144–154.

Vitte, E., Sémont, A. and Berthoz, A. (1994). Repeated optokinetic stimulation in conditions of active standing facilitates recovery from vestibular deficits. *Exp Brain Res*, **102**, 141–148.

Walker, C., Brouwer, B.J. and Cullham, E.G. (2000). Use of visual feedback in retraining balance following acute stroke. *Phys Ther*, **80**, 886–895.

Wall III, C. and Weinberg, M.S. (2003). Balance prostheses for postural control. *IEEE Eng Biol Med Mag*, **22**, 84–90.

Whitney, S.L., Poole, J.L. and Cass, S.P. (1998). A review of balance instruments for older adults. *Am J Occup Ther*, **52**, 666–671.

Whitney, S.L., Sparto, P.J., Brown, K.E., Furman, J.M., Jacobson, J.L. and Redfern, M.S. (2002). The potential use of virtual reality in balance and vestibular rehabilitation: preliminary findings with the BNAVE. *Neurol Report*, **26**, 72–79.

Winstein, C.J., Gardner, E.R., McNeal, D.R., Barto, P.S. and Nicholson, D.E. (1989). Standing balance training: effect on balance and locomotion in hemiparetic adults. *Arch Phys Med Rehabil*, **70**, 755–762.

Winter, D.A. (1990). *Biomechanics and Motor Control of Human Movement*, 2nd edn., Wiley-Interscience, New York.

Wolf, S.L., Barnhart, H.X., Ellison, G.L. and Coogler, C.E. (1997). The effect of Tai Chi Chuan and computerized balance training on postural stability in older subjects. Atlanta FICSIT Group. Frailty and injuries: cooperative studies on intervention techniques. *Phys Ther*, **77**, 371–381.

Woollacott, M. and Shumway-Cook, A. (2002). Attention and the control of posture and gait: a review of an emerging area of research. *Gait Posture*, **16**, 1–14.

Wright, D.L. and Kemp, T.L. (1992). The dual-task methodology and assessing the attentional demands of ambulation with walking devices. *Phys Ther*, **72**, 306–315.

Wu, G. (1997). Real-time feedback of body center of gravity for postural training of elderly patients with peripheral neuropathy. *IEEE Trans Rehabil Eng*, **5**, 399–402.

Zwick, D., Rochelle, A., Choksi, A. and Domowicz, J. (2000). Evaluation and treatment of balance in the elderly: a review of the efficacy of the Berg balance test and Tai Chi Quan. *Neurorehabilitation*, **15**, 49–56.

9

Functional electrical stimulation in neurorehabilitation

Peter H. Gorman[1], Gad Alon[2] and P. Hunter Peckham[3]

[1]Department of Neurology and Rehabilitation, University of Maryland School of Medicine and Spinal Cord Injury Service, Kernan Orthopaedics and Rehabilitation Hospital, Baltimore MD, USA; [2]Department of Physical Therapy and Rehabilitation Science, University of Maryland School of Medicine, Baltimore MD, USA and [3]Department of Biomedical Engineering, Case Western Reserve University and FES Center of Excellence, Cleveland VA Medical Center, Cleveland, OH, USA

9.1 Introduction

Functional electrical stimulation (FES), also known as *functional neuromuscular stimulation (FNS)* or *neuromuscular electrical stimulation (NMES)* is the method of applying safe levels of electric current to activate the damaged or disabled neuromuscular system. The terms FES, FNS, and NMES are often used interchangeably, although NMES typically refers to using surface electrodes. The term *neuroprosthesis* refers to devices that use electrical stimulation to activate the nervous system in order to perform a specific functional task. This chapter will examine both the therapeutic aspects of FES as well as the direct functional applications as it is applied to individuals with neurologic injury.

9.2 Mechanism of FES activation of nervous tissue

Peripheral effects

When a sufficiently strong external electric field is applied to a nerve via a pair of electrodes, depolarization of the axon will occur. If depolarization occurs with sufficient intensity and speed, the membrane will reach threshold and an action potential will fire and propagate bidirectionally. The number of nerve fibers activated during applied stimulation will be related to the amount of phase charge delivered with each pulse (Adams et al., 1993).

Motor units are activated electrically by depolarization of motor axons, or terminal motor nerve branches. Electrical current can directly depolarize muscle fibers, but the amount of current necessary for this to occur is considerably greater than that for depolarization of nerve axons (Crago et al., 1974). Therefore for practical purposes, FES systems stimulate nerves, not muscles. Unlike the normal physiological recruitment order of motor units that follows the size principle, electrically induced recruitment order is neither reversed nor predictable. The number and type of motor units activated depends on motor unit size, the distance of each motor unit from the stimulating electrode, and the relative impedance of intervening tissues (Knaflitz et al., 1990). There has been some literature on electrical stimulation of denervated muscle, but clinical applicability remains controversial. Tetanic contraction can be achieved in denervated muscle so long as long duration and high amplitude stimulation is used via very large surface electrodes (Kern et al., 1999, 2002).

Similar to muscles undergoing voluntary exercise, FES-stimulated muscles will change morphologically and physiologically. Type II glycolytic fibers will convert to Type I oxidative fibers over weeks to months, depending on the intensity and frequency of stimulation. This phenomenon is associated with changes in vascular supply and increased fatigue resistance (Munsat et al., 1976). It is still not clear how much FES "exercise" is adequate to achieve fiber changes and allow for functional use.

Central nervous system effects

Recent evidence affirms the rationale of applying NMES to paralyzed or paretic muscles in order modulate central nervous system (CNS) plasticity. NMES induces transmission of afferent inputs along sensory pathways originating from both muscular and non-contractile structures. Kimberley et al., (2004) Han et al. (2003) and Smith et al. (2003) have presented evidence of increased excitability in the contralateral hemisphere following excitation of selected peripheral nerves of both stroke survivors and healthy subjects (see Volume I, Chapters 6, 14 and 15).

A potential role for NMES in promoting recovery following damage to the brain is derived from the hypothesis of territorial competition. The hypothesis is based on evidence that the cortical representation of body segments is continuously modulated in response to activity, inactivity, and skill acquisition. As part of this ongoing adaptation process there seems to be competition among body segments for territorial representation in the sensorimotor cortex (Muellbacher et al., 2002). Artificial alteration of afferent inputs can be achieved with NMES via amplification and sustaining of afferent vollies from the more deprived distal segments, thus helping those segments compete for territorial representation. NMES treatment groups have shown at least a 50% improvement over controls in Fugl-Meyer (Chae et al., 1998) action research arm (ARA) test scores (Powell et al., 1999), and upper limb advanced distributed learning tests (Popovic et al., 2003) in various populations.

9.3 Components of FES systems

FES systems typically consist of three major components. First, there is a control mechanism. Second, there is an electronic stimulator, which may be external or implanted. Third, there are electrodes that allow for interface between the stimulator and the nervous system. Cabling or other technologies such as radio-frequency coupled telemetry allow for communication between these three components.

Electronic stimulators are usually battery powered. Stimulators range in sophistication and number of channels. Most portable FES neuroprostheses are built around a microprocessor controller, which may allow for software modification of the stimulator output. The number of stimulator channels can vary with the application. Channels can be activated sequentially or in unison to allow for orchestration of complex movements.

Control systems for therapist-operated FES systems consist of dials and switches. For subject-controlled FES systems (i.e., neuroprostheses), control can come in the form of switches, buttons, joysticks, joint position sensors, electromyography (EMG) electrodes, voice activated controls, sip and puff devices, switches, etc. Subject control of an FES system can be either "open loop" or "closed loop". In open loop control, the electrical output of the FES system is not dependent on the muscular force or joint movement produced by the stimulation. In closed loop control, real time information on muscle force and/or joint position or movement is fed back into the FES system to allow for modification of its output (Crago et al., 1991).

Electrodes provide the interface between the electrical stimulator and the nervous system. Different types that have been used include surface, percutaneous intramuscular, implantable intramuscular, epimysial, and nerve cuff electrodes. These electrodes will be discussed separately.

Surface electrodes

Surface electrodes vary in composition, size, and configuration. Electrode materials that dominate in clinical practice are carbon–silicon and stainless steel or silver fibers–fabric mesh. Conduction through the entire electrode surface and the contact pressure should be as uniform as possible. Non-uniformity of the conductive medium can generate loci of high current density that can cause discomfort, skin irritation, or even burns.

Electrode size should be considered a major factor that can help minimize electrode–skin interface impedance and current density. The relationship between electrode size and impedance is non-linear. Larger electrode size enables stronger muscle force generation and less perceived stimulation discomfort (Alon, 1985; Kantor et al., 1994; Alon et al., 1996). However, the increased size is relative to the contractile mass of the target muscle. Small muscles require considerably smaller electrode sizes than larger muscles. Actual effective size of surface electrodes is not determined by simply measuring the diameter of the electrode because the effective size is influenced by the uniformity of conduction and pressure. Both are likely to change over time and with repeated electrode reuse. Clinicians must be aware of the need to continually ascertain the adequacy of the surface electrode–skin interface. Failure to do so may jeopardize treatment effectiveness, increase skin irritation and possibly cause skin burns (Hasan et al., 1996; Burridge et al., 1997b).

Implantable electrodes

Implantable electrodes fall into several subcategories. Electrodes that travel across the skin to insert into muscle are *percutaneous intramuscular* electrodes. They are usually inserted using a hypodermic needle, and have a barbed end to ensure stability once inside the muscle. Percutaneous electrodes have been used primarily in developmental research protocols or temporary applications. Their long-term survival has not been as great as that for implanted electrodes (Memberg et al., 1993). There are also *implantable intramuscular* electrodes that are more robust than the percutaneous versions, mainly because of their thicker lead wires. *Epimysial* electrodes are surgically sewn onto the epimysial surface of muscles. They typically have a conductive metallic alloy core or disc and a surrounding silicone elastomer skirt. *Nerve cuff* electrodes directly stimulate nerves by surrounding them circumferentially. Implanted cables link the stimulator and the stimulating electrodes and are complex in design to

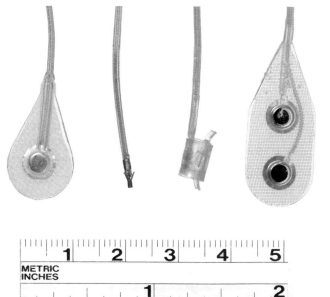

Figure 9.1. Implantable electrodes used in FES applications. The following electrodes are pictured (from left to right): monopolar epimysial, intramuscular, nerve cuff, and bipolar epimysial electrodes.

withstand bending stresses and the body's saline environment. Photographs of several implanted electrodes are found in Fig. 9.1.

9.4 Stimulation parameters

There are several important parameters that can be adjusted during FES application, including pulse waveform, amplitude, duration, frequency, charge, and modulations (Baker et al., 1993). Individual parameters will be discussed below.

Stimulus waveform

Stimulators with a pulsatile current (PC) output typically deliver either monophasic or biphasic waveforms. Monophasic waveforms produce uni-directional current flow and thus cause a net movement of charged ions across the electrode/tissue interface. In contrast, biphasic waveforms are characterized by very rapid reversal of stimulus polarity. The absence of charged ion movement makes the symmetric biphasic waveform preferred because it minimizes skin irritation and is perceived as being more comfortable (Baker et al., 1988; Kantor et al., 1994; Laufer et al., 2001; Bennie et al., 2002). Monophasic stimulation is also less desirable for long-term implanted FES use, since it can cause electrode and tissue breakdown (Mortimer, 1981). Waveforms can be either constant voltage or constant current (Kantor et al., 1994; Alon et al., 1996). Constant current waveforms are used primarily (although not exclusively) in FES systems.

Peak and root mean square current amplitude

Peak current refers to the highest amplitude of each phase. For any biphasic waveform there are two peaks. Knowing the root mean squared (RMS) current is important in order to determine the safety of stimulation because current density (RMS current divided by electrode surface area) may be closely associated with the risk of skin irritation and the risk

of burns (Alon, 1985; Alon et al., 1994; Panescu et al., 1994a, b; Henkin et al., 2003).

Phase duration

Also termed *pulse width*, phase duration indicates how long each phase lasts. It usually ranges between 5 and 400 μs. Short durations minimize the stimulation discomfort, minimize skin–electrode interface impedance, and reduce the chance of electrochemical skin irritation (the latter in the case of monophasic waveforms only) (Rollman, 1975; Iggo, 1978; Friedli and Meyer, 1984; Baker et al., 1988; Frijns et al., 1994; Gold and Shorofsky, 1997; Mulcahey et al., 1999; Wesselink et al., 1999). As either pulse amplitude or duration is increased above threshold, *spatial* recruitment of additional motor units will occur. The product of the amplitude and pulse duration represents the net charge injected into the tissue. The charge injected and the force output of the muscle being stimulated is related by an S-shaped curve within which a portion of the curve has a very high gain. This relationship is important to be aware of when attempting gradual proportional recruitment of motor strength.

Pulse rate (frequency)

Pulse rate or frequency determines the rate of nerve depolarization. Increasing pulse frequency provides for *temporal* summation of force output. A pulse rate that ranges between 1 and 10 pulses per second (pps) induces twitch contractions of skeletal muscles. Faster pulse rates (15–25 pps) induce incomplete tetanic contractions and pulse rates higher than 45–50 pps typically induce fused tetanic contraction. For most applications it is desirable to have a tetanic contraction of muscle. There is considerable inter-subject variability with regard to fusion frequency. Pulse rate is also associated with stimulation comfort during tetanic contractions (Naaman et al., 2000). Increasing pulse rate is known to cause a greater degree of muscle fatigue during tetanic contractions (Binder-Macleod and Guerin, 1990; Cestari et al., 1995; Binder-Macleod and Lee, 1996;

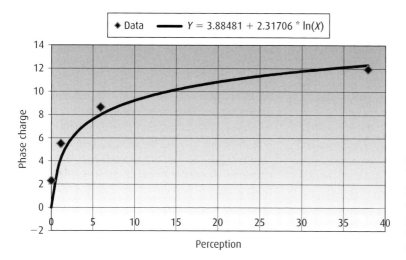

Figure 9.2. Logarithmic relationship between phase charge and perception of stimulus discomfort in a single healthy volunteer. The perception of discomfort was determined by a visual-analog scale from 0% to 100%.

Russ and Binder-Macleod, 1999; Galea, 2001). For FES, the tradeoff as stimulating frequency is increased (in order to obtain a smoother contraction) is more rapid muscle fatigue.

Phase charge (charge per phase)

Phase charge is defined as the current-time integral over the phase duration period. Phase charge has been closely associated with the ability of a stimulus to depolarize the nerve membrane and initiate action potential propagation (Gracanin and Trnkoczy, 1975; Alon et al., 1983; Kantor et al., 1994). As the amount of phase charge increases, more nerve fibers are excited leading to stronger perception (sensory excitation) and stronger muscle contraction (Fig. 9.2) (Adams et al., 1993; Vanderthommen et al., 2000).

Stimulus time modulations

Three basic modulations are common in commercially available stimulators. One is termed inter-pulse interval, the second "burst of pulses" and the third "interrupted pulses" (or "ON and OFF" modes). Modulation of the inter-pulse interval simultaneously modulates pulse (rate) frequency. Binder-Macleod and colleagues identified a pattern of modulation termed catch-like property of human muscle where manipulation of the inter-pulse intervals resulted in greater force production and less muscle fatigue compared to using constant pulse rate (Binder-Macleod and Lee, 1996; Russ and Binder-Macleod, 1999). Having a burst of three pulses decreases the amplitude of peak current at a given level of excitation while concurrently causing a three-fold increase in RMS current amplitude compared to a single biphasic pulse (Kantor et al., 1994). Consequently the use of burst of pulses can be justified only if it makes the stimulation more comfortable.

The option of interrupted pulses is mandatory in most neurorehabilitation clinical applications. Each stimulation program for different clinical applications is likely to require somewhat different contraction (on) and relaxation (off) times, also known as the duty cycle. The greater the duty cycle, the more profound the problem with muscle fatigue, since the time of rest is reduced.

9.5 Applications of FES systems

Management of musculoskeletal impairments

Impairments that dominate the difficulties in neuro-rehabilitation of CNS mediated paralysis/paresis are muscle weakness/atrophy, limited passive and active joint range of motion, loss of motor control, spasticity, pain, and edema. A number of clinical studies in chronic stroke have demonstrated that a daily or three times per week stimulation program over 3–6 weeks strengthens the stimulated muscles and restores some degree of active and passive range of motion of the mobilized joints (Smith, 1990; Hazlewood et al., 1994; Pandyan et al., 1997; Alon et al., 1998; Powell et al., 1999). More recent clinical trials have combined the NMES with task-specific training of the paretic upper limb (Alon, 2003; Cauraugh and Kim, 2002, 2003a, b, c). Significant improvement in motor control as documented by Fugl-Meyer score or EMG has been reported by a number of investigators (Faghri et al., 1994; Chae et al., 1998; Francisco et al., 1998; Powell et al., 1999; Cauraugh et al., 2000; Cauraugh and Kim, 2002, 2003a, b, c; Kimberley et al., 2004). Improved functional ability was limited to improvement in performance speed or increasing number of blocks transferred but not re-learning of hand function or ability lost due to paralysis, however.

Spasticity

Over 50 clinical studies are published on the application of stimulation for modification of spasticity. Three approaches have been used. The first approach uses sensory stimulation over the spastic muscle group. The second approach elicits muscle contraction in the antagonist muscle group for strengthening and simultaneous stretch of the spastic muscles. The third, most recent approach has been to stimulate alternately both agonists and antagonists (Alon et al., 1998, 2003). All three approaches have been statistically equally beneficial. Many patients are likely to experience a long-term reduction in spasticity of about 0.7–1 notch on the 0–5 Ashworth scale, a rather modest effect that may not justify prescribing NMES for the sole purpose of spasticity management. For additional information on the mechanisms and management of spasticity, see Volume II, Chapter 17.

Stroke

Shoulder subluxation

Four clinical trials have been performed investigating whether early initiation of NMES could minimize shoulder subluxation, a problem in 20–40% of stroke survivors (see Volume II, Chapter 36 on stroke rehabilitation). (Faghri et al., 1994; Chantraine et al., 1999; Linn et al., 1999; Wang et al., 2000). The impairments of subluxation and shoulder pain can be minimized in the majority of patients while improving passive joint range and volitional deltoid activation after 4–6 weeks of training. This training is insufficient to yield meaningful reduction if the NMES is delayed for 6–12 months post-subluxation (Wang et al., 2000). It should be noted that these studies used reduction of subluxation as an outcome and not upper limb functional activities.

Upper limb function in hemiparesis

The value of NMES to the training of upper limb function remains controversial. Recent studies have begun to test the contribution of NMES particularly to hand function (Cauraugh et al., 2000; Alon et al., 2002; Cauraugh and Kim, 2002, 2003a, b, c; Alon and Ring, 2003; Alon et al., 2003; Popovic et al., 2003). Outcome measures used in hand function evaluation vary considerably. Cauraugh and colleagues only use the box and blocks test while others also use the Jebsen-Taylor and the nine-hole peg (Alon and Ring, 2003; Alon et al., 2003; Kimberley et al., 2004). Popovic et al. (2003) recently used a comprehensive test battery that included many ADLs that depend on the upper limb collectively termed upper extremity functioning test (UEFT) as well as hand drawing test and patients testimonial statements regarding reduced upper extremity motor activity long (MAL) tests.

Diversity of training programs and the delay of training initiation have contributed to the reluctance of the clinical community to accept FES as a valuable intervention. Most studies that tested true upper limb function and not just impairments enrolled only patients with chronic stroke. Four clinical investigations synchronized clearly described task-specific activities with stimulation. Such synchronization resulted in upper limb functional improvement in 70–80% of participants (Alon and Ring, 2003; Alon et al., 2003; Berner et al., 2004; Ring et al., 2005). The authors added a cautionary note

Table 9.1. Development stages of FES systems for use in spinal cord injury.

| Type of system | Basic research | Clinical research | | FDA regulatory approval |
		Feasibility	Multicenter	
Cardiovascular exercise		√		Yes (Regys, Ergys)
Breathing assist	√	√		Yes (Avery Mark IV) (IDE: Atrotech)
Hand grasp		√	Completed	Yes (Freehand and Handmaster)
Standing	√	√	√	No
Walking		√	Completed	Yes (Parastep)
Bladder/bowel	√	√	√	Yes (Vocare)
Electroejaculation		√	√	Yes

that while the gains of hand functions were both statistically and clinically meaningful, the vast majority of patients improve the time of performance but did not re-learn functional ability.

Ambulation in hemiparesis

Gait performance has been enhanced by FES during ambulation (Malezic et al., 1987). The most common target muscle for stimulation has been the dorsiflexors of hemiparetic patients. The stimulation is typically synchronized with the gait cycle, so that the dorsiflexors are active during the swing phase. The main outcome measures that improve after 4–5 months of use are walking speed (20–27%) and physiological cost index (PCI). Walking speed after the training period without the stimulator only improves 10–14% if the stimulation was limited to the dorsiflexors, however (Burridge et al., 1997b; Taylor et al., 1999; Yan et al., 2005), multisegment stimulation of both plantar flexors and dorsiflexors has been used in stroke. Training involved increasing speed of ambulation as well as stair climbing and walking on different terrains. Using this paradigm, gait velocity improved 36% and cadence by 19% (Alon and Ring, 2003), which represents an improvement from the results with dorsiflexors stimulation alone.

9.6 Spinal cord injury

Functional uses for FES after spinal cord injury (SCI) include applications in standing, walking, hand grasp, bladder and bowel function, respiratory assist, and electroejaculation. Each of these technologies have been developed and implemented to various degrees over the course of the past few decades. These applications will be discussed separately. Table 9.1 lists the applications and indicates for each one the current stage of development.

Therapeutic exercise

The most common system for lower extremity FES exercise is the bicycle ergometer (Glenn and Phelps, 1985). The most common commercially available ergometer is the ERGYS Clinical Rehabilitation System (Therapeutic Technologies, Inc., Tampa, FL). This computer controlled ergometer uses six channels and surface electrodes to sequentially stimulate quadriceps, hamstrings and glutei bilaterally. Some systems also include the capacity for simultaneous voluntary arm crank exercise by paraplegics, thereby permitting *hybrid exercise.*

Cardiac capacity and muscle oxidative capacity (see Volume II, Chapter 21) have both been shown to improve with FES ergometry. Some subjects can train with FES ergometry up to a similar aerobic metabolic rate (measured by peak VO_2) as those achieved in the able-bodied population (Glaser, 1991). Electrical exercise also increases peripheral venous return and fibrinolysis. There are limits to the cardiovascular benefits of FES ergometry, however, especially in those with lesions above T5. In those patients, there is loss of supraspinal sympathetic control, which in turn limits the body's ability to increase heart rate, stroke volume and cardiac output (Ragnarsson, 1991). Evidence is mixed as to whether FES ergometry can retard or reverse the osteoporosis seen in patients with SCI. In one study of 10 spinal cord injured individuals who underwent 12 months of FES cycling 30 min per day, 3 days per week, bone mineral density of the proximal tibia increased 10%. Unfortunately, after a further 6 months of exercise but at a frequency of only one session per week, the bone mineral density reverted to pre-training levels (Mohr et al., 1997).

Breathing assistance in high tetraplegia

Phrenic nerve pacing was developed in the early 1960s by Glenn and colleagues (Glenn and Phelps, 1985). In appropriate candidates (see Volume II, Chapter 37 on Rehabilitation in Spinal Cord Injury), phrenic nerve pacing has the potential to improve mobility, speech, and overall health, as well as to reduce anxiety and the volume of respiratory secretions, improve the level of comfort, and reduce required nursing care in ventilator dependent tetraplegic individuals (DiMarco, 2001). Confirmation of phrenic nerve function via nerve conduction studies or observation of diaphragm movement under fluoroscopy is necessary before considering phrenic nerve stimulation and diaphragmatic pacing (MacLean and Mattioni, 1981).

The implanted components of neuroprosthetic systems for phrenic nerve pacing consist of nerve electrodes placed around or adjacent to the phrenic nerves, radio-frequency receivers, and cabling. The external components are the radio-frequency transmitter and the antenna. There are currently three manufactures of these devices: Avery, Atrotech, and MedImplant. The Avery and Atrotech devices are available in the USA. The Avery device has received pre-market approval by the food and drug administration (FDA), and is the one most widely used. The Atrotech system is available under an FDA Investigational Device Exemption. The Atrotech has a more sophisticated four-pole electrode system, which is thought to reduce the chance for fatigue. All of these systems allow for changes in stimulus frequency, amplitude, and train rate.

Surgically, the electrodes are placed on or around the phrenic nerve in the neck or thorax. The receiver is placed in a subcutaneous pocket on the anterior chest wall, and the leads are tunneled through the third or fourth inter-costal space. Stimulation is initiated approximately 2 weeks post-operatively. Reconditioning is then required to improve the fatigue resistance of the diaphragm. Low-frequency stimulation (7–12 Hz) is required to help convert the diaphragm to primarily oxidative, slow-twitch Type I fibers (Oda et al., 1981). The respiratory rate usually lies within 8–14 breaths/min during initiation of therapy, and then is reduced to 6–12 breaths/min later on.

The possible complications of phrenic nerve pacing include infection, mechanical injury to the phrenic nerve, upper airway obstruction, reduction in ventilation due to altered respiratory system mechanics, and technical malfunctions. Most patients using electrophrenic respiration maintain their tracheostomy stoma to be used at night and for suctioning, although many of them can plug the sites during the day.

Recent advances for respiratory pacing have been contributed by the work of DiMarco and colleagues, who have demonstrated the use of a minimally invasive approach for introducing electrodes into the diaphragm with a laparoscope. This technique significantly reduces the surgical procedure required. Electrodes are placed bilaterally near the motor points to activate the muscles simultaneously for inspiration; expiration is due to passive relaxation. Of five subjects who have been entered into a clinical protocol and are through the exercise period, four have sufficient ventilation for breathing without other aids (e.g., respirator) for many hours per day. Subjects also report the return of smell as a result of the procedure (DiMarco, 2001).

FES for standing and walking in paraplegia

There have been over 24 centers worldwide that have participated over the years in investigation of the use of FES for lower extremity standing and walking in paraplegia (Peckham, 1987; Peckham and Creasey, 1992). Standing alone is a goal of some systems. The potential physiologic benefits of standing include a beneficial effect on digestion, bowel and bladder function. There are also functional standing goals of reaching for high objects and face-to-face interaction with other people, and improved transfer between surfaces. The muscles usually stimulated to provide for standing function are the quadriceps and hip extensors, which provide for knee and hip extension and joint stability in a locked position in a similar biomechanical way as do knee-ankle-foot orthoses. Implanted systems, which provide activation of eight separate muscle groups, also employ trunk extension for greater postural stability (Triolo et al., 1996).

Several different approaches have been used in helping paraplegics walk. Hybrid approaches, such as the reciprocating gait orthosis (RGO) originally developed at Louisiana State University, and modified at Wright State University, use both mechanical bracing and surface FES. Specifically, FES hip extension on one side provides contralateral leg swing through the RGO mechanism (Solomonow et al., 1997). In general, patients with injuries between T4 and T12 with upper body strength and stability as well as intact lower motor neurons are appropriate candidates for consideration, although higher-level patients have been involved in some protocols.

There is one FDA approved class III surface FES walking system available for use in the USA. Made by Sigmetics Inc., the Parastep system is a four- or six-channel surface stimulation device for ambulation with the aide of a walker. The Parastep system uses the triple-flexion response elicited by peroneal nerve stimulation as well as knee and hip extensor surface stimulation to construct the gait cycle. The patient controls the gait with switches integrated into a rolling walker. The electronic controller is housed in a cassette-sized box mounted on the patient's belt. The Parastep System and other similar systems have been used by paraplegics not only for functional standing and walking but also for aerobic exercise (Graupe and Kohn, 1998). In April, 2003, the Centers for Medicare and Medicaid Services (CMS)

started to provide insurance coverage for the purchase of and training with the Parastep.

Implantable lower extremity FES has also been developed. The percutaneous system developed in Cleveland used up to 48 different electrodes to provide reciprocal gait. The considerable effort required for maintenance of percutaneous electrodes has made that type of system impractical for widespread use, however. Implantable eight-channel systems with the more limited goals of standing and transfer are also under investigation.

All of the above mentioned pure FES systems require use of a walker for stability and safety. The energy expenditures required for continuous FES walking using any system is at least twice (if not more) than that for normal upright ambulation. Future directions for lower extremity FES for paraplegia would be to achieve more modest goals than originally envisioned, such as standing, transfer assistance, and possibly short distance (e.g., home) mobility. It is not anticipated that FES for walking in paraplegia will replace the wheelchair as the primary mobility aide.

FES for hand grasp and release

Technology for the restoration of hand function in tetraplegic individuals has been under development for over three decades (Billian and Gorman, 1992) and has now entered the clinical environment (Peckham et al., 2001). The objective of the use of FES in hands of tetraplegic individuals is to restore grasp, hold and release, thereby increasing independence in performance of functional tasks.

Tetraplegic hand grasp systems have focused on the C5 and C6 level SCI patient populations. These individuals have adequate voluntary strength in the proximal muscles (i.e., deltoid, rotator cuff, biceps) to move their hand in a functional space. Those with C4 level injury have also participated in limited laboratory-based investigations of FES systems (Nathan and Ohry, 1990), but the results of these studies have been limited. Patients injured at the C7 and lower levels have multiple voluntarily active forearm muscles which can be used to motor new functions by means of tendon transfer surgery (Keith et al., 1996).

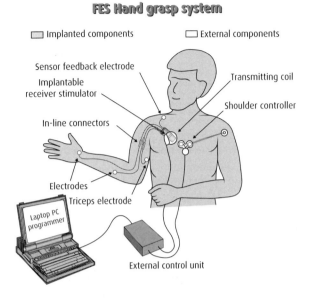

FES Hand grasp system

☐ Implanted components   ☐ External components

Sensor feedback electrode
Implantable receiver stimulator
Transmitting coil
Shoulder controller
In-line connectors
Electrodes
Triceps electrode
Laptop PC programmer
External control unit

Figure 9.3. Components of an implantable upper extremity neuroprosthesis. On the left of the diagram are the implanted components, which include the implant stimulator, electrode leads, epimysial electrodes, and in some cases a sensory electrode to provide a form of sensory feedback. Not shown are implantable intramuscular electrodes which are an available option. On the right are the external components of the neuroprosthesis, which include a shoulder position controller incorporating the device's on/off switch, an ECU, and a transmitting coil.

Two commercially available FDA approved upper extremity neuroprostheses have been developed. One of them is a surface system and one is implanted. These devices will be discussed separately.

Freehand system

The Freehand System® consists of an external joint position transducer/controller, a rechargeable programmable external control unit (ECU) and an implantable eight-channel stimulator/receiver attached via flexible wires to epimysial disc electrodes (Fig. 9.3). The user controls the system through small movements of either the shoulder or wrist. The joint position transducer is typically mounted on the skin from sternum to contralateral shoulder or across the ipsilateral wrist. The ECU uses this signal to power proportional control of hand grasp and release. Communication between the ECU and the implantable stimulator, which is located in a surgical pocket in the upper chest, is through radiofrequency coupling. The system can be programmed through a personal computer interface to individualize the grasps as well as the shoulder control (Kilgore et al., 1997). Individuals can choose to use

either a palmar or lateral prehension grasp pattern. This is helpful in handling either large objects or small objects respectively. The current system is intended to provide unilateral hand grasp only. Results from the multicenter trial that led to FDA approval in 1997 are discussed below (Peckham et al., 2001).

Sixty-one C5 or C6 patients were enrolled. All of the patients had one or more concurrent surgical procedures to augment hand function. A total of 128 cumulative implant years were evaluated. Summary pinch force measurements with and without the neuroprosthesis are shown in Fig. 9.4. Pinch force in both lateral and palmar prehension improved with the neuroprosthesis. The small improvement seen post-operatively with the neuroprosthesis turned off can be attributed to tendon synchronization. All patients realized some improvement in pinch force measurement in at least one grasp pattern with the neuroprosthesis.

A grasp and release test was used to evaluate each subject's ability to grasp, move, and release six standardized objects. The number of completed moves in 30 s achieved by subjects increased significantly for the heavier objects with the neuroprosthesis.

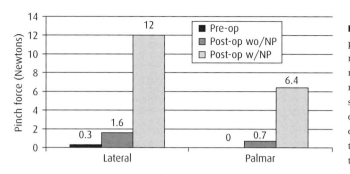

Figure 9.4. Pinch force for lateral and palmar prehension with and without the Freehand® neuroprosthesis. The histogram family on the left represents lateral grasp; palmar grasp is on the right. Force represented in Newtons. There is some increase in force produced post-operatively even with the neuroprosthesis turned off. This is probably related to the increase in tone produced by surgical tightening of the flexor tendons.

No improvement was seen in manipulation of the lightest objects. An ADL abilities test evaluated whether the neuroprosthesis decreased the amount of assistance required to perform various ADLs. Across all patients and tasks, 50% showed an improvement in independence score, and 78% preferred to use the neuroprosthesis to perform the activities. Through a survey instrument, patients reported overall satisfaction with the performance of the system, indicated that it had a positive impact on their lives, and provided them with less dependence on other adaptive equipment. As of January 2004, there are over 200 patients in the world who have received this device.

Adverse events requiring surgical management included receiver repositioning or replacement, skin openings, electrode breakage, infection requiring electrode removal or system explant and tendon adhesion. The major non-surgical adverse events included swelling or discomfort over the implantable components, skin irritation from external products, irritation from incisions or sutures and skin irritation from splints or casts.

Handmaster

The Handmaster, which is produced by the NESS Corporation in Israel (Jjzerman et al., 1996), is composed of a hinged shell with a spiral splint that stabilizes the wrist. Surface electrodes are built into the shell and stimulate the finger flexors and extensors and the thenar musculature. In addition, the company has recently produced a proximal arm segment

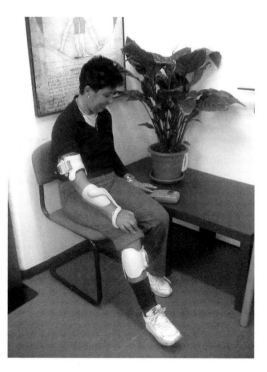

Figure 9.5. The Handmaster System external orthoses, manufactured by NESS Limited. The forearm device incorporates three surface stimulation electrodes into the molded orthosis to provide pinch grip. An additional arm segment and a lower leg segment using the same surface stimulation technology, is also available. The subject controls the device through a controller box, which contains a trigger button to start stimulation and a mode button to choose between pre-programmed patterns of muscle activation.

and a leg segment using the same technology (Fig. 9.5). A trigger button mounted on a separate control unit allows the user to start the stimulation sequence. A separate mode button allows the user to choose different pre-programmed patterns of muscle activation. The device is designed to be used with C5 and C6 tetraplegic individuals as well as individuals with hemiplegia. The NESS device has been studied clinically in pilot investigations (Weingarden et al., 1998; Alon and McBride, 2003). A case study of seven patients with C5 or C6 tetraplegia has been completed, and three ADL activities that could not be performed without the Handmaster were performed successfully with the neuroprosthesis. In addition, improvements in grip strength, finger motion, and Fugl-Meyer scores were documented. The advantages of the Handmaster are its non-invasiveness, cost, and relative ease of application. Disadvantages include its cosmesis, as external splinting is required and the fact that the device is less customizable than the Freehand system.

Future directions for hand grasp neuroprostheses

Future developments and improvements in tetraplegic hand grasp systems include increasing the number of channels, use of implantable controllers (Johnson et al., 1999), closed loop feedback with improved sensor technology, proximal muscle control, control of the prontation/supination axis, addition of finger intrinsics to improve finger extension (Lauer et al., 1999), bilateral implementation, and myoelectric EMG control. Ultimately, technologies such as the development of injectable electrodes and cortical control of movement may impact as well on these devices. The overall objective of these developments is to simplify the control functions by making them more natural, provide enhanced movement of the hand and stronger control of the proximal musculature, and reduce the donning process.

Control of micturition with FES

Electrical stimulation to control bladder function after supra-sacral SCI has been under investigation for several decades. Stimulation at various levels of the neurourologic axis has been attempted. In Great Britain, Brindley and Rushton (1990) has had the most experience and success with S2 through S4 anterior sacral nerve root stimulation in combination with posterior rhizotomy. This system is surgically implanted through lumbar laminectomy and employs either epidural or intradural electrodes. Electrodes are connected via cable to an implanted radio receiver, which couples to an external stimulator/transmitter. Pulsed stimulation is used to take advantage of the differences between activation of the slow response smooth musculature of the detrusor (bladder) and activation of the fast twitch striated sphincter musculature (Fig. 9.6). Bladder pressure gradually increases in a tetanic fashion, while sphincter pressure rapidly falls after the end of each stimulation pulse. This produces short spurts of urination that result in nearly complete bladder emptying.

Potential candidates for the Vocare implant need to have intact parasympathetic efferent neurons to the detrusor musculature (see Volume II, Chapter 24). This can be ascertained by cysometrogram recording of bladder pressure (Creasey, 1999). In order to provide continence of urine with this device, one has to abolish reflex incontinence caused by activation of the sensory reflex pathway. This has been done by performance of a sacral posterior rhizotomy. This procedure abolishes uninhibited reflex bladder contractions and restores bladder compliance. Detrusor-sphincter dyssynergia is also reduced, thereby avoiding the chance of autonomic dysreflexia. The downside of this procedure, however, is loss of perineal sensation in sensory incomplete individuals and loss of reflex erection and ejaculation if present.

Over 1500 sacral anterior root stimulators have been implanted. Of those approximately 90% are in regular use 4–6 times per day. In the USA, the FDA approved the implantation of the device in 1998 under the trade name Vocare™.

In a study of 20 patients, post-void residual volumes were reduced on average from 212 to 22 ml with the Vocare system (Van Kerrebroeck et al., 1993). A significant reduction in the number of

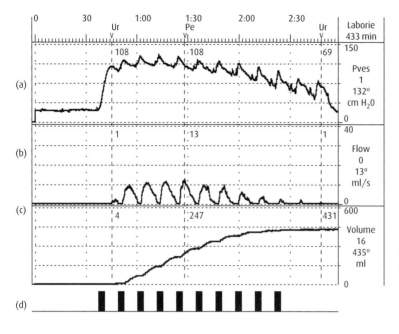

Figure 9.6. Physiology of micturition produced by the Vocare® sacral nerve stimulator as identified by cystometrogram recording. X-axis represents time in minutes and seconds with the total tracing lasting approximately 3 min. (a) Intravesicular pressure in mm water from 0 to 150. (b) Urine flow rate in ml/s with the scale from 0 to 40 ml/s. (c) Cumulated volume of urine voided in ml with the scale from 0 to 600 ml. (d) Approximate timing of the sacral nerve stimulation used to produce this intermittent voiding pattern.

symptomatic urinary tract infections has been seen. Continence has been achieved in more than 85% of implant recipients, probably due to the concurrent posterior rhizotomy (Brindley, 1995). Improved health of the upper urinary tracts has been demonstrated by a decreased incidence of bladder trabeculation and hydronephrosis (Peckham et al., 2001).

The sacral anterior root stimulators have also been shown to improve bowel care (i.e., increased defecation, reduced constipation). About half of implant recipients can use the stimulator to defecate. Even in those patients that cannot, the amount of time spent in bowel evacuation has been shown to be considerably less (MacDonagh et al., 1990). Approximately 60% of men can also produce penile erection with the device.

Long-term follow-up from Europe has documented the safety of this implant device and procedure. Economic analysis of the long-term cost savings due to the decreased use of catheters, antibiotics, medical resources etc. indicate that the implant would pay for itself within 5–7 years (Creasey et al., 2000).

Electroejaculation

Originally developed within veterinary medicine, electroejaculation now provides a mechanism by which spinal cord injured men can father children. Electrically stimulated rectal probes are used to produce seminal emission. After serial electroejaculation procedures, the quality of the semen produced generally improves to the point where artificial insemination or in-vitro fertilization is possible. As the coordination required to achieve successful pregnancies with this technique, multidisciplinary expertise is required (Ohl, 1993). For additional discussion of rehabilitation for sexual dysfunction, see Volume II, Chapter 25.

9.7 Future directions and challenges

The intense scientific research and developmental work in the field of FES that has occurred over the last half century has realized meaningful clinical applications to ameliorate functional deficiencies of

serious neurological injuries. Several neuroprosthetic devices have gone through regulatory review
and have reached the clinical world. Further development and refinement of this technology will likely
enhance the lives of a greater number of patients
with disability.

Technological advancements that are currently
ongoing relate to the interface to nerve structures
and implant stimulator design. The nerve interface
is key to the stimulation or inhibition process.
Considerable progress has been made in the design
of nerve-based electrodes that provide close contact
to the nerve. Advanced stimulator designs are now
also being realized. A newly emerging technology,
called the BION®, now entering clinical trials in
some applications, allows a small single-channel
device to be implanted through a cannula into the
desired location for activation of the nerve. Multiple
units can be controlled through a single encompassing external transmitting coil powered by an external
processor, thus enabling some clinical applications
to be realized without surgery. The advances in
these technologies and the physiological interventions that they enable will make it possible to realize
even greater impact in the lives and function of people with neurological disability.

REFERENCES

Adams, G.R., Harris, R.T., et al. (1993). Mapping of electrical
muscle stimulation using MRI. *J Appl Physiol*, **74(2)**,
532–537.

Alon, G. (1985). High voltage stimulation. Effects of electrode size
on basic excitatory responses. *Phys Ther*, **65(6)**, 890–895.

Alon, G. (2003). Training dosage and timing of electrical stimulation may be the key for maximizing the effects of NMES in
neuro-rehabilitation. *Adv Physical Rehabil Med*, N. Soroker
and H. Ring, Monduzzi Editore, 441–447.

Alon, G., Allin, J., et al. (1983). Optimization of pulse duration
and pulse charge during transcutaneous electrical nerve
stimulation. *Aust J Physiother*, **29**, 195–201.

Alon, G., Dar, A., et al. (1998). Efficacy of a hybrid upper limb
neuromuscular electrical stimulation system in lessening
selected impairments and dysfunctions consequent to
cerebral damage. *J Neuro Rehabil*, **12**, 73–80.

Alon, G., Kantor, G., et al. (1994). Effects of electrode size on
basic excitatory responses and on selected stimulus parameters. *J Orthop Sports Phys Ther*, **20(1)**, 29–35.

Alon, G., Kantor, G., et al. (1996). The effect of three types of surface electrodes on threshold excitation of human motor
nerve. *J Clin Electrophysiol*, **8**, 2–8.

Alon, G. and McBride, K. (2003). Persons with C5 or C6 tetraplegia achieve selected functional gains using a neuroprosthesis. *Arch Phys Med Rehabil*, **84(1)**, 119–124.

Alon, G., McBride, S., et al. (2002). Improving selected hand
functions using upper extremity noninvasive neuroprosthesis in persons with chronic stroke. *J Stroke Cerebrovascul
Dis*, **11**, 99–106.

Alon, G. and Ring, H. (2003). Gait and hand function enhancement following training with a multi-segment hybrid-
orthosis stimulation system in stroke patients. *J Stroke
Cerebrovascul Dis*, **12(5)**, 209–216.

Alon, G., Sunnerhagen, K.S., et al. (2003). A home-based, self-
administered stimulation program to improve selected
hand functions of chronic stroke. *Neurorehabilitation*,
18(3), 215–225.

Baker, L.L., Bowman, B.R., et al. (1988). Effects of waveform on
comfort during neuromuscular electrical stimulation. *Clin
Orthop*, **(233)**, 75–85.

Baker, L.L., Benton, L.A., et al. (1993). *Neuromuscular Electrical
Stimulation: A Practical Guide*. Rancho Los Amigos Medical
Center, Downey, California.

Bennie, S.D., Petrofsky, J.S., et al. (2002). Toward the optimal
waveform for electrical stimulation of human muscle.
Eur J Appl Physiol, **88(1–2)**, 13–19.

Berner, Y.N., Lif Kimchi, O., Spokoiny, V., Finkeltov, B. (2004).
The effect of electric stimulation treatment of the functional rehabilitation of acute geriatric patients with stroke –
a preliminary study. *Arch Gerontol Geriatr*, **39(2)**: 125–132.

Billian, C. and Gorman, P.H. (1992). Upper extremity applications of functional neuromuscular stimulation. *Assist
Technol*, **4(1)**, 31–39.

Binder-Macleod, S.A. and Guerin, T. (1990). Preservation of
force output through progressive reduction of stimulation
frequency in human quadriceps femoris muscle. *Phys Ther*,
70(10), 619–625.

Binder-Macleod, S.A. and Lee, S.C. (1996). Catchlike property of
human muscle during isovelocity movements. *J Appl
Physiol*, **80(6)**, 2051–2059.

Brindley, G.S. (1995). The first 500 sacral anterior root stimulators:
implant failures and their repair. *Paraplegia*, **33(1)**, 5–9.

Brindley, G.S. and Rushton, D.N. (1990). Long-term follow-up
of patients with sacral anterior root stimulator implants.
Paraplegia, **28(8)**, 469–475.

Burridge, J., Taylor, P., et al. (1997a). Experience of clinical use of the Odstock dropped foot stimulator. *Artif Organs*, **21**(3), 254–260.

Burridge, J.H., Taylor, P.N., et al. (1997b). The effects of common peroneal stimulation on the effort and speed of walking: a randomized controlled trial with chronic hemiplegic patients. *Clin Rehabil*, **11**(3), 201–210.

Cauraugh, J.H. and Kim, S. (2002). Two coupled motor recovery protocols are better than one: electromyogram-triggered neuromuscular stimulation and bilateral movements. *Stroke*, **33**(6), 1589–1594.

Cauraugh, J.H. and Kim, S. (2003a). Progress toward motor recovery with active neuromuscular stimulation: muscle activation pattern evidence after a stroke. *J Neurol Sci*, **207**(1–2), 25–29.

Cauraugh, J.H. and Kim, S.B. (2003b). Chronic stroke motor recovery: duration of active neuromuscular stimulation. *J Neurol Sci*, **215**(1–2), 13–19.

Cauraugh, J.H. and Kim, S.B. (2003c). Stroke motor recovery: active neuromuscular stimulation and repetitive practice schedules. *J Neurol Neurosurg Psychiatr*, **74**(11), 1562–1566.

Cauraugh, J., Light, K., et al. (2000). Chronic motor dysfunction after stroke: recovering wrist and finger extension by electromyography-triggered neuromuscular stimulation. *Stroke*, **31**(6), 1360–1364.

Cestari, I.A., Marques, E., et al. (1995). Effects of muscle length, frequency of stimulation, and fatigue on the isometric tension in canine latissimus dorsi. *Artif Organs*, **19**(3), 217–221.

Chae, J., Bethoux, F., et al. (1998). Neuromuscular stimulation for upper extremity motor and functional recovery in acute hemiplegia. *Stroke*, **29**(5), 975–979.

Chantraine, A., Baribeault, A., et al. (1999). Shoulder pain and dysfunction in hemiplegia: effects of functional electrical stimulation. *Arch Phys Med Rehabil*, **80**(3), 328–331.

Crago, P.E., Peckham, P.H., et al. (1974). The choice of pulse duration for chronic electrical stimulation via surface, nerve, and intramuscular electrodes. *Ann Biomed Eng*, **2**(3), 252–264.

Crago, P.E., Nakai, R.J., et al. (1991). Feedback regulation of hand grasp opening and contact force during stimulation of paralyzed muscle. *IEEE Trans Biomed Eng*, **38**(1), 17–28.

Creasey, G. (1999). Restoration of bladder, bowel, and sexual function. *Top Spinal Cord Inj Rehabil*, **5**(1), 21–32.

Creasey, G.H., Kilgore, K.L., et al. (2000). Reduction of costs of disability using neuroprostheses. *Assist Technol*, **12**(1), 67–75.

DiMarco, A.F. (2001). Neural prostheses in the respiratory system. *J Rehabil Res Dev*, **38**(6), 601–607.

Faghri, P.D., Rodgers, M.M., et al. (1994). The effects of functional electrical stimulation on shoulder subluxation, arm function recovery, and shoulder pain in hemiplegic stroke patients. *Arch Phys Med Rehabil*, **75**(1), 73–79.

Francisco, G., Chae, J., et al. (1998). Electromyogram-triggered neuromuscular stimulation for improving the arm function of acute stroke survivors: a randomized pilot study? *Arch Phys Med Rehabil*, **79**(5), 570–575.

Friedli, W.G. and Meyer, M. (1984). Strength-duration curve: a measure for assessing sensory deficit in peripheral neuropathy. *J Neurol Neurosurg Psychiatr*, **47**(2), 184–189.

Frijns, J.H., Mooij, J., et al. (1994). A quantitative approach to modeling mammalian myelinated nerve fibers for electrical prosthesis design. *IEEE Trans Biomed Eng*, **41**(6), 556–566.

Galea, V. (2001). Electrical characteristics of human ankle dorsi- and plantar-flexor muscles. Comparative responses during fatiguing stimulation and recovery. *Eur J Appl Physiol*, **85**(1–2), 130–140.

Glaser, R. (1991). Physiology of functional electrical stimulation-induced exercise: basic science perspective. *J Neuro Rehab*, **5**(1–2), 49–61.

Glenn, W.W. and Phelps, M.L. (1985). Diaphragm pacing by electrical stimulation of the phrenic nerve. *Neurosurgery*, **17**(6), 974–984.

Gold, M.R. and Shorofsky, S.R. (1997). Strength-duration relationship for human transvenous defibrillation. *Circulation*, **96**(10), 3517–3520.

Gracanin, F. and Trnkoczy, A. (1975). Optimal stimulus parameters for minimum pain in the chronic stimulation of innervated muscle. *Arch Phys Med Rehabil*, **56**(6), 243–249.

Graupe, D. and Kohn, K.H. (1998). Functional neuromuscular stimulator for short-distance ambulation by certain thoracic-level spinal-cord-injured paraplegics. *Surg Neurol*, **50**(3), 202–207.

Han, B.S., Jang, S.H., et al. (2003). Functional magnetic resonance image finding of cortical activation by neuromuscular electrical stimulation on wrist extensor muscles. *Am J Phys Med Rehabil*, **82**(1), 17–20.

Hasan, S.T., Robson, W.A., et al. (1996). Transcutaneous electrical nerve stimulation and temporary S3 neuromodulation in idiopathic detrusor instability. *J Urol*, **155**(6), 2005–2011.

Hazlewood, M.E., Brown, J.K., et al. (1994). The use of therapeutic electrical stimulation in the treatment of hemiplegic cerebral palsy. *Dev Med Child Neurol*, **36**(8), 661–673.

Henkin, Y., Kaplan-Neeman, R., et al. (2003). Changes over time in electrical stimulation levels and electrode impedance values in children using the Nucleus 24M cochlear implant. *Int J Pediatr Otorhinolaryngol*, **67**(8), 873–880.

Iggo, A. (1978). The physiological interpretation of electrical stimulation of the nervous system. *Electroencephalogr Clin Neurophysiol Suppl*, **34**, 335–341.

Jjzerman, M.J., in 't Groen, F.A., Klatte, M.A.P., Snock, O.J., Vorsteveld, J.H.C., Nathan, R.H., Hermens, H.J. (1996). The NESS Handmaster orthosis: restoration of hand function in C5 and stroke patients by means of electrical stimulation. *J Rehabil Sci*, **9**, 86–89.

Johnson, M.W., Peckham, P.H., et al. (1999). Implantable transducer for two-degree of freedom joint angle sensing. *IEEE Trans Rehabil Eng*, **7**(3), 349–359.

Kantor, G., Alon, G., et al. (1994). The effects of selected stimulus waveforms on pulse and phase characteristics at sensory and motor thresholds. *Phys Ther*, **74**(10), 951–962.

Keith, M.W., Kilgore, K.L., et al. (1996). Tendon transfers and functional electrical stimulation for restoration of hand function in spinal cord injury. *J Hand Surg [Am]*, **21**(1), 89–99.

Kern, H., Hofer, C., et al. (1999). Standing up with denervated muscles in humans using functional electrical stimulation. *Artif Organ*, **23**(5), 447–452.

Kern, H., Hofer, C., et al. (2002). Denervated muscles in humans: limitations and problems of currently used functional electrical stimulation training protocols. *Artif Organ*, **26**(3), 216–218.

Kilgore, K.L., Peckham, P.H., et al. (1997). An implanted upper-extremity neuroprosthesis. Follow-up of five patients. *J Bone Joint Surg Am*, **79**(4), 533–541.

Kimberley, T.J., Lewis, S.M., et al. (2004). Electrical stimulation driving functional improvements and cortical changes in subjects with stroke. *Exp Brain Res*, **154**(4), 450–460.

Knaflitz, M., Merletti, R., et al. (1990). Inference of motor unit recruitment order in voluntary and electrically elicited contractions. *J Appl Physiol*, **68**(4), 1657–1667.

Lauer, R.T., Kilgore, K.L., et al. (1999). The function of the finger intrinsic muscles in response to electrical stimulation. *IEEE Trans Rehabil Eng*, **7**(1), 19–26.

Laufer, Y., Ries, J.D., et al. (2001). Quadriceps femoris muscle torques and fatigue generated by neuromuscular electrical stimulation with three different waveforms. *Phys Ther*, **81**(7), 1307–1316.

Linn, S.L., Granat, M.H., et al. (1999). Prevention of shoulder subluxation after stroke with electrical stimulation. *Stroke*, **30**(5), 963–968.

MacDonagh, R.P., Sun, W.M., et al. (1990). Control of defecation in patients with spinal injuries by stimulation of sacral anterior nerve roots. *Br Med J*, **300**(6738), 1494–1497.

MacLean, I.C. and Mattioni, T.A. (1981). Phrenic nerve conduction studies: a new technique and its application in quadriplegic patients. *Arch Phys Med Rehabil*, **62**(2), 70–73.

Malezic, M., Bogataj, U., et al. (1987). Evaluation of gait with multichannel electrical stimulation. *Orthopedics*, **10**(5), 769–772.

Memberg, W., Peckham, P.H., Thrope, G.B., Keith, M.W., Kicher T.P. (1993). An analysis of the reliability of percutaneous intramuscular electrodes in upper extremity FNS applications. *IEEE Trans Rehab Eng*, **1**(2), 126–132.

Mohr, T., Podenphant, J., et al. (1997). Increased bone mineral density after prolonged electrically induced cycle training of paralyzed limbs in spinal cord injured man. *Calcif Tissue Int*, **61**(1), 22–25.

Mortimer, J. (1981). Motor Prostheses. In: *Handbook of Physiology – The Nervous System II, Motor Control* (ed. Brooks, V.B.), American Physiology Society, Bethesda, MD, pp. 158–187.

Muellbacher, W., Richards, C., Ziemann, U., Wittenberg, G., Weltz, D., Boroojerdi B., et al. (2002). Improving hand function in chronic stroke. *Arch Neurol*, **59**(8), 1278–1282.

Mulcahey, M.J., Smith, B.T., et al. (1999). Evaluation of the lower motor neuron integrity of upper extremity muscles in high level spinal cord injury. *Spinal Cord*, **37**(8), 585–591.

Munsat, T.L., McNeal, D., et al. (1976). Effects of nerve stimulation on human muscle. *Arch Neurol*, **33**(9), 608–617.

Naaman, S.C., Stein, R.B., et al. (2000). Minimizing discomfort with surface neuromuscular stimulation. *Neurorehabil Neural Repair*, **14**(3), 223–228.

Nathan, R.H. and Ohry, A. (1990). Upper limb functions regained in quadriplegia: a hybrid computerized neuromuscular stimulation system. *Arch Phys Med Rehabil*, **71**(6), 415–421.

Oda, T., Glenn, W.W., et al. (1981). Evaluation of electrical parameters for diaphragm pacing: an experimental study. *J Surg Res*, **30**(2), 142–153.

Ohl, D. (1993). Electroejaculation. *Urol Clin North Am*, **20**(1), 181–188.

Pandyan, A.D., Granat, M.H., et al. (1997). Effects of electrical stimulation on flexion contractures in the hemiplegic wrist. *Clin Rehabil*, **11**(2), 123–130.

Panescu, D., Webster, J.G., et al. (1994a). Modeling current density distributions during transcutaneous cardiac pacing. *IEEE Trans Biomed Eng*, **41**(6), 549–555.

Panescu, D., Webster, J.G., et al. (1994b). A nonlinear finite element model of the electrode–electrolyte–skin system. *IEEE Trans Biomed Eng*, **41**(7), 681–687.

Peckham, P.H. (1987). Functional electrical stimulation: current status and future prospects of applications to the neuromuscular system in spinal cord injury. *Paraplegia*, **25**(3), 279–288.

Peckham, P.H. and Creasey, G.H. (1992). Neural prostheses: clinical applications of functional electrical stimulation in spinal cord injury. *Paraplegia*, **30**(2), 96–101.

Peckham, P.H., Keith, M.W., et al. (2001). Efficacy of an implanted neuroprosthesis for restoring hand grasp in tetraplegia: a multicenter study. *Arch Phys Med Rehabil*, **82**(10), 1380–1388.

Popovic, M.B., Popovic, D.B., et al. (2003). Clinical evaluation of functional electrical therapy in acute hemiplegic subjects. *J Rehabil Res Dev*, **40**(5), 443–454.

Powell, J., Pandyan, A.D., et al. (1999). Electrical stimulation of wrist extensors in poststroke hemiplegia. *Stroke*, **30**(7), 1384–1389.

Ragnarsson, K., Pollack, S.F. and Twist, D. (1991). Lower limb endurance exercise after spinal cord injury: implications for health and functional ambulation. *J. Neuro Rehab*, **5**(1–2), 37–48.

Ring, H. and Rosenthal, N. (2005). Controlled study of neuro-prosthetic functional electrical stimulation in sub-acute post-stroke rehabilitation. *J Rehabil Med*, **37**(1), 32–6.

Rollman, G.B. (1975). Behavioral assessment of peripheral nerve function. *Neurology*, **25**(4), 339–342.

Russ, D.W. and Binder-Macleod, S.A. (1999). Variable-frequency trains offset low-frequency fatigue in human skeletal muscle. *Muscle Nerve*, **22**(7), 874–882.

Smith, L.E. (1990). Restoration of volitional limb movement of hemiplegics following patterned functional electrical stimulation. *Percept Mot Skills*, **71**(**3 Part 1**), 851–861.

Smith, G.V., Alon, G., Roys S.R. and Gullapalli, R.P. (2003). Functional MRI determination of a dose–response relationship to lower extremity neuromuscular electrical stimulation in healthy subjects. *Exp Brain Res*, **150**(1), 33–9.

Solomonow, M., Reisin, E., et al. (1997). Reciprocating gait orthosis powered with electrical muscle stimulation (RGO II). Part II: Medical evaluation of 70 paraplegic patients. *Orthopedics*, **20**(5), 411–418.

Taylor, P.N., Burridge, J.H., et al. (1999). Clinical use of the Odstock dropped foot stimulator: its effect on the speed and effort of walking. *Arch Phys Med Rehabil*, **80**(12), 1577–1583.

Triolo, R.J., Bieri, C., et al. (1996). Implanted functional neuro-muscular stimulation systems for individuals with cervical spinal cord injuries: clinical case reports. *Arch Phys Med Rehabil*, **77**(11), 1119–1128.

Van Kerrebroeck, P.E., Koldewijn, E.L., et al. (1993). Worldwide experience with the Finetech–Brindley sacral anterior root stimulator. *Neurourol Urodyn*, **12**(5), 497–503.

Vanderthommen, M., Depresseux, J.C., et al. (2000). Spatial distribution of blood flow in electrically stimulated human muscle: a positron emission tomography study. *Muscle Nerve*, **23**(4), 482–489.

Wang, R.Y., Chan, R.C., et al. (2000). Functional electrical stimulation on chronic and acute hemiplegic shoulder subluxation. *Am J Phys Med Rehabil*, **79**(4), 385–390; quiz 391–394.

Weingarden, H.P., Zeilig, G., et al. (1998). Hybrid functional electrical stimulation orthosis system for the upper limb: effects on spasticity in chronic stable hemiplegia. *Am J Phys Med Rehabil*, **77**(4), 276–281.

Wesselink, W.A., Holsheimer, J., et al. (1999). A model of the electrical behaviour of myelinated sensory nerve fibres based on human data. *Med Biol Eng Comput*, **37**(2), 228–235.

Yan, T., Hui-Chan, C.W. and Li, L.S. (2005). Functional electrical stimulation improves motor recovery of the lower extremity and walking ability of subjects with first acute stroke: a randomized placebo-controlled trial. *Stroke*, **36**(1), 80–5.

10

Environmental control and assistive devices

Jessica Johnson and William C. Mann

Department of Occupational Therapy, University of Florida, Gainesville, FL, USA

Following a stroke or traumatic brain injury (TBI), a person may have residual deficits even after completing a therapeutic program designed to regain function. The deficits may be physical, cognitive, and/or psychosocial. To overcome these deficits, people frequently use assistive technology (AT). The terms assistive technology, assistive device, and assistive technology device are used synonymously. AT device refers to "any item, piece of equipment, or product system, whether acquired commercially, modified, or customized, that is used to increase, maintain, or improve functional capabilities of individuals with disabilities" (Assistive Technology Act, 2004). Assistive devices include both low-technology items such as a long-handled shoehorn, and higher-technology devices such as computers with special interfaces. Assistive devices range from basic consumer products like a television remote, cordless phone, and microwave oven to more specialized devices such as walkers, assistive listening devices, or dressing sticks.

Environmental control devices provide another example of assistive devices. Environmental control devices can be set up to remotely operate electronic devices in the home (Mann, 1998), including lights, television, radio, phone, furnace, or air conditioner. Light timers, for example, are simple environmental control devices that turn lights on and off at pre-set times of day.

The AT increases a person's level of independence in performing tasks, and it may also have a positive impact on self-esteem. For example, after having a stroke, a woman experiences hemiplegia and becomes dependent on her husband for cutting food. This dependency may make her feel more like a child than a wife. To overcome the dependency, the woman works with an occupational therapist, who shows her how to use a rocker knife. This is an adaptive utensil that allows people to cut food with one hand. With the rocker knife, she no longer needs to rely on her husband. Her newly acquired independence makes her feel more self-reliant.

This chapter focuses on use of AT to address residual deficits resultant from a brain injury. While we recognize psychosocial issues may have an impact on the person's life and their response to AT, use of AT for physical and cognitive deficits is emphasized. Firstly, the chapter will outline considerations for intervening with AT following a neurologic condition resultant from injury or disease. Secondly, we will discuss AT for neuromotor impairments. Thirdly, we will present AT for cognitive impairments. Fourthly, we will address AT for sensory-perceptual impairments. Then, we will cover AT by categories of activities of daily living (ADL) including: bathing, dressing, grooming, toileting, eating/drinking, walking/mobility, telephone use, medication management, food preparation, shopping, and leisure. Finally, the chapter will end with a discussion about future AT.

10.1 AT intervention

Prior to recommending assistive devices, a thorough assessment of the individual should be performed. The assessment must consider the individual's physical deficits and strengths, cognitive status, sensory status, functional status, environment, the tasks the person performs or would like to participate in, caregivers, and others living in the person's environment (Mann, 1998).

Functional status relates to how much assistance an individual requires to complete tasks and activities. Functional status alone is not enough to decide where to intervene with AT. The type of AT to recommend will also depend on what activities the client wishes to accomplish and what device features are important to the client. For some tasks, different devices accomplish the same thing, but each device may offer unique features and a distinctive design.

The assessment must also address the role and needs of informal caregivers. For example, a stroke survivor may be able to put on his pants independently with a dressing stick, but the task could take 40 min and result in fatigue. But if he lives with his wife, who assists as a primary caregiver, her assistance with donning his pants could save him time and energy. In this example, the dressing stick would allow the patient to be independent, but be an inappropriate intervention given his living situation. When AT is prescribed inappropriately, it often ends up unused.

Physical status is also important in prescription of AT. While recognizing deficits, remaining abilities must be considered in recommending AT. Consider a person who is unable to squeeze a fingernail clipper with her left hand to trim the nails on her right hand. With the remaining strength in her left arm, using an adapted nail clipper that can be pressed with a gross motor movement of the left hand, she is able to trim her own nails on her right hand.

Sensory deficits, which are often not obvious, are also important to consider in recommending assistive devices. Intact sensation is important in using many assistive devices safely and effectively. For instance, in using a reacher one must be able to sense how much force is being applied to ensure objects are adequately grasped. A person with decreased sensation may not be able to determine the applied force, and become quickly frustrated in trying to use a reacher to grasp objects.

Cognition is also very important in being able to use assistive devices effectively. If a patient has impaired cognition, he or she may not remember how to use a device, or may forget that they have the device. On the other hand, assistive devices may be used to increase the safety of people with cognitive deficits. Automatic braking systems on wheelchairs lock when an individual moves from sitting to standing without applying the brakes manually, and work well for individuals with both mobility and memory impairment. Wander alerts help caregivers supervise people with impaired cognition by alerting them when the person moves beyond a prescribed environment.

10.2 AT for motor impairments

Common motor deficits resultant from neurologic conditions include impairments in balance, gait, gross and fine motor coordination, and unilateral weakness or paralysis (National Institute of Neurological Disorders and Stroke (NINDS), April 21, 2003).

AT for balance and gait impairments

Patients with balance and gait impairments are at risk for falling (Volume II, Chapter 8). With training in the use of assistive devices, this risk may decrease. During AT intervention for falls, an increase in the frequency and duration of education can positively impact the safe and effective use of the device (Mann et al., 2002). When an individual initially obtains an assistive device, they are still likely to have a fear of falling. Simply moving from place to place within their residence may provoke anxiety, which further increases the person's risk of falling. The individual may rush through a transfer without using the assistive device appropriately and safely. Professional training is essential for safe and effective use of balance and mobility devices.

Grab bars are simple yet important devices that assist with impaired balance. They are usually made from metal but may be covered in a more attractive material. Grab bars are placed in critical locations in the home, such as near the toilet, bathtub, shower, and bed (Fig. 10.1).

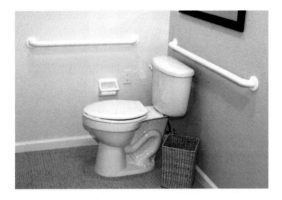

Figure 10.1. Grab bars installed around toilet to assist with impaired balance.

There are several types of bathroom grab bar systems. These systems provide support during transferring on and off the toilet, during clothing management, and during pericare. For use by the toilet, grab bars may be floor mounted, wall mounted, wall to floor mounted, or attached to the toilet itself. A toilet seat with armrests may be installed to offer support (Abledata, 2004).

Grab bars in the shower or by the bathtub assist a person with a balance impairment in transferring safely in and out of the shower, and provide support while standing in the shower. Depending on the individual's needs, grab bars may be installed in several different configurations inside and outside of the shower/tub area. Grab bars can be attached to the shower wall or clamped to the side of the bathtub with a rubber-covered clamp (Abledata, 2004). The number and placement of grab bars will depend on how much support a person requires, and where the support is needed.

An individual with balance or gait impairment may benefit from a variety of devices when transferring in and out of bed including: a vertical pole, trapeze bar, or bed rail. The vertical pole extends from floor to ceiling. Often, a perpendicular arm extends from the vertical pole to facilitate grasping. A trapeze bar can assist a person in moving from a prone to sitting position, and is usually attached to the bed frame. Finally, a half-bed rail may be helpful in

assisting people with rolling onto their side, sitting up, or moving from sitting to standing.

Handrails are also important in compensating for balance impairments. Stairs leading into the house or between floors should have at least one handrail. In some instances, handrails should be placed on both sides of the staircase. For a person with hemiparesis, or weakness on one side of the body, handrails assist on one side when ascending a staircase and on the opposite side when descending the staircase. Moreover, some individuals use both handrails for added stability while climbing up and down stairs.

AT for hemiparesis/hemiplegia

Following a brain injury, such as a stroke, many individuals experience residual weakness or paralysis on one side of the body (NINDS, April 21, 2003; Volume II, Chapter 36). To compensate for lower-extremity weakness, devices such as an ankle-foot orthosis provide extra stability to the affected limb and allow for a safer gait pattern. Similarly, an upper extremity may be weak or paralyzed. Assistive devices can compensate for the functional loss of the impaired limb. These devices enable a person to use one hand to complete tasks that typically require two hands, such as cutting food with a knife, buttoning a shirt, brushing dentures, tying a shoe, flossing teeth, preparing food, using a walker, and using a wheelchair. A variety of devices available to accomplish these tasks using one hand are discussed later in this chapter.

10.3 AT for cognitive impairments

A person who has survived a stroke or TBI may have residual cognitive impairments that include: language impairments, shortened attention span, impaired short-term memory, poor insight to the extent of deficits, unilateral neglect, or difficulty completing tasks from start to finish and following instructions (NINDS, April 21, 2003).

AT for language and cognition

At least 25% of stroke survivors have some form of aphasia (American Speech–Language–Hearing Association (ASHA), 2004) (NINDS, April 21, 2003). There are three major types of aphasia: receptive aphasia, expressive aphasia, and global aphasia (Volume II, Chapter 26). With receptive aphasia a person has difficulty understanding what is said to them. With expressive aphasia the person has difficulty communicating their thoughts to a listener. These symptoms may range from mild to severe depending on the location and extent of brain damage. Expressive and receptive aphasia do not exist in isolation. Often someone who is diagnosed with one form of aphasia will have mild symptoms of the other. When both types of aphasia are severe, it is called "global aphasia."

Currently, there are no assistive devices to help persons with receptive aphasia understand what is being said to them. However, a medical alert tag may be beneficial so that others understand the individual has a language impairment. People with expressive aphasia may use communication boards and computer systems to communicate with others (Mann and Lane, 1995).

AT for memory

Memory impairment is one of the most common residual deficits following a brain injury, such as stroke or TBI (Volume II, Chapter 29). The use of AT to compensate for memory deficits may require that the individual remember to use the memory device, such as a calendar, notebook, memory journal, or date book. Assistive devices for memory are commonly called "cognitive orthotics," which means "a device that supports weakened, aberrant, or deficient cognitive functions" (Bergman, 2002).

Wilson et al. (1997) studied the use of electronic devices to help people with brain injuries remember appointments, medications, and other daily events. With the use of an electronic paging system, Wilson found that participants' rate of success in remembering tasks increased from 37% to 86% in 12 weeks. When the paging system was discontinued for

2–4 weeks, participants continued to be 76% successful. This suggests that some of the participants were able to use the device for a short time and continue to meet daily demands without its use. However, some individuals required long-term use of the electronic device.

In a follow-up study of electronic paging systems, Wilson et al. (2001) conducted a 14-week randomized controlled cross-over trial with 143 participants. Half of the participants (Group A) received the paging system for the first 7 weeks of the study and then discontinued use of the paging system the last 7 weeks. The other group (Group B) did not use the paging system until the last 7 weeks of the study. At the end of the first 7 weeks, Group A was 74% successful in remembering daily tasks compared to 48% for Group B. Similarly, at the end of the last 7 weeks, Group B was 76% successful compared to 62% for Group A. This suggests that the paging system allowed the participants to perform more tasks than they did without the paging system.

Evans et al. (2003) reported that the four most common memory interventions for people with brain injury are a wall calendar/chart, notebook, list, and appointment diary. However, these methods were considered not as effective as less-used electronic systems. Four factors associated with memory-aid usage were found: being less than age 30 at time of injury, having a more recent injury, higher current intellectual ability, and having better attention skills. People who do not possess these characteristics may require more support in learning to use memory aids.

Paging systems appear to work well for people with brain injury. Typically, the system pages the person when a certain task needs to be performed. The prompt displayed on the screen can be worded so that it is meaningful to the user. The user may set the paging system to alert with a beep and/or vibration when a text message is delivered.

An example of a paging system for persons with memory impairment is the NeuroPage (Oliver Zangwell Centre, 2005). The caregiver provides NeuroPage with the appropriate messages and delivery times, which can be updated as needed. After receiving the information from the caregiver,

NeuroPage automatically sends messages to the individual's pager at the appropriate times. The individual presses one button and reads the message.

ISAAC is an example of another cognitive orthosis (Cogent Systems, Inc, 2005). The ISAAC device is wearable and battery powered. This device has a pressure sensitive screen that the user touches when a message is delivered. Like a paging system, ISAAC delivers prompts in the forms of auditory speech, text, checklists, or graphics to the user at the appropriate time of day.

The planning and execution assistant and trainer (PEAT) uses artificial intelligence on a PDA to help people with brain injury function independently (Levinson, 1997). The program helps the individual plan their day, taking into consideration alternative steps in completing tasks. PEAT comes up with a best plan to complete all steps. Then PEAT provides cues to the user assisting them to complete the steps. The user tells PEAT when a step has been completed or if the user requires more time. As a result, PEAT alters the plan based on the user's input.

Current applications and devices that can be used to assist people with a brain injury in completing daily activities have been reviewed recently (LoPresti, 2004). Some of the devices and systems include: customized computer systems adapted to the individual's needs, use of sensors and switches to detect the task the person is performing and providing cues to assist the person in its completion, and paging systems.

Other devices used by people with memory impairments include medical alert tags and personal emergency response systems. The medical alert tag conveys information, such as allergies, when the individual is unable to remember the information. The tag may also provide the person's name and phone number, which is useful if he or she becomes disoriented and lost. A personal emergency response system provides a quick link to help for a person with limited memory or problem solving abilities (Federal Trade Commission for the Consumer and American Association of Retired Persons, 2004). These systems typically include a button on a necklace or bracelet that the individual

wears, and a console that is connected to the person's telephone. When the button is pressed, a call is placed to a response center. The response center operator can answer questions, provide reassurance, or in an emergency, send help.

10.4 AT for sensory perceptual impairments

People who have a neurologic condition resulting from injury or disease may have sensory impairments (NINDS, April 21, 2003). These impairments may include diminished or absent tactile, temperature, pain, or proprioceptive (position of the limb or body in space) sensations (Volume II, Chapter 16). Furthermore, they may experience odd sensations (paresthesias) like numbness, pain, or tingling in the affected limbs. Loss of sensation can cause safety problems. For example, the person may not be able to determine that their hand is on something hot, resulting in a burn. If the person does not feel pain, they could get their hand caught in the wheel of a wheelchair. To decrease the risk of injury due to sensory impairments, equipment for improved positioning can be used, temperature gauges may be employed, no scald shower/bath faucets should be installed, and the individual should be trained to visually inspect the affected body part often.

10.5 AT for ADL and instrumental ADL

ADL refers to basic self-care tasks, such as dressing or eating. Instrumental ADLs (IADLs) refer to more complex tasks, such as using a phone or cooking a meal, and can be affected in less severely impaired individuals than ADLs.

ADLs

AT for bathing

Most homes in the US have a bathtub/shower combination either with glass doors or with a shower curtain (Mann, 1998). This is often a difficult setup for someone with a physical impairment. Getting down into the tub and out again may not be possible due to decreased balance and hemiparesis. If tub bathing is not feasible, other options include showering or sponge bathing.

To shower safely, several types of device can be used. Grab bars are an option, as discussed earlier in this chapter. A transfer bench allows a person to perform a seating transfer into the tub (Mann, 1998). After sitting, the person turns toward the front of the tub and swings one leg and then the other into the tub. One consideration when using a transfer bench is the amount of space in the bathroom as they require space outside of the tub, as well as in the tub. Also, a shower curtain must be used rather than glass doors because glass doors do not allow enough room to sit and swing the legs into the tub. The shower curtain must be positioned so that water does not spill out of the shower and onto the floor creating a safety hazard. Finally, the weight of the bench should be considered if it will be removed when others use the tub/shower.

For people who can safely perform a standing transfer, but are unable to remain standing while showering, a shower chair or bath bench is recommended. These are available in several styles. Some have backs that assist people with compromised sitting balance and some have armrests for additional stability. Again, the weight of the chair must be considered if it has to be removed for others to use the bathtub (Fig. 10.2).

Devices that control the water temperature can be installed. These devices are important for people

with sensation deficits and can prevent burns. Several water temperature control devices are available, as listed at www.abledata.com (Abledata, 2004).

A hand-held shower is useful for rinsing when seated on a bath bench or shower chair. The use of a hand-held shower may also help keep water in the tub when using a transfer bench. If a person has the use of only one-hand and the showerhead does not have an on/off button, the hand-held shower can be set down into the tub while the person washes. However, hand-held showers with an on/off control are relatively inexpensive.

A variety of brushes and sponges can assist with bathing (Abledata, 2004). A long-handled sponge can help a person with impaired balance or range of motion wash their lower legs. A foot sponge is much like the long-handled sponge but narrower for cleaning toes and feet. For hands-free use, foot brushes attach to the bathtub to clean feet and toes. Finally, some back brushes can also be used to wash the lower legs.

Many assistive devices are available for soap and shampoo dispensing. A push button dispenser is useful for an individual who is unable to use both hands to open a shampoo bottle and pour it into the other hand. People who are unable to press buttons could use hands-free motion-activated dispensers. A soap swing can turn any bar of soap into "soap on a rope." Soap is placed in the soft mesh bag that doubles as a bathing sponge. The mesh bag is attached to a long nylon rope that is mounted to the wall.

AT for dressing

Dressing requires body movement and the use of both hands. To put on socks and shoes, a person must have good trunk flexion and be able to maintain balance (Mann, 1998). Furthermore, tying shoes involves the use of two hands and fine motor coordination. Dressing can be challenging when one side of the body is weak and balance is impaired.

A person with decreased balance should have a sturdy chair to sit on while dressing. A chair with arms may be helpful for transferring, but the arms may interfere with putting on a shirt. Beds are not an

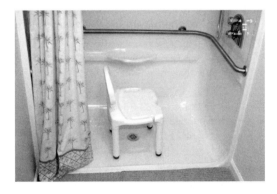

Figure 10.2. Shower chair with backrest.

ideal platform for dressing as they are often too soft for an individual to maintain an upright posture.

A long-handled shoehorn may help in putting on shoes (Fig. 10.3). The person has to point their toe into the shoe and get the shoehorn behind the heel before they begin to push down into the shoe. Sometimes the affected leg will have an ankle-foot orthosis, or AFO, which is already in the shoe and acts like a shoehorn. Similarly, the end of a dressing stick can act as a long-handled shoehorn. The dressing stick can also assist in getting pants over feet and pulling them up to the knees where the hand can take over. Reachers can also be used for donning pants.

Fasteners like buttons, zippers, and snaps are often difficult to manipulate due to hemiparesis or decreased fine motor coordination. For many people with these impairments, pull-on pants and pull-over shirts are easier because there are no closures. Likewise, sport bras in an extra size may be easier for women to pull over than using a rear closure bra with hooks or even a front closure bra. Velcro can also be substituted for hard-to-close fasteners. Elastic cuff links allow a person to slip their hand through cuffs without unbuttoning them. Button extenders enable a person to pull a button-up shirt over the head (Abledata, 2004).

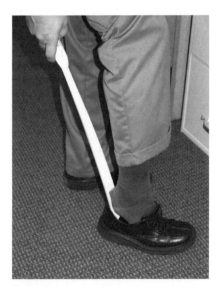

Figure 10.3. Long-handled shoehorn.

Devices are available to assist in fastening clothes that have buttons, zippers, and laces. For garments with buttons, button aids can compensate for fine motor impairment and can be used by one hand. Also, zipper pulls can be added to zippers and allow a person with use of only one hand to zip a garment. They are larger than the typical zipper lever so people with fine motor impairments can grasp the pull as well. Elastic laces can be placed in shoes, which make donning them similar to slip on shoes. The laces come in different colors, widths, and styles. Other devices to fasten shoes include Velcro and shoelace fasteners that can be used to lock shoelaces in position.

For a person with diminished fine motor control or hemiplegia, jewelry can also be challenging to don. Clip-on earrings or earrings with hooks rather than posts are easier to put on with one hand. Necklaces and bracelets with magnetic clasps may be easier than other traditional jewelry clasps (Abledata, 2004).

AT for grooming

Typically, flossing is a two-hand task, but a disposable or non-disposable dental floss holder can make flossing with one hand possible (Mann et al., 1995b, September). Brushing dentures also requires two hands. However, denture brushes with a suction cup make it possible to clean dentures using one hand (Abledata, 2004). A toothpaste dispenser is available that has a slot for the toothbrush: the device dispenses the appropriate amount of paste when the person presses the dispenser lever.

For an individual with decreased fine motor coordination, an electric shaver may prevent cuts. This may be especially helpful for a person who shaves with the non-dominant hand due to hemiplegia.

A few items that make nail care easier for people with hemiplegia or hemiparesis include adapted nail clippers, emery boards, and nail brushes. Fingernail clippers for operation with one hand are available, although for some individuals it may still be difficult to clip the nails on the unaffected hand. A foot-operated nail clipper is also available (Abledata, 2004). An emery board with a suction cup allows one-handed use for filing nails. Nailbrushes with suction bases can be used to clean under nails for people with hemiplegia.

AT for toileting

Several options for hygiene assistance are available. Pre-moistened wipes make it easier to cleanse after toileting if hygiene is difficult (Mann, 1998). Also, use of a bidet rather than toilet paper can be beneficial for people who are unable to maintain balance while wiping themselves. Add-on washing devices serve the same purpose as a bidet at much lower cost.

Raised toilet seats may make it easier for someone with hemiparesis or hemiplegia to get on and off the toilet. If the person requires extra support or something to push on when transferring, raised toilet seats with armrests can be used. The Toilevator is a device that raises the toilet from the bottom up, so the person is still sitting on his or her own toilet seat. The Toilevator adds a section between the floor and the bottom of the toilet.

At night, a person with hemiplegia or impaired balance may require a significant amount of time to get from bed to the bathroom to use the toilet. To avoid an accident on the way to the bathroom, the individual may use a urinal or a bedside commode (Fig. 10.4). Urinals may be gender specific or unisex (Mann, 1998). The weight of the urinal is important for a person with hemiplegia or hemiparesis. The weight of the urinal after it has been used should also be considered. Another option is a bedside commode. These are available in many different styles, including commodes with removable arms, swing away arms, or stationary arms (Abledata, 2004). A consideration when prescribing a bedside commode is how the indi-

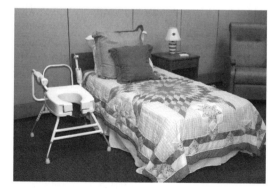

Figure 10.4. Bedside commode.

vidual transfers. A commode with a seat lift helps the person move from sitting to standing.

AT for eating and drinking

Assistive devices are available that make eating with one hand easier. Some of the adaptive utensils that make cutting food with one hand easier include rocker knives, rocker fork-knife combinations, and roller knives (Abledata, 2004). Roller knives look similar to a small pizza cutter. Rocker utensils have an edge the shape of a semi-circle that is used to cut food. To prevent spilling, a person with poor coordination or decreased cognition may use bowls and plates with built up edges, plate guards, dishes with non-skid bottoms, and cups with lids.

AT for walking and mobility

A variety of mobility devices are available for people with impaired balance or gait. Canes support up to 25% of a person's weight (Mann, 1998). Canes are usually single-end or have multiple feet, such as a quad cane. Quad canes offer more support than single-end canes, but are heavier.

Walkers can support up to 50% of a person's body weight (Mann, 1998). Types of walkers include hemi-walkers, platform, standard, front-wheeled, and four-wheeled. Hemi-walkers are used by people with hemiplegia. These walkers offer more support than a quad cane, and are still used with one hand. A platform walker allows the person to put the affected hand and forearm in a trough on the walker and then bear weight through the upper arm to push the walker forward. Standard walkers and front-wheeled walkers provide support to people with impaired balance, but the person must grasp both sides of the walker to use it properly. Finally, four-wheeled walkers provide some support and are able to move faster than standard and two-wheeled walkers. Four-wheeled walkers have a seat that allows the user to rest when needed. Some four-wheeled walkers have a bin under the seat for carrying objects.

Walker accessories can help the user transport items while walking. They include walker bags, baskets, and trays. Bags are useful to transport items that do not have to stay upright. Baskets allow transportation of items in an upright position, but may interfere with the individual approximating counters and cabinets. Trays are another alternative for carrying objects and allow the user to approach counters and cabinets closely, but do not allow the person to use a walker seat to rest.

Wheelchairs are another category of mobility device (Chapter 11 of Volume II). There are many different types of wheelchairs, including manual wheelchairs, power wheelchairs, and power assisted wheelchairs. In positioning someone post-stroke in a wheelchair there are several important considerations. Initially, how will the person propel the chair? Will they use their hands and feet, just one foot and one hand, no feet and two hands? If they are going to use one hand and one foot (or one hand, which is very difficult), then the person needs a wheelchair that can be maneuvered on one side. Additionally, the person may need lateral support to maintain an upright posture in the wheelchair. A tray table, half tray, or arm trough may be used to keep the patient's arm in a safe position. The individual may need a seat alarm or seat belt if he or she does not have good insight into the deficits present and is at risk of trying to walk. Another consideration when positioning someone is the type of wheelchair cushion they should use. If the person is not very mobile and is at risk of developing pressure sores, a pressure-relieving cushion would be best. But if the person is able to shift in the seat and transfers often, a less expensive foam cushion may be appropriate. Finally, a brake extension on the affected side allows the individual to reach with the unaffected hand to lock the opposite brake. If the person has residual memory impairment, an automatic braking system may help prevent falls.

Scooters are a less expensive alternative to power wheelchairs, but they offer less support (Mann, 1998). Often motorized scooters have baskets to allow transportation of objects. Many stores carry motorized scooters with baskets.

People who have a neurologic condition and use a wheelchair or scooter have to consider how they will get around their home, vehicles, and community. Many people who use these devices use wheelchair ramps and lifts.

IADLs

Telephone AT

Cordless telephones allow people with impaired mobility to carry their phone at all times, so they do not have to get up to answer the phone. An answering machine can also limit the need for rising to answer the phone by screening out unwanted calls. Telephones have many features today that can be helpful to someone with physical and cognitive impairments. Phones with large buttons are easier to dial for people with impaired fine motor coordination (Mann, 1998). People who have difficulty holding the receiver can use voice-activated phones, hands-free headsets, or speakerphones. Lastly, the memory dial feature of a phone or a list of frequently called numbers can be especially beneficial for people with impaired memory.

AT for medications

For people who have mild memory impairment, medication organizers can be helpful. Some watches can also be set to sound an alarm at appropriate times to remind the person to take their medication. Paging systems may be used to remind the person to take a specific medication at a certain time. The person with hemiplegia may have to request medications be put in an easy to open container, something other than a childproof container that can be opened with one hand.

Food preparation

Items that will be used for food preparation should be within easy reach. Lazy Susans can make it easier to get to items that would normally be stored in the rear of cabinets. Pull-out racks in lower cabinets can make it easier to get the items stored there (Mann, 1998) (Fig. 10.5).

Several items can be helpful in the kitchen for someone with a neurologic injury or disease. Cutting boards with pins and clamps to hold food in place are helpful for those who need to prepare food with one hand (Abledata, 2004). A pan holder holds

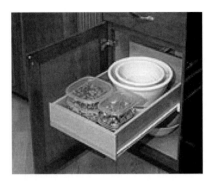

Figure 10.5. Pull out racks.

a hot pan in place while the cook stirs with one hand. Burner guards also help keep pans from sliding off burners. A variety of jar openers make it possible to open a jar using one hand. Electric can openers and power-operated corkscrews make it easier to open cans and bottles with one hand. Lightweight dishes facilitate transporting dishes. An automatic dishwasher will help prevent fatigue from standing and doing dishes by hand.

Microwave ovens can be used to ease food preparation. They may be a better option for those with mild memory impairment who may forget about foods they were cooking on the stove, or forget to turn the stove off. Cooking time in a microwave is significantly less than with a conventional oven or stove, which may be beneficial for someone with diminished activity tolerance. Also, burns from cooking are not as likely with a microwave oven. This is especially important for a person with decreased sensation. Multi-use containers make food preparation and storage easier by allowing the individual to use the same container for cooking and refrigerating leftovers. Often store-bought frozen foods come in a dish that is microwaveable. Countertop devices may be helpful such as: a toaster oven, an automatic shut off coffeepot, or a toaster.

AT for shopping

For people with impaired mobility, some of their shopping can be done over the phone or with a computer.

When the individual travels to a store, scooters with baskets or walkers with baskets and seats are helpful (Mann, 1998). Also, using a cart or backpack may be helpful in carrying items home from the store.

AT for leisure

Mann et al. (1995a, March) found the types of activities most missed by older stroke survivors living at home were sports, crafts, and long walks. The article points out that these are all leisure activities and often leisure is not a focus of intervention. Many devices are available to assist people with leisure activities following a brain injury. Card holders and card shufflers are available for people with decreased fine motor coordination, or who are only able to use one hand (Abledata, 2004). A television remote with large buttons is easier to use for someone with decreased fine motor coordination or visual disturbances. A sewing machine with an attached magnifier may help people with visual disturbances. High-intensity lighting can help people who are having difficulty seeing their project. Crochet and knitting aids are also available to allow for one-handed work.

Several types of writing aids are available for people who have difficulty grasping or controlling a pen. If writing with a pen or pencil is too difficult or impossible, a computer may be used for word processing. Many computer interfaces can be used if a standard keyboard is not feasible. Schweitzer et al. (1999), discussed the case of a man who survived a stroke and used a computer for word processing to compensate for difficulty formulating thoughts and putting them on paper.

10.6 Future assistive devices

Advances in computing power, the Internet, wireless technologies, and battery power are making it possible to design electronic devices that will serve multiple functions: operate appliances, open doors, close and open drapes, provide reminders for medications, and much more (Mann, 2004). At the University of Florida, the Rehabilitation Engineering Research

Center on Technology for Successful Aging (www.rerc.ufl.edu) is developing voice activated computer applications as well as auditory and visual alerts that accomplish all of these tasks and provide alerts, such as when mail is delivered, or doors are left unlocked. Products or applications such as these will be available in the very near future.

Combining these advanced technologies in a home setting provides even more potential applications. For with the neurologically disabled, behavior could be tracked by adding sensors throughout the home. Sensors and "intelligence" programmed into the home will make it possible to determine if the occupant had not risen from bed, had a sleepless night, or had not eaten – all of which could trigger an alert to a family member or a formal care provider. Smart homes such as these will also help a person with a cognitive impairment by providing prompts through everyday activities, reminders to drink, and to take meals or medications.

While the future promises a new generation of assistive devices, and "assistive environments," the basic assistive devices we have described in this chapter can make a very large difference for a person who has a neurologic injury or disease – helping them maintain their independence and quality of life. The need for careful assessment, typically by an occupational therapist, cannot be overly stressed. Selection of appropriate devices, training in their use, and continued follow-up are essential.

REFERENCES

Abledata Database. Retrieved March 22, 2004, from http://www.abledata.com/Site_2/prod_type.htm. For information, telephone 800-227-0216 or write Abledata, 8630 Fenton Street, Suite 930, Silver spring, MD 20910.

American Speech–Language–Hearing Association (n.d.). *Aphasia*. Retrieved March 22, 2004, from http://www.asha.org/public/speech/disorders/Aphasia_info.htm

Assistive Technology Act of 2004, 29 U.S.C. §3002 (2004).

Bergman, M. (2002). The benefits of a cognitive orthotic in brain injury rehabilitation. *J Head Trauma Rehabil*, **17**(5), 431–445.

Evans, J.J., Wilson, B.A., Needham, P. and Brentnall, S. (2003). Who makes good use of memory aids? Results of a survey of people with acquired brain injury. *J Int Neuropsychol Soc*, **9**, 925–935.

Federal Trade Commission for the Consumer & American Association of Retired Persons (2004). *Facts for Consumers: Personal Emergency Response Systems*. Retrieved March 30, 2004, from http://www.ftc.gov/bcp/conline/pubs/services/ pers. htm

Levinson, R. (1997). The planning and execution assistant and trainer (PEAT). *J Head Trauma Rehabil*, **12**(2), 85–91.

LoPresti, E.F., Mihailidis, A. and Kirsch, N. (2004). Assistive technology for cognitive rehabilitation: state of the art. *Neuropsychol Rehabil*, **14**(1–2), 5–39.

Mann, W.C. (1998). Assistive technology for persons with arthritis. In: *Rheumatologic Rehabilitation Series: Volume 1, Assessment and Management of Arthritis in Rehabilitation* (Chapter 16, pp. 369–392), American Occupational Therapy Association, Inc., Bethesda, MD.

Mann, W.C. (2004) *Smart Technology: Aging, Disability and Independence. The State of the Science*, Wiley, Hoboken, NJ (in preparation).

Mann, W.C. and Lane, J.P. (1995). *Assistive Technology for Persons with Disabilities*, 2nd edn., The American Occupational therapy Association, Inc., Bethesda, MD.

Mann, W.C., Hurren, D., Tomita, M. and Charavat, B. (1995a). Assistive devices for home-based older stroke survivors. In: *Topics in Geriatric Rehabilitation*, **10**(3), March, Aspen Publishers, Inc., Gaithersburg, MD, pp. 75–86.

Mann, W.C., Hurren, D., Tomita, M. and Charavat, B. (1995b). A follow-up study of older stroke survivors living at home. In: *Topics in Geriatric Rehabilitation*, **11**(1), September, Aspen Publishers, Inc., Gaithersburg, MD, pp. 52–66.

Mann, W.C., Goodall, S., Justiss, M.D. and Tomita, M. (2002). Dissatisfaction and nonuse of assistive devices among frail elders. *Assist Technol*, **14**, 130–139.

National Institute of Neurological Disorders and Stroke (2003). April 21. *Post-Stroke Rehabilitation Fact Sheet*. Retrieved March 22, 2004, from http://www.ninds.nih.gov/health_and_medical/pubs/poststrokerehab.htm

Schweitzer, J.A., Mann, W.C., Nochajski, S.M. and Tomita, M. (1999). Patterns of engagement in Leisure activity by older adults using assistive devices. *Technol Disabil*, **11**, 103–117.

The Oliver Zangwell Centre (2005). *NeroPage*. Retrieved March 11, 2003 from http://www.neuropage.nhs.uk

Wilson, B.A., Evans, J.J., Emsile, H. and Malinek, V. (1997). Evaluation of NeuroPage: a new memory aid. *J Neurol, Neurosurg, Psychiatr*, **63**(1), 113–115.

Wilson, B.A., Emsile, H.C., Quirk, K. and Evans, J.J. (2001). Reducing everyday memory and planning problems by means of a paging system: a randomized control crossover study. *J Neurol, Neurosurg, Psychiatr*, **70**, 477–482.

Wheelchair design and seating technology

Rory A. Cooper, Rosemarie Cooper and Michael L. Boninger

Departments of Rehabilitation Science and Technology Physical Medicine, and Rehabilitation and VA Pittsburgh Healthcare System Human Engineering Research Laboratories, Pittsburgh, PA, USA

11.1 Introduction

In the USA an estimated 2.2 million people currently use wheelchairs for their daily mobility (Americans with Disabilities, 1994; Shalala et al., 1996). It is likely that more than twice that number use wheelchairs at any given time to augment their mobility. Worldwide, an estimated 100–130 million people with disabilities need wheelchairs, though less than 10% own or have access to one (New Freedom Initiative Act, 2001). While these numbers are staggering, experts predict that the number of people who need wheelchairs will increase by 22% over the next 10 years (Department of Veterans Affairs, 2002). The leading cause of disabilities in the world can be attributed to landmines, particularly in developing nations, leading to 26,000 people injured or killed by landmines each year (Department of Veterans Affairs, 2002).

11.2 Prevention of secondary conditions

Wheelchair and seating biomechanics research includes studies to prevent secondary conditions due to wheelchair and seating use (e.g., pressure ulcers, adverse changes in posture, repetitive strain injuries), and to reduce the incidence of accidental injuries (e.g., injuries from wheelchair tips and falls, injuries from motor vehicle accidents).

Upper extremity repetitive strain injuries

Studies have shown that manual wheelchair propulsion efficiency is between 5% and 18% depending upon the style of the wheelchair and the fit to the user (Bayley et al., 1987; Curtis et al., 1995; Nichols et al., 1979). The low efficiency of manual wheelchairs make them ineffective for some individuals to use during activities of daily living. Manual wheelchair users also experience a high incidence of upper extremity pain and joint degeneration. Between 25% and 80% of long-term manual wheelchair users are reported to have injuries to the wrist, elbow or shoulder (Boninger et al., 1999, 2001). The risk of injury tends to increase with age, while cardiovascular fitness tends to decrease (Boninger et al., 2003a).

The SMART[Wheel] kinetic measurement system was developed to study wheelchair propulsion and to improve clinical assessment of manual wheelchair propulsion (Cooper et al., 1997b, 1998b; Asato et al., 1993). The SMART[Wheels] provides a method for analyzing pushrim force that has proven critical to assess injury mechanisms (Cooper, 1997c, 1999; Boninger et al., 1997). Upper extremity models have been created in order to determine motion as well as net joint forces and moments (Koontz et al., 2002; Boninger et al., 1998b; Robertson et al., 1996). It has been shown that wheelchair pushrim forces are related to nerve conduction studies (NCS) variables (Boninger et al., 2000). NCS are used to diagnose carpal tunnel syndrome (CTS) a common condition that causes pain for wheelchair users. This study found that when controlling for subject weight, NCS was correlated with the cadence of propulsion and the rate of rise of the resultant force. Of particular importance was that the body mass of the wheelchair user was significantly correlated with NCS. Changes can be made to the wheelchair that alter the biomechanics and offer the potential for intervention (Boninger et al., 2000). Research has shown that individuals who sit low and behind the rear wheels had lower propulsive forces and stroke frequency, both shown to be associated with CTS (Cooper and Boninger, 1999).

In a series of magnetic resonance imaging (MRI) and X-ray imaging results for people with paraplegia, a high prevalence of osteolysis of the distal clavicle was revealed (Boninger et al., 2001). Investigations of the propulsive stroke concluded that the recovery phase is an important and modifiable parameter that can impact injurious biomechanics (Shimada et al., 1998; Boninger et al., 2002). A propulsion stroke during which the hand drops below the pushrim results in a greater push angle and lower stroke frequency, both of which likely protect against injury. The way an individual with paraplegia propels a wheelchair at baseline can predict progression of MRI findings 2 years later. Specifically, a large force directed towards the hub (radial force) was correlated with a higher MRI change score over time. Interestingly, almost all of the individuals with progression of MRI findings were women. Women use a larger radial force and are at greater risk of injury. This could be related to wheelchair set up or other gender differences (Boninger et al., 2003a).

Vibration exposure injuries and prevention

While propelling a wheelchair, users encounter obstacles such as bumps, curb descents, and uneven driving surfaces. These obstacles cause vibrations on the wheelchair and in turn, the wheelchair user, which through extended exposure can cause low back pain, disc degeneration and other harmful effects to the body (Seidel et al., 1986). Typically, seating systems are prescribed by clinicians based on the ability of the cushion to reduce pressure and provide proper positioning (Cooper et al., 1996). The primary goals being to reduce the risk of developing an ulcer and ensure adequate seated posture. The ability of a seating system to minimize impact (shock) and repetitive vibrations that an individual experiences is commonly not considered. Whole-body vibration experienced during wheelchair mobility can decrease

an individual's comfort and increase the rate of fatigue (Boninger et al., 2003b; DiGiovine et al., 2000). This may adversely affect the physical performance of the individual. It may also lead to social inactivity. Shock and vibration induced discomfort and fatigue may also lead to poor body mechanics leading to secondary disability.

To date, little research has been conducted to assess the vibrations experienced by wheelchair users (Tai et al., 1998). VanSickle et al. recorded the forces when using the American National Standards Institute (ANSI)/Rehabilitation Engineering and Assistive Technology Society of North America (RESNA) standards double drum and curb drop tests and compared them to the road loads during ordinary propulsion (VanSickle et al., 1996, 2000). VanSickle et al. also showed that wheelchair propulsion produces vibration loads that exceed the ISO 2631-1 standards at the seat of the wheelchair as well as the head of the user (VanSickle et al., 2001). DiGiovine et al. (2000) showed that users prefer ultralight wheelchairs to lightweight wheelchairs while traversing a simulated road course with higher comfort level and better ergonomics. DiGiovine et al. (2003) examined the relationship between the seating systems for manual wheelchairs and the vibrations experienced, showing differences in how seating systems transmit or dampen vibrations. Foam and captured air cushions are best at attenuating the peak and average shocks and vibrations seen during actual wheelchair use. Wolf et al. (2001) concluded that, on average, suspension manual wheelchairs do reduce the transmission of shock vibrations to wheelchair users, but are not yet optimal in their design. Cooper et al. (2003b) have shown that in the natural frequency of humans (4–15 Hz) the addition of suspension caster forks do reduce the amount of vibrations transferred to the user. Wolf et al. (2002) have shown that suspension manual wheelchairs are approaching significance in reducing the amount of shock vibrations transmitted to wheelchair users during curb descents. Kwarciak et al. (2002) revealed that although suspension manual wheelchairs reduce shock vibrations the chairs are not yet ideal, possibly due to the orientation of the suspension elements.

Dobson et al. (2003) and Wolf et al. (2003) conducted evaluations of the vibration exposure during electric-powered wheelchair driving and manual wheelchair propulsion over selected sidewalk surfaces. Their results indicate that all surfaces with an 8 mm gap or less between components surfaces yielded results that were similar to the poured concrete sidewalk, and should be considered acceptable as a pedestrian access route for wheelchair users.

Prevention of accidental injuries while using wheelchairs

Wheelchair-related driving accidents occur frequently and can have devastating effects. Unmat and Kirby (1994) reported that there are about 36,000 serious wheelchair accidents annually. Between 1973 and 1987, 770 wheelchairs-related deaths were reported to the United States Consumer Product Safety Commission (USCPSC), 68.5% of which were attributed to falls and tips (Calder and Kirby, 1990). In 1991 alone there were 50,000 wheelchair-related accidents that required emergency room treatment (Kirby et al., 1994). Wheelchairs accidents are often attributed to improper use or installation of safety systems and/or poor adjustment of the wheelchair (Van Roosmalen et al., 2002; Bertocci et al., 2001, Cooper, 1999).

In some cases, people use their wheelchairs as seats in motor vehicles. While this is necessary to transport some individuals, and to provide independent mobility for others it raises an entire set of safety issues. Only wheelchairs that meet safety criteria should be used regularly as seats in a motor vehicle (Bertocci et al., 1996). Serious injury may occur under typical test conditions, 30 mph at 30 times gravity acceleration frontal collision, as been shown by both simulation and testing (Bertocci et al, 1999a). Injuries are more likely to occur in wheelchairs that are unable to fail gracefully during crash loads (Bertocci et al., 1999b).

The method of braking affects the braking distance, braking time, and braking acceleration (Cooper et al., 1998a). The results indicate that using a seat belt and properly adjusted legrests reduces risk of injury or lowering the speed while driving without legrests may also decrease risk of injury. A video-based analysis of tips and falls shows that proper legrest adjustment and seat belt use offers wheelchair users greater safety when traversing common obstacles (Corfman et al., 2003b). A study of power wheelchair driving revealed that the obstacles most likely to induce a fall or loss of control were ascending a curb cut, ascending a curb (50 mm) at a 45-degree angle, and descending a 5-degree ramp.

Prevention of pressure ulcers

The loss of tissue integrity evidenced by pressure ulcers, diabetic foot ulcers, venous stasis ulcers, and chronically swollen limbs are examples of common, chronic medical conditions (Brienza et al., 1996a). Characterized by chronicity and relapse, these conditions are among the most costly, yet *preventable* of soft tissue injuries. Excessive, unevenly applied or repetitive tissue loading is a common contributory factor in all of these conditions. In-depth knowledge of the interaction between externally applied pressure and the soft tissue is crucial to the prevention, early detection, and management of soft tissue injuries.

Injury depends on the duration and intensity of tissue loading as well as the characteristics of both the tissue and the interfacing support surface. Recent work has resulted in significant findings and developments. Brienza et al. (1996b) developed a system for the analysis of seat support surfaces using shape control and simultaneous measurement of applied pressures. The system has been used to investigate the biomechanical factors for predicting pressure ulcer risk (Wang et al., 1998, 2000). In a randomized control trial pressure-reducing seat cushions for elderly wheelchair users were found to reduce the incidence and severity of pressure ulcers (Geyer et al., 2001). In an investigation of the relationship between pressure ulcer incidence and buttock-seat cushion interface pressure in at-risk elderly wheelchair users showed that lower interface pressures corresponded to fewer pressure ulcers (Brienza et al., 2001).

11.3 Manual wheelchairs

Design characteristics

The Centers for Medicare and Medicaid Services (CMS) is one of the nation's largest purchasers of wheelchairs (CMS, 2003; Shalala et al., 1996). However, neither CMS's coverage nor payment of wheelchairs is always in the best interest of the patients who need them (Collins et al., 2002). Wheelchairs are considered by CMS to be durable medical equipment (DME) and must meet the following criteria: capable of withstanding repeated use; primarily used to serve a medical purpose; not useful to person in absence of illness or injury; and appropriate for in home use (CMS, 2003). The last criterion is often interpreted by Durable Medical Equipment Regional Carriers (DMERC's) to exclude payment of wheelchairs that would provide community mobility and improve function outside the home (Fitzgerald et al., 2001a). Depot wheelchairs represent wheelchairs that are essentially designed for depot (e.g., airport, amusement park) or temporary institutional use (e.g., hospitals) and are generally not appropriate as a long-term mobility device. The obvious attraction of depot wheelchairs is their low purchase price, see Fig. 11.1(c). Lightweight and ultralight wheelchairs provide clinicians and consumers greater ability to select and adjust the wheelchair to the user and accommodate the consumer's functional needs. Ultralight manual wheelchairs are moderately adjustable or selectable manual wheelchairs intended to be used by a single individual, see Fig. 11.1(a). Lightweight manual wheelchairs are minimally adjustable or non-adjustable manual wheelchairs intended for an individual or for institutional use, see Fig. 11.1(b).

All manual wheelchairs are not alike. There are variations in the quality and performance of manual wheelchairs (Cooper et al., 1994a, b, 1995, 1996, 1997a). It is important for clinicians to realize the benefits of a proper wheelchair prescription, not only for the consumer's comfort and mobility needs but also in the quality of the wheelchair that will last with minimal repairs (Cooper and Cooper, 2003c; Cooper et al., 1999a, 1999b; Fitzgerald et al., 2001).

Adjustment and fitting

Ultralight wheelchairs offer to most flexibility in selecting or setting the fit to the user (Cooper, 1991, 1998a). For anyone who will be self-propelling a wheelchair for more then a few months, and ultralight wheelchair should be recommended. For most first-time wheelchair users, and adjustable wheelchair is best (Cooper and Cooper, 2003c). However, for experienced and highly skilled wheelchair users more features may be selected and set by the manufacturer

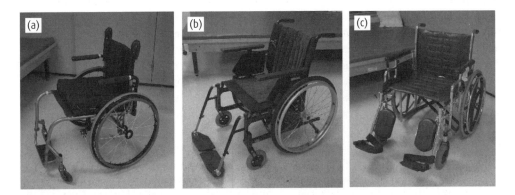

Figure 11.1. Pictures of (a) ultralight, (b) lightweight, and (c) depot manual wheelchairs.

to reduce the overall mass and increase reliability (Cooper, 1996; Whitman et al., 1998).

The seat depth and the seat width are often the best starting points when selecting the wheelchair dimensions. Typically, the seat width should be as narrow as possible. Bringing the rear wheels in close to the user facilitates propulsion as well as negotiation of the built environment (e.g., home, school, work). A simple rule to follow is that one finger should be between the sides of the wheelchair and the greater trochantors of the user. Clothing guards are most useful for allowing the chair to remain narrow and to keep clothing out of the wheels. The seat depth should be selected, so that there is 40–75 mm space between the front edge of the seat and the popliteal area behind the knees.

A tight legrest angle provides smaller maneuvering space for the wheelchair, which makes it easier to get around indoors. Legrest angles commonly vary from 70 to 95 degrees. If the user has good flexibility and low tone, than a higher legrest angle is recommended. Otherwise, the maximum legrest angle that can accommodate the user's range of motion should be specified. The legrest angle will bring the footrests closer or further from the front casters. Therefore, a balance must be struck between the caster size and legrest angle. A larger caster requires a lower legrest angle. Casters are readily available from most manufacturers in sizes ranging from 50–200 mm in diameter. Casters under 100 mm should only be recommended for users who can balance their wheelchair on its rear wheels.

The backrest height and angle effect both balance and the ability to propel the wheelchair. A backrest that is too high may interfere with the arms when propelling the wheelchair. However, if the backrest is not high enough it will not provide adequate support for the user. Most backrests offer some adjustment. The best approach is to start with an adjustable tension backrest or a rigid padded backrest. Either of these designs offers some adjustment for the user. With rigid backrests, the backrest height may be lower than standard upholstery as they tend to provide greater support for the pelvis and lumbar spine. The backrest angle should be set at 90 degrees, and then

it can be reclined to improve balance. The optimal angle is best found having the user attempt a few different driving tasks (e.g., ascend/descend ramps, start/stop quickly, balance on rear wheels).

Probably the most critical feature to set is the axle position with respect to the center of mass (CoM) of the user and wheelchair combination. While there is no agreed upon method of optimizing the rear axle position, research shows that placing the rear axle as close as possible to the CoM is best. Rear axle position near the CoM reduces the efforts required for propulsion, for turning, and decreases the tendency to veer of course on a cross slope. In addition, it tends to make a larger portion of the pushrim accessible for propulsion. Simple method for setting the rear axle position is to set it slightly forward (anterior) for the rearmost position and ask the use to balance on the rear wheels. If the person is unable to balance on the rear wheels, an assistant can tilt the user and wheelchair backwards to find the balance point. The axle should continue to be moved forwards so that the front casters are between 50–100 mm above the ground while balancing. If the user feels uncomfortable in this position, the rear axles can be moved rearwards a few millimeters. Rear anti-tip wheels can be used to assist the operator from becoming more comfortable with the wheelchair set-up and to help prevent rearward falls.

There are two basic rules of thumb for determining seat height. The seat should be high enough to perform typical activities of daily living, but low enough to fit under desks and tables and to efficiently propel the wheelchair. In order the set the seat height, the user should be able to comfortably touch the rear axle with his/her arms at the side, and at the same time the elbow angle should be 90–120 degrees with the upper arm along the trunk and the hand at top dead center on the pushrim. Often the rear wheel size can be selected to provide a wider range of positions.

The angle of the seat with respect to horizontal, also known as seat dump, can effect seat height as well. About 5 degrees of posterior tilt is common; however, larger angles are desirable for some wheelchair users who require more trunk support. A larger seat dump helps to increase stability by pushing the pelvis into the backrest, although one must be cautious not to promote pressure sore on the back. Transferring out of the wheelchair becomes more difficult as seat dump increases.

There are a variety of pushrims available. The most common types are standard anodized aluminum tubing, vinyl coated aluminum tubing, neoprene coated aluminum tubing, protrusion rims, and ergonomic rims. Most people should use ergonomic rims designed to help reduce the loading on the upper extremity joints, and to provide a more natural fit for the hand.

11.4 Pushrim activated power assisted wheelchairs

A pushrim activated power assisted wheelchair uses motors and batteries to augment the power applied by the users to one or both pushrims during propulsion or braking (Cooper et al., 2002c). Some people cannot functionally propel a manual wheelchair while at the same time they may have barriers to be able to use an electric powered wheelchair effectively (Buning et al., 2001). The pushrim activated power-assisted wheelchairs (PAPAW), provides another option that may be most appropriate for some clients. The PAPAW novel control technology amplifies the force applied to the pushrim to propel or brake the wheelchair (Cooper et al., 2001).

A PAPAW can provide mobility similar to a manual wheelchair with less stress on the arm joints, while at the same time offering some of the aerobic exercise benefits of manual wheelchair propulsion (Arva et al., 2001). PAPAWs have been shown to reduce the amount of force required for propulsion, to lower the stroke frequency, and to reduce the range of motion required for efficient propulsion (Corfman et al., 2003a). There are also clients who desire a manual wheelchair, but who have difficulty negotiating ramps, side slopes, soft surfaces (e.g., carpet) and other mobility barriers. These individuals may have impaired upper extremities or their limitation could be due to disease or injury-related reduction in cardiorespiratory capacity. It may be difficult for

the wheelchair user to load a PAPAW into a car or van that is not equipped with a lift or ramp, it is not difficult for an assistant.

People who have severe difficulty walking or who have the inability to walk should be evaluated for a PAPAW. In order to use a PAPAW effectively, the individual must have the coordination and strength to propel a manual wheelchair over a smooth hard floor with at least one arm. The PAPAW is beneficial for reducing the stress on the upper extremities, increasing propulsion efficiency, and lowering the cardiopulmonary demand of wheelchair propulsion. Individuals who experience pain or fatigue negotiating ramps, carpets or outdoor surfaces are ideal candidates for a PAPAW. Individuals with spinal cord injury or dysfunction, people with cerebral palsy, and elderly people may benefit from a PAPAW.

11.5 Electric powered mobility

Electric powered wheelchair designs

Powered wheelchairs can be grouped into several classes or categories (Cooper, 1995a, 1998a). A convenient grouping by intended use is primarily indoor, both indoor/outdoor, and active indoor/outdoor. Indoor wheelchairs have a small footprint (i.e., area connecting the wheels). This allows them to be maneuverable in confined spaces. However, they may not have the stability or power to negotiate obstacles outdoors. Indoor/outdoor powered wheelchairs are used by people who wish to have mobility at home, school, work, and in the community, but who stay on finished surfaces (e.g., sidewalks, driveways, flooring). Both indoor and indoor/outdoor wheelchairs conserve weight by using smaller batteries, which in turn reduces the range for travel.

Some wheelchair users want to drive over unstructured environments, travel long distances, and to move fast (Cooper et al., 2002b). Active indoor/outdoor wheelchairs may be best suited for these individuals. The active indoor/outdoor-use wheelchairs include those with suspension and use of a power-base design. The power base consists of the

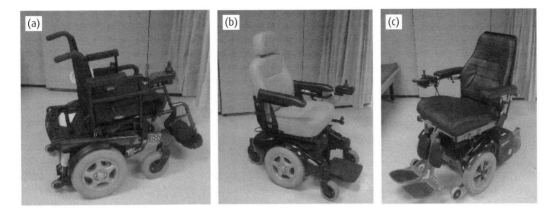

Figure 11.2. Picture of (a) rear wheel, (b) mid wheel, and (c) front wheel drive electric-powered wheelchairs.

motors, drive wheels, castors, controllers, batteries, and frame. The seating system (e.g., seat, backrest, armrests, legrests, footrests) is a separate integrated unit. Often, seating systems from one manufacturer are used on a power base from another manufacturer.

Power wheelchair bases can be classified as rear wheel drive (RWD), mid wheel drive (MWD), or front wheel drive (FWD) (Cooper, 1998a). The classification of these three drive systems is based on the drive wheel location relative to the systems center of gravity (CoG). The drive wheel position defines the basic handling characteristic of any power wheelchair. All three systems have unique driving and handling characteristics. In RWD power bases the drive wheels are behind the user's CoG and the casters are in the front. RWD systems are the traditional design and therefore many long-term power wheelchairs are familiar with their performance and prefer them to other designs. A major advantage of RWD systems is its predictable driving characteristics and stability. A potential drawback to a RWD system is its low maneuverability in tight areas due to a larger turning radius, see Fig. 11.2(a).

In MWD power bases the drive wheels are directly below the user's CoG and generally have a set of casters or anti-tippers in front and rear of the drive wheels, see Fig. 11.2(b). The advantage of the MWD system is a smaller turning radius to maneuver in tight spaces. A disadvantage is a tendency to rock or pitch forward especially with sudden stops or fast turns. When transitioning from a steep slope to a level surface (like coming off a curb cut), the front and rear casters can hang up leaving less traction on the drive wheels in the middle.

A FWD power base has the drive wheels in front of the user's CoG and it tends to be quite stable and provides a tight turning radius, see Fig. 11.2(c). FWD systems may climb obstacles or curbs more easily as the large front wheels hit the obstacle first. A disadvantage is that a FWD system has more rearward CoG, therefore the system may tend to fishtail and be difficult to drive in a straight line especially on uneven surfaces (Guo et al., 2004).

Scooters

Scooters are designed for people with limited walking ability and substantial body control (Cooper, 1998a). They are power bases with a mounted seat and usually a tiller (e.g., handle bar) steering system, see Fig. 11.3. Scooters are primarily characterized by the captain's seat. Most scooter seats swivel to ease ingress and egress. The seats are often removable to simplify transport in a personal automobile. One of the most important distinguishing features of a scooter is that speed is controlled electronically and

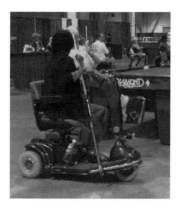

Figure 11.3. Photograph of a three-wheeled scooter.

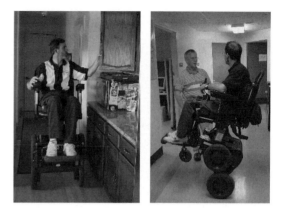

Figure 11.4. An IBOT in balance function.

direction is controlled manually. Most scooters allow the steering column to fold or be removed without tools in order to make the scooter easier to transport in a personal motor vehicle. There are products that use electronic steering by using a motor to change the direction of one or both front wheels.

Robotic wheelchairs

The Independence 3000 IBOT Transporter (IBOT) has probably garnered the most attention for its innovations in dynamic stabilization that provide it with a unique combination of capabilities, Fig. 11.4. The IBOT incorporates a variety of sensors and actuators for dynamic stabilization of the device, speed control, self-diagnosis, and for changing operational functions (Cooper et al., 2003a). In a study by Cooper et al. (2003a), subjects reported using the IBOT to perform a variety of activities including holding eye-level discussions with colleagues and shopping by balancing on two wheels, going up and down steep ramps, traversing outdoor surfaces (e.g., grass, dirt trails) and climbing curbs. Other stair-climbing and curb-negotiating devices have also been investigated. Lawn et al. (2001) reported on an electric powered wheeled mobility device that can negotiate stairs and ingress/egress into a motor vehicle. Wellman et al. (1995) described the investigation into combing the use of robotic legs with a wheeled device to provide increased mobility to people with disabilities. Their device was intended to assist with climbing curbs and uneven terrain. Future advances in controls may benefit from learning from nature and how insects negotiate rough terrain (Jindrich and Full, 2002).

Simpson et al. (2002), Yoder et al. (1996) and Levine et al. (1999) have reported on combing obstacle detection and avoidance with an electric powered wheelchair. They use a combination of ultrasound and infrared sensors to map the environment and provide assistance with guidance and control of an electric powered wheelchair for people who have visual as well as lower limb impairments.

Use assessment, fitting, and training

The mastery and functional use of electric powered wheelchair can be instrumental to self-esteem, activities of daily living, employment and community integration (Spaeth et al., 1998; Jones and Cooper, 1998). Critical for the success of these devices is the link between the consumer and the machine. Interchangeably referred to as the "interface", "man/machine interface" or "access method", all refer to a combination of a technology and a communication paradigm that allows a consumer to independently access and operate a useful system. There are three main elements when examining the usage of an assistive device. The first element is the person who has certain physical, sensory, and cognitive abilities. The second is the machine or technology, which has certain physical input devices, physical output devices and information processing capabilities. Finally, the third element is often simply referred to as the interface. It is through the interface that the person and machine actually interact, transfer information and affect each other. This is the most dynamic, and possibility the most complex element of the system.

In 2000, Fehr et al. (2000) describe the result of a clinical survey of 65 practicing clinicians in a variety of rehabilitation services from 29 states. The clinicians reported that between 10% and 40% of their clients who desired powered mobility could not be fitted with electric powered wheelchairs; because sensory impairments, poor motor function or cognitive deficits made it impossible for them to safely drive a power wheelchair with any of the existing commercial controls. Individuals with *movement disorders* are often the most underserved population. If an individual has partial or complete paralysis but has residual fine motor control either in the affected limb or at an alternative motor site, a technology for control access is commercially available. However, if the consumer has a movement disorder, e.g., *tremor* or other *unintentional* movement pattern, the commercial control options fall off precipitously to devices such as keyguards, expanded keyboards and single switch scanning interfaces.

The analog, armrest mounted, joystick is the traditional method of control for electric powered wheelchairs (Cooper et al., 2000a, c). The commercial offerings have almost no options for personalization (Cooper et al., 2002a). The return spring tension of the stick, axis alignment, template shape, and damping factor are non-adjustable-one size fits all. Manufacturers provide gain adjustments at the motor control power stage but these provide little improvement in a consumer's control capability. Gain adjustments simply slow the chair down (to a crawl if necessary) so that the consumer can obtain a minimal level of mobility. Currently, clinicians only have simple adjustments in the electronic controls to accommodate their clients for electric-powered wheelchairs

(Cooper, 1998a). The maximum speed forward and reverse can be set, as well as acceleration in the fore–aft directions and while turning.

11.6 Specialized seating and mobility

Pressure ulcers, pain management and postural accommodation are critical issues for many individuals with neurological impairments. Tilt-in-space and recline seating functions may be of benefit for ameliorating these conditions. Tilt-in-space can significantly reduce static seating pressure, a key ingredient in the development of pressure sores. Sprigle and Sposato (1997) and Hobson (1992) studied the effects of various seated positions and found that pressure was reduced significantly with 120 degrees of recline. In addition, using recline and tilt-in-space can allow for a change in position in the wheelchair and thus improve comfort. Nachemson (1975) found decreased inter-vertebral disc pressure by reclining the back from 80 to 130 degrees. Others purported advantages of tilt and recline system include better swallowing and decreased leg edema (Schunkewitz et al., 1989). Based on these arguments tilt-in-space and recline are widely prescribe accessories on power wheelchairs.

Reclining wheelchairs allow the user to change sitting posture through the use of a simple interface (e.g., switch), see Fig. 11.5. Changing seating posture can extend the amount of time a person can safely remain seated without damaging tissue or becoming fatigued. Reclining wheelchairs assist in performing pressure relief. Changing seating position redistributes pressure on weight-bearing surfaces, alters the load on postural musculature, and changes circulation. Changing position can also facilitate respiration. Elevating the legs while lowering the torso can improve venous return, and decrease fluid pooling in the lower extremities.

Tilt-in-space systems allow the person to change position with respect to gravity without changing their seated posture (i.e., the joints of the body maintain their seated position) Fig. 11.6. There are some difficulties with tilt-in-space wheelchairs.

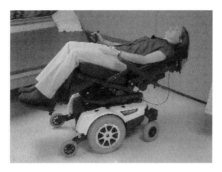

Figure 11.5. Picture of an electric-powered wheelchair with a power seat recline.

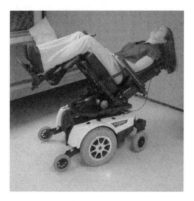

Figure 11.6. Picture of an electric-powered wheelchair with power seat tilt function.

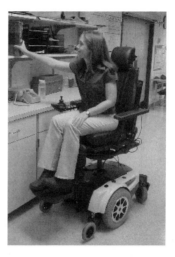

Figure 11.7. Example of an electric-powered wheelchair with powered seat elevation function.

These wheelchairs are heavier than standard wheelchairs, they are less stable, and can require greater turning diameter when reclined. A potential problem with tilt-in-space and reclining seating systems is that the body may not remain in a stable position after transitioning through several seating orientations. Sliding or stretching during reclining or tilting in some individuals may produce undesirable shear forces, excite spasticity, and bunch clothing.

Many activities can be promoted by using a variable seat height wheelchair, Fig. 11.7. Lowering seat height can make it simpler to get under tables and desks. Picking up objects from the floor can also be assisted by an adjustable seat height. Access to the floor is an important feature for promoting the cognitive and social development of children. Children

often play, explore the environment, and interact with other children at ground level. Children who use wheelchairs can benefit from being able to access the ground. As the person is lowered to the floor by the wheelchair stability is affected. Some seat lowering mechanisms alter the legrest angle in order to get closer to the ground. It is important to assure that the rider has suitable range of motion to safely use this feature. Lowering the seat makes access to desks and tables easier. Lowering the seat height tends to make the wheelchair more stable. A lower seat position can be helpful when maneuvering the wheelchair on steep ramps or slopes. The added stability of being able to lower the seat height can be of considerable benefit on cross slopes.

Raising the seat height also offers several benefits. Items on high shelves or in high cabinets can be obtained by using an elevating seat. Elevating the seat height is helpful for viewing people at eye level. Tasks such as cooking and washing can be simplified with an elevated seat height. Many powered wheelchair controllers cause the speed of the wheelchair to decrease as the seat height is raised. Increasing seat height tends to decrease the stability of the wheelchair. Most wheelchair manufacturers do not recommend elevating the seat on a slope or uneven terrain.

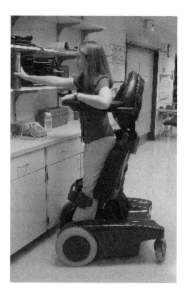

Figure 11.8. Example of an electric-powered stand-up wheelchair.

Stand-up wheelchairs are being produced that are lightweight and transportable. Stand-up wheelchairs offer a variety of advantages over standard wheelchairs, see Fig. 11.8. They provide easy access to cabinets, shelves, counters, sinks, and many windows. Many activities around the home are easier to accomplish by using a stand-up wheelchair, for example, cooking, washing dishes, and ironing clothes. Stand-up wheelchairs can reduce the need for significant home modifications. In the workplace, stand-up wheelchairs may help when making presentations using a "white board", accessing copiers, and interacting with colleagues. The ability to perform some occupations can be enhanced by using a stand-up wheelchair. For example, machine operators or machinists can perform normal job functions with minimal modifications to the worksite and physicians and surgeons can examine patients and perform procedures safely and effectively.

However, specialized technology provides greater flexibility when making individual accommodations (Troy et al., 1997). The rehabilitation team must work with the individual to determine if the stand-up wheelchair should have an electric powered base or

whether it should be manually propelled (Cooper et al., 2000b). Stand-up features are integrated into some power wheelchairs with minimal trade-offs (i.e., no additional weight or size). Manually powered stand-up wheelchairs are heavier than lightweight manual wheelchairs.

11.7 Seating and positioning hardware

Seat cushions

Various densities and types (Polyurethane, Urethane, T-Foam, Sun-Mate) of foam are commonly used in linear seating systems. Foam has been shown to offer the lowest maximum pressure over the seating surface when the appropriate densities and contours are used. However, foam has a tendency to deteriorate at an undesirable rate. A foam cushion may be sculpted or contoured in order to make foam more effective for pressure relief.

Air floatation cushions provide an excellent example of cushion design based upon the interface pressure theory (Fitzgerald et al., 2001b). If one were to simply sit on a balloon full of air, the pressure over the entire seating surface would be equal. Air floatation cushions do an excellent job of distributing the pressure over the entire seating area. In order to better control interface pressure many air floatation cushions use multiple compartments, contouring, and baffling.

Viscous fluid cushions use an electrolyte fluid mixture in a closed plastic or latex pocket. The viscous fluid conforms to the body and provides a nearly even pressure distribution. Viscous fluid cushions work much like air to equalize pressure over the entire seating surface. This is because the viscous fluid moves to come to a constant pressure within its container. Baffles can be used to control to flow of the viscous fluid just as with air cushions. The pressure distribution can be altered by using a stiff base (e.g., plastic or foam) to provide some contouring.

Positioning hardware

With some care and properly adjusted and maintained postural support system can promote good health and maximal function (Engel, 1991). Postural support systems can be customized to meet individual needs. Most systems are available with a variety of covers (e.g., vinyl, lycre-spandex, bare). Plastic, wood or metal can be used to reinforce areas for additional support and control. Special mounting hardware can be provided by manufacturers upon request or developed by local rehabilitation engineers.

People with cerebral palsy, spina Bifida, osteogenesis imperfecta, or advanced muscular dystrophy primarily use postural supports and positioning hardware. However, people who have spinal cord injury, severe multiple sclerosis, arthrogyposis, arthritis, traumatic brain injury, stroke, lower limb amputations, or some severely impaired elderly persons can benefit from postural supports (Boninger et al., 1998a; Cooper, 1998a). More recently, postural control has gained greater attention among active wheelchair users as a means of improving comfort, increasing function, and preventing some of the debilitating effects associated with long-term wheelchair use. Proper positioning can help to improve pulmonary function. The ability to use the hands and arms to perform activities of daily living may be increased through positioning. Positioning helps to orient the skeleton and the distribution of stresses within soft tissues. This can be used to help prevent or control pelvic and spinal deformities, and to prevent pressure sores.

All wheelchair users require some degree of postural support. The simplest form of postural support uses a linear sling back and a linear sling seat. For some people linear systems provide adequate support. Other people who are more severely impaired or who are at risk for developing postural deformities require greater postural support. Greater postural control can be obtained by using off-the-shelf products for most cases. In a few cases, custom fabricated postural support systems are necessary. There are a wide variety of products which are used to promote good seating posture and functional seating for wheelchair users.

Pelvic support and positioning can be achieved using a pelvic belt, lap belt, subasis bar, or anti-thrust cushion. These devices can help to prevent or correct a slouching posture with an unacceptable postural pelvic tilt. In some cases combinations of these devices must be used. Pelvic support for minor cases can be provided by using a seat belt and an anti-thrust seat cushion. The anti-thrust seat helps to maintain posture by positioning the ischial tuberosities. The pelvic belt or subasis bar must be positioned snugly (e.g., about two adult fingers should be able to fit between the belt and abdomen). The pelvic belt or subasis bar should prevent the person from sliding forward on the seat even when the occupant wiggles or squirms. The pelvis should be maintained in a neutral position against the backrest. The latch on the pelvic belt must be selected to meet the physical and cognitive abilities of the user. The pelvic belt should not slip or become unlatched inadvertently. If attached to the wheelchair, the pelvic belt or subasis bar should be used whenever the person is sitting in the wheelchair. For some people the pelvic belt or subasis bar works in concert with thoracic supports. If the pelvic belt or subasis bar is not adjusted properly with the pelvis against the backrest, the child may slump in the seat such that the thoracic supports can bruise or abrade the underarms. In some cases choking may occur which can lead to death. If an anti-thrust seat is used, the step in the seat must be positioned in front of the ischial tuberosities such that the proper pelvic angle is maintained.

Backrests may also be contoured to provide additional support for those people who need it. Two common approaches used are a flat back base with additional supports or a back base with curved sides. The width and height of the back base should be determined based upon the users mode of mobility (e.g., manual, attendant propelled, power) and postural support needs. For people who use manual wheelchairs the backrest should follow the individuals frontal contour and the height should not extend above 4 cm below the scapula. The height should be sufficient to provide comfortable support, and to provide a base to push against. Generally, the higher the degree of impairment the taller the backrest must be to provide adequate support. Contour can be added to backrests via carved foam, foam in place, standard contours, or custom molded/carved contours. People with significant loss of lateral stability may benefit from fixed or adjustable lateral trunk supports. A depth between 125 and 200 mm is sufficient for most people. The height and width depends on the individual's anatomy. When using lateral supports many backrest plates require reinforcement. Scoliosis support systems can provide additional support for proper positioning for greater comfort and better control over the wheelchair. Scoliosis supports should be prescribed or designed to be independently adjustable (i.e., inferior–superior, fore–aft, medial–lateral). Supports can be designed or prescribed to wrap around the trunk anteriorly, and may include a strap which wraps around the trunk for greatest support. Often the wrap around Scoliosis supports incorporate a quick adjust mechanism (e.g., quick release pin, knob head bolt) and a simply operated strap locking mechanism (e.g., Velcro, ring lock, or cam lock) to aid in transferring in and out of the wheelchair. Lateral and Scoliosis supports require padding (i.e., typically 8–25 mm is sufficient depending upon the applied force), and the person should be isolated from all fasteners.

A lumbar support can be added to the backrest or a rigid backrest can be used on many wheelchairs for people who have difficulty maintaining the natural curvature of the spine. Rigid backrest for lumbar support is becoming widely used among wheelchair users. Lumbar support can improve balance with added comfort and mobility. A 25–100 mm thick piece of contoured foam the width of the back is placed in the lumbar area. Custom devices and systems can be designed for people with unusual postural support needs. A properly placed lumbar support can position the head squarely over the shoulders, and improve pelvic alignment. For many wheelchair users a standard sling seat induces sacral seating. This can be corrected with a lumbar support. Spinal extension can be achieved with some people.

Head and neck supports often provide the necessary stability required to control a power wheelchair, environmental control unit, or communication device. Extensions are designed and added to the backrest structure which support the head and neck.

The degree of support required determines the type of head and neck support employed. For people who require minimal head and neck support a simple flat headrest is sufficient. This type of headrest prevents the head from extending beyond the plane of the backrest, which is especially important if the seating system is tilted or reclined. Curvature can be added to the headrest to keep the user's head within the confines of the headrest. A good seating and head support system is unlikely to be a solutions to all of a person's functional limitations. The clinicians must work with the person to develop a plan for how the person will ultimately sit and function. Head control is difficult to evaluate and requires specialized knowledge. A skilled clinician must determine the direction and the amount of force required to place the head in the desired position. Most systems attempt to bring the head to a neutral position. The clinician should be cautious to avoid placing excessive force while positioning the head. Many people who can benefit from head positioning systems can exert active muscle forces in addition to gravitational and passive connective tissue forces. After determining the amount of force and direction of force required, the desired support is duplicated by selecting head support hardware. Head supports should not apply pressure to the temporal area, the mastoid process, or the mandible. In most case, some functional tests with the head support hardware are required to verify improved function.

11.8 Applying evidence-based practice to wheelchairs and seating

Credentialing

In response to the needs of clinicians with specialized knowledge of and experience with assistive technology (AT), the RESNA developed a credentialing program in AT. RESNA offers three levels of credentials. Rehabilitation technology suppliers can be an important part of the wheelchair and seating selection and fitting process. Unfortunately, there are few suppliers who are trained in AT or who have formal rehabilitation training or experience. This has led to wide discrepancies in the quality of the services provided by rehabilitation technology suppliers. Hence, RESNA created the Assistive Technology Supplier (ATS) credential. In order to attain the ATS credential, an individual must demonstrate compensated employment in the field of AT and pass an examination that consists of fundamental elements and case-based scenarios. Suppliers with the ATS credential have demonstrated a minimum level of knowledge and experience in with AT. Clinics should give careful consideration to encouraging the suppliers who work with them to demonstrate that their employees hold the ATS credential.

Some therapists and other licensed clinicians choose to specialize in the delivery of AT services. For example, these individuals typically have a clinical degree and license in occupational therapy, physical therapy, audiology, or speech therapy. In order to identify clinicians whom have specialized in AT service provision, RESNA created the Assistive Technology Provider (ATP) credential. For years engineers and technicians have been supporting AT clinics; however, there was no appropriate clinical credential for these individuals. (Cooper, 1998b) For these individuals, RESNA created the Rehabilitation Engineering Technologist (RET) credential which requires an individual to hold and engineering or technology degree. After a suitable period of clinical AT service delivery experience, individuals are eligible to sit for the ATP examination and the supplemental RET examination. These credentials help consumers to identify individuals who have acquired specialized knowledge of AT and who are committed to providing high-quality services.

Team approach

Medical rehabilitation is a profession that is best practiced as part of a team. The best AT clinics include a team consisting of a therapist, rehabilitation engineer, a credentialed supplier, and a physician. These individuals work with cooperatively with the client to attain the client's rehabilitation goals. Other professionals may also be consulted depending on the needs and goals of the client. Rehabilitation counselors, nurses, personal care assistants and other similar professionals can also make important contributions to the AT service delivery team. During an AT assessment the team must work with the client to assess the client's goals, current abilities, and availability of resources (Cooper, 1995b). Ideally, the team will have ready access to a variety of assistive devices for the client to evaluate during his/her clinic visit and if necessary to try at home. It is absolutely critical for the team to thoroughly discuss each client's circumstances and to prepare detailed documentation supported by scientific and clinical literature. Unfortunately, AT is an area of healthcare that receives undue scrutiny and hence extra diligence is required in ensure that each client's needs are met (HCFA, 1998; Schmeler, 2003).

AT standards

When developing a new mobility device for people with disabilities it is a requirement of the US Food and Drug Administration that the device be both safe and effective. A means of demonstrating safety and efficacy is to use the ANSI and RESNA wheelchair standards (Cooper, 1998a). Wheelchair standards attempt to provide quantitative data to clinicians, engineers, and consumers. ANSI-RESNA and International

Based on the results of wheelchair standards testing, manufacturers can improve their products, particularly because consumers are demanding higher quality products and competition between manufacturers is growing. Improving products can increase the reliability of wheelchairs and reduce the risk to users. Unfortunately, the standards do not require disclosure of most of the results in manufacturer's product literature (Cooper, 1998a). Consumers or clinicians can obtain the information if requested, but this is tedious and makes comparisons difficult.

REFERENCES

Americans with Disabilities. (1994). Bureau of Census Statistical Brief, SB/94-1, US Department of Commerce, January.

Arva, J., Fitzgerald, S.G., Cooper, R.A., Boninger, M.L., Spaeth, D.M. and Corfman, T.J. (2001). Mechanical efficiency and user power reduction with the JWII pushrim activate power assisted wheelchair. *Med Eng Phys*, **23**(**12**), 699–705.

Asato, K.T., Cooper, R.A., Robertson, R.N. and Ster, J.F. (1993). SMART^Wheels: development and testing of a system for measuring manual wheelchair propulsion dynamics. *IEEE Trans Biomed Eng*, **40**(**12**), 1320–1324.

Bayley, J.C., Cochran, T.P. and Sledge, C.B. (1987). The weight-bearing shoulder: the impingement syndrome in paraplegics. *J Bone Joint Surg Am*, **69**(**5**), 676–678.

Bertocci, G.E., Hobson, D.A. and Digges, K. (1996). Development of transportable wheelchair design criteria using computer crash simulation. *IEEE Trans Rehabil Eng*, **4**(**3**), 171–181.

Bertocci, G.E., Szobota, S., Digges, K. and Hobson, D.A. (1999a). Computer simulation and sled test validation of a power-base wheelchair and occupant subjected to frontal crash conditions. *IEEE Trans Neural Syst Rehabil Eng*, **7**(**2**), 234–244.

Bertocci, G., Cooper, R.A., Young, T., Esteireiro, J. and Thomas C. (1999b). Testing and evaluation of wheelchair caster assemblies subjected to dynamic crash loading. *J Rehabil Res Dev*, **36**(**1**), 32–41.

Bertocci, G., Manary, M. and Ha, D. (2001). Wheelchairs used as motor vehicle seats: seat loading in frontal impact sled testing. *Med Eng Phys*, **23**(**10**), 679–685.

Boninger, M.L., Cooper, R.A., Robertson, R.N. and Shimada, S.D. (1997). 3-D pushrim forces during two speeds of wheelchair propulsion. *Am J Phys Med Rehabil*, **76**(**5**), 420–426.

Boninger, M.L., Saur, T., Trefler, E., Hobson, D.A., Burdette, R. and Cooper, R.A. (1998a). Postural changes with aging in tetraplegia. *Arch Phys Med Rehabil*, **79**, 1577–1581.

Boninger, M.L., Cooper, R.A., Shimada, S.D. and Rudy, T.E. (1998b). Shoulder and elbow motion during two speeds of wheelchair propulsion: a description using a local coordinate system. *Spinal Cord*, **36**(**6**), 418–426.

Boninger, M.L., Cooper, R.A., Baldwin, M.A., Shimada, S.D. and Koontz, A. (1999). Wheelchair pushrim kinetics: weight and median nerve function. *Arch Phys Med Rehabil*, **80**(**8**), 910–915.

Boninger, M.L., Baldwin, M., Cooper, R.A., Koontz, A.M. and Chan, L. (2000). Manual wheelchair pushrim biomechanics and axle position. *Arch Phys Med Rehabil*, **81**(**5**), 608–613.

Boninger, M.L., Towers, J.D., Cooper, R.A., Dicianno, B.E. and Munin, M.C. (2001). Shoulder imaging abnormalities in individuals with paraplegia. *J Rehabil Res Dev*, **38**(**4**), 401–408.

Boninger, M.L., Souza, A.L., Cooper, R.A., Fitzgerald, S.G., Koontz, A.M. and Fay, B.T. (2002). Propulsion patterns and pushrim biomechanics in manual wheelchair propulsion. *Arch Phys Med Rehabil*, **83**(**5**), 718–723.

Boninger, M.L., Dicianno, B.E., Cooper, R.A., Towers, J.D., Koontz, A.M. and Souza, A.L. (2003a). Shoulder injury, wheelchair propulsion, and gender. *Arch Phys Med Rehabil*, **84**(**11**), 1615–1620.

Boninger, M.L., Cooper, R.A., Fitzgerald, S.G., Lin, J., Cooper, R., Dicianno, B. and Liu B. (2003b). Investigating neck pain in wheelchair users. *Am J Phys Med Rehabil*, **82**(**3**), 197–202.

Brienza, D.M., Cooper, R.A. and Brubaker, C.E. (1996a). Wheelchairs and seating. *Curr Opin Orthoped*, **7**, 82–86.

Brienza, D., Chung, K., et al. (1996b). System for the analysis of seat support surfaces using surface shape control and simultaneous measure of applied pressures. *IEEE Trans Rehabil Eng*, **4**(**2**), 103–113.

Brienza, D.M., Karg, P.E., et al. (2001). The relationship between pressure ulcer incidence and buttock-seat cushion interface pressure in at-risk elderly wheelchair users. *Arch Phys Med Rehabil*, **82**(**4**), 529–533.

Buning, M.E., Angelo, J.A. and Schmeler, M.R. (2001). Occupational performance and the transition to powered mobility: a pilot study. *Am J Occup Ther*, **55**(**3**), 339–344.

Calder, C.J. and Kirby, R.L. (1990). Fatal wheelchair-related accidents in the United States. *Am J Phys Med Rehabil*, **69**(**4**), 184–190.

CMS (2003). Power wheelchair coverage overview. Center for Medicare and Medicaid Services, Retrieved August 17, 2003: http://www.cms.hhs/medlearn/PowerWheelchair.pdf

Collins, D., Cooper, R., Cooper, R.A. and Schmeler, M. (2002). Strengthening justification for assistive technology with research findings: a case study *RESNA News*, Spring, 1.

Cooper, R.A. (1991). High tech wheelchairs gain the competitive edge. *IEEE Eng Med Biol Mag*, **10**(**4**), 49–55.

Cooper, R.A. (1995a). Intelligent control of power wheelchairs. *IEEE Eng Med Biol Mag*, **15**(**4**), 423–431.

Cooper, R.A. (1995b). Forging a new future: a call for integrating people with disabilities into rehabilitation engineering. *Technol Disabil*, **4**, 81–85.

Cooper, R.A. (1996). A perspective on the ultralight wheelchair revolution. *Technol Disabil*, **5**, 383–392.

Cooper, R.A. (1998a). *Wheelchairs: A Guide to Selection and Configuration*, Demos Medical Publishers, New York, NY.

Cooper, R.A. (1998b). Wheelchair research and development for people with spinal cord injury, guest editorial. *J Rehabil Res Dev*, **35**(**1**), xi.

Cooper, R.A. (1999). Engineering manual and electric powered wheelchairs. *Crit Rev Biomed Eng*, **27**(**1/2**), 27–74.

Cooper, R.A. and Boninger, M.L. (1999). Walking on your hands. *Parapleg New*, **53**(**3**), 12–16.

Cooper, R.A. and Cooper, R. (2003c). Time to mobilize: 21st annual survey of lightweight-wheelchair manufacturers. *Sports 'N' Spokes*, **29**(**2**), 34–42.

Cooper, R.A., Stewart, K.J. and VanSickle, D.P. (1994a). Evaluation of methods for determining rearward static stability of manual wheelchairs. *J Rehabil Res Dev*, **31**(**2**), 144–147.

Cooper, R.A., Robertson, R.N., VanSickle, D.P., Stewart, K.J. and Albright, S. (1994b). Wheelchair impact response to ISO test pendulum and ISO standard curb. *IEEE Trans Rehabil Eng*, **2**(**4**), 240–246.

Cooper, R.A., VanSickle, D.P., Albright, S.J., Stewart, K.J., Flannery, M. and Robertson, R.N. (1995). Power wheelchair range testing and energy consumption during fatigue testing. *J Rehabil Res Dev*, **32**(**3**), 255–263.

Cooper, R.A., Trefler, E. and Hobson, D.A. (1996a). Wheelchairs and seating: issues and practice. *Technol Disabil*, **5**, 3–16.

Cooper, R.A., Robertson, R.N., Lawrence, B., Heil, T., Albright, S.J., VanSickle, D.P. and Gonzalez, J. (1996b). Life-cycle analysis of depot versus rehabilitation manual wheelchairs. *J Rehabil Res Dev*, **33**(**1**), 45–55.

Cooper, R.A., Gonzalez, J., Lawrence, B., Rentschler, A., Boninger, M.L. and VanSickle, D.P. (1997a). Performance of selected lightweight wheelchairs on ANSI/RESNA tests. *Arch Phys Med Rehabil*, **78**(**10**), 1138–1144.

Cooper, R.A., Boninger, M.L., VanSickle, D.P., Robertson, R.N. and Shimada, S.D. (1997b). Uncertainty analysis of wheelchair propulsion dynamics. *IEEE Trans Rehabil Eng*, **5**(**2**), 130–139.

Cooper, R.A., Robertson, R.N., VanSickle, D.P. and Boninger, M.L. (1997c). Methods for determining 3-dimensional wheelchair pushrim forces and moments. *J Rehabil Res Dev*, **34**(**2**), 162–170.

Cooper, R.A., Dvorznak, M.J., O'Connor, T.J., Boninger, M.L. and Jones, D.J. (1998a). Braking electric powered wheelchairs: effect of braking method, seatbelt, and legrests. *Arch Phys Med Rehabil*, **79**(**10**), 1244–1249.

Cooper, R.A., DiGiovine, C.P., Boninger, M.L., Shimada, S.D. and Robertson, R.N. (1998b). Frequency analysis of 3-dimensional pushrim forces and moments for manual wheelchair propulsion. *Automedica*, **16**, 355–365.

Cooper, R.A., Boninger, M.L. and Rentschler, A. (1999). Evaluation of selected ultralight manual wheelchairs using ANSI/RESNA standards. *Arch Phys Med Rehabil*, **80**(**4**), 462–467.

Cooper, R.A., O'Connor, T.J., Gonzalez, J.P., Boninger, M.L. and Rentschler, A.J. (1999a). Augmentation of the 100 kg ISO wheelchair test dummy to accommodate higher mass. *J Rehabil Res Dev*, **36**(**1**), 48–54.

Cooper, R.A., DiGiovine, C.P., Rentschler, A.J., Lawrence, B.M. and Boninger, M.L. (1999b). Fatigue life of two manual wheelchair cross-brace designs. *Arch Phys Med Rehabil*, **80**(**9**), 1078–1081.

Cooper, R.A., Jones, D.K., Boninger, M.L., Fitzgerald, S. and Albright, S.J. (2000a). Analysis of position and isometric joysticks for powered wheelchair driving. *IEEE Trans Biomed Eng*, **47**(**7**), 902–910.

Cooper, R.A., Dvorznak, M.J., Rentschler, A.J. and Boninger, M.L. (2000b). Technical note: displacement between the seating surface and hybrid test dummy during transitions with a variable configuration wheelchair. *J Rehabil Res Dev*, **37**(**3**), 297–303.

Cooper, R.A., Widman, L.M., Jones, D.K. and Robertson, R.N. (2000c). Force sensing control for electric powered wheelchairs. *IEEE Trans Control Syst Technol*, **8**(**1**), 112–117.

Cooper, R.A., Fitzgerald, S.G., Boninger, M.L., Prins, K., Rentschler, A.J., Arva, J. and O'Connor, T.J. (2001). Evaluation of a pushrim activated power assisted wheelchair. *Arch Phys Med Rehabil*, **82**(**5**), 702–708.

Cooper, R.A., Jones, D.K., Spaeth, D.M., Boninger, M.L., Fitzgerald, S.G. and Guo, S.F. (2002a). Comparison of virtual and real electric powered wheelchair driving using a position sensing and an isometric joystick. *Med Eng Phys*, **24**, 703–708.

Cooper, R.A., Thorman, T., Cooper, R., Dvorznak, M.J., Fitzgerald, S.G., Ammer, W., Song-Feng, G. and Boninger, M.L. (2002b). Driving characteristics of electric powered wheelchair users: how far, fast, and often do people drive? *Arch Phys Med Rehabil*, **83**(**2**), 250–255.

Cooper, R.A., Corfman, T.A., Fitzgerald, S.G., Boninger, M.L., Spaeth, D.M., Ammer, W. and Arva, J. (2002c). Performance assessment of a pushrim activated power assisted wheelchair. *IEEE Trans Cont Syst Technol*, **10**(**1**), 121–126.

Cooper, R.A., Boninger, M.L., Cooper, R., Dobson, A.R., Schmeler, M., Kessler, J. and Fitzgerald, S.G. (2003a). Technical perspectives: use of the independence 3000 IBOT transporter at home and in the community. *J Spinal Cord Med*, **26**(**1**), 79–85.

Cooper, R.A., Wolf, E., Fitzgerald, S.G., Boninger, M.L., Ulerich, R. and Ammer, W.A. (2003b). Seat and footrest accelerations in manual wheelchairs with and without suspension. *Arch Phys Med Rehabil*, **84**(**1**), 96–102.

Corfman, T.A., Cooper, R.A., Boninger, M.L., Koontz, A.M. and Fitzgerald, S.G. (2003a). Range of motion and stroke frequency differences between manual wheelchair propulsion and pushrim activated power assisted wheelchair propulsion. *J Spinal Cord Med*, **26**(**2**), 135–140.

Corfman, T.A., Cooper, R.A., Fitzgerald, S.G. and Cooper, R. (2003b). A video-based analysis of "tips and falls" during electric powered wheelchair driving. *Arch Phys Med Rehabil*, **84**(**12**), 1797–1802.

Curtis, K.A., Roach, K.E., Applegate, E.B., Amar, T., Benbow, C.S., Genecco, T.D. and Gualano, J. (1995). Development of the wheelchair user's shoulder pain index (WUSPI). *Paraplegia*, **33**(**5**), 290–293.

Department of Veteran Affairs. Facts about the Department of Veterans Affairs. March 2002. Available at http://www.va.gov/opa/fact/docs/vafacts.htm

DiGiovine, M.M., Cooper, R.A., Boninger, M.L., Lawrence, B.L., VanSickle, D.P. and Rentschler, A.J. (2000). User assessment of manual wheelchair ride comfort and ergonomics. *Arch Phys Med Rehabil*, **81**(**4**), 490–494.

DiGiovine, C.P., Cooper, R.A., Fitzgerald, S.G., Boninger, M.L., Wolf, E. and Guo, S.F. (2003). Whole-body vibration during manual wheelchair propulsion with selected seat cushions and back supports. *IEEE Trans Neural Syst Rehabil Eng*, **11**(**3**), 311–322.

Dobson, A., Cooper, R.A., Wolf, E., Fitzgerald, S.G., Ammer, W.A., Boninger, M.L. and Cooper, R. (2003). Evaluation of vibration exposure of power wheelchair users over selected sidewalk pavement surfaces. *Proceedings 26th Annual RESNA Conference*, Atlanta, GA.

Durable Medical Equipment Regional Carrier (DMERC). *Region D Supplier Manual*, 54–57, 6-1997. CIGNA Health Care (Chapter IX).

Engel, P. (1991). Aspects of wheelchair seating comfort. *Ergo of Manual Wheelchair Prop*, 105–111.

Fass, J.M., Cooper, R.A., Fitzgerald, S.G., Schmeler, M., Boninger, M.L., Algood, S.D., Ammer, W.A., Rentschler, A.J. and Duncan, J. (2004). Durability, value, and reliability of selected electric powered wheelchairs. *Arch Phys Med Rehabil*, **85**(**5**), 805–814.

Fehr, L., Langbein, E. and Skaar, S.B. (2000). Adequacy of power wheelchair control interfaces for persons with severe disabilities: a clinical survey. *J Rehabil Res Dev*, **37**, 353–360.

Fitzgerald, S.G., Yoest, L.M., Cooper, R.A. and Downs, F. (2001). Comparison of laboratory and actual fatigue life for three types of manual wheelchairs. In: *Proceedings of the RESNA 2001 Annual Conference* (ed. Simpson, R.), 2001 June 22–26; RESNA Press, Reno (NV), Arlington (VA), pp. 352–354.

Fitzgerald, S.G., Cooper, R.A., Boninger, M.L. and Rentschler, A.J. (2001a). Comparison of fatigue life for three types of manual wheelchairs. *Arch Phys Med Rehabil*, **82**(**10**), 1484–1488.

Fitzgerald, S.G., Thorman, T., Cooper, R. and Cooper, R.A. (2001b). Evaluating wheelchair cushions. *Rehabil Manage*, **14**(**1**), 42–44.

Geyer, M.D., Brienza, et al. (2001). A randomized control trial to evaluate pressure-reducing seat cushion for elderly wheelchair users. *Adv Skin Wound Care*, **14**(**3**), 120–129.

Guo, S., Cooper, R.A., Corfman, T.A. and Ding, D. (2003). Influence of wheelchair front caster wheel on the reverse driving stability. *Assist Technol*, **15**(**2**), 98–104

Health Care Financing Administration (1998). *Proceedings Rehab Specialities/Wheelchair Documentation, Continuing Education Workshop*, Fall, Baltimore, MD.

Hobson, D. (1992). Comparative effects of posture on pressure and shear at the body seat interface. *J Rehabil Res Dev*, **29**(**4**), 21–31.

Jindrich, D.L. and Full, R.J. (2002). Dynamic stabilization of rapid hexapedal locomotion. *J Exp Biol*, **205**, 2803–2823.

Jones, D.K. and Cooper, R.A. (1998). Electro-mechanical devices for control of powered wheelchairs. *Saudi J Disabil Rehabil*, **4**(**3**), 200–206.

Kirby, R.L., Ackroyd-Stolarz, S.A., Brown, M.G. and Kirkland, S.A. (1994). Wheelchair-related accidents caused by tips and falls among non-institutionalized users of manually propelled wheelchairs in Nova Scotia. *Am J Phys Med Rehabil*, **73**, 319–330.

Koontz, A.M., Boninger, M.L., Cooper, R.A., Souza, A.S. and Fay, B.T. (2002). Shoulder kinematics and kinetics during two speeds of wheelchair propulsion. *J Rehabil Res Dev*, **39**(**6**), 635–650.

Kwarciak, A.M., Cooper, R.A. and Wolf, E. (2002). Effectiveness of rear suspension in reducing shock exposure to manual wheelchair users during curb descents. *Proceedings of the 25th Annual RESNA Conference*, Minneapolis, MN, pp. 365–367.

Lawn, M., Sakai, T., Kuroiwa, M. and Ishimatsu, T. (2001). Development and practical application of a stair-climbing wheelchair in Nagasaki. *Int J Human-Friendly Welfare Robot Syst*, 33–39.

Levine, S., Bell, D., Jaros, L., Simpson, R., Koren, Y. and Borenstein, J. (1999). The NavChair assistive wheelchair navigation system, *IEEE Trans Rehabil Eng*, **7**(**4**), 443–451.

Nachemson, A. (1975). Towards a better understanding of low back pain: a review of the mechanics of the lumbar disc. *Rheumatol Rehabil*, **14**, 129–143.

New Freedom Initiative Act (2001). Available at http://www.whitehouse.gov/news/freedominitiative/freedominitiative.html

Nichols, P.J., Norman, P.A. and Ennis, J.R. (1979). Wheelchair user's shoulder? Shoulder pain in patients with spinal cord lesions. *Scand J Rehabil Med*, **11**, 29–32.

Robertson, R.N., Boninger, M.L., Cooper, R.A. and Shimada, S. (1996). Pushrim forces and joint kinetics during wheelchair propulsion. *Arch Phys Med Rehabil*, **77**, 856–864.

Schmeler, M., Kelleher, A., Cooper, R.A. and Cooper, R. (2003). Show me the money. *Adv Direct Rehabil*, **12(10)**, 31.

Schunkewitz, J., Sprigle, S. and Chung, K.C. (1989). The effect of postural stress on lower limb blood flow in SCI persons. In: *Proceedings of the RESNA 12th Annual Conference*, New Orleans, pp. 77–78.

Seidel, H., et al. (1986). Long term effects of whole-body vibration: a critical review of the literature. *Int Arch Occup Environ Health*, **58**, 1–26.

Shalala, D.E., Vladeck, B.C., Wolf, L.F., et al. (1996). *Health Care Financing Review: Statistical Supplement*, 320–321 (Table 57).

Shimada, S.D., Robertson, R.N., Boninger, M.L. and Cooper, R.A. (1998). Kinematic characterization of wheelchair propulsion stroke patterns. *J Rehabil Res Dev*, **35(2)**, 210–218.

Simpson, R.C., Poirot, D. and Baxter, F. (2002). The hephaetstus smart wheelchair system. *IEEE Trans Neural Syst Rehabil Eng*, **10(2)**, 118–122.

Spaeth, D.M., Jones, D.K. and Cooper, R.A. (1998). Universal control interface for people with disabilities. *Saudi J Disabil Rehabil*, **4(3)**, 207–214.

Sprigle, S. and Sposato, B. (1997). Physiologic effects and design considerations of tilt and recline wheelchairs. *Orthop Phys Ther Clin North Am*, **6(1)**, 99–122.

Tai, C.F., Liu, D., Cooper, R.A., DiGiovine, M.M. and Boninger, M.L. (1998). Analysis of vibrations during manual wheelchair use. *Saudi J Disabil Rehabil*, **4(3)**, 186–191.

Troy, B.S., Cooper, R.A., Robertson, R.N. and Gray, T. (1997). An analysis of working postures of manual wheelchair users in the office environment. *J Rehabil Res Dev*, **34(2)**, 151–161.

Unmat, S. and Kirby, R.L. (1994). Nonfatal wheelchair-related accidents reported to the national electronic injury surveillance system. *Am J Phys Med Rehabil*, **73(3)**, 163–167.

Van Roosmalen, L., Bertocci, G.E., Hobson, D.A. and Karg, P. (2002). Preliminary evaluation of wheelchair occupant restraint system usage in motor vehicles. *J Rehabil Res Dev*, **39(1)**, 83–93.

VanSickle, D.P., Cooper, R.A., Robertson, R.N. and Boninger, M.L. (1996). Determination of wheelchair dynamic load data for use with finite element analysis. *IEEE Trans Rehabil Eng*, **4(3)**, 161–170.

VanSickle, D.P., Cooper, R.A. and Boninger, M.L. (2000). Road loads acting on manual wheelchairs. *IEEE Trans Rehabil Eng*, **8(3)**, 385–393.

VanSickle, D.P., Cooper, R.A., Boninger, M.L. and DiGiovine, C.P. (2001). Analysis of vibrations induced during wheelchair propulsion. *J Rehabil Res Dev*, **38(4)**, 409–422.

Wang, J., Brienza, D., et al. (1998). Biomechanical analysis of buttock soft tissue using computer-aided seating system. *Proceedings of the International Conference of the IEEE Engineering in Medicine and Biology Society*, 2757–2759.

Wang, J., Brienza, D.M., et al. (2000). A compound sensor for biomechanical analyses of buttock soft tissue in vivo. *J Rehabil Res Dev*, **37(4)**, 433–439.

Wellman, P., Krovi, W., Kuma, V. and Harwin, W. (1995). Design of a wheelchair with legs for people with motor disabilities. *IEEE Trans Rehabili Eng*, **3**, pp. 343–353.

Whitman, J.D., Cooper, R.A. and Robertson, R.N. (1998). An automated process to aid in wheelchair selection. *Saudi J Disabil Rehabil*, **4(3)**, 180–185.

Wolf, E.J., Cooper, R.A., DiGiovine, C.P. and Ammer, M.L. (2001). Analysis of whole-body vibrations on manual wheelchair using a hybrid III test dummy. *Proceedings 24th Annual RESNA Conference*, Reno, NV, pp. 346–348.

Wolf, E., Cooper, R,A. and Kwarciak, A. (2002). Analysis of whole body vibrations of suspension manual wheelchairs: utilization of the absorbed power method. *Proceedings of the 25th Annual RESNA Conference*, Minneapolis, MN, pp. 303–305.

Wolf, E., Cooper, R.A., Dobson, A., Fitzgerald, S.G. and Ammer, W.A. (2003). Assessment of vibrations during manual wheelchair propulsion over selected sidewalk surfaces. *Proceedings 26th Annual RESNA Conference*, Atlanta, GA.

Yoder, J.D., Baumgartner, E.T. and Skaar, S.B. (1996). Initial results in the development of a guidance system for a powered wheelchair. *IEEE Trans Rehabil Eng*, **4(3)**, 143–151.

12

Rehabilitation robotics, orthotics, and prosthetics

H.I. Krebs[1], N. Hogan[2], W.K. Durfee[3] and H.M. Herr[4]

[1] Department of Mechanical Engineering, Massachusetts Institute of Technology and Adjunct Assistant Research Professor of Neuroscience, The Winifred Masterson Burke Medical Research Institute, Weill Medical College of Cornell University, New York, USA; [2] Departments of Mechanical Engineering, and Brain and Cognitive Sciences, Massachusetts Institute of Technology, Cambridge, USA; [3] Department of Mechanical Engineering, University of Minnesota, Minnesota, USA and [4] The Media Lab and The Harvard/MIT Division of Health Science and Technology, Cambridge, USA

12.1 Overview

One overarching goal drives our research and development activities: to revolutionize rehabilitation medicine with robotics, mechatronics, and information technologies that can assist movement, enhance treatment and quantify outcomes. In this chapter, we present three fronts of this revolution: rehabilitation robotics, orthotics, and prosthetics.

The first and newest approach, rehabilitation robotics, has grown significantly in the last 10 years (cf. special issue of the *Journal of Rehabilitation Research and Development*, **37**(**6**) of Nov/Dec 2000; *International Conference on Rehabilitation Robotics – ICORR* 2001, 2003 and 2005). Previously, robotics were incorporated into assistive devices to help the physically challenged accommodate their impairment. Rehabilitation robotics, by contrast, fashions a new class of interactive and user-friendly robots that enhance the clinicians' goal of facilitating recovery by not only evaluating but also by delivering measured therapy to patients. Krebs and Hogan review pioneering clinical results in the field, discuss the growing pains of forging a novel technology, and outline the potential for a brilliant future.

Of the other two activities, we will limit our discussion to mechatronic systems. Orthotics and prosthetics may be considered as a category of assistive robotics. While the previous high water mark for mechatronic assistive technology occurred during the Vietnam War decades of 1960s and 1970s, recent advancements in materials, computers, and neuro-connectivity (neuro-prostheses) have reinvigorated research in this field. In fact, the lack of equivalent advances in realm of energy storage represents the only major hurdle preventing the realization of practical versions of Hollywood's fancies such as Star Trek's Commander Data or the Terminator. Durfee reviews pioneering developments in orthotics, Krebs and Hogan review upper-limb prostheses, and Herr reviews lower extremity prostheses. We will also discuss some emerging developments that could render some science fictions into reality.

12.2 Rehabilitation robotics

Rehabilitation robotics encompasses an emerging class of interactive, user-friendly, clinical devices designed to evaluate patients and, also deliver therapy. Robots and computers are being harnessed to support and enhance clinicians' productivity, thereby facilitating a disabled individual's functional recovery. This development represents a shift from earlier uses of robotics as an assistive technology for the disabled. The new focus on mechanisms of recovery and evidence-based treatment together with developments facilitating safe human–machine interaction has paved the way for the surge in academic research, which started in early 1990s.

We can group devices into two main categories for the upper and lower extremity. For upper, extremity, Erlandson et al. (1990) described a patented robotic "smart exercise partner" in which the recovering stroke patient executes general spatial motions specified by the robot. Positive results using that system in a clinical setting were reported (Erlandson, 1995). However, patients had to be capable of moving independently or using the contralateral limb to move and guide the impaired limb (self-ranging). Independent movement is also essential to use of Rosen's 3-D controllable brake device (Maxwell, 1990), Rahman's functional upper limb orthosis (Rahman et al., 2000), and Burdea's pneumatically actuated glove (Merians et al., 2002). Other upper extremity robotic tools differ insofar as they do not require patients to be capable of independent movement; controlled forces can be exerted to move the patient or to measure aspects of motor status such as spasticity, rigidity or muscle tone. Lum et al. (1993, 1995) described the design and application of robotic assistive devices focused on bi-manual tasks to promote motor recovery. More recently, Lum et al. (Burgar et al., 2000; Reinkensmeyer et al., 2000a; Lum et al., 2002) used a commercial PUMA robot augmented by improved sensors to implement the Mirror Image Movement Enabler (MIME) system, in which the robot moves the impaired limb to mirror movements of the contralateral limb. Harwin et al. (2001) is using another commercial robot (Fokker) to move the impaired arm in the recently initiated European Union sponsored project. While attempts to adapt or re-configure industrial robots for use in rehabilitation robotics appears to be a reasonable approach it suffers from a critical drawback: some 20 years of experience with industrial robots shows that low impedance comparable to the human arm cannot practically be achieved with these machines (intrinsically high impedance machines). In contrast to these approaches other groups have developed robotic technology configured for safe, stable and compliant operation in close physical contact with humans. For example, the MIT-MANUS robot developed in the Newman Laboratory for Biomechanics and Human Rehabilitation was specifically designed for clinical neurologic applications and ensures a gentle compliant behavior (Hogan et al., 1995). Other low-impedance rehabilitation devices are Reinkensmeyer's *ARM Guide* (2000) and Furusho's *EMUL* (2003). Operationally, these robots can "get out of the way" as needed. They can therefore be programmed to allow the recovering stroke survivor to express movement, in whole or in part, even when the attempts are weak or uncoordinated. Whether this feature is crucial for effective therapy remains unproven but its importance for obtaining uncorrupted measurements of a patient's sensorimotor function has been established unequivocally (Krebs et al., 1998, 1999a; Reinkensmeyer et al., 2002; Rohrer et al., 2002).

Evolving lower extremity devices are inspired mainly by gym machines and orthoses rather than by re-configured industrial robots. The best examples are Hesse's Elliptical Gait Trainer, Yaskawa's therapeutic exercise machine (TEM), and the Lokomat (Sakaki et al., 1999; Colombo et al., 2000; Hesse and Uhlenbrock, 2000; see Volume II, Chapters 3 and 19). Not unlike their upper-extremity industrial robot counterparts, however, these designs suffer from a high impedance drawback. Most are presently being re-designed to modulate their impedance and to afford an interactive experience similar to the low-impedance lower extremities devices under development at MIT in the Newman Laboratory and at University of California Irvine.

Accompanying the vigorous development of rehabilitation robotic devices is an equivalent growth in clinical evaluations of device performance. Results include new insights into the recovery mechanisms for a variety of conditions, and into the rehabilitation techniques that best engage those mechanisms. Areas of research focus include not only stroke, but also motor deficits associated with diverse neurologic, orthopedic, arthritic conditions. A number of studies demonstrated the exciting opportunities and benefits of integrating robotic technology into patients' daily rehabilitation program (e.g., Aisen et al., 1997; Krebs et al., 1998, 2000; Volpe et al., 1999, 2000, 2001; Burgar et al., 2000; Colombo et al., 2000; Hesse and Uhlenbrock, 2000; Reinkensmeyer et al., 2000, 2002; Lum et al., 2002; Fasoli et al., 2003, 2004; Ferraro et al., 2003).

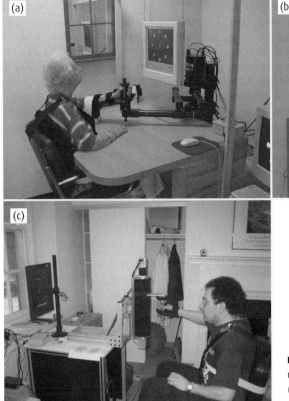

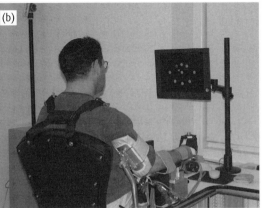

Figure 12.1. Rehabilitation robot modules during clinical trials at the Burke Rehabilitation Hospital (White Plains, NY). (a) and (b) show the shoulder and elbow robot (MIT-MANUS) and the wrist robot, and (c) the anti-gravity spatial module.

This chapter presents only our own results to delineate the potential of the technology and future directions for rehabilitation robotics. To date, we have deployed three distinct robot modules in collaborating clinical institutions[1] for shoulder and elbow, wrist, and spatial movements (Fig. 12.1).

Volpe (2001) reported results of robotic training with 96 consecutive inpatients admitted to Burke Rehabilitation Hospital (White Plains, NY) who met inclusion criteria and consented to participate. Inclusion criteria were diagnosis of a single unilateral stroke within 4 weeks of admission to the study; the ability to understand and follow simple directions;

and upper limb weakness in the hemiparetic arm (i.e., a strength grade of 3/5 or less in muscle groups of the proximal arm) as assessed with the standardized Medical Research Council battery. Patients were randomly assigned to either an experimental or control group. The sensorimotor training for the experimental group consisted of a set of "video games" in which patients were required to move the robot end-effector according to the game's goals. If the patient could not perform the task, the robot assisted and guided the patient's hand. The sensorimotor training group received an additional 4–5 h per week of robot-aided therapy while the control group received an hour of weekly robot exposure.

Although patient groups were comparable on all initial clinical evaluation measures, the robot-trained group demonstrated significantly greater motor

---

[1] Hospitals presently operating one or more MIT-MANUS class robots include Burke (NY), Spaulding (MA), Helen Hayes (NY), Rhode Island (RI) Rehabilitation Hospitals, and the Baltimore (MD) and Cleveland (OH) Veterans Administration Medical Centers.

Table 12.1. Mean interval change in impairment and disability measure for inpatients (significance $P < 0.05$). For all evaluations higher scores indicate better performance. MP was only evaluated for shoulder and elbow movements.

Between group comparisons: final evaluation minus initial evaluation	Robot-trained ($n = 55$)	Control ($n = 41$)	P-value
Impairment measures (±SEM)			
Fugl Meyer shoulder/elbow (FM-se) max/42	6.7 ± 1.0	4.5 ± 0.7	NS
MP max/20	4.1 ± 0.4	2.2 ± 0.3	<0.01
Motor Status shoulder/elbow (MS-se) max/40	8.6 ± 0.8	3.8 ± 0.5	<0.01
Motor Status wrist/hand (MS/wh) max/42	4.1 ± 1.1	2.6 ± 0.8	NS
Disability evaluation			
FIM (upper) max/42	32.0 ± 5.0	25.5 ± 6.5	NS

MP: Motor Power; NS: not significant.

improvement (higher mean interval change ± SEM) than the control group on the impairment scales (see Table 12.1). These gains were specific to motions of the shoulder and elbow, the focus of the robot training. There were no significant between group differences in the mean change scores for wrist and hand function, although there was a trend favoring the robot group. Likewise there were no significant differences in functional independence measure (FIM) performance, used to indicate changes in the level of disability. Use of the FIM to indicate changes in the level of disability that may be associated with robotic therapy is not without limitations. Although the FIM is a well-established, reliable, and valid measure of basic activities of daily living, many of the self-care tasks that comprise the motor subscale of the FIM can be independently accomplished by using only the "unaffected" upper limb (Dodds et al., 1993; Granger et al., 1993). Therefore, a definitive conclusion about the relationship between changes in upper limb motor impairment, increased motor function, and reduction in disability is not possible with the FIM.

Long after stroke, patients still suffer a variety of impairments dependent on the size and location of their individual stroke. Fasoli et al. (2003, 2004) reported results of robotic training described at Spaulding Rehabilitation Hospital (Boston, MA) with 42 consecutive community dwelling volunteers with stroke, who responded to information they had

Table 12.2. Comparison of mean interval change for outpatients at Spaulding Rehabilitation Hospital ($n = 42$, sensorimotor protocol). For all evaluations higher scores indicate better performance. MP was only evaluated for shoulder and elbow movements.

Between group comparisons: final evaluation minus initial evaluation	Robot-trained ($n = 42$)	P-value
Impairment measures (±SEM)		
Fugl Meyer shoulder/elbow (FM-se) max/42	3.4 ± 4.0	<0.01
MP max/40	2.1 ± 1.9	<0.01
Motor Status shoulder/elbow (MS-se) max/40	1.4 ± 2.0	<0.01

obtained from media sources about the robotic training experiments. These patients received the same sensorimotor robotic training used with inpatients (see above). Prior to engaging in robotic therapy, these patients were assessed on three separate occasions to determine baseline function and to establish a within subject control. The primary outcome measures were the Fugl Meyer, Motor Status Scale for the shoulder and elbow, and the Motor Power (MP) score. Our baseline analyses revealed no statistically significant differences among any of the pre-treatment clinical evaluations, indicating the stability of chronic motor impairments in this subject group (Fasoli et al., 2003, 2004). However, after robotic training we found significant reductions in motor impairment of the hemiparetic upper limbs shown in Table 12.2. Results indicated statistically significant increases in each primary measure: Fugl Meyer test, Motor Status Score for shoulder and elbow, and the MP. Clinically, subjects reported greater comfort when attempting to move their hemiparetic limb, and were better able to actively coordinate shoulder and elbow movements when reaching toward visual targets during robotic therapy. This result has demonstrated that task specific robotic therapy can improve upper limb motor abilities and reduce chronic motor impairments, on average, 6 months after stroke. Others have obtained similar results (Lum et al., 1993, 1999, 2002; Burgar et al., 2000; Reinkensmeyer et al., 2000; Kahn et al., 2001; Shor et al., 2001).

A critical aspect of low-impedance rehabilitation robots that often escapes clinicians is that these devices can be programmed to deliver a vast range of different kinds of therapy. For example, the sensorimotor training mentioned earlier can be described in lay terms as a "hand-over-hand" approach. In prior work Hogan (Flash and Hogan, 1985) has shown that normal reaching movements may be accurately described as "optimally smooth" in the sense of minimizing mean-squared jerk. While executing point-to-point movements, the robot controller uses this minimum-jerk profile as the reference hand path. The parameters of these minimum-jerk reference trajectories were obtained from therapists performing the same task at comfortable speed for training. During sensorimotor training, the robot uses a fixed impedance controller while following this fixed minimum-jerk reference trajectory.

To exemplify the potential of delivering different kinds of therapy, let us compare the results of Table 12.2 with those from an innovative robotic therapy modality developed in our laboratory based on motor-learning models. It applies a performance-based progressive algorithm and modulates the parameters of an impedance controller according to patient's performance (Krebs et al., 2003). This approach appears particularly suitable when considering that different stroke lesions can lead to quite different kinematic behavior during reach. For

Table 12.3. Effect of robot training on impairment and disability measures. For 29 outpatients at Burke Rehabilitation Hospital, mean interval changes in performance were calculated between the initial and final evaluations. For all evaluations higher scores indicate better performance. MP was only evaluated for shoulder and elbow movements.

Between group comparisons: final evaluation minus initial evaluation	Robot-trained (n = 29)	P-value
Impairment measures (±SEM)		
Fugl Meyer shoulder/elbow (FM-se) max/42	5.6 ± 0.9	<0.01
MP max/40	3.3 ± 0.7	<0.01
Motor Status shoulder/elbow (MS-se) max/40	2.7 ± 0.6	<0.01
Disability Evaluation: FIM upper max/42 (±SEM)		
All patients (n = 29)	0.9 ± 0.7	NS
Patients with moderate strokes (n = 16)	3.0 ± 0.6	<0.01

NS: not significant.

example, one patient might make rapid but poorly aimed movements, while another might aim well but move slowly. The novel feature of the performance-based progressive algorithm is that it can guide the hand of the patient that aims poorly without holding him/her back and assist the slow patient in making faster movements. Ferraro reported results of performance-based robotic training at Burke Rehabilitation Hospital with consecutive community dwelling volunteers with stroke, who responded to information they had obtained from media sources about the robotic training experiments (Ferraro et al., 2003). This protocol has the same enrollment criteria and lasted the same amount of time and number of sessions as the one reported by Fasoli et al. (2003, 2004), but the outcome of the performance-based protocol represent a significant improvement over the sensorimotor one (see Table 12.3). In fact, if we exclude the severe strokes from the analysis of both protocols, persons with moderate stroke receiving the performance-based protocol improved twice as much as the ones receiving the sensorimotor protocol for both impairment and disability measures (Krebs et al., 2005 manuscript in preparation).

In conclusion, research in rehabilitation robotics has so vibrantly evolved during the last decade that it is now feasible to mingle robots with humans, supporting or participating in therapy activities. We envision a short-term future with a range of natural extensions of the existing rehabilitation robots including novel modules suitable to provide therapy for the fingers, for the ankle, and for over-ground walking. Since it appears that we can influence impairment and disability, the next step is to determine how to tailor therapy to particular patient needs and maximize the stroke survivor's motor outcome. Results to date are statistically strong and reproducible by different groups in different clinical settings, but the reported results are also arguably functionally modest. For the near-term future, we envision a range of clinical and neuroscience-based training paradigms addressing both functional abilities and impairment, harnessing the patient's potential to its limits with just movement-based therapy. It is not far-fetched to predict that by decade's end, we will have a range of rehabilitation robots at home and in the clinic, operating much like a gym. While movement-based therapy may lack the glamor of cure, for the long-term future we envision the combination of rehabilitation robotics working synergistically with novel pharmacological, neuro-regeneration or tissue-regeneration agents to achieve results equivalent to a "cure".

12.3 Orthoses

Orthoses are passive or powered external devices that support loads, or assist or restrict relative motion between body segments. The word orthosis is derived from Greek for making or setting straight, and is a general term that encompasses bracing and splints. Orthotics plays an important role in the rehabilitation of patients with motor impairments. Orthotics include devices for the neck, upper limb, trunk, and lower limb that are designed to guide motion, bear weight, align body structures, protect joints or correct deformities. Unlike prostheses that replace a body part, orthoses are designed to work in cooperation with the intact body, and either control or assist movement.

Common types of lower limb orthoses include foot orthosis (FO) shoe inserts for correcting ankle and foot deformities, ankle–foot orthoses (AFO) for correcting foot drop, functional knee orthoses (KO) for athletic injuries, hip abduction orthoses for limiting range of motion, long leg knee–ankle–foot orthosis (KAFO), and full length hip–knee–ankle–foot orthoses (HKAFO) for standing and gait stability. Trunk and neck orthoses include thoracolumbosacral orthoses (TLSO) for correcting scoliosis, lubrosacral orthoses (LSO) for stabilizing low back fractures, elastic trunk supports for preventing back injuries during lifting, and the common cervical orthoses (neck braces) for whiplash injuries or muscle spasms. Upper limb devices include shoulder and elbow slings for weight support during fracture healing, balanced forearm orthoses (BFO) for feeding assist, and an array of wrist, hand, and wrist–hand orthoses to position the joints or assist in activities of daily living.

Orthoses apply forces to resist or transfer motions and loads. For example, a knee brace restricts motion to the sagittal plane to protect a knee from off-axis forces following surgery or injury (Edelstein and Bruckner, 2002; Seymor, 2002). A hand orthosis can be constructed to provide elastic resistance to finger extension, thus enhancing a strengthening program following stroke (Fess and Philips, 1987). Plaster casts and wrist immobilization splints are orthoses that restrict all motion. In these cases, orthoses act very much like mechanical bearings whose purpose is to restrict motion in some dimensions and allow frictionless motion in others. A sling orthosis transfers loads from one part of the body to another. For example, a simple, single strap shoulder sling off loads the weight of the arm from the ipsilateral shoulder joint and applies it to the contralateral scapula and clavicle, thus preventing ipsilateral shoulder subluxation in those with rotator cuff injuries or paralysis. Foot orthoses are carefully designed to shift load bearing forces on the bottom of the foot from one area to another, typically to reduce pain or to off load pressure ulcers. Other orthoses transfer motion. A prehension orthosis contains a linkage that couples the wrist to the fingers. Extension of the wrist causes the fingers to close enabling patients with spinal cord injury at C6 to grasp objects (Edelstein and Bruckner, 2002).

The fit of orthosis is critical as they must carry loads without interfering with normal skin and tissue function (Fess and Philips, 1987). Of particular concern is excess pressure, particularly over bony prominences, that can lead to pressure ischemia and eventually skin ulcers. This is a particular problem when fitting patients with neuropathies or spinal cord injury who lack conscious sensation. A basic principle for the design and fitting of an orthosis is to spread the load over as large an area as possible. Avoiding bony prominences means the body attachment point for an orthosis is largely over soft tissue. This brings out an inherent tradeoff that continually challenges orthosis designers. The ideal orthosis should be rigidly anchored to the skeleton, while practical orthoses have considerable motion with respect to the skeleton because of the soft tissue that lies between.

Orthotic interventions are prescribed for patients with orthopedic or neurologic impairments (Nawoczenski, 1997). Orthopedic impairments result from chronic musculoskeletal disorders or acute musculoskeletal injuries, including athletic injuries. Ankle taping for athletes is a simple, custom fit orthosis to limit motion in the subtalar joint (Hemsley, 1997). The most common neurologic impairments where orthotic approaches are considered include traumatic brain injury, stroke, and spinal cord injury (Zablotny, 1997).

Lower limb orthotics prescribed for those with neurologic impairments have the function of restoring or improving gait (Zablotny, 1997). Typical objectives for walking orthotics are to establish stable weight bearing, to control the speed or direction of limb motion, or to reduce the energy required to ambulate. Simple AFOs are used to correct the foot drop that is a common byproduct of stroke, while KAFOs can improve gait for those with progressive quadriceps weakness. The challenge with designing and prescribing more involved orthotics is to generate an energy-efficient gait (Waters and Yakura, 1989). Walking with bi-lateral KAFOs and crutches requires five times the energy per meter as normal gait, while gait velocity is about one-third normal. Wheelchairs are a faster, more efficient means of travel, and with the recent explosion in mobility device design and improved accessibility of buildings, wheelchairs are generally the device of choice for those with severe neurologic impairments.

Several HKAFOs have been developed as paraplegic walking systems (Miller, 1997). There are two major walking systems. The first is the hip guidance orthosis (HGO) that locks the knee joint but has freely moving hip and ankle joints (Major et al., 1981; Butler et al., 1984; Stallard et al., 1989). The second is the reciprocating gait orthosis (RGO) that links opposite joints so that extension of the hip on one side leads to flexion on the contralateral side (Jefferson and Whittle, 1990). Although these systems can restore rudimentary gait for some people with spinal cord injury, the energy cost, and the size, weight and unwieldiness of the hardware has resulted in limited use (Stallard et al., 1989; Whittle et al., 1991).

Functional electrical stimulation (FES) is another means of providing assisted gait to those with spinal cord injury (see Volume II, Chapter 9). In an attempt to overcome the limitations of FES and orthotic walking systems alone, hybrid systems that combine FES and orthotics have been developed. Several studies have shown improved gait speeds and lower energy consumption when FES and the RGO are combined (Solomonow et al., 1989; Hirokawa et al., 1990; Petrofsky and Smith, 1991; Isakov et al., 1992; Solomonow et al., 1997). Others have combined stimulation with the HGO (McClelland et al., 1987; Nene and Jennings, 1989); an enhanced AFO (Andrews et al., 1988), the Hybrid Assistive System (Popovic et al., 1989; Popovic 1990; Popovic et al., 1990), the Case Western Hybrid System (Ferguson et al., 1999; Marsolais et al., 2000), the Strathclyde Hybrid System (Yang et al., 1997; Greene and Granat, 2003), and the Controlled Brake Orthosis shown in Fig. 12.2 (Goldfarb and Durfee 1996; Goldfarb et al., 2003).

The addition of power to an orthosis enables the external device to move a limb actively. Most commonly, powered orthoses are designed for use by individuals with spinal cord injury to restore modest function to a paralyzed extremity. Powered exoskeletons have a long and rich history, starting from the

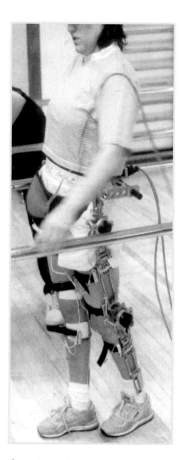

Figure 12.2. Laboratory version of a hybrid orthotic/FES system to enable rudimentary gait for some individuals with complete spinal cord injury at the thoracic level. The controlled brake orthosis combines surface electrical stimulation of the lower limb muscles with an orthotic structure containing computer-controlled brakes that regulate stance and swing phase trajectories (Goldfarb and Durfee, 1996; Goldfarb et al., 2003).

first robotics arm built in the 1960s at Case Western Reserve University, and the early powered walking machines pioneered by Tomovic and colleagues (Tomovic et al., 1973). For example, an electro-myogram (EMG) controlled battery powered hand orthosis can provide grasp for C5 quadriplegics (Benjuya and Kenney, 1990), while more ambitious multi-degree of freedom, upper extremity exoskeletons have been tested in the laboratory (Johnson et al., 2001).

Powered lower limb walking systems have also been designed. Popovic developed a powered knee joint (Popovic et al., 1990), as did Beard (Beard et al., 1991). A hydraulic powered, 5 degree of freedom walking assist device was developed by Seireg and colleagues in the 1970s (Grundman, 1981). More recently, Beleforte et al. have created the pneumatic active gait orthosis (Belforte et al., 2001) and Hiroaki and Yoshiyuki have developed the Hybrid Assistive Leg, a battery and direct current (DC) motor driven powered exoskeleton (Kawamoto, 2002).

Laboratory-based powered exoskeletons have been developed for non-rehabilitation, human power amplification applications. The most famous is the 1965 Hardiman whole-body exoskeleton developed at the General Electric Research and Development Center in Schenectady, NY (Rosheim, 1994). Since then, a variety of human amplification systems have been developed for civilian and military applications, but none have made it out of the laboratory (Kazerooni and Mahoney, 1991; Rosheim, 1994; Kazerooni, 1996; Jansen et al., 2000; Neuhaus and Kazerooni, 2001).

12.4 Prosthetics

Upper-limb amputation prostheses

Despite advances in technology, progress in the development of effective upper-limb amputation prostheses has been modest. This may be partly due to irregular interest in their development, which tends to correlate with major wars. Mann (1981) shows an 1866 Civil War era below-elbow prosthesis with eating utensils and a hook. World War II saw the development by Northrop Aircraft cable-operated "body-powered" arm prosthesis. Mechatronic or "externally powered"[2] prostheses were introduced in the Vietnam War decades. Unfortunately, the resulting devices offer limited benefits. Studies suggested that as few as 50% of upper-limb amputees

---

[2] A "body-powered" prosthesis is powered by the amputee, for example, bi-scapular abduction (shoulder rounding) for elbow flexion; mechatronic prostheses are typically powered by batteries "external" to the amputee.

use any prosthesis at all, versus 75% for lower-limb amputees (LeBlanc, 1973). Unilateral amputees (with one sound arm) overwhelmingly find that a prosthesis offers too little cosmetic or functional benefit to offset its discomfort and inconvenience. LeBlanc (1991) estimated that only 10% of prosthesis users in the USA (5% of the upper-limb amputee population) operate externally powered devices. Thus half of all upper-limb amputees do not use a prosthesis and nine-tenths of those who do use the body-powered type, whose basic design is essentially unchanged in over half a century.

Yet mechatronic prostheses hold substantial promise. It is difficult to transmit significant power from the body to the prosthesis without severely compromising comfort; externally powered devices avoid this problem. It is difficult to control multiple degrees of freedom (e.g., elbow, wrist, thumb, fingers) by recruiting other body motions; mechatronic prostheses may be controlled by bioelectric signals, which can be obtained from a large number of nerves or muscles including, in principle, those originally responsible for controlling the functions of the lost limb. The concept of using bioelectric signals to control a mechatronic device is due to MIT's Norbert Wiener who proposed it in his well-known work *cybernetics* (Wiener, 1948). In founding cybernetics, the "study of automatic control systems formed by the nervous system and brain and by mechanical–electrical communication systems" he had "the idea several years ago to take an amputated muscle, pick up the action potentials, amplify this and make motion of it". Mann implemented this idea in an above-elbow amputation prosthesis controlled by EMG[3] from muscles in the residual limb (Rothchild and Mann, 1966; Mann, 1968), which led to commercial products including the Boston Arm (Jerard et al., 1974; Liberty Mutual, Inc.; Liberating Technologies, Inc.) and the Utah Arm (Jacobsen et al., 1982; Sarcos, Inc.; Motion Control, Inc.). EMG control has been applied to other upper-extremity motions including wrist rotation and grasp and methods for simultaneous control of many

[3] "EMG" refers to the ElectroMyoGram, more correctly "myoelectric activity".

degrees of freedom have been proposed (Jerard and Jacobsen, 1980).

Given the potential advantages of EMG control, the continued overwhelming preference for the body-powered system is remarkable. Although generally lighter and less expensive, a body-powered prosthesis is also considerably less comfortable, mostly due to the harness needed to transmit body motion the prosthesis; its lifting ability is extremely limited; it is less cosmetic than mechatronic models as it requires unnatural body motions for its operation; and independent operation of multiple degrees of freedom is difficult to impossible (LeBlanc, 1991). A clue to this puzzle may be found by studying how an arm amputation prosthesis is used.

Motion control and sensory feedback

One abiding concern is that EMG control may restore "forward path" communication between the central nervous system and the peripheral (bio-)mechanical system but does not restore "feedback" sensory communication from periphery to center. However, whether continuous feedback is essential for unimpaired movement control remains unclear with recent evidence suggesting that neural commands are substantially "pre-computed" from learned internal models (Shadmehr and Mussa-Ivaldi, 1994). Furthermore, substantial feedback information is available through mechanical interaction with the socket and harness that secure the prosthesis to the amputee. Doeringer and Hogan (1995) compared motor performance of unilateral amputees using a body-powered prosthesis with their performance using their unimpaired arm on a series of elbow motion tasks. Motion control with the prosthesis was remarkably good. For the more active and experienced prosthesis users, eyes-closed positioning ability was indistinguishable from unimpaired arm performance.

Interaction control

Most functional tasks for an upper-limb prosthesis are *contact tasks* involving kinematically constrained motions (e.g., opening a drawer, wiping a surface, etc.) or mechanical interaction (e.g., wielding a tool, cooperating with the other arm, etc.). For unilateral amputees (who constitute about 95% of the arm amputee population) a prosthesis will mostly serve as the non-dominant arm, for example, holding or steadying objects while they are manipulated by the unimpaired limb. Controlling interaction is thus a fundamental requirement for arm prosthesis function. However, most mechatronic prostheses have been designed using motion control technology (Klopsteg and Wilson, 1968; Mason, 1972; Jerard et al., 1974; Jacobsen et al., 1982). Unfortunately, robotic experience has shown that motion controllers are poorly suited to controlling interaction.

A comparison with natural motor behavior is informative. Natural arms are compliant, yielding on contact with objects, which makes them less sensitive to the disturbances caused by contact (see Hogan, 2002 for a review). In contrast, a typical mechatronic prosthesis responds little, if at all, to external forces. Furthermore, the natural arm's compliance is under voluntary control (Billian and Zahalak 1983; Humphrey and Reed 1983). Tensing muscles makes the arm less compliant and serves to stabilize it against disturbances. Relaxing the muscles makes the arm more compliant and allows it to accommodate external constraints.

The advantages of the natural arm's behavior may be conferred on a machine using impedance control (Hogan, 1979, 1985), which has proven effective for robot control, especially for contact tasks (see Hogan and Buerger, 2004 for a brief review). Impedance control has been applied to an EMG-controlled mechatronic arm prosthesis, partially mimicking the natural arm's behavior (Abul-Haj and Hogan, 1990): the response to external forces varies with co-activation of agonist and antagonist muscles while differential activation generates motion.

Amputee performance of contact tasks

A study of amputees performing simple contact tasks showed the importance of interaction control. A computer-controlled arm amputation prosthesis (see Abul-Haj and Hogan, 1987; Fig. 12.3) was programmed

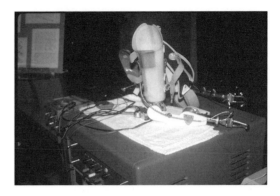

Figure 12.3. Prosthesis emulator.

to emulate (1) a body-powered prostheses in free-swing mode; (2) the Boston elbow; and (3) the New York elbow (two mechatronic prostheses which control elbow velocity from the difference between EMG of remnant arm muscles); and (4) an impedance-controlled prosthesis. The main difference between these cases is that the velocity-controlled prostheses, (2) and (3), are unresponsive to external forces whereas the other two, (1) and (4), move easily under external forces. Unilateral amputee subjects used each prosthesis to turn a crank mounted in a vertical plane at three speeds (low, medium and fast, approximately 2, 4 and 6 rad/s). In almost all cases, motions of prosthesis and crank were similar, the crank handle moving with a smooth, unimodal speed profile, indicating that all prostheses provided comparable motion control. In contrast, the forces exerted on the crank were significantly different in each case. Computation of the power produced by the prosthesis motor showed that for the impedance control system, prosthesis output power was always positive. For the body-powered prosthesis in free-swing mode power was zero. For the Boston elbow and the New York elbow control systems, output power was *negative* for a significant portion of the task. Positive output power from the impedance control system means that it always assisted motion; amputees consistently rated this prosthesis easiest to control. Negative output power means that the Boston elbow and New York elbow prosthesis were behaving as *brakes* and *impeding* performance of the task, not assisting it (Mansfield et al., 1992; Krebs et al., 1999b).

Control and communication are the barriers

The way a mechatronic prosthesis responds to forces (its mechanical impedance) is clearly an important factor determining its usefulness. Unfortunately, most available mechatronic prostheses are unresponsive (they typically have high impedance) and this may be the main reason why, after decades of development, most amputees prefer not to use them, despite their apparent functional advantages such as independent control of different motions (e.g., elbow and terminal device).

Providing an amputee with the ability to adjust impedance (as in the natural limb) yielded superior performance and seems a promising way to improve upper-limb prostheses. However, it requires additional control signals to assess the user's intent (e.g., both reciprocal *and* co-contraction of antagonist muscles). For limited motions EMG may be suitable; activity of two muscles such as the remnant biceps and triceps may be used to command the elbow. However, the ideal mechatronic arm, assuming that one could be built, is not limited to elbow movement, but must also assess the user's intent to drive the wrist and fingers. Recent work on brain-machine interfaces (Nicolelis et al., 1995) shows that in principle the required information may be obtainable directly from the brain (see Chapter 33 of Volume I), though advances in technology for implantable neuro-electric recording in the periphery may be more practical (e.g., Bions, Chapter 32 of Volume I). New ways to communicate and more natural control strategies could reinvigorate research and open a plethora of possibilities to turn Hollywood's mechatronic fancies into reality.

Lower-limb amputation prostheses

Dissipative knees and energy-storing prosthetic feet

Today's prosthetic knees typically comprise a hydraulic and/or pneumatic damper that dissipates mechanical energy under joint rotation (Popovic and Sinkjaer, 2000). In these devices, fluid is pushed through an orifice when the knee is flexed or extended, resulting in a knee torque that increases with increasing knee angular rate. To control knee damping, the size of the fluid orifice is adjusted. Although for most commercial knees the orifice size is controlled passively when weight is applied to the prosthesis, some contemporary knee systems use a motor to actively modulate orifice size. For example, in the Otto Bock C-Leg, hydraulic valves are under microprocessor control using knee position and axial force sensory information (James et al., 1990). Actively controlled knee dampers such as the C-Leg offer considerable advantages over passive knee systems, enabling amputees to walk with greater ease and confidence (Dietl and Bargehr, 1997; Kastner et al., 1998).

Today's prosthetic ankle–foot systems typically employ elastomeric bumper springs or carbon composite leaf springs to store and release energy throughout each walking or running step (Popovic and Sinkjaer, 2000). For example, in the Flex-Foot Vertical Shock Pylon System, carbon composite leaf springs offer considerable heel, toe, and vertical compliance to the below-knee prosthesis, enabling leg amputees to move with greater comfort and speed. Although considerable progress has been made in materials and methods, commercially available ankle–foot devices are passive, and consequently, their stiffnesses are fixed and do not change with walking speed or terrain.

Patient-adaptive prosthetic knee system

Using state-of-the-art prosthetic knee technology such as the C-Leg, a prosthetist must pre-program knee damping levels until a knee is comfortable, moves naturally, and is safe (James et al., 1990; Dietl and Bargehr, 1997; Kastner et al., 1998). However, these adjustments are not guided by biological gait data, and therefore, knee damping may not be set to ideal values, resulting in the possibility of undesirable gait movements. Still further, knee-damping levels in such a system may not adapt properly in response to environmental disturbances. Recently, an external knee prosthesis was developed that automatically adapts knee damping values to match the amputee's gait requirements, accounting for variations in both forward speed and body size (Herr et al., 2001; Herr and Wilkenfeld, 2003). With this technology, knee damping is modulated about a single rotary axis using magnetorheologic (MR) fluid in the shear mode, and only local mechanical sensing of axial force, sagittal plane torque, and knee position are employed as control inputs (see Fig. 12.4). With every step, the controller, using axial force information, automatically adjusts early stance damping. When an amputee lifts a suitcase or carries a backpack, damping levels are increased to compensate for the added load on the prosthesis. With measurements of foot contact time, the controller also estimates forward speed and modulates swing phase flexion and extension damping profiles to achieve biologically realistic lower-limb dynamics. For example, the maximum flexion angle during early swing typically does not exceed 70 degrees in normal walking (Inman et al., 1981). Hence, to achieve a gait cycle that appears

natural or biological, the knee controller automatically adjusts the knee damping levels until the swinging leg falls below the biologic threshold of 70 degrees for each foot contact time or forward walking speed.

To assess the clinical effects of the patient-adaptive knee prosthesis, kinematic gait data were collected on unilateral trans-femoral amputees. Using both the patient-adaptive knee and a conventional, non-adaptive knee, gait kinematics were evaluated on both affected and unaffected sides. Results were compared to the kinematics of age, weight and height-matched normals. The study showed that the patient-adaptive knee successfully controlled early stance damping, enabling amputee to undergo biologically realistic, early stance knee flexion. Additionally, the knee constrained the maximum swing flexion angle to an acceptable biologic limit. In Fig. 12.4, the maximum flexion angle during the swing phase is plotted versus walking speed for a unilateral

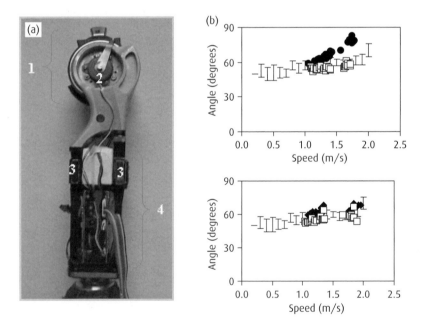

Figure 12.4. An external knee prosthesis for trans-femoral amputees. The damping of the knee joint is modulated to control the movement of the prosthesis throughout each walking cycle. (a) The prosthesis shown on the left comprises MR brake (1), potentiometerangle sensor (2), force sensors (3), and battery and electronic board (4). (b) The right plots show the maximum flexion angle during the swing phase versus walking speed. The patient-adaptive knee affords a greater symmetry between affected and unaffected sides.

trans-femoral amputee using the non-adaptive, mechanical knee (top plot, filled diamonds) and the patient-adaptive knee (bottom plot, filled diamonds). In both plots, the subject's sound side leg is shown (open squares), along with reference data from unimpaired walkers (standard error bars). For the amputee participant, the non-adaptive, mechanical knee produced a maximum flexion angle that increased with increasing speed, far exceeding 70 degrees at the fastest forward walking speed, whereas the patient-adaptive knee gave a maximum flexion angle that was less than 70 degrees and agreed well with the unimpaired, biologic data. These results indicate that a patient-adaptive control scheme and local mechanical sensing are all that is required for amputees to walk with an increased level of biologic realism compared to mechanically passive prosthetic systems.

New horizons for lower-limb prosthetic technology: merging body and machine

Society is at the threshold of a new age when prostheses will no longer be separate, lifeless mechanisms, but will instead be intimate extensions of the human body, structurally, neurologically, and dynamically. Such a merging of body and machine will not only increase the acceptance of the physically challenged into society, but will also enable individuals suffering from leg amputation to more readily accept their new artificial appendage as part of their own body. Several scientific and technological advances will accelerate this mergence. An area of research of considerable importance is the development of improved power supplies and more efficient prosthetic actuator designs where both joint impedance and mechanical power generation can be effectively controlled in the context of a low-mass, high cycle-life, commercially viable prosthesis. Another critical area of research will be to combine local mechanical sensing about an external prosthetic joint with peripheral and/or central neural sensors positioned within the body. Neural prostheses such as the Bion (Loeb, 2001, see Chapter 32 of Volume I), combined with external biomimetic prosthetic systems, may offer important functional advantages to amputees. The fact that only EMG

or local mechanical sensors were employed in prosthetics imposes dramatic limitations in the system's ability to assess user intent. In the advancement of prosthetic systems, we feel that distributed sensory architectures are research areas of critical importance.

REFERENCES

Abul-Haj, C. and Hogan, N. (1987). An emulator system for developing improved elbow-prosthesis designs. *IEEE Trans Biomed Eng*, **34**(**9**), 724–737.

Abul-Haj, C.J. and Hogan, N. (1990). Functional assessment of control systems for cybernetic elbow prostheses. *IEEE Trans Biomed Eng*, **37**(**11**), 1025–1047.

Aisen, M.L., Krebs, H.I., Hogan, N., McDowell, F. and Volpe, B.T. (1997). The effect of robot assisted therapy and rehabilitative training on motor recovery following stroke. *Arch Neurol*, **54**, 443–446.

Andrews, B., Baxendale, R., Barnett, R., Phillips, G., Yamazaki, T., Paul, J. and Freeman, P. (1988). Hybrid FES orthosis incorporating closed loop control and sensory feedback. *J Biomed Eng*, **10**, 189–195.

Beard, J., Conwell, J., Rogers, D. and Lamousin, H. (1995). *Proceedings of the 1995 Applied Mechanics and Robotics Conference.* Design of a Powered Orthotic Device to Aid Individuals with a Loss of Bipedal Locomotion. **2**, Cincinnati, OH.

Belforte, G., Gastaldi, L. and Sorli, M. (2001). Pneumatic active gait orthosis. *Mechatronics*, **11**, 301–323.

Benjuya, N. and Kenney, S. (1990). Myoelectric hand orthosis. *J Prosthet Ortho*, **2**, 149–154.

Billian, C. and Zahalak, G.I. (1983). A programmable limb testing system and some measurements of intrinsic muscular and reflex-mediated stiffnesses. *J Biomech Eng*, **105**.

Burgar, C.G., Lum, P.S., Shor, P.C. and Machiel Van der Loos, H.F. (2000). Development of robots for rehabilitation therapy: the palo alto VA/Stanford experience. *J Rehabil Res Dev*, **37**, 663–673.

Butler, P., Major, R. and Patrick, J. (1984). The technique of reciprocal walking using the hip guidance orthosis (HGO) with crutches. *Prosthet Orthot Int*, **8**, 33–38.

Colombo, G., Joerg, M., Schreier, R., Dietz, V. (2000). Treadmill training of paraplegic patients using a robotic orthosis. *VA J Rehabil Res Dev*, **37**(**6**), 693–700.

Dietl, H. and Bargehr, H. (1997). Der einsatz von elektronik bei prothesen zur versorgung der unteren extremitat. *Med Orth Tech*, **117**, 31–35.

Dodds, T.A., Martin, D.P., Stolov, W.C. and Deyo, R.A. (1993). A validation of the functional independence measurement and its performance among rehabilitation inpatients. *Arch Phys Med Rehabil*, **74**, 531–536.

Doeringer, J.A. and Hogan, N. (1995). Performance of above-elbow body-powered prostheses in visually-guided tasks. *IEEE Trans Biomed Eng*, **42**(6), 1–11.

Edelstein, J. and Bruckner, J. (2002). *Orthotics: A Comprehensive Clinical Approach* SLACK Incorporated, Thorofare, NJ.

Erlandson, R.F. (1995). Applications of robotic/mechatronic systems in special education, rehabilitation therapy, and vocational training: a paradigm shift. *IEEE Trans Rehabil Eng*, **3**, 22–34.

Erlandson, R.F., de Bear, P., Kristy, K., Dilkers, M. and Wu, S. (1990). A robotic system to provide movement therapy. *Proceedings of the 5th International Robot Conference*, Detroit, MI, pp. 7–15.

Fasoli, S.D., Krebs, H.I., Stein, J., Frontera, W.R. and Hogan, N. (2003). Effects of robotic therapy on motor impairment and recovery in chronic stroke. *Arch Phys Med Rehabil*, **84**, 477–482.

Fasoli, S.E., Krebs, H.I., Stein, J., Frontera, W.R., Hughes, R. and Hogan, N. (2004). Robotic therapy for chronic motor impairments after stroke: follow-up results. *Arch Phys Med Rehabil*, **85**, 1106–1111.

Ferguson, K.A., Polando, G., Kobetic, R., Triolo, R.J. and Marsolais, E.B. (1999). Walking with a hybrid orthosis system. *Spinal Cord*, **37**, 800–804.

Ferraro, M., Palazzolo, J.J., Krol, J., Krebs, H.I., Hogan, N. and Volpe, B.T. (2003). Robot-aided sensorimotor arm training improves outcome in patients with chronic stroke. *Neurology*, **61**, 1604–1607.

Fess, E. and Philips, C. (1987). *Hand Splinting: Principles and Methods*, C.V. Mosby, St. Louis, MO.

Flash, T. and Hogan, N. (1985). The coordination of arm movements: an experimentally confirmed mathematical model. *J Neurosci*, **5**, 1688–1703.

Furusho, J., Koyanagi, K., Ryu, U., Inoue, A. and Oda, K. (2003). Development of rehabilitation robot system with functional fluid devices for upper limbs. *ICORR*, 31–34.

Goldfarb, M. and Durfee, W.K. (1996). Design of a controlled-brake orthosis for FES-aided gait. *IEEE Trans Rehabil Eng*, **4**, 13–24.

Goldfarb, M., Korkowski, K., Harrold, B. and Durfee, W. (2003). Preliminary evaluation of a controlled-brake orthosis for FES-aided gait. *IEEE Trans Neural Syst Rehabil Eng*, **11**, 241–248.

Granger, C.V., Hamilton, B.B., Linacre, J.M., Heinemann, A.W. and Wright, B.D. (1993). Performance profiles of the functional independence measure. *Am J Phys Med Rehabil*, **72**, 84–89.

Greene, P.J. and Granat, M.H. (2003). A knee and ankle flexing hybrid orthosis for paraplegic ambulation. *Med Eng Phys*, **25**, 539–545.

Grundman, A.S.a.J. (1981). Design of a multitask exoskeletal walking device for paraplegics. In: *Biomechanics of Medical Devices* (ed. Ghista, D.), Marcel-Dekker, New York, pp. 569–639.

Harwin, W.S., Loureiro, R.C.V., Amirabdollahian, F., Taylor, L.M., Johnson, G., Stokes, E., Coote, S., Topping, M., Collin, C., Tamparis, S., Kontoulis, J., Munih, M., Hawkins, P. and Driessen, B. (2001). The GENTLE/S project: a new method of delivering neuro-rehabilitation. In: *Assistive Technology – Added Value to the Quality of Life*, Vol. 10, IOS Press, Amsterdam, The Netherlands, pp. 36–41.

Hemsley, K. (1997). Protective padding and adhesive strapping. In: *Orthotics in Functional Rehabilitation of the Lower Limb* (eds Nawoczenski, D. and Epler, M.), Saunders, Philadelphia, pp. 157–203.

Herr, H. and Wilkenfeld, A. (2003). User-adaptive control of a magnetorheological prosthetic knee. *Ind Robot*, **30**, 42–55.

Herr, H., Wilkenfeld, A. and Olaf, B. (2003). Speed-adaptive and patient-adaptive prosthetic knee. *US Patent*, 6, 610, 101.

Hesse, S. and Uhlenbrock, D. (2000). A mechanized gait trainer for restoration of gait. *VA J Rehabil Res Dev*, **37**(6), 701–708.

Hirokawa, S., Grimm, M., Le, T., Solomonow, M., Baratta, R., Shoji, H. and D'Ambrosia, R. (1990). Energy consumption in paraplegic ambulation using the reciprocating gait orthosis and electric stimulation of the thigh muscles. *Arch Phys Med Rehabil*, **71**, 687–694.

Hogan, N. (1979). Adaptive stiffness control in human movement. In: *Advances in Bioengineering* (ed. Wells, M.K.), ASME, Amsterdam, The Netherlands, pp. 53–54.

Hogan, N. (1985). Impedance control: an approach to manipulation. *ASME J Dyn Syst Meas Cont*, **107**, 1–24.

Hogan, N. (2002). Skeletal muscle impedance in the control of motor actions. *J Mech Med Biol*, **2**(3 & 4), 359–373.

Hogan, N. and Buerger, S.P. (2004). Impedance and interaction control. In: *Robotics and Automation Handbook* (ed. Kurfess, T.), CRC Press.

Hogan, N., Krebs, H.I., Sharon, A. and Charnnarong, J. (1995). Interactive robot therapist. *MIT Patent #5, 466, 213*, USA.

Humphrey, D.R. and Reed, D.J. (1983). Separate cortical systems for the control of joint movement and joint stiffness: reciprocal activation and coactivation of antagonist muscles. *Adv Neurol*, **39**, 347–372.

Inman, V.T., Ralston, H.J. and Todd, F. (1981). *Human Walking*, Williams and Wilkins, Baltimore.

Isakov, E., Douglas, R. and Berns, P. (1992). Ambulation using the reciprocating gait orthosis and functional electrical stimulation. *Paraplegia*, **30**, 239–245.

Jacobsen, S.C., Knutti, D.G., Johnson, R.T. and Sears, H.H. (1982). Development of the Utah artificial arm. *IEEE Trans Biomed Eng*, **29**(4), 249–269.

James, K., Stein, R.B., Rolf, R. and Tepavac D. (1990). Active suspension above-knee prosthesis. *Goh JC 6th International Conference of Biomechanical Engineering*, 317–320.

Jansen, J.B.R., Pin, F., Lind, R. and Birdwell, J. (2000). *Exoskeleton for Soldier Enhancement Systems: Feasibility Study*, Oak Ridge National Laboratory, Oak Ridge.

Jefferson, R. and Whittle, M. (1990). Performance of three walking orthoses for the paralysed: a case study using gait analysis. *Prosthet Orthot Int*, **14**, 103–110.

Jerard, R.B. and Jacobsen, S.C, (1980). Laboratory evaluation of a unified theory for simultaneous multiple axis artificial arm control. *J Biomech Eng*, **102**(3), 199–207.

Jerard, R.B., Williams, T.W. and Ohlenbusch, C.W. (1974). Practical design of an EMG controlled above-elbow prosthesis. *Proceedings of Conference on Engineering Devices for Rehabilitation*, Boston, MA.

Johnson, G.R., Carus, D.A., Parrini, G., Scattareggia Marchese, S. and Valeggi, R. (2001). The design of a five-degree-of-freedom powered orthosis for the upper limb. *Proc Inst Mech Eng [H]*, **215**, 275–284.

Kahn, L., Averbuch, M., Rymer, W.Z. and Reinkensmeyer, D.J. (2001). Comparison of robot assisted reaching to free reaching in promoting recovery from chronic stroke. In: *Integration of Assistive Technology in the Information Age* (ed. Mokhtari, M.), IOS, Amsterdam, The Netherlands, pp. 39–44.

Kastner, J., Nimmervoll, R., Kristen, H., Wagner, P. (1998). A comparative gait analysis of the C-Leg, the 3R45 and the 3R80 prosthetic knee joints. http://www.healthcare.ottobock.com

Kawamoto, H.Y.S. (2002). Power assist system HAL-3 for gait disorder person. In: *Lecture Notes in Computer Science* (eds Miesenberger, J.K., Zagler, W.), Vol. 2398, Springer-Verlag, Berlin, Heidelberg, pp. 196–203.

Kazerooni, H. (1996). Human power amplifier technology at the University of California, Berkeley. *Robot Auton Syst*, **19**, 179–187.

Kazerooni, H. and Mahoney, S. L. (1991). Dynamics and control of robotic systems worn by humans. *J Dyn Syst Trans ASME*, **113**, 379–387.

Klopsteg, P.E. and Wilson, P.D. (1968). *Human Limbs and Their Substitutes*, Hafner Publishing Co., New York.

Krebs, H.I., Hogan, N., Aisen, M.L. and Volpe, B.T. (1998). Robot-aided neurorehabilitation. *IEEE Trans Rehabil Eng*, **6**, 75–87.

Krebs, H.I., Aisen, M.L., Volpe, B.T. and Hogan, N. (1999a). Quantization of continuous arm movements in humans with brain injury. *Proc Natl Acad Sci*, **96**, 4645–4649.

Krebs, H.I., Volpe, B.T., Aisen, M.L. and Hogan, N. (1999b). Robotic applications in neuromotor rehabilitation. *Topic Spinal Cord Injury Rehabil*, **5**(3), 50–63.

Krebs, H.I., Volpe, B.T., Aisen, M.L. and Hogan, N. (2000). Increasing productivity and quality of care: robot-aided neurorehabilitation, *VA J Rehabil Res Dev*, **37**(6), 639–652.

Krebs, H.I., Palazzolo, J.J., Dipietro, L., Ferraro, M., Krol, J., Rannekleiv, K., Volpe, B.T. and Hogan, N. (2003). Rehabilitation robotics: performance-based progressive robot-assisted therapy. *Auton Robot*, **15**, 7–20.

Krebs, H.I., Volpe, B.T., Stein, J., Bever, C., Palazzolo, J.J., Fasoli, S.E., Hughes, R., Lynch, D., Meister, C., MacClellan, L., Ohlhoff, J., Frontera, W.R. and Hogan, N. (2005). Variations on a Rehabilitation Robotics Theme: Different Training and Intensities Achieve Different Results (in preparation).

LeBlanc, M. (1973). Patient population and other estimates of prosthetics and orthotics in the USA. *Orthotics Prosthet*, **27**, 38–44.

LeBlanc, M.A. (1991). Current evaluation of hydraulics to replace the cable force transmission system for body-powered upper-limb prostheses. *Assist Technol*, **2**, 101–107.

Loeb, J. (2001). Neural prosthetics. In: *The Handbook of Brain Theory and Neural Networks*, 2nd edn., (ed. Arbib, M.A.), MIT Press, Cambridge, M.A.

Lum, P.S., Reinkensmeyer, D.J. and Lehman, S. (1993). Robotic assist devices for bimanual physical therapy: preliminary experiments. *IEEE Trans Rehabil Eng*, **1**, 185–191.

Lum, P.S., Lehman, S.L. and Reinkensmeyer, D.J. (1995). The bimanual lifting rehabilitator: an adaptive machine for therapy of stroke patients. *IEEE Trans Rehabil Eng*, **3**, 166–174.

Lum, P.S., Burgar, C.G., Kenney, D.E. and Van der Loos, H.F. (1999). Quantification of force abnormalities during passive and active-assisted upper-limb reaching movements in post-stroke hemiparesis. *IEEE Trans Biomed Eng*, **46**, 652–662.

Lum, P.S., Burgar, C.G., Shor, P.C., Majmundar, M. and Van der Loos, M. (2002). Robot-assisted movement training compared with conventional therapy techniques for the rehabilitation of upper-limb motor function after stroke. *Arch Phys Med Rehabil*, **83**, 952–959.

Major, R., Stallard, J. and Rose, G. (1981). The dynamics of walking using the hip guidance orthosis (HGO) with crutches. *Prosthet Orthot Int*, **5**, 19–22.

Mann, R.W. (1968). Efferent and afferent control of an electromyographic, proportional-rate, force sensing artificial elbow with cutaneous display of joint angle. *Symposium on* the *Basic Problems of Prehension, Movement and Control of Artificial Limbs, Institute of Mechanical Engineers*, **183**, paper no. 15.

Mann, R.W. (1981). Cybernetic limb prosthesis: the alza distinguished lecture. *Annals Biomed Eng*, **9**, 1–43.

Mansfield, J.M., Hogan, N., Russell, D.L., Clancy, E.A., Popat, R.A. and Krebs, D.E. (1992). Cybernetic prosthesis control systems may degrade amputee performance. *Proceedings of the 7th World Congress of the International Society for Prosthetics and Orthotics*, Chicago, IL.

Marsolais, E.B., Kobetic, R., Polando, G., Ferguson, K., Tashman, S., Gaudio, R., Nandurkar, S. and Lehneis, H.R. (2000). The Case Western Reserve University hybrid gait orthosis. *J Spinal Cord Med*, **23**, 100–108.

Mason, C.P. (1972). Design of a powered arm system for the above-elbow amputee. *Bull Prosthet Res*, **10**, 18–24.

Maxwell, S. (1990). PhD Thesis, Massachusetts Institute of Technology.

McClelland, M., Andrews, B., Patrick, J., Freeman, P. and el Masri, W. (1987). Augmentation of the Oswestry Parawalker orthosis by means of surface electrical stimulation: gait analysis of three patients. *Paraplegia*, **25**, 32–38.

Merians, A.S., Jack, D., Boian, R., Tremaine, M., Burdea, G.C., Adamovich, S., Recce, M., Poizner, H. (2002). Virtual reality-augmented rehabilitation for patients following stroke. *Phys Ther*, **82**(9), 898–915.

Miller, P. (1997). Orthoses for the pelvic and hip region. In: *Orthotics in Functional Rehabilitation of the Lower Limb* (eds Nawoczenski, D. and Epler, M.), Saunders, Philadelphia, pp. 15–30.

Nawoczenski, D. (1997). Introduction to orthotics: rationale for treatment. In: *Orthotics in Functional Rehabilitation of the Lower Limb* (eds Nawoczenski, D. and Epler, M.), Saunders, Philadelphia, pp. 1–14.

Nene, A. and Jennings, S. (1989). Hybrid paraplegic locomotion with the Parawalker using intramuscular stimulation: a single subject study. *Paraplegia*, **27**, 125–132.

Neuhaus, P. and Kazerooni, H. (2001). Industrial-strength human-assisted walking robots. *IEEE Robot Autom Mag*, **8**, 18–25.

Nicolelis, M.A.L., Baccala, L.A., Lin, R.C.S. and Chapin, J.K. (1995). Sensorimotor encoding by synchronous neural ensemble activity at multiple levels of the somatosensory system. *Science*, **268**, 1353–1358.

Petrofsky, J. and Smith, J. (1991). Physiologic costs of computer-controlled walking in persons with paraplegia using a reciprocating-gait orthosis. *Arch Phys Med Rehabil*, **72**, 890–896.

Popovic, D. (1990). Dynamics of the self-fitting modular orthosis. *IEEE Trans Robot Automat*, **6**, 200–207.

Popovic, D. and Sinkjaer, T. (2000). *Control of Movement for the Physically Disabled*, Springer-Verlag, London.

Popovic, D., Tomovic, R. and Schwirtlich, L. (1989). Hybrid assistive system – the motor neuroprosthesis. *IEEE Trans Biomed Eng*, **36**, 729–737.

Popovic, D., Schwirtlich, L. and Radosavljevic, S. (1990). Powered hybrid assistive system. In: *Adv External Contr. Human Extremities* (ed. Popovic, D.), NAUKA. Belgrade, Yugoslavia, pp. 177–186.

Rahman, T., Sample, W., Seliktar, R., Alexander, M. and Scavina, M. (2000). A body-powered functional upper limb orthosis. *VA J Rehabil Res Dev*, **37**(6), 675–680.

Reinkensmeyer, D.J., Cole, A., Kahn, L.E. and Kamper, D.J. (2002). Directional control of reaching is preserved following mild/moderate stroke and stochastically constrained following severe stroke. *Exp Brain Res*, **143**, 525–530.

Reinkensmeyer, D.J., Hogan, N., Krebs, H.I., Lehman, S.L. and Lum, P.S. (2000a). Rehabilitators, robots, and guides: new tools for neurological rehabilitation. In: *Biomechanics and Neural Control of Movement* (eds Winters, J.M. and Crago, P.E.), Springer-Verlag, New York.

Reinkensmeyer, D.J., Kahn, L.E., Averbuch, M., McKenna-Cole, A., Schmit, B.D. and Rymer, W.Z. (2000b). Understanding and treating arm movement impairment after chronic brain injury: progress with the ARM guide. *J Rehabil Res Dev*, **37**, 653–662.

Rohrer, B., Fasoli, S., Krebs, H.I., Hughes, R., Volpe, B.T., Frontera, W., Stein, J. and Hogan, N. (2002). Movement smoothness changes during stroke recovery. *J Neurosci*, **22**(18), 8297–8304.

Rosheim, M. (1994). *Robot Evolution: The Development of Anthrobotics*, Wiley & Sons, New York.

Rothchild, R.A. and Mann, R.W. (1966). An EMG controlled, force sensing, proportional rate elbow prostheses. *Proc Symp on Biomed Eng*, **1**, 106–109.

Sakaki, T., Okada, S., Okajima, Y., Tanaka, N., Kimura, A., Uchida, S., Taki, M., Tomita, Y. and Horiuchi, T. (1999). TEM: therapeutic exercise machine for hip and knee joints of spastic patients, *ICORR*, Palo Alto, CA, pp. 183–186.

Seymor, R. (2002). *Prosthetics and Orthotics: Lower Limb and Spinal*, Lippincott Williams & Wilkins, Baltimore, MD.

Shadmehr, R. and Mussa-Ivaldi, F.A. (1994). Adaptive representation of dynamics during learning of a motor task. *J Neurosci*, **14**, 3208–3224.

Shor, P.C., Lum, P.S., Burgar, C.G., Van der Loos, H.F.M., Majmundar, M. and Yap, R. (2001). The effect of robot aided therapy on upper extremity joint passive range of motion and pain. In: *Integration of assistive technology in the information age* (ed. Mokhtari, M.), IOS Press, Amsterdam, The Netherlands, pp. 79–83.

Solomonow, M., Baratta, R., Hirokawa, S., Rightor, N., Walker, W., Beaudelte, P., Shoji, H. and D'Ambrosia, R. (1989). The

RGO generation II: muscle stimulation powered orthosis as a practical walking system for thoracic paraplegics. *Orthopedics*, **12**, 1309–1315.

Solomonow, M., Aguilar, E., Reisin, E., Baratta, R., Best, R., Coetzee, T. and D'Ambrosia, R. (1997). Reciprocating gait orthosis powered with electrical muscle stimulation (RGO II). Part I. Performance evaluation of 70 paraplegic patients. *Orthopedics*, **20**, 315–324.

Stallard, J., Major, R. and Patrick, J. (1989). A review of the fundamental design problems of providing ambulation for paraplegic patients. *Paraplegia*, **27**, 70–75.

Tomovic, R., Vukobrativic, M. and Vodovnik, L. (1973). Hybrid actuators for orthotic systems: hybrid assistive systems. In: *Adv. External Contr. Human Extremities IV*, Yugoslav Committee for Electronics and Automation, Belgrade, Yugoslavia, pp. 73–80.

Volpe, B.T., Krebs, H.I., Hogan, N., Edelstein, L., Diels, C., Aisen, M.L. (1999). Robot training enhanced motor outcome in patients with stroke maintained over three years. *Neurology*, **53**, 1874–1876.

Volpe, B.T., Krebs, H.I., Hogan, N., Edelstein, L., Diels, C., Aisen, M.L. (2000). A novel approach to stroke rehabilitation: robot-aided sensorimotor stimulation. *Neurology*, **54**, 1938–1944.

Volpe, B.T., Krebs, H.I. and Hogan, N. (2001). Is robot aided sensorimotor training in stroke rehabilitation a realistic option? *Curr Opin Neurol*, **14**(**6**), 745–752.

Waters, R. and Yakura, J. (1989). The energy expenditure of normal and pathologic gait. *Crit Rev hys Rehabil Med*, **1**, 183–209.

Whittle, M., Cochrane, G., Chase, A., Copping, A., Jefferson, R., Staples, D., Fenn, P. and Thomas, D. (1991). A comparative trial of two walking systems for paralysed people. *Paraplegia*, **29**, 97–102.

Wiener, N. (1948). *Cybernetics*, MIT Press, Cambridge, Massachusetts.

Yang, L., Granat, M.H., Paul, J.P., Condie, D.N. and Rowley, D.I. (1997). Further development of hybrid functional electrical stimulation orthoses. *Artif Organs*, **21**, 183–187.

Zablotny, C. (1997). Use of orthoses for the adult with neurologic involvement. In: *Orthotics in Functional Rehabilitation of the Lower Limb* (eds Nawoczenski, D. and Epler, M.), Saunders, Philadelphia, pp. 205–244.

13

Virtual reality in neurorehabilitation

Patrice L. Weiss[1], Rachel Kizony[1,2], Uri Feintuch[2,3] and Noomi Katz[2]

[1]Department of Occupational Therapy, University of Haifa, Haifa; [2]School of Occupational Therapy,
Hadassah-Hebrew University, Jerusalem and [3]Caesarea-Rothschild Institute for Interdisciplinary
Applications of Computer Science, University of Haifa, Haifa, Israel

Imagine the following scenario. Stuck in traffic, you have your digital agent make contact with the secretary at the Rehabilitation Center via your wireless palmtop. You are immediately provided with a verbal listing of your daily schedule. It is clear that you will have a tight timetable, and already anticipate a hectic day filled with clinical rounds, research meetings and an afternoon lecture for third year medical students. You request your digital agent to retrieve last year's lecture presentation on the rehabilitation of patients with Parkinson's disease, and to locate abstracts of the latest research on this topic. These files will be waiting for you on your office computer when you arrive at the Rehabilitation Center. Finally traffic starts to move, and you make it to your office. Clinical rounds have been delayed and you use the opportunity to complete your daily exercise routine on your stationary bike which is facing an omnisurround screen. Viewing a virtual mountain path winding through the Swiss Alps, you are inspired to cycle uphill for a full 15 min. Your digital agent calls you just as you warm down to notify you that ward rounds are about to begin. The first patient is a 45-year-old businessman who is at the Center for intensive rehabilitation following knee arthroscopy. The patient is anxious to return home so you ask your intelligent agent to contact the agents of the surgeon, physiotherapist and occupational therapist who are not currently at the Center. All team members gather around an interactive, collaborative workspace to examine the X-rays, digital probe and ultrasound as well as other clinical outcome measures. The decision is to discharge with a course of telerehabilitation; the patient will sign on daily to a remotely supervised exercise program. You then ask the surgeon

to demonstrate the procedure he used to the ward resident via a virtual knee arthroscopy simulator. The manipulation is somewhat complex but with some practice the resident gains a good sense of what the procedure entails. Upon your return to your office, you log onto your synchronous distance learning platform to connect up with the third year students who are in their classroom on campus. They can each see your slide presentation on their personal tablets and hear you lecture. They each activate emoticons to indicate their response to your lecture as it unfolds. After reviewing the basic concepts of the disease etiology, prevalence and clinical signs and symptoms, you ask them to each don a cyberglove in order to feel the difference between Parkinsonian rigidity and upper motor neuron spasticity. They next put on a miniature liquid crystal display (LCD) lens while you run through a series of simulations that enable them to evaluate the improvement in Parkinsonian gait experienced by these patients when provided with virtual overground cues. The students use their own microphones to participate in an interactive discussion about the advantages and limitations of these and other recent non-invasive interventions. As you complete the class and prepare for the intake of a new patient you reflect in amazement that not a single student fell asleep! This is a certainly different from the days when you went to medical school.

13.1 Introduction

Not so very long ago the "high tech" gadgets of the type used by Dr. McCoy of Star Trek fame were considered to be intriguing but far from attainable. Beaming through space, scanning medical diagnostic "tricorders" and "genetronic replicators" came from the creative imaginations of the hit television shows creators. Although the future has not yet arrived, recent developments in technology have succeeded in changing the practice of today's clinician. Indeed, technology has enhanced a variety of clinical, administrative, academic and personal tasks facing the clinician of the new millennium. Virtual reality (VR) is one of the most innovative and promising of these developments and promises to have a considerable impact on neurorehabilitation over the next 10 years (Schultheis and Rizzo, 2001).

VR typically refers to the use of interactive simulations created with computer hardware and software to present users with opportunities to engage in environments that appear and feel similar to real world objects and events (Sheridan, 1992; Weiss and Jessel, 1998). Users interact with displayed images, move and manipulate virtual objects and perform other actions in a way that attempts to "immerse" them within the simulated environment thereby engendering a feeling of "presence" in the virtual world. One way to achieve a stronger feeling of presence, users are provided with different feedback modalities including visual and audio feedback and, less often, haptic and vestibular feedback of their performance. Depending on the characteristics of hardware, software and task complexity, VR aims to provide users with more than just an engaging experience, and is hence quite different in both scope and intensity than traditional computer simulation games. The purpose of this chapter is to provide an overview of applications of VR to rehabilitation.

13.2 Key concepts related to VR

Presence is widely considered to be the subjective feeling of being present in a simulated environment. Sheridan (1992) has defined it as being "… experienced by a person when sensory information generated only by and within a computer compels a feeling of being present in an environment other than the one the person is actually in" (Sheridan, 1992, p. 6). Presence is believed to be a major phenomenon characterizing a person's interaction within a virtual environment, but the term is used inconsistently by different researchers (Slater, 2003). Slater (1999) suggested that presence includes three aspects – the sense of "being there", domination of the virtual environment over the real world and the user's memory of visiting an actual location rather than a compilation of computer-generated images and sounds. Witmer and Singer (1998) related presence to the concept of selective attention. Despite the numerous studies that have attempted to merge the various definitions of presence, it continues to be viewed as a complex concept that may be influenced by numerous interdependent factors (Schuemie et al., 2001; Mantovani and Castelnuovo, 2003).

One set of factors relates to characteristics of the system that presents the virtual environment (see Fig. 13.1). These include the extent to which the user is encumbered with sensors, the way in which the user is represented within the virtual environment (Nash et al., 2000), whether the platform supports two- (2-D) or three-dimensional (3-D) interactions, and the number and quality of feedback modalities (e.g., Durfee, 2001). Another set of factors relates to a given user's characteristics. These include age, gender, immersive tendencies, prior VR experience and disability (e.g., Stanney et al., 1998). Finally, a third set of factors relates to characteristics of the virtual environment and the task that is being performed within it (Nash et al., 2000). These include the meaningfulness of the task (Hoffman et al., 1998), how realistic it is and the intuitiveness of the interaction (Rand et al., 2005).

A second key concept related to VR is immersion. Immersion relates to the extent to which the VR system succeeds in delivering an environment which refocuses a user's sensations from the real world to a virtual world (Slater, 1999, 2003). Whereas immersion is an objective measure referring to the VR platform, it does not immediately correspond to the level of presence (which is a subjective measure), produced by the system. Immersion is thus dependent, in large part, upon the quality of the technologies used with

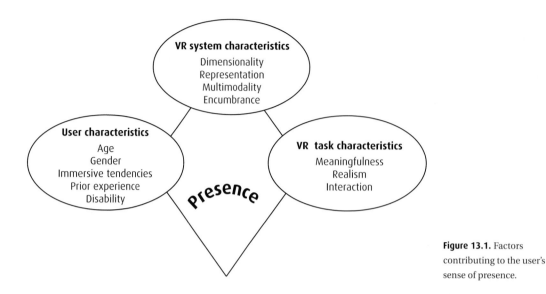

Figure 13.1. Factors contributing to the user's sense of presence.

the VR system (e.g., their resolution and speed of response) (Slater, 2003). Virtual environments may be delivered to the user via a variety of different technologies that differ in the extent to which they are able to "immerse" a user. In contrast to past references to immersive versus non-immersive VR systems, it is preferable to regard immersion as a continuum, ranging from lower to higher degrees of immersion. The relationship between the sense of presence, immersion and performance within the virtual environments is still not fully understood (Mania and Chalmers, 2001; Nash et al., 2000). Nevertheless, there is considerable evidence indicating that a high sense of presence may lead to deeper emotional response, increased motivation and, in some cases, enhanced performance (Schuemie et al., 2001). The use of a more immersive system does not necessarily generate a higher level of presence (Rand et al., 2005) nor does it guarantee clinical effectiveness. Taken together, there are many interwined issues involved in building a successful VR rehabilitation tool.

A third issue is cybersickness which refers to the fact that some users experience side effects during and following exposure to virtual environments delivered by some of the more immersive VR systems, a factor that may limit its usability for all patients under all circumstances (Kennedy and Stanney, 1996; Kennedy et al., 1997). Effects noted while using some VR systems can include nausea, eyestrain and other ocular disturbances, postural instability, headaches and drowsiness. Effects noted up to 12 h after using VR include disorientation, flashbacks and disturbances in hand–eye coordination and balance (e.g., Kennedy and Stanney, 1996; Stanney et al., 1998). Many of these effects appear to be caused by incongruities between information received from different sensory modalities (Lewis and Griffin, 1998). Other factors that may influence the occurrence and severity of side effects include characteristics of the user and the display, the user's ability to control simulated motions and interactivity with the task via movement of the head, trunk or whole body (Lewis and Griffin, 1998). VR systems which include the use of a head mounted display (HMD), have a greater potential of causing short-term side effects, mainly oculomotor symptoms (Lo Priore et al., 2003). The potential hazard of side effects for patients with different neurologic deficits has not been sufficiently explored although there is increasing evidence that their prevalence is minimal with video-capture VR systems (see below) that are growing in popularity for clinical applications (Rand et al., 2005).

13.3 Instrumentation

Virtual environments are usually experienced with the aid of special hardware and software for input (transfer of information from the user to the system) and output (transfer of information from the system to the user). The selection of appropriate hardware is important since its characteristics may greatly influence the way users respond to a virtual environment (Rand et al., 2005). The output to the user can be delivered by different modalities including visual, auditory, haptic, vestibular and olfactory stimuli, although, to date, most VR systems deliver primarily visual auditory feedback. Visual information is commonly displayed by HMDs, projection systems or flat screens of varying size. An HMD, such as Fifth Dimension Technologies (www.5dt.com) unit shown in Fig. 13.2, is essentially composed of two small screens positioned at eye level within special goggles or a helmet. Thus users view the virtual environment in very close proximity. Advanced HMDs even provide stereoscopic 3-D displays of the environment and usually are referred to as more immersive systems. Other VR applications use projection systems whereby the virtual environment is projected onto a large screen located in front of the user. VividGroup's Gesture Xtreme (GX)-VR system (www.vividgroup. com), shown in Fig. 13.3, is an example of a video-capture projection system. The user sees him or herself within the simulated environment, and is able to interact with virtual objects that are presented. Some expensive projection systems, such as the CAVE (http://evlweb.eecs.uic.edu/info/index.php3), are composed of several large screens surrounding users from all sides such that the virtual environment may be viewed no matter where they gaze. A third way of displaying visual information is based on simple desktop monitors, used singly or sometimes in clusters of screens positioned around the user providing a quasi-panoramic view of the virtual environment (Schultheis and Mourant, 2001). This method is the least immersive but its low cost supports wider distribution to clinics and even to patients' homes.

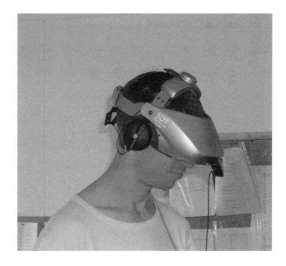

Figure 13.2. Fifth Dimension Technologies (www.5dt.com) HMD.

Sophisticated VR systems employ more than specialized visual displays. Engaging the user in the virtual environment may be enhanced via audio display, either ambient or directed to specific stimuli (Västfjäll, 2003). In recent years, haptic display has been introduced to the field of VR. Haptic feedback enables users to experience the sensation of touch, making the systems more immersive and closer to the real world experience. Haptic gloves, such as the Rutgers Master II shown in Fig. 13.4, may provide force feedback while manipulating virtual objects (Jack et al., 2001) or for strength training (Deutsch et al., 2002). Haptic information may also be conveyed by simpler means such as a force-feedback joystick (Reinkensmeyer et al., 2003) or a force-feedback steering wheel (Kline-Schoder, 2004). Other, less frequently used ways of making the virtual environment more life-like are by letting the user stand on a platform capable of perturbations and thereby providing vestibular stimuli such as that available with Motek's CAREN multisensory system (http://www. e-motek.com/medical/index.htm). Still more rare is the provision of olfactory feedback to add odor to a virtual environment, a feedback channel whose potential is now being investigated (Harel et al., 2003; Bordnick et al., 2005).

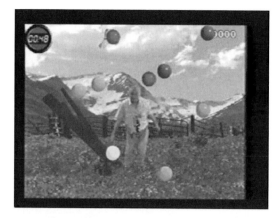

Figure 13.3. VividGroup's GX-VR system
(www.vividgroup.com) video-capture projection VR system.

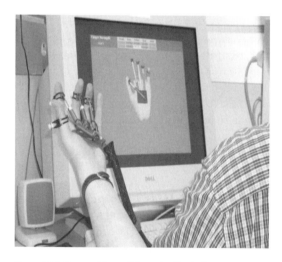

Figure 13.4. Rutgers Master II force-feedback glove.

The technologies mentioned above address only the output aspect of the VR experience. Equally important to achieving a realistic experience within a virtual environment is the ability of the user to navigate and manipulate objects within it. Thus the user must be able to interact (directly or indirectly) with the environment via a wide array of input technologies. One class of input technologies may be considered as direct methods since users behave in a natural way, and the system tracks their actions and

responds accordingly. Generally, this is achieved by using special sensors or by visual tracking. With the sensor approach, such as used by Intersense's (www.isense.com) InterTrax2, a three degree of freedom, inertial orientation tracker used to track pitch, roll and yaw movements, the user wears a tracking device that transmits position and orientation data to the VR system. With the visual tracking approach, such as used by VividGroup's video-capture VR system, the user's motion is recorded by video cameras, where special software processes the video image, extracts the user's figure from the background in real-time, and identifies any motion of the body.

A second class consists of indirect ways for users to manipulate and navigate within a virtual environment. These include activation of computer keyboard keys, a mouse or a joystick or even virtual buttons appearing as part of the environment (Rand et al., 2005).

In addition to specialized hardware, application software is also necessary. In recent years, off-the-shelf, ready-for-clinical-use VR software has become available for purchase. However, more frequently, special software development tools are required in order to design and code an interactive simulated environment that will achieve a desired rehabilitation goal. In many cases, innovative intervention ideas may entail customized programming to construct a virtual environment from scratch, using traditional programming languages.

VR hardware that facilitates the input and output of information, in combination with programmed virtual environments provide the tools for designing tasks that enable users to perform in ways that help them achieve established rehabilitation goals. When creating a specific virtual rehabilitation tool the clinician and technical team face the challenge of choosing and integrating the software and hardware, and the input and the output methods. For example, should one use an HMD, attach to it an orientation tracker and move around the virtual environment with a joystick? Or, should the user be positioned in front of a virtual environment projected onto a large screen and employ visual tracking to capture the user's responses? Such decisions have to take many factors into account including budget, physical space, mobility of the system, the nature of the patient population, the complexity of the task with respect to the patient population and the extent of immersion desired from the system.

13.4 VR attributes for rehabilitation

In recent years, VR technologies have begun to be used as an assessment and treatment tool in rehabilitation. The rationale for using VR in rehabilitation is based on a number of unique attributes of this technology (Riva et al., 1999; Schultheis and Rizzo, 2001). These include the opportunity for experiential, active learning which encourages and motivates the participant (Mantovani and Castelnuovo, 2003). In addition, there is the ability to objectively measure behavior in challenging but safe and ecologically valid environments, while maintaining strict experimental control over stimulus delivery and measurement (Rizzo et al., 2002b). VR also

offers the capacity to individualize treatment needs, while providing increased standardization of assessment and retraining protocols. Virtual environments provide the opportunity for repeated learning trials and offer the capacity to gradually increase the complexity of tasks while decreasing the support and feedback provided by the therapist (Schultheis and Rizzo, 2001). Moreover, the automated nature of stimulus delivery within virtual environments enables a therapist to focus on the provision of maximum physical support when needed without detracting from the complexity of the task. For example, several objects can be displayed simultaneously from different directions while the therapist supports the patient's paretic shoulder. Finally, the ability to change the virtual environments relatively easily enables clinicians to assess more efficiently different environmental modifications, which endeavor to enhance clients' accessibility. A summary of these attributes are listed in Table 13.1 together with some applications taken from the literature.

Table 13.1. VR attributes and some applications taken from the literature.

Attributes	Examples
Safe and ecologically valid environments	Training patients with neglect to safely cross the street (Naveh et al., 2000; Weiss et al., 2003a)
	Assessment of driving with patients following traumatic brain injury (Schultheis and Rizzo, 2001)
Control over delivery of stimuli via adaptation of the environment and task to elicit various levels of performance	Adaptation of the GX-VR system in terms of color, direction, speed and amount of stimulus (Kizony et al., 2003a)
Gradual changes in task complexity while changing extent of therapist intervention	Using video-based VR system with patients following spinal cord injury (Kizony et al., 2003b)
Increased standardization of assessment and treatment protocols	Assessment of cognitive function using a virtual kitchen (Christiansen et al., 1998)
Objective measurement of behavior and performance	Documenting hand function (e.g., range of motion of fingers) after stroke (Jack et al., 2001)
	Analyzing behavior (movements of body parts as well as success in virtual task) of children with ADHD (Rizzo, 2000, 2002a)
Provision of enjoyable and motivating experiences	Providing leisure opportunities using video-based VR with young adults with physical and intellectual disabilities (Weiss et al., 2003)

ADHD: attention deficits hyperacture disorder.

13.5 VR applications in neurologic populations

VR applications in rehabilitation are expanding at a rapid pace and a large variety of platforms and programs are currently being used and developed. Due to limitations in space this review is by no means comprehensive.

Assessment and remediation of cognitive, meta-cognitive and motor deficits

Cognitive deficits

VR has been used as a medium for the assessment and rehabilitation of cognitive processes, such as visual perception, attention, memory, sequencing and executive functioning (Pugnetti et al., 1998; Rizzo et al., 2000). For example, a meal preparation task in a virtual kitchen viewed via an HMD examined the sequencing of 30 steps during a soup preparation task. The evaluation was found to be reliable and valid for the assessment of cognitive functioning of 30 patients with closed head injury (Christiansen et al., 1998). In a second study with the same VR scenario the subtasks were categorized into information processing, problem solving, logic sequence and speed of responding; in all components, participants with brain injury showed significantly worse performance when compared to healthy volunteers (Zhang et al., 2001).

Grealy et al. (1999) combined a bicycle exercise program with three virtual environments (a Caribbean Island, a town and countryside and snowy mountain with ski runs) that were linked to a cycle ergometer and displayed on a screen while steering within the virtual course. The study aimed to improve cognitive abilities via exercise within different virtual environments. An experimental group included 13 patients with traumatic brain injury (TBI) who were treated for 4 weeks with pre- and post-testing of standard cognitive measures such as digit span, trail making and memory (auditory, visual and logic). The control group consisted of 12 patients from the same hospital who did not receive this treatment but were matched for other variables. Results showed significant improvement in auditory and visual learning following the VR treatment but not in complex figure and logic memory tasks. Speed of information processing was also enhanced, suggesting that learning may have been facilitated by an increase in arousal activation level (Grealy et al., 1999).

In a different series of studies, a street crossing virtual environment, run on a desktop VR system, with successively graded levels of difficulty was developed to provide users' with an opportunity to decide when it is safe to cross a virtual street. It was initially tested on 12 subjects, six stroke patients and six matched controls (Naveh et al., 2000; Weiss et al., 2003a). Results showed that the program is suitable for patients with neurologic deficits in both its cognitive and motor demands. Currently, the program is being used in a controlled clinical trial to train patients with right hemisphere stroke and unilateral spatial neglect (USN) in order to improve their attention and ability to scan to the left. Measures included standard paper and pencil cancellation tests, as well as pre- and post-performance within the virtual environment and during actual street crossing. Initial results from 11 patients who used the virtual environment (VR street test) versus a control group of eight patients who used non-VR computer-based scanning tasks showed that both groups improved in their scores, namely the number of correctly canceled items on the star cancellation from the behavioral inattention test (BIT) (Wilson et al., 1987) and Mesulam symbol cancellation test (Weintraub and Mesulam, 1987); however, the VR group completed the tests in less time which may also be an indicator of improvement, while the control group needed longer time to perform (Katz et al., 2005). The performance of the VR group in the VR street test showed training effects, as all patients improved in looking to the left and most of them had fewer accidents during the virtual street crossing at post-test, while the majority of the control group did not change their performance from pre- to post-test on the VR street test.

The GX video-capture VR system has recently been investigated to determine its potential for remediation of cognitive and motor deficits (Kizony et al.,

2002; Reid, 2002; Sveistrup et al., 2003; Weiss et al., 2004) and to provide recreational opportunities for people with severe disabilities (Weiss et al., 2003b). For example, Kizony et al. (2003a) described an example of a patient following a right hemisphere stroke with attention deficits 6 months after the event. During VR treatment he was required to pay attention to the entire visual space as well as moving his affected arm in the neglected space, as for example, he played the role of a soccer goalkeeper whose task was to deflect balls that came towards him from all directions. During the game, he saw himself within the virtual environment, and received immediate visual and auditory feedback to help him improve his performance. The patient expressed enjoyment and motivation to continue with this kind of treatment. The adaptations applied to these VR environments enable the treatment of visual spatial attention and USN common symptoms following brain damage, by controlling the direction, number and color of stimuli and by adding distracters to the scenario (Kizony et al., 2003a). This is an example of where off-the-shelf software has been adapted to make it more applicable for clinical use.

A study is now underway in which the effect of training with this VR system to remediate attention and USN deficits of patients with right hemisphere stroke is being evaluated. Both the street crossing environment as well as the video-capture games (such as soccer) are examples of the use of VR technology as applied to the treatment of stroke patients with attention deficits and USN, a phenomenon described more fully in Chapters 28 and 36 of this volume. The desktop VR system focuses mainly on visual scanning whereas the video-capture system combines visual scanning with motor activation both of which have been shown to be important rehabilitation goals.

Another approach for the assessment and rehabilitation of attention and memory processes is one that makes use of HMD-delivered virtual environments such as the applications developed by Rizzo and colleagues (Rizzo et al., 2000; Schultheis and Rizzo, 2001; Rizzo et al., 2002a). A virtual classroom was developed for the assessment and training of attention in children with attention deficits

hyperactive disorder (ADHD), and a Virtual Office was developed for assessment of memory processes in patients with TBI. The virtual classroom contains the basic objects (e.g., tables, chairs, blackboard, windows) and subjects (e.g., female teacher, pupils) found in a typical classroom. Both visual (e.g., car outside the window, paper airplane flying above the classroom) and auditory (e.g., steps in the hallway) distracters inside and outside the classroom randomly appear, as a child who wears an HMD to view the environment, performs various tasks of selective, sustained and divided attention. The child's performance is measured in terms of reaction time. Behavioral factors such as head turning and gross motor movement related to distractibility and hyperactivity are also recorded. An initial clinical trial compared eight children aged 6–12 years with ADHD and 10 control children on standard tests and VR performance. Results showed that the children with ADHD had slower and more variable reaction times, made more omission and commission errors and showed higher overall body movements than did the control children (Rizzo et al., 2002a). Hyperactive motor movements tracked from the head, arms and legs were greater for the children with ADHD and more pronounced when distractions were presented.

The Virtual Office is modeled on the same principles as the virtual classroom; however, in addition to attention, memory was also tested (Rizzo et al., 2002a). Sixteen objects are placed in the environment; eight of the objects would typically be found in an office environment (e.g., clock) whereas eight would not be (e.g., fire hydrant). The user is asked to scan the office via an HMD for 1 min and then to recall the objects from memory. Both the classroom and office virtual environments have considerable potential to train individuals to improve their attention and memory abilities within a task that is relevant, similar to real world settings, but still controlled with the possibility of systematic and precise measurement.

In a recent review of the use of VR in memory rehabilitation, Brooks and Rose (2003) discussed one example of a virtual four-room bungalow which runs on a desktop computer for the assessment of prospective memory, an ability that is critical for multitasking. Twenty-two patients with stroke and a control group were requested to perform a furniture removal task (using a mouse or a joystick) while they were required to remember certain conditions of cue, activity and timed-based tasks. The differences between the groups indicated that using VR as a rehabilitation intervention enabled a more comprehensive and controlled assessment of prospective memory than did standard memory tests (Brooks et al., 2002).

Executive functions deficits

VR environments have the potential to enhance cognitive neuropsychologic tests of executive function since they generate a better subjective perception of presence and immersion than do artificial laboratory tests (Lo Priore et al., 2002). Moreover, virtual environments appear to offer a way to systematically assess and rehabilitate executive functions, since they have ecologic validity and can be readily designed to simulate the demands found in everyday tasks as noted above (Rizzo et al., 2002b).

Pugnetti et al. (1995; 1998) was one of the first groups to assess executive functions via VR. They developed an HMD-delivered virtual environment that embodied the cognitive challenges that characterize the Wisconsin card sorting test (WCST).

The four-room bungalow environment described above was successfully used to test executive functions by Morris et al. (2002). They defined components of strategy formations, rule breaking and prospective memory for 35 patients with focal prefrontal neurosurgical lesions as compared to 35 matched controls. Their results showed that the VR test procedure was successful in differentiating between the groups on all measures.

Lo Priore et al. (2002) developed the V-store, a desktop VR-based tool for the rehabilitation of executive functions for patients with TBI. This environment requires the patient to choose and place different pieces of fruit in a basket in accordance with verbal commands. Six tasks are graded in complexity with the aim of eliciting the need for executive functions, problem solving, behavioral control,

categorical abstraction, memory and attention. A series of distracting elements are included to generate time pressure and elicit management strategies. An initial study of control subjects who used the V-store environment via an immersive HMD display as well as via a non-immersive flat screen display was carried out (Lo Priore et al., 2003). Outcomes including physiologic, neuropsychologic and presence measures showed no major differences between the VR systems.

In another study, McGeorge et al. (2001) compared real world and virtual world "errand running" performance in five patients with TBI who had poor planning skills and in five normal control subjects. The video taped performance of subjects was coded and compared while performing a series of errands in the University of Aberdeen Psychology Department (real world) and within a flat screen VR scenario modeled after this environment. Performance in both the real and virtual environments, defined as the number of errands completed in a 20-min period, was highly correlated. This finding suggests that performance in the real and virtual worlds was functionally similar, emphasizing the echologic validity of the VR. Finally, measures of both real and virtual world performance showed concordance with staff observations of planning skills (Rizzo et al., 2004). Initial evidence points to the value of VR technology for the rehabilitation of executive functions in TBI. Background material on executive functions and TBI are presented in Chapters 30 and 33 of this volume.

Motor deficits

The majority of VR-based interventions used to train motor deficits have been used with patients who have had a stroke. Piron et al. (2001) used a virtual environment to train reaching movements, Broeren et al. (2002) used a haptic device for the assessment and training of motor coordination, and Jack et al. (2001) and Merians et al. (2002) have developed a force-feedback glove to improve hand strength and a non-haptic glove to improve the range of motion and speed of hand movement. Based on the results of the latter study, which included three patients who had a stroke, it appears that training within a virtual environment may lead to improvements in upper extremity function in this population even when at a chronic stage (Merians et al., 2002).

Since many of the VR applications for rehabilitation have used desktop VR systems wherein the user interacts within the virtual environment via a keyboard, mouse or joystick, the focus of intervention has often been cognitive, meta-cognitive or functional or limited to wrist, digit or ankle movements as illustrated above. More recently the use of other methods of interaction has enabled applications that can also be used for the improvement of motor deficits. For example, individuals with acquired brain injury have been trained to perform specific arm movements within a virtual environment and have then been able to generalize this ability and engage in daily functional use of the affected arm (Holden et al., 2001).

The VividGroup's GX system was used to develop an exercise program for balance retraining in which users see their own mirror image. Following 6 weeks of training at an intensity of three sessions per week, improvement was found for all 14 participants in both the VR and control groups (Sveistrup et al., 2003). However, the VR group reported more confidence in their ability to "not fall" and to "not shuffle while walking". Kizony et al. (2004) presented results of 13 patients who had a stroke and who used a number of virtual games via the GX-VR system. The findings showed that the system is suitable for use with elderly patients who have motor and cognitive deficits. In addition all participants expressed their enjoyment from the experience.

The same VR system has been used to explore its potential to train balance for patients with spinal cord injury (SCI) (Kizony et al., 2003b). Such training for these patients is essential in order to help them achieve maximal independence, namely remediation of motor deficits via compensatory strategies to maintain balance. Initial results from a usability study of nine patients showed that they enjoyed doing the tasks, were highly motivated to participate and asked to have repeated sessions with the VR system. More importantly, they were able to maintain balance under the very dynamic conditions available

within the virtual environment (Kizony et al., 2002) and appeared to make considerably more effort than during conventional therapy (Kizony et al., 2003b). It was also evident that the task was highly motivating for him (Kizony et al., 2003b). This preliminary evidence demonstrates the value of VR technology for balance training and SCI, topics that are presented in Chapters 20 and 37 of this volume.

Functional evaluation and training

Instrumental activities of daily living

VR shows promise for training activities of daily living with different populations. Davies et al. (1999, 2002) developed three desktop applications for rehabilitation of daily tasks – a virtual kitchen, a service and vending machine and a hospital and university way-finding environment. The functional tasks and the 3-D way finding within the virtual environment were carried out using an adapted keyboard or a touch screen. A virtual kitchen was also developed by Gourlay et al. (2000) to enable practice that is safe, controlled and stimulating for patients with stroke and TBI, who have cognitive deficits, prior to practice within an actual kitchen. These researchers developed a "telerehabilitation" system for use at home under supervision by practitioners from a clinic, thus enabling training without having to travel which is difficult for many patients.

Initial support for the ecological value of VR "route finding training" can be found in a case study by Brooks et al. (1999). In this report, a patient with stroke and with severe amnesia showed significant improvements in her ability to find her way around a rehabilitation unit following training within a virtual environment modeled on the unit. This was most notable given that prior to training the patient had resided on the unit for 2 months and was still unable to find her way around, even to places that she visited regularly. Four additional patients were trained on this system using four different routes. Results showed that for all patients virtual training was found to be as successful as real training (Brooks and Rose, 2003).

Another activity of daily living is street crossing. Safe street crossing is a major concern for many patients with neurologic deficits as well as for elderly people, and is thus an important goal in rehabilitation. The VR desktop system of street crossing described above (Katz et al., 2005; Naveh et al., 2000; Weiss et al., 2003a) aimed at testing the effectiveness of virtual training for patients with stroke who had USN or other deficits of spatial perception, and to determine whether these skills transferred to performance in the real world.

Application of VR to driving assessment and training has had, to date, very promising results (Schultheis and Rizzo, 2001). A VR-based driving assessment system using an HMD was developed and tested at Kessler Medical Rehabilitation. The rehabilitation of driving skills following TBI is one example where individuals may begin at a simple level (i.e., straight, non-populated roads) and gradually progress to more challenging situations (i.e., crowded, highway roads, night driving) (Schultheis and Mourant, 2001). The first study compared the VR-based driving system with the behind the wheel (BTW) evaluation, the current "gold standard", and found comparable results for the two approaches (Schultheis and Rizzo, 2001). Next, an analysis of the demands for safe driving was carried out, and the issue of divided attention was studied by adding a task of calling out digits appearing on the screen while maintaining driving at differing speed levels. The comparison of three patients with TBI to matched healthy controls showed that speed of driving was consistent and similar for the two groups, but the patients failed to call the digits, while the healthy performed this task significantly better than the patients. Thus, the patients with TBI showed a serious problem in dual tasking. The results on the divided attention task were highly correlated with neuropsychologic tests, validating the method of testing during VR driving. An extensive research project is underway to test the system for different neurologic populations. As in the case of the street crossing program, described above, both cognitive variables which may explain the difficulty of performing the actual task (crossing streets or driving) and the functional evaluation and training for transfer and generalization to the daily

tasks are combined. This provides for ecologic validity of VR systems which is missing in traditional standard measures.

13.6 A model of VR-based rehabilitation

The VR experience is multidimensional and appears to be influenced by many parameters whose interactions remain to be clarified. A proposed model for VR in rehabilitation is presented in Fig. 13.5. This model was developed within the context of the International Classification of Functioning, Disability and Health (ICF) (World Health Organization, 2001) terminology (Kizony et al., 2002) and consists of three nested circles, the inner "interaction space", the intermediate "transfer phase" and the outer "real world".

When using VR in rehabilitation we construct a virtual environment that aims to simulate real world environments. In contrast to real world settings, the virtual environment can be adapted with relative ease to the needs and characteristics of the clients under our care. The ultimate goal of VR-based intervention is to enable clients to become more able to participate in their own real environments in as independent manner as possible.

As represented schematically in Fig. 13.5, two primary factors within the "interaction space" influence the nature of the interaction between the user and the virtual environment. The first of these factors relates to the user's personal characteristics (body functions and structures). The second factor relates to characteristics of the virtual environment including both the type of VR platform and its underlying technology and the nature and demands of the task to be performed within the virtual environment. The characteristics of the virtual environment may be either barriers or enablers to performance. The client interacts within the virtual environment, performing functional or game-like tasks of varying levels of difficulty. This enables the therapist to determine the optimal environmental factors for the client. Within the "interaction space" sensations and perceptions related to the virtual experience take place (sense of presence, meaning and actual performance).

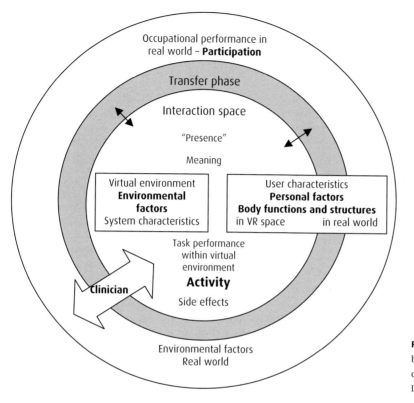

Figure 13.5. A model of VR-based rehabilitation within the context of terminology from the ICF (indicated in bold).

From the interaction space (inner circle) we move to the transfer phase (intermediate circle) since our goal in rehabilitation is to improve daily function in the real world and this requires transfer of the trained skills or tasks as well as environmental modifications from the virtual environment to the real world. Finally, the large, outer circle represents real world environments illustrating that the ultimate goal is to help the client achieve participation in the real world environment by overcoming, adapting to or minimizing the environmental barriers. The entire process is facilitated by the clinician whose expertise helps to actualize the potential of VR as a rehabilitation tool.

13.7 Conclusions

It is clear from the above review that the future holds great promise for the further development of applications of VR to rehabilitation. In addition to the many exciting rehabilitation applications presented above, VR-based therapy has been very effective in other realms of medicine such as in the treatment of phobias (Hodges et al., 2001) and to reduce of pain during burn care (Hoffman et al., 2000) and venipuncture (Reger et al., 2003).

VR has also been shown to be highly effective as a means for providing alternate modes of feedback in cases of sensory impairment such as the substitution of auditory (Sanchez et al., 2000) and/or haptic (Yu and Brewster, 2002) cues for individuals with severe visual impairment via interactive virtual environments.

The cost of equipment is decreasing and the availability of off-the-shelf software is growing such that it is now feasible for many clinical facilities to embrace this new technology. As presented above, the literature to date strongly suggests that these technologies are poised to have a major impact on evaluation and intervention for cognitive, motor and functional rehabilitation due to the unique attributes of VR-based therapy. These attributes make it highly suitable for the achievement of many rehabilitation goals including the encouragement of experiential, active learning, the provision of challenging but safe and ecologically valid environments, the flexibility of individualized and graded treatment protocols, the power to motivate patients to perform to their utmost capability and the capacity to record objective measures of performance.

Nevertheless, further development of VR-based rehabilitation depends, to some extent, on the resolution of certain issues that currently present either technological or financial limitations. The cost of some of the more immersive VR systems is still prohibitive rendering them more suitable to investigative studies rather than to routine clinical applications. Continued development of off-the-shelf, low-cost virtual environments that can be displayed on standard desktop equipment or via dedicated microprocessors (e.g., the Sony PlayStation II's "EyeToy" application, www.eyetoy.com) will make the use of VR affordable to a variety of treatment and educational settings (Rand et al., 2004). Of course, the clinical effectiveness of these less expensive applications must be verified prior to their wide promotion and adoption.

There is also a need to address issues related to the number and quality of feedback channels used with virtual environments. As indicated above, visual and auditory feedback is extensively used; haptic, vestibular and olfactory feedback is far less commonly available. The cost of devices capable to transmitting feedback of high quality is often high and their potential for encumbering users is also significant. The relationship between feedback quality and effectiveness is not certain, nor is the relationship between the number of feedback channels and effect of therapy known. Considerably more research as to impact that VR feedback has on clinical intervention is therefore needed.

Finally, it is encouraging to note that much progress has been made in the demonstration of the transfer of abilities and skills acquired within virtual environments to the real world performance. Although continued efforts are needed to firmly establish that attainments with virtual environments are both the transferable and generalizable to function within the real world, the evidence to date substantiates the initial promise of these dynamic technologies.

REFERENCES

Bordnick, P.S. and Graap, K.M. (2005). Virtual reality applications in addictions treatment and research. In: *Advances in Virtual Environments Technology: Musings on Design, Evaluation, and Applications* (ed. Stanney, K.). Lawrence Erlbaum Associates Proceedings of the 11th International Conference on Human Computer Interactions. Las Vegas. July 22–27.

Broeren, J., Bjorkdahl, A., Pascher, R. and Rydmark, M. (2002). Virtual reality and haptics as an assessment devise in the postacute phase after stroke. *Cyberpsychol Behav*, **5**, 207–211.

Brooks, B.M. and Rose, F.D. (2003). The use of virtual reality in memory rehabilitation: current findings and future directions. *Neurorehabilitation*, **18**, 147–157.

Brooks, B.M., McNeil, J.E., Rose, F.D., Greenwood, R.J., Attree, E.A. and Leadbetter, A.G. (1999). Route learning in a case of amnesia: a preliminary investigation into the efficacy of training in a virtual environment. *Neuropsychol Rehabil*, **9**, 63–76.

Brooks, B.M., Rose, F.D., Potter, E.A., Attree, S., Jayawardena, S. and Morling, A. (2002). Assessing stroke patient's ability to remember to perform actions in the future using virtual reality. In: *Proceeding of the 4th International Conference on Disability, Virtual Reality and Associated Technology* (eds Sharkey, P., Lanyi, C.S. and Stanton, P.), University of Reading, Vresprem, Hungary, pp. 239–245.

Christiansen, C., Abreu, B., Ottenbacher, K., Huffman, K., Masel, B. and Culpepper, R. (1998). Task performance in virtual environments used for cognitive rehabilitation after traumatic brain injury. *Arch Phys Med Rehabil*, **79**, 888–892.

Davies, R.C., Johnsson, G., Boschain, K., Linden, A., Minor, U. and Sonesson, B. (1999). A practical example of using virtual reality in the assessment of brain injury. *Int J Virt Real*, **4**, 3–10.

Davies, R.C., Lofgren, E., Wallergard, M., Linden, A., Boschain, K., Minor, U., Sonesson, B. and Johansson, G. (2002). Three applications of virtual reality for brain injury rehabilitation of daily tasks. *Proceeding of the 4th International Conference on Disability, Virtual Reality and Associated Technology*, University of Reading, Vresprem, Hungary, pp. 93–100.

Deutsch, J.E., Merians, A.S., Burdea, G.C., Boian, R., Adamovich, S.V. and Poizner, H. (2002). Haptics and virtual reality used to increase strength and improve function in chronic individuals post-stroke: two case reports. *Neurol Report*, **26**, 79–86.

Durfee, W. (2001). Multi-modal virtual environments or haptics does not stand alone. *Proceedings of the Haptics, Virtual Reality, and Human Computer Interaction*, Institute for Mathematics and its Applications, Minneapolis, Minnesota.

Gourlay, D., Lun, K.C., Lee, Y.N. and Tay, J. (2000). Virtual reality for relearning daily living skills. *Int J Med Inform*, **60**, 255–261.

Grealy, M.A., Johnson, D.A. and Rushton, S.K. (1999). Improving cognitive function after brain injury: the use of exercise and virtual reality. *Arch Phys Med Rehabil*, **80**, 661–667.

Harel, D., Carmel, L. and Lancet, D. (2003). Towards an odor communication system. Retrieved from the world wide web, January 12, 2004: http://www.wisdom.weizmann.ac.il/~dharel/papers/OdorScheme.pdf

Hodges, L.F., Anderson, P., Burdea, G., Hoffman, H.G. and Rothbaum, B.O. (2001). VR as a tool in the treatment of psychological and physical disorders. *IEEE Comput Graph Appl*, **21**, 25–33.

Hoffman, H.G., Prothero, J., Wells, M. and Groen, J. (1998). Virtual chess: the role of meaning in the sensation of presence. *Int J Hum- Comput Int*, **10**, 251–263.

Hoffman, H.G, Patterson, D.R. and Carrougher, G.J. (2000). Use of virtual reality for adjunctive treatment of adult burn pain during physical therapy: a controlled study. *Clin J Pain*, **16**, 244–250.

Holden, M., Dettwiler, A., Dyar, T., Niemann, G. and Bizzi, E. (2001). Retraining movement in patients with acquired brain injury using a virtual environment. *Proceedings of Medicine Meets Virtual Reality 2001* (eds Westwood, J.D., et al.), IOS Press, Amsterdam, pp. 192–198.

Jack, D., Boian, R., Merians, A., Tremaine, M., Burdea, G.C., Adamovich, S.V., Recce, M. and Poizner, H. (2001). Virtual reality-enhanced stroke rehabilitation. *IEEE Trans Neural Syst Rehabil Eng*, **9**, 308–318.

Katz, N., Ring, H., Naveh, Y., Kizony, R., Feintuch, U. and Weiss, P.L. Effect of interactive virtual environment training on independent safe street crossing of stroke patients with unilateral spatial neglect. *Disabil Rehabil* (in press 2005)

Kennedy, R.S. and Stanney, K.M. (1996). Postural instability induced by virtual reality exposure: development of certification protocol. *Int J Hum- Comput Int*, **8**, 2547.

Kennedy, R.S., Stanney, K.M., Ordy, J.M. and Dunlap, W.P. (1997). Virtual reality effects produced by head-mounted display (HMD) on human eye–hand coordination, postural equilibrium, and symptoms of cybersickness. *Soc Neurosci Abstr*, **23**, 772.

Kizony, R., Katz, N., Weingarden, H. and Weiss, P.L. (2002). Immersion without encumbrance: adapting a virtual reality system for the rehabilitation of individuals with stroke and spinal cord injury. In: *Proceeding of the 4th International Conference on Disability, Virtual Reality and Associated Technology* (eds Sharkey, P., Lanyi, C.S. and Stanton, P.), University of Reading, Vresprem, Hungary, pp. 55–61.

Kizony, R., Katz, N. and Weiss, P.L. (2003a). Adapting an immersive virtual reality system for rehabilitation. *J Visual Comp Animat*, **14**, 261–268.

Kizony, R., Raz, L., Katz, N., Weingarden, H. and Weiss, P.L. (2003b). Using a video projected VR system for patients with spinal cord injury. In: *Proceeding of the Second International Workshop on Virtual Rehabilitation* (eds Burdea, G.C., Thalmann, D. Lewis, J.A.), Piscataway, NJ, USA, pp. 82–88.

Kizony, R., Katz, N. and Weiss, P.L. (2004). A model of VR-based intervention in rehabilitation: Relationship between motor and cognitive abilities and performance within virtual environments for patients with stroke. *Proceedings of the Fifth International Conference on Disability, Virtual Reality and Associated Technologies*, Oxford, UK.

Kline-Schoder, R. (2004). Virtual reality-enhanced physical therapy system. *Proceedings of CyberTherapy*, San Diego.

Lewis, C.H. and Griffin, M.J. (1998). Human factors consideration in clinical applications of virtual reality. In: *Virtual Reality in Neuro-Psycho-Physiology* (ed. Riva, G.), IOS Press, Amsterdam.

Lo Priore, C., Castelnuovo, G. and Liccione, D. (2002). Virtual environments in cognitive rehabilitation of executive functions. In: *Proceeding of the 4th International Conference on Disability, Virtual Reality and Associated Technology* (eds Sharkey, P., Lanyi, C.S., Stanton, P.), University of Reading, Vresprem, Hungary, pp. 165–171.

Lo Priore, C., Castelnuovo, G., Liccione, D. and Liccione, D. (2003). Experience with V-STORE: considerations on presence in virtual environments for effective neuropsychological rehabilitation of executive functions. *Cyberpsychol Behav*, **6**, 281–287.

Mania, K. and Chalmers, A. (2001). The effects of levels of immersion on memory and presence in virtual environments: a reality centered approach. *Cyberpsychol Behav*, **4**, 247–264.

Mantovani, F. and Castelnuovo, G. (2003). Sense of presence in virtual training: enhancing skills acquisition and transfer of knowledge through learning experience in virtual environments. In: *Being There: Concepts, Effects and Measurement of User Presence in Synthetic Environments* (eds Riva, G., Davide, F. and Ijsselsteijn, W.A.). IOS Press, Amsterdam, The Netherlands.

McGeorge, P., Phillips, L.H., Crawford, J.R., Garden, S.E., Della Sala, S., Milne, A.B., Hamilton, S. and Callander, J. (2001). Using virtual environments in the assessment of executive dysfunction. *Presence-Teleop Virt Environ*, **10**, 375–383.

Merians, A., Jack, D., Boian, R., Tremaine, M., Burdea, G.C., Adamovich, S.V., Recce, M. and Poizner, H. (2002). Virtual reality-augmented rehabilitation for patients following stroke. *Phys Ther*, **82**, 898–915.

Morris, R.G., Kotitsa, M., Bramham, J., Brooks, B. and Rose, F.D. (2002). In: *Proceeding of the 4th International Conference on Disability, Virtual Reality and Associated Technology* (eds Sharkey, P., Lanyi, C.S. and Stanton, P.), University of Reading, Vresprem, Hungary, pp. 101–108.

Nash, E.B., Edwards, G.W., Thompson, J.A. and Barfield, W. (2000). A review of presence and performance in virtual environments. *Int J Hum- Comput Int*, **12**, 1–41.

Naveh, Y., Katz, N. and Weiss, P.L. (2000). The effect of interactive virtual environment training on independent safe street crossing of right CVA patients with unilateral spatial neglect. *Proceedings of the 3rd International Conference on Disability, Virtual Reality and Associated Technology*, Algbero, Italy pp. 243–248.

Piron, L., Cenni, F., Tonin, P. and Dam, M. (2001). Virtual reality as an assessment tool for arm motor deficits after brain lesions. *Stud Health Technol Inform*, **81**, 386–392.

Pugnetti, L., Mendozzi, L., Motta, A., Cattaneo, A., Barbieri, E. and Brancotti, A. (1995). Evaluation and retraining of adults' cognitive impairments: which role for virtual reality technology? *Comput Biol Med*, **25**, 213–227.

Pugnetti, L., Mendozzi, L., Attree, E.A., Barbieri, E., Brooks, B.M., Cazzullo, C.L., Motta, A. and Rose, F.D. (1998). Probing memory and executive functions with virtual reality: past and present studies. *Cyberpsychol Behav*, **1**, 151–162.

Rand, D., Kizony, R. and Weiss, P.L. (2004). VR Rehabilitation for all: vivid GX versus Sony Playstation II EyeToy. *Proceedings of the 5th International Conference on Disability, Virtual Reality and Associated technologies*, Oxford, UK, September, pp. 87–94.

Rand, D., Kizony, R., Feintuch, U., Katz, N., Josman, N., Rizzo, A.A. and Weiss, P.L. (2005). Comparison of two VR platforms for rehabilitation: video capture versus HMD. *Presence, Teleop Virt Environ*, **14**, 147–160.

Reger, G.M., Rizzo, A.A., Buckwalter, J.G., Gold, J., Allen, R., Augustine, R. and Mendelowitz, E. (2003). Effectiveness of virtual realty for attentional control to reduce children's pain during venipuncture. *Proceedings of the 2nd International Workshop on Virtual Reality*, Piscattaway, NJ.

Reid, D. (2002).Virtual reality and the person–environment experience. *Cyberpsychol Behav*, **5**, 559–564.

Reinkensmeyer, D.J., Iobbi, M.G., Kahn, L.E., Kamper, D.G. and Takahashi, C.D. (2003). Modeling reaching impairment after stroke using a population vector model of movement control that incorporates neural firing-rate variability. *Neural Comput*, **15**, 2619–2642.

Riva, G., Rizzo, A., Alpini, D., Barbieri, E., Bertella, L., Davies, R.C., Gamberini, L., Johansson, G., Katz, N., Marchi, S., Mendozzi, L., Molinari, E., Pugnetti, L. and Weiss, P.L. (1999). Virtual environments in the diagnosis, prevention, and intervention of age-related diseases: a review of VR scenarios proposed in the EC VETERAN Project. *Cyberpsychol Behav*, **2**, 577–591.

Rizzo, A.A. (2002). Virtual reality and disability: emergence and challenge. *Disabil Rehabil*, **24**, 567–569.

Rizzo, A.A., Buckwalter, J.G., Bowerly, T., van der Zaag, C., Humphrey, L., Neumann, U., Chua, C., Kyriakakis, C., van Rooyen, A. and Sisemore, D. (2000). The virtual classroom: a virtual environment for the assessment and rehabilitation of attention deficits. *Cyberpsychol Behav*, **3**, 483–500.

Rizzo, A.A., Bowerly, T., Buckwalter, J.G., Schultheis, M.T., Matheis, R., Shahabi, C., Neumann, U., Kim, L. and Sharifzadeh, M. (2002a). Virtual environment for the assessment of attention and memory processes: the virtual classroom and office. *Proceeding of the 4th International Conference on Disability, Virtual Reality and Associated Technology*, University of Reading, Vresprem, Hungary, pp. 3–11.

Rizzo, A., Buckwalter, J.C. and Van der Zaag, C. (2002b). Virtual environment applications in clinical neuropsychology. In: *The Handbook of Virtual Environments* (ed. Stanney, K.), Erlbaum Publishing, New York, pp. 1027–1064.

Rizzo, A.A., Schultheis, M.T., Kerns, K. and Mateer, C. (2004). Analysis of assets for virtual reality in neuropsychology. *Neuropsychol Rehabil*, **14**, 207–239.

Sanchez, J., Jorquera, L., Munoz, E. and Valenzuela, E. (2000). Virtual aurea: perception through spatialized sound. *Proceeding of the 3rd International Conference on Disability, Virtual Reality and Associated Technology*, University of Reading, Algbero, Sardnia.

Schultheis, M.T. and Mourant, R.R. (2001). Virtual reality and driving: the road to better assessment of cognitively impaired populations. *Presence Teleop Virt Environ*, **10**, 436–444.

Schultheis, M.T. and Rizzo, A.A. (2001). The application of virtual reality technology for rehabilitation. *Rehabil Psychol*, **46**, 296–311.

Schuemie, M.J., van der Straaten, P., Krijn, M. and van der Mast, C.A.P.G. (2001). Research on presence in virtual reality: a survey. *Cyberpsychol Behav*, **4**, 183–201.

Sheridan, T.B. (1992). Musings on telepresence and virtual presence. *Presence*, **1**, 120–125.

Slater, M. (1999). Measuring presence: a response to the Witmer and Singer questionnaire. *Presence Teleop Virt Environ*, **8**, 560–566.

Slater, M. (2003). A note on presence terminology. *Presence-Connect*, **3**.

Stanney, K.M., Mourant, R.R. and Kennedy, R.S. (1998). Human factors issues in virtual environments: a review of the literature. *Presence*, **7**, 327–351.

Sveistrup, H., McComas, J., Thornton, M., Marshall, S., Finestone, H., McCormick, A., Babulic, K. and Mayhew, A. (2003). Experimental studies of virtual reality-delivered compared to conventional exercise programs for rehabilitation. *Cyberpsychol Behav*, **6**, 245–249.

Västfjäll, D. (2003). The subjective sense of presence, emotion recognition, and experienced emotions in auditory virtual environments. *Cyberpsychol Behav*, **6**, 181–188.

Weintraub, S. and Mesulam, M.M. (1987). Right cerebral dominance in spatial attention: further evidence based on ipsilateral neglect. *Arch Neurol*, **44**, 621–625.

Weiss, P.L. and Jessel, A.S. (1998). Virtual reality applications to work. *Work*, **11**, 277–293.

Weiss, P.L., Naveh, Y. and Katz, N. (2003a). Design and testing of a virtual environment to train stroke patients with unilateral spatial neglect to cross a street safely. *Occup Therapy Int*, **10**, 39–55.

Weiss, P.L., Bialik, P. and Kizony, R. (2003b). Virtual reality provides leisure time opportunities for young adults with physical and intellectual disabilities. *Cyberpsychol Behav*, **6**, 335–342.

Weiss, P.L., Rand, D., Katz, N. and Kizony, R. (2004). Video capture virtual reality as a flexible and effective rehabilitation tool. *J NeuroEng Rehabil*, **1**, 1–12.

Wilson, B.A., Cockburn, J. and Halligan, P. (1987). *Behavioral Inattention Test Manual*, Thames Valley Test Company, UK.

Witmer, B.G. and Singer, M.J. (1998). Measuring presence in virtual environments: a presence questionnaire. *Presence Teleop Virt Environ*, **7**, 225–240.

World Health Organization. (2001). *International Classification of Functioning Disability and Health (ICF)*, World Health Organization, Geneva.

Yu, W. and Brewster, S.A. (2002). Multimodal virtual reality versus printed medium in visualization for blind people. *Proceedings of the Fifth International ACM Conference on Assistive Technologies*, 57–64.

Zhang, L., Abreu, B.C., Masel, B., Scheibel, R.S., Christiansen, C.H., Huddleston, N. and Ottenbacher, K.J. (2001). Virtual reality in the assessment of selected cognitive function after brain injury. *Am J Phys Med Rehabil*, **80**, 597–604.

14

Communication devices

Cheryl Y. Trepagnier[1], Beth Mineo Mollica[2], Sheela Stuart[3] and Carole W. Brown[4]

[1]Department of Psychology, The Catholic University of America, Washington, DC, USA; [2]Center for Applied Science and Engineering and Department of Linguistics, University of Delaware, Newark, Delaware, USA; [3]Children's Hearing and Speech Center, Neurobehavioral Sciences Department, Children's National Medical Center, Washington, DC, USA and [4]Department of Education, The Catholic University of America, Washington, DC, USA

14.1 Introduction

Among the most disabling impairments in patients with neural injuries are those affecting communication. Fortunately, advances in the technology of communication devices and communication training have greatly expanded the proportion of affected individuals who can reacquire the ability to communicate. Even when residual motor control is very limited, or when there are sensory impairments or parasite movements, technology exists to translate something that the would-be communicator can comfortably do into a means of operating a communication device (e.g., Gragnani, 1990; Gryfe, 1996; Kubota et al., 2000; Perring et al., 2003). Techniques also exist to help most persons with cognitive, language or behavioral challenges to enhance their level of participation and control (Trepagnier, 1996; Gorman et al., 2003). Nor is cost a major barrier, since devices and techniques to support communication are generally affordable, and third-party reimbursement has become increasingly available (Smith, 1998; Higdon, 2002).

Communication devices can make an important difference in the quality of life of people affected by disorders that result in impaired speech or writing (Tolley et al., 1995; Diener and Bischof-Rosarioz, 2004). Youngsters with severe movement disorder from cerebral palsy can pursue educational and career goals (McNaughton and Bryen, 2002). Patients with amyotrophic lateral sclerosis (ALS or Lou Gehrig's disease) can continue to communicate with their family, friends and colleagues when they can no longer speak (Doyle and Phillips, 2001). Patients in critical care need not be deprived of a means of interaction with their family members and care providers (Happ, 2001). People with significant core language impairments coupled with severe developmental disabilities can interact socially, communicate preferences, express feelings and conduct their own lives with the help of carefully selected augmentative techniques (Trepagnier, 1996; Happ, 2001; Hadjistavropoulos et al., 2001). There are also devices to facilitate computer access for individuals who have impaired ability to write or keyboard, for example persons with high-level spinal cord injury that reduces their upper limb control (Hurlburt and Ottenbacher, 1992). Finally, very young children for whom development of speech and/or language are at risk can gain a foothold in the communicative world, become active rather than passive agents, and begin to progress in social and communicative skills (Cress and Marvin, 2003).

It is not only possible, but vital, for people across the lifespan to gain the capacity to interact effectively with the people around them. Neither cognitive disabilities, nor absence of literacy skills, nor very young or old age, nor the temporary nature of the impairment, nor being on school vacation, is sufficient justification for any individual to be deprived of a means of communication. Unawareness of the fact that there are means to support communication by people with severe impairments is also not an acceptable justification. The more that healthcare providers, educators, consumers, family members and the general public know about supports for people with severe communication impairments, the more apt they will be to identify the need when it is present, and recognize that it can be addressed.

The people who will communicate with the device-using individual, and everyone who exerts influence on the communication context, are important to the success of the aided communication. This includes the individual's family, friends and colleagues, as well as educators and human services and healthcare providers (Granlund et al., 2001). In order to select the most useful techniques, the individual's needs and abilities, the characteristics of the living and working context, and the symptomatology and prognosis of the disabling condition all need to be taken into account. The physician's information regarding expected disease course will affect the selection of control modalities. The family's awareness of the individual's activities and communication partners will be important in deciding on the particular features the techniques will need to incorporate. Once the devices and techniques are acquired, conversation partners will need to modify their interactive style in order to foster participation by device-users (Russel, 1984).

The growing body of knowledge and clinical experience related to supporting communication by means of assistive devices and techniques is known as "augmentative and alternative communication", or, for (relative) brevity, "augmentative communication" or "AAC" (Beukelman and Mirenda, 1998). The people served are often referred to as "augmentative communicators", and will be referred to here, for convenience, as "communicators". The challenge of evaluating the potential communicator's needs and putting together an optimal means of addressing them is complex. Accordingly it is very important to involve someone with depth and breadth of experience and up-to-date knowledge in the AAC domain. While AAC specialists may come from occupational therapy, rehabilitation engineering, or other professions, it is necessary to obtain an evaluation and recommendation from a speech-language pathologist (an SLP) in order to acquire funding for purchase of a device. Ideally, a speech pathologist who is experienced in AAC will be the one to provide the overall guidance of the process of assessment,

recommendations and integration of the techniques into the communicator's daily life. The SLP may work with other health professionals, such as an occupational or physical therapist and/or a rehabilitation engineer, to resolve questions of seating and positioning for maximum stability and function (Goossens' et al., 1989; McEwen and Karlan, 1990), and to identify the best control options within the individual's repertoire. The SLP will also be concerned with communicators' cognitive and language status, their goals and the contexts in which they will be participating (Beukelman and Ball, 2002). It is of particular importance that whoever manages the evaluation process be independent. Just as one would not ask a salesperson at a General Motors dealership for advice on what make of car to purchase, it is wise to obtain evaluation and recommendation services from professionals who have no financial connection with a particular device manufacturer.

Unfortunately, there is no central registry of AAC specialists. The family member, educator or healthcare provider seeking these services needs to review the human and information resources available in order to meet the communicator's needs as effectively as possible. The community is often a good information source, including associations of individuals with the same disabling condition. Appendix 1 lists some additional resources.

Once recommendations have been made, the communicator may wish to "test-drive" a potential purchase. Manufacturers' representatives can be of great help at this point, as they may be able to arrange for a loaner device, and can provide the necessary technical support for getting started. Manufacturers can also help navigate funding issues, as they have acquired considerable experience in dealing with third-party payers. The best route to obtaining financial help with purchase of communication supports may depend on the individual's circumstances; for example, the school system may provide devices for school-aged children and adolescents, and the state vocational rehabilitation system may be a source of funding for people who wish to work (Smith, 1998).

Simply acquiring a communication device does not in itself equip the individual to be a competent communicator. Training is needed for communicators and for their frequent communication partners. The communicator and family members may need help with technical aspects of device operation, for example, how to maintain calibration when using a device operated by direction of gaze. Training of this type is usually provided by the manufacturer's representatives Parents and teachers may be offered guidance for using the device to support development of a child's language and communication, generally by an SLP or educational specialist (Pebly and Koppenhaver, 2001). It is, unfortunately, difficult to obtain funding to support training, and the gap is often filled by manufacturers' representatives. Of necessity, the cost of this service will already have been folded into the purchase price of the device.

14.2 Control and display

There are many kinds of actions that can be sensed and converted into the equivalent of a switch closure or a computer keystroke. Similarly, there are many types of effects that a switch closure, keystroke or equivalent can produce. Control input, on the one hand, and output, on the other, can be wholly independent of each other. Control inputs can range from tongue contact with switches to a "sip-and-puff" switch; from an eye-blink, as illustrated in Fig. 14.1, to changes in direction of gaze sensed by an infrared eye tracking system; from hitting a large, robust switch by extending a limb or inclining the head, to almost imperceptibly contracting a muscle in the forearm or slightly raising an eyebrow (Soderholm et al., 2001). There are switches that require sustained force, so that accidental bumping would not close them; and there are switches that require no force at all, merely contact. Some individuals with aphasic impairments of written expression have been able to use their residual speech as a control mode, by means of mass-market speech recognition software. Even dysarthric speech can be a viable control option in some cases (Goodenough-Trepagnier et al., 1992; Bruce et al.,

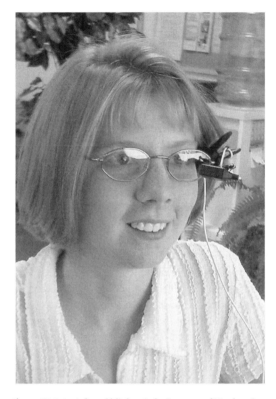

Figure 14.1. An infrared blink switch. Courtesy of Words + Inc. www.words-plus.com

2003; Havstam et al., 2003). Control parameter values may be adjustable to fit the communicator's abilities.

Output is seldom, any longer, robotic-sounding synthetic speech. That has been replaced in most devices either by digitally recordable and re-recordable spoken messages, or by sophisticated text-to-speech software and a variety of more natural-sounding artificial voices, so that the communicator can choose an age- and gender-appropriate one. Of course the output of a computerized device need not be limited to just speech and/or text. Communication may be directed not only to persons in the immediate environment, but also to persons who will receive the communication at a future date, or who are a few miles or a continent away, or it may go out to untold numbers of people who access a web site. People also communicate with electronic and computer-aided devices, in order to control electrical devices in their environment, listen to music, edit photos, shop, seek information, manage finances, play games or take courses, and they will undoubtedly use computers in the near future to carry out other activities that most of us have not yet imagined. The individual with communicative impairment needs access to these capabilities as least as much as, if not more than, people who do not have deficits in motor control, language or cognition.

It can be helpful to think of AAC techniques and devices in terms of three categories. There are techniques that do not require any props, and techniques that involve non-electronic ones. These are sometimes called "no-tech" and "low-tech", respectively. Finally, there are electronic devices, which have for the most part come to involve computers of one type or another, and are sometimes referred to as "hi-tech". It is a misperception that devices that incorporate technology inevitably entail complexity for the people who will use these devices. Difficulty of learning or use is in most cases an indication of poor design or, at the least, poor fit to the consumer's abilities (Norman, 1993; Goodenough-Trepagnier, 1994; Norman, 2002).

In no-tech scanning, the conversation partner not only speaks both parts of the conversation, but also plays the role that a device would fulfill, for example by reciting the alphabet until the communicator indicates which letter is intended, perhaps by a facial movement or eye movement. Signs (borrowed from American Sign Language, the native language of many deaf people in this country) are another no-tech method. They have been useful for some hearing, language-impaired communicators with mental retardation, autism, or both, and can be used in combination with speech (Konstantareas, 1987). There is some evidence that using gesture at the same time as speech is helpful to the speaker (Clibbens, 2001).

In the domain of "low-tech", there are language boards that offer letters, chunks of words, whole words and messages. These are represented by regular or phonetically adapted spelling, pictures and/or symbols of various types (Goodenough-Trepagnier and Prather, 1981; Goodenough-Trepagnier et al., 1982; Musselwhite and Ruscello, 1984). Low-tech

and no-tech have in common that there is no explicit output entirely under the communicator's control. Instead, communication depends on the conversation partner. These methods can be highly effective in many circumstances, and are indeed preferred in some (Doyle and Phillips, 2001). The language board never runs out of batteries. While a device may get left behind, a no-tech method is always available, as long as a knowledgeable communication partner is present, and it can offer greater privacy and intimacy within a conversation dyad. With a skilled familiar conversation partner, these techniques provide more rapid spontaneous communication than current devices, because the familiar partner can use special knowledge of the communicator and the context to guess ahead. At the same time, only an electronic device offers independent communication. Whatever the technique, there are advantages and disadvantages to be considered in the context of individual communicators and their activities and communication partners, and it is often the case that more than one technique is needed.

14.3 Communicative needs of particular clinical populations

Just as devices can be categorized, device-users are often considered in terms of the disability that is at the root of their need for communication support. This is a useful starting point; at the same time, however, it is important to recognize the diversity within any clinical category. A device that proves helpful for one individual with autism, or for one adult with acquired neuromotor impairment, may be wholly unsuitable for others who happen to share the same diagnostic labels. With this caveat, the following portion of the chapter will point out considerations that are often of special concern for particular disability groups.

Individuals with motor impairment

An adult who can no longer speak intelligibly, a young adult with brain injury that impairs speech and makes new learning difficult, and a young student with severe cerebral palsy who has acquired basic literacy skills are some of the people to whom this category applies. Since these are largely people who do not have serious problems understanding language, the problem that shows up here in particularly stark relief is the issue of impoverished communication rate, a drawback that is common across all AAC. While English speakers may converse at rates of 200 and even more words per minute, most users of augmentative devices require as much as 3 minutes and others may take longer still, to produce half a dozen words of real-time output. Despite many ingenious attempts to improve this situation, the problem remains a major stumbling block to the successful integration of augmentative communicators in conversation, education and employment.

Communicators whose impairment is primarily motor in nature need a communication device with which they can express whatever message they intend. This requires combining the sounds of speech, generally by means of the rather complex way of representing speech sounds that standard English spelling provides. Spelling of individual words does not preclude use of software techniques, sometimes implemented in mass-market computers, as illustrated in Fig. 14.2, intended to accelerate and support communication. One such technique is "prediction", by means of which the software anticipates intended words based on letters already typed. With expertise, prediction becomes equivalent to a practised shorthand, and the communicator does not need to exert as much effort. Another approach, of which there are numerous variants, is to compose phrases in advance and store them for quick retrieval. Entire jokes or speeches, one's phone number, a phrase that will capture the listener's attention while a novel message is slowly composed (a "floorholder") or a slogan in support of a favorite team may be stored whole on the device. Retrieval of such pre-constructed messages usually involves some variant of a shift-key strategy. For example, instead of just hitting the "h" key (to produce the letter "h"), the user might first hit a designated shift key (usually called a "level" key, or part of a code) and

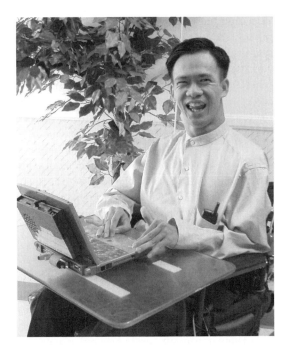

Figure 14.2. Using an orthographical system implemented on a laptop computer. Courtesy of Words + Inc. www. words-plus.com

then the "h," to call up a message that had been constructed in advance. However, if the communicator cannot accomplish the precise verbal task she or he wishes to carry out, the ability to interject "How about them Redsox" at the socially appropriate moment does not suffice (Bedrosian et al., 2003), and communicators whose device does not provide easy access to a spelling mode of some type, or who do not have the skills to utilize spelling, are at a disadvantage.

Usability is important in all cases. Communicators with preserved cognitive and language skills rightfully expect to be able to utilize their device right from the start. While it is to be expected that one would make gains in skill and speed with experience, no communicator should be required to spend a long period as a trainee, as a prerequisite to effective use of a communication device.

As is the case for any group, whether it is a question of augmentative devices, glasses or orthopedic shoes, individual preference and acceptance is key.

The potentially most useful device will not do much good if the individual does not wish to use it, and a given individual may, for a number of reasons, prefer to use speech, however difficult it is to understand, rather than resort to the more intelligible channel offered by augmentative technology.

Young children with cerebral palsy

In the first years of life, typically-developing children use their oral mechanisms to engage in sound play, begin to produce words at around the time of their first birthday, and progress to word combination by 18 months of age. Typically-developing children's intensive vocal exploration is not available to children with significant physical limitations, who are unable to orchestrate the complex movements of the articulators needed to create differentiated word forms and build a basic expressive vocabulary. Absence of intelligible speech often has the secondary effect of relegating children with significant speech and physical impairments (SSPI) to a passive role in social interaction (see Volume II, Chapter 39). As a result of the direct and second-order effects of their deficit, young children with SSPI may experience their prime language-development years in a suboptimal manner, and accrue impairments in development of grammar, phonological awareness and metalinguistic skills that will undermine their literacy development (Wagner and Torgesen, 1987). To these individuals' deficits in mobility and opportunities to engage with their environment are added, then, the additional limitations of reading and writing impairments (Berninger and Gans, 1986; Koppenhaver and Yoder, 1992).

While comparable studies of individuals with motor limitations have not been carried out, the consequences of delay and suboptimality of exposure to language and communication experienced by deaf infants, and their amenability to intervention, may be instructive here. Delayed access to language, as happens with deaf infants who are not taught sign, or whose early exposure to sign is sporadic, has been found to result in language impairments and failure to acquire "native-speaker" level skills (whether in signed or oral language) (Mayberry and Eichen, 1991). Long-term effects on the representation of language in the brain have been documented (Kral et al., 2001; Leybaert and D'Hondt, 2003), and there is evidence of negative effects on other aspects of cognitive development (Mayberry and Eichen, 1991; Woolfe et al., 2002). The unfortunate sequelae of SSPI will, it is hoped, be minimized in children now growing up, with the help of early intervention, the entitlements provided in the *Individuals with Disabilities Education Act*, the new emphasis given to literacy as a metric of schools' educational success and the implementation of novel instructional and assistive technologies, which offer new ways for children to participate and learn.

Current understanding of how language typically develops can usefully inform the facilitation of language development in children with SSPI (Gerber and Kraat, 1992). For example, children's first words tend to be about things and events in the "here and now," with nouns predominating until the vocabulary reaches about 100 words, when the proportion of actions increases (Benedict, 1979; Bates et al., 1994). Function words remain relatively infrequent until the child has passed the 400-word mark. Although there is great variability among children regarding rate of lexical acquisition, the emergence of grammar coincides with mastery of sufficient vocabulary to facilitate word combination. Children initially learn from experience and interaction how to map words to objects, actions and attributes in the environment (Pinker, 1984; Golinkoff et al., 1994). Once they have some knowledge of syntax, they can use the information derived from syntactic relationships to intuit the meaning of unfamiliar words (Gleitman, 1990; Mineo and Goldstein, 1990). Clearly, maximizing the SSPI child's opportunities for interaction and providing a means to address lexical and syntactic development are important considerations in the design of AAC interventions.

AAC can scaffold early language learning and provide the means to engage in language practice and experimentation that otherwise would be unattainable. Augmentative techniques need to be applied to acquisition of morphological and syntactic structures as well as metalinguistic awareness (Paul, 1997;

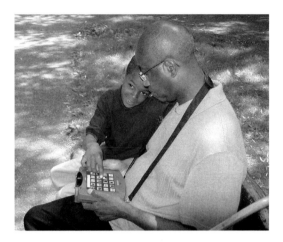

Figure 14.3. An augmented communicative interaction using a large-vocabulary graphical display on a dedicated device. Photo courtesy of DynaVox Systems LLC, Pittsburgh, PA (1-800-344-1778).

Sutton et al., 2002). Voice output may facilitate the development of phonological awareness (Blischak, 1994; Paul, 1997), an effect that might be amplified by incorporating rhyming games and other tasks designed for building phonological awareness. While parents and service providers may find it appealing to offer devices that yield complete sentences from single selections, devices that primarily offer these strategies do not provide children with expressive language experiences that parallel those of their typically-developing peers.

Severe motor impairment from cerebral palsy does not entail severe cognitive impairment. Indeed it can co-exist with superior intellectual abilities. Often training with assistive technology can enable the capacities for independent expression that will in turn make it possible to assess, and thus better serve, the child's potential. Devices that are hardened to survive everyday use, have the numerous characteristics that make them practical (including light weight, small size and long battery-life), and the flexibility and power of a computer, such as the one illustrated in Fig. 14.3, may be considered for a variety of populations, including children with impairments in motor control as well as individuals, discussed below, who also experience cognitive impairments.

Individuals with mental retardation and other developmental cognitive disabilities

Not so long ago individuals with developmental disabilities whose communicative intent was hard to discern were not offered augmentative techniques, and this population continues to be seriously underserved. In part this stems from the complexity of diagnosing and addressing communication disturbances that are secondary to cognitive deficits (Beukelman and Mirenda, 1998; Mollica, 1999). It is also the case that many existing devices and techniques are a poor fit to the needs of people with significant mental retardation. When device operation demands a disproportionate share of the user's cognitive resources, there may be little left to meet the demands of message formulation and partner engagement. There are nevertheless AAC techniques and devices available that can support expression of communicative intent, and that can help introduce to persons with severe cognitive involvement the concept of indicating their preferences and thereby gaining a desirable outcome.

It is unfortunately the case that knowledge and skill barriers still preclude many from accessing augmentative services and supports. A large number of speech language pathologists have had neither academic coursework nor practicum experience in supporting communication development and use by individuals with significant cognitive limitations. Many clinicians lack the confidence and/or expertise necessary to exploit the potential of AAC tools for maximum consumer benefit: they may not understand how to assess communication skills at a pre-intentional or emerging intentional level, or they may be unable or unwilling to explore the range of technology options available, to customize the device to meet consumer needs, and to train individuals and their circles of supports in how to operate the devices or techniques and how to utilize them in the context of real-world exchanges. Since many families are not aware that their loved ones could benefit from communication technologies, they do not become advocates for the inclusion of these services in program planning. Policy and practice barriers, too, often hinder access to communication technology by individuals with cognitive limitations (Mollica, 1998, 1999). The recent position statement of the National Joint Committee for the Communication Needs of Persons with Disabilities clarifies that reliance on a priori eligibility criteria, such as chronological age, diagnosis or the absence of cognitive or other skills purported to be prerequisites, violates recommended practice principles by precluding consideration of individual needs (National Joint Committee for the Communication Needs of Persons with Severe Disabilities, 2003). Historically, many third-party payers, such as Medicaid and school districts, have denied requests on behalf of individuals with mental retardation for communication devices, presuming that such individuals would derive only limited benefits. In practice, however, the growing body of research documenting the efficacy of AAC in enhancing both language development and use (Sevcik and Romski, 1997; Rowland and Schweigert, 2000) reinforces that such discriminatory practices are unjustified. In fact, the availability of dynamic language representations (increasingly in portable and wearable form), voice output and flexible language organization may facilitate language development and communication in ways not possible through other means such as sign language or static picture cards.

Aphasia

Aphasia is the blanket term used for the myriad speech and language disorders that can result from injury to the adult brain, typically from a cerebrovascular accident or stroke, in most cases on the left side of the brain (see Chapter 26 of Volume II). The location, extent and type of lesion, as well as time after stroke or injury, are the main factors determining the type and severity of the aphasia (Pedersen et al., 2004); and these factors, in conjunction with treatment, also affect its course (Pradat-Diehl et al., 2001; Kiran and Thompson, 2003). While gains can be achieved years after onset, in general aphasia that persists after 1 year is considered chronic. In addition to reports by neurology and rehabilitation medical specialists, it is helpful to have a thorough evaluation of expressive and receptive written and auditory language carried out by a speech language

pathologist who specializes in aphasia, and who is cognizant of therapeutic and augmentative techniques that have been of help to individuals with aphasic disorders.

Many individuals who experience aphasia in the period immediately after their stroke recover fully or recover with minor residual deficits. Residual aphasia may be as mild as a difficulty in retrieving names or other precise words in as timely a fashion as one would like. At the other extreme is chronic severe "global" aphasia. Individuals with aphasia of this type can make little sense of what people say to them and their attempts to speak may yield only a couple or at best a few "frozen phrases". Written language, for reading or writing, is also globally impaired in these severe cases. In between the extremes there is a broad range that is not linear. Some individuals may have specific impairments in the context of an otherwise high level of preserved language ability. Others may have some preserved skills that are the more remarkable compared with the severity of their overall level of language impairment. Persons with relatively preserved speech but impaired writing may be able to use augmentative technology in the form of speech recognition, to accomplish writing tasks (Wade et al., 2001; Bruce et al., 2003). Similarly, someone with severely limited speech may be able to convey specific words by pointing to words on a list. Augmentative approaches must accordingly be tailored to their users' profile of preserved and impaired abilities. If the ability to recall the initial letters of words, or subcategories of words, such as names or common nouns, is preserved, it can be a helpful component of a communication system, and visual support may help some individuals with aphasia to engage in conversation and transmit information (Goodenough-Trepagnier, 1995; Linebarger et al., 2000; Linebarger Schwartz et al., 2001; Garrett and Huth, 2002). While computerized systems that enable users to select and string together pictures standing for concepts are useful for some individuals with aphasia both for communication and as therapy (Weinrich, 1995), persons with global language impairment may not be able to relate spatial order of pictures or words to grammatical function, and may be unable to assign verb and preposition meanings to graphical representations at all (Goodenough-Trepagnier, 1989; Shelton et al., 1996).

Unlike individuals with congenital disabilities, who have not had the benefit of typical socialization, many individuals with aphasia retain the ability to read social situations and extract information from non-language cues. Directional skills are also generally retained, such that someone may be an effective navigator without, however, being able to provide verbal directions. Preserved social and spatial abilities may be put to use for communication via gestures, mime and drawing, which are helpful for some individuals, and can improve with training (Sacchett et al., 1999). While it is possible that a communication device designed for an adult with acquired neuromotor disability, or a device developed for young children with cerebral palsy, could be useful for someone with aphasia, that can in no way be assumed. It should also be remembered that unlike the primarily motor-impaired population, many people with aphasic communication difficulties are ambulatory and some may continue to drive a personal vehicle. Accordingly, the range of contexts in which they might benefit from communicative supports can be large, and the need for a repertoire of techniques in keeping with the demands of different situations should be considered (Cress and King, 1999). As with other populations who use augmentative techniques, conversation partners can take steps to improve communicators' participation, with the help of appropriate training (Rayner and Marshall, 2003). A speech-language therapist specializing in aphasia, and who is also familiar with AAC techniques, can be of great help in this regard.

Autism

Autism is a lifelong disability with complex genetic origins (Folstein and Rosen-Sheidley, 2001) whose signal feature is a profound disturbance of social relations (Wing, 1976; Volkmar, 1987). The beginning of modern understanding of autism dates back to the mid-20th century (Kanner, 1943; Rimland, 1964). Scientific study of this spectrum of disorders began to gather momentum as general agreement was reached on diagnostic criteria around 1994 (American Psychiatric Association, 1994). The pace of autism-related research has increased rapidly in recent years, and has yielded improved methods of detection and intervention that can make a major difference in the individual's potential to live a satisfying life (Eikeseth et al., 2002). There is, however, no cure. It is estimated that as many as half of people with autism do not develop speech that is adequate to meet their communication needs (Sigman and Capps, 1997), and language impairment, in addition to the evident pragmatics deficits (Wing and Atwood, 1987; Beukelman and Mirenda, 1998), is present to some degree in most individuals on the spectrum (Rapin and Dunn, 2003). About 70% have mental retardation (La Malfa et al., 2004). While there are movement and motor control anomalies associated with autism, these are minor in relation to the overall picture of profound deficits. Motor impairments do not limit the AAC options for most people with autism, and indeed the fact that these individuals are almost all ambulatory and that many children are especially active puts its own sorts of constraints on augmentative choices.

Despite their mobility, children with autism share with SSPI children a key secondary consequence of their disability: exclusion from communicative interaction. Their limited and idiosyncratic social and communicative repertoire results in their failing to participate in most of the play-based learning in which typically-developing children constantly engage. Children with autism who have not developed speech are not only verbally impaired, they are also profoundly impaired in understanding nonverbal communication: how to interpret the facial expressions, directions of gaze, tones of voice and gestures of the people around them (Trepagnier, 1996). Children whose speech is not emerging at the expected time need augmentative support in order to begin to gain social interaction experience, and to support efforts to foster their language development.

Many people with autism demonstrate strengths in the area of visuo-spatial and visual memory skills, and clinicians and investigators have long advocated multimodal, and especially visual, support for communication, as is frequently used in the TEAACH program (Mesibov, 1995; Helms Tillery et al., 2003). The descriptively-named Picture Exchange Communication System or PECS, (Bondy and Frost, 2001) makes use of the autistic child's mobility to build interaction into the use of the technique, and there is some evidence that its use can have beneficial effects on the child's development (Bondy and Frost, 1995; Charlop-Christy et al., 2002). Printed materials too can appeal even to very young communicatively-impaired children with autism, with positive effects on development of literacy skills (Koppenhaver, 2003). Literacy is important, as it is to any individual, and the more important if speech impairment is severe, since it opens the door to spelling-based communication. Families of children with autism face a myriad of divergent information. They must make life-affecting decisions on the basis of woefully inadequate information, both in regard to the education, management and treatment of their child and in regard to the particular issues involved in communication support. The desperate nature of the problem and the paucity of research have combined to create a vacuum into which many unsubstantiated "treatments" have flowed. Recommended guidelines for augmentative support, similar to the guidelines for autism treatment in general (Simeonsson et al., 1987; Dawson and Osterling, 1997), include intensive intervention that begins as early as possible, involves the family, and pays special attention to generalization across partners and settings (Beukelman and Mirenda, 1998).

14.4 Ongoing and emerging issues

Unmet needs

Communication rate: As noted above, communicating by means of augmentative techniques is terribly slow relative to speech. While the disparity is perhaps most acutely felt by individuals who have had to turn to AAC because of the deterioration of their own motor capabilities, it is a problem for anyone who is attempting to join the flow of human social and communicative interaction by means of a communication device (Goodenough-Trepagnier et al., 1984; Todman and Rzepecka, 2003). This is, of course, the reason for storing pre-constructed messages, since such messages can, in principle, be produced at a normal conversational rate. Investigators have developed numerous strategies for accelerating communication; these have included populating the device's vocabulary, or "selection set" with items chosen for their frequency of occurrence in combination with each other (Goodenough-Trepagnier and Prather, 1981; Goodenough-Trepagnier et al., 1982); using transitional probabilities of letters to "guess" the word once an initial letter or letters have been entered (Koester and Levine, 1994; Hunnicutt, 2001); using multi-letter keys such that the software "disambiguates" by referring to transitional probabilities and a dictionary look-up (Minneman, 1985) and a variety of attempts at mnemonic storage and retrieval schemes. Besides choosing *what* items should be offered in the device's "selection set", attention is also given to *where* they should be placed, in order to make operation of the device as easy and rapid as possible (Levine and Goodenough-Trepagnier, 1990). Whatever the technique, the inherent flaw remains, that communicators are being asked to use their residual, often impaired, motor control to compensate for their motor speech impairment. The challenge of finding some way around this problem in order to achieve responsive communication at conversationally acceptable rates still stands.

Mental load: The additional cognitive demands that device operation places on the communicator are a problem not only for people with cognitive disabilities but for all augmentative users. A useful analogy might be that of speaking a language one does not know very well. It is not difficult to imagine that passing an interview, meeting a new colleague or communicating in an emotionally fraught interaction would be all the more difficult if one had to do so using a language one does not know well. Investigators recognize and are striving to address the need to minimize demands on working memory and attention, so that the augmentative technique can become "second nature" to the communicator (Goodenough-Trepagnier, 1994; Hunnicutt, 2001).

Lifelong use: In the communication history of most children and adults with persistent severe speech impairment, there are stages: first augmentative systems tend to be picture-based, and later ones alphabet-based, with possibly intervening stages using symbols and combinations of all three. To use again the analogy of second language, it is as if the child's education were begun in Chinese, which was then supplanted by Japanese and later still by English. Non-disabled keyboard users have resisted the relatively minor alteration of replacing the QWERTY keyboard arrangement (designed to prevent tangling the typewriter's keys) with the potentially more rapid Dvorak system. Unlearning is undesirable. Yet children with severe communication disorders are as a matter of standard practice asked to give up their communication techniques to move on to techniques that are presumed to be better. Indeed it is the case that the individual who can use written language should have the opportunity to do so, since it is so much more powerful and economical than pictures. The challenge here, then, is to meet the need for conversational rate and transparency and add to it the goal of continuity: devise a way to meet the child's need for more powerful communication and at the same time reduce and ideally obviate the need to learn and then give up earlier, less ultimately useful techniques. This goal also implies providing more powerful and effective communication media for the earliest stages of communicative life, a challenge that is perhaps the area of greatest need, since our failure to meet it deprives the individual of developmental opportunities that will not recur.

Mind over matter

It is conceivable that by the time these words are published there will be a communication device on the market that the communicator can operate by means of electrical events in his or her own brain. At present several groups of investigators around the world are pursuing this goal, as Wolpaw and colleagues (Wolpaw et al., 2002) describe. This work encompasses several different types of brain signals, including evoked potentials in response to the appearance of significant events (e.g., the illumination of an intended letter on a letter matrix); and brain rhythms that change as a function of preparation for movement. Typically, the brain activity of interest is sensed by electrodes in contact with the communicator's scalp. Since the electrodes receive innumerable signals simultaneously, signal processing is required to extract the pertinent information. The limiting factor here is not computing power and speed: the signal processing is carried out in real time. Not surprisingly, it is the interface of the user to the device that continues to be problematic. In virtually all current brain interfaces, control is by means of a two-state switch, adequate only for scanning of some kind, a far from satisfactory means of device operation. Even this level of capability can entail large amounts of training. Furthermore, despite the training, some individuals, including individuals who are not disabled, are unsuccessful. Questions remain as to the extent to which individuals with movement disorders of various types would be capable of controlling signals from somatosensory areas of the brain. It may be that combining information about the type of signal with information about the time relationship between device events and brain events (Schalk et al., 2000) will bring added power to this intriguing interface approach. While at present there are usually more easily acquired techniques with similar power to which a person with severe motor disability can have recourse, recent animal work, in which trained monkeys have rapidly attained the ability to control events on a monitor using a brain interface, strongly suggest that we will have significantly improved interfaces to offer to people with disabilities in the not-too-distant future (Wolpaw et al., 2000; Helms Tillery et al., 2003).

14.5 Conclusion

Recognition of the human right to communication and the many ways in which communication can be supported, whatever the nature of the individual's profile of abilities and deficits, continues to spread rather gradually through the community of health-care providers, human service workers and educators, and even more slowly among the general public. This is troubling because it means that there are children who are losing precious years of communicative, social and intellectual development that they will not recoup, children learning to be helpless or resorting to disruptive behaviors for want of a more effective communication modality, bright minds frustrated by the lack of a way to convey their thoughts and individuals experiencing needless isolation during periods of illness. There is no doubt that effort must be directed to increasing professional and public awareness of AAC.

It must also be recognized that there are knowledge gaps in the AAC "field". The field is relatively new, eclectic and not as well anchored in evidence as we would wish. The problem is compounded by the fact that many health professionals have had little experience with this domain, and little or no formal training. This situation will undoubtedly improve. Consumers and family members will, however, for some time to come, need to exercise careful judgment, whether networking with other affected families, consulting with specialists or trying out products. One of the most useful things an advocate can do is to spend time interacting with other consumers who have similar capabilities and needs, to see how they fare with their AAC supports. Another is to ask questions, and not to be content with unsatisfying answers.

Communication devices can contribute in major ways to the well-being of members of society who would otherwise be virtual prisoners in their own bodies. It could contribute considerably more, and may do so in the near future, in order to enable these citizens to express their full cognitive, social and emotional potential.

REFERENCES

American Psychiatric Association (1994). *Diagnostic and Statistical Manual of Mental Disorders*, Washington, DC, Author.

Bates, E., Marchman, V., et al. (1994). Developmental and stylistic variation in the composition of early vocabulary. *J Child Lang*, **21**(**85–124**).

Bedrosian, J.L., Hoag, L.A., et al. (2003). Relevance and speed of message delivery trade-offs in augmentative communication. *J Speech Lang Hear Res*, **46**(**4**), 800–817.

Benedict, H. (1979). Early lexical development: comprehension and production. *J Child Lang*, **6**, 183–200.

Berninger, V. and Gans, B. (1986). Language profiles of non-speaking individuals of normal intelligence with severe cerebral palsy. *Augment Alternat Commun* (**2**), 45–50.

Beukelman, D.R. and Ball, L.J. (2002). Improving AAC use for persons with acquired neurogenic disorders: understanding human and engineering factors. *Assist Technol*, **14**(**1**), 33–44.

Beukelman, D.R. and Mirenda, P. (1998). AAC for individuals with developmental disabilities. In: *Augmentative and Alternative Communication Management of Severe Communication Disorders in Children and Adults* (eds Beukelman, D.R., Mirenda, P.), Paul H. Brookes Publishing Co, Baltimore, MD, pp. 252–258.

Beukelman, D.R. and Mirenda, P. (1998). *Augmentative and Alternative Communication: Management of Severe Communication Disorders in Children and Adults*, Paul H. Brookes, Baltimore, MD.

Blischak, D. (1994). Phonologic awareness: implications for individuals with little or no functional speech. *Augment Alternat Commun* (**10**), 145–154.

Bondy, A. and Frost, L. (1995). Educational approaches in pre-school: behavior techniques in a public school setting. In: *Learning and Cognition in Autism* (eds Schopler, E. and Mesibov, G.), Plenum Press, New York, pp. 311–333.

Bondy, A. and Frost, L. (2001). The picture exchange communication system. *Behav Modif*, **25**(**5**), 725–744.

Bruce, C., Edmundson, A., et al. (2003). Writing with voice: an investigation of the use of a voice reproduction system as a writing aid for a man with aphasia. *Int J Lang Commun Disorders*, **38**(**2**), 131–148.

Charlop-Christy, M.H., Carpenter, M., et al. (2002). Using the picture exchange communication system (PECS) with children with autism: assessment of PECS acquisition, speech, social-communicative behavior, and problem behavior. *J Appl Behav Anal*, **35**(**3**), 213–231.

Clibbens, J. (2001). Signing and lexical development in children with Down syndrome. *Downs Syndrome Res Pract*, **7**(**3**), 101–105.

Cress, C.J. and King, J.M. (1999). AAC strategies for people with primary progressive aphasia without dementia: two case studies. *Augment Alternat Commun*, **15**(**4**), 248–259.

Cress, C.J. and Marvin, C.A. (2003). Common questions about AAC services in early intervention. *Augment Alternat Commun*, **19**(**4**), 254–272.

Dawson, G. and Osterling, J. (1997). Early intervention in autism. In: *The Effectiveness of Early Intervention* (ed. Guralnick, M.J.), Paul H. Brookes Publishing Co, Baltimore, MD, pp. 307–326.

Diener, B. and Bischof-Rosarioz, J. (2004). Determining decision-making capacity in individuals with severe communication impairments after stroke: the role of augmentative-alternative communication (AAC). *Topics Stroke Rehabil*, **11**(**1**), 84–88.

Doyle, M. and Phillips, B. (2001). Trends in augmentative and alternative communication use by individuals with amyotrophic lateral sclerosis. *Augment Alternat Commun*, **17**(**3**), 167–178.

Eikeseth, S., Smith, T., et al. (2002). Intensive behavioral treatment at school for 4- to 7-year-old children with autism. A 1-year comparison controlled study. *Behav Modif*, **26**(**1**), 49–68.

Folstein, S.E. and Rosen-Sheidley, B. (2001). Genetics of autism: complex aetiology for a heterogeneous disorder. *Nat Rev Genet*, **2**(**12**), 943–955.

Garrett, K.L. and Huth, C. (2002). The impact of graphic contextual information and instruction on the conversational behaviours of a person with severe aphasia. *Aphasiology*, **16**(**4–6**), 523–536.

Gerber, S. and Kraat, A. (1992). Use of a developmental model of language acquisition: applications to children using AAC systems. *Augment Alternat Commun*, **8**, 19–33.

Gleitman, L. (1990). The structural sources of verb meaning. *Lang Acquisit J Develop Linguist*, **1**, 3–55.

Golinkoff, R.M., Mervis, C.B., et al. (1994). Early object labels: the case for a developmental lexical principles framework. *J Child Lang*, **21**, 125–156.

Goodenough-Trepagnier, C. (1989). Computer interface for severe language disability. In: *Designing and Using Human Computer Interfaces and Knowledge Based Systems* (ed. Smith, G.S.M.J.), Elsevier Science Publishers, Amsterdam, pp. 420–427.

Goodenough-Trepagnier, C. (1994). Design goals for augmentative communication devices. *Assist Technol*, **6**(**1**), 3–9.

Goodenough-Trepagnier, C. (1995). Visual analog communication: an avenue of investigation and rehabilitation of severe aphasia. *Aphasiology*, **9**(**4**), 321–341.

Goodenough-Trepagnier, C., Galdieri, B., et al. (1984). *Slow message production rate and receivers' impatience*. Second International Conference on Rehabilitation Engineering, Ottawa, Canada, Rehabilitation Engineering Society of North America.

Goodenough-Trepagnier, C., Hochheiser, H., et al. (1992). Assessment of dysarthic speech for computer control using speech recognition: preliminary results. *RESNA International 1992*, RESNA Press, Toronto, Canada.

Goodenough-Trepagnier, C. and Prather, P. (1981). Communication systems for the nonvocal based on frequent phoneme sequences. *J Speech Lang Hearing Res*, **24**, 322–329.

Goodenough-Trepagnier, C., Tarry, E., et al. (1982). Derivation of an efficient nonvocal communication system. *Hum Factors*, **24**(**2**), 163–172.

Goossens' C., et al. (1989). Aided communication intervention before assessment: a case study of a child with cerebral palsy. *Augment Alternat Commun*, **5**(**1**), 14–26.

Gorman, P., Dayle, R., et al. (2003). Effectiveness of the ISAAC cognitive prosthetic system for improving rehabilitation outcomes with neurofunctional impairment. *Neurorehabilitation*, **18**(**1**), 57–67.

Gragnani, J.A. (1990). A lighted joystick control for a quadriparetic child with impaired visual awareness. *Archiv Phys Med Rehabil*, **71**(**9**), 709–710.

Granlund, M., Bjorck-Akesson, E., et al. (2001). Working with families to introduce augmentative and alternative communication systems. In: *Communicating Without Speech: Practical Augmentative and Alternative Communication. Clinics in Development Medicine* (eds Cockerill, H.E.C.-F. and Lesley), Cambridge University Press, New York, pp. 88–102.

Gryfe, P.K.I., Gutmann, M., et al. (1996). Freedom through a single switch: coping and communicating with artificial ventilation. *J Neurol Sci*, **139**(**Suppl.**), 132–133.

Hadjistavopoulos, T., von Baeyer, C., et al. (2001). Pain assessment in persons with limited ability to communicate. In: *Handbook of Pain Assessment* (eds Turk, D.C. and Melzack, R.), Guilford Press, New York, pp. 134–149.

Happ, M.B. (2001). Communicating with mechanically ventilated patients: state of the science. *AACN Clin Issues*, **12**(**2**), 247–258.

Havstam, C., Buchholz, M., et al. (2003). Speech recognition and dysarthria: a single subject study of two individuals with profound impairment of speech and motor control. *Logoped Phoniatr Vocol*, **28**(**2**), 81–90.

Helms Tillery, S.I., Taylor, D.M. et al. (2003). Training in cortical control of neuroprosthetic devices improves signal extraction from small neuronal ensembles. *Rev Neurosci*, **14**(**1–2**), 107–119.

Higdon, C.W. (2002). The medicare payment process for AAC devices. *RESNA News*.

Hunnicutt, S. and Johan, C. (2001). Improving word prediction using Markov models and heuristic methods. *Augment Alternat Commun*, **17**(**4**), 255–264.

Hurlburt, M. and Ottenbacher, K. (1992). An examination of direct selection typing rate and accuracy for persons with high-level spinal cord injury using QWERTY and default on-screen keyboards. *J Rehabil Res Develop*, **29**(4), 54–63.

Kanner, L. (1943). Autistic disturbances of affective contact. *Nerv Child*, **3**, 217–250.

Kiran, S. and Thompson, C. (2003). The role of semantic complexity in treatment of naming deficits: training semantic categories in fluent aphasia by controlling exemplar typicality. *J Speech Lang Hearing Res*, **46**(3), 608–622.

Koester, H. and Levine, S. (1994). Learning and performance of able-bodied individuals using scanning systems with and without word prediction. *Assist Technol*, **6**(1), 42–53.

Konstantareas, M.M. (1987). Autistic children exposed to simultaneous communication training: a follow-up. *J Autism Develop Disorders*, **17**(1), 115–131.

Koppenhaver, D. and Yoder, D. (1992). Literacy issues in persons with severe physical and speech impairments. In: *Issues and Research in Special Education* (ed. Gaylord-Ross, R.), Vol. 2, Teacher's College Press, New York, NY, pp. 156–201.

Koppenhaver, D.A.E. and Karen, A. (2003). Natural emergent literacy supports for preschoolers with Autism and severe communication impairments. *Topics Lang Disorders*, **23**(4), 283–292.

Kral, A., Hartmann, R., et al. (2001). Delayed maturation and sensitive periods in the auditory cortex. *Audiol Neuro-Otol*, **6**(6), 346–362.

Kubota, M., Sakahira, Y., et al. (2000). New ocular movement detector system as a communication tool in ventilator-assisted Werdnig–Hoffmann disease. *Develop Med Child Neurol*, **42**(1), 61–64.

La Malfa, G., Lassi, S., et al. (2004). Autism and intellectual disability: a study of prevalence on a sample of the Italian population. *J Intellect Disabil Res*, **48**(Pt 3), 262–267.

Levine, S.H. and Goodenough-Trepagnier, C. (1990). Customized text-entry devices for motor-impaired users. *Appl Ergonom*, **23**(1), 55–62.

Leybaert, J. and D'Hondt. (2003). Neurolinguistic development in deaf children: the effect of early language experience. *Int J Audiol*, **42**(Suppl. 1:S), 34–40.

Linebarger, M.C., Schwartz, M.F., et al. (2000). Grammatical encoding in aphasia: evidence from a "processing prosthesis". *Brain Lang*, **75**(3), 416–427.

Linebarger, M.L., Schwartz, M.F., et al. (2001). Computer-based training of language production: an exploratory study. *Neuropsychol Rehabil*, **11**(1), 57–96.

Mayberry, R.I. and Eichen, E.B., (1991). The long-lasting advantage of learning sign language in childhood: another look at the critical period for language acquisition. *J Memory Lang*, **30**(4), 486–512.

McEwen, I.R. and Karlan, G.R. (1990). Assessment of effects of position on communication board access by individuals with cerebral palsy. *Augmentat Alternat Commun*, **5**(4), 235–242.

McNaughton, D. and Bryen, D.N. (2002). Enhancing participation in employment through AAC technologies. *Assist Technol*, **14**(1), 58–70.

Mesibov, G.B. (1995). *What is TEACCH*, University of North Carolina.

Mineo, B.A. and Goldstein, H. (1990). Generalized learning of receptive and expressive action–object responses by language-delayed preschoolers. *J Speech Hear Res*, **55**, 665–678.

Minneman, S.L. (1985). A simplified touch-tone telecommunication aid for deaf and hearing impaired individuals. *Eighth Annual Conference on Rehabilitation Technology*, Memphis TN, The Rehabilitation Engineering Society of North America.

Mollica, B. (1999). Field of assistive and rehabilitation technology. *Assist Technol*, **11**(2), 79–80.

Mollica, B.M. (1998). *Assessment of the Need for Assistive Technology Among Consumers of Division of Mental Retardation Services*, University of Delaware, Wilmington, DE.

Mollica, B.M. (1999). Emerging technologies in augmentative and alternative communication: restorative and compensatory approaches to acquired disorders of communication. *NeuroRehabilitation*, **12**, 27–37.

Musselwhite, C.R. and Ruscello, D.M. (1984). Transparency of three communication symbol systems. *J Speech Hear Res*, **27**(3), 436–443.

National Joint Committee for the Communication Needs of Persons with Severe Disabilities. (2003). Position statement on access to communication services and supports: concerns regarding the application of restrictive "eligibility" policies. *ASHA Suppl*, **23**, 19–23.

Norman, D. (1993). Things that make us smart. In: *Things That Make Us Smart: Defending Human Attributes in the Age of the Machine*, Perseus Publishing, Cambridge, MA.

Norman, D. (2002). *The Design of Everyday Things*, Basic Books, New York (Perseus).

Paul, R. (1997). Facilitating transitions in language development for children who use AAC. *Augment Alternat Commun*, **13**, 139–140.

Pebly, M. and Koppenhaver, D.A. (2001). Emergent and early literacy interventions for students with severe communication impairments. *Semin Speech Lang*, **22**(3), 221–230.

Pedersen, P.M., Vinter, K., et al. (2004). Aphasia after stroke: type, severity and prognosis. The Copenhagen aphasia study. *Cerebrovas Dis*, **17**(1), 35–43.

Perring, S., Summers, A., et al. (2003). A novel accelerometer tilt switch device for switch actuation in the patient with profound disability. *Archiv Phys Med Rehabil*, **84**(**6**), 921–923.

Pinker, S. (1984). *Language Learnability and Language Development*, Harvard University Press, Cambridge, MA.

Pradat-Diehl, P., Tessier, C., et al. (2001). [Long term outcome of a severe non fluent aphasia. The effect of prolonged rehabilitation] [Article in French]. *Ann Readapt Med Phys*, **44**(**8**), 525–532.

Rapin, I. and Dunn, M. (2003). Update on the language disorders of individuals on the autistic spectrum. *Brain Develop*, **25**(**3**), 166–172.

Rayner, H. and Marshall, J. (2003). Training volunteers as conversation partners for people with aphasia. *Int J Lang Commun Disorders*, **38**(**2**), 149–164.

Rimland, B. (1964). *Infantile Autism: The Syndrome and its Implications for a Neural Theory of Behavior*, Appleton-Century-Crofts, New York.

Rowland, C. and Schweigert, P. (2000). Tangible symbols, tangible outcomes. *Augment Alternat Commun*, **16**, 61–78.

Russel, M. (1984). Assessment and intervention issues with the nonspeaking child. *Except Child*, **51**(**1**), 64–71.

Sacchett, C., Byng, S., et al. (1999). Drawing together: evaluation of a therapy programme for severe aphasia. *Int J Lang Commun Disorders*, **34**(**3**), 265–289.

Schalk, G., Wolpaw, J.R., et al. (2000). EEG-based communication: presence of an error potential. *Clin Neurophysiol*, **111**(**2**), 2138–2144.

Sevcik, R.A. and Romski, M.A. (1997). Comprehension and language acquisition: evidence from youth with severe cognitive disabilities. In: *Communication and Language Acquisition: Discoveries from Atypical Development* (eds Adamson, L.B. and Romski, M.A.), Brookes, Baltimore, MD, pp. 187–2002.

Shelton, J.R., Weinrich, M., et al. (1996). Differentiating globally aphasic patients: data from in-depth language assessments and production training using C-VIC. *Aphasiology*, **10**(**4**), 319–342.

Sigman, M. and Capps, L. (1997). *Children with Autism: A Developmental Perspective*. Harvard University Press, Cambridge, MA.

Simeonsson, R., Olley, J., et al. (1987). Early intervention for children with autism. In: *The Effectiveness of Early Intervention for at-Risk and Handicapped Children* (eds Guralnick, M. and Bennett, F.), Academic Press, New York, pp. 275–293.

Smith, D.C. (1998). Assistive technology: Funding options and strategies. *Ment Phys Disabil Law Report*, **22**(**1**), 115–123.

Soderholm, S., Meinander, M., et al. (2001). Augmentative and alternative communication methods in locked-in syndrome. *J Rehabil Med*, **33**(**5**), 235–239.

Sutton, A., Soto, G., et al. (2002). Grammatical issues in graphic symbol communication. *Augment Alternat Commun*, **18**, 192–204.

Todman, J.R. and Rzepecka, H. (2003). Effect of pre-utterance pause length on perceptions of communicative competence in AAC-aided social conversations. *Augment Alternat Commun*, **19**(**4**), 222–234.

Tolley, K., Leese, B., et al. (1995). Communication aids for the speech impaired. Cost and quality-of-life outcomes of assessment programs provided by specialist Communication Aids Centers in the United Kingdom. *Int J Technol Assess Health Care*, **11**(**2**), 196–213.

Trepagnier, C. (1996). Initial assessment of individuals with severe cognitive disabilities for augmentative communication. *RESNA 1996 Annual Conference*, RESNA Press, Arlington, Virginia.

Trepagnier, C. (1996). A possible origin for the social and communicative deficits of autism. *Focus Autism Other Develop Disabil*, **11**(**3**), 170–182.

Volkmar, F.R. (1987). Social development. In: *Handbook of Autism and Pervasive Developmental Disorders* (ed. Donnellan, D.J.C.A.M.), Wiley/Winston, New York, pp. 41–60.

Wade, J., Petheram, B., et al. (2001). Voice recognition and aphasia: can computers understand aphasic speech? *Disabil Rehabil*, **23**(**14**), 604–613.

Wagner, R.K. and Torgesen, J.K. (1987). The nature of phological processess and its causal role in the acquisition of reading skills. *Psychol Bull*, **101**, 192–212.

Weinrich, M.M.D., Weber, C., et al. (1995). Training on an iconic communication system for severe aphasia can improve natural language production. *Aphasiology*, **9**(**4**), 343–364.

Wing, L. (1976). *Early Childhood Autism*, Pergamon Press, Elmsford, NY.

Wing, L. and Atwood, T. (1987). Syndromes of autism and atypical development. In: *Handbook of Autism and Pervasive Developmental Disorders* (eds Cohen, D. and Donnellan, A.), John Wiley & Sons, New York, pp. 3–19.

Wolpaw, J.R., Birbaumer, N., et al. (2000). Brain–computer interface technology: a review of the first international meeting. *IEEE Trans Rehabil Eng*, **8**(**2**), 164–173.

Wolpaw, J.R., Birbaumer, N., et al. (2002). Brain–computer interfaces for communication and control. *Clin Neurophysiol*, **113**(**6**), 767–791.

Woolfe, T., Want, S.C., et al. (2002). Signposts to development: theory of mind in deaf children. *Child develop*, **73**(**3**), 768–778.

Appendix: web resources

ABLEDATA is an on-line database project funded by the National Institute on Disability and Rehabilitation Research (NIDRR), part of the Office of Special Education and Rehabilitative Services (OSERS) of the US Department of Education to provide information on assistive technology. http://www.abledata.com/

The Rehabilitation Engineering Research Center (RERC) on Communication Enhancement, is an AAC research and development center also funded by NIDRR and competitively renewed every 5 years. http://www.AAC-rerc.com/

The Communication Aid Manufacturers Association (CAMA) is a non-profit organization representing manufacturers of AAC software and hardware technology that provides information workshops in locations that rotate around the country. http://www.AACproducts.org/index.lasso

RESNA, the Rehabilitation Engineering and Assistive Technology Society of North America, is an interdisciplinary association of people with an interest in technology and disability that sponsors conferences and certifies assistive technology providers. http://www.resna.org/index.php

The International Society for Augmentative and Alternative Communication (ISAAC), with its American chapter, the United States Society for Alternative and Augmentative communication (USSAC) is an organization of AAC service providers, manufacturers and people who use the techniques, and their families. This society provides educational and networking opportunities. http://www.ussAAC.org/ pages/membership.html

ASHA, The American Speech, Hearing and Language Association, is the professional organization of Speech Pathologists and Audiologists. http://www.asha.org/default.htm

Symptom-specific neurorehabilitation

CONTENTS

Sensory and motor dysfunctions

CONTENTS

Chronic pain

Herta Flor[1] and Frank Andrasik[2]

[1]Department of Clinical and Cognitive Neuroscience, University of Heidelberg, Central Institute of Mental Health, Mannheim, Germany and [2]Institute for Human and Machine Cognition, University of West Florida, Pensacola, FL, USA

15.1 Introduction

Despite the many advances in the pathophysiology and treatment of pain, chronic pain still remains elusive to treat. Once the pain problem has exceeded the acute and subacute stage, peripheral factors seem to loose their importance and central changes become much more important (Sandkühler, 2000; Ji et al., 2003). One major factor that seems to contribute to chronicity are memory traces that occur as a consequence of ongoing and/or very intense pain and that are enhanced by learning processes designed to imprint and consolidate these pain-related memory traces. In this chapter we will review the evidence on plastic changes along the neuraxis and their relationship to pain in humans and then delineate treatment approaches that are designed less towards analgesia but more towards reversing maladaptive plasticity with the hypothesis that this would consequently also reduce chronic pain and extinguish pain memories.

15.2 Pain and plasticity

Chronic musculoskeletal pain

In the last two decades our understanding of the modifiability of the primary sensory and motor areas of the brain has greatly changed (see Chapters 6–8 of Volume 1). Animal models have shown that long-lasting and/or intense states of pain (e.g., when an inflammation is present) lead to the sensitization of spinal cord neurons (e.g., Sandkühler, 2000) as well

as an altered representation of the painful area in the brainstem (Tinazzi et al., 2000), thalamus (Vos et al., 2000) and cortex (Benoist et al., 1999). In chronic pain patients both perceptual and cerebral hyper-reactivity to tactile or noxious stimuli have been observed. For example, Kleinböhl et al. (1999) showed that patients with back pain as well as patients with tension headache sensitize more than healthy controls, that is, they show steeper increases in perceived pain intensity with repetitive painful stimulation. In addition, perception and pain thresholds as well as pain tolerance levels were found to be significantly lower in patients with chronic back pain compared to persons with episodic headaches and healthy controls, and these thresholds varied as a function of chronicity (the more chronic pain, the lower the threshold) (Flor et al., 2004). This chronicity distinction is particularly important when considering tension-type headache. Chronic forms of tension-type headache consistently reveal evidence of central sensitization to thermal, electrical and pressure stimulation (Langemark et al., 1989; Schoenen et al., 1991; Bendtsen et al., 1996), whereas patient groupings whose diagnoses are episodic or episodic mixed with chronic do not (Bovim, 1992; Jensen et al., 1993; Jensen, 1996). In fibromyalgia syndrome, hypervigilance and exaggerated perception of both painful and non-painful tactile stimuli has been reported (Staud et al., 2001), however, this sensitivity has not been observed with respect to auditory stimuli (Lorenz, 1998).

Elevated responses to painful and non-painful tactile stimulation as assessed by magnetoencephalography were reported in chronic back pain patients (Flor et al., 1997). Stimulation at the affected back but not at the finger led to a significantly higher magnetic field in the time window <100 ms whereas both types of stimulation caused higher fields in the later time windows (>200 ms) in the patients compared to the controls. When the source of this early activity was localized, it was shown to originate from primary somatosensory cortex (SI). Whereas the localization of the fingers was not significantly different between patients and controls, the localization of the back was more inferior and medial in the patients indicating a shift and expansion toward the cortical representation of the leg. These data suggest that chronic pain leads to an expansion of the cortical representation zone related to nociceptive input much like the expansions of cortical representations that have been documented to occur with other types of behaviorally relevant stimulation (Braun et al., 2000). Nociceptive input is of high relevance for the organism and it might be useful to enhance the representation of this type of stimulation to prepare the organism for the adequate response. The amount of expansion of the back region was positively correlated with chronicity suggesting that this pain-related cortical reorganization develops over time. Using functional magnetic resonance imaging (fMRI), Gracely et al. (2002) reported a similar hyperreactivity to painful stimulation in a number of brain regions including SI cortex in fibromyalgia patients. In a continuous pain rating in the scanner it was shown that patients with fibromyalgia displayed an increasing level of pain across several stimulation trials and failed to return to baseline. This was true for both the affected (trapezius muscle) and the non-effected body part (finger muscle). In patients with chronic upper back pain it was shown that the stimulation of the trapezius but not the flexor digitorum muscle showed sensitization, suggesting site-specificity. The accompanying fMRI measurements revealed enhanced activation in somatosensory cortex but reduced activation in anterior cingulate cortex compared to the healthy controls (see Fig. 15.1). The cerebral activation was also site-specific in the back pain patients but generalized in the fibromyalgia patients.

This type of central alteration may correspond to what Katz and Melzack (1990) have termed a somatosensory pain memory in patients with phantom limb pain. Although they referred mainly to explicit memories, that is, the patients' recollection that the phantom pain was similar to previously experienced pains, somatosensory memories can also be implicit as already stated by them. Implicit pain memories are based on changes in the brain that are not open to conscious awareness but lead to behavioral and perceptual changes – such as hyperalgesia and allodynia – the patient is not aware of. It is therefore impossible for the patient to counteract these pain memories. This type of memory trace may lead to pain perception in the absence of peripheral stimulation since an expansion of a representational zone is related to higher acuity in the perception of tactile input (Merzenich et al., 1984).

Implicit pain memories can be established and altered by learning processes such as habituation and sensitization, operant and classical conditioning or priming. There is now ample evidence that learning not only affects pain behaviors and the subjective experience of pain but also the physiologic processing of painful stimulation. For example, a spouse who habitually reinforces pain can also influence the pain-related cortical response. When chronic back pain patients were stimulated with electric impulses at either the finger of the back in either the presence or absence of the spouse, spouse presence influenced the electroencephalographic potentials that were recorded from the patients' skull. Whereas the spouses who habitually ignored the pain or punished their partners for expressing pain had no effect, spouses who habitually reinforced pain behaviors caused a 2.5-fold increase in the patients' brain response to pain applied to the back. At the finger no difference for the presence or the absence of the spouse was observed nor was there a difference for the healthy controls (see Fig. 15.2). The main difference between these conditions was observed in an area that corresponds to the location of the anterior cingulate cortex that has been shown to be involved in the processing of the emotional aspects of pain (Rainville et al., 1997).

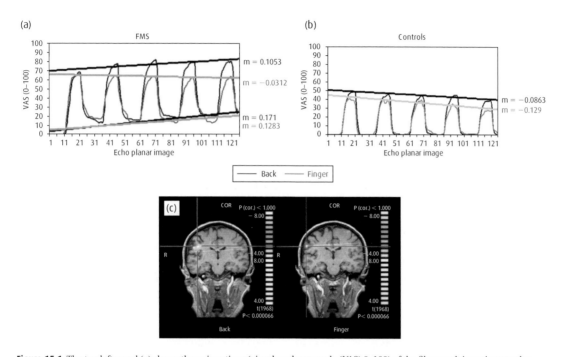

Figure 15.1. The top left panel (a) shows the pain ratings (visual analogue scale (VAS) 0–100) of the fibromyalgia patients to the stimulation of the back (black) or the finger (grey). The patients were stimulated in blocks of 20s with 20-s rest intervals. The top right (b) panel shows the same ratings for the healthy controls. The straight lines show the slope of the ratings. A negative slope indicates a reduction in pain rating and thus habituation and a positive slope indicates sensitization and increased pain ratings. The numbers to the right give the slope. The bottom panel (c) shows the difference in activation between the fibromyalgia patients (FMS) and the healthy controls related to the secondary somatosensory cortex. Note that the FMS patients show more activation both during the back and finger stimulation.

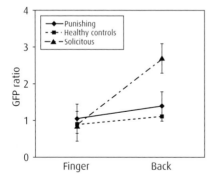

Figure 15.2. This figure shows the enhanced brain response in the chronic back pain patients with solicitous spouses to the back but not the finger stimulation. The brain activity was computed as the global field power related to the EEG gathered with 90 surface electrodes.

Direct verbal reinforcement of pain has been identified as an additional important modulator of the pain response. When patients and healthy controls were reinforced for increasing or decreasing their verbal pain responses both groups learned this task equally well, however, the patients showed a delay in the extinction of the response. When the somatosensory evoked potentials to the pain stimuli were examined, the late event-related responses (>200 ms) were unaltered and showed mainly habituation. However, the early response (N150) was affected by the conditioning procedure and remained high in the chronic pain group that had been reinforced for higher pain ratings thus indicating a direct effect of verbal reinforcement on the early cortical processing of nociceptive information (Flor et al., 2002b).

This lack of extinction in the cortical domain suggests that learning processes related to verbal and behavioral conditioning may exert long-lasting influences on the cortical response to pain-related stimuli and form implicit pain memories.

In addition to operant, classical conditioning has been identified as an important modulator of pain-related responses. This effect pertains not only to the ascending nociceptive system but also to descending pain-modulatory systems (Dubner and Ren, 1999). The fact that stress positively influences the pain response and activates the descending pain-inhibitory system has commonly been described by the term stress-induced analgesia or hypoalgesia. Animal studies have shown that stress analgesia can be conditioned and that some forms of both conditioned and unconditioned stress analgesia are mediated by the endogenous opioid system (Maier, 1989). It was recently shown that stress analgesia can also be classically conditioned in humans and that this conditioned analgesia is mediated by the release of endogenous opioids (Flor and Grüsser, 1999; Flor et al., 2002a). To what extent deficient descending pain inhibition is involved in chronic pain has not yet been established nor do we know enough about the role of learning and memory process in the inhibition of pain. In an elegant study, Wunsch and colleagues (Wunsch et al., 2003) used pain as an conditioned and affective pictures as unconditioned stimuli (US) and showed that a classical conditioning procedure modified the pain ratings to a more or less intense perception depending on the nature of the US (aversive versus appetitive).

In summary, chronic pain states lead to the development of somatosensory pain memories that manifest themselves in alterations in the somatotopic map in somatosensory cortex as well as other brain areas related to the processing of pain. These plastic changes may contribute to hyperalgesic and allodynic states in the absence of or the presence of only minor peripheral nociceptive stimulation. These pain memories can be influenced by psychologic processes such as operant and classical conditioning that may establish additional and potentially more widespread implicit memories and may enhance existing memories. In addition to local representational changes, chronic states of pain are associated with increased cortical excitation that may significantly contribute to cortical reorganization. Pain-inhibitory systems are also influenced by learning and memory processes and may be altered in chronic pain.

Neuropathic pain

As noted above, not only enduring nociceptive input but also the loss of input, for example, subsequent to amputation or nerve injury, can alter the cortical map. Several studies examined cortical reorganization after amputation in humans. These studies were instigated by the report of Ramachandran et al. (1992) that phantom sensation could be elicited in upper extremity amputees when they were stimulated in the face. There was a point-to-point correspondence between stimulation sites in the face and the localization of sensation in the phantom. Moreover, the sensations in the phantom matched the modality of the stimulation, for example warmth was perceived as a warm phantom sensation, painful touch was perceived as pain. The authors assumed that this phenomenon might be the perceptual correlate of the type of reorganization previously described in animal experiments. The invasion of the cortical hand or arm area by the mouth representation might lead to activity in the cortical amputation zone which would be projected into the no longer present limb. Subsequently, Elbert et al. (1994) and Yang et al. (1994) used a combination of magnetoencephalographic recordings and structural magnetic resonance imaging – neuromagnetic source imaging – to test this hypothesis. They observed a significant shift of the mouth representation into the zone that formerly represented the now amputated hand or arm, however, this shift occurred in patients with and without phantom sensation referred from the mouth. Flor et al. (1995) showed that phantom limb pain rather than referred sensation was the perceptual correlate of these cortical reorganizational changes. Patients with phantom limb pain displayed a significant shift of the mouth into the hand representation whereas this was not the case in patients without phantom limb pain. The intensity of phantom limb pain was significantly positively correlated with the amount of displacement of the mouth representation. It was later shown that referred sensations as those described by Ramachandran et al. (1992) can also be elicited from areas far removed from the amputated limb (e.g., from the foot in arm amputees). Therefore, it was concluded that alterations in the organization of SI, where arm and foot are represented far apart, are most likely not the neuronal substrate of referred phantom sensations (Borsook et al., 1998; Grüsser et al., 2001, 2004).

Similar results were obtained when the motor cortex was investigated. For example, an fMRI study where upper extremity amputees had to perform pucking lip movements showed that the representation of the lip in primary motor cortex had also shifted into the area that formerly occupied the amputated hand (Lotze et al., 2001; see Fig. 15.3). The magnitude of this shift was also highly significantly correlated with the amount of phantom limb pain experienced by the patients thus suggesting parallel processes in the somatosensory and motor system. A high concordance of changes in the somatosensory and the motor system was reported by Karl et al. (2001) who used transcranial magnetic stimulation to map the motor cortex and neuroelectric source

imaging (that combines the determination of cortical sources by evoked potential recordings with structural magnetic resonance imaging) to map the somatosensory cortex. This close interconnection of changes in the somatosensory and motor system suggests that rehabilitative efforts directed at one modality may also affect the other.

The close association between cortical alterations and phantom limb pain was further underscored in a study by Birbaumer et al. (1997). In upper limb amputees, anesthesia of the brachial plexus lead to the elimination of phantom limb pain in about 50% of the amputees whereas phantom limb pain remained unchanged in the other half. Neuroelectric source imaging revealed that cortical reorganization was also reversed in those amputees that showed a reduction of phantom limb pain. Patients who continued to have phantom limb pain during the elimination of sensory input from the residual limb had an even more reorganized mouth representation. These data suggest that in some patients peripheral factors might be important in the maintenance of phantom limb pain whereas in others pain and reorganizational processes might have become independent of peripheral input. The importance of pain experiences prior to amputation was confirmed by a study of Nikolajsen et al. (2000a) who reported a close association between mechanical sensitivity

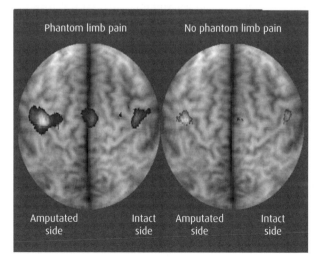

Figure 15.3. Reorganization in the motor cortex related to chronic phantom limb pain. The patients had to puck their lips. Note the more medial/superior and more widespread activation in the phantom limb pain patients.

prior to amputation and early phantom limb pain. However, the authors only tested thresholds and not sensitization. Further research is needed to better clarify these relationships.

As Devor and Seltzer (1998), and others have pointed out it is to date not clear on which level of the neuraxis the cortical changes that have been observed in imaging studies originate. In addition to intracortical changes alterations might be present in the dorsal root ganglion, the dorsal horn, the brain stem or the thalamus. Several imaging studies (e.g., Willoch et al., 2000) have also shown that not only the primary and secondary somatosensory cortex and the posterior parietal cortex but also regions such as the insula and the anterior cingulate cortex are involved in the processing of phantom phenomena.

Similar alterations in the cortical processing of sensory information have recently also been reported in patients with complex regional pain syndromes (CRPS). In a magnetoencephalographic investigation, Juottonen et al. (2002) showed that in patients with CRPS the localization of the fingers of the affected hand had shifted closer together and that the magnitude of the magnetic response on the affected side was positively correlated with the amount of pain experienced by the patients. They also observed altered activity in the motor cortex suggesting a change of inhibition. Similarly, Pleger et al. (2004) found that CRPS patients revealed a marked hemispheric difference in the representation of the hand with the affected hand also being smaller in extent than the intact hand. The amount of hemispheric asymmetry was positively correlated with the amount of pain they experienced. Thus, both in phantom limb pain and in CRPS a smaller representation of the affected and completely or partially deafferented body part was associated with more pain whereas in chronic musculoskeletal pain, a larger representation was found to be associated with more pain. We do not yet fully understand the mechanisms underlying these types of relationship, however, the amount of use of the limb as well as the type of input from the limb or adjacent territory might play an important modulatory role.

Based on these findings and the results obtained on somatosensory memories in chronic back pain it can be assumed that prior pain memories might also be important in the development of phantom limb pain although they are surely not the only factors. Thus, when pain has occurred prior to the amputation, alterations in somatosensory cortex and other brain areas might have occurred that would later – when activated by neighboring input subsequent to the amputation – lead to the sensation of phantom limb pain (Flor, 2002). Initial evidence from a longitudinal study (Huse et al., in press) suggests that chronic pain before the amputation is a much more important predictor of later phantom limb pain than acute pain at the time of the amputation thus supporting this assumption. In addition, peripheral changes related to the amputation may contribute to enhanced cortical reorganization and phantom limb pain. To summarize, somatosensory pain memories represented by alterations in the topographic map of SI cortex may underlie the development of phantom limb pain and may contribute to other neuropathic pain syndromes such as CRPS. Longstanding states of chronic pain prior to the amputation may be instrumental in the formation of these pain memories by inducing representational and excitability changes. Deafferentation does not alter the original assignment of cortical representation zones to peripheral input zones but leads to double coding. Peripheral factors such as loss of C-fiber activity, spontaneous activity from neuroma or psychophysiologic activation may also influence the cortical representational changes (Calford and Tweedale, 1991; Spitzer et al., 1995). Learning processes are instrumental in the development and maintenance of these cerebral changes.

Migraine and cluster headache

Whereas tension headache seems to have some similarity to musculoskeletal pain disorders, migraine headache and cluster headache are distinct categories of pain with different etiologies. In migraine headache, a consistent feature has been an inability to habituate to various types of sensory stimulation in the pain-free interval. For example, in migraine headache a lack of habituation to auditory or visual stimuli was observed for the pain-free interval (Gerber and Schoenen, 1998; Evers et al., 1999; see Ambrosini et al., 2003, for a review). This was assessed either by visual evoked potentials or by changes in the contingent negative variation, a slow cortical potential that is typically present in an S1–S2 task where S1 signals the occurrence of a second signal, S2 that is the sign for a response to be made by the subject. Usually, multiple presentations of the S1–S2 stimuli lead to habituation of the CNV, which was not found in migraine headache. In addition, a brainstem migraine generator has been proposed because alterations in brain stem activity have repeatedly been found during migraine attacks (Weiller et al., 1995; for a review see Sanchez del Rio and Linera, 2004). In cluster headache, several functional and structural imaging studies have identified a cluster headache-specific alteration in the hypothalamus (May et al., 1998, 1999; for a review see Goadsby et al., 2002). It is, however, not clear to what extent these changes are a cause or a consequence or merely an epiphenomenon of the pain that is experienced.

15.3 Influencing chronic pain and brain plasticity

Behavioral interventions

The discussion in the preceding sections suggests that the alteration of somatosensory pain memories might be an influential method to reduce both chronic musculoskeletal and neuropathic pain. This could be achieved by altering the peripheral input that enters the brain region that coded a pain memory, for example by using electromyogram (EMG) or temperature biofeedback or other types of standard behavioral interventions (for reviews see Andrasik, 2003, 2004; Flor et al., 1992; Sherman, 1997) or by employing a sensory stimulation protocol that provides relevant correlated sensory input to the respective brain region. It would also be possible to directly alter the brain response to pain by providing feedback of event-related potential components or electroencephalogram (EEG) rhythms (Kropp et al.,

2002). Most of these methods have not yet been tested in a systematic manner and their effects on cortical reorganization are so far unknown. Alternatively, pharmacologic interventions could be used that prevent or reverse the establishment of central memory traces.

In phantom limb pain, it was assumed that the pain is maintained by cortical alterations fed by peripheral random input. In this case the provision of correlated input into the amputation zone might be an effective method to influence phantom limb pain. fMRI was used to investigate the effects of prosthesis use on phantom limb pain and cortical reorganization (Lotze et al., 1999). Patients who systematically used a myoelectric prosthesis that provides sensory and visual as well as motor feedback to the brain showed much less phantom limb pain and cortical reorganization than patients who used either a cosmetic or no prosthesis. The relationship between phantom limb pain and use of a myoelectric prosthesis was entirely mediated by cortical reorganization. When it was partialled out from the correlation, phantom limb pain and prosthesis use were no longer associated. This suggests that sensory input to the brain region that formerly represented the now absent limb may be beneficial in reducing phantom limb pain. These studies were performed in chronic phantom limb pain patients. An early fitting and training with a myoelectric prosthesis would probably be of great value not only in the rehabilitation of amputees but also in preventing or reversing phantom limb pain.

These assumptions were further confirmed in an intervention study where the patients received feedback on sensory discrimination of the residual limb (Flor et al., 2001). Eight electrodes were attached to the residual limb and provided high-intensity non-painful electric stimulation of varying intensity and location that led to the experience of intense phantoms. The patients were trained to discriminate the location or the frequency of the stimulation (alternating trials) of the stimulation and received feedback on the correct responses. The training was conducted for 90 min per day and was spread over a time of 2 weeks (10 days of training). Compared to a medically

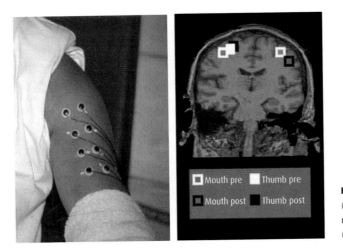

Figure 15.4. Changes in cortical reorganization (distance of the hand and lip representation in millimeter) during the discrimination training (electrode montage is depicted on the left side).

treated control group that received an equal amount of attention the trained patients showed significantly better discrimination ability on the stump. They also experienced a more than 60% reduction of phantom limb pain and a significant reversal of cortical reorganization with a shift of the mouth representation back to its original location. The alterations in discrimination ability, pain and cortical reorganization were highly significantly correlated (see Fig. 15.4).

In a related study (Huse et al., 2001b) asynchronous tactile stimulation of the mouth and hand region was used over a time period of several weeks. This training was based on the idea that synchronous stimulation leads to fusion and asynchronous stimulation leads to a separation of cortical representation zones. In this case it was postulated that input from the mouth representation that would now activate the region that formerly represented the now amputated hand and arm would be eliminated and with it the phantom phenomena that would be projected to the amputated limb. This intervention also showed a reduction in phantom limb pain and cortical reorganization.

Pharmacologic interventions

In addition to behavior, pharmacologic interventions may also be useful in the treatment of both chronic musculoskeletal and neuropathic pain. The prevention of pain memories might be possible by using pharmacologic agents that are known to also prevent or reverse cortical reorganization. Among these substances, gamma amino butyric acid (GABA) agonists, N-methyl-D-aspartate (NMDA) and alpha-amino-3-hydroxy-5methyl-4-isoxazole propionic acid (AMPA) receptor antagonists and anticholinergic substances seem to be the most promising. A recent double-blind placebo-controlled study that used the NMDA receptor antagonist memantine in the perioperative phase in acute amputations reported a decrease of the incidence of phantom limb pain from 72% to 20% 1 year after the amputation (Wiech et al., 2001; see Fig. 15.5). The pharmacologic intervention was most effective in those patients where treatment had begun before or immediately after the amputation. This study could explain why the results of different controlled prospective studies about the effect of preemptive analgesia initiated at least 24 h before the amputation on the incidence of phantom limb pain are inconsistent. For example, a well-controlled study by Nikolajsen et al. (1997) showed no effect of preemptive analgesia on phantom limb pain. If a preexisting pain memory is important in the development of phantom limb pain, the use of preemptive analgesia, that eliminates afferent barrage in the perioperative phase but will not alter previously formed neuronal changes may be ineffective.

Treatment of chronic phantom limb pain with pharmacologic agents has also yielded inconsistent

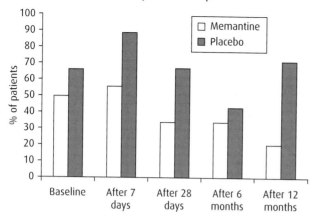

Incidence of phantom limb pain

Figure 15.5. Here the results of the NMDA receptor antagonist memantine on acute phantom limb pain are shown in amputees who participated in a double-blind randomized study with either memantine or placebo. Note the significantly lower incidence of phantom limb pain at the 12-month follow-up in the memantine condition.

results. Pharmacologic interventions include a host of agents and although tricyclic antidepressants and sodium channel blockers have been indicated as treatments of choice for neuropathic pain (see Sindrup and Jensen, 1999 for a review), there are few controlled studies for phantom limb pain. Controlled studies have been performed for opioids (Huse et al., 2001a), calcitonin (Jaeger and Maier, 1992), ketamine (Nikolajsen et al., 1996) and gabapentin (Bone et al., 2002) all of which were found to effectively reduce phantom limb pain. Memantine, an NMDA receptor antagonist like ketamine, was, however, not effective in three studies (Nikolajsen et al., 2000b; Maier et al., 2003; Wiech et al., 2004). Antidepressants yielded no pain relief (Robinson et al., 2004). We found positive effects of both opioids (Huse et al., 2001a) and memantine (Koeppe et al., 2003) on both chronic phantom limb pain and cortical reorganization suggesting that more work is necessary to determine under which circumstances which pharmacologic agents can effectively reverse the maladaptive plastic changes that are a consequence of amputation and chronic pain.

15.4 Conclusions and summary

The empiric evidence discussed above suggests that neuroplastic changes in the central nervous system

play an important role in the development and maintenance of chronic pain. It is so far not clear to what extent changes in the spinal cord, the brain stem or the thalamus contribute to the changes in cortical reorganization and to what extent cortical reorganization affects the lower levels. Longitudinal studies and controlled outcome studies would also be needed to elucidate in greater detail the efficacy and mechanisms of feedback-based interventions designed to alter cortical pain memories.

Functional reorganization in both the somatosensory and the motor system was observed in neuropathic and musculoskeletal pain. In chronic low back pain and fibromyalgia patients the amount of reorganizational change increases with chronicity, in phantom limb pain and other neuropathic pain syndromes cortical reorganization is correlated with the amount of pain. A complicating factor is that in chronic pain syndromes lack of use of an affected body part may contribute to the central changes that are observed. These central alterations may be viewed as pain memories that alter the processing of both painful and non-painful input to the somatosensory system as well as its effects on the motor system. Cortical plasticity related to chronic pain can be modified by behavioral interventions that provide feedback to the brain areas that were altered by somatosensory pain memories or by pharmacologic agents that prevent or reverse maladaptive memory formation. Future research needs to focus on emotional changes that contribute to and interact with the sensory and motor changes described here.

ACKNOWLEDGEMENTS

The completion of this article was supported by the Deutsche Forschungsgemeinschaft (Fl 156/26), by the German Research Network on Neuropathic Pain (BMBF 01EM0103) and the Max-Planck Award for International Cooperation.

REFERENCES

Ambrosini, A., de Noordhout, A.M., Sándor, P.S. and Schoenen, J. (2003). Electrophysiological studies in migraine: a comprehensive review of their interest and limitations. *Cephalalgia*, **23**(**Suppl. 1**), 13–31.

Andrasik, F. (2003). Behavioral treatment approaches to chronic headache. *Neurol Sci*, **24**(**Suppl. 2**), S80–S85.

Andrasik, F. (2004). Behavioral treatment of migraine: current status and future directions. *Expert Rev Neurotherapeutics*, **4**, 403–413.

Bendtsen, L., Jensen, R. and Olesen, J. (1996). Decreased pain detection and tolerance thresholds in chronic tension-type headache. *Arch Neurol*, **53**, 373–376.

Benoist, J.M., Gautron, M. and Guilbaud, G. (1999). Experimental model of trigeminal pain in the rat by constriction of one infraorbital nerve: changes in neuronal activities in the somatosensory cortices corresponding to the infraorbital nerve. *Exp Brain Res*, **126**, 383–398.

Birbaumer, N., Lutzenberger, W., Montoya, P., Larbig, W., Unertl, K., Töpfner, S., Grodd, W., Taub, E. and Flor, H. (1997). Effects of regional anesthesia on phantom limb pain are mirrored in changes in cortical reorganization. *J Neurosci*, **17**, 5503–5508.

Bone, M., Critchley, P. and Buggy, D.J. (2002). Gabapentin in postamputation phantom limb pain: a randomized, double-blind, placebo-controlled, cross-over study. *Reg Anesth Pain Med*, **27**, 481–486.

Borsook, D., Becerra, L., Fishman, S., Edwards, A., Jennings, C.L., Stojanovic, M., et al. (1998). Acute plasticity in the human somatosensory cortex following amputation. *NeuroReport*, **9**(**6**), 1013–1017.

Bovim, G. (1992). Cervicogenic headache, migraine, and tension-type headache: pressure-pain threshold measurements. *Pain*, **51**, 169–173.

Braun, C., Schweizer, R., Elbert, T., Birbaumer, N. and Taub, E. (2000). Differential activation in somatosensory cortex for different discrimination tasks. *J Neurosci*, **20**(**1**), 446–450.

Calford, M.B. and Tweedale, R. (1991). C-fibres provide a source of masking inhibition to primary somatosensory cortex. *Proc Roy Soc London B Biol Sci*, **243**(**1308**), 269–275.

Devor, M.S. and Seltzer, Z. (1998). Pathophysiology of damaged nerves in ralation to chronic pain. In: *Textbook of Pain* (eds Wall, P.O. and Malzack, R.A.), Churchill-Livingstone, NY, pp. 129–164.

Dubner, R. and Ren, K. (1999). Endogenous mechanisms of sensory modulation. *Pain*, **82**(**Suppl. 1**), S45–S53.

Elbert, T.R., Flor, H., Birbaumer, N., Knecht, S., Hampson, S., Larbig, W., et al. (1994). Extensive reorganization of the somatosensory cortex in adult humans after nervous system injury. *NeuroReport*, **5**, 2593–2597.

Evers, S., Quibeldey, F., Grotemeyer, K.H., Suhr, B. and Husstedt, I.W. (1999). Dynamic changes of cognitive habituation and serotonin metabolism during the migraine interval. *Cephalalgia*, **19**(**5**), 485–491.

Flor, H. (2002). Phantom limb pain: characteristics, causes and treatment. *Lancet Neurol*, **3**, 182–189.

Flor, H. and Grüsser, S.M. (1999). Conditioned stress-induced analgesia in humans. *Eur J Pain*, **3**, 317–324.

Flor, H., Fydrich, T. and Turk, D.C. (1992). Efficacy of multidisciplinary pain treatment centers: a meta-analytic review. *Pain*, **49**, 221–230.

Flor, H., Elbert, T.R., Knecht, S., Wienbruch, C., Pantev, C., Birbaumer, N., et al. (1995). Phantom limb pain as a perceptual correlate of massive cortical reorganization in upper extremity amputees. *Nature*, **357**, 482–484.

Flor, H., Braun, C., Elbert, T. and Birbaumer, N. (1997). Extensive reorganization of primary somatosensory cortex in chronic back pain patients. *Neurosci Lett*, **224**(**1**), 5–8.

Flor, H., Denke, C., Schäfer, M. and Grüsser, S. (2001). Effects of sensory discrimination training on cortical reorganization and phantom limb pain. *Lancet*, **357**, 1763–1764.

Flor, H., Birbaumer, N., Schulz, R., Mucha, R.F. and Grüsser, S.M. (2002a). Opioid mediation of conditioned stress analgesia in humans. *Eur J Pain*, **6**, 395–402.

Flor, H., Knost, B. and Birbaumer, N. (2002b). The role of operant conditioning in chronic pain: an experimental investigation. *Pain*, **95**, 111–118; **3**(**4**), 317–324

Flor, H., Diers, M. and Birbaumer N. (2004). Peripheral and electrocortical responses to painful and non painful stimulation in chronic pain patients, tension headache patients and healthy controls. *Neurosci Lett*, **361**, 147–150.

Gerber, W.D. and Schoenen, J. (1998). Biobehavioral correlates in migraine: the role of hypersensitivity and information-processing dysfunction. *Cephalalgia*, **18**(**Suppl. 21**), 5–11.

Goadsby, P.J. (2002). Pathophysiology of cluster headache: a trigeminal autonomic cephalgia. *Lancet Neurol*, **1**, 251–257.

Gracely, R.H., Petzke, F., Wolf, J.M. and Clauw, D.J. (2002). Functional magnetic resonance imaging evidence of augmented pain processing in fibromyalgia. *Arthritis Rheum*, **46**(5), 1333–1343.

Grüsser, S.M., Mühlnickel, W., Schaefer, M., Villringer, K., Christmann, C., Koeppe, C. and Flor, H. (2004). Remote activation of referred phantom sensation and cortical reorganization in human upper extremity amputees. *Exp Brain Res*, **154**, 97–102.

Grüsser, S., Winter, C., Mühlnickel, W., Denke, C., Karl, A., Villringer, K. and Flor, H. (2001). The relationship of perceptual phenomena and cortical reorganization in upper extremity amputees. *Neuroscience*, **102**, 263–272.

Huse, E., Larbig, W., Flor, H. and Birbaumer, N. (2001a). The effect of opioids on phantom limb pain and cortical reorganization. *Pain*, **90**, 47–55.

Huse, E., Preissl, H., Larbig, W. and Birbaumer, N. (2001b). Phantom limb pain. *Lancet*, **358**, 1015.

Huse, E., Larbig, W., Gerstein, J., Lukaschewski, T., Montoya, P., Birbaumer, N. and Flor, H. (in press). Pain-related and psychological predictors of phantom limb and residual limb pain and non-painful phantom phenomena. *Pain*.

Jaeger, H. and Maier, C. (1992). Calcitonin in phantom limb pain: a double-blind study. *Pain*, **48**, 21–27.

Jensen, R. (1996). Mechanisms of spontaneous tension-type headaches: an analysis of tenderness, pain thresholds and EMG. *Pain*, **64**, 251–256.

Jensen, R., Rasmussen, B.K., Pedersen, B. and Olesen, J. (1993). Muscle tenderness and pressure pain thresholds in headache. A population study. *Pain*, **52**, 193–199.

Ji, R.R., Kohno, T., Moore, K.A. and Woolf, C.J. (2003). Central sensitization and LTP: do pain and memory share similar mechanisms? *Trend Neurosci*, **26**(12), 696–705.

Juottonen, K., Gockel, M., Silen, T., Hurri, H., Hari, R. and Forss, N. (2002). Altered central sensorimotor processing in patients with complex regional pain syndrome. *Pain*, **98**(3), 315–323.

Karl, A., Birbaumer, N., Lutzenberger, W., Cohen, L. and Flor, H. (2001). Reorganization of motor and somatosensory cortex in upper extremity amputees with phantom limb pain. *J Neurosci*, **21**, 3609–3618.

Katz, J. and Melzack, R. (1990). Pain "memories" in phantom limbs: review and clinical observations. *Pain*, **43**, 319–336.

Kleinböhl, D., Hölzl, R., Möltner, A., Rommel, C., Weber, C. and Osswald, P.M. (1999). Psychophysical measures of sensitization to tonic heat discriminate chronic pain patients. *Pain*, **81**(1–2), 35–43.

Koeppe, C., Fritzsche, K., Schaefer, M., Christmann, C. and Flor, H. (2003). The effect of the NMDA-receptor antagonist

memantine on cortical reorganization and phantom phenomena. *Soc Neurosci Abstr*, **29**, 813.

Kropp, P., Siniatchkin, M. and Gerber, W.D. (2002). On the pathophysiology of migraine – links for "empirically based treatment" with neurofeedback. *Appl Psychophysiol Biof*, **27**, 203–213.

Langemark, M., Jensen, K., Jensen, T.S. and Olesen, J. (1989). Pressure pain thresholds and thermal nociceptive thresholds in chronic tension-type headache. *Pain*, **38**, 203–210.

Lorenz, J. (1998). Hyperalgesia or hypervigilance? An evoked potential approach to the study of fibromyalgia syndrome. *Z Rheumatol*, **57**(**Suppl. 2**), 19–22.

Lotze, M., Flor, H., Grodd W., Larbig, W. and Birbaumer, N. (2001). Phantom movements and pain. An fMRI study in upper limb amputees. *Brain*, **124**(**Pt 11**), 2268–2277.

Lotze, M., Grodd, W., Birbaumer, N., Erb, M., Huse, E. and Flor, H. (1999). Does use of a myoelectric prosthesis reduce cortical reorganization and phantom limb pain? *Nat Neurosci*, **2**, 501–502.

Maier, C., Dertwinkel, R., Mansourian, N., Hosbach, I., Schwenkreis, P., Senne, I., Skipka, G., Zenz, M. and Tegenthoff, M. (2003). Efficacy of the NMDA-receptor antagonist memantine in patients with chronic phantom limb pain – results of a randomized double-blinded, placebo-controlled trial. *Pain*, **103**, 277–283.

Maier, S.F. (1989). Determinants of nature of environmentally induced hypoalgesia. *Behav Neurosci*, **103**(1), 131–143.

May, A., Bahra, A., Büchel, C., Frackowiak, R.S. and Goadsby, P.J. (1998). Hypothalamic activation in cluster headache attacks. *Lancet*, **352**, 275–278.

May, A., Ashburner, J., Büchel, C., et al. (1999). Correlation between structural and functional changes in brain in an idiopathic headache syndrome. *Nat Med*, **5**, 836–838.

Merzenich, M.M., Nelson, R.J., Stryker, M.P., Cynader, M.S., Schoppmann, A. and Zook, J.M. (1984). Somatosensory cortical map changes following digit amputation in adult monkeys. *J Comp Neurol*, **224**(4), 591–605.

Nikolajsen, L., Hansen, C.L., Nielsen, J., Keller, J., Arendt-Nielsen, L. and Jensen, T.S. (1996). The effect of ketamine on phantom limb pain: a central neuropathic disorder maintained by peripheral input. *Pain*, **67**, 69–77.

Nikolajsen, L., Ilkjaer, S., Christensen, J.H., Kroner, K. and Jensen, T.S. (1997). Randomised trial of epidural bupivacaine and morphine in prevention of stump and phantom pain in lower-limb amputation. *Lancet*, **350**, 1353–1357.

Nikolajsen, L., Ilkjaer, S. and Jensen, T.S. (2000a). Relationship between mechanical sensitivity and post-amputation pain: a perspective study. *Eur J Pain*, **4**, 327–334.

Nikolajsen, L., Gottrup, H., Kristensen, A.G.D. and Jensen, T.S. (2000b). Memantine (an *N*-methyl D-aspartate receptor antagonist) in the treatment of neuropathic pain following amputation or surgery – a randomised, double-blind, cross-over study. *Anesth Analg*, **91**, 960–966.

Pleger, B., Tegenthoff, M., Schwenkreis, P., Janssen, F., Ragert, P., Dinse, H.R., Volker, B., zenz, M. and Maier, C. (2004). Mean sustained pain levels are linked to hemispherical side-to-side differences of primary somatosensory cortex in the complex regional pain syndrome I. *Exp Brain Res*, **155**(1), 115–119.

Rainville, P., Duncan, G.H., Price, D.D., Carrier, B. and Bushnell, M. C. (1997). Pain affect encoded in human anterior cingulate but not somatosensory cortex. *Science*, **277**(**5328**), 968–971.

Ramachandran, V.S., Rogers-Ramachandran, D. and Stewart, M. (1992). Perceptual correlates of massive cortical reorganization. *Science*, **258**, 1159–1160.

Robinson, L.R., Czerniecki, J.M., Ehde, D.M., Edwards, W.T., Judish, D.A., Goldberg, M.L., Campbell, K.M., Smith, D.G. and Jensen, M.P. (2004). Trial of amitriptyline for relief of pain in amputees: results of a randomized controlled study. *Arch Phys Med Rehabil*, **85**, 1–6.

Sanchez del Rio, M. and Linera, J.A. (2004). Functional neuroimaging of headaches. *Lancet Neurol*, **3**, 645–651.

Sandkühler, J. (2000). Learning and memory in pain pathways. *Pain*, **88**(2), 113–118.

Schoenen, J., Bottin, D., Hardy, F. and Gerard, P. (1991). Cephalic and extracephalic pressure pain thresholds in chronic tension–type headache. *Pain*, **47**, 145–149.

Sherman, R.A. (ed.) (1997). *Phantom Limb Pain*, Plenum, New York.

Sindrup, S.H., Jensen, T.S. (1999). Efficacy of pharmacological treatments of neuropathic pain: an update and effect related to mechanism of drug action. *Pain*, **83**, 389–400.

Spitzer, M., Böhler, P., Weisbrod, M. and Kischka, U. (1995). A neural network model of phantom limbs. *Biol Cyber*, **72**, 197–206.

Staud, R., Vierck, C.J., Cannon, R.L., Mauderli, A.P. and Price, D.D. (2001). Abnormal sensitization and temporal summation of second pain (wind-up) in patients with fibromyalgia syndrome. *Pain*, **91**(1–2), 165–175.

Tinazzi, M., Fiaschi, A., Rosso, T., Faccioli, F., Grosslercher, J. and Aglioti, S.M. (2000). Neuroplastic changes related to pain occur at multiple levels of the human somatosensory system: a somatosensory-evoked potentials study in patients with cervical radicular pain. *J Neurosci*, **20**, 9277–9283.

Vos, B.P., Benoist, J.M., Gautron, M. and Guilbaud, G. (2000). Changes in neuronal activities in the two ventral posterior medial thalamic nuclei in an experimental model of trigeminal pain in the rat by constriction of one infraorbital nerve. *Somatosens Mot Res*, **17**, 109–122.

Weiller, C., May, A., Limmroth, V., Juptner, M., Kaube, H., Schayck, R.V., Coenen, H.H. and Diener, H.C. (1995). Brain stem activation in spontaneous human migraine attacks. *Nat Med*, **1**, 658–660.

Wiech, K., Preissl, H., Kiefer, T., Töpfner, S., Pauli, P., Grillon, C., Flor, H. and Birbaumer, N. (2001). Prevention of phantom limb pain and cortical reorganization in the early phase after amputation in humans. *Society for Neuroscience, Abstract*, **28**, 163.9.

Wiech, K., Kiefer, R.T., Töpfner, S., Preissl, H., Unertl, K., Flor, H. and Birbaumer, N. (2004). A placebo-controlled randomized crossover trial of the *N*-methyl-D-aspartic acid receptor antagonist, memantine, in patients with chronic phantom limb pain. *Anesth Analg*, **98**, 408–413.

Willoch, F., Rosen, G., Tölle, T.R., Oye, I., Wester, H.J., Berner, N., et al. (2000). Phantom limb pain in the human brain: unraveling neural circuitries of phantom limb sensations using positron emission tomography. *Ann Neurol*, **48**(6), 842–849.

Wunsch, A., Philippot, P. and Plaghki, L. (2003). Affective associative learning modifies the sensory perception of nociceptive stimuli without participant's awareness. *Pain*, **102**(1–2), 27–38.

Yang, T.T., Schwartz, B., Gallen, C., Bloom, F.E., Ramachandran, V.S. and Cobb, S. (1994). Sensory maps in the human brain. *Nature*, **368**, 592–593.

16

Loss of somatic sensation

Leeanne Carey

School of Occupational Therapy Faculty of Health Sciences, LaTrobe University, Bundoora, Victoria, Australia

Evidence of behavioral recovery of somatic sensations following peripheral and central nervous system lesions challenges therapists to not only understand the nature and extent of the change, but the conditions under which the recovery can be maximized and the mechanisms underlying. This challenge requires input from basic sciences and rehabilitation fields. Integration of these fields will provide direction for the development and testing of scientific-based interventions designed to maximize recovery by driving and shaping neural reorganization.

The focus of this chapter will be on loss of somatic sensations, treatments currently available to address this problem, and the potential application of theories of perceptual learning and neural plasticity. More detail will be given to therapies following central nervous system (CNS) lesions, with particular reference to stroke. Comparisons will also be made in relation to loss following peripheral nervous system (PNS) lesions.

16.1 Nature of impairment and functional implications of loss

Definition and processing within the somatosensory system

Somatosensory function is the ability to interpret bodily sensation (Puce, 2003). Sensory systems are organized to receive, process and transmit information obtained from the periphery to the cerebral cortex. Within the *somatosensory* system submodalities of touch, proprioception, temperature sense, pain and itch are identified. (Gardner and Martin, 2000). Detailed description of the system involved in sensory processing is provided in seminal texts

such as Kandel, Schwartz and Jessell (Gardner and Martin, 2000). Further, neuroimaging studies are complementing and extending information gained from animal and lesion studies in humans (Schnitzler et al., 2000).

Two features of the structure and function of the system have particular implication for understanding the nature of impairment and neurorehabilitation. First is the high degree of specificity in the organization and processing of information. Specialized sensory receptors, modality-specific line of communication (Gardner and Martin, 2000), specific columnar organization and sub-modality-specific neurons in primary (SI) and secondary (SII) somatosensory areas (Mountcastle, 1997) support this specificity. Second, the opportunity for convergence of somatosensory information within the CNS (Mesulam, 1998), as well as the presence of distributed sensory networks and multiple somatotopic representation (Gardner and Kandel, 2000), impact on the scope for neural plastic changes (Volume I, Chapter 6) and rehabilitation outcome.

Loss of somatic sensation following interruption to central and peripheral nervous systems

Loss of somatic sensations can be sustained due to damage at various levels of the sensory system, for example from receptors to peripheral nerves, spinal cord, brainstem and cerebral cortex. This may result from disease or trauma associated with a wide range of conditions (see Section E Disease-specific Neurorehabilitation Systems of Volume II). Somatosensory impairment may be in the form of anesthesia (total loss of one or more sensory submodalities in the region), hyposensitivity (reduced ability to perceive sensations, including poor localization, discrimination and integration), or hypersensitivity (non-noxious stimuli become irritating, for example dyesthesia, paraesthesia or causalgia). Clinical description of loss should include identification of body part and submodalities affected as well as the level of processing impairment, for example detection, discrimination and integration of information across submodalities.

There are differences in the nature of the loss following peripheral and CNS lesions. For example, injury to the PNS involves well-defined loss of specific modalities that can be mapped relative to the nerve distribution or receptor location. In comparison, loss following CNS lesions such as stroke can result in very different patterns of deficit, from complete hemianaesthesia of multiple modalities to dissociated loss of sub-modality specificity in a particular body location (see Carey, 1995 for review). Loss of discriminative sensibilities is most characteristic (Bassetti et al., 1993; Carey, 1995; Kim and Choi-Kwon, 1996), thresholds for primary sensory qualities (e.g., touch) are often indefinable (Head and Holmes, 1911–1912), qualitative alterations, response variability (Carey, 1995) and dissociated sensory loss (Roland, 1987; Bassetti et al., 1993) are observed, and hypersensitivity may be present initially or develop over time (Holmgren et al., 1990). Typically the loss is contralateral to the injury, although ipsilateral deficits are also reported (Carey, 1995; Kim and Choi-Kwon, 1996). The early and chronic pattern of deficit may be influenced by the site of lesion, relative sparing and redundancy within the distributed sensory system and neural plastic changes that may occur with recovery.

Functional implications of loss

Impairment of body sensations poses a significant loss in its own right and has a negative impact on effective exploration of the environment, personal safety, motor function, and quality of life (Rothwell et al., 1982; Carey, 1995). Everyday tasks such as searching for a coin in a pocket, feeling if a plate is clean when washing dishes, maintaining the grip of an object without crushing or dropping it, using cutlery, fastening buttons, writing and walking on uneven ground become difficult and often frustrating (Carey, 1995). The important role of sensation in motor function is particularly evident in: control of pinch grip (Johansson and Westling, 1984); ability to sustain and adapt appropriate force without vision (Jeannerod et al., 1984); object manipulation (Johansson, 1996); combining component parts of movement such as transport and grasp (Gentilucci et al., 1997); discrimination of surfaces at end of hand-held objects (Chan and Turvey, 1991); restraint of moving objects (Johansson et al., 1992); and adjustment to sensory conflict conditions such, as a rough surface (Wing et al., 1997). Moreover, the affected limb may not be used spontaneously, despite adequate movement abilities. This may contribute to a learned non-use of the limb and further deterioration of motor function after stroke (Dannenbaum and Dykes, 1988). These activity limitations impact on life roles, social communication, safety and participation in personal and domestic activities of daily living as well as sexual and leisure activities (Carey, 1995).

The personal and functional implications of sensory loss are highlighted in the words of a client who experienced sensory loss after stroke: "… my right side cannot discriminate rough, smooth, rigid or malleable, sharp or blunt, heavy or light. It cannot tell whether that which touches it as hand or tennis racket…it is frustratingly difficult to control or feel relaxed about any right-sided movement…. How does one trust a foot that "feels" as though it has no real connection with the earth? It is difficult to pick up or hold a pair of glasses or a sheet of paper when one's right hand/fingers feel uncontrollably strong and very big and clumsy, capable of crushing objects with one's grip yet incapable of letting go or throwing off even the lightest objects (e.g. a tissue)…. better to feel something-however bizarre-than nothing."

Loss of somatic sensations also negatively impacts on rehabilitative and functional outcomes, as indicated in a review of stroke outcome studies (Carey, 1995). It has a cumulative impact on functional deficits beyond severity of motor deficits alone (Patel et al., 2000) and negatively impacts on reacquisition of skilled movements of the upper limb (Kusoffsky et al., 1982; Jeannerod et al., 1984), postural control and ambulation (Reding and Potes, 1988). The importance of the sensory system as an early indicator of motor recovery after stroke has been suggested in neuroimaging (Weiller, 1998) and clinical (Kusoffsky et al., 1982) studies. It has been suggested that sensory reorganization may precede motor reorganization and may, in fact, trigger the latter (Weiller, 1998).

16.2 Assessment of somatic sensation

Guidelines for the selection of measures for use in clinical settings

The directive to follow evidence-based practice demands that clinicians employ quantitative measures that are valid and reliable. Numerous tests have been developed to evaluate the various qualities of sensibility, including touch, pressure, temperature, pain, proprioception and tactual object recognition (Carey, 1995; Dellon, 2000). In clinical settings we need information not only on thresholds of detection, but also on the ability to make accurate discriminations and recognize objects with multiple sensory attributes. Selection of suitable measures should be based on the following criteria: valid measurement of the sensory outcome of interest, for example discrimination; quantitative measurement; objectively defined stimuli; control for test bias and other clinical deficits; standardized protocol; adequate scale resolution to monitor change; good reliability and age-appropriate normative standards. For a critique of routine clinical and quantitative measures refer to Carey (1995), Dellon (2000) and Winward et al. (1999).

The need for standardized measures for use following stroke has been highlighted (Carey, 1995; Winward et al., 1999). Measures commonly used are largely subjective, lack standardized protocol (Lincoln et al., 1991; Carey, 1995;), use gross scales such as

"normal", "impaired" or "absent" (Wade, 1992), have variable reliability (Winward et al., 1999), no defined criterion of abnormality, and are often insensitive or inaccurate (Carey et al., 2002c). Kim and Choi-Kwon found that discriminative sensation remained in only 3 of 25 stroke patients who were reported as having no sensory impairment on the basis of conventional sensory tests (Kim and Choi-Kwon, 1996).

Over the past decade new measures have been developed for use post-stroke. Clinical test batteries developed are the Nottingham Sensory Assessment (NSA) (Lincoln et al., 1991; Lincoln et al., 1998) and the Rivermead Assessment of Somatosensory Performance (RASP) (Winward et al., 2002). The RASP is standardized, uses seven quantifiable subtests of touch and proprioceptive discrimination and includes three new instruments, the neurometer, neurotemp and two-point neurodiscriminator. Intra and inter-rater reliability are high ($r = 0.92$). The NSA employs methods consistent with clinical practice, but are more detailed and standardized. Intra and inter-rater reliability are variable, with most tests showing relatively poor agreement across raters. The revised NSA reports acceptable ($k > 0.6$) agreement in only 12 of 86 items (Lincoln et al., 1998), and inter-rater reliability of 0.38–1.00 for the stereognosis component (Gaubert and Mockett, 2000).

New tests of specific sensory functions commonly impaired post-stroke have also been achieved. A test of sustained touch-pressure, based on the need to appreciate sustained contact of an object in the hand during daily manual tasks, was developed and impairment demonstrated in six patients with severe sensory deficit (Dannenbaum and Dykes, 1990). Empirical foundations for the test are required. New measures of tactile (Carey et al., 1997) and proprioceptive (Carey et al., 1996) discrimination provide quantitative measurement of the characteristic discriminative loss post-stroke. They are founded on strong neurophysiological and psychophysical evidence (Clark and Horch, 1986; Darian-Smith and Oke, 1980; Morley, 1980) and perception of the grid surfaces has been associated with cerebral activation in multiple somatosensory areas in unimpaired (Burton et al., 1997) and impaired (Carey et al., 2002a) humans. The measures are quantitative, reliable, standardized, measure small changes in ability, have empirically demonstrated ability to differentiate impaired performance relative to normative standards (Carey et al., 1996, 1997) and advance current clinical assessment (Carey et al., 2002c). Tests of fabric discrimination and discrimination of finger and elbow position sense have also been developed (Carey, 1995) and are being empirically tested by us.

In addition to quantitative measures of sensibility, it is important to evaluate the presence and impact of the impairment in daily activities. This may involve structured interview and/or observation of occupational performance difficulties in tasks relevant to the patient. Focus of observations may include impact of loss on unilateral and bilateral tasks, level of independence, nature of difficulties (e.g., clumsy) and use of compensatory techniques. Tasks with varying sensory demands may be structured to systematically assess the impact of sensory loss. As yet there is no standardized test of the impact of sensory loss on daily activities.

16.3 Potential for recovery

The potential for recovery of somatosensory abilities has been demonstrated, following lesions to peripheral (Dellon, 2000) and central (Carey, 1995) nervous systems under both spontaneous and training-induced recovery conditions.

The natural history of recovery

The potential for recovery depends on regeneration of structures within the somatosensory system as well as the capacity for neural plasticity and reinterpretation of altered stimuli. These factors are further influenced by the level at which the system is interrupted, extent of injury, progression of disease, age, prior and intervening experience (Callahan, 1995; Carey, 1995; Dellon, 2000; see also Chapters 12, 13, and 27 of Volume I). Regeneration and recovery following damage to PNS has been relatively well described (Callahan, 1995; Dellon, 2000). In

comparison, few studies have systematically investigated the natural history of spontaneous recovery of somatosensations post-stroke. Improvements have been reported across a range of measures including touch detection, texture and proprioceptive discrimination and object recognition (see Carey, 1995 for review). However, the extent of recovery is varied (Kusoffsky et al., 1982), ranging from lasting deficits (Wadell et al., 1987) to "quite remarkable" improvement in capacities such as stereognosis (Schwartzman, 1972). The temporal aspects of recovery are also relatively unknown. Recovery appears most marked within the first 3 months (Newman, 1972), although ongoing recovery has been observed at 6 months and later (Kusoffsky, 1990). It has been suggested that persistent deficit may be associated with particular lesion site (Corkin et al., 1970).

Evidence of training-induced recovery

Evidence of training-induced sensory improvements further highlights the potential for recovery following PNS (Dellon, 2000) and CNS (Carey, 1995) lesions. Moreover, improvements have been observed months and years post-injury, after the period of expected nerve regeneration (Dellon, 2000). Dellon (2000) asserts that results of sensory rehabilitation must be due to higher CNS functions and that cortical plasticity is the underlying mechanism. Similarly following stroke, task-specific and generalized training effects have been observed across tactile, proprioceptive and object recognition tasks, under quasi-experimental and controlled conditions (see Section Review of documented programs in relation to basic science and empirical foundations of documented of this chapter for review). In most instances the improvements have been observed after the period of expected spontaneous recovery. Neural plastic changes have also been proposed as the likely mechanism underlying these improvements.

Neural plastic changes associated with recovery of somatic sensations

Neural plastic changes occur in response to injury, but also as part of normal learning and development (refer to Section A on Neural plasticity in Volume I). The cellular, physiological and behavioral mechanisms operating in adaptive brain plasticity are discussed in this section. Changes can occur immediately post-lesion or months and years later and can involve multiple levels of the somatosensory system (Jones and Pons, 1998). Longer-term stable changes, likely linked with change in synaptic connections and learning, are the most relevant for rehabilitation. Investigations in humans confirm reorganization in somatosensory regions following extensive use (Pascual-Leone and Torres, 1993), transient anesthesia (Rossini et al., 1994) and injury to the PNS (Merzenich and Jenkins, 1993) and CNS (Carey et al., 2002a; Wikström et al., 2000; see also Chapters 6, 14 and 15 of Volume I).

Studies of change in human brain activation, suggestive of neural reorganization, are providing new insights into the mechanisms underlying stroke recovery (Weiller, 1998; see also Chapter 5 of Volume II). Evolution of change over time and a potential relationship with recovery has been demonstrated in the motor system (e.g., Carey et al., 2005; Small et al., 2002; Ward et al., 2003). Findings indicate involvement of cortical and subcortical sites primarily within the pre-existing motor network and include recruitment of sites not typically used for the task and return to a more "normal" pattern of activation. Changes in SI (Rossini et al., 1998; Wikström et al., 2000), SII (Carey et al., 2002a) and thalamus (Ohara and Lenz, 2001) have been reported in the few studies of somatosensory recovery post-stroke. In serial pilot functional magnetic resonance imaging (fMRI) studies we found re-emergence of activation in ipsilesional SI and bilateral SII in a stroke patient who had marked sensory loss followed by good recovery (Fig. 16.1, Patient 1; Carey et al., 2002a). In comparison, only very limited recruitment in non-primary sensory areas was observed in the second patient who showed poor spontaneous recovery.

As yet little is known about neural mechanisms underlying functional recovery associated with *specific training* post-stroke in humans. Animal models highlight the benefit of experience in facilitating brain reorganization within motor and sensory systems. Controlled studies in primates suggest that both

positive and negative patterns of brain reorganization can occur and that these can be "strongly influenced by appropriate rehabilitation programs after brain damage" (Nudo et al., 1996b; Nudo, 1999). Brain plasticity related to treatment-induced *motor* recovery has been suggested in the sensorimotor system of humans post-stroke (Liepert et al., 2000; Nelles et al., 2001; Carey J.R. et al., 2002). In addition, we have recently demonstrated good clinical recovery and changes in ipsilesional SI, bilateral SII and premotor areas following *somatosensory* training in a patient who showed poor spontaneous recovery in the 6 months prior (see Fig. 16.1, Patient 2). Investigation of changes in brain activation associated with training-induced recovery of somatosensations under randomized control conditions is now required.

16.4 Approaches to retraining impaired sensory function

Review of documented programs in relation to basic science and empirical foundations

Neurorehabilitation needs to be founded on a rigorous basic and clinical science platform and include cure in its mission (Seltzer, introduction to this text). Sensory re-education has been an integral part of the rehabilitation of patients with peripheral nerve disorders for many years. Some of the most influential programs are those developed by Wynn Parry and Salter (1976) and expanded by Dellon (1981; 2000). These programs employ principles of direct, repeated sensory practice, feedback through vision, subjective grading of stimuli such as texture and objects, verbalization of sensations and comparison of sensations experienced across hands. Evidence for the effectiveness of sensory training following peripheral lesions is reviewed in (Dellon, 2000, Chapter 11). Whilst some programs are directed to localized somatosensory deficits and regeneration of specific nerve fibers, Dellon (2000) highlights the need to focus on interpretation of altered stimuli at a cortical level based on evidence of neural plasticity.

There are a relatively limited number of documented sensory retraining programs designed for

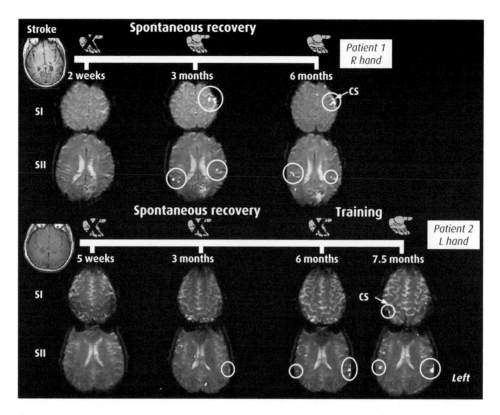

Figure 16.1. Serial fMRI pilot studies of touch discrimination during the interval of spontaneous recovery (non-specific rehabilitation) and following specific sensory retraining post-stroke. The functional echoplanar axial slices shown sample two brain regions of interest, that is primary somatosensory cortex (SI) posterior to the central sulcus (CS), and secondary somatosensory cortex (SII). Significant brain activation (Puncorrected < 0.0001) in ipsilesional SI and bilateral SII observed during stimulation of the affected hand is circled.

use with stroke patients (Carey, 1995). Early studies suggesting improvement of sensory abilities (Vinograd et al., 1962; De Jersey, 1979) have lacked controls and a sound theoretical basis. The program by Vinograd et al. involved repeated exposure to test stimuli with 3D feedback from a box lined with mirrors while DeJersey used bombardment with multiple sensory stimuli. The only early study with a controlled design (Van Deusen Fox, 1964) also did not employ current theories of perceptual learning and neurophysiology and failed to obtain a therapeutic effect (see Carey, 1995 for review).

In comparison, Dannenbaum and Dykes (1988) described a therapeutic rationale based on neurophysiologic concepts and "rules governing somatosensory cortical reorganization after trauma". Their program involved stimulation of "important sensory surfaces" at an intensity sufficient for appreciation and in a task that was motivating to the patient. Subjects were encouraged to attend to the input and given reinforcement. Electric stimulation and velcro were used in the early stages, followed by finger localization, exploration of velcro shapes and use of utensils taped with velcro. Improvement was reported in the case study presented.

Yekutiel and Guttman (1993) reported significant gains following sensory retraining in 20 stroke patients with chronic sensory impairment under controlled conditions. Principles of training were derived initially from peripheral nerve injury training programs (Wynn Parry and Salter, 1976), with contributions from psychology (Yekutiel, 2000). The essential principles included focus on the hand, attention and motivation, guided exploration of the tactics of perception and use of the "good" hand. The findings confirm that sensory discriminations are trainable after stroke and suggest a potential for generalized sensory gains. The authors reported variation in results across patients and noted that, the method used – although aimed at higher brain centers – may still be too "peripheral" (Yekutiel and Guttman, 1993) (p. 243).

We have developed and investigated the effectiveness of two different approaches to training sensory discrimination: Stimulus Specific Training (SST) (Carey, 1993; Carey et al., 1993) and Stimulus Generalization Training (SGT) (Carey and Matyas, 2005). The programs employ principles derived from theories of perceptual learning (Gibson, 1991; Goldstone, 1998), recovery following brain damage (Bach-y-Rita, 1980; Weiller, 1998) and neurophysiology of somatosensory processing (Gardner and Kandel, 2000). SST was designed to maximize improvement in specific stimuli trained. It involves repeated presentation of targeted discrimination tasks; progression from easy to more difficult discriminations; attentive exploration of stimuli with vision occluded; use of anticipation trials; feedback on accuracy, method of exploration and salient features of the stimuli; and use of vision to facilitate calibration of sensory information (Carey, 1993; Carey et al., 1993). In comparison, the SGT approach was designed to facilitate transfer of training effects to untrained, novel stimuli and included additional principles of variation in stimulus and practice conditions, intermittent feedback and tuition of training principles (Carey and Matyas, 2005; Gibson, 1991; Schmidt and Lee, 1999).

SST effects were replicated in 37 of 41 time-series across 30 single-case experiments. Stimulus Generalization effects were found in 8 of 11 time-series across 11 subjects. Marked improvements, to within normal performance standards, were achieved within ten or fewer training sessions and maintained over follow-up periods of 3–5 months, suggesting a long-term therapeutic effect. SST effects were specific to the trained sensory perceptual dimension (tactile or proprioceptive) and stimulus type (e.g., texture gratings or fabrics). Generalized improvements in touch discrimination, that is *untrained* fabric surfaces, were achieved by the program deliberately oriented to enhance transfer (Carey and Matyas, 2005), as shown in Fig. 16.2. Meta-analysis of SST effects (tactile $z = -8.6$, $P < 0.0001$; proprioception $z = -4.3$, $P < 0.0001$) and SGT effects (tactile $z = -5.7$; $P < 0.0001$) supports the overall conclusion that tactile and proprioceptive discriminations are retrainable following stroke and that both modes of training are effective. Finally, we have also applied the SGT approach to training friction discrimination and investigated its effect on the fundamental pinch grip task in pilot studies, with positive results (Carey et al., 2002b)

Two further retraining programs have been documented recently. These programs are in part derived from earlier programs, employ principles consistent with perceptual learning and neural plasticity and focus on training sensory *and* motor functions. Smania et al. (2003) describe a program of sensory and motor exercises for patients with pure sensory stroke. The program involved graded exercises, reported to be challenging for the patient, and feedback on accuracy and execution of task for each trial. Exercises focused on tactile discrimination using different textured surfaces, object recognition, joint position sense, weight discrimination, blindfolded motor tasks involving reach and grasp of different objects, as well as practice of seven daily life activities. Improvement in sensory and motor outcomes, as well as increased use of the affected arm in daily activities, was reported in the four cases studied.

Byl et al. (2003) described a program aimed to improve accuracy and speed in sensory discrimination and sensorimotor feedback. Principles, derived from studies of neural adaptation, included: matching tasks to ability of the subject, attention, repetition, feedback on performance and progression in difficulty. Sensory training focused on improving

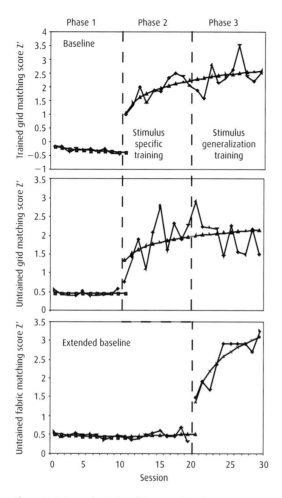

Figure 16.2. Example single-subject case chart demonstrating SST effects on trained grids and untrained grids. Improvement in *untrained* fabric discriminations is evident only following introduction of the program designed to enhance generalization. Baseline conditions of repeated exposure to the stimuli were not sufficient to effect clinically significant improvement. The raw time-series data (×) and predicted time-series models (■ ▲ ♦) are shown. Higher scores represent an improvement in texture matching ability. The criterion of normality for the Grid Matching Test is 0.62 z' score (mean = 1.47) and for the Fabric Matching Test is 1.61 z' score (mean = 2.46). Statistical time-series analyses of trend and level effects (*P* < 0.01) confirm the training effects shown for this subject.

sensory discriminations through games and fine motor activities, use of velcro on objects, retrieving objects from a box filled with rice and exercises in graphesthesia, localization, stereognosis and kinesthesia. Movements of the hand, mental rehearsal to reinforce learning and tasks to quiet the nervous system were also used. Patients were educated regarding the potential for improvement in neural processing and the unaffected hand was constrained through wearing of a glove. Training was investigated in 21 subjects with order of sensory or motor training crossed, although no placebo intervention period was employed. Improvements in sensory discrimination, fine motor function and musculoskeletal measurements of the upper limb were reported following sensory training. Gains were hemispheric and training specific.

In summary, recent training programs with successful outcomes have included a number of common principles consistent with theories of learning and neural plasticity. These include: attention to the sensory stimulus; repetitive stimulation with and without vision; use of tasks that are challenging and motivating; focus on the hand; graded progression of tasks and feedback on accuracy and execution. A more detailed discussion of principles of training related to perceptual learning and neural plasticity follows with suggestions for their application.

16.5 Principles of neural plasticity and learning as they apply to rehabilitation of sensation

Identification and application of principles to optimize perceptual learning and brain adaptation

Evidence of neural plasticity provides a strong foundation for restorative sensory retraining post-injury, both in acute and chronic phases. Review of theories of perceptual learning and the conditions under which neural plastic changes occur suggests a number of principles that have potential application in retraining somatosensations following PNS or CNS injury.

Table 16.1. Summary of principles of sensory training derived from theories of perceptual learning, neural plasticity and physiology of the somatosensory system.

Principle of training	Derived from and/or consistent with theories of		
	Perceptual learning	Neural plasticity	Physiology
Repeated stimulation of specific stimuli	√ improvement maximal for specific stimulus	√ modification of sensory map is task-dependent	√ specificity of processing within the system
Attentive exploration	√ attention important in learning	√ modulation of neural plasticity	√ component of sensory processing
Vision occluded		√ force use of somatosensory system	√ vision may dominate
Motivating/ meaningful task	√ link with attention, learning and success	√ brain responds to meaningful goals	
Use of anticipation trials (and imagery)		√ activation of similar sites as for direct stimulation.	√ consistent with normal processing
Feedback on – accuracy – method of exploration and summary feedback	√ extrinsic and summary feedback may enhance learning	√ enhance new connections	
Calibration of sensation: within and across modalities	√ improved perception	√ cross-modal plasticity	√ pre-existing connections within system
Progression from easy to more difficult discriminations	√ required for learning within and across sensory dimensions	√ progressively challenge system	
Intensive training	√ improved performance and retention	√ forced use, competitive use	
Variation in stimuli, intermittent feedback and tuition of training principles	√ facilitates transfer of training effects		

Most of the principles identified from these fields are complementary, consistent with the knowledge that neural plasticity underlies learning and recovery following injury. In addition, the physiology of processing somatosensory information must be considered in application to the sensory system. More recent sensory retraining approaches have begun to base their training on these principles (see Section Review of documented programs in relation to basic science and empirical foundations of this chapter for review). Key principles that have been successfully applied, or have potential for application, are discussed below. Their application is summarized in Table 16.1.

Neural plastic changes are experience-dependent (see Section A on Neural plasticity in Volume I; Nudo

et al., 1996a) and the system is competitive (Merzenich and Jenkins, 1993; Weinreich and Armentrout, 1995). Functional reorganization has been demonstrated after behaviorally controlled tactile stimulation in intact animals (Recanzone et al., 1992). Forced use of the system, for example using constraint induced movement therapy, has also been associated with neural plastic changes in post-stroke motor recovery (Liepert et al., 2000). Even less intensive programs based on principles of motor learning found training-induced changes (Carey J.R. et al., 2002). Importantly, repetitive use alone may not be sufficient to effect changes in cortical representation. Rather changes are associated with specific skill learning, consistent with a "learning-dependent" hypothesis of neural plasticity (Karni et al., 1995; Plautz et al., 2000). Sensory neurorehabilitation should therefore challenge the sensory system using repeated stimulation of targeted sensory tasks coupled with an intensive perceptual-learning based training program.

Learning is reported to be maximal for the specific task trained (Gibson, 1969; Goldstone, 1998; Sathian and Zangaladze, 1997), consistent with highly specific organization of the system (see Section Definition and processing within the somatosensory system of this chapter for review) and evidence that functional reorganization is directly linked with changes in cortical regions engaged by these inputs (Recanzone et al., 1992). Repetition over time with an increasing number of coincident events serves to strengthen synaptic connections (Byl and Merzenich, 2000). However, competition between afferent inputs for connections in the sensory cortex (Merzenich and Jenkins, 1993) suggests the need for caution with overstimulation of a specific site at the expense of related areas. Consequently to maximize task-specific learning, training stimuli and the method of processing the information should match targeted discrimination tasks (Carey et al., 1993). Training of important sites normally responsible for the sensation, for example the hand (Dannenbaum and Dykes, 1988; Yekutiel and Guttman, 1993), and discriminations characteristically impaired and important for daily function (Carey et al., 1993) have been recommended.

Motivation is important in learning (Goldstone, 1998) and recovery after brain injury (Bach-y-Rita, 1980), and the brain responds to meaningful goals (Nudo et al., 1996b). Training should therefore be goal directed, interesting and demanding if it is to tap into the brain's potential for functional reorganization (Byl and Merzenich, 2000; Yekutiel, 2000). It should provide regular opportunities for success, with reinforcement to encourage motivation and participation (Carey, 1993; Yekutiel, 2000).

Attention is crucial in perceptual learning. Attentive exploration of stimuli allows purposeful feedback within the sensory-perceptual system (Epstein et al., 1989) and perception becomes adapted to tasks by increasing the attention paid to important features (with less noticing of irrelevancies) (Gibson, 1969; Goldstone, 1998). Perceptual learning (Goldstone, 1998) and neurophysiological (Johnson and Hsiao, 1992) evidence propose that "distinctive features of difference" are learned and form the basis of transfer of training. Attention is also important in the modulation of cortical plasticity (see Chapter 12 of Volume I), particularly in early stages of plastic changes and learning (Karni et al., 1995). Thus patients should actively (where possible) and purposively explore sensory stimuli with attention directed to distinctive features of difference. This may be facilitated through requiring a response and guiding the patient to search for distinctive features (Carey et al., 1993). Further, as vision may dominate tactile and proprioceptive senses in some instances (Clark and Horch, 1986; Lederman et al., 1986), exploration of stimuli with vision occluded should be included to allow subjects to focus specifically on the somatic sensations (Carey et al., 1993).

Anticipation may facilitate recruitment of existing or new sensory sites in the brain. Similar brain sites are active under direct stimulation and anticipated stimulation conditions (Roland, 1981). Further, prior and subjective experience can influence early stages of information processing and facilitate stimulus differentiation (Goldstone, 1998). Anticipation trials, in which the patient is informed that a limited set of previously experienced stimuli will be used (Carey et al., 1993), may tap into this capacity and encourage new neural connections. A patient may also be encouraged to imagine what a stimulus should feel like, based on evidence that haptic (tactile and proprioceptive) information is represented through imagery (Klatzky et al., 1991).

Augmented feedback on accuracy of response outcome and on performance is important in skill acquisition (Schmidt and Lee, 1999) and may enhance perceptual learning (Gibson, 1969). Although improvement in perceptual discriminations may be experienced in unimpaired subjects without extrinsic feedback in some cases (Epstein et al., 1989), practice with correction can enhance learning

(Gibson, 1969). We found that repeated exposure alone was insufficient to effect a positive training outcome in the majority of cases post-stroke (Carey et al., 1993; Carey and Matyas, 2005). Thus feedback on accuracy of response and performance, for example method of exploration (Lederman and Klatzky, 1993), should be provided. Feedback should be immediate, precise and quantitative to maximize acquisition (Salmoni et al., 1984). Summary feedback also enhances learning (Salmoni et al., 1984) and should be provided at the end of each training session.

Calibration of perceptions would also appear to be important. This may involve comparison of the sensation with the other hand (Gibson, 1969) and use of vision to facilitate cross-modal calibration (Lederman et al., 1986), consistent with activity in visual cortical regions during tactile perception (Zangaladze et al., 1999). Computational neural models indicate that when two modalities are trained at the same time and provide feedback for each other, a higher level of performance is possible than if they remained independent (Becker, 1996). Moreover, cross-modal plasticity in sensory systems (see Chapter 11 of Volume I) may facilitate alternate and new neural connections.

Finer perceptual differences are able to be distinguished through exposure to a series of graded stimuli (Ahissar and Hochstein, 1997; Goldstone, 1998). Graded progression facilitates perceptual differentiation, especially of complex stimuli, as presentation of an easy discrimination first allows the subject to allocate attention to the relevant dimension (Goldstone, 1998). Further, transfer from one stimulus to another within a unidimensional sensory quality requires presentation in a graded manner (Gibson, 1969). Thus training should progress from easy to more difficult discriminations across stimuli and within a unidimensional sensory quality.

Performance is better on frequently presented items than rare items (Allen and Brooks, 1991). In addition, best available evidence suggests that training should continue for some time after "mastery" to increase retention (Lane, 1987). This further suggests the need for repetition and intensive training.

Specificity of learning and principles to facilitate learning transfer

Whilst the above principles have been associated with positive perceptual learning, there are limits on the generality of perceptual learning. Perceptual learning is usually highly specific to the task, receptor location and method of processing (Sathian and Zangaladze, 1997; Goldstone, 1998). Similarly, we found highly specific training effects in tasks employing the same sensory dimension (tactile or proprioceptive), sub-modality (grid or fabric textures) and body location (fingertip or wrist) with SST post-stroke (Carey et al., 1993; Carey and Matyas, 2005). However, perceptual transfer is possible in some instances with unimpaired subjects (Epstein et al., 1989; Ettlinger and Wilson, 1990; Spengler et al., 1997). Similarity between original and transfer tasks is an important factor influencing the degree of transfer (Gibson, 1969). It has been suggested that transfer should be more prominent where the stimuli are more complex and potentially share a number of distinctive features (Gibson, 1991; Goldstone, 1998). Transfer across body sites has also been reported in unimpaired systems (Sathian and Zangaladze, 1997; Spengler et al., 1997), and may be influenced by the attention demands and complexity of the task (Ahissar and Hochstein, 1997).

Principles of learning that facilitate transfer of training effects in unimpaired subjects have potential application following injury. Transfer of training effects is more effective when variation in stimuli is employed (Gibson, 1991; Goldstone, 1998; Schmidt and Lee, 1999). Optimally this should include training across a variety of stimuli with a wide range of distinctive features, for example roughness characteristics, as well as variation in tasks and environments (Carey and Matyas, 2005). To achieve grading, progressive difficulty should be defined across stimuli sets as well as within sets (Carey and Matyas, 2005).

Intermittent feedback on accuracy of response (Winstein and Schmidt, 1990) and specific instruction on principles of training and how these apply across tasks (Cormier and Hagman, 1987) have also been associated with enhanced transfer and retention. Further, an important part of learning transfer tasks is acquiring the capacity to cope with novel situations (Schmidt and Lee, 1999). This suggests the need to provide exposure to novel stimuli with opportunity to get feedback on the act of generalization (Carey and Matyas, 2005).

In summary, positive findings from studies of sensory retraining (see section Review of documented programs in relation to basic science and empirical foundations of this chapter for review) support the application of principles of training derived from literature on perceptual learning and neural plasticity. Further, the nature of training, that is stimulus specific versus generalization optimized, appears crucial to outcome. Evidence of a learning phenomenon associated with sensory retraining post-stroke has been quantified in the intervention time-series data of our patients (Carey, 1993; see also Fig. 16.2). The improvement curve was consistent with that described in the learning literature (Lane, 1987; Epstein et al., 1989) and in studies of neural plasticity (Recanzone et al., 1992). However, in contrast to unimpaired subjects (Epstein et al., 1989), the characteristic learning curve was only achieved under supervised training conditions (Carey et al., 1993). The potential for generalization of training within a sensory dimension has also been demonstrated post-stroke, provided a program designed to enhance transfer is used (Carey and Matyas, 2005). Other programs that have employed training across a variety of tasks have also found generalized training effects (Byl et al., 2003; Smania et al., 2003; Yekutiel and Guttman, 1993).

16.6 Future directions for the integration of basic science in clinical practice, as applied to neurorehabilitation of somatic sensation

Brain networks may reorganize to optimize stroke recovery. However, despite evidence of behavioral improvement, it is not known to what extent training-induced recovery is associated with changes in the functional neuroanatomy of sensation in humans. In particular it is unknown whether sites different to those typically used are involved in the recovery process, possibly suggestive of different behavioral strategies. Clinically effective sensory training programs, derived from theories of perceptual learning and recovery following brain damage, may be used to test for outcomes related to brain adaptation. Confirmation of the prediction that neural plastic changes occur primarily within the pre-existing somatosensory system (Weinreich and Armentrout, 1995), will highlight the importance of sparing and dynamic adaptation within pre-existing sensory sites. Evidence of recruitment of different sites may identify involvement of other systems important in recovery, such as attention (see Chapter 12 of Volume I) and visual (see Chapters 9 and 11 of Volume I) systems. This will advance our understanding of whether training is operating at a level of restitution or substitution within the system and provide insight into behavioral strategies associated with training. Comparison with motor recovery findings will help determine if there is a common model of neural plasticity associated with motor and somatosensory recovery.

Systematic investigation of the conditions under which behavioral improvement and neural repair is most effectively achieved is required to provide ongoing direction for the development of science-based interventions. For example, the timing (post-injury) and intensity of training requires investigation, given evidence of possible maladaptive changes (Merzenich and Jenkins, 1993; Nudo et al., 1996b). Investigation of the need for specific training, compared to non-specific exposure, and the neural outcomes of learning transfer (Spengler et al., 1997) will help elucidate the mechanisms and brain regions involved in different training methods. Similarly, different principles of training (e.g., cross-modality matching and feedback on accuracy) require systematic investigation of their contribution as they may involve different neural structures and mechanisms. Paradigms that permit investigation of component stages in neural processing need to be conducted and interpreted using models of analysis that focus on connectivity within the system.

Knowledge of the relationship between brain activation and recovery will have predictive significance in relation to identifying patients who are likely to show spontaneous recovery and/or who are able to benefit from training. Potential explanations for individual differences in the nature and extent of recovery may relate to lesion site (Zemke et al., 2003) and remote changes in structure, including diaschisis (Seitz et al., 1999). Investigation of the association between structural brain changes and the brain's capacity for reorganization is indicated.

Further development of current training programs is also indicated. Programs reviewed (see Section Review of documented programs in relation to basic science and empirical foundations of this chapter for review) have incorporated principles consistent with perceptual learning and neural plasticity. However, individual features of the training protocols have not been dissected. This is necessary to identify the critically important elements associated with successful learning and transfer. Previous studies have provided some insight into the boundaries of spontaneous and facilitated transfer with stroke patients (Carey et al., 1993; Carey and Matyas, 2005). Investigation of similarity of trained and transfer tasks, method of information processing, level of task difficulty and relative body location on learning transfer is needed to guide clinical training programs and clarify the nature of what is being learnt.

The most optimal combination of principles may also vary with individual patient characteristics including the nature of loss (e.g., detection versus discrimination versus multisensory integration), the phase of recovery (acute versus chronic) and the site of lesion (PNS versus CNS or specific location within these). Systematic investigation of these is indicated. The focus of training could also be expanded to include training in discrimination of size, shape and weight of objects, detection of slip when holding objects, regulation of pressure during grasp and spontaneous use of the limb. Finally, the ability to modify sensory abilities experimentally opens up an experimental paradigm for future investigations of the relationship between sensation and other abilities, such as pinch grip, and the effect of improving sensation on motor function and activities of daily living.

ACKNOWLEDGEMENTS

I wish to acknowledge the contribution of collaborators who have worked with me on various aspects of research related to sensory recovery and retraining following stroke. In particular Ass/Prof Thomas Matyas and Ms Lin Oke have collaborated on the clinical studies investigating methods of assessing and training somatosensations post-stroke. Ongoing clinical studies are being conducted also in collaboration with Prof Derek Wade and Dr Richard Macdonnell. Investigation of neural outcomes associated with motor and sensory recovery under spontaneous and training-induced recovery conditions is being conducted in collaboration with a number of researchers including Prof Geoffrey Donnan, Dr David Abbott, Dr Gary Egan, Prof Aina Puce and Prof Rüdiger Seitz.

REFERENCES

Ahissar, M. and Hochstein, S. (1997). Task difficulty and the specificity of perceptual learning. *Nature*, **387**, 401–406.

Allen, S.W. and Brooks, L.R. (1991). Specializing the operation of an explicit rule. *J Exp Psychol Gen*, **120**, 3–19.

Bach-y-Rita, P. (1980). Brain plasticity as a basis for therapeutic procedures. In: *Recovery of function: theoretical considerations for brain injury rehabilitation* (ed. Bach-y-Rita, P.), Hans Huber, Vienna, pp. 225–263.

Bassetti, C., Bogousslavsky, J. and Regli, F. (1993). Sensory syndromes in parietal stroke. *Neurology*, **43**, 1942–1949.

Becker, S. (1996). Mutual information maximization: models of cortical self-organization. *Network Comp Neural Syst*, **7**, 7–31.

Burton, H., MacLeod, A.M., Videen, T.O. and Raichle, M.E. (1997). Multiple foci in parietal and frontal cortex activated by rubbing embossed grating patterns across fingerpads: a positron emission tomography study in humans. *Cereb Cortex*, **7**, 3–17.

Byl, N., Roderick, J., Mohamed, O., Hanny, M., Kotler, J., Smith, A., Tang, M. and Abrams, G. (2003). Effectiveness of sensory and motor rehabilitation of the upper limb following the principles of neuroplasticity: patients stable poststroke. *Neurorehab Neural Re*, **17**, 176–191.

Byl, N.N. and Merzenich, M.M. (2000). Principles of neuroplasticity: implications for neurorehabilitation and learning. In: *Downey and Darling's Physiological Basis of Rehabilitation Medicine* (eds. Gonzalez, E.S., Myers, S., Edelstein, J., Liebermann, J.S. and Downey, J.A.), Butterworth-Heinemann, Boston, pp. 609–628.

Callahan, A.D. (1995). Methods of compensation and reeducation for sensory dysfunction. In: *Rehabilitation of the Hand: Surgery and Therapy* (eds. Hunter, J.M., Mackin, E.J. and Callahan, A.D.), Mosby, St Louis, pp. 701–714.

Carey, J.R., Kimberley, T.J., Lewis, S.M., Auerbach, E.J., Dorsey, L., Rundquist, P. and Ugurbil, K. (2002). Analysis of fMRI and finger tracking training in subjects with chronic stroke. *Brain*, **125**, 773–788.

Carey, L.M. (1993). *Tactile and Proprioceptive Discrimination Loss After Stroke: Training Effects and Quantitative Measurement*, LaTrobe University, Melbourne.

Carey, L.M. (1995). Somatosensory loss after stroke. *Crit Rev Phys Rehabil Med*, **7**, 51–91.

Carey, L.M. and Matyas, T.A. (2005). Training of somatosensory discrimination after stroke: facilitation of stimulas generalization. *Am J Phys med Rehabil*, **88**, 428–442.

Carey, L.M., Abbott, D.F., Egan, G.F., Bernhardt, J., Donnan, G.A. (2005). Motor impairment and recovery in the upper limb after stroke: behavioral and neuroanatomical correlates. *Stroke*, **36**, 625–629.

Carey, L.M., Abbott, D.F., Puce, A., Jackson, G.D., Syngeniotis, A. and Donnan, G.A. (2002a). Reemergence of activation with poststroke somatosensory recovery: a serial fMRI case study. *Neurology*, **59**, 749–752.

Carey, L.M., Matyas, T.A. and Morales, G. (2002b). Influence of touch sensation and its retraining on finger grip after stroke. In: *13th World Congress of Occupational Therapists*, Stockholm, Sweden.

Carey, L.M., Matyas, T.A. and Oke, L.E. (1993). Sensory loss in stroke patients: effective tactile and proprioceptive discrimination training. *Arch Phys Med Rehabil*, **74**, 602–611.

Carey, L.M., Matyas, T.A. and Oke, L.E. (2002c). Evaluation of impaired fingertip texture discrimination and wrist position sense in patients affected by stroke: comparison of clinical and new quantitative measures. *J Hand Ther*, **15**, 71–82.

Carey, L.M., Oke, L.E. and Matyas, T.A. (1996). Impaired limb position sense after stroke: a quantitative test for clinical use. *Arch Phys Med Rehabil*, **77**, 1271–1278.

Carey, L.M., Oke, L.E. and Matyas, T.A. (1997). Impaired touch discrimination after stroke: a quantitative test. *J Neurol Rehabil*, **11**, 219–232.

Chan, T.-C. and Turvey, M.T. (1991). Perceiving the vertical distances of surfaces by means of a hand-held probe. *J Exp Psychol Hum Percept Perform*, **17**, 347–358.

Clark, F.J. and Horch, K.W. (1986). Kinesthesia. In: *Handbook of Perception and Human Performance*, Vol. 1. Sensory Processes and Perception (eds. Boff, K.R., Kaufman, L. and Thomas, J.P.), John Wiley, New York, (chapter. 13).

Corkin, S., Milner, B. and Rasmussen, T. (1970). Somatosensory thresholds: contrasting effects of post-central gyrus and posterior parietal-lobe excisions. *Arch Neurol*, **23**, 41–58.

Cormier, S.M. and Hagman, J.D. (eds) (1987). *Transfer of Learning: Contemporary Research and Applications*, Academic Press, San Diego.

Dannenbaum, R.M. and Dykes, R.W. (1988). Sensory loss in the hand after sensory stroke: therapeutic rationale. *Arch Phys Med Rehabil*, **69**, 833–839.

Dannenbaum, R.M. and Dykes, R.W. (1990). Evaluating sustained touch-pressure in severe sensory deficits: meeting an unanswered need. *Arch Phys Med Rehabil*, **71**, 455–459.

Darian-Smith, I. and Oke, L.E. (1980). Peripheral neural representation of the spatial frequency of a grating moving across the monkey's finger pad. *J Physiol*, **309**, 117–133.

De Jersey, M.C. (1979). Report on a sensory programme for patients with sensory deficits. *Aust J Physiother*, **25**, 165–170.

Dellon, A.L. (1981). *Evaluation of Sensibility and Re-education of Sensation in the Hand*, Williams & Wilkins, Baltimore.

Dellon, A.L. (2000). *Somatosensory Testing and Rehabilitation*, Institute for Peripheral Nerve Surgery, Baltimore.

Epstein, W., Hughes, B., Schneider, S.L. and Bach-y-Rita, P. (1989). Perceptual learning of spatiotemporal events: evidence from an unfamiliar modality. *J Exp Psychol: Hum Percept Perform*, **15**, 28–44.

Ettlinger, G. and Wilson, W.A. (1990). Cross-modal performance: behavioural processes, phylogenetic considerations and neural mechanisms. *Behav Brain Res*, **40**, 169–192.

Gardner, E.P. and Kandel, E.R. (2000). Touch. In: *Principles of Neural Science* (eds. Kandel, E.R., Schwartz, J.H. and Jessell, T.M.), McGraw-Hill, New York, pp. 451–471.

Gardner, E.P. and Martin, J.H. (2000). Coding of sensory information. In: *Principles of neural science*. (eds. Kandel, E.R., Schwartz, J.H. and Jessell, T.M.), McGraw-Hill, New York, pp. 412–429.

Gaubert, C.S. and Mockett, S.P. (2000). Inter-rater reliability of the Nottingham method of stereognosis assessment. *Clin Rehabil*, **14**, 153–159.

Gentilucci, M., Toni, I., Daprati, E. and Gangitano, M. (1997). Tactile input of the hand and the control of reaching to grasp movements. *Exp Brain Res*, **114**, 130–137.

Gibson, E.J. (1969). *Principles of Perceptual Learning and Development*, Meredith Corporation, New York.

Gibson, E.J. (1991). *An odyssey in learning and perception*, Massachusetts Institute of Technology Press, Cambridge.

Goldstone, R.L. (1998). Perceptual learning. *Annu Rev Psychol*, **49**, 585–612.

Head, H. and Holmes, G. (1911–1912). Sensory disturbances from cerebral lesions. *Brain, 34*, 102–271.

Holmgren, H., Leijon, G., Boivies, J., Johansson, I. and Ilievska, L. (1990). Central post-stroke pain: somatosensory evoked potentials in relation to location of the lesion and sensory signs. *Pain*, **40**, 43–52.

Jeannerod, M., Michel, F. and Prablanc, C. (1984). The control of hand movements in a case of hemianaesthesia following a parietal lesion. *Brain*, **107**, 899–920.

Johansson, R.S. (1996). Sensory control of dexterous manipulation in humans. In: *Hand and Brain: the Neurophysiology and Psychology of Hand Movements* (eds. Wing, A.M., Haggard, P. and Flanagan, J.R.), Academic Press, San Diego, pp. 381–414.

Johansson, R.S. and Westling, G. (1984). Roles of glabrous skin receptors and sensorimotor memory in automatic control of precision grip when lifting rougher or more slippery objects. *Exp Brain Res*, **56**, 550–564.

Johansson, R.S., Häger, C. and Bäckström, L. (1992). Somatosensory control of precision grip during unpredictable pulling loads: III. Impairments during digital anesthesia. *Exp Brain Res*, **89**, 204–213.

Johnson, K.O. and Hsiao, S.S. (1992). Neural mechanisms of tactual form and texture perception. *Annu Rev Neurosc*, **15**, 227–250.

Jones, E.G. and Pons, T.P. (1998). Thalamic and brainstem contributions to large-scale plasticity of primate somatosensory cortex. *Science*, **282**, 1121–1125.

Karni, A., Meyer, G., Jezzard, P., Adams, M.M., Turner, R. and Ungerleider, L.G. (1995). Functional MRI evidence for adult motor cortex plasticity during motor skill learning. *Nature*, **377**, 155–158.

Kim, J.S. and Choi-Kwon, S. (1996). Discriminative sensory dysfunction after unilateral stroke. *Stroke*, **27**, 677–682.

Klatzky, R.L., Lederman, S.J. and Matula, D.E. (1991). Imagined haptic exploration in judgments of object properties. *J Exp Psychol Learn, Memory Cognit*, **17**, 314–322.

Kusoffsky, A. (1990). *Sensory Function and Recovery After Stroke*, Karolinska Institute, Stockholm.

Kusoffsky, A., Wadell, I. and Nilsson, B.Y. (1982). The relationship between sensory impairment and motor recovery in patients with hemiplegia. *Scand J Rehabil Med*, **14**, 27–32.

Lane, N.E. (1987). *Skill Acquisition Rates and Patterns: issues and Training Implications*. Springer-Verlag, New York.

Lederman, S.J. and Klatzky, R.L. (1993). Extracting object properties through haptic exploration. *Acta Psychol*, **84**, 29–40.

Lederman, S.J., Thorne, G. and Jones, B. (1986). Perception of texture by vision and touch: multidimensionality and intersensory integration. *J Exp Psychol: Human Percept Perform*, **12**, 169–180.

Liepert, J., Bauder, H., Miltner, W.H.R., Taub, E. and Weiller, C. (2000). Treatment-induced cortical reorganization after stroke in humans. *Stroke*, **31**, 1210–1216.

Lincoln, N.B., Crow, J.L., Jackson, J.M., Waters, G.R., Adams, S.A. and Hodgson, P. (1991). The unreliability of sensory assessments. *Clin Rehabil*, **5**, 273–282.

Lincoln, N.B., Jackson, J.M. and Adams, S.A. (1998). Reliability and revision of the Nottingham Sensory Assessment for stroke patients. *Physiotherapy*, **84**, 358–365.

Merzenich, M.M. and Jenkins, W.M. (1993). Reorganization of cortical representations of the hand following alterations of skin inputs induced by nerve injury, skin island transfers, and experience. *J Hand Ther*, April–June, 89–104.

Mesulam, M.-M. (1998). From sensation to cognition. *Brain*, **121**, 1013–1052.

Morley, J.W. (1980). *Tactile Perception of Textured Surfaces*, University of Melbourne, Australia.

Mountcastle, V.B. (1997). The columnar organization of the neocortex. *Brain*, **120**, 701–722.

Nelles, G., Jentzen, W., Jueptner, M., Muller, S. and Diener, H.C. (2001). Arm training induced brain plasticity in stroke studied with serial positron emission tomography. *Neuroimage*, **13**, 1146–1154.

Newman, M. (1972). The process of recovery after hemiplegia. *Stroke*, **3**, 702–710.

Nudo, R.J. (1999). Recovery after damage to motor cortical areas. *Curr Opin Neurobiol*, **9**, 740–747.

Nudo, R.J., Milliken, G.W., Jenkins, W.M. and Merzenich, M.M. (1996a). Use-dependent alterations of movement representations in primary motor cortex of adult squirrel monkeys. *J Neurosci*, **16**, 785–807.

Nudo, R.J., Wise, B.M., SiFuentes, F. and Milliken, G.W. (1996b). Neural substrates for the effects of rehabilitative training on motor recovery after ischemic infarct. *Science*, **272**, 1791–1794.

Ohara, S. and Lenz, F.A. (2001). Reorganization of somatic sensory function in the human thalamus after stroke. *Ann Neurol*, **50**, 800–803.

Pascual-Leone, A. and Torres, F. (1993). Plasticity of the sensorimotor cortex representation of the reading finger in Braille readers. *Brain*, **116**, 39–52.

Patel, A.T., Duncan, P.W., Lai, S.-M. and Studenski, S. (2000). The relation between impairments and functional outcomes poststroke. *Arch Phys Med Rehabil*, **81**, 1357–1363.

Plautz, E.J., Milliken, G.W. and Nudo, R.J. (2000). Effects of repetitive motor training on movement representations in adult squirrel monkeys: role of use versus learning. *Neurobiol Learn Mem*, **74**, 27–55.

Puce, A. (2003). Somatosensory function. In: *The Concise Corsini Encyclopedia of Psychology and Neuroscience* (eds. Criaghead, W.E. and Nemeroff, C.B.), John Wiley & Sons, New York.

Recanzone, G.H., Merzenich, M.M. and Jenkins, W.M. (1992). Frequency discrimination training engaging a restricted skin surface results in an emergence of a cutaneous response zone in cortical area 3a. *J Neurophysiol*, **67**, 1057–1070.

Reding, M.J. and Potes, E. (1988). Rehabilitation outcome following initial unilateral hemispheric stroke: life table analysis approach. *Stroke*, **19**, 1354–1358.

Roland, P.E. (1981). Somatotopical tuning of postcentral gyrus during focal attention in man: a regional cerebral blood flow study. *J Neurophysiol*, **46**, 744–754.

Roland, P.E. (1987). Somatosensory detection of microgeometry, macrogeometry and kinesthesia after localized lesions of the cerebral hemispheres in man. *Brain Res Rev*, **12**, 43–94.

Rossini, P.M., Martino, G., Narici, L., Pasquarelli, A., Peresson, M., Pizzella, V., Tecchio, F., Torrioli, G. and Romani, G.L. (1994). Short-term brain "plasticity" in humans: transient finger representation changes in sensory cortex somatotopy following ischemic anesthesia. *Brain Res*, **642**, 169–177.

Rossini, P.M., Tecchio, F., Pizzella, V., Lupoi, D., Cassetta, E., Pasqualetti, P., Romani, G.L. and Orlacchio, A. (1998). On the reorganization of sensory hand area after mono-hemispheric lesion: a functional (MEG)/anatomical (MRI) integrative study. *Brain Res*, **782**, 153–166.

Rothwell, J.C., Traub, M.M., Day, B.L., Obeso, J.A., Thomas, P.K. and Marsden, C.D. (1982). Manual motor performance in a deafferented man. *Brain*, **105**, 515–542.

Salmoni, A.W., Schmidt, R.A. and Walter, C.B. (1984). Knowledge of results and motor learning: a review and critical reappraisal. *Psychol Bull*, **95**, 355–386.

Sathian, K. and Zangaladze, A. (1997). Tactile learning is task specific but transfers between fingers. *Percept Psychophys*, **59**, 119–128.

Schmidt, R.A. and Lee, T.D. (1999). *Motor Control and Learning: A Behavioral Emphasis*, Human Kinetics, Illinois.

Schnitzler, A., Seitz, R.J. and Freund, H.-J. (2000). The somatosensory system. In: *Brain Mapping: The Systems* (eds. Toga, A.W. and Mazziotta, J.C.), Academic Press, San Diego.

Schwartzman, R.J. (1972). Somatesthetic recovery following primary somatosensory projection cortex ablations. *Arch Neurol*, **27**, 340–349.

Seitz, R.J., Azari, N.P., Knorr, U., Binkofski, F., Herzog, H. and Freund, H.-J. (1999). The role of diaschisis in stroke recovery. *Stroke*, **30**, 1844–1850.

Small, S., Hlustik, P., Noll, D., Genovese, C. and Solodkin, A. (2002). Cerebellar hemispheric activation ipsilateral to the paretic hand correlates with functional recovery after stroke. *Brain*, **125**, 1544–1557.

Smania, N., Montagnana, B., Faccioli, S., Fiaschi, A. and Aglioti, S.M. (2003). Rehabilitation of somatic sensation and related deficit of motor control in patients with pure sensory stroke. *Arch Phys Med Rehabil*, **84**, 1692–1702.

Spengler, F., Roberts, T.P., Poeppel, D., Byl, N., Wang, X., Rowley, H.A. and Merzenich, M.M. (1997). Learning transfer and neuronal plasticity in humans trained in tactile discrimination. *Neurosci Lett*, **232**, 151–154.

Van Deusen Fox, J. (1964). Cutaneous stimulation: effects on selected tests of perception. *Am J Occup Ther*, **18**, 53–55.

Vinograd, A., Taylor, E. and Grossman, S. (1962). Sensory retraining of the hemiplegic hand. *Am J Occup Ther*, **16**, 246–250.

Wade, D.T. (1992). *Measurement in Neurological Rehabilitation*, Oxford University Press, Oxford.

Wadell, I., Kusoffsky, A. and Nilsson, B.Y. (1987). A follow-up study of stroke patients 5–6 years after their brain infarct. *Int J Rehabil Res*, **10**, 103–110.

Ward, N., Brown, M., Thompson, A. and Frackowiak, R. (2003). Neural correlates of motor recovery after stroke: a longitudinal fMRI study. *Brain*, **126**, 2476–2496.

Weiller, C. (1998). Imaging recovery from stroke. *Exp Brain Res*, **123**, 13–17.

Weinreich, M. and Armentrout, S. (1995). A neural model of recovery from lesions in the somatosensory system. *J Neurol Rehabil*, **9**, 25–32.

Wikström, H., Roine, R.O., Aronen, H.J., Salonen, O., Sinkkonen, J., Ilmoniemi, R.J. and Huttunen, J. (2000). Specific changes in somatosensory evoked fields during recovery from sensorimotor stroke. *Ann Neurol*, **47**, 353–360.

Wing, A.M., Flanagan, J.R. and Richardson, J. (1997). Anticipatory postural adjustments in stance and grip. *Exp Brain Res*, **116**, 122–130.

Winstein, C.J. and Schmidt, R.A. (1990). Reduced frequency of knowledge of results enhances motor skill learning. *J Exp Psychol Learn Memory Cognit*, **16**, 677–691.

Winward, C.E., Halligan, P.W. and Wade, D.T. (1999). Somatosensory assessment after central nerve damage: the need for standardized clinical measures. *Phys Ther Rev*, **4**, 21–28.

Winward, C.E., Halligan, P.W. and Wade, D.T. (2002). The Rivermead assessment of somatosensory performance (RASP): standardization and reliability data. *Clin Rehabil*, **16**, 523–533.

Wynn Parry, C.B. and Salter, M. (1976). Sensory re-education after median nerve lesions. *The Hand*, **8**, 250–257.

Yekutiel, M. (2000). *Sensory Re-education of the Hand After Stroke*, Whurr Publishers, London.

Yekutiel, M. and Guttman, E. (1993). A controlled trial of the retraining of the sensory function of the hand in stroke patients. *J Neurol Neurosurg Psychiat*, **56**, 241–244.

Zangaladze, A., Epstein, C.M., Grafton, S.T. and Sathian, K. (1999). Involvement of visual cortex in tactile discrimination of orientation. *Nature*, **401**, 587–590.

Zemke, A.C., Heagerty, P.J., Lee, C. and Cramer, S.C. (2003). Motor cortex organization after stroke is related to side of stroke and level of recovery. *Stroke*, **34**, e23–e28.

17

Management of spasticity

David A. Gelber

Springfield Clinic Neuroscience Institute, Springfield, IL, USA

Spasticity is commonly defined as excessive motor activity characterized by a velocity-dependent increase in tonic stretch reflexes. It is often associated with exaggerated tendon jerks, and is often accompanied by abnormal cutaneous and autonomic reflexes, muscle weakness, lack of dexterity, fatigability, and co-contraction of agonist and antagonist muscles (Young, 1987; Young, 2002; Sanger et al., 2003). It is a common complication of central nervous system disorders, including stroke, traumatic brain injury, cerebral palsy, multiple sclerosis, anoxic brain injury, spinal cord injury, primary lateral sclerosis, and hereditary spastic paraparesis (Young, 2002).

In many individuals, the presence of spasticity has negative consequences, interfering with mobility and activities of daily living. Disability may result from spasticity-related impairment of posture, abnormal quality of movement, painful spasms, and poor hygiene. In these patients treatment of spasticity is often considered. This chapter will review the pathophysiology of spasticity, outline the rationale for treatment and the development of treatment goals. In addition, pharmacologic and surgical management strategies will be discussed.

17.1 Physiology

Muscle tone, defined as the resistance to externally imposed muscle movement, is modulated by central nervous system influences on the alpha motor neuron in the spinal cord (Rossi, 1994). The pathways that regulate tone are similar to those that regulate voluntary and involuntary motor movements and, as a final common pathway, involve the spinal reflex arc. Alpha motor neurons that innervate muscle fibers are located in the ventral horns of the spinal cord, and comprise the efferent limb of this reflex arc. Afferent sensory impulses from muscle spindles are relayed to the spinal cord via Ia fibers. Some of these fibers synapse directly on alpha motor neurons that innervate agonist muscles. This is a monosynaptic reflex pathway and allows for sensory feedback necessary for motor movements. Collateral fibers from the Ia afferents also synapse on inhibitory interneurons in the dorsal horn, which in turn synapse on alpha motor neurons of antagonist muscles to inhibit their contraction; this is a polysynaptic reflex (Rossi, 1994). These pathways allow for coordinated action of agonist and antagonist muscles necessary for fine and gross motor movements.

There are several descending central nervous system pathways that synapse directly or indirectly (via internuncial pathways) on motor neurons and allow for suprasegmental control of movement (Volume II, Chapter 2). The corticospinal tract synapses directly on motor neurons and is responsible for voluntary control of the extremities, as well as inhibition of antigravity muscles of the trunk and limbs (Rossi, 1994). The reticulospinal tract has two components that influence motor movement. The pontine reticulospinal tract is excitatory to alpha motor neurons, while the medullary reticulospinal tract is inhibitory. The vestibulospinal tract is excitatory to the motor neurons of antigravity muscles (Merritt, 1981).

Upper motor neuron lesions result in spasticity from a number of mechanisms. Collateral branches from these descending motor pathways excite inhibitory presynaptic interneurons. With an upper motor neuron lesion this excitation is removed leading to decreased "presynaptic inhibition" of the motor neuron pool and overactivity of the spinal reflex pathways (Young, 2002).

Ia inhibitory interneurons to antagonist muscles are also activated by descending motor pathways (reciprocal inhibition) (Young, 2002). Removal of this excitation by an upper motor neuron insult leads to overactivity of antagonist muscle motor neurons, resulting in co-contraction of agonist–antagonist muscles commonly seen in association with spasticity.

Alpha motor neurons send collateral axons to internuncial Renshaw cells that normally act to inhibit the motor neuron pool (feedback or recurrent inhibition). Descending motor pathways typically activate Renshaw cells; supraspinal lesions often result in decreased recurrent inhibition with subsequent overactivity of spinal reflex pathways (Katz and Pierrot-Deseilligny, 1982).

In summary, lesions of the brain and spinal cord that interfere with the descending motor pathways often result in spasticity. Removal, in particular, of these descending inhibitory influences leads to an overactivity of the spinal reflex arc resulting in an increase in muscle tone, hyperreflexia, extensor plantar response (Babinski sign), flexor spasms, clonus, and co-contraction of agonist and antagonist muscles. Lesions that specifically involve the corticospinal tract may also cause concurrent motor weakness and decreased dexterity (Rossi, 1994).

17.2 Pharmacology

A number of neurotransmitters are involved in the sensory and motor pathways that regulate muscle tone. Acetylcholine is released by motor neuron axons that terminate on Renshaw interneurons (Young, 2002). Glutamate, an excitatory neurotransmitter, is released by the descending corticospinal tract and by primary spinal cord Ia afferent fibers (Davidoff, 1985). Gamma aminobutyric acid (GABA), the predominant inhibitory neurotransmitter in the spinal cord, is contained in interneurons in the dorsal and intermediate grey matter of the spinal cord and acts to mediate presynaptic inhibition of primary Ia afferent inputs on motor neurons (Young and Delwaide, 1981). Presynaptic inhibition acts to suppress sensory signals from skin and muscle receptors and to decrease the amount of glutamate released by the primary afferent fibers (Davidoff, 1985). Glycine interneurons (Renshaw cells) are also inhibitory, and mediate postsynaptic recurrent inhibition of alpha motor neurons and reciprocal Ia fiber inhibition, discussed above (Davidoff, 1985).

Substance P is released by small, predominantly unmyelinated sensory afferent fibers that mediate pain, and enhances the postsynaptic effect of glutamate (Young, 2002). Nociceptive stimuli can result in an increase in flexor reflexes causing painful flexor spasms that often accompany spasticity (Rossi, 1994). Enkephalins, which modulate pain, are located in the dorsal horn of the spinal cord and may also play a role in the pain-spasticity interaction (Young, 2002).

Descending pathways containing catecholamines and serotonin are also involved in the regulation of spinal cord reflexes. These pathways primarily affect the transmission of impulses from primary sensory afferent fibers and affect the excitability of interneurons (Merritt, 1981).

17.3 Clinical manifestations of spasticity

Spasticity is one of the components of the "upper motor neuron syndrome," which includes both positive and negative phenomena (Table 17.1). Injury to the corticospinal tract, which has facilatory influence on motor neurons in the spinal cord, causes the "negative" manifestations including muscle weakness, fatigability, and decreased dexterity (Rossi, 1994). These features are the major determinant of motor disability associated with upper motor neuron lesions. Conversely, injury to the reticulospinal or vestibulospinal tracts, which normally inhibit

Table 17.1. Positive and negative symptoms of spasticity.

Negative symptoms	Positive symptoms
Muscle weakness	Increased muscle tone
Fatigue	Co-contraction of agonist and
Decreased dexterity	antagonist muscles
Slowed initiation of	Flexor and extensor muscle spasms
movement	Hyperreflexia
	Clonus

spinal reflex pathways, results in "positive" symptoms including spasticity, hyperactive muscle stretch reflexes, abnormal cutaneous and autonomic reflexes, and co-contraction of agonist and antagonist muscles (dystonia).

Immediately after an acute brain or spinal cord injury muscles generally become weak and hypotonic (O'Brien et al., 1996). This is referred to as "spinal shock" and is accompanied by loss of muscle stretch reflexes and impaired F-wave responses on nerve conduction testing (Hiersemenzel et al., 2000). Spasticity then often develops days to weeks after the acute injury; this is thought to be due to upregulation of spinal cord receptors and synaptic reorganization (McGuire and Harvey, 1999). Patients with cerebral lesions tend to recover reflexes and tone within a few days of injury, while patients with spinal cord injuries may have a period of spinal shock last for weeks (Calancie et al., 2002). Generally, the longer it takes for tone to return the worse the prognosis is for meaningful motor recovery (Young, 2002).

The pattern of spasticity often differs depending on the location of the upper motor neuron lesion. For example, spasticity tends to preferentially involve upper extremity flexors and lower extremity extensor groups following cerebral injuries, and flexor groups in both the upper and lower extremities following spinal cord injuries. Although not seen following cerebral injury, patients with spinal lesions often have grossly exaggerated cutaneous reflexes, such as a "triple flexion" lower extremity withdrawal reflex following cutaneous stimulation (Young, 2002).

Spasticity is not always detrimental and relief of spasticity does not ensure improvement in clinical disability. In patients with severe muscle weakness an increase in muscle tone, especially in the antigravity muscles of the trunk and lower extremities, may actually facilitate transfers, standing, and ambulation. The spastic posture of the upper extremity, with the adducted arm held close to the body, may help with balance. A spastic urinary sphincter may help maintain continence. As well, spasticity may help prevent muscle atrophy, decrease peripheral edema, and reduce the risk of deep venous thrombosis (Gelber and Jozefczyk, 1999).

However, in many patients with brain and spinal cord disorders, spasticity can interfere with functional mobility and activities of daily living. For example, in stroke patients, spasticity of the lower extremity extensor muscles can result in a stifflegged gait with toe dragging (Riley and Kerrigan, 1999). Excessive ankle plantarflexion spasticity can affect the ability to comfortably wear an ankle foot orthosis. Spasticity of the upper extremity musculature can lead to difficulties with self-feeding, grooming, and hygiene. Other spasticity-related factors, which often contribute to overall disability, include impairment of posture (e.g., affecting wheelchair seating), and painful spasms. The presence of spasticity also increases skin friction, especially over extensor surfaces of limbs; if severe this can lead to the development of decubitus skin ulcers (Peerless et al., 1999).

17.4 Evaluation of spasticity

Spasticity can be evaluated at bedside during the physical examination. Manual muscle stretch should be assessed at different rates of movement. When spasticity is mild it often takes high velocities of movement to elicit resistance. With moderate spasticity, resistance to passive movement may be noted with slower rates of stretch. With severe spasticity, the resistance to passive stretch may be so marked as to stop movement entirely, the so-called clasp-knife phenomenon (Dimitrijevic, 1995).

Table 17.2. Modified Ashworth and Spasm Scales (Ashworth, 1964; Bohannon and Smith, 1987).

Score	Degree of muscle tone
0	No increase in muscle tone
1	Slight increase in tone, elicit a "catch when affected part is moved in flexion or extension"
2	Moderate increase in tone, passive movement difficult
3	Considerate increase in tone, passive movement difficult
4	Affected part rigid in flexion or extension

Spasticity can be more formally assessed using quantitative scales and laboratory measures. This can be of particular benefit in assessing response to spasticity treatment. The most commonly used semi-quantitative clinical scale to assess spasticity is the Modified Ashworth Scale (Ashworth, 1964) (Table 17.2). The examiner rates the resistance on a scale of 0–4 when muscles are passively lengthened. This scale has been found to be a reliable and reproducible method of measuring spasticity with good interrater reliability (Bohannon and Smith, 1987; Brashear et al., 2002).

For research trials spasticity can also be measured in the laboratory by biomechanical methods. The Pendulum Drop Test quantitates spasticity in knee muscles by recording a ratio of two angles of knee angular displacement. The patient sits with their hanging over the edge of a table. The leg is held at full extension and then dropped, allowing free swinging of the extremity. The flexion angle of the first swing of the leg is defined as the acute angle. The final resting angle is then determined and the ratio of these angles is calculated (Jamshidi and Smith, 1996). Measurements can be made by videotape, electrogoniometry, or with an isokinetic dynamometer (Bohannon, 1986). Other laboratory measurements of spasticity include assessment of the H-reflex and the tonic vibratory reflex (Allison and Abraham, 1995). Variable correlation has been demonstrated between these measures and the Modified Ashworth Scale (Leslie et al., 1992; Bohannon, 1999; Prandyan et al., 2003).

17.5 Treatment general principles

Treatment for spasticity is generally initiated when the increase in muscle tone interferes with functional activities, such as positioning in bed or wheelchair, mobility (walking or transfers), activities of daily living, or hygiene (e.g., if excessive hip adductor tone impairs the ability to catheterize). Furthermore, treatment should be considered when spasticity causes discomfort or painful spasms, or if excessive tone leads to complications such as decubitus ulcers or early contractures.

Again, it is important to recognize that in some patients spasticity may actually be of benefit, especially in those with marginal strength; in these individuals the increase in tone may actually allow them to stand or walk. Reducing tone in these patients may be functionally detrimental and should either be avoided or done cautiously.

When planning treatment the patient's underlying neurologic and medical conditions should always be considered. For example, spinal cord injured patients with autonomic dysreflexia, patients on antihypertensive medications, or elderly patients often do not tolerate antispasticity medications with hypotensive side effects. Patients with traumatic brain injury, stroke, or multiple sclerosis who have significant cognitive impairments may not tolerate drugs that are sedating. Furthermore, patients with marginal strength may lose functional abilities if treated with medications that cause muscle weakness. Therefore, the pros and cons of the various treatments must always be considered for each individual patient. An algorithm for the management of spasticity is presented in Fig. 17.1. This is by no means exhaustive.

It is important that the specific goals of treatment always be discussed in detail with the patient, family, and caregivers so all understand fully what the targeted outcomes of management are. As an example, spasticity treatment goals for a spinal cord injured patient with paraplegia might include a reduction in painful spasms and more comfortable positioning in a wheelchair, but not be expected to improve strength in the lower extremities or facilitate the ability to walk.

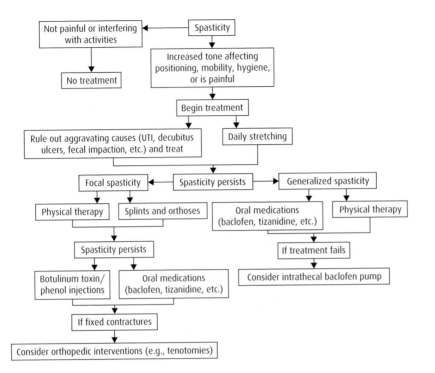

Figure 17.1. Spasticity treatment algorithm.

Realistic expectations must be carefully reviewed for all those involved in the patient's care.

17.6 General medical and nursing care

In all patients with spasticity, medical conditions or extrinsic factors that can worsen spasticity should always be sought. For example, fever can worsen spasticity. Certain medications, such as the interferons, commonly used in multiple sclerosis management, can result in an increase in spasticity (Walther and Hohfield, 1999). The most common precipitants of a sudden worsening in spasticity and spasms are painful stimuli, especially those involving the lower extremities. This is thought to be mediated by nociceptive sensory afferents (that release substance P), which increase segmental spinal reflex activity. Initial evaluation of a spastic patient, or one in whom spasticity or flexor spasms suddenly worsens should

always include a search for potential noxious stimuli, including urinary tract infections, bladder distension, bowel impaction, ingrown toenails, decubitus ulcers, and deep venous thrombosis (Merritt, 1981). Treatment of these underlying conditions will often improve tone and spasms.

17.7 Physical therapy

There are alterations that occur in muscles and connective tissue associated with chronic spasticity. Spastic muscles have been shown to have shorter resting sarcomere length with evidence of changes in connective tissue constituents, such as collagen and titin (Friden and Lieber, 2003). Biomechanical interventions, including range of motion exercises and splinting, may help minimize these changes.

Passive range of motion of spastic muscles, performed at least 2–3 times a day, should be an integral part of any treatment regimen for spasticity. Although the improvement in tone is only temporary (several hours), routine range of motion exercises may help prevent the development of contractures (Nuyens et al., 2002).

There are certain physical therapy philosophies that stress the inhibition of spasticity in their treatment approach. For example, the neurodevelopmental technique is based on the attempt to inhibit tonic reflexes by passively bringing patients into reflex inhibitory postures (Kabat and Knott, 1954). The techniques of proprioceptive neuromuscular facilitation (PNF) emphasizes the instruction of normal patterns of movement to spastic patients (Pierson, 2002). Although studies have not demonstrated better functional outcomes in patients treated with this particular technique compared to others, patients with marked spasticity might be ones to benefit from these therapy approaches (Gelber et al., 1995).

Anecdotal reports suggest that other therapy modalities might help reduce muscle tone. Vibration, especially of antagonist muscles, may help reduce tone in a spastic limb (Lee et al., 2002). Topical cold and anesthetics may reduce tone by decreasing the sensitivity of cutaneous receptors and slowing nerve conduction (Miglietta, 1973; Sabbahi et al., 1981). There are also case reports of improved spasticity following magnetic stimulation of the spinal cord and acupuncture (Nielsten 1995; Moon et al., 2003).

Orthotic devices may also be considered in the management of spasticity, to reduce tone, improve range of motion, prevent contractures, and reduce pain. Orthoses also control joint instability and may alter the loading of a limb to prevent stretch reflex activity in antagonist muscles. The theory behind tone inhibiting orthoses suggests that prolonged stretch may actually change the mechanical properties of spastic muscles, perhaps by reducing muscle spindles' reaction to stretch (Kogler, 2002). Although clinical observations suggest tone to be reduced with splints, experimental evidence is scarce and studies have not determined the most effective splint design (Langlois, et al., 1989). However, most commonly splints are fabricated to position affected joints opposite to the tonal response (Kogler, 2002).

Ankle–foot orthoses (AFO's) are commonly prescribed in patients with spastic lower extremity paresis to inhibit tone, and if possible, improve ambulation (Lehmann et al., 1987, Sankey et al., 1989). Rarely, knee–ankle–foot orthoses (KAFO's) are used in the management of young patients with cerebral palsy (Kogler, 2002).

The goals of upper extremity splinting are to reduce tone, improve range of motion, and prevent palm maceration. Some of the commonly used wrist–hand–finger orthoses include the Snook splint (Snook, 1979), cone splint, Bobath splint, and finger-abductor splint. Static or dynamic orthoses can also be considered for management of elbow flexion spasticity (Kogler, 2002).

Serial casting is an effective means for managing early soft tissue contractures resulting from spasticity, and is often combined with the use of botulinum toxin or medications (Mortenson and Eng, 2003). This process involves positioning an extremity at the end of passive range of motion and casting in that position. The cast is left in place for several days and is then removed (Pohl et al., 2002). The patient undergoes range of motion therapy between castings and is then recast at the new (reduced) angle; this is repeated 4–5 times until as close as possible to a normal range of motion can be reestablished. It is suggested that serial casting is most effective when initiated within 6 months of acute neurologic injury, while neurologic recovery is still possible. Once the cast is removed, if the overall spasticity has not been reduced the likelihood of maintaining the improvement in range of motion without further splinting or bracing is poor (Conine et al., 1990).

Electrical stimulation has also been used to reduce spasticity in patients with hemiplegia and spinal cord injury, often as adjunctive therapy with other physical therapy modalities (Armutulu et al., 2003; Scheker and Ozer, 2003). The most common technique is to stimulate antagonist muscles; this causes activation of polysynaptic spinal cord pathways resulting in inhibition of agonist muscle activity and tone (Alfieri, 1982). The decrease in spasticity generally lasts from 15 min to 3 h, allowing the therapists to do more aggressive range of motion and strengthening exercises during this time. However, the long-term benefit of electrical stimulation in reducing muscle tone is probably limited (Dali et al., 2002).

17.8 Pharmacologic interventions

A number of medications are effective in the treatment of spasticity (Table 17.3). These drugs all decrease the excitability of spinal reflexes, but act through different mechanisms. Such mechanisms of action include a reduction in the release of excitatory neurotransmitters from presynaptic terminals of primary Ia afferent fibers, facilitation of the action of inhibitory interneurons involved in reflex pathways, interference with the contractile mechanism of skeletal muscle, and inhibition of supraspinal influences on the spinal reflex arc (Davidoff, 1985). The choice of drug should take into account the patient's underlying neurologic disease, concurrent medications, and medical conditions.

Baclofen is a GABA agonist, active primarily at $GABA_B$ fibers, that inhibits monosynaptic extensor and polysynaptic flexor reflexes (Davidoff, 1985).

Baclofen acts presynaptically to reduce the release of excitatory neurotransmitters from the descending corticospinal tracts and primary spinal cord Ia afferent fibers, and possibly of substance P from afferent nociceptive fibers (Young and Delwaide, 1981). At high concentrations, baclofen also acts postsynaptically to decrease the effects of the excitatory neurotransmitters, thus inhibiting activation of motor neurons in the ventral horn (Rossi, 1994).

Baclofen is most effective for the treatment of spasticity secondary to spinal cord injuries, but is also approved for the treatment of spasticity of cerebral origin (Albright et al., 1993). The advantages of baclofen are that it is less sedating than the benzodiazepines, especially when started at a low dose and titrated slowly upward and works extremely well in treating painful flexor and extensor muscle spasms (Fromm, 1994). Its major drawback is that it can cause muscle weakness at moderate and high doses, although much less than dantrolene (Roussan et al., 1985). Less common side effects include ataxia, confusion, headache, hallucinations, dyskinesias, respiratory, and cardiovascular depression (Young and Delwaide, 1981). Baclofen can also lower seizure threshold and should be used cautiously in epileptic

Table 17.3. Pharmacologic treatment of spasticity.

Drug	Action	Major adverse effects
Baclofen	Reduces release of excitatory neurotransmitters and substance P in the spinal cord Decreases postsynaptic effects of excitatory neurotransmitters	Sedation Weakness Seizures
Tizanidine	Reduces release of excitatory neurotransmitters and substance P in the spinal cord Decreases neuronal firing in locus ceruleus	Sedation Dry mouth Dizziness
Benzodiazepines	Enhances presynaptic and postsynaptic inhibition in the spinal cord through GABA pathways	Sedation Fatigue Habituation
Dantrolene	Inhibits release of calcium from muscle sarcoplasmic reticulum	Weakness Hepatotoxicity
Clonidine	Similar to tizanidine	Orthostatic hypotension
Phenothiazines	Reduce gamma motor neuron excitability	Extrapyramidal side effects Sedation

patients (Hansel et al., 2003). Baclofen is generally started at a low dose (5–10 mg qd-bid) and titrated upward to a maximum of 80–120 mg/day (divided tid-qid). Abrupt withdrawal should be avoided as this can precipitate rebound flexor spasms and hallucinations (Merritt, 1981).

Tizanidine is an alpha$_2$-adrenergic agonist and binds to both alpha$_2$-adrenergic and imidazoline receptors in the spinal cord. Tizanidine has been shown to decrease polysynaptic reflex activity, probably by reducing release of excitatory neurotransmitters from presynaptic neurons (Lastate et al., 1994). It also inhibits the release of substance P from nociceptive sensory afferents, and may also decrease neuronal firing at the level of the locus ceruleus (Wagstaff and Bryson, 1997).

Tizanidine has been shown to be effective in the treatment of spasticity caused by multiple sclerosis, spinal cord injury, stroke, traumatic brain injury, and cerebral palsy (Wallace, 1994; Nance et al., 1994; Wagstaff and Bryson, 1997; Gelber et al., 2001). Overall, the data from multiple series have shown that tizanidine has efficacy similar to baclofen and diazepam (Wallace, 1994). However, in contrast to baclofen, tizanidine has not been shown to cause muscle weakness, and, therefore, may be advantageous in patients with marginal strength (Gelber et al., 2001). The sedative side effects are somewhat equivalent to that of baclofen, but less than the benzodiazepines (Wallace, 1994). Since tizanidine is an alpha$_2$-adrenergic agonist it can cause hypotension, which is generally dose-related (Wagstaff and Bryson, 1997). The risk is minimized by slow titration of drug. Caution should be used when administering tizanidine to patients taking antihypertensive medications and in spinal cord injured patients with autonomic dysfunction. Slight elevation of liver enzymes have been noted in 5% of patients; these generally normalize with a decrease in dosage or discontinuation of medication. It is recommended that liver enzymes be monitored during the first 6 months of treatment and that the drug should be avoided in patients with liver disease. Other side effects of tizanidine include dry mouth, asthenia, dizziness, and visual hallucinations (Wallace, 1994). Initial dosage is 2–4 mg/d

and is slowly titrated upwards in 2–4 mg increments every 3–4 days to a maximum of 36 mg/d divided tid-qid. Peak effect is in 1–2 h with 3–6 h duration of action (Wagstaff and Bryson, 1997).

Benzodiazepines enhance presynaptic and postsynaptic inhibition in the spinal cord by enhancing the affinity of GABA receptors for endogenous GABA (Merritt, 1981; Rossi, 1994). These drugs are effective in reducing spasticity from both spinal cord and cerebral injuries and work well in the treatment of painful spasms (Dahlin et al., 1993). Although benzodiazepines have similar efficacy to baclofen their use is limited by side effects, including habituation and tachyphylaxis, sedation, fatigue, and paradoxical agitation (Rossi, 1994). Due to this, benzodiazepines are probably best used as adjunctive therapy, especially in patients who have nocturnal spasms and in who can benefit from the sedative/anxiolytic side effects. The usual dosage of diazepam is 2–10 mg bid-qid, and 0.5–2 mg bid-tid for clonazepam.

Dantrolene interferes with the excitation–coupling reaction in skeletal muscle by inhibiting depolarization-induced release of calcium from the sarcoplasmic reticulum (Pinder et al., 1997). It is effective in the treatment of spasticity of both cerebral and spinal origin. Since dantrolene acts directly on the muscle it causes weakness in addition to reduction of tone; this is its biggest limiting feature. This drug may be best used to manage spasticity in quadriplegic patients in whom spasticity interferes with positioning and hygiene; in these patients increasing their weakness should have no deleterious effect on their functional abilities (Young and Delwaide, 1981). Since dantrolene has no cognitive side effects it may also be of benefit at low doses in brain injured patients in whom the sedation associated with baclofen, tizanidine, or benzodiazepines may not be tolerated. The most serious potential side effect of dantrolene is liver damage; there is a 1% incidence of hepatotoxicity and 0.1% incidence of fatal hepatitis (Rossi, 1994). Liver function tests should be monitored closely and the dosage should be decreased or the medication discontinued if the liver enzymes are elevated. Dantrolene is typically started at 25–50 mg/d and slowly increased to a maximum of 100 mg qid.

There are other medications that can be considered in patients with refractory spasticity. Clonidine is an alpha$_2$-adrenergic agonist similar to tizanidine ans is also effective in reducing muscle tone, but is limited in its use by orthostatic hypotension. Given orally it is begun at 0.05 mg bid and increased by 0.1 mg/d weekly to a maximum of 0.4 mg/d. It may also be administered transdermally via a patch at doses of 0.1 to 0.3 mg (Weingarden and Belen, 1992). Phenothiazines, such as chlorpromazine, have been shown to decrease spasticity probably due to their alpha-adrenergic blocking properties. They reduce gamma motor neuron excitability and antagonize the postsynaptic actions of dopamine (Merritt, 1981; Davidoff, 1985). Their use is limited by sedation and development of extrapyramidal side effects, including tardive dyskinesia (Rossi, 1994). Several studies have also reported improvement in spasticity following treatment with valproic acid, gabapentin, and cyproheptadine although benefits need to be confirmed in large clinical trials (Finke, 1978; Barbeau et al., 1982; Priebe et al., 1997). A number of recent studies have reported cannabanoids to be effective in the management of spasticity and spasms in patients with multiple sclerosis (Killestein et al., 2002; Russo et al., 2003; Zajicek et al., 2003).

17.9 Intrathecal medications

Approximately 30% of patients do not achieve adequate control of their spasticity with oral medications, or are unable to tolerate them due to side effects (Zajicek et al., 2003). In these patients, intrathecal administration of baclofen via an implantable pump may be an alternative. Numerous studies demonstrate the efficacy of intrathecal baclofen in the treatment of spasticity in patients with cerebral palsy, traumatic brain injury, multiple sclerosis, and spinal cord injury with intrathecal baclofen (Ochs et al., 1989; Penn et al., 1989; Lazorthes et al., 1990; Loubser et al., 1991; Meythaler et al., 1992; Albright et al., 1993; Coffey et al., 1993; Rifici et al., 1994;

Meythaler et al., 1996; Francisco and Boake, 2003), and is approved for treatment in patients as young as 4 years (Murphy et al., 2002).

Prior to placement of a baclofen pump most third-party payors require that patients respond favorably to a screening trial of intrathecal baclofen. A baseline Modified Ashworth Scale Score (MAS) is recorded for hip abductors, hip flexors, knee flexors, and ankle dorsiflexors bilaterally. A 50 µg test dose of baclofen is then administered intrathecally via lumbar puncture. The onset of drug action is within 30–60 min, peaks in 4 h, and lasts up to 8 h (Pohl et al., 2003). The MAS score is repeated at 1, 2, 4, and 8 h; a positive response is defined as an average of a 1-point drop in the average MAS score (calculated by adding the scores and dividing by the number of muscles assessed) (Parke et al., 1992). If the 50 µg dosage is ineffective the test bolus should be repeated at 75 or 100 µg the following day. If there is a positive response an intrathecal pump is implanted. If there is no significant improvement alternative treatment strategies should be sought.

The pump is surgically implanted subcutaneously in the abdominal wall and connected to a catheter that is passed intrathecally at the L3–L4 level. The catheter tip is threaded rostrally ending at approximately the T10 level.

The starting intrathecal daily dosage is usually twice the test bolus that produced a positive effect (e.g., if 50 µg test bolus was effective the pump is started at 100 µg/d). The dosage can then be titrated upwards by 5–15% daily until a satisfactory response is obtained. The pump can be programmed to administer baclofen on a continuous basis, and/or to provide boluses at specific times during the day. The pump requires refilling every 4–12 weeks depending on the reservoir used and the dosage administered.

Complications of the surgical procedure include wound infections and erosion of the pump pocket. Mechanical pump failure and catheter malfunctions can occur, leading to worsening spasticity (Meythaler et al., 1996). Side effects of intrathecal baclofen include orthostatic hypotension, sedation, and loss of erection. There are also reports of seizures occurring as a result of baclofen overdosage (Francisco et al., 2003). For intrathecal overdoses physostigmine may reverse the associated respiratory depression and somnolence. Abrupt withdrawal of intrathecal baclofen can result in profound worsening of spasiticity and spasms and in severe cases can cause fever and mental status changes (Kao et al., 2003). In approximately 5% of patients tolerance to baclofen develops, perhaps due to downregulation of GABA receptors (Kroin et al., 1993). Tolerance may respond to a brief drug holiday (Meythaler et al., 1996).

Morphine inhibits polysynaptic reflexes in the spinal cord through its action at opiate receptors (Barres et al., 2003). Intrathecal morphine, administered alone, or in combination with baclofen via an implantable pump, has been shown to improve pain and spasticity associated with spinal cord injuries (Soni et al., 2003). Due to the potential development of habituation use of intrathecal morphine should be used judiciously. However, it is an reasonable option for patients with refractory spasticity, especially when there is severe concurrent pain.

17.10 Nerve blocks and botulinum toxin injections

For patients who have spasticity that is particularly severe in one or a few muscle groups, focal treatment of their spasticity may be considered. Clinical examples would include a patient with severe ankle plantar flexor and invertor tone that impairs the ability to wear an ankle–foot orthosis, excessive wrist and finger flexor spasticity that cannot be adequately managed with a resting hand splint, or severe hip adductor spasticity that interferes with hygiene and nursing care. For focal spasticity, treatment with botulinum toxin or nerve blocks may of benefit.

Chemodenervation or neurolysis may also be considered during the acute "recovery phase" from a central nervous system injury, such as traumatic brain injury, often in combination with other modalities, such as serial casting. Relief of spasticity during this time may allow for more complete range of motion exercises and prevention of contractures.

Phenol is the most commonly used agent for nerve blocks. Injection causes a chemical axonotmesis by destroying neuronal axons but preserving endoneurial tubes (Felsenthal et al., 1974). This results in a reduction of muscle tone, but also causes muscle weakness if a motor nerve is injected. Fortunately the effect of phenol is temporary, typically lasting for a period of weeks to months. Regenerating axons eventually reinnervate motor endplates, allowing for a return in strength.

There are a variety of techniques for phenol nerve blocks. One of the original techniques performed was a closed perineural injection of nerve trunks. This technique does result in decreased muscle tone but because mixed nerves are injected it is often complicated by development of painful paresthesias; for this reason this method is used only rarely (Khalil and Betts, 1967).

Closed motor branch blocks involve injection of a nerve terminal's motor branch after identification of the branch using electrical stimulation. Commonly blocked nerves using this technique include the recurrent branch of the median, obturator, and musculocutaneous nerves. An advantage of closed motor branch blocks is that this technique does not cause dysesthesias; however, the response is generally not as long lasting or predictable as an open motor point block (Keenan et al., 1990).

The technique of open motor point blocks requires surgical isolation of the motor nerve branch. Injections of the motor nerve branches with 3–5% phenol in glycerin have shown a decrease in spasticity lasting 2–8 months (Botte et al., 1995). Nerves commonly blocked with this method include the motor branches of the median and ulnar nerves in the forearm, deep motor branch of the ulnar nerve at the wrist, obturator nerve, sciatic motor branch in the posterior thigh, and posterior tibial nerve. The obvious drawback to this procedure is that surgery is required.

Most commonly used today is the technique of intramuscular motor point blocks. This involves injection of specific motor points within muscle, the areas where there is a high concentration of motor endplates. The motor points are identified using a needle stimulator. Multiple motor points in chosen muscles can be injected allowing for a "graded response," that is a desired degree of spasticity reduction can be achieved depending on the amount of phenol injected and number of individual motor points injected. Although this technique results in decreased spasticity of shorter duration than open branch blocks, the major advantages are ease of administration and that no surgery is required (Awad and Dykstra, 1990). Phenol nerve blocks can be safely performed on children but it is generally recommended that general anesthesia or deep conscious sedation be used due to the discomfort associated with the procedure.

Phenol can be prepared in aqueous or oil solution. Aqueous solution of 3–5% is the choice for percutaneous injections, while 3% glycerin is generally used for open blocks: 1–5 cc are used for percutaneous injections; <0.5 cc is required for open blocks. The most common side effects are lightheadedness, nausea and vomiting immediately after an injection, thrombophlebitis, or peripheral nerve injury (Gracies et al., 1997). Contraindications to the use of phenol blocks include poor general health, and severe or excessive contractures.

Botulinum toxin is a thermolabile exotoxin produced by the *Clostridium botulinum* bacteria (Brin, 1997). There are seven immunologically distinct serotypes, types A–G. Both botulinum toxins type A (BTX-A) (Botox^R and Dysport^R) and type B (BTX-B) (Myobloc^R) are available for clinical use.

BTX-A inhibits the release of acetylcholine from presynaptic nerve terminals; this causes a functional denervation of muscle fibers resulting in muscle weakness and a decrease in muscle tone. After injection into muscle at motor endpoint regions, the toxin is internalized within the neuron and interferes with calcium-mediated acetylcholine release from the vesicles, by disrupting the protein that is involved in the docking of acetylcholine containing vesicles to the cell membrane (Brin, 1997). Different BTX serotypes bind to different constituents of this protein complex. BTX-A binds to synapse-associated protein-25, while BTX-B binds to vesicle-associated membrane protein (Snow et al., 1990).

A number of studies have shown BTX to be effective in reducing upper and lower limb spasticity and painful spasms in both adults and children with stroke, multiple sclerosis, cerebral palsy, spinal cord injury, and traumatic brain injury (Snow et al., 1990; Schiavo et al., 1992; Cosgrove et al., 1994; Hesse et al., 1994; Dunne et al., 1995; Grazko et al., 1995; Gooch and Sandell, 1996; Pullman et al., 1996; Simpson et al., 1996; Simpson, 1997; Bakheit et al., 2001; Bakheit, 2003; Brashear et al., 2003; Wong, 2003). In addition to a reduction in spasticity, several studies have also reported an improvement in functional abilities, such as walking and the ability to perform daily cares, in patients treated with BTX (Sarioglu et al., 2003; Slawek and Klimont, 2003; Woldag and Hummelsheim, 2003). Treatment is often combined with other spasticity modalities, such as oral or intrathecal medications, physical therapy modalities including serial casting (Bottos et al., 2003). Injection of botulinum toxin directly into the detrusor muscle or urinary sphincter may be considered for the management of patients with neurogenic bladders (Schulte-Baukloh et al., 2003).

The clinical indications for BTX are similar to those noted for nerve blocks. Specific spastic muscles that are to be injected are identified by electromyogram (EMG) guidance. The toxin is diluted to the desired concentration and a decision is made regarding the number of units to be used; this varies depending on the particular muscle and degree of weakness desired (O'Brien, 1997).

After an intramuscular injection of the toxin a decline in motor endplate potentials can be identified within a few hours, although there is a delay in the onset of clinical effect for 24–72 h. With time, nerve sprouting occurs with reinnervation of muscle fibers resulting in a gradual wearing off of the effect. Duration of action averages 12–16 weeks; BTX-B may have a slightly longer duration of benefit than BTX-A (Lew et al., 1997; Brashear et al., 1999; Brin et al., 1999). Repeat injections are not recommended any more frequently than 12 weeks as neutralizing antibodies are more likely to develop in these instances, potentially leading to a poor treatment response (Jankovic and Brin, 1991). Neutralizing antibodies may be serotype specific; several studies have suggested that patients who become resistant to treatment with BTX-A may respond to treatment with BTX-B (Lew et al., 1997; Brin et al., 1999).

Side effects of botulinum toxin injections include local skin reactions and pain at the site of injection. Weakness can occur both in injected muscles and adjacent non-injected muscles.

Advantages to use of phenol injections include an immediate response (in contrast to botulinum toxin), low cost, and ease of sterilization and preparation. The major advantages of BTX is the relative ease of administration and availability at many centers.

17.11 Orthopedic procedures

Several orthopedic surgical procedures are available for the management of focal spasticity, and include tenotomies, tendon transfers, and tendon lengthening procedures. Tenotomies involve the release of muscle tendons of severely spastic muscles. Since the tendon is completely severed this procedure is generally reserved for spastic muscles without voluntary movement. Tendon lengthening may be performed on spastic muscles to position joints at a more natural and functional angle. Tendon transfers allow weakened muscles to perform more functional movements. These procedures are most successful in the lower extremities and may help improve ambulation (Sanger et al., 2003).

The most often performed orthopedic procedures include hamstring tendon lengthening for knee flexion contractures, Achilles tenotomy or lengthening for equinus deformity, adductor tenotomy for hip adductor spasticity, iliopsoas tenotomy for hip flexor spasms, and toe flexor tenotomies for claw foot deformities. Split posterior tibial tendon transfers are often useful in improving gait patterns in patients with posterior tibialis spasticity (Kagaya et al., 1996). A split anterior tibialis tendon transfer may help correct equinovarus posturing and excessive subtalar supination (Waters et al., 1982). Similar orthopedic procedures for upper extremity deformities, such as thumb-in-palm posturing or wrist contractures may

be considered, although typically do not improve function to the degree that the lower extremity surgeries do (Sakellarides and Kirvin, 1995; Sakellarides et al., 1995), and are prescribed less frequently.

17.12 Dorsal rhizotomy

An increase in the activity of Ia afferent fibers in monosynaptic spinal cord reflex pathways can often be demonstrated in spastic patients (Fasano et al., 1979). The theory behind selective dorsal rhizotomy is that by ablating the specific dorsal rootlets (levels L2–S2) that are overactive and involved in these abnormal reflex circuits, muscle tone can be lessened (Kim et al., 2003). Strength is preserved as the ventral roots are left intact. In the typical dorsal rhizotomy surgery 40–50% of rootlets at each level are sectioned, thus preserving at least some lower extremity sensation. This procedure has been shown to be efficacious in children with cerebral palsy; a number of studies have demonstrated improvement in lower extremity spasticity, standing, sitting, and ambulation with benefit persisting for at least 10 years (Peters and Arens, 1993; Nishida et al., 1995; Moroto et al., 2003). Several studies have also reported improvement in upper extremity function and speech following lumbosacral dorsal rhizotomy (Mittal et al., 2002; Salame et al., 2003). This is thought to be due to the fact that dorsal root neurons have collaterals that ascend to the cervical cord and brainstem nuclei; sectioning lumbar dorsal rootlets could, therefore, reduce facilatory influences at more rostral levels (Peacock et al., 1987). The most common side effects of the procedure are paresthesias and dysesthesias in the lower extremities.

Intraoperative nerve conduction recording is required. During the surgery individual dorsal rootlets are stimulated electrically; compound muscle action potentials are recorded from leg muscles representing the L2–S2 myotomes. Electrophysiologic criteria have been described which identify which of the specific rootlets are hyperexcitable and should therefore be sectioned (Fasano et al., 1979). These criteria include a low threshold to a single stimulus, a sustained response to a 50-Hz tetanic stimulation, and spread of the response (with muscle contraction) to muscle groups outside the rootlet's segmental distribution (often with spread to the contralateral limb). However, subsequent studies have questioned these criteria, since many control patients (without spasticity) demonstrate similar electrophysiologic findings with dorsal root stimulation (Cohen and Webster, 1991; Steinbok et al., 1994). The most effective means to identify hyperexcitable nerve rootlets, and the lumbosacral levels and extent to which the dorsal rootlets should be ablated remains controversial.

17.13 Invasive neurosurgic procedures

For severe refractory cases of spasticity neurosurgical procedures can be considered. This includes a myelotomy, or the severing of tracts within the spinal cord, interrupting the segmental reflex arc in the grey matter (Laitinen and Singounas, 1971). Recent modifications of the procedure allow for preservation of lateral column and white matter tract function (Livshits et al., 2002). Side effects include potential permanent loss of bowel and bladder function.

Cordectomy, which involves sectioning part of the cord, is also an irreversible procedure, reserved for only extreme cases of spasticity. This procedure results in flaccid paraplegia, and permanent bowel and bladder dysfunction (White et al., 2000).

17.14 Summary

Spasticity is a common consequence of neurologic disorders affecting the central nervous system. Treatment of spasticity is considered when the increase in muscle tone affects functional activities, including positioning, transfers, ambulation, or the ability to perform daily cares, or causes complications such as pain or contractures. A multidisciplinary approach, including nursing approaches, physical and occupational therapy, modalities such as splinting or casting, pharmacologic interventions, and surgical options should be considered in patient management.

REFERENCES

Albright, A.L., Barron, W.B., Fasick, M.P., Polinko, P. and Janosky, J. (1993). Continuous intrathecal baclofen infusion for spasticity of cerebral origin. *J Am Med Assoc*, **270**, 2475–2477.

Alfieri, V. (1982). Electrical treatment of spasticity. *Scand J Rehabil Med*, **14**, 177–182.

Allison, S.C. and Abraham, L.D. (1995). Correlation of quantitative measures with the modified Ashworth scale in the assessment of plantar flexor spasticity in the patients with traumatic brain injury. *J Neurol*, **242**, 699–706.

Armutulu, K., Meric, A., Kiodi, N., Yakut, E. and Karabudak, R. (2003). The effect of transcutaneous electrical nerve stimulation in spasticity in multiple sclerosis. *Neurorehabit Neural Repair*, **17**, 79–82.

Ashworth, B. (1964). Preliminary trial of carisoprodol in multiple sclerosis. *Practitioner*, **192**, 540–542.

Awad, E.A. and Dykstra, D. (1990). Treatment of spasticity by neurolysis. In: *Krusen's Handbook of Physical Medicine and Rehabilitation* (eds Kottke, F.J. and Leahmann, J.F.), 4th edn., Saunders, Philadelphia, pp. 1154–1161.

Backheit, A.M., Pittock, S., Moore, A.P., Wurker, M., Otto, S., Erbguth, F. and Coxon, L. (2001). A randomized, double-blind, placebo-controlled study of the efficacy and safety of botulinum toxin type A in upper limb spasticity in patients with stroke. *Eur J Neurol*, **8**, 559–565.

Bakheit, A.M. (2003). Botulinum toxin in the management of childhood muscle spasticity: comparison of clinical practice of 17 treatment centers. *Eur J Neurol*, **10**, 415–419.

Barbeau, H., Richards, C.L. and Bedard, P.J. (1982). Action of cyproheptadine in spastic paraparetic patients. *J Neurol Neurosurg Psychiatr*, **45**, 923–926.

Bohannon, R. (1999). Usefulness of the pendulum test. *Neurorehabil Neural Repair*, **13**, 259–260.

Bohannon, R.W. (1986). Variability and reliability of the pendulum test for spasticity using a Cybex II isokinetic dynamometer. *Phys Ther*, **67**, 659–661.

Bohannon, R.W. and Smith, M.B. (1987). Interrater reliability of a modified Ashworth scale of muscle spasticity. *Phys Ther*, **67**, 206–207.

Botte, M.J., Abrams, R.A. and Bodine-Fowler, S.C. (1995). Treatment of acquired muscle spasticity using phenol peripheral nerve blocks. *Orthopedics*, **18**, 151–159.

Bottos, M., Benedetti, M., Salucci, P., Gasparroni, V. and Giannini, S. (2003). Botulinum toxin with and without casting in ambulant children with spastic diplegia: a clinical and functional assessment. *Dev Med Child Neurol*, **45**, 758–762.

Brashear, A., Lew, M.F., Dykstra, D.D., Comella, C.L., Factor, S.A. and Rodnitzky, R.L. (1999). Safety and efficacy of NeuroBloc (botulinum toxin type B) in type A-responsive cervical dystonia. *Neurology*, **53**, 1439–1446.

Brashear, A., Zalonte, R., Coccoran, M., Galvez-Jimenez, N., Gracies, J.M., Gordon, M.F., McAfee, A., Ruffing, K., Thompson, B., Williams, M., Lee, C.H. and Turkel, C. (2002). Inter- and intrarater reliability of the Ashworth scale and the disability assessment scale in patients with upper-limb post stroke spasticity. *Arch Phys Med Rehabil*, **83**, 1349–1354.

Brashear, A., McAfee, A.L., Kuhn, E.R. and Ambrosius, W.T. (2003). Treatment with botulinum toxin type B for upper limb spasticity. *Arch Phys Med Rehabil*, **84**, 103–107.

Brin, M.F. (1997). Botulinum toxin: chemistry, pharmacology, toxicity, and immunology. *Muscle Nerve*, **20(Suppl. 6)**, S146–S168.

Brin, M.F., Lew, M.F. and Adler, C.H. (1999). Safety and efficacy of NeuroBloc (botulinum toxin type B) in type A-resistant cervical dystonia. *Neurology*, **53**, 1431–1438.

Calancie, B., Molano, M.R. and Broton, J.G. (2002). Interlimb reflexes and synaptic plasticity become evident months after human spinal cord injury. *Brain*, **125**, 1150–1161.

Coffey, R.J., Cahill, D., Steers, W. and Park, T.S. (1993). Intrathecal baclofen for intractable spasticity of spinal origin: results of long-term multicenter study. *J Neurosurg*, **78**, 226–232.

Cohen, A.R. and Webster, H.C. (1991). How selective is selective posterior rhizotomy? *Surg Neurol*, **35**, 267–272.

Conine, T.A., Sullivan, T., Mackie, T. and Goodman, M. (1990). Effect of serial casting for the prevention of equinus in patients with acute head injury. *Arch Phys Med Rehabil*, **71**, 310–312.

Cosgrove, A.P., Corry, I.S. and Graham, H.K. (1994). Botulinum toxin in the management of lower limb spasticity in cerebral palsy. *Dev Med Child Neurol*, **36**, 386–396.

Dahlin, M., Knutsson, E. and Nergardh, A. (1993). Treatment of spasticity in children with low dose benzodiazepine. *J Neurol Sci*, **117**, 54–60.

Dali, C., Hansen, F.J., Pedersen, S.A., Skov, L., Hilden, J., Bjornskov, I., Strandberg, C., Jeite, C., Ulla, H., Herbst, G. and Ulla, L. (2002). Threshold electrical stimulation (TES) in ambulent children with CP: a randomized double-blind placebo-controlled clinical trial. *Dev Med Child Neurol*, **44**, 364–369.

Davidoff, R.A. (1985). Antispasticity drugs: mechanisms of action. *Ann Neurol*, **17**, 107–116.

Dimitrijevic, M.R. (1995). Evaluation and treatment of spasticity. *J Neurol Rehabil*, **9**, 97–110.

Dunne, J.W., Heye, N. and Dunne, S.L. (1995). Treatment of chronic limb spasticity with botulinum toxin A. *J Neurol Neurosurg Psych*, **58**, 232–235.

Fasano, V.A., Barolat-Romana, G., Zeme, S. and Sguazzi, A. (1979). Electrophysiological assessment of spinal circuits in spasticity by direct dorsal root stimulation. *Neurosurgery*, **4**, 146–151.

Felsenthal, G. (1974). Pharmacology of phenol in peripheral nerve blocks: a review. *Arch Phys Med Rehabil*, **55**, 13–16.

Finke, J. (1978). Therapy of spasticity using sodium valproate. *J Medizinischewelt*, **29**, 1579–1581.

Francisco, G.E. and Boake, C. (2003). Improvement in walking speed in poststroke spastic hemiplegia after intrathecal baclofen in therapy: a preliminary study. *Arch Phys Med Rehabil*, **84**, 1194–1199.

Friden, J. and Lieber, R.L. (2003). Spastic muscle cells are shorter and stiffer than normal cells. *Muscle Nerve*, **27**, 157–164.

Fromm, G.H. (1994). Baclofen as an adjuvant analgesic. *J Pain Symptom Manag*, **9**, 500–509.

Gelber, D.A. and Jozefczyk, P.B. (1999). Therapeutics in the management of spasticity. *Neurorehabil Neural Repair*, **13**, 5–14.

Gelber, D.A., Jozefczyk, P.B., Herrmann, D., Good, D.C. and Verhulst, S.J. (1995). Comparison of two therapy approaches in the rehabilitation of the pure motor hemiparetic stroke patient. *J Neurol Rehabil*, **9**, 191–196.

Gelber, D.A., Good, D.C., Dromerick, A., Sergay, S. and Richardson, M. (2001). Open-label dose-titration safety and efficacy study of tizanidine hydrochloride in the treatment of spasticity associated with chronic stroke. *Stroke*, **32**, 1841–1846.

Gooch, J.L. and Sandell, T.V. (1996). Botulinum toxin for spasticity and athetosis in children with cerebral palsy. *Arch Phys Med Rehabil*, **77**, 598–611.

Gracies, J.M., Elovic, E., McGuire, J. and Simpson, D. (1997). Traditional pharmacological treatments for spasticity part I: local treatments. *Muscle Nerve*, **20(Suppl. 6)**, S61–S91.

Grazko, M.A., Polo, J.B. and Jabbari, B. (1995). Botulinum toxin A for spasticity, muscle spasms, and rigidity. *Neurology*, **45**, 712–717.

Hansel, D.E., Hansel, C.R., Shindle, M.K., Reinhardt, E.M., Madden, L., Levey, E.B., Johnston, M.V. and Hoon, A.H. (2003). Oral baclofen in cerebral palsy: possible seizure potentiation. *Pediatr Neurol*, **29**, 203–206.

Hesse, S., Lucke, D., Malezic, M., Bertelt, C., Friedrich, H., Gregoric, M. and Mauritz, K.H. (1994). Botulinum toxin treatment for lower limb extensor spasticity in chronic hemiparetic patients. *J Neurol Neurosurg Psych*, **57**, 1321–1324.

Hiersemenzel, L.P., Curt, A. and Dietz, V. (2000). From spinal shock to spasticity: neuronal adaptations to a spinal cord injury. *Neurology*, **54**, 1574–1582.

Jamshidi, M. and Smith, A.W. (1996). Clinical measurement of spasticity using the pendulum test: comparison of electrogoniometric and videotape analyses. *Arch Phys Med Rehabil*, **77**, 1129–1132.

Jankovic, J. and Brin, M.F. (1991). The therapeutic uses of botulinum toxins. *New Engl J Med*, **324**, 1186–1194.

Kabat, H. and Knott, M. (1954). Proprioceptive facilitation therapy for paralysis. *Physiotherapy*, **40**, 171.

Kagaya, H., Yamada, S., Nagasawa, T., Ishihara, Y., Kodama, H. and Endoh, H. (1996). Split posterior tibial tendon transfer for varus deformity of hindfoot. *Clin Ortho Rel Res*, **323**, 254–260.

Kao, L.W., Amin, Y., Kirk, M.A. and Turner, M.S. (2003). Intrathecal baclofen withdrawal mimicking sepsis. *J Emerg Med*, **24**, 423–427.

Katz, R. and Pierrot-Deseilligny, E. (1982). Recurrent inhibition of alpha-motorneurones in patients with upper motorneurone lesions. *Brain*, **105**, 103–124.

Keenan, M.A., Tomas, E.S., Stone, L. and Gersten, L.M. (1990). Percutaneous phenol block of the musculocutaneous nerve to control elbow flexor spasticity. *J Hand Surg*, **15A**, 340–346.

Khalil, A.A. and Betts, H.B. (1967). Peripheral nerve block with phenol in the management of spasticity. *J Am Med Assoc*, **200**, 1155–1157.

Killestein, J., Hoogervorst, E.L.J., Kalkers, N.F., vanLoenen, A.C., Staats, P.G.M., Gorter, R.W., Uitdehaag, B.M.J. and Poiman, C.H. (2002). Safety, tolerability, and efficacy of orally administered cannabanoids in MS. *Neurology*, **58**, 1404–1407.

Kim, D.S., Choi, J.U., Yang, K.H., Park, C.I. and Park, E.S. (2003). Selective posterior rhizotomy for lower extremity spasticity: how much and which of the posterior rootlets should be cut? *Surg Neurol*, **57**, 87–93.

Kogler, G.F. (2002). Orthotic management. In: *Clinical Evaluation and Management of Spasticity* (eds. Gelber, D.A. and Jeffery, D.R.), Humana Press, Totowa, NJ, pp. 67–91.

Kroin, J.S., Bianchi, G.D. and Penn, R.D. (1993). Intrathecal baclofen down regulates $GABA_B$ receptors in the rat substantia gelatinosa. *J Neurosurg*, **79**, 544–549.

Laitinen, L. and Singounas, E. (1971). Longitudinal myelotomy in the treatment of spasticity of the legs. *J Neurosurg*, **35**, 536–540.

Langlois, S., MacKinnon, J.R. and Pederson, L. (1989). Hand splints and cerebral spasticity: a review of the literature. *Canad J Occup Ther*, **56**, 113–119.

Lazorthes, Y., Sallerin-Caute, B., Verdie, J., Bastide, R. and Carillo, J. (1990). Chronic intrathecal baclofen administration for control of severe spasticity. *J Neurosurg*, **72**, 393–402.

Lee, S.U., Bang, M.S. and Han, T.R. (2002). Effect of cold air therapy in relieving spasticity: applied to spinalized rabbits. *Spinal Cord*, **40**, 67–73.

Lehmann, J.F., Condon, S.M., Price, R. and deLateur, B.J. (1987). Gait abnormalities in hemiplegia: their correction by ankle–foot orthoses. *Arch Phys Med Rehabil*, **68**, 763–771.

Leslie, G.C., et al. (1992). A comparison of the assessment of spasticity by the Wartenberg pendulum test and the Ashworth grading scale in patients with multiple sclerosis. *Clin Rehabil*, **6**, 41–48.

Lew, M.F., Adornato, B.T., Duane, D.D., et al. (1997). Botulinum toxin type B: a double-blind, placebo-controlled, safety and efficacy study in cervical dystonia. *Neurology*, **49**, 701–707.

Livshits, A., Rappaport, Z.H., Livshits, V. and Gepstein, R. (2002). Surgical treatment of painful spasticity after spinal cord injury. *Spinal Cord*, **40**, 167–173.

Loubser, P.G., Narayan, R.K., Sandin, K.J., Donovan, W.H. and Russell, K.D. (1991). Continuous infusion of intrathecal baclofen: long-term effects on spasticity in spinal cord injury. *Paraplegia*, **29**, 48–52.

McGuire, J.R. and Harvey, R.L. (1999). The prevention and management of complications after stroke. *Phys Med Rehabil Clin N Am*, **10**, 857–874.

Merritt, J.L. (1981). Management of spasticity in spinal cord injury. *Mayo Clin Proc*, **156**, 614–622.

Meythaler, J.M., Steers, W.D., Tuel, S.M., Cross, L.L. and Haworth, C.S. (1992). Continuous intrathecal baclofen in spinal cord spasticity. *Am J Phys Med Rehabil*, **71**, 321–327.

Meythaler, J.M., DeVivo, M.J. and Hadley, M. (1996). Prospective study on the use of bolus intrathecal baclofen for spastic hypertonia due to acquired brain injury. *Arch Phys Med Rehabil*, **77**, 461–466.

Miglietta, O. (1973). Action of cold on spasticity. *Am J Physical Med*, **52**, 198–205.

Mittal, S., Farmer, J.P., Al-Atassi, B., Montpetit, K., Gervais, N., Poulin, C., Cantin, M.A. and Benaroch, T.E. (2002). Impact of selective posterior rhizotomy in fine motor skills: long-term results using a validated evaluative measure. *Pediatr Neurosurg*, **36**, 133–141.

Moon, S.K., Whang, Y.K., Park, S.U., Ko, C.N., Kim, Y.S., Bae, H.S. and Cho, K.H. (2003). Antispastic effect of electroacupuncture and moxibustion in stroke patients. *Am J Clin Med*, **31**, 467–474.

Moroto, N., Kameyama, S., Masuda, M., Uishi, M., Aguni, A., Yehara, T. and Dagamine, K. (2003). Functional posterior rhizotomy for severely disabled children with mixed type cerebral palsy. *Acta Neurochir* (**Suppl. 87**), S99–S102.

Mortenson, P.A. and Eng, J.J. (2003). The use of casts in the management of mobility and joint hypertonia following brain injury in adults: a systemic review. *Phys Therapy*, **83**, 648–658.

Murphy, N.A., Irwin, M.C. and Hoff, C. (2002). Intrathecal baclofen therapy in children with cerebral palsy: efficacy and complications. *Arch Phys Med Rehabil*, **83**, 1721–1725.

Nance, P.W., Bugaresti, J., Shellenberger, K., Sheramata, W., Martinez-Arizala, A. and the North American Tizanidine Study Group. (1994). Efficacy and safety of tizanidine in the treatment of spasticity in patients with spinal cord injury. *Neurology*, **44(Suppl. 9)**, S44–S52.

Nielsten, J.F. (1995). A new treatment of spasticity with repetitive magnetic stimulation in multiple sclerosis. *J Neurol Neurosurg Psych*, **58**, 254–255.

Nishida, T., Thatcher, S.W. and Marty, G.R. (1995) .Selective posterior rhizotomy for children with cerebral palsy: a 7-year experience. *Child Nerv Sys*, **11**, 374–380.

Nuyens, G.E., DeWeerdt, W.J., Spaepen, A.J., Kiekens, C. and Feys, H.M. (2002). Reduction of spastic hypertonia during repeated passive knee movements in stroke patients. *Arch Phys Med Rehabil*, **83**, 930–935.

O'Brien, C.F. (1997). Injection techniques for botulinum toxin using electromyography and electrical stimulation. *Muscle Nerve*, **20(Suppl. 6)**, S176–S180.

O'Brien, C.F., Seeberger, L.C. and Smith, D.B. (1996). Spasticity after stroke, epidemiology and optimal treatment. *Drugs Aging*, **9**, 332–340.

Ochs, G., Struppler, A., Meyerson, B.A., Linderoth, B. and Gybels, J. (1989). Intrathecal baclofen for long-term treatment of spasticity: a multicentre study. *J Neurol Neurosurg Psychiatr*, **52**, 933–939.

Peacock, W.J., Arens, L.J. and Berman, B. (1987). Cerebral palsy spasticity. Selective posterior rhizotomy. *Pediatr Neurosci*, **13**, 61–66.

Peerless, J.R., Davies, A., Klein, D. and Yu, D. (1999). Skin complications in the intensive care unit. *Clin Chest Med*, **20**, 453–467.

Penn, R.D., Savoy, S.M., Corcos, D., Latash, M., Gottlieb, G., Parke, B. and Kroin, J.S. (1989). Intrathecal baclofen for severe spinal spasticity. *New Engl J Med*, **320**, 517–521.

Peter, J.C. and Arens, L.J. (1993). Selective posterior lumbosacral rhizotomy for the management of cerebral palsy spasticity. *S Afr Med J*, **83**, 745–747.

Pierson, S.H. (2002). Physical and occupational therapy approaches. In: *Clinical Evaluation and Management of Spasticity* (eds Gelber, D.A. and Jeffery, D.R.), Humana Press, Totowa, NJ, pp. 47–66.

Pinder, R.M., Brogden, R.N., Speight, T.M. and Avery, G.S. (1997). Dantrolene sodium: a review of its pharmacological properties and therapeutic efficacy in spasticity. *Drugs*, **13**, 3–23.

Pohl, M., Ruckreim, S., Mehrholz, J., Ritschel, C., Strik, H. and Pause, M.R. (2002). Effectiveness of serial casting in patients with severe cerebral spasticity: a comparison study. *Arch Phys Med Rehabil*, **83**, 784–790.

Pohl, M., Rockstroh, G., Ruckriem, S., Mehrholz, J., Pause, M., Kock, R. and Strik, H. (2003). Peak time course of the effect of a bolus dose of intrathecal baclofen on severe cerebral spasticity. *J Neurol*, **250**, 1195–2000.

Prandyan, A.D., Price, C.I., Barme, M.D. and Johnson, G.R. (2003). A biomechanical investigation into the validity of the modified Ashworth scale as a measure of elbow spasticity. *Clin Rehabil*, **17**, 290–293.

Priebe, M.M., Sherwood, A.M., Graves, D.E., Mueller, M. and Olson, W.H. (1997). Effectiveness of gabapentin in controlling spasticity: a quantitative study. *Spinal Cord*, **35**, 171–175.

Pullman, S.L., Greene, P., Fahn, S. and Pedersen, S.F. (1996). Approach to the treatment of limb disorders with botulinum toxin A. *Arch Neurol*, **53**, 617–624.

Rifici, C., Kofler, M., Kronenberg, M., Kofler, A., Bramanti, P. and Saltuari, L. (1994). Intrathecal baclofen application in patients with supraspinal spasticity secondary to severe traumatic brain injury. *Funct Neurol*, **9**, 29–34.

Riley, P.O. and Kerrigan, D.C. (1999). Kinetics of stiff-legged gait: induced acceleration analysis. *IEEE Trans Rehabil Eng*, **7**, 420–426.

Rossi, P.W. (1994). Treatment of spasticity. In: *The Handbook of Neurorehabilitation* (eds. Good, D.C. and Couch, J.R.), Marcel Dekker, Inc., New York, pp. 197–218.

Roussan, M., Terrence, C. and Fromm, G. (1985). Baclofen versus diazepam for the treatment of spasticity and long-term follow-up of baclofen therapy. *Pharmatherapeutics*, **4**, 278–284.

Russo, E.B., Killestein, J., Uitdehaag, B.M.J. and Pohlman, C.H. (2003). Safety, tolerability, and efficacy of orally administered cannabanoids in MS. *Neurology*, **66**, 729–730.

Sabbahi, M.A., DeLuca, C.J. and Powers, W.R. (1981). Topical anesthesia: a possible treatment for spasticity. *Arch Phys Med Rehabil*, **62**, 310–314.

Sakellarides, H.T. and Kirvin, F.M. (1995). Management of the unbalanced wrist in cerebral palsy by tendon transfer. *Ann Plast Surg*, **35**, 90–94.

Sakellarides, H.T., Mital, M.A., Matza, R.A. and Dimakopoulos, P. (1995). Classification and surgical treatment of thumb-in palm deformity in cerebral palsy and spastic paralysis. *J Hand Surg*, **20**, 428–431.

Salame, K., Ouaknine, G.E., Rochkind, S., Constantin, S. and Razon, N. (2003). Surgical treatment of spasticity by selective posterior rhizotomy: 30 years experience. *Isr Med Assoc J*, **5**, 546–549.

Sanger, J.D., Delgado, M.R., Gaebler-Spira, D., Hallett, M. and Mink, J.W. (2003). Clinical practice guideline: classification and definition of disorders causing hypertonia in childhood. *Pediatrics*, **111**, 98–97.

Sankey, R.J., Anderson, D.M. and Young, J.A. (1989). Characteristics of ankle-foot orthoses for management of the spastic lower limb. *Dev Med Child Neurol*, **31**, 466–470.

Sarioglu, B., Serdaroglu, G., Tutuneuogle, S. and Ozer, E. (2003). The use of botulinum toxin type A treatment in children with spasticity. *Pediatr Neurol*, **29**, 299–301.

Scheker, L.R. and Ozer, K. (2003). Electrical stimulation in the management of spastic deformity. *Hand Clinics*, **19**, 601–606.

Schiavo, G., Benfenati, F. and Poulain, B. (1992). Tetanus and botulinum-B neurotoxins block neurotransmitter release by a proteolytic cleavage of synaptobrevin. *Nature*, **359**, 832–835.

Schulte-Baukloh, H., Michael, T., Sturzebeeher, B. and Knispel, H. (2003). Botulinum-a toxin detrusor injection as a novel approach in the treatment of bladder spasticity in children with neurogenic bladder. *Eurol Urol*, **44**, 139–143.

Simpson, D.M. (1997). Clinical trials of botulinum toxin in the treatment of spasticity. *Muscle Nerve*, **20(Suppl. 6**), S169–S175.

Simpson, D.M., Alexander, D.N., O'Brien, C.F., Tagliati, M., Aswad, A.S., Leon, J.M., Gibson, J., et al. (1996). Botulinum toxin type A in the treatment of upper extremity spasticity: a randomized double-blind placebo-controlled trial. *Neurology*, **46**, 1306–1310.

Slawek, J. and Klimont, L. (2003). Functional improvement in cerebral palsy patients treated with botulinum toxin A injections – preliminary results. *Eur J Neurol*, **10**, 313–317.

Snook, J.H. (1979). Spasticity reduction splint. *Am J Occup Ther*, **33**, 648–651.

Snow, B.J., Tsui, J.K., Bhatt, B.H., Varelas, M., Hashimoto, S.A. and Calne, D.B. (1990). Treatment of spasticity with botulinum toxin: a double blind study. *Ann Neurol*, **28**, 512–515.

Soni, B.M., Mani, R.M., Oo, T. and Vaidyanatharis, S. (2003). Treatment of spasticity in a spinal-cord-injured patient with intrathecal morphine due to intrathecal baclofen tolerance – a case report and review of the literature. *Spinal Cord*, **41**, 58–69.

Steinbok, P., Keyes, R., Langill, L. and Cochrane, D.D. (1994). The validity of electrophysiological criteria used in selective functional posterior rhizotomy for treatment of spastic cerebral palsy. *J Neurosurg*, **81**, 354–361.

Wagstaff, A.J. and Bryson, H.M. (1997). Tizanidine: a review of its pharmacology, clinical efficacy and tolerability in the management of spasticity associated with cerebral and spinal disorders. *Drugs*, **53**, 435–452.

Wallace, J.D. (1994). Summary of combined clinical analysis of controlled clinical trials with tizanidine. *Neurology*, **44(Suppl. 9**), S60–S69.

Walther, E.U. and Hohlfield, R. (1999). Multiple sclerosis: side effects of interferon beta therapy and their management. *Neurology*, **53**, 1622.

Waters, R.L., Frazier, J., Garland, D.E., Jordon, C. and Perry, J. (1982). Electromyographic gait analysis before and after operative treatment for hemiplegic equinus and equinovarus deformity. *J Bone Joint Surg*, **64A**, 284–288.

Weingarden, S.I. and Belen, J.G. (1992). Clonidine transdermal system for treatment of spasticity in spinal cord injury. *Arch Phys Med Rehabil*, **73**, 876–877.

White, K.D., Ince, P.G., Lusher, M., Lindsey, J., Cookson, M., Bashir, R., Shaw, P.J. and Bughby, K.M.D. (2000). Clinical and pathological findings in hereditary spastic paraparesis with spastin mutation. *Neurology*, **55**, 89–94.

Woldag, H. and Hummelsheim, H. (2003). Is the reduction of spasticity by botulinum toxin A beneficial for the recovery of motor function of arm and hand in stroke patients. *Eur Neurol*, **50**, 165–171.

Wong, V. (2003). Evidence-based approach to the use of botulinum toxin type A (BTX) in cerebral pasy. *Pediatr Rehabil*, **6**, 85–96.

Young, R.R. (1987). Physiologic and pharmacological approaches to spasticity. *Neurologic Clinics*, **5**, 529–539.

Young, R.R. (2002). Physiology and pharmacology of spasticity. In: *Clinical Evaluation and Management of Spasticity* (eds Gelber, D.A. and Jeffery, D.R.), Humana Press, Totowa, NJ, pp. 3–12.

Young, R.R. and Delwaide, P.J. (1981). Drug therapy: spasticity. *New Engl J Med*, **304**, 28–33.

Zajicek, J., Fox, P., Santos, H., Wright, D., Vickery, J., Nunn, A., Thompson, A. and UK MS Research Group. (2003). Cannabinoids for treatment of spasticity and other symptoms related to multiple sclerosis (CAMS Study): multicentre randomised placebo controlled trial. *Lancet*, **362**, 1517–1526.

Arm and hand weakness

Sarah Blanton and Steven L. Wolf

Department of Rehabilitation Medicine, Emory University, Atlanta, GA, USA

18.1 Introduction

The generation of controlled and precise contractile forces in our skeletal muscles is what fundamentally allows us to maintain posture, manipulate objects, and interact with our environment (Ghez, 1991). In this context, what we generally term "weakness" is often a major reason for loss of control in the genesis of a muscular contraction. Muscle weakness can occur from lesions at various levels of the nervous system that impact the output of either the upper motor neuron (UMN) or lower motor neuron (LMN). Disorders of LMNs refer to lesions that occur in the cells of the ventral gray column (or "horn") of the spinal cord or brain stem or in their axons (Waxman, 2003) and are discussed in more detail in Chapter 40 of Volume II, "Neuromuscular Rehabilitation: Diseases of Motor Neuron, Peripheral Nerve and Neuromuscular Junction". UMN lesions, occurring as a result of damage to the cerebral hemispheres or lateral white columns of the spinal cord (Waxman, 2003), are typically caused by strokes, traumatic brain injuries, infections, or tumors. Muscle weakness is considered one of the major causes of disability in patients with UMN lesion (Sahrmann and Norton, 1977; Gowland et al., 1992; Fellows et al., 1994). In light of this fact and considering that the primary symptom of cerebral injury is manifested in impairments of strength and motor control, the concept of weakness can be viewed in the context of stroke and traumatic brain injury.

Accordingly, the purpose of this chapter is to identify and describe weakness of the upper extremity (UE) through exploration of impairment in movements following cerebral injury. The present perspective of weakness is presented with respect to strength and the consequent relationship of strength to function. Weakness involves many factors and is discussed by addressing features of UMN, secondary muscular adaptations, and finally age related changes in the motor system. The extent to which weakness is a factor in determining a prognosis of motor recovery is explored, followed by aspects of therapeutic intervention. In concluding, limitations in our current knowledge about UE weakness are identified and suggestions for future study are provided.

18.2 Definitions of weakness and strength

Ng and Shepherd (2000) define strength as "the capacity of a muscle or group of muscles to produce the force necessary for initiating, maintaining, and controlling movement". Weakness, defined as the diminution of strength, would therefore reflect the reduced capacity of muscles to produce the necessary tension during conditions of voluntary loading of the musculoskeletal system (Smidt and Rogers, 1982; Bourbonnais and Vanden Noven, 1989). The measurement of strength is often recorded as the maximal amount of force exerted in a single attempt.

Factors contributing to inadequate strength as a basis for weakness

Several major determinants of strength include: recruitment, cross-sectional area, fiber type, length–force and force–velocity relationship, and kinesiology (Frontera et al., 2001b).

A coordinated, properly sequenced recruitment of motor units is an important precursor to the development of strength. The force generated by a normal muscle contraction depends on the number and type of motor units recruited, and the characteristics of that motor unit discharge. Tension is increased when either the number or rate of active motor units is increased.

The size of a muscle cross-sectional area is proportional to force generation and is related to the number and size of muscle fibers (Maughan et al., 1983). The length–force relationship of a muscle corresponds structurally with the number of cross-bridges, which are determined by the overlap of actin and myosin. Maximum force occurs with muscle length that offers maximum overlap between actin and myosin. Taking into account that muscle length is limited by the anatomy of joint motions, maximum force of a muscle is typically found to occur during the middle of the joint range of motion (ROM) (Frontera et al., 2001b).

Velocity and type of muscle contraction can also affect force generation, with the greatest force developing with a rapid eccentric contraction, compared to a slow concentric contraction. Moreover, torque generation is affected by the origin/insertion of a muscle relative to the axis of rotation about a joint. Insertions closer to the center of rotation produce a great arc of movement, but a lower maximal force. A greater force but smaller arc is generated when the insertion of the muscle is farther from the joint center.

Other functional constituents of the neuromuscular system relevant to strength include local muscular endurance (the ability to resist muscular fatigue) and muscular power (force applied multiplied by the velocity of movement) (Deschenes and Kraemer, 2002). Limitations in endurance often interfere with completion of functional activities. For example, individuals with stroke may have enough strength to initiate gripping forces, but cannot maintain adequate force to continue to hold an object during transport. As many common movements take place in less than 0.2 ms, the ability to produce force quickly is also vital in daily activities. Consequently, muscular power, a function of speed and strength, should be another perspective to consider in evaluation of the impairment of weakness.

In summary, weakness can result from inadequate strength caused by limitations in force production. In addition, the resultant weakness is affected by architectural characteristics of muscle and how the generation of muscle torque changes over time (endurance) because of the task-specific demands upon the speed of movement (power).

18.3 The weakness–disability connection

Relationship between muscle strength and function

Weakness is recognized as a major impairment causing disability (Gowland et al., 1992; Canning et al., 1999; Ng and Shepherd, 2000) and thus a primary obstacle to stroke recovery. The magnitude of joint torque generated in the hemiplegic UE may be impaired by as much as 53% compared to the non-dominant arm of healthy individuals (McCrea et al., 2003). Strength is also impaired in the arm ipsilateral to the lesion (Colebatch and Gandevia, 1989; Andrews and Bohannon, 2000; Jung et al., 2002) by as much as 15% (McCrea et al., 2003).

To date, findings from studies of the hemiplegic UE suggest a moderate to strong correlation existing between muscle weakness and impaired motor function in patients after stroke (Ng and Shepherd, 2000). Torques measured during hand grip have been correlated with some hand function tests among patients in the acute and sub-acute post-stroke stages (Sunderland et al., 1989). In addition, isometric strength of elbow flexors strongly correlates with functional hand to mouth movements (Bohannon et al., 1991). Completion of the hand to mouth maneuver (simulating eating) relates positively to actual elbow flexor muscle strength (Spearman correlation = 0.829) and inversely to elbow flexion active ROM deficits (−0.853). Indeed, Bohannon et al. noted that patients with less than 3.0 kg of elbow flexion force cannot fully bring their hands to their mouths. Weakness in muscle contraction and the degree of co-contraction in paretic wrist flexors and extensors also correlate significantly with upper limb motor impairment and physical disability measures (Chae et al., 2002b). Muscle strength as reflected by electromyographic (EMG) activity correlates positively with UE scores on the Fugl-Meyer motor assessment (FMA) and the arm motor ability test (AMAT), while the presence of co-contraction of the antagonist muscles (as represented by the ratio of agonist to antagonist EMG activity) is inversely related to these outcome measures.

However, as Ng and Shepherd caution, correlations from these cross-sectional studies only indicate a level of association, not an actual causal relationship. Data from Alberts and colleagues (2004) indicate that absolute strength is not a predictor of dexterity in the UE, and that the ability to control grip forces has a greater impact on UE function than maximal strength. Indeed, patients who have sustained strokes are able to show improved control of force and torque generation in a functional activity, such as turning a key (Fig. 18.1), after repetitive task training without necessarily demonstrating large changes in UE strength. Accordingly, more research is required to explore the mechanisms by which an increase in strength may cause an increase in function as a basis for providing better justification in the treatment of UE weakness.

18.4 Pathophysiology of weakness

Figure 18.2, adapted from Ng and Shepherd (2000), outlines mechanisms contributing to impairment of muscle weakness. It is chosen as a model to discuss UE weakness to illustrate the multi-factorial aspects

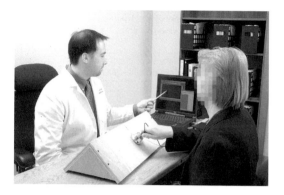

Figure 18.1. Patient turning key instrumented with force transducer following intense rehabilitation to her more impaired upper extremity.

of this impairment. These mechanisms may be classified into three primary categories:

1 features of UMN;
2 features of secondary muscular adaptation due to altered patterns of use (immobility and inactivity);
3 features associated with age-related changes in motor system.

Features of the UMN include:

1 lack of excitation arising in descending pathways,
2 direct changes in the agonist motor units,
3 active restraints of agonist motor activation,
4 passive restraints of agonist activation.

Features resulting from secondary muscular adaptation include:

1 length associated changes of muscle fibers and connective tissues in shortened position;
2 specific disuse weakness (atrophy of muscle fibers and impairments in motor unit activation).

Additionally, features associated with the aging process are possible contributing factors to weakness of a limb. Collectively these changes result in deficiencies in generating force and sustaining force output. Recognition of the many factors contributing to weakness allows the clinician to identify areas of movement impairment that may be amendable

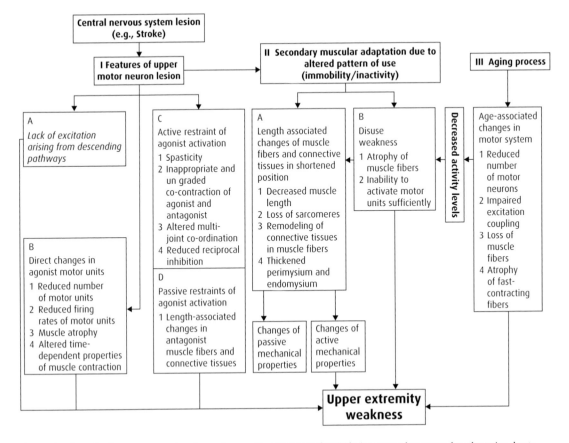

Figure 18.2. Contributions to upper extremity weakness – direct features of UMN lesion, secondary muscular adaptation due to altered pattern of use, and the aging process (modified after Ng and Shepherd, 2000; with permission).

to change through appropriate therapeutic interventions.

Features of upper motor neuron lesion

Lack of excitation arising in descending pathways

Corticospinal pathways can be interrupted at different anatomical locations following a stroke. Typically, patterns of weakness are due to the involvement of these pathways, however corticospinal tracts may not be the only ones involved (Chae et al., 2002b). More than likely, UMN weakness is due to the decreased supraspinal input from several descending fiber systems. The apparent weakness found in the less impaired side maybe in fact due to the small percentage of descending cortical tracts that originate from the lesion site and remain ipsilateral (Davidoff, 1990).

Direct changes in motor units

Changes in motor units may result in deficiencies in generating force and sustaining force output. These changes include: loss of agonist motor units, reduced firing rates of agonist motor units, atrophy of fast-contracting fibers, hypertrophy of slow-contracting fibers, and prolonged agonist contraction time.

Reduced number of motor units

McComas (1973) estimated that the number of motor units are reduced by 50% between the 2nd and 6th months after stroke. Hara and colleagues (2004) found that thenar muscle motor unit loss on the hemiparetic side is present as early as the 2nd week after stroke onset. This physiologic change correlates with hemiparesis severity, with the motor unit loss present at 3–4 months remaining unchanged at 1 year. This persistent change may be due to trans-synaptic degeneration of alpha motor neurons precipitated by the reduction of trophic inputs typically received through the descending motor pathways.

Reduced firing rates of motor units

Evidence strongly suggests that there is a reduction in motor unit firing rates after stroke (Rosenfalck and Andreassen, 1980; Dengler et al., 1990; Gemperline et al., 1995) resulting in a less effective generation of tension (Rack and Westbury, 1969; Bourbonnais and Vanden Noven, 1989) and directly contributing to muscle weakness (Rosenfalck and Andreassen, 1980; Tang and Rhymer, 1981). Thus, more units must be recruited to achieve a given force level and consequential limb movement (Bourbonnais and Vanden Noven, 1989).

Force production in normal muscle is length-dependent (Rassier et al., 1999). Ada and colleagues (2003) found that patients with stroke have particular difficulty in generating torque in shortened ranges. For maximum torque to be produced at shortened muscle lengths, motor unit firing rates need to be increased. Consequently, this selective weakness maybe related to reduced firing rates after stroke.

Muscle atrophy

There is no unanimity on the factors contributing to muscle atrophy in hemiplegic extremities. Frontera et al. (1997) found atrophy in both type I and IIA

fibers in the paretic tibialis anterior contributing to the presence of weakness. However, other studies have shown selective atrophy of type II fibers in UE muscles (Edstrom, 1970; Edstrom et al., 1973; Chokroverty et al., 1976). This selective atrophy may be muscle-specific depending upon the function of the muscle and the degree of spasticity (Frontera et al., 1997). Furthermore, the weakness seen in paretic muscles may also be due to a reduction in cross-bridges and lower force generation per cross-bridge.

Altered time-dependent properties of muscle contraction

An important aspect of muscle contraction involves the speed with which the torque profiles rise and fall. Typically peak torque is achieved in healthy individuals within 1 s of the initiation of a maximum voluntary contraction. In patients after stroke, the time to develop torque is impaired by 61% in the more affected arm and by 22% in the less affected arm (McCrea et al., 2003). The time to reduce torque was also impaired by 22% in the more affected arm as compared to the less affected arm and non-dominant arm. Delays in both initiation and termination of muscle contraction correlate positively with measures of impairment and disability (Chae et al., 2002a). A typical example of the prolonged time to reduce torque is the stroke survivor's difficulty releasing a grasp ("letting go") of an object. The time-alteration in torque reduction maybe related to changes in the motoneuron membrane firing behavior (McCrea et al., 2003), described as the "plateau potential" (Hounsgaard et al., 1988). This shift in the synaptic current–frequency relationship driven by neuro-modulator changes results in a cell that can maintain a prolonged tonic firing rate following a brief period of excitation (Kiehn and Eken, 1998).

Active restraints of agonist motor activation

Spasticity

Spasticity is arguably one of the most debated aspects of motor control in neurorehabilitation.

A more detailed discussion is provided in Chapter 17 of Volume II, "Management of spasticity". Here, spasticity is considered a component of UE movement dysfunction that is differentiated from the other symptoms contributing to weakness. In this section, spasticity will be referred to as muscular hyperactivity resulting from an exaggerated velocity-dependent passive stretch reflex. However, spasticity is a movement disorder and not an independent phenomenon (Lance, 1980). Consequently, altered reflex behavior should be acknowledged for its influence on movement control (Levin et al., 2000). Other interrelated factors that impact neuronal activity, such as inappropriate co-activation of flexors and extensors, altered joint coordination, and reduced reciprocal inhibition are addressed subsequently, as they may also participate in the production of limb weakness.

Inappropriate/ungraded co-contraction of agonist and antagonist

Excessive agonist–antagonist co-contraction of muscles during voluntary movement is a frequent and troublesome clinical phenomenon in patients post-stroke. Although both weakness and co-contraction are known to cause movement deficits, the relative contribution of each of these factors to impaired function of the UE remains inconclusive. Gowland et al. (1992) found that inadequate recruitment in the agonist muscles, not abnormal co-contraction of the agonist and antagonist muscles was the significant factor differentiating patients who could or could not complete tasks. However, Chae and colleagues (2002b) recently showed that abnormal co-contraction of wrist flexors and extensors in addition to the degree of muscle weakness positively correlated with the amount of motor impairment and disability in the post-stroke upper limb. Evaluating the relative contributions of neural mechanisms to finger extension deficits following stroke, Kamper and colleagues (2003) described a combination of factors, including: inappropriate co-contraction of the flexors and extensor of the metacarpophalangeal (MCP) joint during voluntary

MCP extension; difficulty in terminating excitation of the flexor digitorum superficialis (FDS) and first dorsal interosseous (FDI); and profound weakness of the MCP extensor muscles. Additional research is needed to further elucidate the relative contribution of abnormal co-contraction both within and across patients and in relation to completion of functional tasks.

Altered multi-joint coordination/ abnormal co-activation of synergistic muscles

In healthy individuals, co-activation of muscles about a joint contributes to motor control (Lamontagne et al., 2000), by regulating joint stiffness (Simmons and Richardson, 1988; Solomonow et al., 1988), and assisting in stability (Cholewicki et al., 1997; Levin and Dimov, 1997). Typically, fractionation of movement is thought to be due to selective activation of components with the corticospinal pathways (Buys et al., 1986; Colebatch et al., 1990; Dewald et al., 1995). If a loss of corticospinal projections provokes an increased reliance on residual undamaged pathways, these alternative descending projections (with more extensive branching at the spinal cord) may result in an obligatory co-activation of muscle groups not normally activated together and a dysregulation of fractionated movements (Dewald et al., 1995). The deficit of selective muscle activation required for complex tasks causes a tight coupling between movements at adjacent joints, characterized by stereotypic movement patterns, or "synergies". Multiple components may contribute to the underlying mechanisms resulting in these synergistic movements. Examining post-stroke hand function, Li et al. (2003) observed that both decreases in general finger force and limitations in multi-finger interactions contributed to impaired movement. This reduction in individual finger control was related to the gross flexor synergy as described by Brunnstrom (1970).

Dewald et al. (1995) evaluated abnormal muscle co-activation patterns at the elbow and shoulder during isometric torque generation. Both healthy and post-stroke subjects exhibited consistent co-activation patterns. However, in the subjects post-stroke, additional novel patterns were noted between elbow flexors/shoulder abductors and elbow extensors/shoulder adductors. These patterns may represent a reduction in the number of possible muscle combinations (or "synergies") during movement of the hemiplegic limb. Additionally, these patterns appear to be task-dependent and relate to the mechanics of the upper limb. Subsequent studies from this group (Beer et al., 1999) indicate that abnormal synergies between the shoulder and elbow reflect a weakness of paretic elbow musculature that is strongly task dependent. In short, multiple joint movements that appear as a synergy may be due to selective activation of muscle groups that collectively demonstrate the flexion or extensor patterns seen in the UEs of patients with stroke. The extent to which these multi-joint "patterns" are driven by selective activation of specific muscle groups in the absence of cortical drive to antagonist muscles or impaired reciprocal inhibition is still a source of intense study.

Reduced reciprocal inhibition

Reciprocal inhibition refers to the relaxation of antagonistic muscles when a prime mover is activated (Pyndt et al., 2003). In patients with spastic hemiplegia, a reduction of elements contributing to reciprocal inhibition has been reported (Nakashima et al., 1989; Baykousheva-Mateva and Mandaliev, 1994); however, studies primarily in lower extremities (LEs) of patients with stroke, have shown limited evidence for correlations between the amount of Ia reciprocal inhibition and clinical deficits. Okuma and Lee (1996) found that in patients with a poor recovery after stroke, disynaptic Ia inhibition from peroneal nerve afferents to soleus motoneurones was diminished or unchanged; whereas in those patients with a good recovery of function with mild spasticity, Ia inhibition had actually increased. The investigators postulate that an increased Ia inhibition onto soleus motoneurones during recovery may be a mechanism to compensate for loss of descending motor commands.

Passive restraints of agonist activation

Length associated changes in antagonist muscle fibers and connective tissues

Adaptive length-associated changes in muscles and connective tissue can alter passive mechanical properties (including stiffness and decrease in extensibility) of antagonist muscles. When antagonists are in a typically shortened position, a passive restraint to the agonists during dynamic movement is generated (Williams and Goldspink, 1978; Herbert, 1988) resulting in a decreased net agonist torque (Knuttson and Martensson, 1980; Dietz et al., 1981; Hammond et al., 1988).

Improvements in passive and active elbow extension ROM despite biceps co-contraction have been demonstrated in patients post-stroke (Wolf et al., 1994). These ROM improvements through function biofeedback training indicated that passive biomechanical (peripheral) rather than active central mechanisms may have been limiting joint movement.

Features of secondary muscular adaptation due to altered patterns of use (immobility and inactivity)

Length associated changes of muscle fibers and connective tissues in shortened position

The limited capacity for voluntary movement after a UMN lesion contributes the altered patterns of use of the hemiplegic UE. This immobility and inactivity result in secondary morphologic adaptations that can further contribute to the perception of weakness during functional tasks. In animal studies, these changes include: decreased muscle length (Tabary et al., 1972; Williams and Goldspink, 1978; Williams, 1988); decreased tendon length (Herbert and Crosbie, 1995); decrease in sarcomeres in a series (Tabary et al., 1972; Williams and Goldspink, 1978; Williams, 1988); increase in proportion of connective tissue to muscle fiber within the muscle (Williams and Goldspink, 1984; Williams, 1988); decreases in extensibility of periarticular connective tissue (Akeson et al., 1974), alterations in the orientation of the intramuscular connective tissue (Williams and Goldspink, 1984); and thickened perimysium and endomysium (Jozsa et al., 1990). In fact, cellular muscle changes have been shown to occur in animals after as little as 24 h of disuse or bed rest (Williams and Goldspink, 1978; Tardieu et al., 1981).

Disuse weakness

Disuse from any pathology will result in muscle weakness (see also Volume II, Chapter 21). Results from human studies have shown atrophy of muscle fibers (Rose and Rothstein, 1982) and the inability to activate motor units sufficiently (Duchateau and Hainaut, 1987, 1990) after decreased patterns of use and immobility. In the stroke population, disuse plays a major role in the development of atrophy and weakness in LEs (Hachisuka et al., 1997). Unfortunately, patients in rehabilitation endure long hours of inactivity or in the performance of tasks unrelated to rehabilitative goals (Lincoln et al., 1996; Mackey et al., 1996; Esmonde et al., 1997). Many factors besides the primary motor dysfunction may contribute to inactivity after stroke (Ng and Shepherd, 2000). Dementia and arthritis are primary examples of medical conditions limiting mobility, as well as co-morbid heart disease (Roth and Green, 1996), learned non-use (Taub and Wolf, 1997), learned helplessness (Peterson et al., 1993), and a non-stimulating rehabilitative environment (Mackey et al., 1996).

Features associated with age-related changes in motor system

Age is considered significant risk factors for stroke. Since stroke incidence increases with age (Hollander et al., 2003), especially in the very old, age-related changes in the motor system become important factors to consider in diagnosis and treatment of weakness after a UMN injury. Even in healthy individuals, the force-generating capacity of skeletal muscles is reduced with age (Frontera et al., 2000; Williams et al., 2002). This loss in strength may be due to alterations in the amount of contractile tissue within the muscle and muscle atrophy (Lexel et al., 1988; Frontera et al., 2000; Kent-Braun et al., 2000) more than actual deficits in motor unit recruitment and firing rates (Kent-Braun and Ng, 1999; Connelly et al., 1999; Roos et al., 1999). The decrease in skeletal muscle cross-sectional area, is primarily a result of decreased fiber number (Lexel et al., 1988), although there is some decrease in fiber size. The effects of aging on the motor unit characteristics include: a decrease in the number of motor neurons and consequently motor units (Campbell et al., 1973); possible decrease or variability in firing rates (Connelly et al., 1999; Laidlaw et al., 2000); and impaired excitation coupling (Delbono et al., 1997). Consequently, these physiologic and morphologic changes in the motor system combine with disuse weakness to produce the age-related decline in strength.

To summarize, because muscle weakness is compounded by a mosaic of mechanical and neural constraints, the evaluation and treatment of upper functional limitations can be a complex endeavor. A thorough knowledge of the possible pathophysiology contributing to UMN weakness will enable the clinician to choose the most appropriate and effective intervention.

18.5 Prognosis of motor recovery

Prognosis of UE motor recovery after UMN lesions remains difficult and uncertain. In light of reduced health care reimbursement, development of accurate prognostic indicators is essential for the delivery of cost-efficient rehabilitation services and to guide clinicians in appropriate allocation of patients' resources.

Lesion type and location

Estimates from studies indicate that only 5% to 20% of patients demonstrate full recovery (Heller et al., 1987; Nakayama et al., 1994) at 6 months post-stroke. At this subacute stage, at least 30% (Heller et al., 1987) to 60% (Wade et al., 1983; Sunderland et al., 1989) of stroke survivors will be forced to adapt to a non-functional UE. Neuroimaging studies indicate that involvement of the supratentorial corticospinal pathways may predict the presence or absence of arm weakness after stroke (Knopman and Rubens, 1986). Recovery is also influenced by lesion locations that implicate involvement of cortical or subcortical structures associated with primary and or secondary motor systems (Shelton and Reding, 2001). Recovery of upper limb capabilities is strongly related to the extent the primary-motor corticospinal input remains intact (Shelton and Reding, 2001). Shelton and colleagues found that patients with purely cortical strokes were likely to recover UE isolated movement (75%); however motor recovery declined progressively as lesions involved the corona radiata and the posterior limb of the internal capsule.

Stroke severity and minimal motor criteria

Most stroke survivors have sensory loss; however the presence of gross sensory deficiencies is an indicator of poor future function (Broeks et al., 1999). Other factors that complicate motor recovery in UE hemiplegia include: shoulder pain, limited shoulder ROM, and increased muscle tone (Twitchell, 1951; Andrews et al., 1981; Olsen, 1990). However, the initial grade of paresis may be the most important predictor of motor recovery (Hendricks et al., 2002), with initial lack of movement within the 1st month after stroke associated a very poor prognosis for subsequent recovery (Broeks et al., 1999). Conversely, the presence of grip strength at 1 month post-stroke indicates at least partial functional recovery may occur at 6 months (Sunderland et al., 1989).

For the most part, this initial level of UE impairment after stroke appears to be a "moderating variable" (Winstein et al., 2003) in recovery. Typically the less impaired stroke survivors with at least initial UE movement respond better to treatment because they can begin to voluntarily engage the limb in activities. This active participation is the foundation for motor skill learning and consequent improved function. Using transcranial magnetic stimulation (TMS) and functional magnetic resonance imaging (fMRI),

Lotze and colleagues (2003) demonstrated neurophysiologic differences between passive training of wrist extension and active, voluntary motor training. Although changes did occur with passively elicited movements, motor performance and cortical reorganization were greater with the active movement paradigm. Appropriately then, the ability to initiate distal active movement of the UE is a potent indicator for potential re-acquisition of meaningful function.

These observations have been supported by analyses of outcomes from the Kansas City Stroke Study (Duncan et al., 2003), involving subacute patients with stroke. This investigation showed that a multifaceted approach to UE rehabilitation, including strengthening, yielded the best results among those least impaired (based upon their Orpington scores). Collectively, these data suggest that lesion type, location, and severity help to define the magnitude of impairment and the potential role that strengthening might offer toward improving upon weakness and enhancing ability.

18.6 Elements of the interventional process and the role of strengthening

The value in treating UE weakness as a symptom of neuropathology resides in the clinician's ability to recognize the magnitude of the weakness and how it must be overcome within the context of several considerations, all of which must be addressed to achieve maximal "ability in manipulating the environment" with the more impaired limb. To treat weakness in isolation as though other critical factors including changes in viscoelastic properties of muscle and connective tissue, spasticity, fatigue, endurance, and cognition are not an integral aspect of clinical decision making and treatment planning would be erroneous. Accordingly, our ability to differentiate recovery from imposition of compensatory behavior; evaluate aspects of treatment intensity, duration, and frequency; consider the need for specificity of training; assess the long-term effects of any intervention that includes improving strength; address patient and caregiver compliance with treatment prescription; and identify fundamental differences between changes in strength and existing spasticity can make the difference between successful outcomes and failure. This statement is particularly true in the context of constricting numbers of treatment sessions and the need to provide best evidence in considering each of these important matters.

Recovery versus compensation – determining the appropriateness of an intervention

Evidence supporting the efficacy of neurorehabilitative approaches to improve UE function is limited. Inevitably, reductions in coverage for health care treatments of neurorehabilitation patients are manifest in decreasing inpatient lengths of stays and total therapy visits. Constraints in time and resources have produced a general shift in therapeutic focus to the basic needs of a patient upon returning home. The drive to quickly achieve the primary rehabilitative goal of safety with general mobility (i.e., transfers and gait) fosters development of one-handed behavioral compensatory techniques to achieve function, often at the expense of treating motoric impairments in the more affected UE.

Both clinician and patient would prefer interventions to improve function through remediation of underlying motor impairments and to do so by determining those interventions for which evidence for efficacy has been demonstrated (Logigian et al., 1983; Dickstein et al., 1986; Basmajian et al., 1987; Gelber et al., 1995; Kwakkel et al., 1997; van der Lee et al., 1999; Barreca et al., 2003).

Several recent reviews of evidenced-based neurorehabilitative approaches for improving arm and hand function have yielded mixed results. Two have concluded that there is insufficient evidence to make a definitive conclusion regarding the effectiveness of exercise therapy on arm function (van der Lee et al., 2001; Woldag and Hummelsheim, 2002). However, a recent systematic review driven by the calculation of predictive equations was able to determine appropriate treatment recommendations for the impaired UE based upon phases of recovery (Barreca et al.,

2003). Sensorimotor training; motor learning training that includes the use of imagery; electrical stimulation alone, or combined with biofeedback; and engaging the client in repetitive novel tasks can all be effective in reducing motor impairment after stroke. These are all approaches for which measurable benefits can be derived based upon the analyses of studies among patients less than 9 months post-stroke and with a minimal to moderate level of impairment at the time treatment is rendered. Conversely, among patients with less functional ability, careful positioning and handling, electrical stimulation, movement with elevation, strapping, and the avoidance of overhead pulleys are recommended treatments. Evidence suggests these interventions can effectively reduce or prevent pain; however, with respect to impacting weakness, the relationship of each of these treatment approaches to UE outcomes is unclear.

Intensity, duration, and frequency of treatment

Mounting evidence continues to support the notion that increased intensity, structure, and progression may be critical components in effective therapy. Findings from sub-human primate studies indicate that use-dependent cortical reorganization is a key element in functional recovery after UMN lesions (Nudo, 1997; Nudo and Friel, 1999; Kleim et al., 2002; Nudo, 2003). Several human studies indicate that intensive UE task practice appears to drive an adaptive response contributing to the experience driven-changes of the neural representations underlying trained tasks (Liepert et al., 1998; Kopp et al., 1999; Liepert et al., 2000; Levy et al., 2001; Liepert et al., 2001; Carey et al., 2002; Johansen-Berg et al., 2002; Schaechter et al., 2002; Wittenberg et al., 2003; Kimberley et al., 2004). Although studies indicate that intensity of rehabilitation can influence outcome (Kwakkel et al., 1997, 2002) the exact nature of this relationship and the extent of its veracity require considerable exploration (Stein, 2004).

The affects of UMN are broad reaching; however, few studies have evaluated a comprehensive intervention that incorporates multiple components addressing several impairments, such as balance and endurance as well as UE strength and function. Typically a therapeutic treatment session may address several impairments of a stroke survivor, but the possibility of diluting the effectiveness of the intervention on a specific impairment, including UE weakness, is not known. For example, the Kansas City Stroke Study cited previously (Duncan et al., 2003) evaluated a structured, progressive exercise program focusing on strength, balance, endurance, and UE function (36 sessions of 90 min treatments over 3 months). The intervention produced improvements in balance, endurance, peak aerobic capacity, and mobility. However, motor control and strength gains did not reach statistical significance. These results may indicate that greater total practice time, repetition, and intensity may be necessary to influence these parameters in the UE.

Specificity of training

The effectiveness of strength training is task related and specific to the particular muscle length, movement velocity, or position in which muscles are being exercised (Rutherford, 1988). With severely weak muscles, any exercise that may provoke muscle contraction or generate force maybe appropriate. However, once sufficient force can be generated, strengthening programs aimed at improving functional performance may be more effective if the task or a subpart of the task itself is practiced (Ng and Shepherd, 2000). In evaluating UE rehabilitation strategies in acute stroke, Winstein et al. (2004) compared strength training to functional task practice and standard care. An extra 20 h of UE specific training (1h/day) over a period of 4–6 weeks significantly affected functional outcomes, with the immediate benefits of task practice similar to the strengthening approach. However, at the 9 month follow-up the functional task practice group outperformed the strength group in UE isometric torque output, indicating that functional practice through daily activity may provide a more meaningful environment to maintain strength over the long term in individuals

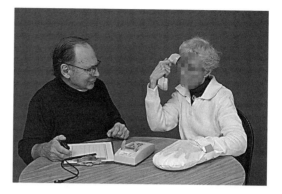

Figure 18.3. Patient undergoing repetitive trials to reduce time required to pick up phone receiver and dial a number while receiving CIT. Note restricted use of patient's less affected UE (left) hand and charting of performance by therapist.

with distal UE movement. This rationale is consistent with motor learning and skill acquisition principles where the individual is challenged to solve movement impairments through practice of functional and meaningful tasks (Winstein et al., 2004). An activity such as constraint-induced therapy (CIT) (Taub et al., 2002; Wolf et al., 2002) that is characterized by components including repetitive task practice and adaptive task practice or "shaping" (Fig. 18.3) may promote reacquisition of functional skills. Neuroimaging techniques provide evidence for cortical reorganization with primarily task-specific training (Jang et al., 2003). In addition some studies using TMS have concluded that massed practice cortical reorganization can occur using CIT (Liepert et al., 1998; Liepert et al., 2001; Cramer et al., 2002; Schaechter et al., 2002; Taub et al., 2003). However, it has been suggested that the interpretation of the actual extent of these neuroplastic changes should be carefully reassessed (see Wolf et al., 2004).

Long-term effects of treatment

Although many publications have evaluated treatment methods, evidence for sustained effects on a long-term basis are limited. Feys and colleagues (2004) examined the effect of repetitive sensorimotor training of the arm after stroke at a 5 years follow-up evaluation. Significant improvements from the early, repetitive targeted stimulation were still evident as measured by the Brunnstrom–Fugl-Meyer test and the Action Research Arm test, but not by the Barthel Index. The continued trend of improvement may be due to patients acquiring basic movement capabilities as the foundation for further activities during functional activities as well as early provision of one or more strategies through which patients could take responsibility for their own therapy. This approach is part of CIT as well, and may contribute to why improvements have been noted to last up to 2 years after intervention in stroke survivors (Taub et al., 2003).

Compliance and role of caregiver support

Family and caregiver participation plays a vital role in the rehabilitation process. Little is known about the effect caregiver support may have on strength or functional performance. Maeshima and colleagues (2003) evaluated the influence of family involvement on non-paretic lower limb strength and ambulation. Patients' strength and mobility improved more in the group that received further strength and gait training provided by family members. Kalra and colleagues (2004) demonstrated that training caregivers in basic skills of moving and handling, facilitation of activities of daily living, and simple nursing tasks during inpatient rehabilitation reduces cost of care and caregiver burden while improving quality of life in caregivers and patients. In addition to traditional family education, enlisting family members as therapeutic partners during early stages of rehabilitation is a promising area for future research.

Relationship between strength training and spasticity

Traditional treatment approaches, such as neurodevelopmental therapy (referred to as NDT or Bobath) (Bobath, 1990), do not recommend strength training for patients with UMN disorders. Resistance training is thought to increase reflex activity and reinforce abnormal movement patterns. Recent reviews of clinical evidence do not support this assumption (Ng and Shepherd, 2000; Riolo and Fisher, 2003). Several studies involving the LE (Engardt et al., 1995; Sharp and Brouwer, 1997; Teixeira-Salmela et al., 1999) and also in the UE (Butefisch et al., 1995; Badics et al., 2002) show that strength training can improve muscle torque without affecting reflex activity. In fact, we are unaware of any studies that indicate strength training interferes with function.

To summarize, progressive, resisted strength training may be an appropriate intervention for weakness in UMN lesions in order to improve motor performance and participation in functional activities of daily living. In the context of improving UE motor control in functional activities, evidence also supports the practice of task-specific skills with at least a moderate amount of challenge and intensity, using progressive amounts of voluntary control in a meaningful and motivating context.

18.7 Future areas of investigation

The previous review discussed the interface between strengthening and spasticity, fatigue, and other "traditional" clinical concerns. Clearly strengthening in and of itself is not the answer to improving functional capability. Inevitably, the ambivalence in findings on strengthening studies in UE rehabilitation approaches among patients with stroke is reinforced through our collective inability to control for the magnitude of impairment or chronicity, let alone cognition and home-based compliance among these patients and their families. The need to exercise more precise controls over these key variables is important. Until that time, we will continue to deduce that those patients who can best benefit from any strengthening or general functional UE program following stroke are those who show at least a minimal level of voluntary control of the arm and hand and minimal impedance from active restraints of agonist/antagonist motor activation.

At the same time, considerable attention is now being directed toward the application of robotics and virtual environments (Volpe et al., 2000; Holden et al., 2001; Lum et al., 2002; Merians et al., 2002; Ferraro et al., 2003). While these interfaces herald the advance of phenomenal technologies, there is need to impose the same considerations for interfacing patients with these peripherals as there has been when providing other interfaces, such as muscle monitoring or functional electrical stimulation. Thus, robotic applications to overcome impairments are only of value if they can be utilized in a cost-efficient manner in the clinic, as well as demonstrate a linkage to function while concurrently demonstrating changes in impairment variables, including strength.

In the absence of considerations and measurements of: inter-limb coordination, imposed voluntary control, compliance, and response burden, the impact that novel approaches might have on strength or spasticity may be no greater than present alternatives. What the precision inherent in both the hardware and software dimensions of virtual training and robotic controls bring to clinician and researcher alike, is an opportunity to measure degrees of freedom of movement with greater spatial and temporal resolution and processing speed than we have as yet experienced. Such exposure will lend more insight into both measurements of mobility and exploration of mechanisms underlying movement control. With respect to the relationship of UE strength and function, the precision of measurement should facilitate greater understanding between multiple joint positioning, rates of change in movement, accuracy of target acquisition, and forces/torques required to capture and control objects in the environment with the more impaired UE.

Ultimately, the primary outcome of a UE weakness intervention should be improved quality of life. However, the few studies that link improvements in strength with functional performance and quality of life measurements in patients with UMN are inconclusive and only address LE strengthening (Sharp and Brouwer, 1997; Teixeira-Salmela et al., 1999; Weiss et al., 2000; Ouellette et al., 2004). Future clinical outcome research studies should evaluate the degree to which the UE treatment intervention that

affects weakness will also affect functional outcomes as well as family functioning and quality of life. This constellation of data will inevitably lend greater insight into the role and value of UE strengthening in neurorehabilitation.

REFERENCES

Ada, L., Canning, C.G., et al. (2003). Stroke patients have selective muscle weakness in shortened range. *Brain*, **126**(**Pt 3**), 724–731.

Akeson, W.H., Woo, S.L.Y., Amiel, D. and Matthews, J.V. (1974). Biomechanical and biochemical changes in the periarticular connective tissue during contracture development in the immobilized rat knee. *Connect Tissue Res*, **2**, 315–323.

Alberts, J., Butler, A., and Wolf, S. (2004). The effects of constraint-induced therapy on force-control: a preliminary study. (submitted).

Andrews, A.W. and Bohannon, R.W. (2000). Distribution of muscle strength impairments following stroke. *Clin Rehabil*, **14**(**1**), 79–87.

Andrews, K., Brockhurst, J.C., Richards, B. and Laycock, P.J. (1981). The rate of recovery from stroke and its measurement. *Int Rehabil Med*, **3**, 155–161.

Badics, E., Wittmann, A., et al. (2002). Systematic muscle building exercises in the rehabilitation of stroke patients. *Neurorehabilitation*, **17**(**3**), 211–214.

Barreca, S., Wolf, S.L., et al. (2003). Treatment interventions for the paretic upper limb of stroke survivors: a critical review. *Neurorehabil Neural Repair*, **17**(**4**), 220–226.

Basmajian, J.V., Gowland, C.A., et al. (1987). Stroke treatment: comparison of integrated behavioral–physical therapy vs traditional physical therapy programs. *Arch Phys Med Rehabil*, **68**(**5 Pt 1**), 267–272.

Baykousheva-Mateva, V. and Mandaliev, A. (1994). Artificial feedforward as preparatory motor control in postical hemiparesis. *Electromyogr Clinl Neurophysiol*, **34**(**7**), 445–448.

Beer, R.F., Given, J.D. and Dewald, J.P.A. (1999). Task-dependent weakness at the elbow in patients with hemiparesis. *Arch Phys Med Rehabil*, **80**, 766–772.

Bobath, B. (1990). *Adult Hemiplegia: Evaluation and Treatment*, Butterworth-Heinemann, London.

Bohannon, R.W., Warren, M.E., et al. (1991). Motor variables correlated with the hand-to-mouth maneuver in stroke patients. *Arch Phys Med Rehabil*, **72**(**9**), 682–684.

Bourbonnais, D. and Vanden Noven, S. (1989). Weakness in patients with hemiparesis. *Am J Occup Ther*, **43**(**5**), 313–319.

Broeks, J.G., Lankhorst G.J., et al. (1999). The long-term outcome of arm function after stroke: results of a follow-up study. *Disabil Rehabil*, **21**(**8**), 357–364.

Brunnstrom, S. (1970). *Movement Therapy in Hemiplegia. A Neurophysiological Approach,* Harper and Row, New York, NY.

Butefisch, C., Hummelsheim, H., et al. (1995). Repetitive training of isolated movements improves the outcome of motor rehabilitation of the centrally paretic hand. *J Neurol Sci*, **130**(**1**), 59–68.

Buys, E.J., Lemon, R.N., et al. (1986). Selective facilitation of different hand muscles by single corticospinal neurones in the conscious monkey. *J Physiol*, **381**, 529–549.

Campbell, M., McComas, A.J. and Petito, F. (1973). Physiological changes in aging muscles. *J Neurol Neurosurg Psychiatr*, **36**, 174–182.

Canning, C.G., Ada, L., et al. (1999). Slowness to develop force contributes to weakness after stroke. *Arch Phys Med Rehabil*, **80**(**1**), 66–70.

Carey, J.R., Kimberley, T.J., et al. (2002). Analysis of fMRI and finger tracking training in subjects with chronic stroke. *Brain*, **125**(**Pt 4**), 773–788.

Chae, J., Yang, G., et al. (2002a). Delay in initiation and termination of muscle contraction, motor impairment, and physical disability in upper limb hemiparesis. *Muscle Nerve*, **25**(**4**), 568–575.

Chae, J., Yang, G., et al. (2002b). Muscle weakness and cocontraction in upper limb hemiparesis: relationship to motor impairment and physical disability. *Neurorehabil Neural Repair*, **16**(**3**), 241–248.

Chokroverty, S., Reyes, M.G., et al. (1976). Hemiplegic amyotrophy. Muscle and motor point biopsy study. *Arch Neurol*, **33**(**2**), 104–110.

Cholewicki, J., Panjabi, M.M., et al. (1997). Stabilizing function of trunk flexor–extensor muscles around a neutral spine posture. *Spine*, **22**(**19**), 2207–2212.

Colebatch, J.G. and Gandevia, S.C. (1989). The distribution of muscular weakness in upper motor neuron lesions affecting the arm. *Brain*, **112**(**Pt 3**), 749–763.

Colebatch, J.G., Rothwell, J.C., et al. (1990). Cortical outflow to proximal arm muscles in man. *Brain*, **113**(**Pt 6**), 1843–1856.

Connelly, D.M., Rice, C.L., et al. (1999). Motor unit firing rates and contractile properties in tibialis anterior of young and old men. *J Appl Physiol*, **87**(**2**), 843–852.

Cramer, S.C., Weisskoff, R.M., et al. (2002). Motor cortex activation is related to force of squeezing. *Hum Brain Mapp*, **16**(**4**), 197–205.

Davidoff, R.A. (1990). The pyramidal tract [see comment]. *Neurology*, **40**(**2**), 332–339.

Delbono, O., Renganathan, M., et al. (1997). Excitation-Ca^{2+} release–contraction coupling in single aged human skeletal muscle fiber. *Muscle Nerve Supp*, **5**, S88–S92.

Dengler, R., Konstanzer, A., Hesse, W., Wolf, W. and Struppler, A. (1990). Abnormal behaviour of single motor units in central weakness. In: *Motor Disturbances II* (eds Berardelli, A., Benecke, R., Manfredi, M. and Marsden, C.D.), Academic Press, London, pp. 379–384.

Deschenes, M.R. and Kraemer, W.J. (2002). Performance and physiologic adaptations to resistance training. *Am J Phys Med Rehabil*, **81**(**Suppl. 11**), S3–S16.

Dewald, J.P., Pope, P.S., et al. (1995). Abnormal muscle coactivation patterns during isometric torque generation at the elbow and shoulder in hemiparetic subjects. *Brain*, **118**(**Pt 2**), 495–510.

Dickstein, R., Hocherman, S., Pillar, T. and Shaham, R. (1986). Stroke rehabilitation. Three exercise therapy approaches. *Phys Ther*, **66**, 1233–1238.

Dietz, V., Quintern, J. and Berger, W. (1981). Electrophysiological studies of gait in spasticity and rigidity: evidence that altered mechanical properties of muscle contribute to hypertonia. *Brain*, **104**, 431–439.

Duchateau, J. and Hainaut, K. (1987). Electrical and mechanical changes in immobilized muscle. *J Appl Physiol* (**62**), 168–173.

Duchateau, J. and Hainaut, K. (1990). Effects of immobilization on contractile properties, recruitment and firing rates of human motor units. *J Physiol*, **422**, 55–65.

Duncan, P., Studenski, S., et al. (2003). Randomized clinical trial of therapeutic exercise in subacute stroke. *Stroke*, **34**(**9**), 2173–2180.

Edstrom, L. (1970). Selective changes in the sizes of red and white muscle fibers in upper motor neuron lesions and Parkinsonism. *J Neurol Sci*, **11**, 537–550.

Edstrom, L., Grimby, L., et al. (1973). Correlation between recruitment order of motor units and muscle atrophy pattern in upper motoneurone lesion: significance of spasticity. *Experientia*, **29**(**5**), 560–561.

Engardt, M., Knutsson, E., et al. (1995). Dynamic muscle strength training in stroke patients: effects on knee extension torque, electromyographic activity, and motor function. *Arch Phys Med Rehabil*, **76**(**5**), 419–425.

Esmonde, T., McGinley, J., Wittwer, J., et al. (1997). Stroke rehabilitation: patient activity during non-therapy time. *Aust J Physiother*, **43**, 43–51.

Fellows, S., Kaus, C., et al. (1994). Voluntary movement at the elbow in spastic hemiparesis. *Ann Neurol*, **36**, 397–406.

Ferraro, M., Palazzolo, J.J., et al. (2003). Robot-aided sensorimotor arm training improves outcome in patients with chronic stroke. *Neurology*, **61**(**11**), 1604–1607.

Feys, H., De Weerdt, W., et al. (2004). Early and repetitive stimu-lation of the arm can substantially improve the long-term outcome after stroke: a 5-year follow-up study of a random-ized trial. *Stroke*, **35**, 924.

Frontera, W.R., Grimby, L., et al. (1997). Firing rate of the lower motoneuron and contractile properties of its muscle fibers after upper motoneuron lesion in man. *Muscle Nerve*, **20**(8), 938–947.

Frontera, W.R., Hughes, V.A., et al. (2000). Aging of skeletal muscle: a 12-yr longitudinal study. *J Appl Physiol*, **88**(4), 1321–1326.

Frontera, W.R., Hughes, V.A., et al. (2001a). Contractile proper-ties of aging skeletal muscle. *Int J Sport Nutr Exe Metabol*, (**Suppl.11**), S16–S20.

Frontera, W.R., Moldover, J.R., Borg-Stein, J. and Watkins, M.P. (2001b). Exercise. In: *Downey and Darling's Physiological Basis of Rehabilitation Medicine* (eds Gonzalez, E.G., Myers, S.J., Edelstein, J.E, Lieberman, J.S. and Downey, J.A.), Butterworth-Heinemann, Boston, pp. 379–396.

Gelber, D., Josefczyk, P.B., Herrman, D. and Good, D.C. (1995). Comparison of two therapy approaches in the rehabilita-tion of the pure motor hemiparetic stroke patient. *J Neurol Rehabil*, **9**, 191–196.

Gemperline, J., Allen, S., Walk, D. and Rymer, W.Z. (1995). Characteristics of motor unit discharge in subjects with hemiparesis. *Muscle Nerve*, **18**, 1101–1114.

Ghez, C. (1991). Muscles: effectors of the motor systems princi-ples of neural science (eds Kandell, E.R., Schwartz, J.H. and Jessell, T.M.), Appleton and Lange, Norwalk, p. 548.

Gowland, C., deBruin, H., et al. (1992). Agonist and antagonist activity during voluntary upper-limb movement in patients with stroke. *Phys Ther*, **72**(9), 624–633.

Hachisuka, K., Umezu, Y., et al. (1997). Disuse muscle atrophy of lower limbs in hemiplegic patients. *Arch Phys Med Rehabil*, **78**(1), 13–18.

Hammond, M., Fitts, S.S., Kraft, G.H., et al. (1988). Cocontrac-tion in the hemiparetic forearm: quantitative EMG evalua-tion. *Arch Phys Med Rehabil*, **69**, 348–351.

Hara, Y., Masakado, Y., et al. (2004). The physiological functional loss of single thenar motor units in the stroke patients: when does it occur? Does it progress? *Clin Neurophysiol*, **115**(1), 97–103.

Heller, A., Wade, D.T., et al. (1987). Arm function after stroke: measurement and recovery over the first three months. *J Neurol Neurosurg Psychiatry*, **50**(6), 714–719.

Hendricks, H.T., van Limbeek, J., et al. (2002). Motor recovery after stroke: a systematic review of the literature. *Arch Phys Med Rehabil*, **83**(11), 1629–1637.

Herbert, R. (1988). The passive mechanical properties of mus-cle and their adaptations to altered patterns of use. *Aust J Physiother*, **34**, 141–149.

Herbert, R.D. and Crosbie, J. (1995). Rest length and passive com-pliance of immobilised rabbit soleus muscle and tendon. *XVth Congress of the International Society of Biomechanics: Book of Abstracts*, Gummerus Printing, Jyvaskyla, Finland.

Holden, M.K., Dettwiler, A., et al. (2001). Retraining movement in patients with acquired brain injury using a virtual envi-ronment. *Stud Health Technol Inform*, **81**, 192–198.

Hollander, M., Koudstaal, P.J., et al. (2003). Incidence, risk, and case fatality of first ever stroke in the elderly population. The Rotterdam Study. *J Neurol Neurosurg Psychiatr*, **74**(3), 317–321.

Hounsgaard, J., Hultborn, H., et al. (1988). Bistability of alpha-motoneurones in the decerebrate cat and in the acute spinal cat after intravenous 5-hydroxytryptophan. *J Physiol*, **405**, 345–367.

Jang, S.H., Kim, Y.H., et al. (2003). Cortical reorganization induced by task-oriented training in chronic hemiplegic stroke patients. *NeuroReport*, **14**(1), 137–141.

Johansen-Berg, H., Dawes, H., et al. (2002). Correlation between motor improvements and altered fMRI activity after rehabilitative therapy. *Brain*, **125**(Pt 12), 2731–2742.

Jozsa, L., Kannus, P., Thoring, J., et al. (1990). The effect of teno-tomy and immobilization on intramuscular connective tis-sues. *J Bone Joint Surg*, **72B**, 293–297.

Jung, H.Y., Yoon, J.S., et al. (2002). Recovery of proximal and dis-tal arm weakness in the ipsilateral upper limb after stroke. *Neurorehabilitation*, **17**(2), 153–159.

Kalra, L., Evans, A., et al. (2004). Training carers of stroke patients: randomised controlled trial. *Br Med J*, **328**(7448), 1099.

Kamper, D.G., Harvey, R.L., et al. (2003). Relative contributions of neural mechanisms versus muscle mechanics in pro-moting finger extension deficits following stroke. *Muscle Nerve*, **28**(3), 309–318.

Kent-Braun, J.A. and Ng, A.V. (1999). Specific strength and vol-untary muscle activation in young and elderly women and men. *J Appl Physiol*, **87**(1), 22–29.

Kent-Braun, J.A., Ng, A.V., et al. (2000). Skeletal muscle contrac-tile and noncontractile components in young and older women and men. *J Appl Physiol*, **88**(2), 662–668.

Kiehn, O. and Eken, T. (1998). Functional role of plateau poten-tials in vertebrate motor neurons. *Curr Opin Neurobiol*, **8**(6), 746–752.

Kimberley, T.J., Lewis, S.M., Auerbach, E.J., Dorsey, L.L., Lojovich, J.M. and Carey, J.R. (2004). Electrical stimulation driving functional improvements and cortical changes in subjects with stroke. *Exp Brain Res*, **154**, 450–460.

Kleim, J.A., Barbay, S., et al. (2002). Motor learning-dependent synaptogenesis is localized to functionally reorganized motor cortex. *Neurobiol Learn Mem*, **77**(1), 63–77.

Knopman, D.S. and Rubens, A.B. (1986). The validity of computed tomographic scan findings for the localization of cerebral functions. The relationship between computed tomography and hemiparesis. *Arch Neurol*, **43**(4), 328–332.

Knuttson, E. and Martensson, A. (1980). Dynamic motor capacity in spastic paresis and its relation to prime mover dysfunction, spastic reflexes and antagonist co-activation. *Scand J Rehabil Med*, **12**, 93–106.

Kopp, B., Kunkel, A., et al. (1999). Plasticity in the motor system related to therapy-induced improvement of movement after stroke. *NeuroReport*, **10**(4), 807–810.

Kwakkel, G., Wagenaar, R.C., et al. (1997). Effects of intensity of rehabilitation after stroke. A research synthesis. *Stroke*, **28**(8), 1550–1556.

Kwakkel, G., Kollen, B.J., et al. (2002). Long term effects of intensity of upper and lower limb training after stroke: a randomised trial [see comment]. *J Neurol Neurosurg Psychiatr*, **72**(4), 473–479.

Laidlaw, D.H., Bilodeau, M., et al. (2000). Steadiness is reduced and motor unit discharge is more variable in old adults. *Muscle Nerve*, **23**(4), 600–612.

Lamontagne, A., Richards, C.L., et al. (2000). Coactivation during gait as an adaptive behavior after stroke. *J Electromyogr Kines*, **10**(6), 407–415.

Lance, J.W. (1980). The control of muscle tone, reflexes and movement: the Robert Wattenburg Lecture. *Neurology*, **30**, 1303–1313.

Levin, M.F. and Dimov, M. (1997). Spatial zones for muscle coactivation and the control of postural stability. *Brain Res*, **757**(1), 43–59.

Levin, M., Selles, R.W., et al. (2000). Deficits in the coordination of agonist and antagonist muscles in stroke patients: implication for normal motor control. *Brain Res*, **853**, 352–369.

Levy, C.E., Nichols, D.S., et al. (2001). Functional MRI evidence of cortical reorganization in upper-limb stroke hemiplegia treated with constraint-induced movement therapy. *Am J Phys Med Rehabil*, **80**(1), 4–12.

Lexel, J., Tayor, C.C. and Sjostrom, M. (1988). What is the cause of aging atrophy? Total number, size and proportion of different fiber types studied in whole vastus lateralis muscle from 15–83-year-old men. *J Neurol Sci*, **84**, 275–294.

Li, S., Latash, M.L., et al. (2003). The effects of stroke and age on finger interaction in multi-finger force production tasks. *Clin Neurophysiol*, **114**(9), 1646–1655.

Liepert, J., Miltner, W.H., et al. (1998). Motor cortex plasticity during constraint-induced movement therapy in stroke patients. *Neurosci Lett*, **250**(1), 5–8.

Liepert, J., Bauder, H., et al. (2000). Treatment-induced cortical reorganization after stroke in humans. *Stroke*, **31**(6), 1210–1216.

Liepert, J., Uhde, I., et al. (2001). Motor cortex plasticity during forced-use therapy in stroke patients: a preliminary study. *J Neurol*, **248**(4), 315–321.

Lincoln, N.B., Willis, D., et al. (1996). Comparison of rehabilitation practice on hospital wards for stroke patients. *Stroke*, **27**(1), 18–23.

Logigian, M., Samuels, M.A., Falconer, J. and Zagar, R. (1983). Clinical exercise trial for stroke patients. *Arch Phys Med Rehabil*, **64**, 364–367.

Lotze, M., Braun, C., et al. (2003). Motor learning elicited by voluntary drive. *Brain*, **126**(Pt 4), 866–872.

Lum, P.S., Burgar C.G., et al. (2002). Robot-assisted movement training compared with conventional therapy techniques for the rehabilitation of upper-limb motor function after stroke. *Arch Phys Med Rehabil*, **83**(7), 952–959.

Mackey, F., Ada, L., et al. (1996). Stroke rehabilitation: are highly structured units more conducive to physical activity than less structured units? *Arch Phys Med Rehabil*, **77**(10), 1066–1070.

Maeshima, S., Ueyoshi, A., et al. (2003). Mobility and muscle strength contralateral to hemiplegia from stroke: benefit from self-training with family support. *Am J Phys Med Rehabil*, **82**(6), 456–462.

Maughan, R.J., Watson, J.S., et al. (1983). Strength and cross-sectional area of human skeletal muscle. *J Physiol*, **338**, 37–49.

McComas, A., Sica, R.E.P., Upton A.R.M., et al. (1973). Functional changes in motor neurons of hemiparetic patients. *J Neurol Neurosurg Psychiatr*, **36**, 183–193.

McCrea, P.H., Eng, J.J., et al. (2003). Time and magnitude of torque generation is impaired in both arms following stroke. *Muscle Nerve*, **28**(1), 46–53.

Merians, A.S., Jack, D., et al. (2002). Virtual reality-augmented rehabilitation for patients following stroke. *Phys Ther*, **82**(9), 898–915.

Nakashima, K., Rothwell, J.C., et al. (1989). Reciprocal inhibition between forearm muscles in patients with writer's cramp and other occupational cramps, symptomatic hemidystonia and hemiparesis due to stroke. *Brain*, **112**(Pt 3), 681–697.

Nakayama, H., Jorgensen, H.S., et al. (1994). Recovery of upper extremity function in stroke patients: the Copenhagen Stroke Study. *Arch Phys Med Rehabil*, **75**(4), 394–398.

Ng, S. and Shepherd, R. (2000). Weakness in patients with stroke: implications for strength training in neurorehabilitation. *Phys Ther Rev*, **5**, 227–238.

Nudo, R.J. (1997). Remodeling of cortical motor representations after stroke: implications for recovery from brain damage. *Mol Psychiatr*, **2**(**3**), 188–191.

Nudo, R.J. (2003). Functional and structural plasticity in motor cortex: implications for stroke recovery. *Phys Med Rehabil Clin N Am*, **14**(**Suppl. 1**), S57–S76.

Nudo, R.J. and Friel, K.M. (1999). Cortical plasticity after stroke: implications for rehabilitation. *Rev Neurol*, **155**(**9**), 713–717.

Okuma, Y. and Lee, R.G. (1996). Reciprocal inhibition in hemiplegia: correlation with clinical features and recovery. *Can J Neurol Sci*, **23**(**1**), 15–23.

Olsen, T.S. (1990). Arm and leg paresis as outcome predictors in stroke rehabilitation. *Stroke*, **21**(**2**), 247–251.

Ouellette, M.M., LeBrasseur, N.K., et al. (2004). High-intensity resistance training improves muscle strength, self-reported function, and disability in long-term stroke survivors. *Stroke*, **35**(**6**), 1404–1409.

Peterson, C., Maier, S.F. and Seligman, M.E.P. (1993). *Learned Helplessness: A Theory for the Age of Personal Control*, Oxford University Press, Oxford.

Pyndt, H.S., Laursen, M., et al. (2003). Changes in reciprocal inhibition across the ankle joint with changes in external load and pedaling rate during bicycling. *J Neurophysiol*, **90**(**5**), 3168–3177.

Rack, P., and Westbury, D.R. (1969). The effect of length and stimulus rate on tension in the isometric cat muscle. *J Neurophysiol*, **204**, 443–460.

Rassier, D., MacIntosh, B.R. and Herzog, W. (1999). Length dependence of active force production in skeletal muscle [Review]. *J Appl Physiol*, **86**, 1445–1457.

Riolo, L. and Fisher, K. (2003). Evidence in practice. Is there evidence that strength training could help improve muscle function and other outcomes without reinforcing abnormal movement patterns or increasing reflex activity in a man who has had a stroke? *Phys Ther*, **83**(**9**), 844–851.

Roos, M.R., Rice, C.L., et al. (1999). Quadriceps muscle strength, contractile properties, and motor unit firing rates in young and old men. *Muscle Nerve*, **22**(**8**), 1094–1103.

Rose, S. and Rothstein, J. (1982). Part I: general concepts and adaptations to altered patterns of use. *Phys Ther*, **62**, 1773–1787.

Rosenfalck, A. and Andreassen, S. (1980). Impaired regulation of force and firing pattern of single motor units in patients with spasticity. *J Neurol Neurosurg Psychiatr*, **43**, 907–916.

Roth, E. and Green, D.G. (1996). Cardiac complications during inpatient stroke rehabilitation. *Top Stroke Rehabil*, **3**, 86–92.

Rutherford, O.M. (1988). Muscular coordination and strength training: implications for rehabilitation. *Sports Med*, **5**, 196–202.

Sahrmann, S. and Norton, B. (1977). The relationship of voluntary movement to spasticity in the upper motor neuron syndrome. *Ann Neurol*, **2**, 460–465.

Schaechter, J.D., Kraft, E., et al. (2002). Motor recovery and cortical reorganization after constraint-induced movement therapy in stroke patients: a preliminary study. *Neurorehabil Neural Repair*, **16**(**4**), 326–338.

Sharp, S.A. and Brouwer, B.J. (1997). Isokinetic strength training of the hemiparetic knee: effects on function and spasticity. *Arch Phys Med Rehabil*, **78**(**11**), 1231–1236.

Shelton, F.N. and Reding, M.J. (2001). Effect of lesion location on upper limb motor recovery after stroke. *Stroke*, **32**(**1**), 107–112.

Simmons, R.W. and Richardson, C. (1988). Peripheral regulation of stiffness during arm movements by coactivation of the antagonist muscles. *Brain Res*, **473**(**1**), 134–140.

Smidt, G. and Rogers, M. (1982). Factors contributing to the regulation and clinical assessment of muscular strength. *Phys Ther*, **62**, 1283–1290.

Solomonow, M., Baratta, R., et al. (1988). Electromyogram coactivation patterns of the elbow antagonist muscles during slow isokinetic movement. *Exp Neurol*, **100**(**3**), 470–477.

Stein, J. (2004). Motor recovery strategies after stroke. *Top Stroke Rehabil*, **11**(**2**), 12–22.

Sunderland, A., Tinson, D., et al. (1989). Arm function after stroke. An evaluation of grip strength as a measure of recovery and a prognostic indicator. *J Neurol Neurosurg Psychiatr*, **52**(**11**), 1267–1272.

Tabary, J., Tabary, C. and Tardieu, C. (1972). Physiological and structural changes in the cat's soleus muscle due to immobilization at different lengths by plaster casts. *J Physiol*, **224**, 231–244.

Tang, A. and Rhymer, W.Z. (1981). Abnormal force–EMG relations in paretic limbs of hemiparetic human subjects. *J Neurol Neurosurg Psychiatr*, **44**, 690–698.

Tardieu, C., Tabary, J.C., Tabary, C., et al. (1981). Adaptation of sarcomere numbers to the length imposed on muscle. In: *Mechanism of Muscle Adaptation to Functional Requirements* (eds Guba, F., Marechal, G. and Takacs, O.), Pergamon Press, Elmsford, NY, pp. 99–114.

Taub, E. and Wolf, S.L. (1997). Constraint-induced movement techniques to facilitate upper extremity use in stroke patients. *Top Stroke Rehabil*, **3**, 38–61.

Taub, E., Uswatte, G., et al. (2002). New treatments in neurorehabilitation founded on basic research. *Nat Rev Neurosci*, **3**(**3**), 228–236.

Taub, E., Uswatte, G., et al. (2003). Improved motor recovery after stroke and massive cortical reorganization following constraint-induced movement therapy. *Phys Med Rehabil Clin N Am*, **14**(**1 Suppl.**), S77–S91.

Teixeira-Salmela, L.F., Olney, S.J., et al. (1999). Muscle strengthening and physical conditioning to reduce impairment and disability in chronic stroke survivors. *Arch Phys Med Rehabil*, **80**(**10**), 1211–1218.

Twitchell, T.E. (1951). The restoration of motor function following hemiplegia in man. *Brain*, **74**, 443–480.

van der Lee, J.H., Wagenaar, R.C., et al. (1999). Forced use of the upper extremity in chronic stroke patients: results from a single-blind randomized clinical trial [see comment]. *Stroke*, **30**(**11**), 2369–2375.

van der Lee, J.H., Snels, I.A., et al. (2001). Exercise therapy for arm function in stroke patients: a systematic review of randomized controlled trials. *Clin Rehabil*, **15**(**1**), 20–31.

Volpe, B.T., Krebs, H.I., et al. (2000). A novel approach to stroke rehabilitation: robot-aided sensorimotor stimulation. *Neurology*, **54**(**10**), 1938–1944.

Wade, D.T., Langton-Hewer, R., et al. (1983). The hemiplegic arm after stroke: measurement and recovery. *J Neurol Neurosurg Psychiatr*, **46**(**6**), 521–524.

Waxman, S.G. (2003). *Clinical Neuroanatomy*, Lange Medical Books/McGraw-Hill, New York City.

Weiss, A., Suzuki, T., et al. (2000). High intensity strength training improves strength and functional performance after stroke. *Am J Phys Med Rehabil*, **79**(**4**), 369–376; quiz 391–394.

Williams, G.N., Higgins, M.J., et al. (2002). Aging skeletal muscle: physiologic changes and the effects of training. *Phys Ther*, **82**(**1**), 62–68.

Williams, P. and Goldspink, G. (1978). Changes in sarcomere length and physiological properties in immobilized muscle. *J Anat*, **127**, 459–468.

Williams, P. and Goldspink, G. (1984). Connective tissue changes in immobilized muscle. *J Anat*, **138**, 343–350.

Williams, P.E. (1988). Effect of intermittent stretch on immobilised muscle. *Ann Rheum Dis*, **47**, 1014–1016.

Winstein, C., Wing, A. and Whitall, J. (2003). Motor control and learning principles for rehabilitation of upper limb movements after brain injury. In: *Handbook of Neuropsychology* (eds Grafman, J. and Robertson, I.H.), Vol. 9, Elsevier Science BV, New York, pp. 77–137.

Winstein, C., Rose, D., et al. (2004). A randomized controlled comparison of upper extremity rehabilitation strategies in acute stroke: a pilot study of immediate and long-term outcomes. *Arch Phys Med Rehabil*, **85**(**4**), 620–628.

Wittenberg, G.F., Chen, R., et al. (2003). Constraint-induced therapy in stroke: magnetic-stimulation motor maps and cerebral activation [erratum appears in *Neurorehabil Neural Repair*, 2003 Sep; **17**(**3**), 197]. *Neurorehabil Neural Repair*, **17**(**1**), 48–57.

Woldag, H. and Hummelsheim, H. (2002). Evidence-based physiotherapeutic concepts for improving arm and hand function in stroke patients: a review [see comment]. *J Neurol*, **249**(**5**), 518–528.

Wolf, S.L., Catlin, P.A., et al. (1994). Overcoming limitations in elbow movement in the presence of antagonist hyperactivity. *Phys Ther*, **74**(**9**), 826–835.

Wolf, S.L., Blanton, S., et al. (2002). Repetitive task practice: a critical review of constraint-induced movement therapy in stroke. *Neurologist*, **8**(**6**), 325–338.

Wolf, S., Butler, A.J., Campana, G.I., Struys, D.M., Winstein, S.R. and Parris, T.A. (2004). Intra-subject reliability of parameters contributing to maps generated by transcranial magnetic stimulation in able-bodied adults. *Clin Neurophysiol*, **115**, 1740–1747.

Gait disorders and rehabilitation

V. Dietz

Spinal Cord Injury Center, University Hospital Balgrist, Zurich, Switzerland

19.1 Summary

This chapter deals with the neuronal mechanisms underlying impaired gait as a paradigm of movement disorder with the aim of first, a better understanding the underlying pathophysiology and second, the selection of an adequate treatment and rehabilitation. For the patient usually one of the first symptoms of a lesion within the central motor system represents the movement disorder, which is most characteristic during locomotion in patients with spasticity or Parkinson's disease. The clinical examination reveals changes in tendon tap reflexes and muscle tone, typical for an impairment of the motor system. However, there exists only a weak relationship between the physical signs obtained during the clinical examination in a passive motor condition and the impaired neuronal mechanisms being in operation during an active movement such as locomotion. By the recording and analysis of electrophysiological and biomechanical signals during a movement, the significance of impaired reflex behaviour or muscle tone and its contribution to the movement disorder can reliably be assessed. Consequently, an adequate treatment should not be restricted to the correction of an isolated clinical parameter but should be based on the pathophysiology and the mechanisms underlying the disorder of movement which impairs the patient. Actual therapy should be directed to take advantage of the plasticity of the central nervous system (CNS). In the future a combination of repair and functional training will further improve mobility of severely disabled patients.

19.2 Introduction

The study of movement control has relevance to our understanding of brain and spinal cord function. However, it also has implications for various fields, such as neurology, cognitive neuroscience, rehabilitation medicine and robotics. The understanding of movement disorders and their appropriate treatment critically depends on the knowledge of the neuronal mechanisms underlying functional movements. Movement disorders are one of the most expanding fields in medicine, leading to increasing costs for treatment and rehabilitation. This chapter will focus on the role of neuronal mechanisms underlying gait disorders and the therapeutic consequences.

Locomotion is a subconciously performed everyday movement with a high reproducibility. It is automatically adapted to the actual conditions, such as ground irregularities with a large security range. Characteristic locomotor disorders are frequently the first sign of a central or peripheral lesion of the motor system. The neurological examination in such cases is characterised by changes in reflex excitability and muscle tone and leads to an appropriate diagnosis underlying the gait disorder. The physical signs obtained during the clinical examination can, however, give little information about the pathophysiology underlying the movement disorder: stretch reflex excitability and muscle tone are basically different in the passive (clinical examination) compared to an active motor condition (movement). In addition, during a movement such as gait, several reflex systems are involved in its execution and control. Therefore, for an adequate treatment of a movement disorder, we have to know about the function of reflexes and supraspinal motor centres involved in the respective motor task (see Volume II, Chapter 2). A movement such as locomotion is determined by the strength of electromyographical (EMG; Volume II, Chapter 4) activation of antagonistic leg muscles as well as intrinsic and passive muscle properties. The EMG activity recorded from the leg muscles reflects the action and interaction between central programs and afferent inputs from various sources, which can only be separated to a limited degree. For an assessment of the neuronal control of locomotion we have to record the EMG activity from several antagonistic leg muscles and the resulting biomechanical parameters such as joint movements and, eventually, of muscle tension. By such an approach it is possible to evaluate the behaviour of neuronal and biomechanical parameters during a gait disorder. Any changes in the neuronal or biomechanical systems may lead to a movement disorder.

Furthermore, impaired movement is not only the consequence of a defective central programme or proprioception. Rather, the movement disorder also reflects secondary compensatory processes induced by the primary lesion. In many cases, the altered motor response can be considered as an optimal outcome for a given lesion of the motor system (cf. Latash and Anson, 1996). The complexity of primary and secondary effects of a lesion requires a detailed analysis of movement disorder to define the target of any treatment.

19.3 Physiological basis of locomotion in humans

Leg muscle activation during locomotion is produced by spinal neuronal circuits within the spinal cord, the spinal pattern generator (central pattern generator (CPG), for reviews see Dietz, 1992a and Volume I, Chapter 13 of this textbook). For the control of human locomotion, afferent information from a variety of sources within the visual, vestibular and proprioceptive systems is utilized by the CPG. The convergence of spinal reflex pathways and descending pathways on common spinal interneurons seem to play an integrative role (for review see Dietz, 2002a), similar as in the cat (Schomburg, 1990). The generation of an appropriate locomotor pattern depends on a combination of central programming and afferent inputs as well as the instruction for a respective motor condition. This information determines the mode of organization of muscle synergies (Horak and Nashner 1986) which are designed to meet multiple conditions of stance and gait (Dietz, 1992a, for review see Mackay-Lyons, 2002).

Central mechanisms and afferent inputs interact in such a way that the strength of a reflex in a muscle or a synergistic group of muscles follows a programme that is dependent on the actual task. The actual weighting of proprioceptive, vestibular and visual inputs to the equilibrium control is context-dependent and can profoundly modify the central programme. Through this weighting, inappropriate responses are largely eliminated (for review see Mackay-Lyons, 2002). Any evaluation of reflex function has to be assessed in connection with the actual motor programme, the bio-mechanical events, including their needs and their restraints.

19.4 Gait disorder in Parkinson's disease

Evidence is accumulating that different regions of the basal ganglia have direct descending output connections to different parts of brainstem motor regulating centres: to the locomotor drive centres in the subthalamic area and in the mesencephalon, and to the centres involved in posture regulation in the pontine reticular formation (Marsden, 1990; Murray and Clarkson, 1996). The mesencephalic locomotor system exerts its descending control via bulbopontine and reticulospinal pathways. Studies on the activity in reticulospinal pathways indicate an inadequate function of these systems in Parkinson's disease (Delwaide et al., 1999).

Pathophysiologically, an impaired neuronal control of gait associated with rigid and poorly modulated motor performance represents a major deficit of Parkinson's disease (Martin, 1967). These abnormalities are thought to result from varying combinations of hypokinesia, rigidity, and from deficits of posture and equilibrium (Murray, 1967; Knutsson, 1972). Furthermore, by quantitative gait analysis distinct differences can be evaluated between the gait pattern of patients with vascular or idiopathic Parkinson's disease (Zijlmans et al., 1996), or of those with normal pressure hydrocephalus (Stolze et al., 2001). Little, however, is known about the extent to which such postural instability reflects deficits in the programmed adjustments or alternatively, in reflex mechanisms or compensation. Figure 19.1 shows the mechanisms that are suggested to be

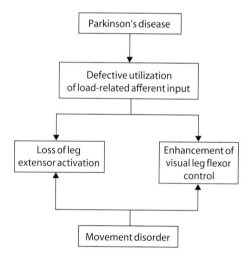

Figure 19.1. Schematic diagram of the mechanisms involved in the movement disorder in Parkinson's disease. The disease of the extrapyramidal system leads to a defective utilisation of afferent input by the CPG. The consequence is a loss of leg extensor activation during the stance phase of gait, associated with an enhanced leg flexor activity, which control strongly depends on visual input. The combination of all sequels of impaired supraspinal control leads to the typical movement disorder (from Dietz, 2003).

involved in the movement disorder in patients with Parkinson's disease. For additional details on the pathophysiology, clinical features and rehabilitation of Parkinson's disease, see Volume II, Chapter 35.

Central mechanisms

In patients with Parkinson's disease several studies on gait indicate an impaired programming (for review see Dietz, 1992a). The electrophysiological gait analysis of patients with Parkinson's disease, in addition to showing slow and reduced movements, reveals a characteristic pattern of leg muscle activation with a reduced amplitude and little modulated EMG activity in the leg extensor muscles during the stance phase and an increased tibialis anterior activity during swing. Furthermore, the characteristic coordination of normal plantigrade gait is lost (Forssberg et al., 1984). The close similarity of gait between parkinsonian patients and children who had not yet developed a plantigrade gait has led to the suggestion that an immature pattern may reappear in Parkinson's disease as a result of deficits in the neuronal circuits controlling plantigrade locomotion (Forssberg et al., 1984).

Furthermore, coordination between lower limbs during walking is impaired in parkinsonian patients compared to age-matched healthy subjects (Dietz et al., 1996): 1. In the patients leg muscle EMG activity is less modulated and gastrocnemius EMG amplitude is small during normal and split-belt walking; 2. The amount of co-activation of antagonistic leg muscles during the support phase of the stride cycle is greater in the patients compared to healthy subjects. It was suggested that reduced EMG modulation and recruitment in the leg extensors may contribute to the impaired walking of the patient (Dietz et al., 1996).

This is in line with observations made on the leg muscle EMG pattern induced by feet displacement which also indicates an impairment of leg muscle activation (Dietz et al., 1988; 1993). In such a condition, the polysynaptic compensatory gastrocnemius EMG responses are smaller than those obtained in an age-matched group of healthy subjects due to a reduced reflex sensitivity (Dietz et al., 1988). This impaired function of polysynaptic reflexes confirms earlier suggestions of alterations in central responseness (Berardelli et al., 1983) and defective utilization of sensory input (Tatton et al., 1984b) in these patients. The reduced sensitivity of polysynaptic reflexes in the leg extensor muscles appears to be a direct consequence of the dopamine deficiency in Parkinsonian patients, as it is also observed in young normal subjects following intake of a single dose of haloperidol (Dietz et al., 1990). Conversely, only some gait parameters (kinematic) are L-Dopa-sensitive, while others (temporal) are L-Dopa-resistant (Blin et al., 1991).

The diminished gastrocnemius activation is followed by a significantly stronger tibialis anterior activation in Parkinsonian patients, which might correspond to the so-called shortening reaction (for review see Angel, 1983; Berardelli and Hallett, 1984; Westphal, 1987). This may be a result of an impaired proprioceptive feedback control that was suggested to be partially compensated in Parkinsonian patients by a greater amount of leg flexor activation which leads to a higher degree of co-activation. Visual input plays a role in the control of this increased activation (Brouwer and Ashby, 1992; Dietz et al., 1997). In addition, Parkinsonian patients are inflexible in adapting and modifying their postural responses to changing support conditions (Schieppati and Nardone, 1991). The idea of an impaired central regulation is an agreement with the concept of an overcompensated and faulty predictive feedback system suggested elsewhere (Tatton et al., 1984a).

The changes in the behaviour of central mechanisms and reflexes described for Parkinsonian patients do not require the introduction of a qualitatively new pattern. These changes also characterize differences between elderly and young normal subjects, although they are more pronounced in Parkinsonian patients (Dietz et al., 1997).

Proprioceptive reflexes and muscle tone

Several observations indicate an impaired function of proprioceptive reflexes in Parkinsonian patients,

which additionally contributes to the instability of Parkinsonian patients during gait (for review see Abbruzzese and Berardelli, 2003). This may be a major reason why these patients rely more on visual information for the regulation of gait (Bronstein et al., 1990).

Furthermore, there is evidence for associated changes of inherent muscle stiffness in Parkinson's disease (Dietz et al., 1988), which was attributed to altered mechanical properties of gastrocnemius muscle in Parkinson's disease and may contribute to rigid muscle tone. Such changes in muscle stiffness may be advantageous in so for as a higher resistance to stretch helps to compensate for a perturbation. Changes of inherent mechanical properties of muscle in Parkinson's disease have also been reported in upper limb muscles (Berardelli et al., 1983; Watts et al., 1986).

The differences in reflex function depend on the condition of the investigation. A great number of electrophysiological studies in Parkinson's disease are concerned with the reflex function during limb displacement in a sitting position. In contrast to the compensatory responses described for perturbations of stance or gait, most of these investigations show an increase in the amplitude of the long-latency EMG response (Chan et al., 1979; Berardelli et al., 1983; Cody et al., 1986). An increase of reflex gain at a central site has been postulated (Burke et al., 1977). The discrepant finding of a reduced stretch sensitivity of proprioceptive postural reflexes may arise primarily from the difference in motor tasks investigated. Locomotion represents a functional condition, with a convergence of several afferent inputs and an interaction with central mechanisms.

Load receptor function

Several studies on motor control in patients with Parkinson's disease are in line with the assumption of a defective load control in these patients (Stelmach, 1991; Burne and Lippold, 1996). The low activation of the leg extensor muscles during conditions of stance and locomotion was assumed to be due to a impaired proprioceptive feedback input

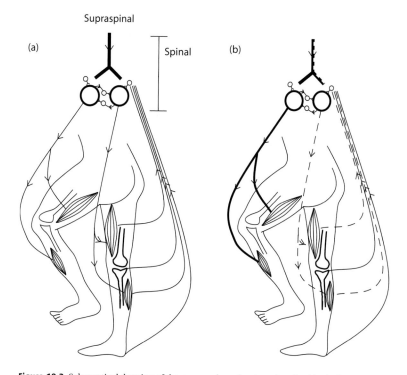

Figure 19.2. Schematical drawing of the neuronal mechanisms involved in the human gait. (a) *Physiological condition.* Leg muscles become activated by a programmed pattern that is generated in spinal neuronal circuits. This pattern is modulated by multi-sensory afferent input, which adapts the pattern to meet existing requirements. Both the programmed pattern and the reflex mechanisms are under supraspinal control. In addition, there is differential neuronal control of leg extensor and flexor muscles. Whereas extensors are mainly activated by proprioceptive feedback, the flexors are predominantly under central control. (b) *Proposed situation in Parkinson's disease.* In this condition, a load-related impairment of proprioceptive feedback can be assumed (dotted lines). This leads to reduced leg extensor activation during the stance phases, which is poorly adapted to actual requirements (e.g., ground conditions) (from Dietz, 2002a).

from extensor load receptors (Dietz et al., 1993). This defective control is illustrated in Fig. 19.2. It may be partially compensated for in Parkinsonian patients by a greater amount of leg flexor activation.

Furthermore, when body becomes unloaded during treadmill locomotion the leg extensor muscles show a load sensitivity in both Parkinsonian patients and healthy subjects (Dietz et al., 1997). However, the absolute level of leg extensor EMG amplitude during the stance phase is smaller in patients with Parkinson's disease than in the age-matched healthy subjects. This suggests that in Parkinson's disease the threshold of load receptor reflex loop is maladjusted or biased. This leads to a

changed magnitude of this reflex response which is essential for the maintenance of body equilibrium.

19.5 Spastic gait disorder

Spasticity produces numerous physical signs such as exaggerated reflexes, clonus and muscle hypertonia (Volume II, Chapter 17). Clinically spastic hypertonia has been defined as a resistance of passive muscle to stretch in a velocity-dependent manner following activation of tonic stretch reflexes (Lance, 1980). On the basis of clinical observations a widely accepted conclusion was drawn for the pathophysiology and treatment of spasticity such that exaggerated reflexes are responsible for the observed muscle hypertonia, and therefore the movement disorder. The function of these reflexes during natural movements and the relationship between exaggerated reflexes and movement disorder is usually not considered (cf. Dietz, 2003a).

The physical signs of spasticity bear, however, little relationship to the patient's disability which is due to a movement disorder. In patients with spinal cord or brain lesions, a characteristic gait impairment is seen. This can be evaluated by the recording of electrophysiological and biomechanical parameters. There is some difference between spasticity of cerebral and of spinal origin, but the main features, such as leg muscle activation during locomotion and the pathophysiology of spastic muscle tone are quite similar (Dietz, 1992b). An overview about the mechanisms that are suggested

to be involved in spastic movement disorder are shown in Fig. 19.3.

Reflexes and muscle tone

It has been suggested that neuronal reorganization occurs following central lesions in both cat (Mendell, 1984) and man (Carr et al., 1993). Novel connections (e.g. sprouting, functional strengthening of existing connections, removed depression of previously inactive connections) may cause changes in the strength of inhibition among neuronal circuits. In addition, supersensitivity caused by the denervation may occur (Mendell, 1984). Although recent observations have indicated that spinal cord lesions do not cause sprouting of primary afferents in either cat (Nacimiento et al., 1993) or man (Ashby, 1989), changes in the reduction of pre-synaptic inhibition of group Ia fibres occur (Burke and Ashby, 1972) which correlate with the enhanced excitability of tendon tap reflexes. In addition, reduction of pre-synaptic inhibition is stronger in patients with paraplegia compared to those with hemiplegia (Faist et al., 1994). However, no correlation is seen between decreased presynaptic inhibition of Ia terminals and the degree of spasticity measured by Ashworth's scale (Faist et al., 1994). Probably also change in transmission in group II pathways may play a role in the pathophysiology of spasticity (Rémy-Néris et al., 2003).

The treatment of spasticity is usually directed towards reducing stretch reflex activity as it was thought that exaggerated reflexes are responsible for increased muscle tone and therefore the movement disorders. Studies on muscle tone and reflex activity have usually been performed under passive motor conditions (Thilmann et al., 1990; 1991; Ibrahim et al., 1993). In such a condition, increased elbow torque following a displacement is associated with an increased EMG activity in the flexor muscles of the spastic side compared to the unaffected side in patients with spastic hemiparesis. Nevertheless, in patients with spastic hemiparesis following stroke, muscle hypertonia was found to be more closely associated with muscle fibre contracture than with reflex hyperexcitability (O'Dwyer et al., 1996).

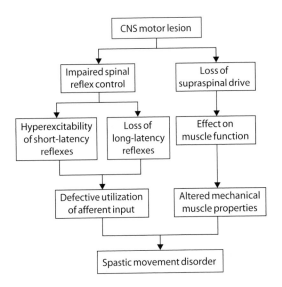

Figure 19.3. Schematic diagram of the mechanism that contribute to spastic paresis and spastic movement disorder. A central motor lesion leads to an impaired reflex control by the CPG and to a loss of supraspinal drive. The consequence is a hyperexcitability of short-latency reflexes and a loss of long-latency reflexes, as well as changes in muscle properties. The combination of all sequels of the primary lesion leads to spastic movement disorder. (from Dietz, 2002a).

Investigations on functional movements of leg (Dietz et al., 1981; Dietz and Berger, 1983; Berger et al., 1984) and arm (Powers et al., 1989; Dietz et al., 1991; Ibrahim et al., 1993) muscles have not revealed any causal relationship between exaggerated reflexes and movement disorder. In adult patients with cerebral or spinal lesions the reciprocal mode of leg muscle activation during gait is preserved in spasticity. Exaggerated short-latency stretch reflexes in spasticity are associated with an absence or reduction of functionally essential polysynaptic (long-latency) reflexes. In addition, both cutaneous (Jones and Yang, 1994) and stretch (Sinkjaer et al., 1993; 1996) reflex modulation are impaired in patients with spinal cord lesion during walking. It was proposed that impaired modulation of the stretch reflex along with increased ankle joint stiffness contribute to the impaired walking ability in these patients.

In spastic patients the EMG activity in the calf muscles during gait is smaller in amplitude compared to healthy subjects, which is most probably due to the impaired function of polysynaptic reflexes in EMG activity. The reduction corresponds to the degree of paresis observed during both gait (Berger et al., 1984) and elbow movements (Dietz et al., 1991). Fast regulation of motoneuron discharge, which characterizes the normal muscle, is absent in spasticity (Rosenfalck and Andreassen, 1980; Dietz et al., 1986). This corresponds to a loss of EMG modulation during gait.

In spastic paresis (acquired at an early or later stage), a fundamentally different development of tension of the triceps surae takes place during the stance phase of the stride cycle (Berger et al., 1984). In the unaffected leg, the tension development correlates with the modulation of EMG activity (the same is true in healthy subjects), while in the spastic leg tension development is connected to the stretching period of the tonically activated (with small EMG amplitude) muscle. During gait there is no visible influence of short-latency reflex potentials on the tension developed by the triceps surae. A similar discrepancy between the resistance to stretch and the level of EMG activity has been described for flexor muscles of the upper limb in spastic patients (Lee et al., 1987; Powers et al., 1988).

Muscle tone during functional movements in patients with spastic paresis cannot be explained by an increased activity of motoneurons. Instead, a transformation of motor units such that a higher tension to EMG activity relationship occurs during the stretching phase of the triceps surae. This has the consequence that regulation of muscle tension takes place at a lower level of neuronal organization. The changed regulation of spastic gait can be considered as optimal for the given state of the motor system (e.g. Latash and Anson, 1996).

Motor unit transformation

There are several findings which support the suggestion that changes in mechanical muscle fibre properties occur in spasticity. Torque motor experiments applied to lower limb muscles indicate a major, non-reflex contribution to the spastic muscle tone in the antigravity muscles, that is in the leg extensors (Hufschmidt and Mauritz, 1985; Sinkjaer et al., 1993). Histochemistry and morphometry studies of spastic muscle have revealed neurogenical changes of the muscle fibres (Edström, 1970; Dietz et al., 1986). A significant part of changes of mechanical muscle fibre properties might, however, be attributed to a shortening of muscle length as a result of a decrease in the number of sarcomeres in series along the myofibrils accompanied by an increase in resistance to stretch (O'Dwyer and Ada, 1996). Such muscle contracture can be produced in experimental animal by plaster cast immobilization of muscles in shortened positions.

The alteration to a simpler regulation of muscle tension following paresis due to spinal or supraspinal lesions is basically advantageous for the patient as it enables him to support the body during gait and, consequently, to achieve mobility (Dietz et al., 1981). However, rapid movements are no longer possible. Following a severe spinal or supraspinal lesion, these transformative processes can overshoot with unwelcome consequences, (i.e. painful spasms and involuntarily movements).

Consequently, in mobile patients primarily physiotherapeutic approaches should be applied, while antispastic during therapy represents a second tool. Only in immobilized patients antispastic drugs may be of benefit to relieve muscle spasms and improve nursing care (cf. Dietz, 2003a).

In children with cerebral palsy, that is when the central nervous lesion is acquired at an early stage, the leg-muscle activity during functional movements, such as locomotion, has characteristic signs of impaired maturation of the normal gait pattern (Berger et al., 1982). This pattern consists of a co-activation of antagonistic leg muscles during the stance phase of a gait cycle and a general reduction in EMG amplitude. In contrast, when the cerebral lesion is acquired at a later stage and the reciprocal mode of leg muscle activity is already established (i.e. at around 4 years), reciprocal activation of antagonistic leg muscles is preserved during spastic gait.

19.6 Target for rehabilitation: plasticity of the CNS

There is increasing evidence that a defective utilization of afferent input, in combination with secondary compensatory processes is involved in typical central movement disorders, such as spasticity and Parkinson's disease. Furthermore, cat (for review see Pearson, 2000) and human (for review see Dietz, 2002a; 2003b) experiments show that neuronal networks underlying the generation of motor patterns are quite flexible after central or peripheral neural lesions (see Volume I, Chapters 8 and 14). Therefore, the aim of rehabilitation should concentrate on the improvement of function by taking advantage of the plasticity of neuronal centres, and should less be directed to the correction of isolated clinical signs, such as the reflex excitability.

There is convincing evidence in spinal animals that a use-dependent plasticity of the spinal cord exists (Edgerton et al., 1997; Pearson, 2000). When stepping is practiced in spinal cat, this task can be performed more successfully than when it is not practiced (Lovely et al., 1986; 1990). The training of any motor task provides sufficient stimulation to initiate a reorganization of neural networks within the spinal cord and, for

example, to generate locomotion. Consequently, the loss of motor capacity following neural injury can become enhanced when locomotor networks are no longer used, for example following a stroke (Edgerton et al., 1997). In contrast, a much greater level of functional recovery might be possible if the concept of use-dependence is applied in both the clinical and rehabilitative settings (Edgerton et al., 1997).

A considerable degree of locomotor recovery in mammals with a spinal cord injury (SCI) can be attributed to a reorganization of spared neural pathways (Curt and Dietz, 1997; Curt et al., 1998; for review see Curt and Dietz, 1999). It has been estimated that if as little as 10–15% of the descending spinal tracts are spared, some locomotor function can recover (Basso, 2000; Metz et al., 2000). If the loss of supraspinal input to the spinal cord is complete, these neuronal networks that exist below the level of the lesion adapt to generate locomotor activity even in the absence of supraspinal input (De Leon et al., 1998a, b; Wirz et al., 2001).

19.7 Locomotor function after SCI

Neuronal capacity of spinal cord from cat to humans

In the cat, recovery of locomotor function following spinal cord transsection can be improved using regular training even in adult animals (Barbeau and Rossignol, 1987; see Volume I, Chapter 13). When stepping was not stimulated, the cat lost the ability to step spontaneously. During such a locomotor training the animal was supported and thus only beared a part of its body weight. Locomotor movements of the hindlimbs were induced by a treadmill while the forelimbs stood on a platform. With ongoing training the body support was decreased associated with improving locomotor abilities. Later on the cat was able to completely take over body weight and perform well-coordinated stepping movements (Barbeau and Rossignol, 1994). The locomotor pattern at this stage closely resembled the pattern of the normal adult cat. Furthermore, hindlimb exercise in adult rats after spinal cord transection can normalize the excitability of spinal reflexes (Skinner et al., 1996). Thus, it can be concluded that the training represents an important factor for the recovery of locomotor function. Recently, stepping movements could also be demonstrated in a monkey after transection of the spinal cord, suggesting that also the isolated primate spinal cord is capable of generating hindlimb stepping movements (Vilensky and O'Connor, 1988).

Human locomotion is not basically different from that described for the cat but is based on a quadrupedal neuronal co-ordination (for review see Dietz, 2002b). Step-like movements are present at birth and can be initiated spontaneously or by peripheral stimuli. The EMG activity underlying this newborn stepping is centrally programmed and, as it has also been observed in anencephalic children, it is likely that spinal mechanisms generate the EMG activity (Forssberg, 1992). The apparent loss of locomotor movements in accidentally spinalized humans has been suggested to be due to a greater predominance of supraspinal over spinal neuronal mechanisms (Kuhn, 1950). Nevertheless, there are indications that in humans spinal interneuronal circuits exist which are involved in the generation of locomotor EMG activity (Calancie et al., 1994) similar to those described for the cat (Barbeau and Rossignol, 1994). Furthermore, involuntary step-like leg movements described in a patient with an incomplete injury to the spinal cord (Nicol et al., 1995; Harkema et al., 1997), as well as the behaviour of a propriospinal clonus released after cervical trauma (Brown et al., 1994), are indicative for a spinal pattern generator in humans.

Effect of locomotor training in paraplegic patients

In patients with incomplete or complete paraplegia a bilateral leg muscle activation combined with coordinated stepping movements can be induced in partially unloaded patients standing on a moving treadmill (Dietz et al., 1994, 1995). The leg movements have to be assisted during the first phases of the training (dependent upon the severity of paresis), in incomplete and during the whole training period in complete paraplegic patients. Walking in incomplete SCI patients is usually achieved only at a low speed (Pépin et al., 2003). While the pattern of leg muscle EMG activity is similar to that seen in healthy subjects, the EMG amplitude is considerably smaller in complete paraplegics compared to incomplete paraplegis. Both patient groups have smaller EMG levels compared to the healthy subjects. Despite the reduced EMG activity, spastic symptoms (e.g. increased muscle tone, exaggerated reflexes) are present in both patient groups. This supports earlier suggestions claiming that alterations of mechanical muscle fibre properties are mainly responsible for the clinical signs of spasticity (see "Spastic gait disorder").

When the EMG of tibialis anterior and gastrocnemius muscles is analysed over the step cycle, it becomes evident that leg muscle EMG activity is about equally distributed during muscle lengthening and shortening in both healthy subjects and patients during locomotion. Furthermore, imposing locomotor movements in complete paraplegic patients with full body unloading does not lead to a significant leg muscle activation (Dietz et al., 2002). This indicates that stretch reflexes are unlikely to play a major role in the generation of the leg muscle EMG pattern in these patients, but that it is rather programmed at a spinal level.

During the course of a daily locomotor training programme, the amplitude of gastrocnemius EMG activity increases significantly during the stance phase, while an inappropriate tibialis anterior activation decreases (Dietz et al., 1994, 1995). This is associated with a greater weight bearing function of the extensors (i.e. body unloading during treadmill locomotion can be reduced). These training effects are seen in both incomplete and complete paraplegic patients. Only patients with incomplete paraplegia benefit from the training programme in so far as they learn to perform unsupported stepping movements on solid ground. Patients with complete paraplegia experience positive effects upon the cardiovascular and musculo-skeletal systems (i.e. they suffer less from the spastic symptoms). Successive reloading of the body during the training may serve as a stimulus for extensor load receptors, which have been shown to be essential for leg extensor activation during locomotion in both cat (Pearson and Collins, 1993) and man (Dietz et al., 1992; Dietz and Colombo, 1996). The generally smaller EMG amplitude in patients with complete paraplegia may be due to a loss of input from descending noradrenergic pathways to spinal locomotor centres (Barbeau and Rossignol, 1994).

For an improved locomotor training during the last years special devices were developed. A driven gait orthosis (DGO) was designed primarily for the training of patients with a SCI (Colombo et al., 2000; 2001) and an electromechanical gait trainer for the restoration of gait in stroke patients (Werner et al., 2002).

Relevant afferent input

For a successful training of patients with a spinal or cerebral lesion, the appropriate afferent input has to be provided to activate spinal neuronal circuits. In healthy subjects during locomotion multi-sensory proprioceptive feedback is continuously weighted and selected. According to recent observations made in healthy subjects (Dietz et al., 1989a, b; 1992), small children (Pang and Yang, 2000) and patients with paraplegia (Harkema et al., 1997; Dietz et al., 2002) afferent inputs from load receptors and hip joints essentially contribute to the activation pattern of leg muscles during locomotion.

It is suggested that proprioceptive input from extensor muscles, and probably also from mechano-receptors, in the foot sole provide load information (Dietz and Duysens, 2000). The signals arising from load receptors are likely to be integrated into the polysynaptic spinal reflex pathway, which adapts the programmed locomotor pattern to the actual ground condition. The afferents that signal hip joint position are suggested to come from muscles around the hip. The role of this afferent activity is to shape the loco-motor pattern, to control phase-transitions and to reinforce ongoing activity. Short-latency stretch- and cutaneous reflexes may be involved in the compensation of irregularities and in the adaptation to the actual ground conditions.

19.8 Assessment of function during rehabilitation

Owing to the exquisite task-dependent regulation of nervous-system function clinical tests must be functional and specific. At present it is a common, well-accepted approach to score isolated clinical measures, such as reflex excitability, muscle tone, or voluntary force of single muscles. For example, muscle tone and spasm frequency can be assessed by the Ashworth scale and Penn spasm frequency scale, respectively (Priebe et al., 1996). For patients with SCI, the American Spinal Injury Association (ASIA) has developed a standardised neurological assessment, that is the ASIA-classification of motor and sensory deficits (Maynard et al., 1997). The question is first, whether such scoring systems can serve as a sensitive outcome measure for new interventional therapies and second, whether they can reflect the functional impairment, which is the most important aspect in terms of the patients' quality of life (see Volume II, Chapter 37 on rehabilitation in spinal cord injury).

Only recently a score has been developed which relates to function. Locomotor ability has been classified into 19 items (Ditunno et al., 2000). A current study indicates that a close relationship between motor scores and locomotor ability exists only in patients with moderately impaired motor function. Patients with a low motor score undergoing a locomotor training can achieve an improved locomotor function without a change in motor score (Dietz, 2002a; Maegele et al., 2002). In these cases, relatively little voluntary force in the leg muscles (reflected in the ASIA score) is required to achieve the ability to walk (cf. Fig. 19.4).

For the future, the effectiveness of any new interventional therapy should be assessed by functional scores in combination with motor scores of selected limb muscles. Motor and sensory scores are most likely to reflect the spontaneous recovery of function, as they depend on the integrity of cortico-spinal connections. In contrast, improvement of locomotor function after SCI also reflects the plasticity of neuronal circuits below the level of lesion. With the combined assessment of voluntary force and automatic

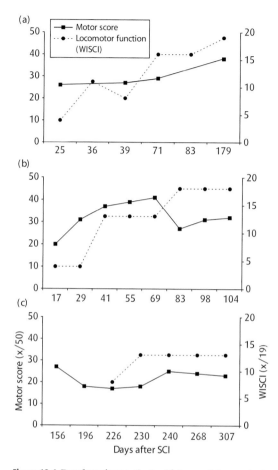

Figure 19.4. Data from three patients with incomplete paraplegia after SCI. In three individual patients (a–c) undergoing locomotor training, there is a differential course of motor score, which reflects the ability to voluntary contract selected muscles, and locomotor function with respect to time. The motor score is assigned according to ASIA standards, with a maximum score of 50. The WISCI (walking index for SCI) score ranges from 0 (no walking ability) to 19 (full walking ability) (from Dietz, 2002a).

function, the superiority of any new interventional therapy on functional movements might reliably be assessed (see also Volume II, Chapter 3).

19.9 Outlook

The advantage of gait analysis represents the quantitative assessment of a functional movement with its underlying neuronal mechanisms and biomechanical consequences. In the future, this approach may further be developed to extract the factors responsible for a movement disorder. For future application in the rehabilitation field, gait analysis may help to select the most effective pharmacological and physiotherapeutical approaches. This may not only be of benefit for the patient but also could lead to reduced health care costs as most physiotherapeutic approaches are not based on controlled studies and their effectiveness was never convincingly demonstrated. For future application in the clinical diagnosis, gait analysis may help to achieve an early diagnosis and detection of subtypes of a movement disorder with the consequence of an early onset of an appropriate training (for review see Dietz, 2002a).

With the gait analysis of patients with a central motor lesion, the best therapeutical approach and the effect of any treatment on the locomotor can be determined. Such an analysis has revealed, for example, that the development of spastic muscle tone can be advantageous, in that it provides body support during stepping movements. This knowledge has, of course, consequences for physiotherapy and drug application.

In severely affected paretic patients the strength of leg muscle activation is not sufficient to build up enough muscle tone or to control limb movements for locomotion. One approach to enhance spinal locomotor activity in the patients with incomplete and complete paraplegia represents the search for substances which influence the gain of leg extensor EMG activity. The most promising approach for the future may be to induce partial regeneration of the lesioned spinal cord tract fibres. Recent experiments in the rat have indicated that after inhibition of neurite growth inhibitors, partial regeneration can occur (for review see Schwab, 1991; Schwab and Bartholdi, 1996). Connected with appropriate locomotor training this approach may improve functional mobility even that of almost completely paraplegic patients. Electrophysiological and biomechanical recordings of locomotion in rats with spinal cord lesions has provided information that this model can be applied in humans with SCI (Metz et al., 2000).

ACKNOWLEDGMENTS

Work is included in this article which was supported by the "Swiss National Science Foundation" (Grant No. 31-64792.01) and the NCCR Neural Plasticity and Regeneration.

REFERENCES

Abbruzzese, G. and Berardelli, A. (2003). Sensorimotor integration in movement disorders (Review). *Mov Disord*, **18**, 231–240.

Angel, R.W. (1983). Muscular contractions elicited by passive shortening. In: *Advances in Neurology* (ed. Desmedt, J.E.), Vol. **39**, Raven Press, New York, pp. 555–563.

Ashby, P. (1989). Spasticity. Discussion I. In: *The Current Status of Research and Treatment* (eds. Emre, M. and Benecke, R.), Partheno, Carnforth, pp. 68–69.

Barbeau, H. and Rossignol, S. (1987). Recovery of locomotion after chronic spinalization in the adult cat. *Brain Res*, **412**, 84–95.

Barbeau, H. and Rossignol, S. (1994). Enhancement of locomotor recovery following spinal cord injury. *Curr Opin Neurol*, **7**, 517–524.

Basso, D.M. (2000). Neuroanatomical substrates of functional recovery after experimental spinal cord injury: implications of basic science research for human spinal cord injury. *Phys Ther*, **80**, 808–817.

Berardelli, A. and Hallett, M. (1984). Shortening reaction of human tibialis anterior. *Neurology*, **34**, 242–246.

Berardelli, A., Sabra, A.F. and Hallett, M. (1983). Physiological mechanisms of rigidity in Parkinson's disease. *J Neurol Neurosurg Psychiatr*, **46**, 45–53.

Berger, W., Quintern, J. and Dietz, V. (1982). Pathophysiological aspects of gait in children with cerebral palsy. *Electroenceph Clin Neurophysiol*, **53**, 538–548.

Berger, W., Quintern, J. and Dietz, V. (1984).Tension development and muscle activation in the leg during gait in spastic hemiparesis: the independence of muscle hypertonia and exaggerated stretch reflexes. *J Neurol Neurosurg Psychiatr*, **47**, 1029–1033.

Blin, O., Fernandez, A.M., Pailhouse, J. and Searratrice, G. (1991). Dopa-sensitive and Dopa-resistant gait parameters in Parkinson's disease. *J Neurol Sci*, **103**, 51–54.

Bronstein, A.M., Hoo, J.D., Gresty, M.A. and Panagi, C. (1990). Visual control of balance in cerebellar and parkinsonian syndromes. *Brain*, **113**, 767–779.

Brouwer, B. and Ashby, P. (1992). Corticospinal projections to lower limb motoneurons in man. *Exp Brain Res*, **89**, 649–654.

Brown, P., Rothwell, J.C., Thompson, P.D. and Marsden, C.D. (1994). Propriospinal myoclonus: evidence for spinal "pattern" generators in humans. *Mov Disord*, **9**, 571–576.

Burke, D. and Ashby, P. (1972). Are spinal "presynaptic" inhibitory mechanisms suppressed in spasticity? *J Neurol Sci*, **15**, 321–326.

Burke, D., Hagbarth, K.E. and Wallin G. (1977). Reflex mechanisms in parkinsonian rigidity. *Scand J Rehabil Med*, **9**, 15–23.

Burne, J.A. and Lippold, O.C.J. (1996). Loss of tendon organ inhibition in Parkinson's disease. *Brain*, **119**, 1115–1121.

Calancie, B., Needham-Shropshire, B., Jacobs, P., Willer, K., Zych, G. and Green, B.A. (1994). Involuntary stepping after chronic spinal cord injury. Evidence for a central rhythm generator for locomotion in man. *Brain*, **117**, 1143–1159.

Carr, L.J., Harrison, L.M., Evans, A.L. and Stephen, J.A. 1993. Patterns of central motor reorganization in hemiplegic cerebral palsy. *Brain*, **116**, 1223–1247.

Chan, C.W.Y., Kearney, R.E. and Melvill-Jones, G. (1979). Tibialis anterior response to sudden ankle displacements in normal and parkinsonian subjects. *Brain Res*, **173**, 303–314.

Cody, F.W.J., Macdermott, N., Matthews, P.B.C. and Richardson, H.C. (1986). Observations on the genesis of the stretch reflex in Parkinson's disease. *Brain*, **109**, 229–249.

Colombo, G., Joerg, M., Schreier, R. and Dietz, V. (2000). Treadmill training of paraplegic patients using a robotic orthosis. *J Rehabil Res Dev*, **17**, 35–42.

Colombo, G., Wirz, M. and Dietz, V. (2001). Driven gait orthosis for improvement of locomotor training in paraplegic patients. *Spinal Cord*, **39**, 693–700.

Curt, A. and Dietz, V. (1997). Ambulatory capacity in spinal cord injury: significance of ASIA protocol and SSEP recordings in predicting outcome. *Arch Phys Med Rehabil*, **78**, 39–43.

Curt, A. and Dietz, V. (1999). Electrophysiological recordings in patients with spinal cord injury: significance for predicting outcome (Review). *Spinal Cord*, **37**, 157–165.

Curt, A., Keck, M. and Dietz, V. (1998). Functional outcome following spinal cord injury. Significance of motor evoked potentials and ASIA scores. *Arch Phys Med Rehabil*, **79**, 81–86.

De Leon, R.D., Hodgson, J.A., Roy, R.R. and Edgerton, V.R. (1998a). Locomotor capacity attributable to step training versus spontaneous recovery following spinalisation in cats. *J Neurophysiol*, **79**, 1329–1340.

De Leon, R.D., Hodgson, J.A., Roy, R.R. and Edgerton, V.R. (1998b). Full weight bearing hindlimb standing following stand training in the adult spinal cat. *J Neurophysiol*, **80**, 83–91.

Delwaide, P.J., Pepin, J.L. and Maertens de Noordhout, A. (1999). The audiospinal reaction in parkinsonian patients reflects functional changes in reticular nuclei. *Ann Neurol*, **33**, 63–69.

Dietz, V. (1992a). Human neuronal control of automatic functional movements: interaction between central programs and afferent input. *Physiol Rev*, **72**, 33–69.

Dietz, V. (1992b). Spasticity: exaggerated reflexes or movement disorder? In: *Medicine Sport Science Vol. 36, Movement Disorders in Children* (eds. Forssberg, H. and Hirschfeld, H.), Karger, Basel, pp. 225–233.

Dietz, V. (2002a). Proprioception and locomotor disorders. *Nat Rev Neurosci*, **3**, 781–790.

Dietz, V. (2002b). Do human bipeds use quadrupedal co-ordination? *Trends Neurosci*, **25**, 462–467.

Dietz, V. (2003a). Spastic movement disorders: what is the impact of research on clinical practice? *J Neurol Neurosurg Psychiatr*, **74**, 820–821.

Dietz, V. (2003b). Spinal pattern generators for locomotion. *Clin Neurophysiol*, **114**, 1379–1389.

Dietz, V. and Berger, W. (1983). Normal and impaired regulation of stiffness in gait: a new hypothesis about muscle hypertonia. *Exp Neurol*, **79**, 680–687.

Dietz, V. and Colombo, G. (1996). Effects of body immersion on postural adjustments to voluntary arm movements in humans: role of load receptor input. *J Physiol (Lond)*, **497**, 849–856.

Dietz, V. and Duysens, J. (2000). Modulation of reflex mechanisms by load receptors. *Gait Post*, **11**, 102–110.

Dietz, V., Quintern, J. and Berger, W. (1981). Electrophysiological studies of gait in spasticity and rigidity. Evidence that altered mechanical properties of muscle contribute to hypertonia. *Brain*, **104**, 431–449.

Dietz, V., Ketelsen, U.P., Berger, W. and Quintern, J. (1986). Motor unit involvement in spastic paresis: relationship between leg muscle activation and histochemistry. *J Neurol Sci*, **75**, 89–103.

Dietz, V., Berger, W. and Horstmann, G.A. (1988). Posture in Parkinson's disease: impairment of reflexes and programming. *Ann Neurol*, **24**, 660–669.

Dietz, V., Horstmann, G.A. and Berger, W. (1989a). Interlimb coordination of leg muscle activation during perturbation of stance in humans. *J Neurophysiol*, **62**, 680–693.

Dietz, V., Horstmann,G.A., Trippel, M. and Gollhofer, A. (1989b). Human postural reflexes and gravity – an underwater simulation. *Neurosci Lett*, **106**, 350–355.

Dietz, V., Feuerstein, T.J. and Berger, W. (1990). Significance of dopamine receptor antagonists in human postural control. *Neurosci Lett*, **117**, 81–86.

Dietz, V., Trippel, M. and Berger, W. (1991). Reflex activity and muscle tone during elbow movements of patients with spastic paresis. *Ann Neurol*, **30**, 767–784.

Dietz, V., Gollhofer, A., Kleiber, M. and Trippel, M. (1992). Regulation of bipedal stance: dependence on "load" receptors. *Exp Brain Res*, **89**, 229–231.

Dietz, V., Zijlstra, W., Assaiante, C., Trippel, M. and Berger, W. (1993). Balance control in Parkinson's disease. *Gait Posture*, **1**, 77–84.

Dietz, V., Colombo, G. and Jensen, L. (1994). Locomotor activity in spinal man. *Lancet*, **344**, 1260–1263.

Dietz, V., Colombo, G., Jensen, L. and Baumgartner, L. (1995). Locomotor capacity of spinal cord in paraplegic patients. *Ann Neurol*, **37**, 574–582.

Dietz, V., Zijlstra, W., Prokop, T. and Berger, W. (1996). Leg muscle activation during gait in Parkinson's disease: adaptation and interlimb coordination. *Electroenceph Clin Neurophysiol*, **97**, 408–415.

Dietz, V., Leenders, K.L. and Colombo, G. (1997). Leg muscle activation during gait in Parkinson's disease: influence of body unloading. *Electroenceph Clin Neurophysiol*, **105**, 400–405.

Dietz, V., Müller, R. and Colombo, G. (2002). Locomotor activity in spinal man: significance of afferent input from joint load receptors. *Brain*, **125**, 226–2634.

Ditunno, J.F., et al., (2000). Walking index for spinal cord injury (WISCI). An international multicenter validity and reliability study. *Spinal Cord*, **38**, 234–243.

Edgerton, V.R., De Leon, R.D., Tillakaratne, N., Recktenwald, M.R., Hodgson, J.A. and Roy, R.R. (1997). Use-dependent plasticity in spinal stepping and standing. In: *Neuronal Regeneration, Reorganization and Repair. Advances in Neurology* (ed. Seil F.J.), Vol. **72**, Lippincott-Raven, Philadelphia, pp. 233–247.

Edström, L. (1970). Selective changes in the sizes of red and white muscle fibres in upper motor lesions and parkinsonism. *J Neurol Sci*, **11**, 537–550.

Faist, M., Mazevet, D., Dietz, V. and Pierrot-Deseilligny, E. (1994). A quantitative assessment of presynaptic inhibition of Ia afferents in spastics: differences in hemiplegics and paraplegics. *Brain*, **117**, 1449–1455.

Forssberg, H. (1992). Preface. In: Medicine Sport Science Vol. 36, *Movement Disorders in Children* (eds Forssberg, H. and Hirschfeld, H.), Karger, Basel, pp. 7–8.

Forssberg, H., Johnels, B. and Steg, G. (1984). Is Parkinsonian gait caused by a regression to an immature walking pattern? In: *Advances in Neurology* (eds. Hassler, R.G. and Christ, J.F.), Vol. **40**, Raven Press, New York, pp. 375–379.

Harkema, S.J., Requejo, P.S., Hurley, S.L., Patel, U.K., Dobkin, B.H. and Edgerton, V.R. (1997). Human lumbosacral spinal cord interprets loading during stepping. *J Neurophysiol*, **77**, 797–811.

Hufschmidt, A. and Mauritz, K.H. (1985). Chronic transformation of muscle in spasticity: a peripheral contribution to increased tone. *J Neurol Neurosurg Psychiatr*, **48**, 676–685.

Ibrahim, I.K., Berger, W., Trippel, M. and Dietz, V. (1993). Stretch-induced electromyographic activity and torque in spastic elbow muscles. *Brain*, **116**, 971–989.

Jones, C.A. and Yang, J.F. (1994). Reflex behavior during walking in incomplete spinal-cord-injured subjects. *Exp Neurol*, **128**, 239–248.

Knutsson, E. (1972). An analysis of parkinsonian gait. Brain, **95**, 475–486.

Kuhn, R.A. (1950). Functional capacity of the isolated human spinal cord. *Brain*, **73**, 1–51.

Lance, J.W. (1980). Symposium synopsis. In: *Spasticity: Disordered Motor Control* (eds Feldman, R.G., Young, R.R. and Koella, W.P.), Year Book Publisher, Chicago, pp. 485–495.

Latash, M.L. and Anson, J.G. (1996). What are "normal movements" in atypical populations. *Behav Brain Sci*, **19**, 55–106.

Lee, W.A., Boughton, A. and Rymer, W.Z. (1987). Absence of stretch reflex gain enhancement in voluntarily activated spastic muscle. *Exp Neurol*, **98**, 317–335.

Lovely, R.G., Gregor, R.J., Roy, R.R. and Edgerton, V.R., (1986). Effects of training on the recovery of full weight bearing stepping in the adult spinal cat. *Exp Neurol*, **9**, 421–435.

Lovely, R.G., Gregor, R.J., Roy, R.R. and Edgerton, V.R. (1990). Weight-bearing hindlimb stepping in treadmill-exercised adult spinal cat. *Brain Res*, **51**, 206–218.

Mac Kay-Lyons, M. (2002). Central pattern generation of locomotion: a review of the evidence. *Phys Ther*, **82**, 69–83.

Maegele, M., Müller, S., Wernig, A., Edgerton, V.R. and Harkema, S.J. (2002). Recruitment of spinal motor pools during voluntary movements versus stepping after human spinal cord injury. *J Neurotraum*, **19**, 1217–1229.

Marsden, C.D. (1990). Neurophysiology. In: *Parkinson's Disease* (ed. Stern, G.), Chapman and Hall, London, pp. 57–98.

Martin, J.P. (1967). *The Basal Ganglia and Posture*, Pitman, London.

Maynard, F.M., et al., (1997). International standards for neurological and functional classification of spinal cord injury. *Spinal Cord*, **35**, 266–274.

Mendell, L.M. (1984). Modifiability of spinal synapses. *Physiol Rev*, **64**, 260–324.

Metz, G., Curt, A., Van De Meent, H., Klusman, I., Schwab M.E. and Dietz, V. (2000). Validation of the weight-drop contusion model in rats: a comparative study to human spinal cord injury. *J Neurotraum*, **17**, 1–17.

Murray, M.P. (1967). Gait as a total pattern of movement. *Am J Phys Med*, **46**, 290–332.

Murray, M.P. and Clarkson, B.H. (1996). The vertical pathways of the foot during level walking. II. Clinical examples of distorted pathways. *J Am Phys Ther Ass*, **46**, 590–599.

Nacimiento, W., Mautes, A., Töpper, R., Oestreicher, A.B., Gispen, W.H., Nacimiento, A.C., Noth, J. and Kreutzberg, G.W. (1993). B-50 (GAP-42) in the spinal cord caudal to hemisection: indication for lack of intraspinal sprouting in dorsal root axons. *J Neurosci Res*, **35**, 603–617.

Nicol, D.J., Granat, M., Baxendale, R.H. and Tison, S.J.M. (1995). Evidence for a human spinal stepping generator. *Brain Res*, **9**, 451–455.

O'Dwyer, N.J. and Ada, L. (1996). Reflex hyperexcitability and muscle contracture in relation to spastic hypertonia. *Curr Opin Neurol*, **9**, 451–455.

O'Dwyer, N.J., Ada, L. and Neilson, P.D. (1996). Spasticity and muscle contracture following stroke. *Brain*, **119**, 1737–1749.

Pang, K.G. and Yang, J.F. (2000). The initiation of the swing phase in human infant stepping: importance of hip position and leg loading. *J Physiol (Lond)*, **528**, 389–404.

Pearson, K.G. (2000). Neural adaption in the generation of rhythmic behavior. *Annu Rev Physiol*, **62**, 723–753.

Pearson, K.G. and Collins, D.F. (1993). Reversal of the influence of group Ib-afferents from plantaris on activity in medial gastrocnemius muscle during locomotor activity. *J Neurophysiol*, **70**, 1009–1017.

Pépin, A., Norman, K.E. and Barbeau, H. (2003). Treadmill walking in incomplete spinal cord-injured subjects: 1. Adaptation to changes in speed. *Spinal Cord*, **41**, 257–270.

Powers, R.K., Marder-Meyer, J. and Rymer, W.Z. (1988). Quantitative relations between hypertonia and stretch reflex threshold in spastic hemiparesis. *Ann Neurol*, **23**, 115–124.

Powers, R.K., Campbell, D.L. and Rymer, W.Z. (1989). Stretch reflex dynamics in spastic elbow flexor muscles. *Ann Neurol*, **25**, 32–42.

Priebe, M.M., Sherwood, A.M., Thomby, J.I., Kharas, N.F. and Markowski, J. (1996). Clinical assessment of spasticity in spinal cord injury: a multidimensional problem. *Arch Phys Med Rehabil*, **77**, 713–716.

Rémy-Néris, O., Denys, P., Daniel, O., Barbeau, H. and Bussel, B. (2003). Effect of intrathecal clonidine on group I and II oligosynaptic excitation in paraplegics. *Exp Brain Res*, **148**, 509–514.

Rosenfalck, A. and Adreassen, S. (1980). Impaired regulation of force and firing pattern of single motor units in patients with spasticity. *J Neurol Neurosurg Psychiatr*, **43**, 907–916.

Schieppati, M. and Nardone, A. (1991). Free and support stance in Parkinson's disease: the effect of posture and "postural set" on leg muscle responses to perturbation and its relation to the severity of the disease. *Brain*, **114**, 1227–1244.

Schomburg, E.D. (1990). Spinal sensory systems and their supraspinal control. *Neurosci Res*, **7**, 265–340.

Schwab, M.E. (1991). Regeneration of lesioned CNS axons by neutralisation of neurite growth inhibitors: a short review. *Paraplegia*, **29**, 294–298.

Schwab, M.E. and Bartholdi, D. (1996). Degeneration and regeneration of axons in the lesioned spinal cord. *Physiol Rev*, **76**, 319–370.

Sinkjaer, T., Toft, E., Larsen, K., Andreassen, S. and Hansen, H. (1993). Non-reflex and reflex mediated ankle joint stiffness in multiple sclerosis patients with spasticity. *Muscle Nerve*, **16**, 69–76.

Sinkjaer, T., Andersen, J.B. and Nielsen, J.F. (1996). Impaired stretch reflex and joint torque modulation during spastic gait in multiple sclerosis patients. *J Neurol*, **243**, 566–574.

Skinner, R.D., Houle, J.D., Reese, N.B., Berry, C.L. and Garcia-Rill, E. (1996). Effects of exercise and fetal spinal cord implants on the H-reflex in chronically spinalized adult rats. *Brain Res*, **729**, 127–131.

Stelmach, G.E. (1991). Basal ganglia impairment and force control. In: *Tutorials in Motor Neuroscience* (eds Requin, J. and Stelmach, G.E.), Kluwer, Dordrecht, pp. 137–148.

Stolze, H., Kutz-Buschbeck, J.P., Drucke, H., John, K.K., Illert, M. and Deuschl, G. (2001). Comparative analysis of the gait disorder of normal pressure hydrocephalus and Parkinson's disease. *J Neurol Neurosurg Psychiatr*, **70**, 289–297.

Tatton, W.G., Bedingham, W., Verrier, M.C. and Blair, R.D.G. (1984a). Characteristic alterations in response to imposed wrist displacement in parkinsonian rigidity and dystonia musculo-rum deformans. *Can J Neurol Sci*, **11**, 281–287.

Tatton, W.G., Eastman, M.J., Bedingham, W., Vierrier, M.C. and Bruce, I.C. (1984b). Defective utilization of sensory input as the basis for bradykinesia, rigidity, and decreased movement repertoire in Parkinson's disease a hypothesis. *Can J Neurol Sci*, **11**, 136–143.

Thilmann, A.F., Fellows, S.J. and Garms, E. (1990). Pathological stretch reflexes on the "good" side of hemiparetic patients. *J Neurol Neurosurg Psychiatr*, **53**, 208–214.

Thilmann, A.F., Fellows, S.J. and Garms, E. (1991). The mechanism of spastic muscle hypertonus: variation in reflex gain over the time course of spasticity. *Brain*, **114**, 233–244.

Vilensky, J.A. and O'Connor, B.L. (1988). Stepping in non-human primates with a complete spinal cord transection: old and new data, and implications for humans. *Ann NY Acad Sci*, **860**, 528–530.

Watts, R.L., Wiegner, A.W. and Young, R.R. (1986). Elastic properties of muscles measured at the elbow in man. II. Patients with parkinsonian rigidity. *J Neurol Neurosurg Psychiatr*, **49**, 1177–1181.

Werner, C., Von Frankenberg, S., Treig, T., Konrad, M. and Hesse, S. (2002).Treadmill training with partial body weight support and an electromechanical gait trainer for restoration of gait in subacute stroke patients. A randomized crossover study. *Stroke*, **33**, 2895–2901.

Westphal, E. (1987). Unterschenkelphänomen und Nervendehnung. *Arch Psychiat Nervenkr*, **7**, 666–670.

Wirz, M., Colombo, G. and Dietz, V. (2001). Long term effects of locomotor training in spinal man. *J Neurol Neurosurg Psychiatr*, **71**, 93–96.

Zijlmans, J.C.M., Poels, P.J.E., Duysens, J., Van der Straaten, J., Thien, T., Van't Hof, M.A., Thijssen, H.O.M. and Horstink, M.W.M. (1996). Quantitative gait analysis in patients with vascular parkinsonism. *Mov Disord*, **11**, 501–508.

Balance, vestibular and oculomotor dysfunction

C.D. Hall[1,2,*] and S.J. Herdman[1,2,3]

[1]Atlanta Veterans Administration, Rehabilitation Research and Development, Decatur, GA; [2]Department of Rehabilitation Medicine, Emory University, and [3]Department of Otolaryngology-Head and Neck Surgery, Emory University, Atlanta, GA

20.1 Introduction

Upright posture is inherently unstable in human beings: a heavy upper body must be balanced over a smaller lower body. The maintenance of upright balance requires that the center of mass be positioned within the base of support, either of which may be moving. Furthermore, in order to meet the demands of a constantly changing environment, body position and movement must be continuously monitored and updated with information received from the visual, somatosensory and vestibular systems. This multimodal sensory information is integrated within the central nervous system and, based on the perception of current demands on postural stability, an appropriate motor response is generated. The motor response must be accurately timed and scaled in order to prevent a fall. Failure in any one of the sensory or motor systems results in impaired ability to control posture and may result in a fall. The effect of sensory or motor system loss on maintaining balance varies with the degree of challenge to stability. For example, the balance challenge to an individual is very different when standing still compared to standing on a bus that suddenly lurches. This chapter will focus on:

1 vestibular contributions to postural stability;
2 the effect of peripheral vestibular loss on balance and postural control;

*Supported in part by Research Career Development Award C3249V awarded by the Veterans Administration.

3 the effect of eye movements on balance;
4 the role of vestibular rehabilitation (VR) in the remediation of imbalance and gaze instability.

20.2 Methods of examination of postural stability

In order to study the unique contribution of the visual and somatosensory systems during quiet stance, researchers systematically reduce or alter the input of each. Using current technology, it is a relatively trivial problem to remove or alter visual or somatosensory information used for postural control. Briefly, postural sway can be measured under conditions in which somatosensory and visual feedback is altered (see Chapter 8 of Volume II for details). As a person stands on a force platform, changes in vertical pressure produced by body sway is used to move either the support surface or visual surround in synchrony with the individual's sway (referred to as "sway-referenced"; Baloh et al., 1998). Movement of the support surface in parallel with the individual alters somatosensory cues normally used for postural stability. For example, in quiet stance we normally have a small amount of anterior and posterior (AP) sway, which results in changes in ankle angle. If the support surface moves with body sway, the change in the ankle angle is minimized. This alters the somatosensory feedback, rendering it less effective as a signal in the maintenance of upright posture. Similarly, if the visual surround is moved in parallel with postural sway, the visual feedback cues are novel and cannot be used as effectively to maintain postural stability. In reality, movement of the support surface and of the visual surround in parallel with body sway occurs only at low frequencies of sway (<0.3 Hz) because of the mechanical constraints of the equipment. At higher frequencies of body sway, support surface and visual surround movement is out of sink with the body. The result, however, is still novel sensory feedback that cannot be used as effectively for postural stability. The test is organized into a series of six conditions of increasing difficulty. The first three conditions are performed on a firm surface with eyes open, eyes closed and finally with vision sway-referenced. The final three conditions are performed with the support surface sway-referenced with eyes open, eyes closed and with vision sway-referenced.

Manipulating vestibular inputs cannot be accomplished so easily because we are bound by the earth's gravitational field (Nashner, 1982). Thus, most of our knowledge about the role of the vestibular system in postural control is derived from studies of individuals with loss of vestibular function. Interpretation of information garnered from these studies is confounded by the fact that the findings reflect both the loss of vestibular function and the compensation for that loss.

Additionally, until recently researchers and clinicians have judged vestibular loss by measuring the function of the horizontal semicircular canals. We could not measure the function of the vertical semicircular canals, the saccule and the utricle until the development of methods such as off-axis rotational testing, vestibular evoked myogenic responses and measurement of subjective visual vertical (Colebatch and Halmagyi, 1992; Halmagyi and Colebatch, 1995; Bohmer and Mast, 1999; Li et al., 1999; Shepard and Howarth, 1999; Vibert et al., 1999; Welgampola and Colebatch, 2001). Thus studies of people with bilateral vestibular loss may be muddled by remaining otolith or even posterior canal function in some but not all subjects. These caveats should be kept in mind as we explore the contribution of vestibular system to postural stability.

Another method utilized to study the role of vestibular inputs is to directly stimulate the vestibular system. This has been accomplished via small, direct electrical current applied to the mastoid processes (galvanic vestibular stimulation, GVS; Nashner and Wolfson, 1974) or by direct head displacement (Horak et al., 1994). GVS has been shown to directly affect posture by increasing activation of distal ankle musculature, thereby increasing postural sway and ankle torque (Nashner and Wolfson, 1974; Magnusson et al., 1990). Finally, postural reactions have been examined using different techniques to perturb balance. The perturbations include translational and pitch perturbations of the support surface, sinusoidal rotation of the support surface at different frequencies and sudden movement or flow of the visual world. These methods both perturb balance and manipulate sensory cues.

20.3 Overview of sensory contributions to postural control

The three systems (visual, somatosensory and vestibular) that provide the main sensory inputs for postural control each contribute unique information regarding body posture and motion. This information is used to generate automatic postural responses and also contributes to voluntary postural control. No single sensory system, however, provides us with sufficient information to definitively determine body position and movement.

Visual information is used to orient the body relative to the visual world and provides information used to determine whether the person is moving or the visual world is moving. There are several different visual cues used for postural stability. One long-held concept has been that, as a person sways, even during quiet standing, retinal slip information is used to determine body movement relative to environmental movement. This concept has been challenged by the recent studies of Jahn et al. (2002) who suggest that efference copy of ocular motor signals, rather than retinal slip, is used to regulate postural sway. Other visual cues include changes in image size and retinal disparity, which would occur with fore-to-aft sway. Visual stabilization of balance appears to be primarily dependent on central vision and is related to the distance from the eyes to the visual target (Brandt et al., 1973; Paulus et al., 1984; Brandt et al., 1985). As distance to a visual target increases, relative changes in visually mediated cues used for balance (eye movement, retinal slip and retinal disparity) decrease and become less effective in maintaining postural stability. It is only when the distance decreases from 100 to 10 cm that postural stability improves. Visual signals by themselves provide ambiguous information about postural stability. We have all had the experience of quickly putting our foot on the brake when a car pulls up next to us at a stoplight. Input from either the somatosensory or vestibular system is required to resolve this sensory conflict and determine the correct locus of the movement.

The somatosensory system provides information concerning body position and movement relative to the support surface. In addition, the somatosensory system provides information regarding the position and movement of body segments relative to each other. Signals from skin, muscle and joint receptors affect postural responses in several ways. Shifts in alignment alter which pressure receptors in the feet are firing; joint receptors may send signals about the absolute position of the joint, about velocity of joint movement or about the direction of joint movement. Even in quiet stance, we normally have a small amount of AP sway, which results in changes in ankle angle and in foot pressure. This alteration in somatosensory feedback is an effective signal in the maintenance of upright posture. One of the more important roles of somatosensory cues in postural stability appears to be the prevention of falls. The majority of falls occur as a result of an external perturbation, such as a slip or trip. In order to prevent a loss of balance or fall, the automatic postural responses must be appropriately timed and scaled. Through use of sudden translations or rotations of the surface upon which the subject stands, researchers simulate the conditions under which a fall might occur. Through these studies, we have gained considerable insight into the role of the sensory cues in automatic postural responses. The weight of evidence identifies the role of somatosensory input as triggering and selecting postural responses to platform perturbations (Keshner et al., 1987; Horak et al., 1990; Allum and Honegger, 1995).

Vestibular input is used to determine head position relative to gravity and to provide information regarding linear and angular head acceleration to detect self-motion. The vestibular system can detect even the small head movements resulting from body sway during quiet stance. Motor responses to head acceleration are then mediated through the vestibulospinal system. Direct stimulation of the vestibular system (via GVS) results in the perception of movement with a resultant increase in leg muscle activation and body sway (Nashner and Wolfson, 1974; Magnusson et al., 1990). Direct stimulation of the vestibular system (via head displacement) results in activation of the same trunk and leg muscles as seen following surface translation (Horak et al., 1994). For example, forward displacement of either the head or body results in activation of the gastrocnemius, hamstrings and paraspinals to maintain upright posture. The amplitude of the muscle response to direct vestibular stimulation is very small (approximately one-third) compared to the response following surface translation initiated through somatosensory input. Therefore, while the vestibular system can trigger appropriate balance responses in the trunk and legs, the primary role of vestibular inputs appears to be stabilization of the head in space.

Vestibular inputs become more critical when visual or somatosensory inputs are absent, reduced or under more challenging balance conditions. When the surface is firm, somatosensory inputs from trunk and legs dominate. When surface is altered (narrow or compliant), input from vision and vestibular dominates. When somatosensory information is reduced (e.g., with sway-referenced surface) the amplitude of muscle response following head displacement is increased (Horak et al., 1994). When the surface is unstable so that the upper extremity is necessary to maintain upright balance, direct stimulation of the vestibular system (via GVS) results in activation of the upper extremity musculature (Britton et al., 1993).

Simultaneous translation of the support surface and GVS results in exaggerated responses (Inglis et al., 1995; Horak and Hlavacka, 2002). Final postural alignment is significantly altered such that subjects have much greater trunk leans than can be accounted for by either stimulus alone or in combination. It may be that the automatic postural responses were triggered by somatosensory input from the platform perturbation and that the vestibular system contributed the internal representation of vertical used to adjust final postural alignment, in this case, increased lean. Ultimately, input from the lower extremity (somatosensory) is integrated with information from the head (vision and vestibular) to provide an accurate internal representation of body position and movement (Mergner and Rosemeier, 1998).

Redundancy: not substitution

There is a certain amount of redundancy in the contributions of the different sensory systems to postural stability. Although this is important to remember, it is equally important to note that each sensory signal appears to have optimal conditions and frequencies over which it works (Dichgans et al., 1976; Berthoz et al., 1979; Diener et al., 1982; Diener et al., 1984; Tokita et al., 1984). For example, when healthy subjects are standing in a normal environment (flat, stable surface), the somatosensory and visual systems have more influence on posture than does the vestibular system (Nashner, 1982). However, as will be discussed later, vestibular information becomes more important in stabilizing head and trunk motion in space under more challenging conditions such as standing on a moving surface or walking and running (Buchanan and Horak, 2001–2002; Creath et al., 2002). Furthermore, Xerri et al. (1988) demonstrated that the control of posture at lower frequencies ($<0.25\,Hz$) is dominated by visual input while at higher frequencies, vestibular inputs (from otoliths) dominate. The end result is that the different sensory systems cannot fully substitute for each other when there is a loss of function. Healthy subjects can maintain balance without vision or somatosensory input, however postural

sway increases when either input is removed (Lee and Lishman, 1975; Diener et al., 1984). When somatosensory and visual information are present but novel, the vestibular system still provides appropriate inputs to resolve the sensory conflict and maintain upright posture but again there is an increase in sway (Nashner, 1982). Conversely, visual and somatosensory cues would only partially compensate for lost vestibular function.

In spite of this, studies show that visual cues help maintain balance in patients with bilateral vestibular hypofunction (BVH; Bles et al., 1983, 1984). Bles et al. (1984) have shown that during the course of recovery following BVH, patients change how they rely on sensory cues. Initially, they rely on visual cues as a substitute for the lost vestibular cues but over a 2-year period they increase their reliance on somatosensory cues to maintain balance. The use of proprioceptive cues would not fully compensate for vestibular function, however. When postural stability is perturbed by viewing a sinusoidal lateral tilt of the visual surround, body sway recovered to within normal limits at lower frequencies but not at higher frequencies (Bles et al., 1983). Thus neither visual nor somatosensory cues fully substitutes for the range of frequencies over which the vestibular system works.

20.4 What vestibular hypofunction tells us about the role of the vestibular system in postural stability

Ankle musculature responses to support surface perturbation

It is interesting to note that bilateral vestibular loss has no effect on the latency, sequence and timing of ankle musculature in response to perturbation of the support surface. That is, individuals with BVH respond with normal muscle onset latencies of the ankle musculature, muscle activation patterns, rate of change of force applied to the surface and symmetry of response between legs (Allum et al., 1988, 1994; Herdman et al., 1994). However, vestibular inputs do appear to modulate the amplitude of muscle activation. Individuals with BVH exhibit reduced stabilization at the ankle as measured by decreased amplitude of ankle muscle activity (to 30% of normal) and a concomitant reduction in ankle torque (Keshner et al., 1987; Allum et al., 1988, 1994). An additional problem that occurs with loss of vestibular function is that ankle muscle torque develops more slowly in patients with bilateral vestibular loss than in healthy subjects. Keshner et al. (1987) found that for random pitch perturbations of the support surface, the slope of ankle muscle torque (i.e., rate of change) was less steep for BVH than healthy controls. This suggests that patients with BVH are at risk of developing too little torque too slowly, which may result in an increased risk for falling.

The effect of vestibular loss on the amplitude of muscle response at the ankle is related to several factors, the most important being the degree of deficit. For example, subjects with unilateral vestibular loss have similar muscle onset latencies and amplitudes to translational perturbations as do normal controls (Nashner et al., 1982; Black et al., 1983). However, if you look at patients with acute unilateral vestibular hypofunction (UVH) separate from those with chronic UVH, there is a gradation of muscle response amplitude and resultant ankle muscle torque developed to pitch rotations of the support surface (Allum et al., 1988). Individuals with chronic UVH have the largest amplitude of muscle response, followed by those with acute UVH and individuals with BVH had the smallest amplitude of responses.

Trunk musculature responses to support surface perturbations

While responses in lower extremity muscles are reduced in BVH subjects, the responses of trunk muscles, particularly paraspinal muscles, are enhanced (Allum et al., 1994; Allum and Honegger, 1995). Thus, subjects with BVH exhibited increased trunk angular velocity during balance recovery. This increase trunk velocity is evidence of greater instability. As individuals with BVH do not generate adequate ankle torque following a balance perturbation, they may have difficulty maintaining upright posture following an external perturbation.

Balance strategies following support surface perturbations

Based on early work, Horak et al. (1990) proposed that individuals with BVH are unable to perform a hip strategy. Individuals with BVH exhibited normal balance responses except when standing on a narrow beam (Black et al., 1988; Horak et al., 1990). Individuals with chronic BVH did not alter muscle activation or shear forces under shortened surface condition. Controls, on the other hand, significantly increased early abdominal and quadricep activation on the shortened surface as well as shear forces (indicative of a hip strategy). More recent work by Runge et al. (1998) demonstrated that individuals with chronic BVH can use a hip strategy (defined by early hip torques) in response to larger perturbations on a normal support surface. These results highlight the importance of vestibular information in balance responses in the presence of reduced somatosensory inputs.

Modulation of response to support surface perturbations

Healthy individuals quickly learn to maintain their balance and are able to decrease the amplitude of response to repeated, identical perturbations of the support surface. Loss of balance is unusual except during the initial trial in younger subjects (Wolfson et al., 1992). Several studies have suggested that the vestibular system is not part of this modulation of motor responses. Herdman et al. (1994) demonstrated that subjects with BVH modulate the response to a series of identical pitch perturbations of the support surface as well as do healthy subjects. Although more subjects with BVH had an inappropriate response on the initial trial than did healthy subjects of the same age, the patients with BVH quickly reduced the amplitude of response on subsequent trials as do healthy subjects. Keshner et al. (1987)

studied the role of the vestibular and visual systems in adaptation. They compared muscle amplitude of trials 1–3 with trials 4–10 and found that both healthy controls and BVH exhibited a decrease (or adaptation)

in response amplitude of ankle and neck muscles in the second set of trials with and without vision. Thus, adaptation is not dependent on either an intact vestibular or visual system.

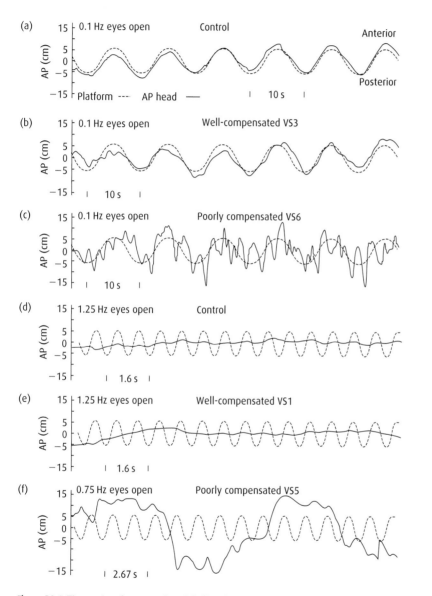

Figure 20.1. Time series of an exemplar trial of head (solid line) and platform (dashed line) AP displacement with vision available (eyes open). (a) Age-matched control at 0.1 Hz; (b) well-compensated subject at 0.1 Hz; (c) poorly compensated subject at 0.1 Hz; (d) control subject at 1.25 Hz; (e) well-compensated subject at 1.25 Hz (f) poorly compensated subject at 0.75 Hz. VS: vestibular subject. (Reprinted from Buchanan and Horak , 2001–2002, with permission from IOS Press.)

Stabilization of head and trunk

Vestibular information is important in stabilizing head and trunk motion in space (Buchanan and Horak, 2001–2002; Creath et al., 2002). When the support surface is moved sinusoidally in pitch at low frequencies, healthy subjects maintain their balance by moving their head and center of mass in phase with the platform movement (Buchanan and Horak, 2001–2002). At higher frequencies, healthy subjects switch to a "head-fixed-in-space" strategy with the result that there is little head displacement. Unlike healthy subjects, however, subjects with BVH have greater head and trunk pitch displacement and center of mass movement is coupled to platform movement regardless of the frequency of platform movement. These findings support the hypothesis that sensory information is re-weighted according to frequency of movement: at low frequencies, somatosensory information is weighted more heavily and at high frequencies of movement, vestibular information is weighted more heavily (Creath et al., 2002). Interestingly, three BVH subjects who were able to maintain balance at all frequencies were identified as being well compensated. These subjects demonstrated the same strategies as the healthy subjects at both low and high frequency of support surface rotation suggesting that some other mechanism has compensated for the lost vestibular function (Fig. 20.1; Buchanan and Horak, 2001–2002).

The role of the vestibular system in stabilizing head and trunk motion in space becomes more obvious during activities such as walking and hopping. Healthy subjects have similar gait speed and vertical amplitude of the head in the light as in the dark (Pozzo et al., 1990; Pozzo et al., 1991). In contrast, subjects with BVH modify their gait in the dark by decreasing walking speed, shortening stride length, decreasing arm swing, widening their base of support and increasing stance phase. These subjects also hold their head stiffly relative to the trunk and have a downward tilt of the head. Healthy subjects demonstrate an out-of-phase relationship between vertical head amplitude and head angular displacement. During hopping, when the head translates upward, it simultaneously rotates downward and vice versa. This acts to stabilize gaze during gait activities. Subjects with BVH do not show a clear phase relationship between head rotation and translation and the majority of BVH report oscillopsia during hopping.

20.5 The role of the vestibulo-ocular reflex in balance

It is well known that certain eye movements affect balance. For the most part, it has been assumed that the interaction between eye movements and postural stability is related to the manner in which eye movements affect the visual cues used for postural stability (Iwase et al., 1979; White et al., 1980; Oblak et al., 1983). When small saccadic eye movements are made, during which visual cues that would disturb balance are suppressed, there is little or no change in stability (Iwase et al., 1979; White et al., 1980; Oblak et al., 1983). Pursuit eye movements against a stationary background, which results in the perception of movement of the visual scene, cause an increase in sway (Strupp et al., 2003). More recent studies suggest that efference copy of the oculomotor signal may also affect postural stability (Jahn et al., 2002; Strupp et al., 2003). For example, smooth pursuit eye movements *in the dark* produce significant increases in postural sway (Strupp et al., 2003). Although it is well known that vestibular loss affects postural stability, it is less clear whether the loss of the vestibulo-ocular reflex (VOR) itself contributes to balance deficits in people with vestibular hypofunction. Logically it seems that it should – without the VOR, gaze stabilization during head movement is poor. The use of visual cues to help maintain postural stability would not be particularly useful in patients with bilateral vestibular loss because without the VOR, the eyes are not stable during head movement and visual acuity is degraded. Even at a static visual acuity of 20/40, postural stability is decreased. The issue of the degradation of visual cues during head movement coupled with our awareness that people with bilateral vestibular loss have an increased incidence and risk for falls led us to explore the possible relationship between gaze stabilization and fall risk in people with vestibular loss.

Measurement of gaze stability during head movement

One of the primary roles of the vestibular system is to stabilize gaze during head movement. When the eyes are stable in space, the image of the target of visual interest falls on the fovea of the retina and the person sees clearly while the head is moving. Patients with vestibular loss frequently complain of oscillopsia – a visual blurring or jumping of the environment during head movement (Gresty et al., 1977; Chambers et al., 1985; Bhansali et al., 1993). It is a serious problem that can result in decreased activity levels and avoidance of driving with resultant diminished independence, limited social interactions and increased isolation. Studies of people with vestibular loss typically focus on the problems of postural stability and do not address the functional problems associated with poor gaze stability. Recent methodology, a computerized test of visual acuity during head movement (dynamic

visual acuity or DVA), controls for periods in which head movement slows and fixation or pursuit eye movements, rather than the VOR, could be used to enable target identification. In the computerized DVA test, a single optotype (the letter E) is displayed on the computer monitor only when horizontal head velocity is between 120 and 180 degree/s (as measured by a Watson rate sensor). The subject is required to identity the orientation of the "E". The reliability of the computerized DVA test has been determined for both normal subjects (intraclass correlation coefficient (ICC) $r = 0.87$) and for patients with vestibular deficits (ICC $r = 0.83$; Herdman et al., 1998). Measurement of visual acuity during head movement, therefore, provides the clinician with a way of assessing the functional impact of vestibular loss.

Patients with vestibular hypofunction have a significantly greater decrement in vision during head movements than do age-matched healthy subjects (Fig. 20.2). The computerized DVA test distinguishes between both normal subjects and patients with unilateral vestibular loss and normal subjects and patients with bilateral vestibular loss. There is

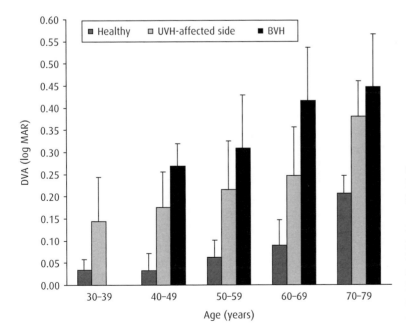

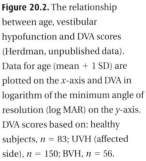

Figure 20.2. The relationship between age, vestibular hypofunction and DVA scores (Herdman, unpublished data). Data for age (mean + 1 SD) are plotted on the x-axis and DVA in logarithm of the minimum angle of resolution (log MAR) on the y-axis. DVA scores based on: healthy subjects, $n = 83$; UVH (affected side), $n = 150$; BVH, $n = 56$.

considerable overlap in DVA scores between patients with unilateral and bilateral vestibular loss. Patients with unilateral loss, however, show an asymmetry in DVA scores for head movements toward affected and unaffected sides, which is not found in the majority of patients with bilateral vestibular deficits. This asymmetry may aid in distinguishing between unilateral and bilateral vestibular loss.

DVA scores in patients with vestibular deficits reflect functional compensation as well as the degree of vestibular loss. In a series of 168 people with UVH who were seen in our clinic, 65 (38.7%) had normal DVA for age at the time of their initial clinic visit (unpublished data). There were no differences between those patients with normal DVA and those with abnormal DVA in age, gender or whether the deficit was complete or incomplete (ANOVA). The difference between groups for time from onset, however, approached significance ($P = 0.054$) with those patients with abnormal DVA having a more recent onset than those patients with normal DVA. We found a similar pattern in a series of 62 patients with BVH, 10% of whom had normal DVA on their initial visit.

20.6 The role of vestibular rehabilitation in recovery of function

Prospective, controlled studies provide evidence that the use of vestibular rehabilitation (VR) is beneficial in improving postural stability, gaze stability and in decreasing subjective complaints of disequilibrium and oscillopsia for patients with unilateral or bilateral vestibular loss (Horak et al., 1992; Krebs et al., 1993; Herdman et al., 1995; Yardley et al., 1998). Vestibular adaptation exercises evoke the error signal (retinal slip and head movement) needed to induce changes in gain in the vestibular system (Gauthier and Robinson, 1975; Zee, 1985; Herdman, 1989; Shelhamer et al., 1994; Herdman et al., 1995). VR accelerates recovery of postural stability and subjective symptoms following acute vestibular loss (Herdman et al., 1995). The VR group reported significantly less disequilibrium than the control group by the 5th day post-surgery and displayed significantly less gait ataxia than controls.

Even in individuals with chronic dizziness, VR has been found to reduce symptoms and improve postural stability (Telian et al., 1990; Horak et al., 1992; Szturm et al., 1994; Yardley et al., 1998; Black et al., 2000). Horak et al. (1992) found that 6 weeks of VR has improved balance and reduced symptoms of dizziness, while medication and general exercise only reduced symptoms. Szturm et al. (1994) compared a home program of standard vestibular habituation exercises versus customized supervised VR. The VR group demonstrated significant improvement in postural stability, whereas the home exercise group did not exhibit any significant changes. In addition, VOR asymmetry improved for the VR group, but not for home exercise group. Yardley et al. (1998) demonstrated that VR results in significant improvements in anxiety and depression, disability, motion sensitivity and performance on static tests of balance compared to standard medical care. Individuals with BVH improve following VR, but to a lesser extent than those with UVH (Krebs et al., 1993).

Vestibular exercises can influence recovery of visual acuity during head movement in patients with UVH (Herdman et al., 2003). As a group, patients who performed vestibular exercises showed a significant improvement in visual acuity during head movement ($P = 0.00001$), while those performing placebo exercises did not ($P = 0.07$). Based on stepwise regression analysis, the leading factor contributing to improvement was vestibular exercise ($P = 0.0009$).

Treatment approach to vestibular rehabilitation

Patients with vestibular hypofunction frequently complain of disequilibrium, oscillopsia and head-movement-induced dizziness, in addition to exhibiting measurable deficits of balance and mobility. Successful treatment requires careful assessment of subjective symptoms, gaze and postural stability during head movements, and use of sensory information for balance. This assessment allows establishment of a customized VR program targeted to improve the identified impairments. The goals of VR are to reduce subjective symptoms, reduce fall risk, improve gaze stability during head movements and to return the patient to normal activities, including regular physical activity, driving and work.

Vestibular rehabilitation includes exercises to promote vestibular adaptation and substitution, exercises to habituate symptoms such as dizziness with head movement, exercises to improve balance and decrease risk for falls and exercises to improve general conditioning. The exercises have the advantage of combining vestibular, visual and somatosensory cues as well as the possibility of central pre-programming to improve gaze and postural stability. Vestibular adaptation exercises are designed to increase gaze stability through long-term changes in the gain of the remaining vestibular system in response to input. The stimulus that induces adaptation is retinal slip. Substitution exercises are designed to foster the use of the visual and somatosensory systems, and of central pre-programming to substitute for lost vestibular function in order to maintain visual fixation.

Adaptation exercises

Adaptation exercises typically require that the patient attempt to fixate on a visual target during either horizontal or vertical head movement. We use brief periods of exercises, performed several times daily to attempt to induce recovery of gaze and postural stability and to improve visual acuity. Consistent head movements are maintained for between 1 and 2 min and the exercises are repeated five times throughout the day. The subject is instructed to make head movements at a velocity that is at the upper limit of their ability to see the target clearly. In the initial exercises, placement of the target on a plain wall eliminates the apparent movement of the background that would occur if the target were held in the hand. More advanced exercises are performed with the target held in the hand. Finally, some exercises will mimic the X2 magnification paradigm used in classical VOR adaptation studies (Istl-Lenz et al., 1985). That is, the target and the head are moved in opposite directions while the patient keeps the target in focus. Target distances are varied from "near" (<0.5 m) to "distant" (3 m) to simulate the range of functional challenges

of normal daily activities. Both foveal and full-field stimuli are used because they stimulate different portions of the visual field.

Substitution exercises

These exercises may act to improve gaze stability through central pre-programming. The emphasis is on having the patient perform different combinations of eye and head movements with the goal of seeing clearly during those tasks. For example, in one paradigm, the patient performs active eye and head movements between two stationary targets. In another paradigm, the patient has to try to maintain "fixation" on a remembered target while making a head movement with eyes closed. These exercises do not require that the patient make continuous head movements (as do the "adaptation" exercises). The patient performs the exercises 2–5 times daily. The following are examples of instructions used in vestibular exercises to improve gaze stability (see Table 20.1 for a sample progression of vestibular adaptation and substitution exercises):

1 To improve remaining vestibular function (X1 viewing; Fig. 20.3a):
   (a) Tape a card with a single letter or word onto the wall at eye level while you are standing 6–10 ft away.
   (b) Move your head from side to side horizontally while focusing on the letter. You should move your head as fast as you can as long as the letter stays in focus.
   (c) Repeat the exercise moving head up and down.

2 To improve remaining vestibular function (X2 viewing; Fig. 20.3b):
   (a) While standing hold a card with a single letter or word on it at arms length.
   (b) Move your head and the card back and forth in opposite directions keeping the word in focus. You should move your head and the card as fast as you can as long as the letter stays in focus. The movements will be small.

Table 20.1. Sample exercise progression.

	Exercise	Duration (min)	Frequency (times/day)	Total time*
Week 1	X1 viewing, foveal target, distant, horizontal/vertical	1	5	20
	X1 viewing, foveal target, near, horizontal/vertical	1	5	
Week 2	X1 viewing, foveal target, distant, horizontal/vertical	1	5	40
	X1 viewing, foveal target, near, horizontal/vertical	1	5	
	Active eye–head, near, horizontal/vertical	2	5	
Week 3	X1 viewing, foveal target, distant, horizontal/vertical	1.5	5	50
	X1 viewing, foveal target, near, horizontal/vertical	1.5	5	
	X1 viewing paradigm, full-field target, near, horizontal	1	5	
	Active eye–head, near, horizontal/vertical	2	3	
	Remembered targets, near, horizontal	1	3	
Week 4	X1 viewing paradigm, full-field target, near, horizontal/vertical	1	4	40
	X2 viewing paradigm, foveal target, near, horizontal/vertical	1	4	
	Active eye–head, near, horizontal/vertical	2	2	
	Remembered targets, near, horizontal/vertical	2	2	
	Walk with head turns, horizontal/vertical	2–3	2	
Week 5	X1 viewing, foveal target, near, horizontal/vertical	1	4	40
	X1 viewing paradigm, full-field target, near, horizontal/vertical	1	4	
	X2 viewing paradigm, foveal target, near, horizontal/vertical	1	4	
	Active eye–head, distant, horizontal/vertical	1	2	
	Remembered targets, near, horizontal/vertical	1	2	
	Walk with head turns, horizontal/vertical	2–3	2	
Week 6	X1 viewing paradigm, full-field target, near, horizontal/vertical	1	5	55
	X2 viewing paradigm, foveal target, near, horizontal/vertical	1.5	5	
	Active eye–head, distant, horizontal/vertical	1	5	
	Remembered targets, near, horizontal/vertical	1	5	
	Walk with head turns, horizontal/vertical, cognitive task	5	5	

* Time in minutes plus walking as an exercise.

   (c) Repeat the exercise moving head and hand up and down.

3 To improve central pre-programming (eye–head exercise):
   (a) Tape two targets ("X" and "Z") on the wall at eye level while you are sitting.
   (b) Look at the "X" with your eyes and face the "X" with your nose. Without moving your head, look directly at the "Z" with your eyes. Then while keeping your eyes on the "Z" turn your head to face the "Z". Now without moving your head look directly at the "X" with your eyes. Then while keeping your eyes on the "X" turn your head to face the "X".
   (c) Keep repeating the eye and head movements between the "X" and "Z."
   (d) Repeat the eye–head movement exercise using two targets one above the other so that you have to move your eyes and head up and down.

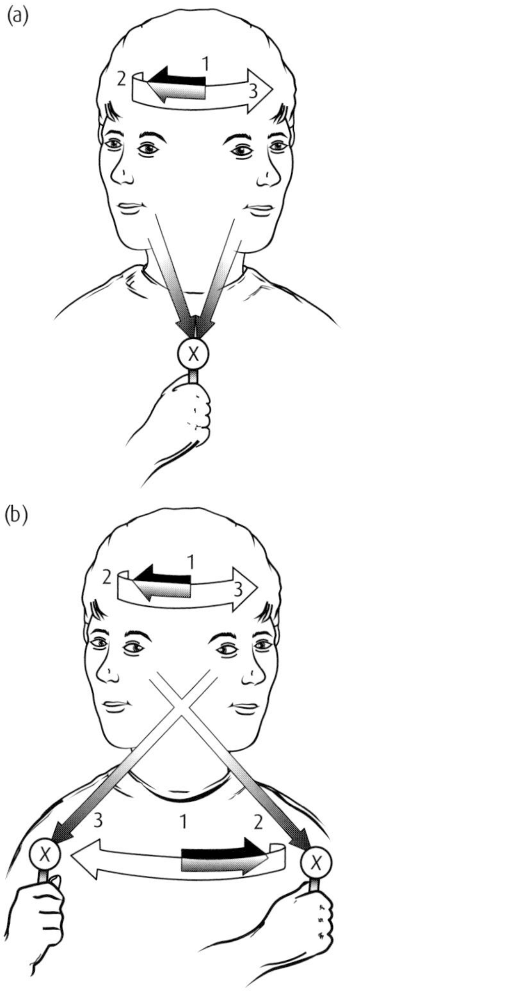

(a)

(b)

Figure 20.3. Exercises to improve remaining vestibular function require that the patient attempt to fixate on a visual target either (a) stationary, or (b) moving during either horizontal or vertical head movement. (Modified from *Vestibular Rehabilitation*, 2nd edn., Herdman, S.J. 2000, p. 437, with permission from F.A. Davis Company.)

4 To improve central pre-programming by producing a retinal position error signal (remembered target):

(a) Tape a letter on the wall 1–2 ft from you and look at it.

(b) Close your eyes and turn your head slightly imagining that your eyes are still looking at the letter. When you stop moving your head, open your eyes and check to see if you are still looking at the letter.

(c) If you had to move your eyes, you were not looking at the target anymore.

Habituation exercises

The goal of habituation exercises is to decrease symptoms of movement-induced dizziness through repeated exposure to the specific stimulus that provokes dizziness. Habituation exercises are chosen based on particular movements that provoke symptoms. The motion sensitivity quotient (MSQ) is a standardized assessment in which the patient rates intensity and duration of dizziness following each of a series of 16 position changes (Smith-Wheelock et al., 1991). A typical home program with the goal of habituation involves performance of 2–3 position changes that induce moderate intensity dizziness for 3–5 repetitions 2 times/day.

Exercise parameters

Exercise parameters that need to be monitored include intensity, frequency and duration. For example, intensity of the adaptation exercise can be modified by changing head or target velocity. Patients are encouraged to perform the exercises at the upper limit of head velocity while maintaining fixation on the target. Frequency of exercise performance varies from study to study and may vary depending on type of exercise. Significant improvements in subjective symptoms as well as improvements in postural stability have been demonstrated in several studies using a home program of vestibular adaptation and substitution exercises at a frequency of 1–5 times/day (Horak et al., 1992; Krebs et al., 1993; Herdman et al., 1995; Yardley et al., 1998). The only study to examine improvements of gaze stability and subjective complaints of oscillopsia (Herdman et al., 2003) found a significant improvement in DVA with an exercise regimen frequency of 4–5 times/day. Duration of individual exercises for the majority of studies examined was 1–2 min for each exercise. These studies found changes in outcome measures in as little as 4 weeks

(Herdman et al., 2003) in individuals with UVH and 8 weeks for individuals with BVH (Krebs et al., 1993).

Balance and gait exercises

In addition to exercises specifically geared to the vestibular system, balance exercises under challenging sensory and dynamic conditions are typically included as part of VR. Static exercises include balancing under conditions of altered somatosensory input (e.g., on a foam cushion) and reduced visual input (e.g., vision distracted by turning head or removed by closing eyes). The tasks are made more challenging by narrowing the base of support from normal stance to Romberg (feet together) to sharpened Romberg. Challenging dynamic conditions include walking with head turns, walking with quick turns to the right or left, or performing a secondary motor task while walking: for example, tossing a ball from hand to hand or to a partner or kicking a ball. As balance competence improves, adding a secondary cognitive task, such as counting backwards by threes, further increases the task challenge.

Many individuals with vestibular hypofunction limit regular physical activities; thus, while general conditioning alone does not reduce symptoms or improve postural stability (Horak et al., 1992), including physical activity is an important element of rehabilitation. We recommend that every patient start a progressive walking program, ideally outside, and increase to 20–30 min on a daily basis.

To our knowledge there is no research evidence upon which to base recommendations regarding the continuation of specific vestibular exercises beyond the typical 4–8-week rehabilitation period in order to maintain gains in gaze and postural stability. Based on our clinical experience, we recommend that individuals with BVH or sedentary individuals with UVH continue with selected exercises once or twice a day.

Falls and fall risk in people with vestibular hypofunction

Individuals with vestibular hypofunction have a greater incidence of falls than their age-matched healthy counterpart (Herdman et al., 2000). The degree of deficit appears to impact the incidence of falling: individuals with BVH have a greater incidence of falls than those with UVH (51% versus 30%). This increased incidence of falls suggests that vestibular inputs are a necessary component to adequate postural reactions to recover from a loss of balance. It supports the general concept that visual and somatosensory cues do not completely substitute for the lost vestibular signals and are unable to generate fully compensatory motor responses.

Very little research has examined the role of VR in reducing fall risk. One retrospective study of patients with bilateral vestibular loss revealed a limited reduction in fall risk as measured by dynamic gait index (DGI) scores following VR (Brown et al., 2001). Subjects exhibited significant improvements in a number of outcome measures, yet there was no difference in number of falls or use of assistive device following VR. In addition, the majority of those initially at risk for falls were still at risk at discharge following VR. In contrast, a retrospective study of individuals with UVH found evidence for significant fall risk reduction following VR (Hall et al., 2004). As a group, individuals who were initially at risk for falls improved their DGI score by 42%, from an initial DGI score of 13.8 ($\pm$3.7) out of a possible 24 to a final DGI score of 19.6 ($\pm$3.2). Furthermore, the majority of the subjects (32/47 or 68%) were at low risk for falls following rehabilitation (Fig. 20.4). The difference in results between these two studies suggests that the degree of vestibular loss influences VR outcome: an individual with bilateral vestibular loss will most likely continue to be at risk for falls while an individual with unilateral loss will most likely be at low risk for falls.

Hall et al. (2004) found that initial DGI score and initial DVA score together could be used to predict the degree of fall risk reduction that an individual would have after rehabilitation. This is the only study that has identified visual acuity during head movements as an important predictor of fall risk in people with vestibular deficits. In people with vestibular hypofunction, visual acuity degrades as a consequence of head movement, presumably

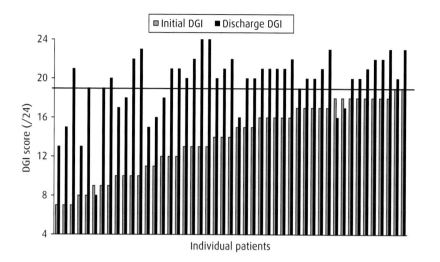

Figure 20.4. Initial DGI and discharge DGI scores are plotted for individual patients. The line is positioned at a DGI score of 19/24, which is considered at risk for falls. Scores falling above the line indicate patients who are at low risk for falls. (Adapted from Hall et al., 2004, with permission.)

because the VOR cannot effectively keep the eyes stationary in space (Herdman et al., 2001; Schubert et al., 2002; Herdman et al., 2003). In these circumstances, visual cues such as retinal target displacement, changes in image size or retinal disparity would not be as useful to maintain balance while walking (Paulus et al., 1989).

20.7 Summary

Vision, somatosensory and vestibular inputs each contribute unique information regarding body position and motion contributing to postural control. No single sensory system provides us with sufficient information to definitively determine body position and movement; therefore, the different sensory systems cannot fully substitute for each other when there is a loss of function.

The vestibular system can trigger appropriate balance responses to an external perturbation, but the primary role of vestibular inputs appears to be stabilization of the head in space. The functional outcomes of loss of vestibular function are decrements in postural stability under more challenging conditions and degradation of vision during head movements. Prospective, controlled studies provide evidence that the use of VR is beneficial in improving postural and

gaze stability as well as decreasing subjective complaints for patients with vestibular hypofunction.

REFERENCES

Allum, J.H.J. and Honegger, F. (1995). The role of proprioceptive and vestibular inputs in triggering human balance corrections. In: *Multisensory Control of Posture* (eds Mergner, T. and Hlavacka, F.), Plenum Press, New York, pp. 69–82.

Allum, J.H.J., Keshner, E.A., Honegger, F. and Pfaltz, C.R. (1988). Organization of leg–trunk–head equilibrium movements in normals and patients with peripheral vestibular deficits. *Prog Brain Res*, **76**, 277–290.

Allum, J.H., Honegger, F. and Schicks, H. (1994). The influence of a bilateral peripheral vestibular deficit on postural synergies. *J Vestibul Res*, **4**, 49–70.

Baloh, R.W., Jacobson, K.M., Enrietto, J.A., Corona, S. and Honrubia, V. (1998). Balance disorders in older persons: quantification with posturography. *Otolaryngol Head Neck Surg*, **119**, 89–92.

Berthoz, A., Lacour, M., Soechting, J.F. and Vidal, P.P. (1979). The role of vision in the control of posture during linear motion. *Prog Brain Res*, **50**, 197–209.

Bhansali, S.A., Stockwell, C.W. and Bojrab, D.I. (1993). Oscillopsia in patients with loss of vestibular function. *Otolaryngol Head Neck Surg*, **109**, 120–125.

Black, F.O., Wall, C. and Nashner, L.M. (1983). Effects of visual and support surface orientation references upon postural control in vestibular deficient subjects. *Acta Otolaryngol*, **95**, 199–201.

Black, F.O., Shupert, C.L., Horak, F.B. and Nashner, L.M. (1988). Abnormal postural control associated with peripheral vestibular disorders. *Prog Brain Res*, **76**, 263–275.

Black, F.O., Angel, C.R., Pesznecker, S.C. and Gianna, C. (2000). Outcome analysis of individualized vestibular rehabilitation protocols. *Am J Otol*, **21**, 543–551.

Bles, W., Vianney de Jong, J.M. and de Wit, G. (1983). Compensation for labyrinthine defects examined by use of a tilting room. *Acta Otolaryngol*, **95**, 576–579.

Bles, W., de Jong, J.M. and de Wit, G. (1984). Somatosensory compensation for loss of labyrinthine function. *Acta Otolaryngol*, **97**, 213–221.

Bohmer, A. and Mast, F. (1999). Chronic unilateral loss of otolith function revealed by the subjective visual vertical during off center yaw rotation. *J Vestibul Res*, **9**, 413–422.

Brandt, T., Dichgans, J. and Koenig, E. (1973). Differential effects of central verses peripheral vision on egocentric and exocentric motion perception. *Exp Brain Res*, **16**, 476–491.

Brandt, T., Paulus, W.M. and Straube, A. (1985). Visual acuity, visual field and visual scene characteristics affect postural balance. In: *Vestibular and Visual Control on Posture and Locomotor Equilibrium* (eds Igarashi, M. and Black, F.O.), Karger, Basel, pp. 93–98.

Britton, T.C., Day, B.L., Brown, P., Rothwell, J.C., Thompson, P.D. and Marsden, C.D. (1993). Postural electromyographic responses in the arm and leg following galvanic vestibular stimulation in man. *Exp Brain Res*, **94**, 143–151.

Brown, K.E., Whitney, S.L., Wrisley, D.M. and Furman, J.M. (2001). Physical therapy outcomes for persons with bilateral vestibular loss. *Laryngosc*, **111**, 1812–1817.

Buchanan, J.J. and Horak, F.B. (2001–2002). Vestibular loss disrupts control of head and trunk on a sinusoidally moving platform. *J Vestibul Res*, **11**, 371–389.

Chambers, B.R., Mai, M. and Barber, H.O. (1985). Bilateral vestibular loss, oscillopsia, and the cervico-ocular reflex. *Otolaryngol Head Neck Surg*, **93**, 403–407.

Colebatch, J.G. and Halmagyi, G.M. (1992). Vestibular evoked potentials in human neck muscles before and after unilateral vestibular deafferentation. *Neurology*, **42**, 1635–1636.

Creath, R., Kiemel, T., Horak, F. and Jeka, J.J. (2002). Limited control strategies with the loss of vestibular function. *Exp Brain Res*, **145**, 323–333.

Dichgans, J., Mauritz, K.H., Allum, J.H. and Brandt, T. (1976). Postural sway in normals and atactic patients: analysis of the stabilising and destabilizing effects of vision. *Agressologie*, **17**, 15–24.

Diener, H.C., Dichgans, J., Bruzek, W. and Selinka, H. (1982). Stabilization of human posture during induced oscillations of the body. *Exp Brain Res*, **45**, 126–132.

Diener, H.C., Dichgans, J., Guschlbauer, B. and Mau, H. (1984). The significance of proprioception on postural stabilization as assessed by ischemia. *Brain Res*, **296**, 103–109.

Gauthier, G.M. and Robinson, D.A. (1975). Adaptation of the human vestibuloocular reflex to magnifying lenses. *Brain Res*, **92**, 331–335.

Gresty, M.A., Hess, K. and Leech, J. (1977). Disorders of the vestibulo-ocular reflex producing oscillopsia and mechanisms compensating for loss of labyrinthine function. *Brain*, **100**, 693–716.

Hall, C.D., Schubert, M.C. and Herdman, S.J. (2004). Prediction of fall risk reduction as measured by dynamic gait index in individuals with unilateral vestibular hypofunction. *Otol Neurotol*, **25**, 746–751.

Halmagyi, G.M. and Colebatch, J.G. (1995). Vestibular evoked myogenic potentials in the sternomastoid muscle are not of lateral canal origin. *Acta Otolaryngol Sup*, **520**, 1–3.

Herdman, S.J. (1989). Exercise strategies for vestibular disorders. *Ear Nose Throat J*, **68**, 961–964.

Herdman, S.J., Sandusky, A.L., Hain, T.C., Zee, D.S. and Tusa, R.J. (1994). Characteristics of postural stability in patients with aminoglycoside toxicity. *J Vestibul Res*, **4**, 71–80.

Herdman, S.J., Clendaniel, R.A., Mattox, D.E., Holliday, M.J. and Niparko, J.K. (1995). Vestibular adaptation exercises and recovery: acute stage after acoustic neuroma resection. *Otolaryngol Head Neck Surg*, **113**, 77–87.

Herdman, S.J., Tusa, R.J., Blatt, P., Suzuki, A., Venuto, P.J. and Roberts, D. (1998). Computerized dynamic visual acuity test in the assessment of vestibular deficits. *Am J Otol*, **19**, 790–796.

Herdman, S.J., Blatt, P., Schubert, M.C. and Tusa, R.J. (2000). Falls in patients with vestibular deficits. *Am J Otol*, **21**, 847–851.

Herdman, S.J., Schubert, M.C. and Tusa, R.J. (2001). Role of central preprogramming in dynamic visual acuity with vestibular loss. *Arch Otolaryngol Head Neck Surg*, **127**, 1205–1210.

Herdman, S.J., Schubert, M.C., Das, V.E. and Tusa, R.J. (2003). Recovery of dynamic visual acuity in unilateral vestibular hypofunction. *Arch Otolaryngol Head Neck Surg*, **129**, 819–824.

Horak, F.B. and Hlavacka, F. (2002). Vestibular stimulation affects medium latency postural muscle responses. *Exp Brain Res*, **144**, 69–78.

Horak, F.B., Nashner, L.M. and Diener, H.C. (1990). Postural strategies associated with somatosensory and vestibular loss. *Exp Brain Res*, **82**, 167–177.

Horak, F.B., Jones-Rycewicz, C., Black, F.O. and Shumway-Cook, A. (1992). Effects of vestibular rehabilitation on dizziness and imbalance. *Otolaryngol Head Neck Surg*, **106**, 175–180.

Horak, F.B., Shupert, C.L., Dietz, V. and Horstmann, G. (1994). Vestibular and somatosensory contributions to responses to head and body displacements in stance. *Exp Brain Res*, **100**, 93–106.

Inglis, J.T., Shupert, C.L., Hlavacka, F. and Horak, F.B. (1995). Effect of galvanic vestibular stimulation on human postural responses during support surface translations. *J Neurophysiol*, **73**, 896–901.

Istl-Lenz, Y., Hyden, D. and Schwartz, D.W.F. (1985). Response of the human vestibulo-ocular reflex following long-term 2x magnified visual input. *Exp Brain Res*, **57**, 448–455.

Iwase, Y., Uchida, T., Hashimoto, M., Suzuki, N., Takemori, T. and Yamamoto, Y. (1979). The effect of eye movements on upright standing in man. *Agressologie*, **20**, 193–194 (abstract).

Jahn, K., Strupp, M., Krafczyk, S., Schuler, O., Glasauer, S. and Brandt, T. (2002). Suppression of eye movements improves balance. *Brain*, **125**, 2005–2011.

Keshner, E.A., Allum, J.H. and Pfaltz, C.R. (1987). Postural coactivation and adaptation in the sway stabilizing responses of normals and patients with bilateral vestibular deficit. *Exp Brain Res*, **69**, 77–92.

Krebs, D.E., Gill-Body, K.M., Riley, P.O. and Parker, S.W. (1993). Double-blind, placebo-controlled trial of rehabilitation for bilateral vestibular hypofunction: preliminary report. *Otolaryngol Head Neck Surg*, **109**, 735–741.

Lee, D.N. and Lishman, J.R. (1975). Visual proprioceptive control of stance. *J Hum Move Stud*, **1**, 87–95.

Li, M.W., Houlden, D. and Tomlinson, R.D. (1999). Click evoked EMG responses in sternocleidomastoid muscles: characteristics in normal subjects. *J Vestibul Res*, **9**, 327–334.

Magnusson, M., Johansson, R. and Wiklund, J. (1990). Galvanically induced body sway in the anterior–posterior plane. *Acta Otolaryngol (Stockholm)*, **110**, 11–17.

Mergner, T. and Rosemeier, T. (1998). Interaction of vestibular, somatosensory and visual signals for postural control and motion perception under terrestrial and microgravity conditions – a conceptual model. *Brain Res Rev*, **28**, 118–135.

Nashner, L.M. (1982). Adaptation of human movement to altered environments. *Trend Neurosci*, **5**, 358–361.

Nashner, L.M. and Wolfson, P. (1974). Influence of head position and proprioceptive cues on short latency postural reflexes evoked by galvanic stimulation of the human labyrinth. *Brain Res*, **67**, 255–268.

Nashner, L.M., Black, F.O. and Wall, C. (1982). Adaptation to altered support and visual conditions during stance: patients with vestibular deficits. *J Neurosci*, **2**, 536–544.

Oblak, B., Gregoric, M. and Gyergyek, L. (1983). Effects of voluntary saccades on body sway. In: *Vestibular and Visual Control on Posture and Locomotor Equilibrium* (eds Igarashi, Black), Karger, Basel, pp. 122–126.

Paulus, W.M., Straube, A. and Brandt, T. (1984). Visual stabilization of posture physiological stimulus characteristics and clinical aspects. *Brain*, **107**, 1143–1163.

Paulus, W., Straube, A., Krafczyk, S. and Brandt, T. (1989). Differential effects of retinal target displacement, changing size and changing disparity in the control of anterior/posterior and lateral body sway. *Exp Brain Res*, **78**, 243–252.

Pozzo, T., Berthoz, A. and Lefort, L. (1990). Head stabilization during various locomotor tasks in humans. I. Normal subjects. *Exp Brain Res*, **82**, 97–106.

Pozzo, T., Berthoz, A., Lefort, L. and Vitte, E. (1991). Head stabilization during various locomotor tasks in humans. II. Patients with bilateral peripheral vestibular deficits. *Exp Brain Res*, **85**, 208–217.

Runge, C.F., Shupert, C.L., Horak, F.B. and Zajac, F.E. (1998). Role of vestibular information in initiation of rapid postural responses. *Exp Brain Res*, **122**, 403–412.

Schubert, M.C., Herdman, S.J. and Tusa, R.J. (2002). Vertical dynamic visual acuity in normal subjects and patients with vestibular hypofunction. *Otol Neurotol*, **23**, 372–377.

Shelhamer, M., Tiliket, C., Roberts, D., Kramer, P.D. and Zee, D.S. (1994). Short-term vestibulo-ocular reflex adaptation in humans. II. Error signals. *Exp Brain Res*, **100**, 328–336.

Shepard, N.T. and Howarth, A.E. (1999). Vestibulocollic auditory evoked potentials: normative ranges. *Midwinter Research Meeting of the ARO*, Clearwater, Florida.

Smith-Wheelock, M., Shepard, N.T. and Telian, S.A. Physical therapy program for vestibular rehabilitation. *Am J Otol*, **12**, 218–225.

Strupp, M., Glasauer, S., Jahn, K., Schneider, E., Krafczyk, S. and Brandt, T. (2003). Eye movements and balance. *Ann NY Acad Sci*, **1004**, 352–358.

Szturm, T., Ireland, D.J. and Lessing-Turner, M. (1994). Comparison of different exercise programs in the rehabilitation of patients with chronic peripheral vestibular dysfunction. *J Vestibul Rehabil*, **4**, 461–479.

Telian, S.A., Shepard, N.T., Smith-Wheelock, M. and Kemink, J.L. (1990). Habituation therapy for chronic vestibular dysfunction: preliminary results. *Otolaryngol Head Neck Surg*, **103**, 89–95.

Tokita, T., Miyata, H. and Fujiwara, H. (1984). Postural response induced by horizontal sway of a platform. *Acta Otolaryngol Sup*, **406**, 120–124.

Vibert, D., Hausler, R. and Safran, A.B. (1999). Subjective visual vertical in peripheral unilateral vestibular diseases. *J Vestibul Res*, **9**, 145–152.

Welgampola, M.S. and Colebatch, J.G. (2001). Characteristics of tone burst-evoked myogenic potentials in the sternocleido-mastoid muscles. *Otol Neurotol*, **22**, 796–802.

White, K.D., Post, R.B. and Leibowitz, H.W. (1980). Saccadic eye movements and body sway. *Science*, **208**, 621–623.

Wolfson, L., Whipple, R., Derby, C.A., Amerman, P., Murphy, T., Tobin, J.N. and Nashner, L.M. (1992). A dynamic posturography study of balance in healthy elderly. *Neurology*, **42**, 2069–2075.

Xerri, C., Borel, L., Barthelemy, J. and Lacour, M. (1988). Synergistic interactions and functional working range of the visual and vestibular systems in postural control: neuronal correlates. *Prog Brain Res*, **76**, 193–203.

Yardley, L., Beech, S., Zander, L., Evans, T. and Weinman, J. (1998). A randomized controlled trial of exercise therapy for dizziness and vertigo in primary care. *Br J Gen Prac*, **48**, 1136–1140.

Zee, D.S. (1985). Vertigo. In: *Current Therapy in Neurologic Disease* (eds Johnson, R.T. and Griffin, J.), C.V. Mosby, St. Louis, pp. 8–13.

Deconditioning and energy expenditure

Marilyn MacKay-Lyons

School of Physiotherapy, Dalhousie University, Halifax, Nova Scotia, Canada

21.1 Introduction

The relative contributions of restoration of basic physiologic processes, neuroplasticity, and behavioral compensation to functional recovery after neurologic insult are unknown. Traditionally, the extent of recovery was viewed as being almost exclusively dependent on the state of the neuromuscular system. As a consequence, intervention strategies have focused primarily on improving the capacity of that system – an approach that has met with limited success in terms of restoring functional independence. It is now becoming clear that recovery cannot be explained solely on the basis of improved neuromuscular function. For example, Roth and colleagues (1998) determined that less than a third of the variance in disability following stroke can be explained by the extent of neurologic impairment. Recently, attention has turned to multi-system approaches to neurorehabilitation that address the interaction of neuromuscular, cardiorespiratory, and musculoskeletal systems and the environment. With growing evidence of a high prevalence of deconditioning among individuals with neurologic involvement, the interaction between the neuromuscular and cardiorespiratory systems is of particular interest.

Both primary effects of upper motor neuron damage (e.g., paralysis, spasticity, sensory-perceptual impairments) and secondary effects (e.g., contractures, inactivity, disuse muscle atrophy, fatigue) contribute to the deconditioned state of individuals with neurologic lesions. Frequently, these effects are superimposed on an already compromised cardiorespiratory system resulting from co-morbid cardiovascular disease (Kennedy, 1986; Roth, 1993) as well as lifestyle- and age-related declines in cardiorespiratory fitness (Bouchard et al., 1990). Cardiovascular and neuromuscular impairments adversely affect exercise capacity – they limit the ability to respond to physiologic stresses induced by prolonged physical effort. For people with neurologic impairment, the detrimental effects of low exercise capacity on human function are compounded by the high metabolic cost of using paretic limbs to respond to the physical demands of everyday life. The increased energy expenditure limits the cardiac reserve for other meaningful activities, with negative consequences on resistance to fatigue and quality of life.

In this chapter, an overview of basic principles of exercise metabolism is presented and acute and adaptive responses to exercise are reviewed. Factors that limit exercise capacity and contribute to the deconditioned state of people with neurologic disability are described. Biomechanical and metabolic mechanisms that help to explain the elevated energy costs of movement typical of this population are outlined, with a particular focus on pathologic gait.

21.2 Exercise capacity

Physical activity poses the greatest physiologic stress to the cardiorespiratory and neuromuscular systems. Maximal oxygen consumption (VO_{2max}), the highest oxygen (O_2) intake an individual can attain during physical work (Wasserman et al., 1999), is generally considered the definitive index of exercise capacity (Foster et al., 1996). Exercise requires increased energy metabolism to fuel skeletal, cardiac, and respiratory muscle activity. At rest, skeletal muscle accounts for less than 20% of the body's total energy expenditure; the brain, comprising only 2% of body weight, also consumes 20% of the available O_2 (Zauner et al., 2002). During exercise, most of the increased energy metabolism occurs within the active muscles (American College of Sports Medicine, 2000). Interaction of the cardiorespiratory and neuromuscular systems is needed to respond to the energy demands of contracting muscle and increased concentrations of carbon dioxide (CO_2) and hydrogen ions (H^+) – by-products of muscle metabolism.

Physiologic responses to acute exercise

The relationship between cardiovascular function and VO_{2max} is described by the Fick equation (Rowell, 1974):

$$VO_{2max} = Q_{max} \times AVO_{2max} \text{ difference} \qquad (21.1)$$

where Q_{max} is maximal cardiac output and AVO_{2max} difference is maximal arteriovenous O_2 difference. Given that Q_{max} equals the product of maximal heart rate (HR_{max}) and maximal stroke volume (SV_{max}),

$$VO_{2max} = HR_{max} \times SV_{max} \times AVO_{2max} \text{ difference}$$
$$(21.2)$$

Thus, VO_{2max} reflects both O_2 transport to the tissues and O_2 utilization by the tissues. Increases in VO_{2max} during exercise are due to both increased Q_{max} and AVO_2 difference, with Q_{max} at VO_{2max} rising three to six times above resting levels, HR increasing 200–300%, and SV about 50%. Over the lower third of the workload range, both HR and SV increase progressively; thereafter, HR continues to increase while SV remains essentially constant (Hartley et al., 1969; Higginbotham et al., 1986). The increase in SV is due to enhanced myocardial contractility and increased venous return, secondary to compression of the veins

by contracting muscles and reduced intrathoracic pressure (Camm, 1996). At low-intensity exercise, increases in HR are mainly the result of decreased vagal tone but, as exercise intensifies, sympathetic stimulation and circulating catecholamines become progressively more important (Whipp, 1994).

Selective distribution of the increased blood flow to regions with heightened metabolic demands – the working muscles – is due to local vasodilation mediated mainly by metabolites acting on the vascular smooth muscle (e.g., CO_2/H^+, nitric oxide, potassium ions, adenosine) and vasoconstriction in tissue with low metabolic demand (Saltin, 1985). Blood flow to other vascular beds either is unchanged or decreases (e.g., renal and splanchnic bed) through active vasoconstriction resulting primarily from increased sympathetic discharge. Cerebral blood flow and O_2 delivery during exercise have been found to either remain stable (Madsen et al., 1993; Hellstrom et al., 1996) or increase slightly (Linkis et al., 1995; Pott et al., 1997). As exercise intensity increases, systolic blood pressure increases markedly while diastolic blood pressure either remains unchanged or lowers slightly, resulting in a moderate increase in mean arterial pressure (Wasserman et al., 1999). The process of cerebral autoregulation ensures that regional and total cerebral blood flow and normal tissue oxygenation are maintained over a wide range of blood pressures (Busija and Heistad, 1984).

O_2 extraction from the muscle capillary blood to mitochondria is dependent on an adequate O_2 diffusion gradient. During a progressive increase in workload, arterial hemoglobin saturation and arterial O_2 content remain relatively constant, whereas the venous O_2 content decreases substantially due to increased O_2 extraction in the active muscles (Wasserman et al., 1967). As the metabolic rate rises, the minute ventilation (VE) increases to remove CO_2 and to regulate pH balance. At low-intensity exercise, increases in VE are mainly due to increased tidal volume whereas at higher intensities the respiratory rate increases without substantial change in tidal volume (Wasserman et al., 1999). At maximal workloads the O_2 cost of breathing may be as much as 10% of VO_{2max}, with the accessory inspiratory muscles and the abdominal muscles sharing the mechanical work of breathing with the diaphragm (Clausen, 1977).

Measurement of exercise capacity

Under standardized conditions that assure: (i) adequate duration and work intensity by at least 50% of total muscle mass; (ii) independence from motivation or skill of the subject; and (iii) standardized environmental conditions (Rowell, 1974), VO_{2max} is a stable and highly reproducible measure of maximal aerobic capacity with variability of repeated measurements being 2–4% (Taylor et al., 1955). Values for VO_{2max} can be expressed in absolute terms (l of O_2/min) or relative to body mass (ml of O_2/kg/min). The optimal duration of a graded exercise test is 8–17 min (Buchfuhrer et al., 1983).

The exercise modality can affect VO_{2max} values. In comparison to the cycle ergometer, the treadmill increases the potential to recruit sufficient muscle mass to elicit a maximal metabolic response, particularly in deconditioned populations (Rowell, 1974). With bike ergometry 85–90% of the VO_{2max} achieved with treadmill testing can be attained while only 70% can be achieved with either arm or supine ergometry (Rowell, 1974). The treadmill is the preferred modality for measuring exercise capacity, not only because it yields higher VO_{2max} values but also because the pattern of muscle activation in treadmill walking is consistent with that used for the majority of mobility tasks and is, therefore, the most functionally relevant mode of testing. However, in patients with neuromuscular conditions, balance and motor control problems often preclude the use of standard treadmill testing protocols. Recently, we devised an exercise protocol to permit safe and valid testing of VO_{2max} early after stroke. The protocol incorporates the use of a body weight-support system, a device originally designed to offset a percentage of body mass and to provide external balance support, thereby permitting treadmill walking of people in the early stages of neurologic recovery (Fig. 21.1). A validation study demonstrated that unweighting of 15% of body mass did not affect VO_{2max} values and, thus, did not

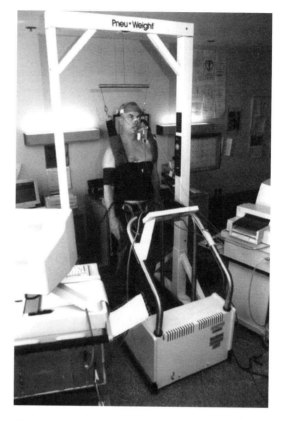

Figure 21.1. Body weight-supported treadmill set-up for measuring exercise capacity early after neurologic insult. The support system consists of a harness, overhead suspension and a pneumatic compressor to vertically displace a prescribed amount of body mass. The electrocardiograph is to the left and the metabolic cart to measure O_2 consumption is to the right.

confound interpretation of the test results (MacKay-Lyons et al., 2001).

The principal criterion to indicate maximal effort during VO_{2max} testing is attainment of a plateau in VO_{2max} beyond which there is less than 150 ml/min increase in VO_2 despite increases in workload (Taylor et al., 1955). When a VO_{2max} plateau is not observed, as is common in deconditioned or elderly individuals (Howley et al., 1995) or in patients with heart disease, the preferred term for the value obtained is peak VO_2 (VO_{2peak}). The essentially linear relationship between VO_2 and HR permits the estimation of VO_{2max} from

HR measurements taken during submaximal exercise. However, unlike VO_{2max}, HR is markedly affected by many stresses (e.g., dehydration, changes in body temperature, acute starvation), thus limiting the accuracy of the estimation (Rowell, 1974).

Factors affecting exercise capacity

The main factors contributing to individual differences in exercise capacity are sex, age, and level of physical activity. Absolute and relative VO_{2max} of women is about 77% of that of men, after adjusting for body weight and activity level (Bruce et al., 1973). Age-associated structural and functional changes, increased inactivity and body fat, loss of co-ordination and flexibility, and co-morbidities (e.g., arthritis, cardiovascular disease) restrict physical work capacity. The decline in VO_{2max} – approximately 1% per year (0.4–0.5 ml/kg/min/year) between 25 and 75 years of age (Åstrand and Rodahl, 1986) – is due to the reduced O_2-transporting and utilization capacity associated with cardiac, respiratory, and muscular changes. Increasing myocardial stiffness and decreased contractility are manifested by reductions in ejection fraction and HR_{max} – hallmarks of cardiovascular aging (Stratton et al., 1994). In addition, reduced elastic recoil of the lung, and calcification and stiffening of the cartilagenous articulations of the ribs restrict compliance of the lungs, thus limiting increases in VE during exercise (Frontera and Evans, 1986). Age-related decline in oxidative capacity of the working muscles has been attributed to alterations in mitochondrial structure and distribution, changes in skeletal muscle microcirculation, and sarcopenia due to reduced number and size of fibers, particularly type II fibers (Jackson et al., 1995).

Cardiovascular alterations resulting from physical inactivity parallel, in many ways, the changes that occur with aging, including reduced VO_{2max} and Q_{max}. Lack of physical activity explains a significant proportion of the age-related decline in VO_{2max}. In fact, if physical activity levels and body composition remain constant over time, the expected rate of decline in aerobic power is reduced by almost 50% (Jackson et al., 1995). Significant reductions in

VO_{2max} following short periods of bedrest have been reported – a 15% reduction in healthy, middle-aged men after 10 days of recumbency (Convertino, 1982) and a 28% reduction in healthy young subjects after 3 weeks (Saltin et al., 1968). Such rapid loss of aerobic capacity has been attributed to both central changes (decreased SV due to impaired myocardial function and increased venous pooling) and peripheral changes (decreases in oxidative enzyme concentrations, mitochondria, and capillary density) (Whipp, 1994).

Exercise capacity of patients with neurologic impairment

A major obstacle to documenting exercise capacity of individuals with neurologic impairments has been the lack of testing protocols that can accommodate motor and balance disturbances. Table 21.1 summarizes VO_{2peak} data from studies of common neurologic conditions. Despite differences in subject characteristics and testing protocols across studies, it is apparent that most individuals are significantly deconditioned. Levels of VO_{2max} less than 84% of normative values are considered pathologic (Wasserman et al., 1999); the minimum VO_{2max} needed to meet the physiologic demands of independent living is about 15 ml/kg/min (Convertino, 1982). Further, for patients with coronary artery disease – a co-morbidity common in people with neuromuscular impairments – VO_{2max} levels less than 21 ml/kg/min place them in a high mortality group whereas those with levels greater than 35 ml/kg/min are in the excellent survival group (Morris et al., 1991).

A diversity of variables contributes to the deconditioned state of individuals with neuromuscular impairment. Factors that explain differences in exercise capacity across all populations (e.g., age and physical activity level) are confounded by the primary effects of upper motor neuron damage. For example, Stanghelle and Festvåg (1997) reported that deterioration in VO_{2peak} in individuals with postpolio syndrome over a 3–5 year period was 12% greater than the decline predicted from increasing age. Physical activity among persons with multiple

Table 21.1. Acute cardiovascular responses to dynamic exercise in individuals with neuromuscular impairments.

Diagnosis	n	Sex (M/F)	Age (years)	Time since diagnosis	Test modality	VO_{2peak} (ml/kg/min)	VO_{2peak} (% normal)	Reference
Stroke	100	56/44	70 ± 10	76 ± 3 days	Cycle ergometer	11.4 ± 3	NR	Duncan et al. (2003)
	42	23/19	56 ± 12	>6 months	Cycle ergometer	15.8 ± 5	NR	Potempa et al. (1995)
	29	22/7	65 ± 14	26 ± 9 days	Treadmill	14.4 ± 5	61	MacKay-Lyons and Makrides, (2002)
	26	22/4	66 ± 9	>6 months	Treadmill	15.6 ± 4	NR	Ryan et al. (2000)
	17	13/4	61 ± 16	29 ± 10 days	Semirecumbent cycle ergometer	14.7 ± 4	51	Kelly et al. (2003)
	12	12/0	59 ± 10	15 ± 7 days	Cycle ergometer	8.3 ± 2	NR	da Cunha Filho et al. (2001)
Multiple sclerosis	46	15/31	40 ± 2	7 ± 1 years	Arm–leg ergometer	25.2 ± 1	79	Petajan et al. (1996)
	10	4/6	39 ± 6	3 ± 5 years	Arm–leg ergometer	39.0 ± 8	87	Ponichtera-Mulcare et al. (1995)
Paraplegia	46	46/0	33 ± 9	>3 years	Wheelchair ergometer	23.9 ± 5	NR	Paré et al. (1993)
	39	39/0	30 ± 1	6 months	Arm ergometer	19.4 ± 1	69	Lin et al. (1993)
	9	9/0	30 ± 7	21 ± 8 years	Arm ergometer	30.5 ± 8	71	Price and Campbell (1999)
	6	6/0	36 ± 10	7 ± 5 years	Arm ergometer	23.7 ± 3	NR	Jacobs et al. (2002)
Tetraplegia	8	8/0	24 ± 4	7 ± 6 years	Arm ergometer	12.1 ± 1	NR	DiCarlo (1988)
Traumatic brain injury	40	29/11	33 ± 11	2 ± 4 years	Treadmill	23.5 ± 7	NR	Mossberg et al. (2002)
	36	28/8	32 ± 10	17 ± 17 months	Cycle ergometer	22.3 ± 9	65	Bhambhani et al. (2003)
	14	13/1	29 ± 2	NR	Treadmill	31.3 ± 2	67	Jankowski and Sullivan (1990)
Parkinson disease	20	13/7	64 ± 7	9 ± 4 years	Cycle ergometer	22.0 ± 7	100	Stanley et al. (1999)
	16	13/3	54 ± 5	6 ± 3 years	Cycle ergometer	27.6 ± 5	93	Canning et al. (1997)
Guillain Barré syndrome	1	1/0	57	3 years	Leg-arm ergometer	27	NR	Pitetti et al. (1993)
Postpolio syndrome	68	23/45	53 ± 11	11 ± 8 years	Cycle ergometer ($n = 37$), arm ergometer ($n = 31$)	23.1 ± 5 15.3 ± 5	63 65	Stanghelle et al. (1993)
	32	16/16	50 ± 10	46 ± 3 years	Cycle ergometer	20.5 ± 7	74	Willén et al. (1999)
	20	10/10	43 ± 6	11–45 years	Cycle ergometer	17.7 ± 6	73	Kriz et al. (1992)

VO_{2peak}: peak oxygen consumption; VO_{2peak} % normal: peak oxygen consumption expressed as a percentage of normative values; NR: not reported.

sclerosis is often avoided in order to prevent elevated body temperature and minimize symptoms of fatigue (Ng and Kent-Braun, 1997). Pathologic changes in paretic muscle increase the likelihood of abnormally low exercise capacity. Reduction in the number of recruitable motor units available for physical work (Dietz et al., 1986), altered muscle fiber distribution and recruitment patterns (Jakobsson et al., 1991), and diminished capacity for oxidative metabolism in paretic muscles (Landin et al., 1977) lower the oxidative potential. In addition, central nervous system trauma, particularly involving the spinal cord, may disrupt the autonomic reflexes and sympathetic vasomotor outflow required for normal cardiovascular responses to exercise (Glaser, 1986). Resulting "circulatory hypokinesis" – reduced cardiac output at a given VO_2 resulting from reduced venous return – impairs delivery of O_2 and nutrients to and removal of metabolites from working muscles, intensifying muscle fatigue (Davis and Shephard, 1988).

Cardiovascular co-morbidity, prevalent in neurologic populations, can restrict exercise capacity. About 75% of patients poststroke have underlying cardiovascular dysfunction (Roth, 1993). Cardiorespiratory complications are the leading causes of death in persons with stroke (Matsumoto et al., 1973), multiple sclerosis (Sadovnick et al., 1991), and spinal cord injury (Kennedy, 1986). Cardiac dysfunction contributes to lower aerobic capacity through two principal mechanisms: ischemia-induced reductions in ejection fraction and SV with exercise (Clausen et al., 1973) and chronotropic incompetence – the inability to increase HR in proportion to the metabolic demands of exercise (Camm, 1996). Respiratory impairment, either as a direct complication of neuromuscular condition (e.g., muscle weakness, impaired breathing mechanics) or secondary to cardiovascular dysfunction or lifestyle factors (e.g., physical inactivity, smoking habits), may limit O_2 availability for exercise (Vingerhoets and Bogousslavsky, 1994; Wiercisiewski and McDeavitt, 1998). Neu et al. (1967) reported an 87% incidence of obstructive pulmonary dysfunction in patients with Parkinson disease; however, despite respiratory compromise

in this patient group, VO_{2peak} levels tend to be within the range of normal values (Canning et al., 1997; Stanley et al., 1999).

Long-term adaptations to exercise training

Endurance training using dynamic exercises of adequate intensity, duration, and frequency provokes central and peripheral adaptations in proportion to the stress imposed on the heart and working skeletal muscles, respectively (Clausen et al., 1973). To induce central adaptations, training must incorporate large muscle mass activities in order to attain high levels of VO_2. The principal indicator of a training effect during maximal exercise is attainment of a higher VO_{2max} than was achieved in the pre-trained state. Healthy individuals with similar pre-training exercise capacity demonstrate comparable exercise trainability regardless of age or sex (Lewis et al., 1986). However, the greatest increments in VO_{2max} occur with the lowest initial values of VO_{2max} (Saltin, 1969).

Training-induced increases in VO_{2max} are due primarily to improved cardiac output (Hartley et al., 1969). Maximal HR remains unchanged with training; thus, higher SV secondary to enhanced myocardial contractility accounts for the higher output (Clausen, 1977). With training, there is decreased vasoconstriction in the non-working muscles and improved venous return, thus, a training-induced increase in Q_{max} can occur without a concomitant increase in mean arterial pressure (Clausen, 1977). Training does not, however, have a substantial effect on blood hemoglobin content and coronary blood flow (Clausen et al., 1973). Its effect on ejection fraction remains unclear (Franklin et al., 1992). Improved AVO_2 difference in the exercising muscle tissue has been attributed to increases in size and number of mitochondria, myoglobin levels, Krebs' cycle enzymes (e.g., succinate dehydrogenase), and respiratory chain enzymes (e.g., cytochrome oxidase) (Whipp, 1994), as well as increased capillary density (Saltin, 1985).

The mechanisms underlying the training-induced bradycardic response at a fixed submaximal workload may be explained by a concomitant elevation in total blood volume (Wilmore et al., 1996), an increase in vagal activity, a reduction in sympathetic-adrenergic drive, or a reduction in resting HR (Casaburi, 1994). However, Wilmore et al. (1996) reported that the small decrease in resting HR is of minimal physiologic significance. Although arterial blood pressure at a given work rate is often unchanged with training, there is lowering of the rate-pressure product (Ogawa et al., 1992), reflecting improved cardiac efficiency (Nelson et al., 1974). In addition, demand for increased anaerobic metabolism is delayed due to the improved capacity for aerobic exercise; thus the lactate threshold is elevated and the VE at a given submaximal workload is reduced (Casaburi, 1994). After training, O_2 consumption at a given submaximal workload is either unchanged (Hartley et al., 1969) or modestly reduced (Gardner et al., 1989) because the increased AVO_2 difference in trained muscles is offset by reduced blood flow to the working muscles and a less pronounced decrease in blood flow to the non-exercising muscles resulting from depressed sympathetic reflex activity (Clausen, 1977).

Factors limiting the capacity of healthy individuals to respond to physical work have not been identified conclusively. The respiratory system, AVO_2 difference, and metabolic capacity of the muscles have not been implicated as principal limiting factors (Rowell, 1974; Andersen and Saltin, 1985); thus, the main limitation appears to be cardiac output.

Long-term adaptations in individuals with neurologic conditions

Controlled trials of the adaptability of the cardiorespiratory system to exercise after neurologic insult are lacking; hence effective training regimens remain unclear. In the past, emphasis in neurorehabilitation was placed on neuromuscular impairments because motor and postural control was considered the main factor limiting functional recovery. Also, clinicians were apprehensive about increased risk of falls, detrimental cardiac responses, and aggravation of spasticity to the overload needed to achieve a training effect; however, such concerns have not been substantiated (Smith et al., 1999; Teixeira-Salmela et al., 1999; Saunders et al., 2004). In fact, there is evidence from studies of spinal cats (Coté et al., 2003) and humans with spinal cord injury (Trimble et al., 1998) that treadmill training may reduce spasticity by improving stretch reflex modulation.

Traditional modes of aerobic training have been used for patients with neuromuscular conditions – leg ergometer, arm ergometer, and arm–leg ergometer (Fig. 21.2.). In addition, innovative approaches have recently been introduced to overcome limitations to exercise training imposed by upper motor neuron damage. For example, a combination of electric stimulation of lower-extremity muscles and voluntary upper extremity rowing has been applied to patients post spinal cord injury to augment the muscle activation needed to achieve a training effect (Wheeler et al., 2002). Body weight-supported treadmill training, originally designed for early gait retraining poststroke (Barbeau and Visitin, 2003), has been pilot tested as a training mode for patients early poststroke (da Cunha Filho et al., 2001) (Fig. 21.3). To enhance attention to the task of exercising in patients post traumatic brain injury, Grealy and colleagues (1999) used a virtual reality recumbent ergometer. The authors postulated that the interaction between the training apparatus and the participant might potentiate structural changes in the brain.

The findings of the few training studies that measured VO_{2peak} suggest that improvements in cardiovascular adaptation to physical work are possible in neurologic populations (Table 21.2). In some studies, the magnitude of change in VO_{2peak} was comparable to the 15% gain reported for healthy, sedentary adults (Samitz and Bachl, 1991) and the 13–15% gains for participants in cardiac rehabilitation (Franklin et al., 1978; Mertens and Kavanagh, 1996). Variability in the results is attributable to many factors, including differences in mode and intensity of training, disparities in level of compliance with exercise regime, and variation in neurologic condition, severity and time post insult. The largest increments in VO_{2peak} tended to occur with the most deconditioned subjects, consistent with findings for people without impairments (Saltin, 1969).

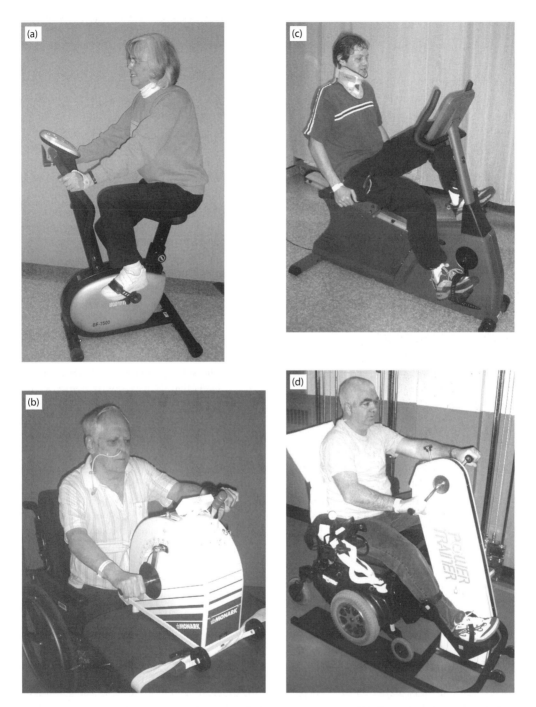

Figure 21.2. Examples of modes of exercise training used in neurorehabilitation. (a) The leg ergometer is appropriate for people with adequate lower-extremity control and sitting balance. (b) The arm ergometer may be used when lower-extremity strength is insufficient for leg ergometry; however, a disadvantage with the arm ergometer is the smaller muscle mass activated when movement is restricted to the upper extremities. (c) The recumbent leg ergometer can be used in place of the standard leg ergometer if sitting balance is impaired. (d) The arm–leg ergometer can be propelled by a combination of lower and upper extremities and therefore is suitable for individuals with hemiparesis or quadriparesis.

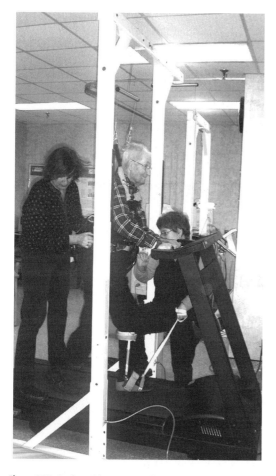

Figure 21.3. Body weight-supported treadmill walking has been introduced as an aerobic training mode for patients in the early stages of neurologic recovery. This patient is walking at a low treadmill speed (0.6 km/h) with 30% body weight support, and manual guidance by two physiotherapists – one to assist advancement of the hemiparetic lower extremity and one to stabilize the pelvis to achieve symmetry of the gait pattern.

Most of the training studies in Table 21.2 involved patients with chronic neurologic impairments; however, the optimal time to introduce training is unknown. Macko et al. (1997) expressed caution about training in the early poststroke period, reasoning that abnormal cardiovascular responses to exercise (e.g., hypotension, dysrhythmia) may impede perfusion of ischemic brain tissue during the period

when cerebral autoregulation is most often impaired. Nevertheless, in a recent study da Cunha Filho and colleagues (2001) training was initiated 8–21 days after stroke without complications.

In addition to improved exercise capacity, other benefits of training realized by healthy populations are also attainable for individuals with neuromuscular impairments. For example, a 15-week training program for patients with multiple sclerosis resulted in decreases in skinfold thickness, triglycerides, and very-low-density lipoprotein and improvements in upper- and lower-extremity strength and quality-of-life measures (i.e., depression, fatigue, social interaction) (Petajan et al., 1996). An 8-week training program for patients early after spinal cord injury led to improved lipid profiles, with more pronounced changes in response to high-intensity training (de Groot et al., 2003). Gordon et al (1998) speculated that the improved cognitive function observed in individuals with traumatic brain injury who exercised on a regular basis may be attributed to exercise-induced increases in brain-derived neurotrophic factor (BDNF) or other growth factors. Neeper and colleagues (1995) were the first to note upregulation of BDNF in the cerebral cortex of rats with free access to a running wheel. Since then, several investigators have demonstrated in rodent models that voluntary running induces BDNF production and synaptic plasticity in the brain (Molteni et al., 2002; Farmer et al., 2004) and spinal cord, (Gomez-Pinilla et al., 2002) and that these responses appear to be dose dependent (Tong et al., 2001). Moreover, Van Praag and colleagues (1999) found *in vitro* evidence of neurogenesis in the dendate gyrus of adult mice exposed to an enriched environment that included voluntary wheel running.

There is a possibility that "spontaneous" increases in exercise capacity can occur during neurologic recovery. Recently, we reported a mean increase of 17% in VO_{2peak} over the course of a stroke rehabilitation program that lacked a specific aerobic training component (MacKay-Lyons and Makrides, 2004). Similar findings of cardiovascular adaptations without formal exercise training have been reported in patients recovering from myocardial infarction

Table 21.2. Long-term cardiorespiratory adaptations to aerobic exercise training programs in individuals with neuromuscular impairments.

Diagnosis	n	Training mode	Duration (weeks)	Frequency (x/week)	Duration (min)	Intensity	Change in VO_{2peak} %	Reference
Stroke	44 E 48 C	Stationary bicycle	12	3	20–30	40 rpm	+9 +0.5	Duncan et al. (2003)
	19 E 23 C	Stationary bicycle	10	3	30	50–70 rpm	+13 +1	Potempa et al. (1995)
	29 E	Aerobic exercise	12	3	30	Target HR = [(HR at RER = 1) − 15]	+8	Rimmer et al. (2000)
	23 E	Treadmill	26	3	20	60% of HRR	+10	Macko et al. (2001)
	6 E 6 C	Treadmill with BWS	2–3	5	20	NR	+35 +1	da Cunha Filho et al. (2001)
Multiple sclerosis	21 E 25 C	Arm–leg ergometry	15	3	30	60% of VO_{2peak}	+22 +1	Petajan et al. (1996)
C_7–T_{12} spinal cord injury	6 E	FES-assisted rowing	6	3	30	75–80% of VO_{2peak}	+11	Wheeler et al. (2002)
Spinal cord injury	18 E	FES-assisted ergometry	12–16	3	30	0–31 W	+23	Hooker et al. (1992)
Tetraplegia	8 E	Arm ergometer	8	3	30	50–60% of HRR or 60 rpm	+94	DiCarlo, (1988)
Traumatic brain injury	40 E	Low-intensity aerobic exercises	16	3	15–20	"Low"	+3	Mossberg et al. (2002)
	14 E	Circuit training	16	3	45	70% of VO_{2peak}	+15	Jankowski and Sullivan (1990)
Guillain Barré syndrome	1 E	Arm–leg ergometer	16	3	20	75–85% HR_{max}	+9	Pitetti et al. (1993)
Postpolio syndrome	16 E 21E	Cycle ergometer	16	3	15–30	70% HR_{max}	+15 +4	Jones et al. (1989)
	10 E 10 C	Arm ergometer	16	3	20	70–75% HRR or 50–60 rpm or RPE_{6-20} = 13	+19 −1	Kriz et al. (1992)

E: experimental; C: control; rpm: revolutions per minute; BWS: body weight support; FES: functional electrical stimulation; HRR: HR reserve; RPE: rating of perceived exertion.

(De Busk et al., 1979; Savin et al., 1981; Sheldahl et al., 1984). Dressendorfer and colleagues (1995) hypothesized that the metabolic demands of unregulated daily activities after myocardial infarction may result in an insidious training effect. Bjuro et al. (1975) provided indirect support for that notion by demonstrating that VO_2 levels of patients poststroke performing household chores were almost twice the normative values.

Whether improvements in exercise capacity in neurologic populations result from central or peripheral mechanisms involved in O_2 transport and utilization has not been determined. For patients with coronary artery disease and an intact nervous system, central adaptations (e.g., reduced myocardial VO_2 demand, increased maximal coronary blood flow) have been shown to be more highly correlated with changes in exercise capacity than skeletal muscle adaptations (e.g., increased succinate dehydrogenase activity and muscle hypertrophy) (Fergueson et al., 1982).

21.3 Energy expenditure

Bjuro et al. (1975) reported that the O_2 consumption of patients poststroke performing household activities was 75–88% of VO_{2peak}, almost twice that of the healthy control subjects. Not surprisingly, a quality-of-life study of patients poststroke reported that poor energy levels outranked mobility limitations, pain, emotional reactions, sleep disturbances, and social isolation as the area of greatest personal concern (Johansson et al., 1992). Most studies of energy expenditure after neuromuscular impairment have focused on locomotion since it is the principal form of human physical activity, and for many people, the only departure from a sedentary life (Passmore and Durnin, 1955). Although there are countless strategies possible to produce locomotion, the dominant influences that shape gait kinetics and kinematics appear to be the minimization of metabolic energy costs and the reduction of musculoskeletal stresses. In this section, biomechanical and metabolic factors will be discussed in relation to the energy expenditure of normal gait and that of individuals with neurologic conditions.

Biomechanical and metabolic factors

From a mechanical perspective, the total muscular work of walking equals the sum of the *external work* (i.e., the work to accelerate and lift the center of mass at each step) and *internal work* (i.e., the work

of sustaining basal metabolic rate and moving the limbs relative to the trunk), both of which require metabolic energy (Dean, 1965; Cavagna and Kaneko, 1977). Energy changes in leg segments account for about 80% of the energy costs of the forward translation of the body (i.e., external work), with the remaining 20% due energy changes resulting from vertical and lateral displacement of the center of gravity of the head, arms, and trunk (Winter et al., 1976). In an idealized "inverted pendulum" model of locomotion, all kinetic energy would be converted into potential energy during the first half of stance and stored until needed as kinetic energy during the second half of stance. In human gait, however, the lower extremities do not behave exactly as rigid struts and complete recovery of mechanical energy is not achieved. Therefore, only 60–70% of the mechanical energy required to lift and accelerate the COM is conserved (Cavagna et al., 1976), resulting in a net expenditure of energy (Saunders et al., 1953).

Concentric and eccentric muscular contractions during walking exert moments of force about the joints, generating substantial internal work (Williams, 1985), whereas the contributions from elastic storage and limitations in joint range to internal work are minimal (Dean, 1965; Cavagna and Kaneko, 1977). Significant net muscle moments occur during the stance phase, particularly the plantarflexion moment at pre-swing (Winter, 1983; Olney et al., 1991). While net muscle moments at hip and knee vary dramatically, limb kinematics are similar, supporting the notion that different motor strategies produce kinematically normal gait provided that the overall objective of minimizing the total muscular effort is attained (Winter, 1980). Despite this flexibility, a dominant feature of human locomotion is its stereotypical pattern, which has been attributed to the automaticity bestowed by pre-programmed central locomotor commands (Knutsson, 1981).

The metabolic demands of walking or other dynamic exercise are determined by the amount of work done and the efficiency of the muscles (Wasserman et al., 1967). Muscular efficiency, the ratio of the work accomplished to the energy expended during steady-state work (Stainsby et al.,

1980), is dependent on the efficiency of both phosphorylative-coupling and contraction-coupling processes (Whipp and Wasserman, 1969). Widely divergent values of muscular efficiency ratios for walking have been reported, ranging from 31% (Donovan and Brooks, 1977) to 67% (Pierrynowski et al., 1980). The metabolic cost of level walking is typically expressed as VO_2 per kilogram of body weight per unit distance traveled (ml O_2/kg/m) (Waters and Yakura, 1989) or in units of kcal/min (de V. Weir, 1949).

Factors affecting energy expenditure

Factors that help to explain differences in the economy of movement in healthy populations include age, walking environment, and walking speed (Martin and Morgan, 1992). Gender does not affect energy costs after adjusting for differences in resting metabolic rate, percent body fat, physical activity level, and walking speed (Davies and Dalsky, 1997; Morio et al., 1997). Older, healthy individuals not only have reduced muscular efficiency and higher relative energy costs of walking but also smaller aerobic reserves, and consequently, decreased ability to accommodate additional physiologic penalties such as a neurologic gait disorder. Walking on a compliant surface results in energy-consuming deformation of the surface, thereby increasing energy expenditure (Dean, 1965). The overall efficiency of uphill walking decreases as grade increases, primarily due to increases in external work (Minetti et al., 1993). Studies comparing energy costs of overground and treadmill walking have reported no differences (Ralston, 1960) or slightly reduced costs on the treadmill (Pearce et al., 1983).

Preferred speed of walking approximates the most economical speed, reflecting the tendency of biologic systems to self-optimize. At the speed where the aerobic demand is the lowest, the magnitudes of the fluctuations in kinetic and gravitational potential energy are similar; thus energy exchange is maximized and the muscular work minimized (Cavagna and Kaneko, 1977; Mansour et al., 1982). A U-shaped speed–energy relationship is apparent for normal gait, with minimum aerobic demands occurring at

1.2–1.4 m/s (Corcoran and Brengelmann, 1970; Pearce et al., 1983). Most individuals with neurologic impairment are unable to walk at optimal speed due to poor motor control, decreased power, instability, fear of falling, and avoidance of musculoskeletal stress. Moreover, the slopes of the U-shaped speed–energy curve of hemiparetic gait are steeper than normal, resulting in a higher rise in VO_2 for a given change in speed (Corcoran and Brengelmann, 1970).

Overt pathologic disturbances can have surprisingly little influence on the fundamental gait pattern (Winter, 1980), but ineffective compensatory strategies can result in high energy costs of locomotion, increased cardiovascular burden, and limitations in the type and duration of daily activities (Saunders et al., 1953). The cost of walking has been reported to be two times (Dasco et al., 1963; da Cunha Filho et al., 2003) to three times (Hash, 1978) higher than control values for people poststroke, four times greater for persons with incomplete spinal cord injuries (da Cunha Filho et al., 2003) and two times (Olgiati et al., 1988) to three times (Olgiati et al., 1986) normal values for people with multiple sclerosis.

The mechanisms underlying the elevated energy costs characteristic of neurologic lesions have not been fully investigated. Hypermetabolism – elevated basal metabolic rates reflecting increased O_2 consumption associated with injury – could contribute to higher energy expenditures. The resting energy expenditure of people with Parkinson disease has been reported to be 22% above normal when on medications and 51% above normal when off medications (Markus et al., 1992). In contrast, following stroke increases in resting metabolic rates are minimal (Finestone et al., 2003) and after traumatic brain injury are observed only in the early recovery stages (Young et al., 1992). Reductions in the oxidative capacity of paretic musculature could explain part of the increased cost; however, Francescato and associates (1995) postulated that mechanical impairments contribute more than metabolic impairments. Olney and associates (1986, 1991) reasoned that the walking speed of hemiparetic gait is too slow to generate the kinetic energies required for optimal energy transfer, thus reducing the efficiency of the pendular mechanism. In addition, loss of the normal phasic pattern of activity of paretic lower-extremity muscles (Peat et al., 1976) and prolonged muscle activation and increased co-activation in muscles of the contralateral extremity (Shiavi et al., 1987) contribute to mechanical inefficiencies.

In addition to altered muscle activation, decreased excursion of lower-extremity joints may contribute to higher energy costs of walking. In patients with hemiplegia, plantarflexion shortening has been shown to obstruct the potential-to-kinetic energy transfer during the second half of stance (Olney et al., 1986) and stride length may be compromised by the inability to simultaneously extend the knee and flex the hip in terminal swing (Perry, 1969). Lack of reciprocal arm swing may adversely affect the motion of the pelvis required for optimal energy exchange; however, extent of arm swing does not significantly affect the energy cost of walking in healthy individuals (Dean, 1965).

The prominent role that spasticity was thought to play in elevating the energy cost of neurologic gait has been downplayed. Whereas Knutsson and Richards (Knutsson and Richards, 1979; Ponichtera-Mulcare, 1993) attributed premature plantarflexor electromyography (EMG) activity in the stance phase to excessive stretch activation of the plantarflexors, others suggest that plantarflexor spasticity contributes minimally to gait dysfunction poststroke (Ada et al., 1998). Biomechanical studies of hemiparetic gait have shown that the pattern of motion of the paretic lower extremity is more strongly correlated with muscle weakness than with spasticity or balance control (Kramers de Quervain et al., 1996), and that walking speed is not correlated with the extent of quadriceps spasticity (Norton et al., 1975; Bohannon and Andrews, 1990).

Relationship between exercise capacity and energy expenditure

For many individuals with neurologic conditions, the co-existence of neuromuscular and cardiovascular impairments increases the complexity of the physiologic adaptations to training. The relationship between exercise capacity and energy expenditure is illustrated in Fig. 21.4. Training-induced

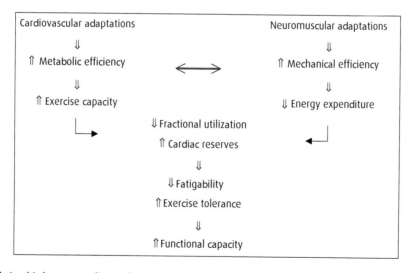

Figure 21.4. Relationship between cardiovascular and neuromuscular adaptations to exercise. Training enhances metabolic and mechanical efficiencies, resulting in increased exercise capacity and reduced energy expenditure, respectively. Fractional utilization is the percentage of peak exercise capacity required to exercise at a fixed submaximal workload. When the numerator (energy expenditure) decreases and the denominator (exercise capacity) increases, fractional utilization is reduced, resulting in greater resistance to fatigue and exercise tolerance.

cardiovascular adaptations enhance metabolic efficiency, which results in increased exercise capacity. Neuromuscular adaptations (e.g., changes in motor unit recruitment and timing resulting from training and motor learning) improve mechanical efficiency, which lowers the energy costs of physical activity. Improvements in metabolic and neuromuscular efficiencies together contribute to reduced fractional utilization – the percentage of peak exercise capacity required to exercise at a fixed submaximal workload. As a consequence, the cardiac reserves available for other activities are greater, thereby enhancing resistance to fatigue and exercise tolerance.

Changes in energy expenditure with neurorehabilitation

To achieve immediate reductions in the energy cost of hemiparetic gait, Hesse et al. (2001) recommended that patients increase locomotor efficiency by walking at speeds higher than their preferred speeds. Also, use of ankle–foot orthoses has been shown to reduce energy costs of hemiparetic gait from 10% (Dasco et al., 1963; Corcoran and Brengelmann, 1970) to 35% (Franceschini et al., 2003). In contrast, paraplegic gait with support from crutches requires 43% greater energy expenditure than does wheelchair propulsion (Waters and Lunsford, 1985).

Few investigators have studied training-induced changes in the energy cost of neurologic gait. An exercise training program designed to improve ambulatory efficiency of patients with traumatic brain injury failed to reduce energy costs despite a 15% improvement in VO_{2peak} (Jankowski and Sullivan, 1990). In contrast, a pilot study involving subjects with incomplete spinal cord injuries reported a 32% reduction in the energy cost of walking after 12 weeks of body weight-supported treadmill training (Protas et al., 2001). Two early studies on the effects of stroke rehabilitation reported mean reductions in energy expenditure of walking of 30% (Dasco et al., 1963) and 23% (Hash, 1978). In the first clinical trial of aerobic training after stroke, the magnitude of improvements in peak workload (43%) and exercise time (40%) exceeded that of VO_{2max} (13%),

intimating that muscular efficiency improved to a greater extent than aerobic capacity (Potempa et al., 1995). In a subsequent training study of patients poststroke, Macko and associates (2001) interpreted gains observed in ambulatory workload capacity as a reflection of both improved exercise capacity and greater gross motor efficiency. The investigators postulated that central neural motor plasticity, mediated by the repetitive, stereotypic training, underlie these adaptations.

21.4 Recommendations for conditioning programs in neurorehabilitation

Specific guidelines for training neurologic populations are lacking. However, the general principles of exercise training outlined by the American College of Sports Medicine (2000) appear to be applicable to aerobic conditioning programs for individuals with upper motor neuron damage. The recommendations outlined in Table 21.3 are derived mainly from the clinical and research experiences of the author.

21.5 Conclusions

Primary and secondary neuromuscular and cardiorespiratory impairments associated with most neurologic conditions adversely affect both exercise capacity and muscular efficiency, giving rise to unfavorable consequences on mobility, energy costs, and quality of life. Despite the pervasive deconditioned state in individuals with neurologic patients and the unequivocal benefits of exercise on health status, details regarding effective strategies to improve endurance and efficiency of movement are lacking. Research, albeit limited, suggests that patients with neurologic impairments respond to exercise training in essentially the same manner as individuals without impairments. These findings have been a catalyst for the introduction of more aggressive, multisystem approaches to neurorehabilitation designed to interrupt the cycle of debilitation and enhance neurologic recovery.

Table 21.3. Recommendations for exercise training of individuals with neurologic impairments.

Screening: Thorough review of the health record of potential participants is critical to identify cardiorespiratory and musculo-skeletal problems that may limit participation in a training program. Cardiac screening, including an exercise stress test with continuous ECG and periodic blood pressure monitoring, is essential for those with cardiac co-morbidities.

Preparation of participants: Participants should be advised to avoid eating 2 h before training and to empty bowel and bladder prior to training. Comfortable clothing and supportive footwear, conducive to dynamic exercise, prepare the participant both physically and psychologically for training.

Program design

- *Setting*: When training high-risk individuals, such as patients in the early phases of neurologic recovery or with significant cardiac co-morbidities, an adverse event protocol and emergency medical equipment and trained personnel during training sessions must be available. For lower-risk individuals, supervised community (Eng et al., 2003) or home-based (Duncan et al., 2003) aerobic exercise programs may be a safe option. Since thermal dysregulation is common in patients with neurologic impairment – particularly multiple sclerosis (Ponichtera-Mulcare, 1993) and spinal cord injuries (Price and Campbell, 1999) – careful control of ambient temperature and provision of fans, spray bottles, towels, and a water cooler are recommended. A water bottle with volumetric indicators is useful to monitor hydration prior to exercise and rehydration following exercise. The training environment should be wheelchair accessible, with adequate space to permit transfer to/from exercise equipment.

- *Scheduling*: Many patients with neurologic involvement report a decline in energy level in the afternoon. If fatigue is a concern, training should be scheduled for morning hours, when circadian body temperature is at its lowest. For certain patient groups, including people with Parkinson disease, timing of medication use to optimize performance during training is an important consideration.

- *Frequency*: Although fitness can improve with twice-weekly sessions, optimal training requires 3–5 sessions per week (American College of Sports Medicine, 2000). Very deconditioned individuals may benefit from multiple brief daily exercise sessions.

- *Duration*: A minimum of 20 min of exercise within the target zone for training per session is required to elicit a training effect (American College of Sports Medicine, 2000). For those with low fitness levels, training may be initiated with 5-min exercise "bouts" with rest periods between bouts. Two additional 5-min periods are required for warm-up and cool-down; hence, the minimal time required to complete a training session is 30 min.

- *Mode of training*: Training modes include treadmill walking with or without body weight support, bicycle ergometer with toe clips and heel-straps, arm–leg ergometer, wheelchair ergometer, stepping machine. Although arm ergometry activates a small portion of total muscle mass, its effectiveness in the aerobic training of patients with quadriplegia has been demonstrated (DiCarlo, 1988). Muscle strengthening exercises should also be prescribed since the combination of physical conditioning and muscle strengthening (e.g., abdominals, hip and knee flexors and extensors, hip abductors, ankle dorsiflexors and plantarflexors) improves outcome (Teixeira-Salmela et al., 1999).

- *Intensity*: Initial exercise intensity and progression must be individualized. Deconditioned individuals can benefit from intensities as low as 55–64% of maximal HR (American College of Sports Medicine, 2000). Continuous HR monitoring and periodic blood pressure readings are recommended. Rating of perceived exertion can serve as a valid proxy to more physiologic measures (Borg, 1982). Evidence suggests that music, properly timed to rhythmic motor events such as walking or cycling, potentiates muscle activation and may be beneficial in pacing movement (Rossignol and Jones, 1976, McIntosh et al., 1997).

- *Adherence to program*: Benefits of training are reversible unless some form of training stimulus is maintained. Strategies to enhance long-term exercise adherence include gradually progressing the exercise intensity, establishing regularity of training sessions, minimizing the risk of muscular soreness, exercising in groups, emphasizing enjoyment in the program, providing on-going positive reinforcement, and using activity logs and charts to record participation and progress. Training sessions should be scheduled at a convenient time and in an accessible location, and if feasible, assistance with transportation and childcare should be offered.

Outcome measures: Walking speed over 10 m and the 6-min walk are clinical measures used to determine functional capacity and are reliable, valid, and easily executed. Blood pressure and HR should be recorded at initiation and termination of the 6-min walk (Eng et al., 2002).

Lifestyle modifications: To sustain improvements in fitness level, education and counseling regarding the daily physical activity, nutrition, energy conservation techniques, and coping strategies are essential.

REFERENCES

Ada, L., Vattanasilp, W., O'Dwyer, N.J. and Crosbie, C. (1998). Does spasticity contribute to walking dysfunction after stroke? *J Neurol Neurosurg Psychiatry*, **64**, 628–635.

American College of Sports Medicine (2000). *Guidelines for Exercise Testing and Prescription*. Williams and Wilkins, Baltimore.

Andersen, P. and Saltin, B. (1985). Maximal perfusion of skeletal muscle in man. *J Physiol*, **366**, 233–249.

Åstrand, P.O. and Rodahl, K. (1986). *Textbook of Work Physiology*. McGraw-Hill, New York.

Barbeau, H. and Visitin, M. (2003). Optimal outcomes obtained with body-weight support combined with treadmill training in stroke patients. *Arch Phys Med Rehabil*, **84**, 1458–1465.

Bhambhani, Y., Rowland, G. and Farag, M. (2003). Reliability of peak cardiorespiratory responses in patients with moderate to severe traumatic brain injury. *Arch Phys Med Rehabil*, **84**, 1629–1636.

Bjuro, T., Fugl-Meyer, A.R., Grimby, G., Hook, O. and Lundgren, B. (1975). Ergonomic studies of standardized domestic work in patients with neuromuscular handicap. *Scand J Rehabil Med*, **7**, 106–113.

Bohannon, R.W. and Andrews, A.W. (1990). Correlation of knee extensor muscle torque and spasticity with gait speed in patients with stroke. *Arch Phys Med Rehabil*, **71**, 330–33.

Borg, G.A. (1982). Psychophysical bases of perceived exertion. *Med Sci Sports Exerc*, **14**, 377–381.

Bouchard, C., Shephard, R.J., Stephens, T., Sutten, J.R. and McPherson, B.D. (1990). *Exercise, Fitness and Health: A Consensus of Current Knowledge*, Human Kinetics, Champaign, Illinois.

Bruce, R.A., Kusumi, F. and Hosmer, D. (1973). Maximal oxygen intake and nomographic assessment of functional aerobic impairment in cardiovascular disease. *Am Heart J*, **85**, 546–562.

Buchfuhrer, M.J., Hansen, J.E., Robinson, T.E., Sue, D.Y., Wasserman, K. and Whipp, B.J. (1983). Optimizing the exercise protocol for cardiopulmonary assessment. *J Appl Physiol*, **55**, 1558–1564.

Busija, D.W. and Heistad, D.D. (1984). Factors involved in the physiological regulation of the cerebral circulation. *Rev Physiol Biochem Pharmacol*, **101**, 161–211.

Camm, A.J. (1996). Chronotropic incompetence. Part 1. Normal regulation of the heart rate. *Clin Cardiol*, **19**, 424–428.

Canning, C.G., Alison, J.A., Allen, N.E. and Groeller, H. (1997). Parkinson's disease: an investigation of exercise capacity, respiratory function, and gait. *Arch Phys Med Rehabil*, **78**, 199–207.

Casaburi, R. (1994). Physiologic responses to training. *Clin Chest Med*, **15**, 215–227.

Cavagna, G.A. and Kaneko, M. (1977). Mechanical work and efficiency in level walking and running. *J Physiol (London)*, **268**, 647–681.

Cavagna, G.A., Thys, H. and Zamboni, A. (1976). The sources of external work in level walking and running. *J Physiol (Lond)*, **262**, 639–657.

Clausen, J.P. (1977). Effect of physical training on cardiovascular adjustments to exercise in man. *Physiol Rev*, **57**, 779–815.

Clausen, J.P., Klausen, K., Rasmussen, B. and Trap-Jensen, J. (1973). Central and peripheral circulatory changes after training of the arms and legs. *Am J Physiol*, **225**, 675–682.

Convertino, V. (1982). Cardiovascular response to exercise in middle-aged men after 10 days of bedrest. *Circulation*, **65**, 134–140.

Corcoran, P.J. and Brengelmann, G.L. (1970). Oxygen uptake in normal and handicapped subjects in relation to speed of walking beside a velocity-controlled cart. *Arch Phys Med Rehabil*, **51**, 78–87.

Coté, M.P., Ménard, A. and Gossard, J.P. (2003). Spinal cats on the treadmill: changes in load pathways. *J Neurosci*, **23**, 2789–2796.

da Cunha Filho, I.T., Lim, P.A., Quershy, H., Henson, H., Monga, T.N. and Protas, E.J. (2001). A comparison of regular rehabilitation with supported treadmill ambulation training for acute stroke patients. *J Rehabil Res Develop*, **38**, 245–255.

da Cunha Filho, I.T., Henson, H., Quershy, H., Williams, A.L., Holmes, S.A. and Protas, E.J. (2003). Differential responses to measures of gait performance among healthy and neurologically impaired individuals. *Arch Phys Med Rehabil*, **84**, 1774–1779.

Dasco, M.M., Luczak, A.K., Haas, A. and Rusk, H.A. (1963). Bracing and rehibilitation training. Effect on the energy expenditure of elderly hemiplegic: A preliminary report. *Postgrad Med*, **34**, 42–47.

Davies, M.J. and Dalsky, G.P. (1997). Economy of mobility in older adults. *J Orthop Sports Phys Ther*, **26**, 69–72.

Davis, G.M. and Shephard, R.J. (1988). Cardiorespiratory fitness in highly active versus inactive paraplegics. *Med Sci Sports Exerc*, **20**, 463–468.

de Groot, P.C.E., Hjeltnes, N., Heijboer, A.C., Stal, W. and Birkeland, K. (2003). Effect of training intensity on physical capacity, lipid profile, and insulin sensitivity in early rehabilitation of spinal cord injured individuals. *Spinal Cord*, **41**, 673–679.

de V. Weir, J.B. (1949). New methods for calculating metabolic rate with special reference to protein metabolism. *J Physiol*, **109**, 1–9.

Dean, G.A. (1965). An analysis of the energy expenditure in level and grade walking. *Ergonomics*, **8**, 31–47.

DeBusk, R.F., Houston, N., Haskell, W., Fry, G. and Parker, M. (1979). Exercise training soon after myocardial infarction. *Am J Cardiol*, **44**, 1223–1229.

DiCarlo, S.E. (1988). Effect of arm ergometry training on wheelchair propulsion endurance of individuals with quadriplegia. *Phys Ther*, **68**, 40–44.

Dietz, V., Ketelsen, U., Berge, W. and Quintern, J. (1986). Motor unit involvement in spastic paresis: relationship between leg muscle activation and histochemistry. *J Neurol Sci*, **75**, 89–103.

Donovan, C.M. and Brooks, G.A. (1977). Muscular efficiency during steady-rate exercise II. Effects of walking speed and work rate. *J Appl Physiol*, **43**, 431–439.

Dressendorfer, R.H., Franklin, B.A., Cameron, J.L., Trahan, K.J., Gordon, S. and Timmis, G.C. (1995). Exercise training frequency in early post-infarction cardiac rehabilitation: influence on aerobic conditioning. *J Cardiopulmonary Rehabil*, **15**, 269–276.

Duncan, P., Studenski, S., Richards, L., Gollub, S., Min Lai, S., Reker, D.M., Perera, S., Yates, J., Koch, V., Rigler, S. and Johnson, D. (2003). Randomized clinical trial of therapeutic exercise in subacute stroke. *Stroke*, **34**, 2173–2180.

Eng, J.J., Chu, K.S., Dawson, A.S., Kim, C.M. and Hepburn, K.E. (2002). Functional walk tests in individuals with stroke. Relation to perceived exertion and myocardial exertion. *Stroke*, **33**, 756–761.

Eng, J.J., Chu, K.S., Kim, C.M., Dawson, A.S., Carswell, A. and Hepburn, K.E. (2003). A community-based group exercise program for persons with chronic stroke. *Med Sci Sports Exerc*, **35**, 1271–1278.

Farmer, J., Zhao, X., Van Praag, H., Woodtke, K., Gage, F.H. and Christie, B.R. (2004). Effects of voluntary exercise on synaptic plasticity and gene expression in the dentate gyrus of adult male Sprague–Dawley rats in vivo. *Neuroscience*, **124**, 71–79.

Fergueson, R.J., Taylor, A.W., Coté, P., Charlebois, J., Dinelle, Y., Péronnet, F., De Champlain, J. and Bourassa, M.G. (1982). Skeletal muscle and cardiac changes with training in patients with angina pectoris. *Am J Physiol*, **243**, H830–H836.

Finestone, H.M., Greene-Finestone, L.S., Foley, N.C. and Woodbury, M.G. (2003). Measuring longitudinally the metabolic demands of stroke patients. *Stroke*, **32**, 502–507.

Foster, C., Crowe, A.J., Daines, E., Dumit, M., Green, M., Lettau, S., Thompson, N.N. and Weymier, J. (1996). Predicting functional capacity during treadmill testing independent of exercise protocol. *Med Sci Sports Exerc*, **28**, 752–756.

Francescato, Z.P., De Luca, G., Lovati, L. and di Prampero, P.E. (1995). The energy cost of level walking in patients with hemiplegia. *Scand J Med Sci Sports*, **5**, 348–352.

Franceschini, M., Massucci, M., Ferrari, L., Agosti, M. and Paroli, C. (2003). Effects of an ankle–foot orthosis on spatiotemporal parameters and energy cost of hemiparetic gait. *Clin Rehabil*, **17**, 368–372.

Franklin, B.A., Besseghini, I. and Goldn, L.H. (1978). Low intensity physical conditioning: effects on patients with coronary heart disease. *Arch Phys Med Rehabil*, **59**, 276–280.

Franklin, B.A., Gordon, S. and Timmis, G.C. (1992). Amount of exercise necessary for the patient with coronary artery disease. *Am J Cardiol*, **69**, 1426–1431.

Frontera, W.R. and Evans, W.J. (1986). Exercise performance and endurance training in the elderly. *Topics Geriat Rehabil*, **2**, 17–32.

Gardner, A.W., Poehlman, E.T. and Corrigan, D.L. (1989). Effect of endurance training on gross energy expenditure during exercise. *Human Biol*, **61**, 559–569.

Glaser, R.M. (1986). Physiologic aspects of spinal cord injury and functional neuromuscular stimulation. *Cent Nerv Syst Trauma*, **3**, 49–62.

Gomez-Pinilla, F., Ying, Z., Roy, R.R., Molteni, R. and Edgerton, R. (2002). Voluntary exercise induces a BDNF-mediated mechanism that promotes neuroplasticity. *J Neurophysiol*, **88**, 2187–2195.

Gordon, W.A., Sliwinski, M. and Echo, J. (1998). The benefits of exercise in individuals with traumatic brain injury: a retrospective study. *J Head Trauma Rehabil*, **134**, 58–67.

Grealy, M.A., Johnson, D.A. and Rushton, S.K. (1999). Improving cognitive function after brain injury: the use of exercise and virtual reality. *Arch Phys Med Rehabil*, **80**, 661–667.

Hartley, L.H., Grimby, G., Kilbom, Å., Nilsson, N.J., Åstrand, I., Bjure, J., Ekblom, B. and Saltin, B. (1969). Physical training in sedentary middle-aged and older men: III. Cardiac output and gas exchange at submaximal and maximal exercise. *Scand J Clin Lab Invest*, **24**, 335–344.

Hash, D. (1978). Energetics of wheelchair propulsion and walking in stroke patients. *Orthop Clin North Am*, **9**, 372–374.

Hellstrom, G., Fischer-Coltrie, W., Wahlgrin, N.G. and Jogestrand, T. (1996). Carotid artery blood flow and middle cerebral artery blood flow velocity during physical exercise. *J Appl Physiol*, **81**, 413–418.

Hesse, S., Werner, C., Paul, T., Bardelben, A. and Chaler, J. (2001). Influence of walking speed on lower limb muscle activity and energy consumption during treadmill walking of hemiparetic patients. *Arch Phys Med Rehabil*, **82**, 1547–1550.

Higginbotham, M.B., Morris, K.C. and Williams, R.S. (1986). Regulation of stroke volume during submaximal and maximal upright exercise in normal man. *Circ Res*, **58**, 281–291.

Hooker, S.P., Figoni, S.F. and Rodgers, M.M. (1992). Physiologic effects of electrical stimulation leg cycle exercise training in human tetraplegia. *Arch Phys Med Rehabil*, **73**, 470–476.

Howley, E.T., Bassett, D.R. and Welch, H.G. (1995). Criteria for maximal oxygen uptake: review and commentary. *Med Sci Sports Exerc*, **27**, 1292–1301.

Jackson, A.S., Beard, E.F., Wier, L.T., Ross, R.M., Stuteville, J.E. and Blair, S.N. (1995). Changes in aerobic power of men ages 25–70 yr. *Med Sci Sports Exerc*, **27**, 113–120.

Jacobs, P.L., Mahoney, E.T., Nash, M.S. and Green, B.A. (2002). Circuit resistance training in persons with complete paraplegia. *J Rehabil Res Develop*, **39**, 21–28.

Jakobsson, F., Edstrom, L. and Grimby, L. (1991). Disuse of anterior tibial muscle during locomotion and increased proportion of type II fibers in hemiplegia. *J Neurol Sci*, **105**, 49–56.

Jankowski, L.W. and Sullivan, S.J. (1990). Aerobic and neuromuscular training: effect on the capacity, efficiency, and fatigability of patients with traumatic brain injury. *Arch Phys Med Rehabil*, **71**, 500–504.

Johansson, B.B., Jadback, G., Norrving, B. and Widner, H. (1992). Evaluation of long-term functional status in first-ever stroke patients in a defined population. *Scand J Rehabil Med*, **(Suppl. 26)**, 105–114.

Jones, D.R., Spier, J., Canine, K., Owen, R.R. and Stiull, G.A. (1989). Cardiorespiratory responses to aerobic training by patients with postpoliomyelitis sequelae. *J Am Med Assoc*, **261**, 3255–3258.

Kelly, J.O., Kilbreadth, S.L., Davis, G.M., Zeman, B. and Raymond, J. (2003). Cardiorespiratory fitness and walking ability in subacute stroke patients. *Arch Phys Med Rehabil*, **84**, 1780–1785.

Kennedy, E.J. (1986). *Spinal Cord Injury: Facts and Figures*, University of Alabama Pr, Birmingham (AL).

Knutsson, E. (1981). Gait control in hemiparesis. *Scand J Rehabil Med*, **13**, 101–108.

Knutsson, E. and Richards, C. (1979). Different types of disturbed motor control in gait of hemiparetic patients. *Brain*, **102**, 405–430.

Kramers de Quervain, I.A., Simon, S.R., Leurgans, S., Pease, W.S. and McAllister, D. (1996). Gait pattern in the early recovery period after stroke. *J Bone Joint Surg*, **78-A**, 1506–1514.

Kriz, J.L., Jones, D.R., Speirer, J.L., Canine, J.K., Owen, R.R. and Serfass, R.C. (1992). Cardiorespiratory responses to upper extremity aerobic training by postpolio subjects. *Arch Phys Med Rehabil*, **73**, 49–54.

Landin, S., Hagenfeldt, L., Saltin, B. and Wahren, J. (1977). Muscle metabolism during exercise in hemiparetic patients. *Clin Sci Mol Med*, **53**, 257–269.

Lewis, D.A., Kamon, E. and Hodgson, J.L. (1986). Physiological differences between genders. Implications for sports conditioning. *Sports Med*, **3**, 357–369.

Lin, K.H., Lai, J.S., Kao, M.J. and Lien, I.N. (1993). Anaerobic threshold and maximal oxygen consumption during arm cranking exercise in paraplegia. *Arch Phys Med Rehabil*, **74**, 515–520.

Linkis, P., Jorgensen, L.G., Olesen, H.L., Madsen, P.L., Lassen, N.A. and Secher, N.H. (1995). Dynamic exercise enhances regional cerebral artery mean flow velocity. *J Appl Physiol*, **78**, 12–16.

MacKay-Lyons, M. and Makrides, L. (2002). Exercise capacity early after stroke. *Arch Phys Med Rehabil*, **83**, 1697–1702.

MacKay-Lyons, M. and Makrides, L. (2004). Longitudinal changes in exercise capacity after stroke. *Arch Phys Med Rebil*, **85**, 1608–1612.

MacKay-Lyons, M., Makrides, L. and Speth, S. (2001). Effect of 15% body weight support on exercise capacity of adults without impairments. *Phys Ther*, **81**, 1790–800.

Macko, R.F., Katzel, L.I., Yataco, A., Tretter, L.D., DeSouza, C.A., Dengel, D.R., Smith, G.V. and Silver, K.H. (1997). Low-velocity graded treadmill stress testing in hemiparetic stroke patients. *Stroke*, **28**, 988–992.

Macko, R.F., Smith, G.V., Dobrovolny, C.L., Sorkin, J.D., Goldberg, A.P. and Silver, K.H. (2001). Treadmill training improves fitness reserve in chronic stroke patients. *Arch Phys Med Rehabil*, **82**, 879–884.

Madsen, P.L., Sperling, B.K., Warming, T., Schmidt, J.F., Secher, N.H., Wildschiodtz, G., Holm, S. and Lassen, N.A. (1993). Middle cerebral artery blood velocity and cerebral blood flow and O_2 uptake during dynamic exercise. *J Appl Physiol*, **74**, 245–250.

Mansour, J.M., Lesh, M.D., Nowak, M.D. and Simon, S.R. (1982). A three dimensional multi-segmental analysis of the energetics of normal and pathological human gait. *J Biomechanics*, **15**, 51–59.

Markus, H., Cox, M.H. and Tomkins, A.M. (1992). Raised resting energy expenditure in Parkinson's disease and its relationship to muscle rigidity. *Clin Sci*, **83**, 199–204.

Martin, P.E. and Morgan, D.W. (1992). Biomechanical considerations for economical walking and running. *Med Sci Sports Exerc*, **24**, 467–474.

Matsumoto, N., Whisnant, J.P., Kurland, L.T. and Okazaki, H. (1973). Natural history of stroke in Rochester, Minnesota, 1955 through 1969: an extension of a previous study, 1945 through 1954. *Stroke*, **4**, 20–29.

McIntosh, G.C., Brown, S.H. and Rice, R.R. (1997). Rhythmic auditory-motor facilitation of gait patterns in patients with Parkinson's disease. *J Neurol Neurosurg Psych*, **62**, 22–26.

Mertens, D.J. and Kavanagh, T. (1996). Exercise training for patients with chronic atrial fibrillation. *J Cardiopulmonary Rehabil*, **16**, 193–196.

Minetti, A.E., Ardigo, L.P. and Saibene, F. (1993). Mechanical determinants of gradient walking energetics in man. *J Physiol*, **471**, 725–735.

Molteni, R., Ying, Z. and Gomez-Pinilla, F. (2002). Differential effects of acute and chronic exercise on plasticity-related genes in the rat hippocampus revealed by microarray. *Eur J Neurosci*, **16**, 1107–1116.

Morio, B., Beaufrere, B., Montaurier, C., Verdier, E., Ritz, P., Fellman, N., Boire, Y. and Vermorel, M. (1997). Gender differences in energy expended during activities and in daily energy expenditure of elderly people. *Am J Physiol*, **273(2 Pt 1)**, E321–E327.

Morris, C.K., Ueshima, K., Kawaguchi, T., Hideg, A. and Froelicher, V.F. (1991). The prognostic value of exercise capacity: a review of the literature. *Am Heart J*, **122**, 1423–1430.

Mossberg, K.A., Kuna, S. and Masel, B. (2002). Ambulatory efficiency in persons with acquired brain injury after a rehabilitation intervention. *Brain Injury*, **16**, 789–797.

Neeper, S.A., Gomez-Pinilla, F., Choi, J. and Cotman, C. (1995). Exercise and brain neurotrophins. *Nature*, **373**, 109.

Nelson, R.R., Gobel, F.L., Jorgenson, C.R., Wang, K., Wang, Y. and Taylor, H.L. (1974). Hemodynamic predictors of myocardial oxygen consumption during static and dynamic exercise. *Circulation*, **50**, 1179–1189.

Neu, H.C., Connolly, J., Schwertley, F., Ladwig, H. and Brody, A. (1967). Obstructive respiratory dysfunction in Parkinson's patients. *Am Rev Respir Dis*, **95**, 33–47.

Ng, A.V. and Kent-Braun, J.A. (1997). Quantification of lower physical activity in persons with multiple sclerosis. *Med Sci Sports Exerc*, **29**, 517–523.

Norton, B.J., Bomze, H.A., Sahrmann, S.A. and Eliasson, S.G. (1975). Correlation between gait speed and spasticity at the knee. *Phys Ther*, **55**, 355–359.

Ogawa, T., Spina, R.J., Martin, W.H., Kohrt, W.M., Schechtman, K.B., Holloszy, J.O. and Ehsani, A.A. (1992). Effects of aging, sex, and physical training on cardiovascular responses to exercise. *Circulation*, **86**, 494–503.

Olgiati, R., Jacquet, J. and Di Prampero, P.E. (1986). Energy cost of walking and exertional dyspnea in multiple sclerosis. *Am Rev Respir Dis*, **134**, 1005–1010.

Olgiati, R., Burgunder, J.-M. and Mumenthaler, M. (1988). Increased energy cost of walking in multiple sclerosis: effect of spasticity, ataxia, and weakness. *Arch Phys Med Rehabil*, **69**, 846–849.

Olney, S., Monga, T.N. and Costigan, P.A. (1986). Mechanical energy of walking of stroke patients. *Arch Phys Med Rehabil*, **67**, 92–98.

Olney, S.J., Griffin, M.P., Monga, T.N. and Mcbride, I.D. (1991). Work and power in gait of stroke patients. *Arch Phys Med Rehabil*, **72**, 309–314.

Paré, G., Noreau, L. and Simard, C. (1993). Prediction of maximal aerobic power from a submaximal exercise test performed by paraplegics on a wheelchair ergometer. *Paraplegia*, **31**, 584–592.

Passmore, R. and Durnin, J.V. (1955). Human energy expenditure. *Physiol Rev*, **35**, 801–840.

Pearce, M.E., Cunningham, D.A., Donner, P.A., Rechnitzer, G.M., Fullerton, G.M. and Howard, J.H. (1983). Energy cost of treadmill and floor walking at self-selected paces. *Eur J Appl Physiol*, **52**, 115–119.

Peat, M., Dubo, H.I.C., Winter, D.A., Quanbury, A.O., Steinke, T. and Grahame, R. (1976). Electromyographic temporal analysis of gait: hemiplegic locomotion. *Arch Phys Med Rehabil*, **57**, 421–425.

Perry, J. (1969). The mechanics of walking in hemiplegia. *Clin Orthop Rel Res*, **63**, 23–31.

Petajan, J.H., Gappmaier, E., White, A.T., Spencer, M.K., Mino, L. and Hicks, R.W. (1996). Impact of aerobic training on fitness and quality of life in multiple sclerosis. *Ann Neurol*, **39**, 432–441.

Pierrynowski, M.R., Winter, D.A. and Norman, R.W. (1980). Transfers of mechanical energy within the total body and mechanical efficiency during treadmill walking. *Ergonomics*, **23**, 147–156.

Pitetti, K.H., Barrett, P.J. and Abbas, D. (1993). Endurance exercise training in Guillain–Barre syndrome. *Arch Phys Med Rehabil*, **74**, 761–765.

Ponichtera-Mulcare, J.A. (1993). Exercise and multiple sclerosis. *Med Sci Sports Exerc*, **25**, 451–465.

Ponichtera-Mulcare, J.A., Mathews, T., Glaser, R.M. and Gupta, S. (1995). Maximal aerobic exercise of individuals with multiple sclerosis using three modes of ergometry. *Clin Kinesiol*, **48**, 4–13.

Potempa, K., Lopez, M., Braun, L.T., Szidon, P., Fogg, L. and Tincknell, T. (1995). Physiological outcomes of aerobic exercise training in hemiparetic stroke patients. *Stroke*, **26**, 101–105.

Pott, F., Ray, C.A., Olesen, H.L. and Secher, N.H. (1997). Middle cerebral artery blood velocity, arterial diameter and muscle sympathetic nerve activity during post-exercise muscle ischemia. *Acta Physiol Scand*, **160**, 43–47.

Price, M.J. and Campbell, I.G. (1999). Thermoregulatory responses of spinal cord injured and well-bodied athletes to prolonged upper body exercise and recovery. *Spinal Cord*, **37**, 772–779.

Protas, E.J., Holmes, S.A., Quereshy, H., Johnson, A., Lee, D. and Sherwood, A.M. (2001). Supported treadmill ambulation training after spinal cord injury: a pilot study. *Arch Phys Med Rehabil*, **82**, 825–831.

Ralston, H.J. (1960). Comparison of energy expenditure during treadmill walking and floor walking. *J Appl Physiol*, **15**, 1156.

Rimmer, J.H., Riley, B., Creviston, T. and Nicola, T. (2000). Exercise training in a predominantly African–American group of stroke survivors. *Med Sci Sport Exerc*, **32**, 1990–1996.

Rossignol, S. and Jones, G.M. (1976). Audio-spinal influence in man studied by the H-reflex and its possible role on rhythmic movements synchronized to sound. *Electroenceph Clin Neurophysiol*, **41**, 83–92.

Roth, E. (1993). Heart disease in patients with stroke. Part 1. Classification and prevalence. *Arch Phys Med Rehabil*, **74**, 752–760.

Roth, E.J., Heinemann, A.W., Lovell, L.L., Harvey, R.L., McGuire, J.R. and Diaz, S. (1998). Impairment and disability: their relation during stroke rehabilitation. *Arch Phys Med Rehabil*, **79**, 329–335.

Rowell, L.B. (1974). Human cardiovascular adjustments to exercise and thermal stress. *Physiol Rev*, **54**, 75–103.

Ryan, A.S., Dobrovolny, C.L., Silver, K.H., Smith, G.V. and Macko, R.F. (2000). Cardiovascular fitness after stroke: role of muscle mass and gait deficit severity. *J Stroke Cerebrovasc Dis*, **9**, 185–191.

Sadovnick, A.D., Eisen, K., Ebers, G.C. and Paty, D.W. (1991). Cause of death in patients attending multiple sclerosis clinics. *Neurology*, **41**, 1193–1196.

Saltin, B. (1969). Physiological effects of physical conditioning. *Med Sci Sport*, **1**, 50–56.

Saltin, B. (1985). Hemodynamic adaptations to exercise. *Am J Cardiol*, **55**, 42D–47D.

Saltin, B., Blomquist, G., Mitchell, J.H., Johnson, R.L., Wildenthal, K. and Chapman, C.B. (1968). Response to exercise after bed rest and after training. A longitudinal study of adaptive changes in oxygen transport and body composition. *Circulation*, **38**(**Suppl. 7**), 1–78.

Samitz, G. and Bachl, N. (1991). Physical training programs and their effects on aerobic capacity and coronary risk profile in sedentary individuals. *J Sports Med Phys Fitness*, **31**, 283–293.

Saunders, D.H., Greig, C.A., Young, A. and Mead, G.E. (2004). Physical fitness training for stroke patients. *Cochrane Database Syst Rev*. (**1**), CD003316.

Saunders, J.B., Inman, V.T. and Eberhart, H.D. (1953). The major determinants in normal and pathological gait. *J Bone Joint Surg*, **35**, 543–558.

Savin, W.M., Haskell, W.L., Houston-Miller, N. and DeBusk, R.F. (1981). Improvements in aerobic capacity soon after myocardial infarction. *J Cardiac Rehabil*, **1**, 337–342.

Sheldahl, L.M., Wilke, N.A., Tritani, F.E. and Hughes, C.V. (1984). Heart rate responses during home activities soon after myocardial infarction. *J Cardiac Rehabil*, **4**, 327–333.

Shiavi, R., Bugle, H.J. and Limbird, T. (1987). Electromyographic gait assessment. Part 2. Preliminary assessment of hemiparetic synergy patterns. *J Rehabil Res*, **24**, 24–30.

Smith, G.V., Silver, K.H.C., Goldberg, A.P. and Macko, R.F. (1999). "Task-oriented" exercise improves hamstring strength and spastic reflexes in chronic stroke patients. *Stroke*, **30**, 2112–2118.

Stainsby, W.N., Gladden, L.B., Barclay, J.K. and Wilson, B.A. (1980). Exercise efficiency: validity of base-line subtractions. *J Appl Physiol*, **48**, 518–522.

Stanghelle, J.K. and Festvåg, L. (1997). Postpolio syndrome: a 5 year follow-up. *Spinal Cord*, **35**, 503–508.

Stanghelle, J.K., Festvag, L. and Aksnes, A.K. (1993). Pulmonary function and symptom-limited exercise stress testing in subjects with late sequelae of poliomyelitis. *Scand J Rehabil*, **25**, 125–129.

Stanley, R.K., Protas, E.J. and Jankovic, J. (1999). Exercise performance in those having Parkinson's disease and healthy normals. *Med Sci Sports Exerc*, **31**, 761–766.

Stratton, J.R., Levy, W.C., Cerqueira, M.D., Schwartz, R.S. and Abrass, I.B. (1994). Cardiovascular responses to exercise: effects of aging and exercise training in healthy men. *Circulation*, **89**, 1648–1655.

Taylor, H.L., Buskirk, E. and Henschel, A. (1955). Maximal oxygen uptake as an objective measure of cardiorespiratory performance. *J Appl Physiol*, **8**, 73–80.

Teixeira-Salmela, L.F., Olney, S.J., Nadeau, S. and Brouwer, B. (1999). Muscle strengthening and physical conditioning to reduce impairment and disability in chronic stroke survivors. *Arch Phys Med Rehabil*, **80**, 1211–1218.

Tong, L., Shen, H., Perreau, V.M., Balazs, R. and Cotman, C. (2001). Effects of exercise on gene-expression profile in the rat hippocampus. *Neurobiol Dis*, **8**, 1046–1056.

Trimble, M.H., Kukulka, C. and Behrman, A.L. (1998). The effect of treadmill gait training on low-frequency depression of the soleus H-reflex: comparison of a spinal cord injured man to normal subjects. *Neurosci Lett*, **246**, 186–188.

Van Praag, H., Kemperman, G. and Gage, F.H. (1999). Running increases cell proliferation and neurogenesis in the adult mouse dentate gyrus. *Nature Neurosci*, **2**, 266–270.

Vingerhoets, F. and Bogousslavsky, J. (1994). Respiratory dysfunction in stroke. *Clin Chest Med*, **15**, 729–737.

Wasserman, K., van Kessel, A. and Burton, G.G. (1967). Interaction of physiological mechanisms during exercise. *J Appl Physiol*, **22**, 71–85.

Wasserman, K., Hansen, J.E., Sue, D.Y., Casaburi, R. and Whipp, B.J. (1999). *Principles of Exercise Testing and Interpretation*, Lippincott Williams and Wilkins, Philadelphia.

Waters, R.L. and Lunsford, B.R. (1985). Energy cost of paraplegic locomotion. *J Bone Joint Surg*, **67**, 1245–1250.

Waters, R.L. and Mulroy, S. (1999). The energy expenditure of normal and pathologic gait. *Gail Posture*, **9**, 207–231.

Wheeler, G.D., Andrews, B., Ledere, R., Davoodi, R., Natho, K., Weiss, C., Jeon, J., Bhambhani, Y. and Steadward, R.D. (2002). Functional electric stimulation-assisted rowing: increasing cardiovascular fitness through functional electric stimulation rowing training in persons with spinal cord injury. *Arch Phys Med Rehabil*, **83**, 1093–1099.

Whipp, B.J. (1994). The bioenergetic and gas exchange basis of exercise testing. *Clin Chest Med*, **15**, 173–192.

Whipp, B.J. and Wasserman, K. (1969). Efficiency of muscular work. *J Appl Physiol*, **26**, 644–648.

Wiercisiewski, D.R. and McDeavitt, J.T. (1998). Pulmonary complications in traumatic brain injury. *J Head Trauma Rehabil*, **13**, 28–35.

Willén, C., Cider, A. and Stibrant Sunnerhagen, K. (1999). Physical performance in individuals with late effects of polio. *Scand J Rehab Med*, **31**, 244–249.

Williams, K.R. (1985). The relationship between mechanical and physiological energy estimates. *Med Sci Sports Exerc*, **17**, 317–325.

Wilmore, J.H., Stanford, P.R., Gagnon, J., Leon, A.S., Rao, D.C., Skinner, J.S. and Bouchard, C. (1996). Endurance exercise training has a minimal effect on resting heart rate: the HERITAGE study. *Med Sci Sports Exerc*, **28**, 829–835.

Winter, D.A. (1980). Overall principle of lower limb support during stance phase of gait. *J Biomech*, **13**, 923–927.

Winter, D.A. (1983). Energy generation and absorption of ankle and knee during fast, natural, and slow cadences. *Clin Orthop*, **175**, 147–154.

Winter, D.A., Quanbury, A.O. and Reimer, G.D. (1976). Analysis of instantaneous energy of normal gait. *J Biomech*, **9**, 253–257.

Young, B., Yingling, B. and McCain, C. (1992). Nutrition and brain injury. *J Neurotrauma*, **9**, S375–S383.

Zauner, A., Daugherty, W.P., Bullock, M.R. and Warner, D.S. (2002). Brain oxygenation and energy metabolism. Part 1. Biological function and pathophysiology. *Neurosurgery*, **51**, 289–302.

Vegetative and autonomic dysfunctions

CONTENTS

22

Rehabilitation of the comatose patient

Francesco Lombardi[1] and Antonio De Tanti[2]

[1]*Riabilitazione Intensiva Neurologica, Ospedale di Correggio, AUSL Reggio Emilia, Via Mandriolo Superiore Correggio, Reggio, Emilia, Italy and* [2]*Responsabile U.O. Gravi Cerebrolesioni e Disturbi Cognitivi, Centro Riabilitativo "Villa Beretta", Costamasnaga, Lecco, Italy*

The main objective in the rehabilitation of the comatose patient is the regaining of consciousness. This is the first step in a life of relationship. After this objective has been achieved, the quality of the rehabilitation project is heightened, and the therapeutic relationship between the therapist and the patient is transformed from a one-way to a two-way relationship. The patient begins to participate, to seek to communicate, to move autonomously, and to take up an independent daily life. Failing to achieve contact with the surroundings, on the other hand, means being doomed to a life of vegetative perceptions and expression, and a negative rehabilitation prognosis.

Due precisely to this aspect of "promotion" or "failure", the definition of the state of consciousness of an individual recovering from a coma is a potential source of conflict between rehabilitation staff and the patient's family. Staff must avoid the formulation of superficial judgments, judgments based on hasty observations, or worst of all, judgments made by inexpert personnel (Zasler, 1997). Currently, a vegetative state (VS) diagnosis is based essentially on clinical observation (Andrews, 1996), and requires the clinical experience of a multidisciplinary team that works well together and that places adequate importance on the family's observations (Giacino et al., 2002; Jennet, 2002). In this realm of extremely complex interests, significant errors of misdiagnosis are still made today (Andrews et al., 1996; Cranford, 1996).

The joint work of several authors has allowed the formulation over time of a more precise definition of the evolution of the state of consciousness beginning from the coma. The definitions for coma, VS, Minimally Responsive State or Minimally Conscious State, A kinetic Mutism and Locked-in Syndrome (American Congress of Rehabilitation Medicine, 1995; Giacino et al., 2002) have been more clearly defined in operative terms, and on the basis of behavioral observation (Table 22.1).

A clearer definition has been provided as well for prognostic terms such as Persistent VS, and Irreversible VS. According to some authors, a VS that persists 3 months after an anoxic event or 1 year after a severe cranial trauma can be defined as permanent (The Multi-Society Task Force on persistent vegetative state (PVS), 1994). Other authors suggest using an interval of 6 months for patients with post-anoxic damage (Working group Royal College of Physicians and Conference of Medical Royal Colleges, 1996). The scientific community is also divided over the possibility of considering a post-traumatic VS permanent after 1 year (American Congress of Rehabilitation Medicine, 1995).

22.1 The natural history of the coma

The comatose state is widely perceived as a serious clinical prognosis. The early literature dealing with the comatose prognosis spoke of the risk of severe disability or the VS for 79% of patients who remained in a non-traumatic coma for at least 1 week (Bates et al., 1977). More recent data paints a less disastrous picture. According to the Traumatic Coma Data Bank (TCDB), "good recovery" or

Table 22.1. Behavioral features associated with coma, vegetative state, minimally responsive state, a kinetic mutism and locked-in syndrome.

	Coma	Vegetative state	Minimally responsive state	Akinetic mutism	Locked-in syndrome
Consciousness	Absent	Absent	Partial	Partial	Present
Sleep/awake	Absent	Present	Present	Present	Present
Motor activity	Reflexive movement Posturing	Spontaneous eyes opening Reflexive movement Posturing Non-purposeful movement	Localizes noxious stimuli Can reach, touch and hold objects in a correct way in respect to their size and shape Inconsistent command following	Minimal degree of movement and command following, depending on the nature and intensity of the stimuli	Quadriplegia Vertical eyes movement and blinking on command
Sensory activity	Absent	Startle to auditive and visual stimuli	Localizes sound location Sustained visual fixation and tracking	Intact visual tracking	Preserved
Communication	Absent	Absent	Contingent vocalization Inconsistent intelligible verbalization or gesture	Minimal degree of speech , depending on the nature and the intensity of the stimuli	Aphonia or anarthria Communication by means of vertical eyes movement and blinking

"moderate disability was observed in 43% of patients 674 days after the event on the average, as compared to 16% that were considered "severely disabled", 5% that were declared to be in "VSs", and 36% that were deceased (Marshall et al., 1991).

The likelihood of recovery varies in relation to the cause that generated the coma. Thirty-three percent of the patients discharged from intensive care in post-traumatic VS achieve contact with the environment 3 months after the trauma. Forty-six percent achieve contact after 6 months, and 52% after a year. Seven percent of these patients achieve the good recovery category described by the Glasgow Outcome Scale (GOS), and 17% reach a state of moderate disability (The Multi-Society Task Force on PVS, 1994). The prognostic picture is considerably less optimistic for post-anoxic encephalopathies, where 11% of patients reach a state of consciousness after 3 months, and 15% achieve consciousness after 6 months. This percentage remains unchanged at follow-up examinations. The prospect for good recovery for these patients is 1%, while 3% of them recover with moderate disability (The Multi-Society Task Force on PVS, 1994; Sazbon et al., 1993).

The anatomical lesions generated in these two conditions are different, and this is the clear reason for the differing prognoses. Severe hypoxia causes multifocal or diffuse extensive laminar cortical necrosis, with constant involvement of the hippocampus. These lesions may be accompanied by small infarcted areas or neuronal loss in the basal ganglia, hypothalamus, or brain stem, with the effect extending to the gray and the white matter (Graham et al., 1993). Diffuse axonal damage, the typical result of traumatic brain injury (TBI), is characterized by extensive subcortical axonal lesions that virtually cut off the cerebral cortex from the other parts of the brain. These lesions are localized in the white matter, and do not greatly affect the gray matter of the cortex (Gennarelli, 1993). In both cases, the lesions in the acute phase are sufficiently widespread to cause the comatose state. However, while anatomical lesions related to axonal damage are theoretically "reparable" since the neuronal bodies are preserved (see Volume I, Chapter 24), the neuronal destruction caused by hypoxia makes the potential for regeneration extremely low. The theory of synaptic plasticity helps provide an explanation for neural repair when axonal damage is involved (Albensi and Janigro, 2003). According to this theory, the central nervous system reacts to external or internal stimuli by modifying its synapses (Hebb, 1949). A high frequency stimulus produces an increase of efficiency in synaptic transmission that continues and lasts in time (Bliss and Lomo, 1973). This phenomenon, which is called long-term potentiation (LTP), is thought to be the normal neurobiological mechanism underlying the learning or memorization processes. The opposite phenomenon was also described, wherein negative stimuli may produce a long-term depression (LTD) that may interfere with stable learning processes (for a detailed discussion of LTP and LTD, see Volume I, Chapter 4). The LTP and LTD responses are manifestations of synaptic plasticity that last in time and which are related to memory consolidation (Bliss and Collingridge, 1993; Izquierdo and Medina, 1997; Holscher, 1999). The LTP and LTD processes are thought to function in the exact opposite way. The factors that modulate the balance between the LTP and LTD responses are the patient's synaptic history, learning, development, age, stress level, type of illness, and brain injury (Stanton, 1996; Foster, 1999). It has been stated that cerebral trauma causes a decrease in LTP responses, while there is no concurring information about LTD responses (Albensi and Janigro, 2003).

In light of physiological learning mechanisms, considering that axonal damage – the anatomical condition underlying the post-traumatic VS – is compatible with the conservation of vitality in the neuronal bodies in the gray matter, it is logical to think of the neurobiological recovery process in these patients as the recovery of the neurophysiological mechanisms underlying the normal learning process. The borderline for neurobiological recovery is represented essentially by the degree of axonal degeneration and by the number of neuronal connections that are saved. Patients in irreversible VS are those that have sustained such widespread axonal degeneration as to no longer regenerate axons or re-establish new synapses.

Axonal damage is by definition a primary lesion. It is determined at the moment the trauma takes place. In serious cases, where there is a risk of irreversible VS, the only strategy that will theoretically limit axonal damage is to prevent the process of extensive degeneration that takes place during the first few months after the trauma (Graham et al., 1993).

What has been said about diffuse axonal damage does not apply to diffuse hypoxic cerebral lesions characterized by extensive loss of gray and white matter. The degree of seriousness of the prognosis for this type of diffuse brain injury is proportionate to the degree of seriousness of the anatomical–pathological lesion. Unlike diffuse axonal damage, hypoxia is a secondary lesion. The severity and the extension of the hypoxic lesion can be limited through appropriate, timely cardio-pulmonary resuscitation during the acute phase (Graham et al., 1993).

22.2 Analyses of prognostic factors

The use of prognostic indicators is of fundamental importance in planning the rehabilitation treatments that will be necessary after the acute phase. Scientifically valid prognostic factors will allow us to offer the family correct information about the patient's chance of recovery, and will help foresee the need for long-term care. Most important, these factors will allow choices to be made in terms of programming finances and health care, and in seeking out effective, appropriate treatment in a system where resources are limited. Finally, we must not forget that a strong demand for scientific evidence comes from the world of bio-ethics and jurisprudence, in relation to the ever-increasing request to stop treatment if the VS can be defined as irreversible (American Academy of Neurology, 1989; May and McGivney, 1998; Diamond, 1999; O'Rourke, 1999).

An analysis of the literature relating to this subject unfortunately leaves us partially unsatisfied. Several authors found that the signs of hypothalamic damage (e.g. generalized sweating) and flaccid motor response most clearly differentiated the recovered from non-recovered patients (Sazbon and Grosswasser, 1990). Others reported that age, pupillary reactivity to light and the best motor response were the most useful prognostic factors for death or continued VS (Braakman et al., 1988). Data from the TCDB unfortunately has not confirmed the existence of any useful prognostic indicator for recovery from VS (Levin et al., 1991).

Other studies have concentrated on the possibility of cerebral magnetic resonance imaging (MRI) being used to help define prognostic indicators. A series of 80 consecutive severe cranial trauma patients in VS was subjected to cerebral MRI within 6–8 weeks from the outset (Kampfl et al., 1998). From an analysis of the results, it was evident that lesions located on the posterior part of the corpus callosum, in the dorsal-lateral cranial areas of the brain stem, and in the corona radiata are strongly indicative of a risk of prolonged VS to 1 year from the trauma (The risk was respectively 132 times greater for lesions on the corpus callosum, 7 times greater for the brain stem, and 4 times greater for the corona radiata). These lesions are typical of diffuse axonal damage. The same authors however, warn us not to consider this pattern to be a sure prediction of irreversible VS in the separate patients we examine. Twenty-four percent of the patients with lesions on the corpus callosum and 26% of those with dorsal-lateral lesions on the brain stem were not in VS 1 year after the trauma, even if none of them reached the "good recovery" stage on the GOS.

Neurophysiological exams have proven so far to be rather unreliable in making predictions concerning traumatic etiology, while they are a powerful tool in the precocious prognosis of anoxic encephalopathies

and ischemia. A systematic review of the literature analyzed 33 studies with a total of 4500 patients examined (Zandbergen et al., 1998). Four variables were found to predict an unfavorable outcome (death or VS), with a specificity of 100%. These four factors are: mydriatic pupils that do not react to light, the absence of motor reflexes as a reaction to pain, a flat electroencephalogram with burst-suppression, and bilateral absence of somatosensory evoked potential (SSEP). The first two factors are reliable within 3 days from the beginning of the coma, and the last two factors within 7 days from the outset. The absence of SSEP is the variable that yields the most accurate prognosis.

Following these results, the authors propose a step-by-step procedure for coming to a decision, which calls for suspending treatment at the end of the first week when the four factors all indicate an unfavorable prognosis. The authors also analyze the predictive value of the SSEP separately, and conclude that the bilateral absence of cortical SSEP 1 month from the beginning of a post-anoxic coma constitutes a sure prognosis for severe and irreversible brain damage (Krieger, 1998; Zandbergen et al., 1998).

Studies of functional imaging, such as single photon emission computed tomography imaging (SPECT) and positron emission tomography (PET) scanning, have not provided sure prognostic elements for predicting the probability of regaining consciousness (Oder et al., 1996). As we have previously pointed out, the duration of the VS is a negative prognostic factor, and criteria for defining a VS as permanent have been recorded in literature (The Multi-Society Task Force on PVS, 1994; Working group Royal College of Physicians and Conference of Medical Royal Colleges, 1996). The currently available data allow us to define a post-anoxic VS as irreversible 6 months after the trauma (Zandbergen et al., 1998; Latronico et al., 2000), while the scientific community is still divided over the possibility of considering a post-traumatic VS permanent after 1 year (American Congress of Rehabilitation Medicine, 1995). Statistics have confirmed the possibility of regaining consciousness after more than 1 year from the trauma, with seven individuals out of

434 (1.6%) regaining consciousness after 1 year in the figures reported by the Task Force. According to other authors, the percentage of late awakenings is about 14% (Childs and Mercer, 1996).

Many projects have been carried out to study the relationship between the length of the period in which the patient does not respond and the quality of the functional recovery after a long period of time. In all cases, a longer duration of the coma/VS is related to worse outcome (The Multi-Society Task Force on PVS, 1994). This is probably due both to the fact that protraction of the coma indicates more severe brain damage, and that the longer the patient is in a coma, the greater the risk of secondary damage.

A retrospective analysis of 134 patients that remained in a coma for more than 30 days showed that 54% regained consciousness within a year of the trauma. Seventy-two percent of these went home, and 48% regained their independence in daily life (Sazbon and Grosswasser, 1990). But in a previous paper, in 1985, Sazbon yet outlined that most of the patients, who recovered from a period of coma of more than 1 month, regained consciousness by 6 months; by 1 year only 4% more of traumatic patients and none of non-traumatic had recovered (Sazbon, 1985). According to the Task Force, progressive protraction of the VS leads to a more serious prognosis, to the extent that after 6 months from the trauma, one finds only patients that are severely disabled according to the GOS (The Multi-Society Task Force on PVS 1994).

In conclusion, at the moment there is no single prognostic factor or model of prediction that will allow us to make an early-on forecast for individual patients in post-traumatic VS. In most cases, no reliable elements are available for formulating a negative recovery prognosis that would justify denying access to rehabilitation facilities (Italian Consensus Conference, 2002). Limiting access to rehabilitation facilities on the basis of uncertain prognostic indicators carries a risk of losing a certain number of patients with neurobiological recovery potential, even though that recovery is delayed. The risk that an unfavorable prognosis may turn into a self-fulfilling prophecy is a real one. Patients will move towards a negative outcome precisely because the prematurely formulated negative prognosis has prohibited access to treatment that could have improved their outcome. The one and the most important exception is that of severe anoxic cerebral lesions where it is possible to formulate a shared, reliable negative prognosis even several weeks after the patient has gone into a coma (Zandbergen et al., 1998).

22.3 Effectiveness of multisensory stimulation programs

In order to facilitate regaining contact with the environment for patients in a coma or VS, many authors have maintained that rehabilitation programs including multisensory stimulation are useful. Such a rehabilitation approach is supported both by a demonstration that sensory deprivation produces loss of neurological functions in animals – as the first authors who proposed this theory believed (Le Winn and Dimancescu, 1978) – and by the theory involving synaptic plasticity and LTP and linguistic data processing (LDP) phenomena (Albensi and Janigro, 2003). It is necessary to point out however, that according to the theory of neuronal plasticity, not all sensory stimuli by nature have a positive effect on the production of stable synaptic bonds. In fact, negative stimuli may produce synaptic depression that will influence learning negatively (Izquierdo and Medina, 1997; Holscher, 1999). To summarize, part of the criticism about multisensory stimulation programs – meaning intensive (15–20 min, repeated every hour for 12–14 h per day, 6 days a week), simultaneous administration of maximum intensity stimuli (all five senses), applied in succession to sensory receptors (Doman et al., 1993) – regards the risk that intense, prolonged and indiscriminate stimulation may produce a temporary increase in the level of arousal during the initial phase, which is not sufficient to lead to or to increase the possibility of full awakening. Prolonging such stimulation rapidly leads to a phenomenon known as psychological "noise habituation", where the patient is psychologically accustomed to background noise, with a corresponding decrease

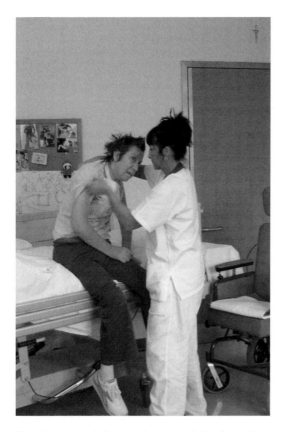

Figure 22.1. Arousal of patients by positional stimulation. The sitting position generates maximal arousal and alertness in a minimally responsive patient.

in the ability to elaborate information (Wood, 1991; see Volume I, Chapters 2 and 5). In light of these considerations, an opposite approach to multisensory stimulation has been proposed, called a "Sensory Regulation Program". It is characterized by single brief sessions of stimulation in a quiet environment completely free of noise (Wood et al., 1993).

Studies dealing with the administration of D-amphetamine to facilitate neurological recovery in animals (see below) have shown that the experience the animal has while under the effect of the drug is essential to producing the desired effect (Feeney et al., 1993). If the rat is confined to a small cage to prevent more energetic movements, the positive effect on neurological recovery is canceled (Feeney et al., 1982). The same thing happens if the major motor-sensory experience is carried out before administering the drug (Hovda and Feeney, 1984). This underlines the fact that the drug is a sort of fuel for rehabilitative exercise (see Volume I, Chapter 15 for more details).

These results have been confirmed by a second experiment, in which the effects of bilateral ablation of cortical areas 17 and 18 on the stereoscopic vision of a cat were studied. The produced impairment regresses completely and definitively after the administration of D-amphetamine, provided the animal's sight is preserved. If the animal is placed in a completely dark place with a total deafferentation, the positive effect on recovery will be completely canceled (Feeney and Hovda, 1985). Unfortunately, the effectiveness of sensory-motor exercise on neurological recovery has not yet been demonstrated in studies carried out on humans. No studies have even been conducted on the combined effect of neurotransmitter therapy and sensory-motor exercise.

A systematic review of the literature on the effectiveness of multisensory stimulation for facilitating awakening from a coma has led to the selection of 25 studies in which the rehabilitation methods used and the system for checking for clinical effectiveness were described in sufficient detail (Lombardi, 2002a,b). Out of these studies, 22 have been excluded from our review for various reasons: fourteen of them were series of cases without a control group (Rosadini and Sannita, 1982; Boyle and Greer, 1983; Weber, 1984; De Young and Grass, 1987; Johnson et al., 1989; Rader et al., 1989; Sisson, 1990; Wilson et al., 1991; 1993; 1996a, b; Hall et al., 1992; Doman et al., 1993; Schinner et al., 1995), five were studies with a historical control group (Cooper et al., 1999; Le Winn and Dimancescu, 1978; Pierce et al., 1990; Wood et al., 1992; 1993), two were case reports (Jones et al., 1994; Guina et al., 1997), and one was a comparative cervical test (CCT) study, and included in the experimental group other types of intervention in addition to multisensory stimulation (Mackay et al., 1992). The remaining three studies, which were considered valid from a methodological point of view, unfortunately did not provide valid results confirming the effectiveness of

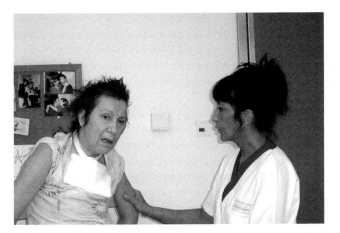

Figure 22.2. Arousal of patients by verbal stimulation. With the patient of figure 1 in the sitting position, which is best for stimulating her to obey simple commands, the therapist asks the patient to look toward her.

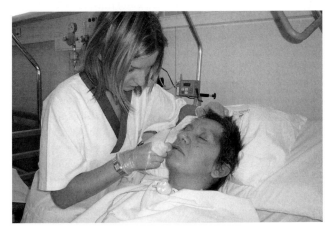

Figure 22.3. Arousal of patients by oral stimulation. Although patients can be aroused by oral stimulation when they are in a sitting position, the same patient as in Figure 22.1 fails to be aroused when orally stimulated in a supine, relaxed position.

multisensory stimulation techniques on patients in a coma (Kater, 1989; Mitchell, 1990; Johnson et al., 1993). The review concludes that there is no reliable evidence to support the effectiveness of multisensory stimulation programs in patients in coma or VS, and that – in order to improve our knowledge of this field – the effectiveness of multisensory stimulation programs should be evaluated through adequately dimensioned randomized, controlled studies (Lombardi, 2002a,b). Given the lack of evidence, the authors suggest that any delivery of treatment interventions based on the concept of "sensory stimulation" should be provided only in the context of properly designed and adequately sized Randomized Controlled Trials, in rehabilitation environments specialized in the care of this type of patient. The precocious, formalized rehabilitation program aimed at facilitating interaction with the environment should be conducted by a multidisciplinary team of experts made up of nurses, physiotherapists and speech therapists, who are able to carry out structured monitoring of patients' responsiveness (Figs 22.1–22.3).

22.4 The influence of drugs on awakening from a coma

Various authors claim that correct use of drugs facilitates regaining contact with the environment (Haig and Ruess, 1990; Wroblewski et al., 1993; Wroblewski

1996; Plenger et al., 1996; Reinhard et al., 1996; Matsuda et al., 1999; Passler and Riggs, 2001; Meythaler et al., 2002). The most widely shared opinion is that some drugs produce an inhibiting effect, while others facilitate neurological recovery (Feeney et al., 1993; Goldstein, 1999). To summarize very briefly, pro-monoaminergic drugs have been credited with a "favorable effect", while anti-monoaminergic drugs cause "inhibition". This opinion has been fairly widely spread in literature and clinical practice in spite of the fact that no concrete evidence of this positive or negative effect has ever been found in studies on humans (Forsyth and Jayamoni, 2003). The only evidence we have is the opinion of experts.

Although there is no scientific evidence from randomized, controlled clinical studies on humans, the neurophysiological knowledge of neuronal plasticity (Goldstein, 1999; Albensi and Janigro, 2003) and of the importance of neurotransmitters in physiology and pathology has grown in time, and the body of doctrine has become more and more substantial and precise, with extremely promising realms of research like the one on the possibility that neurotransmitter drugs may provide neuronal protection or that they may stimulate neuronal plasticity. As we await more substantial scientific evidence, drugs for rehabilitation are prescribed mainly on the basis of neurophysiological knowledge and upon demonstration of reduced cerebral concentration of aminergic neurotransmitters in severe TBI (Gualtieri, 1988). The administration of drugs to speed up neurological recovery has produced and is producing surprising results in selected cases, with clear acceleration of contextual functional recovery upon administration of the drug, as has also been demonstrated in anecdotal studies and experiments by the authors of this review (Haigand Ruess, 1990; Matsuda et al., 1999).

This type of experience is in some ways similar to what has been observed in laboratory animals by the authors who were the first to study the effectiveness of D-amphetamine for facilitating neurological recovery (Feeney et al., 1982). The administration of D-amphetamine, combined for a short period with significant sensory-motor experience, facilitates functional recovery measured by a particular ability

called beam-walking (BW), even when the experience is begun days or weeks after a unilateral ablation has been practiced on the rat's sensory-motor cortex. The animals are able to spontaneously regain BW, but only over a long period of time. The effect of the drug plus the significant experience is so rapid that it would seem that the animal's difficulty in walking is not caused by a neuro-anatomical impairment, but by remote functional depression (RFD) (Feeney et al., 1993). Clinical cases of rapid and contextual clinical and functional improvement in patients in VS or minimally responsive patients treated with activator drugs shows the same results as those described in the animals, and may be explained as a condition of functional inhibition (Haig and Ruess, 1990; Matsuda et al., 1999).

In other cases reported in the literature, the results are modest from a functional point of view, but they have been received positively by health care personnel, therapists, and/or family members, who are able to interact better when they see that the patient is more aware or responsive (Wolf and Gleckman, 1995). In clinical practice however, there are patients that do not receive any benefit from pharmacological manipulation with neurotransmitter drugs. Obviously, these cases have not been published, but they can be perceived through an analysis of the results from observational studies (Passler and Riggs, 2001; Wolf and Gleckman, 1995).

In studies carried out on animals as well, neurological conditions have been found that cannot be modified and that are not consistently affected by multisensory-motor manipulation and drug therapy. This is the case with the placing reflex, which disappears totally in a cat with a unilateral ablation of the sensory-motor cortex (Feeney et al., 1993). It is important not to forget that neurobiological recovery is not possible where there is considerable anatomical brain injury, without transplanting new cerebral tissue. There are also patients in VS who – due to extensive degeneration of the white matter because of severe, diffuse axonal damage or extensive degeneration of the gray and white matter because of diffuse hypoxic lesions – have injuries that will not allow the recovery of neurobiological functions. These patients are defined as being insensitive to both neurotransmitter drugs and to multisensory-motor exercise.

During a rehabilitation project, it is necessary to ask oneself if the individual patient in VS is affected by functional inhibition, or if the patient has an extensive and irreversible neurobiological lesion. It is an integral part of the project to make clear whether the individual patient still has neurobiological potential for recovery through the manipulation of the variables at our disposal: multisensory-motor exercise and available drugs. In the absence of scientific evidence, the clinical experience of those who use neurotransmitter drugs to facilitate awakening carries the risk of remaining in the superficial realm of anecdotal trial and error, without contributing to the necessary evolution of scientific knowledge in this field. It is necessary for reliable models of experimentation to be created in this field too, in spite of all the real methodological difficulties that are often encountered in rehabilitation (Phipps et al., 1997; White et al., 1999).

22.5 Catabolism and neurotransmitter imbalance in severe TBI

Studies that have been conducted to analyze the concentration of neurotransmitters and their metabolites in the fluid after traumatic brain damage have revealed a reduction in these levels as compared to the norm (Minderhoud et al., 1976; van Woerkom et al., 1977; 1982; Vecht et al., 1975a, b; 1976). In particular, the levels of catecholamine in the fluid increase during the first few hours after the traumatic lesion, while their production is chronically reduced during the following phases, with consequent reduction in the concentration in the fluid (Bakay et al., 1986).

The cause of depauperation of neurotransmitters can be traced initially to the massive, acute release of neurotransmitters from neuronal cells in the so-called excitotoxicity phase. Following this, depauperation is maintained by the condition of hypercatabolism to which the traumatized organism is subject (Aquilani, 2000; 2003). This process

characterized by an initial excess of neurotransmitters followed by a deficiency in neurotransmitters, has been pointed out in literature and has even been thought to be a possible cause of failure for clinical trials with antagonists to N-Methyl-D-Asperate (NMDA) receptors (Ikonomidou and Turski, 2003). According to this hypothesis, while the blockage of receptors is initially oriented to preventing the excitotoxicity cascade, this later works as a negative factor for the survival of neurons.

Severe encephalic cranial trauma causes hypercatabolism that is manifested by an increased loss of nitrogen in the urine and destruction of muscle proteins, which are used as the groundwork for producing energy, repairing proteins, cytokines, hormones, and cells. In spite of nutritional efforts to obtain a stable condition, in most patients a balanced level of nitrogen is not reached until 2 or 3 weeks after the trauma (Clifton et al., 1984; Young et al., 1985; Bivins et al., 1986; Bruder et al., 1991). A hypercatabolic condition and failure to reach a positive balance of nitrogen has been demonstrated even 60 days after a severe encephalic cranial trauma (Fugazza et al., 1998). Consuming a larger amount of proteins in the diet produces greater nitrogen balance, but the difference is not statistically significant (Clifton et al., 1985). Since over-feeding is damaging, it is not correct to continue increasing the protein in-take in order to balance the nitrogen level (Roberts, 1995). Administering supplementary ramificated amino acids and arginine has been shown in two different studies to improve the nitrogen balance (Rowlands et al., 1986; Ott et al., 1988), even if the influence on the outcome has not been established.

Studies conducted with patients in the rehabilitation phase have shown considerable reduction in the plasmatic aminogram even 60 days after a severe cranial trauma. In particular, the concentration of essential amino acids was found to be reduced by 60%, and non-essential amino acids were found reduced by more than 50% (Aquilani, 2000). The authors observed the persistence of the hypercatabolic state even in patients in rehabilitation, along with an increase in plasmatic carnitine (which indicates muscular destruction) and reduced concentration of essential amino acids – in particular ramificated chain amino acids – which suggests selective use of the latter. According to various authors, the depauperation of amino acids (in particular, arginine and glutamine) has an effect on immunocompetence (Ziegler et al., 1993; Jensen et al., 1996; Griffiths, 1997; Houdijk et al., 1998) as well as on the balance of neurotransmitters in the central nervous system. In particular, this regards glutamate, aspartate, tyrosine, and tryptophan, the precursors of monoaminergic neurotransmitters (Aquilani, 2000; 2003).

For this reason, it is important that future studies on humans concentrate on a real "nutritional therapy" approach, in the hopes that nutritional manipulation might facilitate and stimulate neurobiological recovery in trauma patients (Aquilani, 2003). It is interesting to point out here that both the nutritional therapy approach and pharmacological manipulation using neurotransmitter drugs work in the same direction. The former approach constitutes the underlying activity for the therapeutic strategy, while the pharmacological approach serves as a temporary support until the patient regains autonomous metabolism. The combined action of these two approaches might constitute a reasonable treatment for facilitating neurobiological recovery in patients in the VS, provided the anatomical potential for recovery exists, or in other words that there is not diffuse axonal or neuronal degeneration (Graham et al., 1993).

22.6 Neurobiological recovery may be interrupted by interfering factors

The outcome of a patient in the VS actually often depends on a combination of various factors. It is possible for these factors to intervene in sequential order, producing situations that inhibit neurobiological recovery. The axonal or hypoxic lesion is the pathognomonic pathological element causing the VS, but these lesions may be accompanied by other lesions that overlap later on. In the following paragraphs, we will discuss a couple of potential secondary causes for the primary rehabilitation prognosis becoming progressively more negative.

Post-traumatic hydrocephalus

It is practically impossible to clinically detect the onset of post-traumatic hydrocephalus in a patient in the VS, since it is impossible for the usual signs of hydrocephalus–cognitive disturbance, gait apraxia, or bladder incontinence–to be manifested (Zasler and Marmarou, 1992; Narayan et al., 1990). One way to make an alteration in fluid circulation visible is to carry out a series of CT brain scans, that will show over a month's time the progressive increase in the dimensions of the cerebral ventricles (Narayan et al., 1990; Chesnut et al., 1992).

Unfortunately, simply noting ventricular enlargement is not sufficient for detecting hydrocephalus, since progressive cerebral atrophy is also characterized by an increase in the dimensions of the ventricles (Zasler and Marmarou, 1992; Marmarou et al., 1996). As we know, both severe diffuse axonal damage and severe hypoxic encephalopathy cause cerebral atrophy and chronic VS (The Multi-Society Task Force on PVS, 1994). Supplementary methods have been defined to allow for the different diagnoses of the two conditions: cerebral spinal fluid (CSF) dynamics studies (Marmarou et al., 1996) and SPECT imaging (Mazzini et al., 2003). However, the use of these diagnostic instruments has not become widespread, and they are not easy to procure in many hospital settings.

The uncertainty in terms of diagnosis, whether clinical or instrumental, is probably one of the reasons the results of ventricular peritoneal shunt operations have been unsatisfactory so far (Chesnut et al., 1993; Cardosa and Galbright, 1985). Data from the TCDB shows that 27 patients were found to have post-traumatic ventricular Enlargement (PTVE) 1 month after the acute event, or 5.4% of the total number of 498 in a sample group of patients with severe cranial trauma. All of the patients in the group were assessed by computerized axial tomography (CAT) scan at 3 days, 7–10 days, 3 months and 6 months from the event, and none of them had shown ventriculomegaly when admitted (Chesnut et al., 1993). This incidence is fairly near to the 3.9% observed by Grosswasser out of a sampling of 335 patients affected with severe cranial trauma, for whom hydrocephalus had been

Table 22.2. Outcome of patients with post traumatic ventricular enlargement in the TCDB.

Status of ventricles	Number of patients	% Total patients	Outcome number (%)		
			Good	Moderate or severe	Vegetative or dead
Total cases	498	100	28	40	32
PTVE	27	5	4	70	26
No PTVE	471	95	29	38	33

Reproduced with permission from Chesnut et al. (1993).

Table 22.3. Outcome of patients with post traumatic ventricular enlargement in the TCDB. A comparison between shunted and not shunted patients.

Presence of shunt	Number of patients	% Total patients	Outcome number (%)		
			Good	Moderate or severe	Vegetative or dead
PTVE	27	100	4	70	26
Shunted	17	63	6	65	29
Not shunted	10	37	0	80	20

Reproduced with permission from Chesnut et al. (1993).

diagnosed through serial CAT scans and radionuclide cisternographies (Grosswasser et al., 1988). Other authors have found very different rates of occurrence of post-traumatic hydrocephalus, ranging from 20% in a sampling of 237 patients with severe cranial trauma – of which 44% showed ventriculomegaly (Marmarou et al., 1996) – to 45% in a series of 240 individuals (Mazzini et al., 2003). From the TCDB data, we know that the prognosis for patients that show PTVE as assessed by the GOS is clearly more serious than that of the total cases in the sample group (see Table 22.2): Chi^2 = 13.04; P = 0.0015 (Chesnut et al., 1993).

Of the 27 patients that showed ventricular enlargement, only 17 were given a CSF shunt. The treatment did not generate a statistically significant difference in outcome in GOS points (see Table 22.3): Chi^2 = 0.338; P = 0.561 (Chesnut et al., 1993).

The small number of patients studied, the insufficient number of subjects in several of the boxes in the

table, and the obvious lack of randomization oblige us to maintain a certain amount of caution in assuming that this study really did not produce statistically significant results. One aspect is interesting however, and provides food for thought: the authors themselves have underlined the following sentence twice in the article. "In various individual patients, the shunt treatment produced considerable and contextual clinical improvement" (Chesnut et al., 1993). This emphasis corresponds to the experience we have had as well.

If we consider that patients affected by ventricular dilation are in any case subject to a negative prognosis (see Table 22.1), and that the "good recovery" category in the table has only one individual (estimated number based on the percentages reported) treated with CSF shunt, we may conclude that for the 27 subjects of the study, the only chance to enter the good recovery category was through surgery. The clinical observation of clear-cut benefit following a

CSF shunt operation was observed in 52.1% of a group of 48 severely traumatized patients that were all treated surgically (Tribl and Oder, 2000).

There are various ways to discuss the usefulness of a CSF shunt in post-traumatic ventricular enlargement. We could speak about the complications the patients are subject to, of the cost-benefit ratio, or of the low degree of effectiveness of the operation. However, from a point of view considering the individual patient in the VS, it is highly likely that "non-treatment" corresponds to a standstill in neurobiological recovery, while "treatment" is the only chance for the individual to express his full neurobiological recovery potential on the basis of the primary neurological lesions alone.

Generalized spasticity

The risk of misdiagnosis among disorders of consciousness in severe brain injuries is well known (Childs et al., 1993). In most cases, the possible diagnostic mistake is usually associated with the presence of significant sensory impairment. For instance, in Andrew's reported cases, 65% of misdiagnosed subjects were either blind or severely visually impaired (Andrews et al., 1996).

In one published case report regarding spasticity which did not respond to treatment by oral drugs (Palumbo, 2004, in press), spasticity was found to be a factor leading to a mistaken diagnosis of the VS. For this individual, treatment by intrathecal baclofen therapy (IBT) 258 days after the trauma brought a rapid change in the patient's response level, going from a minimal response level that continued from the third month after the trauma, to a state of full response, although conditioned by evident cognitive impairment and severe motor disability. The patient, who had episodes of autonomic disorder, showed rapid improvement 7 days after surgery. This result had already been observed by previous authors (Becker et al., 2000; Cuny et al., 2001). In the case described by Palumbo, solving the severe spasticity problem led to an improvement in nutritional methods and the capacity to respond to environmental stimuli, improving the level of participation in the rehabilitation program, with further improvement – albeit slow – in the outcome at check-ups that were carried out 385 and 453 days after the acute event.

22.7 Conclusions

Although there is no substantial scientific evidence, rehabilitation of the comatose patient, and in particular of the patient in a VS, is a process that is geared towards assessing the individual patient's neurobiological potential for recovery. This assessment should be based on a series of different behaviors that make up a step-by-step procedure on which to base the rehabilitation process.

1 In order to conduct the process correctly, it is necessary that it be carried out by a team of experts who are able to sensitively and effectively evaluate every change in the patient's state of response, however small.
2 In order to draw out the patient's residual neurobiological recovery potential, it is necessary to carry out an active assessment process to detect the presence or absence of every possible negative or mistakable factor (sedative drugs, hydrocephalus, spasticity, malnutrition) and to follow up with specific treatment to manage or correct the factor.
3 Standstills in neurobiological recovery come in addition to the primary lesions. They differ by nature, severity, and the time at which they arise, and it is possible for an individual patient to demonstrate more than one inhibiting factor at a time.
4 Once the negative factors that are interfering have been eliminated or put under control, it is necessary to check to see if the introduction of facilitative factors will produce real improvement in the patient's response level:
    – stimulating drugs,
    – nutrients to foster amino acid metabolism,
    – postural variations,
    – changes in the environmental context,
    – stimulating sensory experiences.

5 The improvement in the patient's response level is the basic element on which a prognosis is made at a suitable amount of time after the acute event.

Although there is agreement on the idea that regaining contact with the environment is a multifactorial problem, many studies carried out up until now on single therapeutic approaches may have failed to be in any way effective due to the lack of a holistic vision of the problem, in addition to other reasons. Many of the factors involved are difficult to diagnose, both because of the patient's clinical condition, and because of unsatisfactory instruments. Until more precise diagnostic instruments are available, the only approach that will allow us to raise the number of patients that regain contact with the environment is to operate "by exclusion".

It is important that the clinical attitude of the rehabilitation team be self-determined, and not geared to the patient's clinical progress. This will prevent the risk of considering negative progress predetermined or unavoidable. The clinical behavior of the team must also be analytical and periodically concentrated on checking for possible interfering factors and on the impact of possible favorable factors. Given the uncertainty in detecting interfering factors, it is reasonable to act as though the factor were present, and to carry out the correct treatment, considering the advantages and the risks the patient will be subject to in each particular situation as it arises.

ACKNOWLEDGEMENTS

The authors wish to thank:
Sharon Peachey and Multilab-Holden Language School di Rossi Linda for the translation;
Dr. G. Vezzosi, Head of the Rehabilitation Department in Azienda Sanitaria Locale (AUSL) of Reggio Emilia and Head Physician in the Correggio Hospital;
Dr. R. Brianti, Head of the Intensive Rehabilitation Unit in the Correggio Hospital;
The Local Health Authority (AUSL) of Reggio Emilia, for supporting and financing the project;

Dr. Chesnut for granting us permission to publish data tables from his research.

REFERENCES

Albensi, B.C. and Janigro, D. (2003). Traumatic brain injury and its effects on synaptic plasticity. *Brain Injury*, **17**(8), 653–663.

American Academy of Neurology. (1989). Position of the American Academy of Neurology on certain aspects of the care and management of the PVP patients. *Neurology*, **39**, 125–126.

American Congress of Rehabilitation Medicine (ACRM). (1995). Neurobehavioral criteria in recommendations for use of uniform nomenclature pertinent to patients with severe alterations in consciousness. *Arch Phys Med Rehabil*, **76**, 205–209.

Andrews, K. (1996). International working party on the management of the vegetative state: summary report. *Brain Injury*, **10**(11), 797–806.

Andrews, K., Murphy, L., Munday, R., et al. (1996). Misdiagnosis of the vegetative state: retrospective study in a rehabilitation unit. *Brit Med J*, **313**(7048), 13–16.

Aquilani, R., Viglio, S., Iadarola, P., Guarnaschelli, C., Arrigoni, N., Fugazza, G., Catapano, M., Boschi, F., Dossena, M. and Pastoris, O. (2000). Peripheral plasma amino acid abnormalities in rehabilitation patients with severe brain injury. *Arch Phys Med Rehabil*, **81**, 176–181.

Aquilani, R., Iadarola, P., Boschi, F., Pistarini, C., Arcidiaco, P. and Contardi. (2003). Reduced plasma levels of tyrosine, precursor of brain catecholamines, and of essential amino acids in patients with severe traumatic brain injury after rehabilitation. *Arch Phys Med Rehabil*, **84**(9), 1258–1265.

Bakay, R.A., Sweeney, K.M. and Wood, J.H. (1986). Pathophysiology of cerebrospinal fluid in head injury: part I; pathological changes in cerebrospinal fluid solute composition after brain injury. *Neurosurgery*, **18**, 234–243.

Bates, D., Caronna, J.J., Cartlidge, N.E., Knill-Jones, R.P., Levy, D.E. and Shaw Plum, F. (1977). A prospective study of nontraumatic coma: methods and results in 310 patients. *Ann Neurol*, **2**(3), 211–220.

Becker, R., Benes, L., Sure, U., Hellwig, D. and Bertalanffy, H. (2000). Intrathecal baclofen alleviates autonomic dysfunction in severe brain injury. *J Clin Neurosci*, **7**(4), 316–319.

Bivins, B., Twyman, D. and Young, B. (1986). Failure of non-protein calories to mediate protein conservation in brain-injured patients. *J Trauma*, **26**, 980–986.

Bliss, T.V.P. and Lomo, T. (1973). Long-lasting potentiation of synaptic transmission in the dentate area of the anaesthetized rabbit following stimulation of the perforant path. *J Physiol*, **232**, 331–356.

Bliss, T.V.P. and Collingridge, G.L. (1993). A synaptic model of memory: long-term potentiation in the hippocampus. *Nature*, **361**, 31–39.

Boyle, M.E.M. and Greer, R.D. (1983). Operant procedures and the comatose patient. *J Appl Behav Anal*, **16**, 3–12.

Braakman, R., Jennett, W.B. and Minderhoud, J.M. (1988). Prognosis of the posttraumatic vegetative state. *Acta Neurochir*, **95**, 49–52.

Bruder, N., Dumon, J.C. and Francois, G. (1991). Evolution of energy expenditure and nitrogen excretion in severe head-injured patients. *Crit Care Med*, **19**, 43–48.

Cardosa, E.R. and Galbright, S. (1985). Posttraumatic hydrocephalus – a retrospective review. *Surg Neurol*, **23**, 261–264.

Chesnut, R.M., Luerssen, T.G., van Berkum-Clark, M., Marshall, L.F., Klauber, M.R. and Blunt, B.A. (1992). Determinants of posttraumatic ventriculomegaly in the Traumatic Coma Data Bank. *J Neurosurg*, **6**, 396A–397A.

Chesnut, R.M., Luerssen, T.G., van Berkum-Clark, M., Marshall, L.F., Klauber, M.R., Blunt, B.A. and the TCDB Investigators. (1993). Post-traumatic ventricular enlargement in the Traumatic Coma Data Bank: incidence, risk factors, and influence on outcome. In: *Intracranial Pressure VIII* (eds Avezaat, C.J.J., et al.), Springer-Verlag, New York, pp. 503–506.

Childs, N.L. and Mercer, W.N. (1996). Late improvement in consciousness after post-traumatic vegetative state. *New Engl J Med*, **334**, 24–25.

Childs, N.L., Mercer, W.N. and Childs, H.W. (1993). Accuracy of diagnosis of the persistent vegetative state. *Neurology*, **43(8)**, 1457–1458.

Clifton, G.L., Robertson, C.S., Grossman, R.G., et al. (1984). The metabolic response to severe head injury. *J Neurosurg*, **60**, 687–696.

Clifton, G.L., Robertson, C.S. and Contant, C.F. (1985). Enteral hyperalimentation in head injury. *J Neurosurg*, **62**, 186–193.

Cooper, J.B., Jane, J.A., Alves, W.M. and Cooper, E.B. (1999). Right median nerve electrical stimulation t hasten awakening from coma. *Brain Injury*, **13**, 261–267.

Cranford, R. (1996). Misdiagnosing the persistent vegetative state. *British Med J*, **313**, 5–6.

Cuny, E., Richer, E. and Castel, J.P. (2001). Dysautonomia syndrome in the acute recovery phase after traumatic brain injury: relief with intrathecal baclofen therapy. *Brain Injury*, **15(10)**, 917–925.

De Young, S. and Grass, R.B. (1987). Coma recovery program. *Rehabil Nursing*, **12(3)**, 121–124.

Diamond, E.F. (1999). A note on the "vegetative" state. *Ethics & Medics*, **7**, 3.

Doman, G., Wilkinson, R., Dimancescu, M.D. and Pelligra, R. (1993). The effect of intense multisensory stimulation on coma arousal and recovery. *Neuropsychol Rehabil*, **3(2)**, 203–212.

Feeney, D.M. and Hovda, D.A. (1985). Reinstatement of binocular depth perception by amphetamine and visual experience after visual cortex ablation. *Brain Res*, **342**, 352–356.

Feeney, D.M., Gonzales, A. and Law, W.A. (1982). Amphetamine, haloperidol and experience interact to affect rate of recovery after motor cortex injury. *Science*, **217**, 855–857.

Feeney, D.M., Weisend, M.P. and Kline, A.E. (1993). Noradrenergic pharmacotherapy, intracerebral infusion and adrenal transplantation promote functional recovery after cortical damage. *J Neural Transplant Plast*, **4(3)**, 199–213.

Forsyth, R. and Jayamoni, B. (2003). Noradrenergic agonists for acute traumatic brain injury. *Cochrane Database Syst Rev*, **1**, CD003984.

Foster, T.C. (1999). Involvement of hippocampal synaptic plasticity in age-related memory decline. *Brain Res Rev*, **30**, 236–249.

Fugazza, G., Aquilani, R., Iadarola, P., Dossena, M., Catapano, M., Boschi, F., Cobianchi, A. and Pastoris, O. (1998). The persistence of hypercatabolic state in rehabilitation patients with complicated head injury. *Eur Med Phys*, **34**, 125–129.

Gennarelli, T.A. (1993). Cerebral concussion and diffuse brain injuries. In: *In Head Injury* (ed. Cooper, P.R.), 3rd edn., Williams & Wilkins, Baltimore, USA, pp. 137–158.

Giacino, J.T., Ashwal, M.D. and Childs, M.D. (2002). The minimally conscious state. Definition and diagnostic criteria. *Neurology*, **58**, 349–353.

Goldstein, L.B. (1999). Pharmacological approach to functional reorganization: the role of norepinephrine. *Rev Neurol*, **9(155)**, 731–736.

Graham, D.I., Adams, H. and Gennarelli, T.A. (1993). Pathology of brain damage in head injury. In: *Head Injury* (ed. Cooper, P.R.), 3rd edn., Williams & Wilkins, Baltimore, USA, pp. 91–113.

Griffiths, R.D. (1997). Outcome of critically ill patients after supplementation with glutamine. *Nutrition*, **13**, 752–754.

Grosswasser, Z., Cohen, M., Reider-Grosswasser, I. and Stern, M.J. (1988). Incidence, CT findings and rehabilitation outcome of patients with communicative hydrocephalus following severe head injury. *Brain Injury*, **2(4)**, 267–272.

Gualtieri, C.Y. (1988). Review: pharmacotherapy and the neurobehavioural sequelae of traumatic brain injury. *Brain Injury*, **2**, 101–129.

Guina, F.D., Cosic, T., Kracun, L. and Dimic, Z. (1997). Sensorimotor stimulation of comatose patients. *Acta Medica Croatica*, **51**, 101–103.

Haig, A.J. and Ruess, J.M. (1990). Recovery from vegetative state of six months' duration associated with Sinemet (levocopa/carbidopa). *Arch Phys Med Rehabil*, **71**, 1081–1083.

Hall, M.E.M., MacDonald, S. and Young, G.C. (1992). The effectiveness of directed multisensory stimulation versus non-directed stimulation in comatose CHI patients: pilot study of a single subject design. *Brain Injury*, **6**(5), 435–445.

Hebb, D.O. (1949). *The Organization of Behaviour*. Wiley, New York.

Holscher, C. (1999). Synaptic plasticity and learning and memory: LTP and beyond. *J Neurosci Res*, **58**, 62–75.

Houdijk, A.P.J., Rijnsburger, E.R., Jansen, J., Wesdorp, R.I.C., et al. (1998). Randomised trial of glutamine-enriched enteral nutrition on infectious morbidity in patients with multiple trauma. *Lancet*, **352**, 772–776.

Hovda, D.A. and Feeney, D.M. (1984). Amphetamine and experience promote recovery of function after motor cortex injury in the cat. *Brain Res*, **298**, 358–361.

Ikonomidou, C. and Turski, L. (2002). Why did NMDA receptor antagonists fail clinical trials for stroke and traumatic brain injury? *Lancet Neurol*, **1**(6), 383–386.

Italian Consensus Conference. (2002). Rehabilitation interventions in patients with traumatic brain injury (TBI) during the acute stage, criteria for transfer to rehabilitation facilities and recommendations for adequate rehabilitation practices. *Giorn Ital Med Riabil*, **15**(1), 23–83.

Izquierdo, I. and Medina, J.H. (1997). Memory formation: the sequence of biochemical events in the hippocampus and its connection to activity in other brain structures. *Neurobiol Learn Mem*, **68**, 285–316.

Jennet, B. (2002). *The Vegetative State, Medical Facts, Etichal and Legal Dilemmas*. Cambridge University Press, Cambridge, UK, pp. 7–32.

Jensen, G.L., Miller, R.H., Talabiska, D.G., Fish, J. and Gianferante, L. (1996). A double-blind, prospective, randomized study of glutamine-enriched compared with standard peptide-based feeding in critically ill patients. *Am J Clin Nutr*, **64**, 615–621.

Johnson, D.A., Roething-Johnston, K. and Richards, D. (1993). Biochemical and physiological parameters of recovery in acute severe head injury: responses to multisensory stimulation. *Brain Injury*, **7**(6), 491–499.

Johnson, M.J., Omery, A. and Nikas, D. (1989). Effects of conversation on intracranial pressure in comatose patients. *Heart Lung*, **18**, 56–63.

Jones, R., Hux, K., Morton-Anderson, A. and Knepper, L. (1994). Auditory stimulation effect on a comatose survivor of traumatic brain injury. *Arch Phys Med Rehabil*, **75**, 164–171.

Kampfl, A., Schmutzhard, E., Franz, G., Pfausler, B., Haring, H.P. and Ulmer, H. (1998). Prediction of recovery from post-traumatic vegetative state with cerebral magnetic-resonance imaging. *Lancet*, **351**, 1763–1767.

Krieger, D.W. (1998). Evoked potentials not just to confirm hopelessness in anoxic brain injury. *Lancet*, **352**, 1796–1797.

Latronico, N., Alongi, S., Facchi, E., et al. (2000). Approach to the patient in a vegetative state. Part III: Prognosis. *Miner Anestesiol*, **66**(4), 241–248.

Levin, H.S., Saydjari, C., Eisenberg, H.M. and Foulkes, M. (1991). Vegetative state after closed head injury: a traumatic coma data bank report. *Arch Neurol*, **48**, 580–585.

Le Winn, E.B. and Dimancescu, M.D. (1978). Environmental deprivation and enrichment in coma. *Lancet*, **2**, 156–157.

Lombardi, F., Taricco, M., De Tanti, A., Telaro, E. and Liberati, A. (2002a). Sensory stimulation of brain injured individuals in coma or vegetative state. *Cochrane Database Syst Rev*, **2**, CD001427.

Lombardi, F., Taricco, M., De Tanti, A., Telaro, E. and Liberati, A. (2002b). Sensory stimulation of brain injured individuals in coma or vegetative state. *Clin Rehabil*, **16**, 465–473.

Mackay, L.E., Bernstein, B.A., Chapman, P.E., Morgan, A.S. and Milazzo, L.S. (1992). Early intervention in severe head injury: long-term benefits of a formalized program. *Arch Phys Med Rehabil*, **73**, 635–641.

Marmarou, A., Montasser, A., Foda, A.E., Bandoh, K., Toshihara, M., Yamamoto, T., Tsuji, O., Zasler, N., Ward, T. and Younf, H.F. (1996). Posttraumatic ventriculomegaly: hydrocephalus or atrophy? A new approach for diagnosis using CSF dynamics. *J Neurosurg*, **85**, 1026–1035.

Marshall, L.F., Gautille, T., Klauber, M.R., Eisenberg, H.M., Jane, J.A., Luerssen, T.G., Marmarou, A. and Foulkes, M.A. (1991). The outcome of severe closed head injury. *J Neurosurg*, **75**, S28–S36.

Matsuda, W., Sugimoto, K., Sato, N., Watanabe, T., Yanaka, K., Matsumu Nose, T. (1999). A case of primary brain stem injury recovered from persistent vegetative state after L-dopa administration. *No To Shinkey*, **51**(12), 1071–1074.

May, W.E. and McGivney, W.J. (1998). Tube feeding and the "vegetative". *Ethics & Medics*, **12**, 1–2.

Mazzini, L., Campini, R., Angelino, E., Rognone, F., Pastore, I., Oliveri, G. (2003). Posttraumatic hydrocephalus: a clinical, neuroradiologic, and neuropsychologic assessment of long-term outcome. *Arch Phys Med Rehabil*, **84**(11), 1637–1641.

Meythaler, J.M., Brunner, R.C., Johnson, A. and Novack, T.A. (2002). Amantadine to improve neurorecovery in traumatic brain injury-associated diffuse axonal injury: a pilot double-blind randomized trial. *J Head Trauma Rehabil*, **17**(**4**), 300–313.

Minderhoud, J.M., van Woerkom, T.C. and van Weerden, T.W. (1976). On the nature of brain stem disorders in severe head injured patients. II. A study on caloric vestibular reactions and neurotransmitter treatment. *Acta Neurochir (Wien)*, **34**, 23–35.

Narayan, R.K., Goskaslan, Z.L., Bontke, C.F. and Berrol, S. (1990). Neurologic sequelae of head injury. In: *Rehabilitation of the Adult and Child With Traumatic Brain Injury* (eds Rosenthal, M., Griffith, E.R., Bond, M.R. and Miller, J.D.), 2nd edn., Davis Company, Philadelphia, pp. 98–101.

Oder, W., Podreka, I., Spatt, J., et al. (1996). Cerebral function following catastrophic brain injury: relevance of single photon emission tomography and positron emission tomography. In: *Catastrophic Brain Injury* (eds Levin, H.S. and Muiozelaar, J.P., et al.), Oxford University Press, New York., Chapter 4.

O'Rourke, K. (1999). On the care of the "vegetative" patients. *Ethics Medics*, **4**, 3–4.

Ott, L.G., Schmidt, J.J., Young, A.B., et al. (1988). Compatison of administration of two standard intravenous amino acid formulas to severely brain injured patients. *Drug Intell Clin Pharm*, **22**, 763–768.

Palumbo, G., De Tanti, A., Molteni, F. and Carda, S. (2004). Intrathecal baclofen therapy on severe traumatic brain injury: clinical and managerial perspectives. A case study. 2004 (in press).

Passler, M.A. and Riggs, V.R. (2001). Positive outcomes in traumatic brain injury-vegetative state: patients treated with bromocriptine. *Arch Phys Med Rehabil*, **82**, 311–315.

Phipps, E.J., DiPasquale, M.D., Blitz, C.L. and Whyte, J. (1997). Interpreting responsiveness in persons with severe traumatic brain injury: beliefs in families and quantitative evaluations. *J Head Trauma Rehabil*, **12**(**4**), 52–69.

Pierce, J.P., Lyle, D.M., Quine, S., Evans, N.J., Morris, J. and Fearnside, M.R. (1990). The effectiveness of coma arousal intervention. *Brain Injury*, **4**(**2**) 191–197.

Plenger, P.M., Dixon, C.E., Castillo, R.M., Frankowski, R.F., Yablon, S.A. and Levin, H.S. (1996). Subacute methylphenidate treatment for moderate to moderate severe traumatic brain injury: a preliminary double–blind placebo-controlled study. *Arch Phys Med Rehabil*, **77**(**6**), 536–540.

Rader, M.A., Alston, J.B. and Ellis, D.W. (1989). Sensory stimulation of severely brain-injured patients. *Brain Injury*, **3**(**2**), 141–147.

Reinhard, D.L., Whyte, J. and Sandel, E. (1996). Improved arousal and initiation following tricyclic antidepressant use in severe brain injury. *Arch Phys Med Rehabil*, **77**, 80–83.

Roberts, P.R. (1995). Nutrition in the head-injured patient. *New Horizons*, **3**(**3**), 506–517.

Rosadini, G. and Sannita, W.G. (1982). Inter- and intra-hemispheric topographic analyses of quantitative EEG in patients in coma. *Res Comm Psychol, Psychatr Behav*, **7**(**1**), 97–107.

Rowlands, B., Hunt, D., Roughneen, P., et al. (1986). Intravenous and enteral nutrition with branched chain amino acid enriched products following multiple trauma with closed head injury. *J Parent Enter Nutrit*, **10**(**Suppl.**), 4S.

Sazbon, L. (1985). Prolonged coma. *Prog clin Neurosci*, **2**, b65–b81.

Sazbon, L. and Grosswasser, Z. (1990). Outcome in 134 patients with prolonged posttraumatic unawareness, I: parameters determining late recovery of consciousness. *J Neurosurg*, **72**, 75–80.

Sazbon, L., Zagreba, F., Ronen, J., Solzi, P. and Costeff, H. (1993). Course and outcome of patients in vegetative state of nontraumatic aetiology. *J Neurol Neurosur Psychiatr*, **56**, 407–409.

Schinner, K.M., Chisolm, A.H., Grap, M.J., Siva, P., Hallinan, M. and LaVoice-Hawkins, A.M. (1995). Effects of auditory stimuli on intracranial pressure and cerebral perfusion pressure in traumatic brain injury. *J Neurosci Nurs*, **27**(**6**), 348–354.

Sisson, R. (1990). Effects of auditory stimuli on comatose patients with head injury. *Heart Lung*, **19**, 373–378.

Stanton, P.K. (1996). LTD, LTP and the sliding threshold for long-term synaptic plasticity. *Hippocampus*, **6**, 35–42.

The Multi-Society Task Force on PVS. (1994). Medical aspects of the persistent vegetative state (second of two parts). *New Engl J Med*, **330**, 1572–1579.

Tribl, G. and Oder, W. (2000). Outcome after shunt implantation in severe head injury with traumatic hydrocephalus. *Brain Injury*, **14**(**4**), 345–354.

van Woerkom, T.C., Teelken, A.W. and Minderhoud, J.M. (1977). Difference in neurotransmitter metabolism in frontotemporal lobe contusion and diffuse cerebral contusion. *Lancet*, **I**, 812–813.

van Woerkom, T.C., Minderhoud, J.M., Gottschal, T. and Nicolai, G. (1982). Neurotransmitters in the treatment of patients with severe head injuries. *Eur J Neurol*, **21**, 227–234.

Vecht, C.J., van Woerkom, C.A., Teelken, A.W. and Minderhoud, J.M. (1975a). Homovanillic acid and 5-hydroxyindoleacetic acid cerebrospinal fluid levels. A study with and without probenecid administration of their relationship to the state of consciousness after head injury. *Arch Neurol*, **32**, 792–797.

Vecht, C.J., van Woerkom, T.C., Teelken, A.W. and Minderhoud, J.M. (1975b). 5-hydroxy indoleacetic acid (5-HIAA) levels in the cerebrospinal fluid in consciousness and unconsciousness after head injury. *Life Sci*, **16**, 1179–1185.

Vecht, C.J., van Woerkom, T.C., Teelken, A.W. and Minderhoud, J.M. (1976). On the nature of brain stem disorders in severe head injured patients. *Acta Neurochir (Wien)*, **34**, 11–21.

Weber, P.L. (1984). Sensorimotor therapy: its effect on electroencephalograms of acute comatose patients. *Arch Phys Med Rehabil*, **65**, 457–462.

Whyte, J., DiPasquale, M. and Vaccaro, M. (1999). Assessment of command-following in minimally conscious brain injured patients. *Arch Phys Med Rehabil*, **80**, 653–660.

Wilson, S.L., Powell, G.E., Elliot, K. and Thwaites, H. (1991). Sensory stimulation in prolonged coma: four single case studies. *Brain Injury*, **5**(**4**), 393–400.

Wilson, S.L., Powell, G.E., Elliot, K. and Thwaites, H. (1993). Evaluation of sensory stimulation as a treatment for prolonged coma – seven single experimental case studies. *Neuropsychol Rehabil*, **3**(**2**), 191–201.

Wilson, S.L., Brock, D., Powell, G.E., Thwaites, H. and Elliot, K. (1996a). Constructing arousal profiles for vegetative state patients – a preliminary report. *Brain Injury*, **10**(**2**), 105–113.

Wilson, S.L., Powell, G.E., Brock, D. and Thwaites, H. (1996b). Behavioural differences between patients who emerged from vegetative state and those who did not. *Brain Injury*, **10**(**7**), 509–516.

Wolf, A.P. and Gleckman, A.D. (1995). Sinemet and brain injury: functional versus statistical change and suggestions for future research designs. *Brain Injury*, **9**(**5**), 487–493.

Wood, R.L. (1991). Critical analysis of the concept of sensory stimulation for patients in vegetative states. *Brain Injury*, **4**, 401–410.

Wood, R.L., Winkowski, T. and Miller, J. (1993). Sensory regulation as a method to promote recovery in patients with altered states of consciousness. *Neuropsychol Rehabil*, **3**(**2**), 177–190.

Wood, R., Winkowski, T.B., Miller, J.L., Tierney, L. and Goldman, L. (1992). Evaluating sensory regulation as a method to improve awareness in patients with altered states of consciousness: a pilot study. *Brain Injury*, **6**, 411–418.

Working group convened by the Royal College of Physicians and endorsed by the Conference of Medical Royal Colleges and their faculties of the United Kingdom (1996). The permanent vegetative state (review). *J R Coll Physicians London*, **30**, 119–121.

Wroblewski, B., Glenn, M.B., Cornblatt, R., Joseph, A.B. and Suduikis, S. (1993). Protriptyline as an alternative stimulant medication in patients with brain injury: a series of case reports. *Brain Injury*, **7**(**4**), 353–362.

Wroblewski, B., Joseph, A.B. and Cornblatt, R. (1996). Antidepressant pharmacotherapy and the treatment of depression in patients with severe traumatic brain injury: a controlled, prospective study. *J Clin Psychiatry*, **57**(**12**), 582–587.

Young, B., Ott, L., Norton, J., et al. (1985). Metabolic and nutritional sequelae in the non-steroid treated head injury patient. *Neurosurgery*, **17**, 784–791.

Zandbergen, E.G.J., de Haan, R.J., Stoutenbeek, C.P., Koelman, J.H.T.M. and Hijdra, A. (1998). Systematic review of early prediction of poor outcome in anoxic-ischaemic coma. *Lancet*, **352**, 1808–1812.

Zasler, N.D. (1997). Prognostic indicators in medical rehabilitation of traumatic brain injury: a commentary and review. *Arch Phys Med Rehabil*, **78**, S12–S16.

Zasler, N.D. and Marmarou, A. (1992). Posttraumatic hydrocephalus. In: *TBI Transmit* Vol. (III). N.3, Summer.

Ziegler, T.R., Smith, R.J., Byrne, T.A. and Wilmore, D.W. (1993). Potential role of glutamine supplementation in nutrition support. *Clinical Nutrition*, **12**(**Suppl.**), S82–S90.

23

Plasticity in the neural pathways for swallowing: role in rehabilitation of dysphagia

John C. Rosenbek and Neila J. Donovan

Department of Communicative Disorders, VA RR&D Brain Rehabilitation Research Center, University of Florida, Gainesville, FL, USA

Dysphagia is defined as difficulty moving food and liquid from the mouth into the stomach. Traditionally this condition is divided into oropharyngeal and esophageal dysphagia to identify the locus of involvement. Oropharyngeal dysphagia is the focus of this chapter. It results when the structures or functions of the face, mouth, palate, pharynx, rostral esophagus, or larynx are altered by disease. For decades a feeding tube was the treatment of choice. Beginning in the 1960s and 1970s an array of clinical and instrumental evaluative techniques and medical, surgical, and behavioral approaches to its rehabilitation began appearing (Carrau and Murray, 1999; Huckabee and Pelletier, 1999). The evaluative approaches, including videofluoroscopy of the swallowing structures in action (Logemann, 1997) and endoscopic visualization during swallowing (Langmore, 2000), have increased understanding of the disturbed biomechanics responsible for impaired swallowing. Similarly the treatments for these biomechanical abnormalities have become increasingly powerful influences on the swallowing mechanism and on its neural controls in the nervous system.

This chapter's main purpose is to discuss the notion of neural plasticity in relation to dysphagia rehabilitation. The relative infancy of dysphagia science and the relatively short modern duration of excitement about the nervous system's plastic response to systematic stimulation mean that the data on changes in brain in response to swallowing treatment are in very short supply. They are, however, emerging, and

the extant data will be reviewed. That review requires a context comprising brief discussion of the:

1 structures and neural controls on which swallowing depends,
2 causes of dysphagia,
3 approaches to evaluation, including measurement of treatment effect,
4 classification and description of the most frequently employed treatment approaches.

These brief reviews will acquaint the reader with the clinical science of dysphagia and make the subsequent discussion of the plasticity data easier to evaluate.

23.1 Anatomy

Multiple structures of the head and neck are critical to normal oropharyngeal swallowing which traditionally is divided into oral and pharyngeal stages. During the oral stage the jaw contributes to mouth closure and stabilizes and helps raise the tongue toward the hard and soft palates as the swallow is triggered. The lips and teeth form a cavity with the tongue to contain the bolus of food or liquid in the mouth. The tongue moves the bolus around to mix it with saliva and then propels it posteriorly through the anterior and posterior faucial pillars and into the pharynx. This posterior movement triggers what has come to be called the swallow's pharyngeal stage. Simultaneously, or somewhat ahead of this

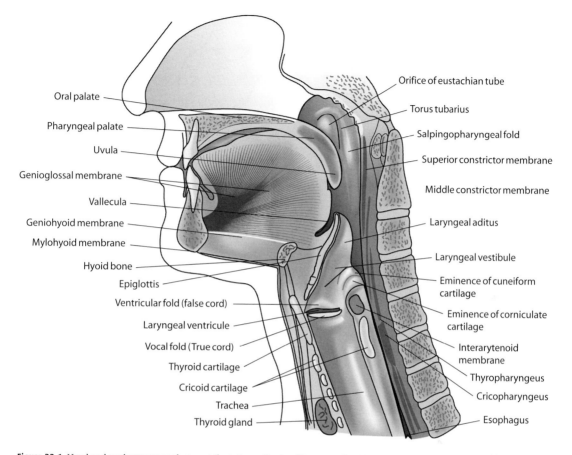

Figure 23.1. Head and neck structures that contribute to swallowing (Bosma et al., 1986, reprinted with permission).

posterior movement, the soft palate elevates toward the posterior pharyngeal wall thereby preventing passage of bolus into the nose. Simultaneously as well, the larynx squeezes shut so material cannot fall into the airway and begins – along with the hyoid bone to which it is connected – to move anteriorly and superiorly in the neck. It is this elevation that both contributes to airway protection and to the opening of the rostral esophagus, called the upper esophageal sphincter (UES). UES opening occurs prior to the bolus's arrival at the rostral esophagus and is made possible by the muscle and tendon connections of the hyoid bone, larynx, and UES. This elevation also causes the epiglottis to tilt down over the opening into the larynx, thereby offering further protection to the airway. These structures are shown in Fig. 23.1.

23.2 Neurophysiology

Predictably this complex set of activities requires complex neural controls. Motor fibers of cranial nerves V, VII, IX, X, XI, and XII innervate jaw, face, palate, pharynx, larynx, and tongue, respectively. As the motor system depends on sensory information if swallowing is to occur normally, sensory fibers from these same cranial nerves, with the exception of XI and XII, which are motor only, are also critical. These sensory components transport taste, temperature,

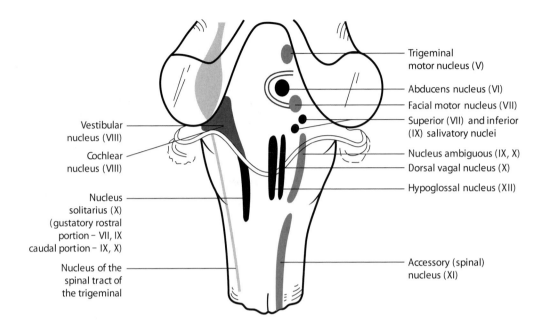

Figure 23.2. Brainstem structures involved in the central pattern generator for swallowing Crary and Groher, 2003, p. 29, reprinted with permission.

touch, and pressure from critical structures in the mouth, pharynx, and larynx.

Central pattern generator

Miller (1986, 1999) has written the most thorough description of the central pattern generator in the medulla where this sensory and motor information is mixed and controlled. Central pattern generator structures are displayed in Fig. 23.2.

The dorsal region of the central pattern generator contains the sensory components comprising nucleus tractus solitarius and the surrounding reticular activating system with additional input from the sensory nucleus of the Vth cranial nerve and from more rostral cortical and subcortical structures. Taste, temperature, touch, and pressure are integrated in this sensory portion of the pattern generator. The resulting cascade of sensations has a twofold effect. First, the cascade facilitates the initiation and repeated activation of the muscles involved in the pharyngeal phase of swallowing. Second, it activates the interneurons that modify the motor output to the swallowing musculature.

The ventral region comprises the nucleus ambiguous and surrounding reticular activating system with additional motor influences from the Vth and XIIth cranial nerves. The ventral motor complex contributes to swallowing by coordinating the complex movements needed to complete the swallow. In addition, according to Miller, this area contains neurons with special properties. Specifically, the neurons in this area produce cyclic bust patterns that allow for timed and sequential discharges, thereby supporting the complex coordinations essential to normal swallowing.

Subcortical and cortical influences

The oropharyngeal swallow is more profitably viewed as a highly patterned response than as a reflex. However, the unfolding swallowing response is increasingly more automatic as one moves from the mouth's chewing, bolus formation, and posterior bolus movement functions to the functions of the pharyngeal stage. Nonetheless, some control can be extended even over the pharyngeal component of the swallow. This control is possible because of inter-actions of subcortical and cortical centers with the central pattern generator. Relevant subcortical and cortical areas include left and right basal ganglia, insula, sensorimotor cortex, and the supplementary and premotor areas of both frontal lobes. Martin and Sessle (1993) suggest that the cerebral cortex is impor-tant to initiation and modulation of the stages of swal-lowing, as well as to integration of swallowing with other sensorimotor functions, including alimenta-tion and respiration.

23.3 Causes of dysphagia

Any abnormality of critical swallowing structures or neural controls can disrupt swallowing with the nature of the deficit being at least in part the result of the locus and type of involvement. Major structural abnormalities are, of course, head and neck tumors such as a cancer invading the floor of the mouth. Surgical and radiation for these tumors can also con-tribute to the swallowing dysfunction. In the latter case a major cause is fibrotic change to otherwise healthy tissue. Reduced saliva from surgery, radia-tion, or medications is another negative influence on swallowing. The full panoply of neurologic diseases can also make swallowing difficult or impossible depending on the site of neurologic involvement. These include stroke, tumor, trauma, infectious dis-ease, movement disorders, and other degenerative diseases. In addition muscle and connective disease such as polymyositis can cause dysphagia. Finally deconditioning as when a geriatric person fractures a hip and is immobilized and nourished via tube during the period before and after surgery can cause swallowing to deteriorate.

23.4 Evaluation

The purposes of evaluation in dysphagia are to:

1 determine the presence of a dysphagia by identi-fying signs of abnormality,

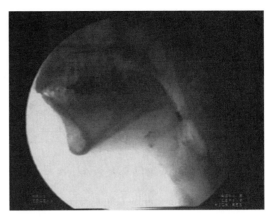

Figure 23.3. Videofluoroscopic image of the swallowing structures Crary and Groher, 2003, p. 190A, reprinted with permission.

2 support hypotheses about the underlying patho-physiology, whether it is weakness, abnormal tone, or discoordination for example,
3 provide guidance to an appropriate treatment,
4 measure change with time, disease, or treatment.

A clinical examination such as the MASA (Mann assessment of swallowing ability; Mann, 2000) is the usual first step and because sensitivity and speci-ficity of signs from this examination are known, especially for stroke patients, it may be the only examination administered. Frequently, however, an instrumented examination follows. The two most frequently employed are the videofluoroscopic swal-lowing examination (VFSE) and the endoscopic swal-lowing examination. A videofluoroscopic image of the swallowing structures appears in Fig. 23.3.

23.5 Treatment

Surgical, medical, and behavioral treatments for dys-phagia are now available (Carrau and Murray, 1999; Huckabee and Pelletier, 1999). Surgical and medical treatments may be curative, palliative, or result in improvements that are nonetheless inadequate to adequate, safe nutrition. The behavioral treatments, which may precede, follow, or be administered concurrently with medical and surgical ones are traditionally divided into compensatory and rehabilitative. Only the rehabilitative treatments will be discussed, because their influence on the person with dysphagia provides the greatest contribution to what is known about plasticity in dysphagia.

Rehabilitative treatments

Treatments to improve tongue function, pharyngeal muscle activity, laryngeal closure, and anterior and superior movement, UES opening, to heighten sensory input, and to improve the coordination of movements among all these structures have been developed. Data documenting their effects on swallowing movements and functional status including improved rate of eating and drinking have also begun to appear. Table 23.1 comprises a listing of the most commonly used methods, brief descriptions of how they are to be performed, indications for use, references, and levels of evidence in support of application.

23.6 Treatment effects

The two principle classes of outcome measurement in the majority of treatment studies are:

1 biomechanical measures of durational relationships between test boluses (material swallowed whether liquid, semi-solid, or solid) and structural movements,
2 measures of bolus flow abnormality.

An example of a traditional durational measure is duration of swallow initiation defined as the time from the bolus' arrival at the posterior mouth to the beginning of pharyngeal stage activity. A traditional and critical bolus flow measure is aspiration defined as bolus passing through the larynx and into the trachea either before, during, or after the swallow. These and other biomechanical measures are usually influenced in positive ways by the treatments previously described. Delays are reduced or eliminated and bolus flow is improved so that aspiration is eliminated or reduced in amount and frequency. These findings are consistent with the hypothesis

that the nervous system's potential plasticity can be activated by treatment.

23.7 Evidence for plasticity

Filipek (2000) defines plasticity as "the brain's ability to recover function that was lost as a result of a defined insult that produced a discrete lesion" (p. 265). The effort to establish the central or plastic effects of treatment for dysphagia is in its infancy. The seminal data are arriving primarily from a single laboratory in Manchester, England (Hamdy et al., 1998, 1999; Fraser et al., 2002; Power et al., 2004). Transcranial magnetic stimulation (TMS) has been the primary method of determining changes in brain (see Volume I, Chapter 15), although positron emission tomography (PET) data are also available (see Volume II, Chapter 5). The only treatment studied in any detail is electrical stimulation applied either to the faucial pillars or pharynx. The population has been limited to stroke, usually unilateral hemispheric stroke in particular. Despite these limitations, the data are informative and are kindling a worldwide effort at replication and expansion of the findings.

Cortical swallowing control

Using TMS and PET, Hamdy and colleagues (1996) were the first to demonstrate the bilateral asymmetric cortical modulation of the oropharyngeal swallow, asymmetric modulation that is independent of handedness. They identified relatively distinct, but overlapping regions of control for oral, pharyngeal, and esophageal stages of swallowing. The oral stage region, as determined by the mylohyoid muscle which shares responsibility for the lingual triggering of the swallow, was more anterolateral than the pharyngeal stage region, which in turn was more anterolateral than the region for the esophagus. More specifically the region for the mylohyoid was located in lateral precentral and inferior frontal gyri. For the pharynx the area was in the anterolateral precentral and middle frontal gyri, and for the esophagus the locus was similar except it involved the superior frontal gyri. As they say in summary: "the mylohyoid locus, therefore,

Table 23.1. Rehabilitative treatments, methodology, indications, and *levels of evidence.

Target	Treatment	Methodology	Indications	*Levels of evidence
Improved tongue function	Showa maneuver (Hirano et al., 1999)	Subject instructed to take a deep breath and hold it while pressing the tongue to the roof of the mouth and performing an effortful swallow	For individuals with decreased posterior tongue movement	Level 3 (n = 8): Case–control design
	Lee Silverman voice treatment (Sharkawi et al., 2002)	Valsalva maneuver with vowel prolongation at maximum performance level	For individuals with dysphagia secondary to Parkinson's disease	Level 4 (n = 8): observational studies without controls
Improved posterior pharyngeal wall movement	Masako maneuver (Fujiu et al., 1995; Fujiu and Logemann, 1996)	Subject protrudes tongue maximally and holds it comfortably between central incisors while performing an effortful swallow	For individuals with reduced or restricted posterior pharyngeal wall movement	Level 4 (n = 10): observational studies without controls
Increased laryngeal closure	Supraglottic swallow (Logemann et al., 1997)	Subject takes a breath and holds it before and during the swallow, and coughs immediately after the swallow but before inhaling	For individuals with inadequate laryngeal closure	Level 4 (n = 9): observational studies without controls
Improved UES opening	Mendelsohn maneuver (Mendelsohn and Martin, 1993)	Subject is asked to swallow normally and when the larynx reaches the highest point, to hold it there for a short time	For individuals with inadequate UES opening	Level 4 (n = 10): observational studies without controls
	Shaker head raise (Shaker et al., 2002)	Subject lies supine on a firm surface and lifts head keeping shoulders down.	For individuals with inadequate UES opening	Level 2 (n = 27): non-randomized controlled trial
Heightened sensory input	Tactile thermal stimulation (Rosenbek et al., 1996, 1998)	Therapist rubs both of the patient's faucial pillars three to four times with an ice stick with firm strokes and asks the subject to swallow hard (300–450 trials)	For individuals with delayed swallow response secondary to decreased sensation	Level 2 (n = 45): non-randomized controlled trial
	Electrical stimulation of pharynx (Hamdy et al., 1998)	Electrical stimulation of the pharynx at midline is administered via a swallowed electrode. Stimulation occurs for 10 min at 5 Hz	For individuals with delayed swallow response and general pharyngeal dysphagia	Level 3 (n = 10): observational studies without controls
	Electrical stimulation of faucial pillars (Power et al., 2004)	Electrical stimulation of the faucial pillars may inhibit the swallow and do more harm than good	For individuals with delayed swallow response and general pharyngeal dysphagia	Level 3 (n = 10): observational studies with controls

* Agency for Healthcare Research and Quality, 2001.

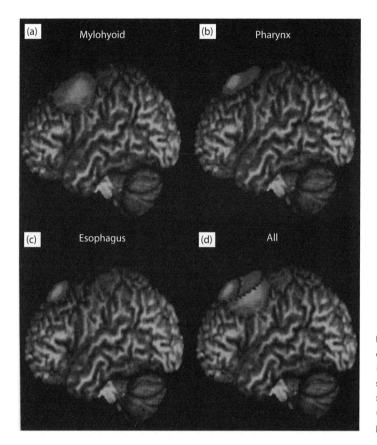

Figure 23.4. Location of regions of cortical control for (a) mylohyoid, (b) pharyngeal, (c) esophageal, and (d) all three states of swallowing in the left hemispheres of normal subjects, as determined by TMS (Hamdy et al., 1996, reprinted with permission).

appeared to be sited predominantly on primary motor cortex, whereas the pharyngeal locus was sited both on primary motor cortex and premotor cortex, and the esophageal locus was sited predominantly on the premotor cortex, but extended onto the primary motor cortex" (p. 1220). The locus of these areas is similar in the two hemispheres but largest in the swallowing dominant hemisphere for the pharyngeal response. The oral stage as represented by the mylohyoid tends to be symmetric. The cortical representation of these three stages is shown in Fig. 23.4.

Dysphagia after cortical insult

Estimates of the proportion of patients with dysphagia after unilateral hemispheric lesion vary, with 30% being a reasonable estimate (Hamdy et al.,

1997). The best extant hypothesis about why is that dysphagia is most likely if the stroke is in the swallowing dominant hemisphere. However, the notion of hemispheric dominance remains controversial (Kelly and Huckabee, 2003). Hamdy and colleagues (1997) studied 20 stroke patients, 8 of whom had dysphagia, in reaching this conclusion. One subtlety in these data is the difference in oral and pharyngeal stage control. They consider mylohyoid control to be bilateral and symmetric, whereas pharyngeal control is asymmetric. If they are correct, their hemispheric dominance hypothesis explains the presence of pharyngeal dysphagia in their sample. Deficits in the oral stage such as preparation, formation, and movement of the bolus may be equally likely from damage to either hemisphere. Studies using VFSE will be needed to resolve this issue.

Recovery from dysphagia

Recovery from the dysphagia resulting from cortical stroke is usually faster and more complete than for that resulting from bilateral cortical, and unilateral and bilateral brain stem lesions (Horner et al., 1991). Hamdy and colleagues (1998) explored the mechanisms of recovery in 28 stroke patients. The participant's swallowing was measured with serial VFSEs at 1 week, 1 month, and 3 months. Bilateral swallowing center control was measured by TMS on the same schedule. Most of these patients had recovered by 1 month and only the severely dysphagic patients had persisting dysphagia at 3 months. In the recovered patients, the size of the cortical swallowing areas for the pharynx increased in the healthy hemisphere. The expansion was in an anterolateral direction. In some instances this expansion occurred before changes in swallowing performance, suggesting that changes in brain are influential in recovery rather than merely reflecting recovery that occurs for some other reason. These findings lead the authors to conclude: "there remains in the intact hemisphere the capacity for reorganization, which can then develop sufficient control over brain stem centers for swallowing recovery to occur" (p. 1112). A review of the individual patient data reveals one other observation critical to thinking about treatment. A small number of patients did not recover, despite having large pharyngeal control areas in the intact hemisphere. This suggests that a patient with dysphagia but a normal region of pharyngeal modulation in the intact hemisphere be given a high treatment priority because there is a low probability for that patient's recovery.

Recovery with treatment

Enhanced sensory input is a traditional treatment for enhancing the swallowing response (Rosenbek et al., 1991, 1996, 1998). The Manchester group (Hamdy et al., 1998; Fraser et al., 2002) has published their experience with electrical stimulation to the pharynx in normal and dysphagic subjects. The method requires each subject to swallow a small diameter catheter to which electrodes are attached for delivery of the stimulation to the pharynx at the midline. A variety of stimulus intensities and durations were studied. TMS was completed prior to, immediately after, and 30 min after stimulation. Ten minutes of stimulation at 5 Hz resulted in increased cortical excitability and an expansion of the area of cortical representation for the pharyngeal stage of swallowing which persisted for 30 min, accompanied by improved swallow. Said another way, the effects of the electrical stimulation produced changes in brain similar to those seen in spontaneously recovering persons. See Fig. 23.5 for cortical representation before and after pharyngeal stimulation in normal swallowers.

In another study (Power et al., 2004), electrical stimulation was administered to the anterior faucial pillars of normal swallowers. Stimulation at 5 Hz at this site inhibited the cortical response and decreased the responsiveness of the functional swallow. Stimulation at 0.2 Hz facilitated the cortical response but had no effect on the functional swallow. These findings are especially interesting to swallowing scientists because faucial pillar stimulation with touch, cold, pressure, and now electrical stimulation has been a staple of clinical practice for three decades (Lazzara et al., 1986; Rosenbek et al., 1991, 1998). For the first time in the swallowing literature data suggesting that negative effects are possible have appeared. These data do not mean that treatments should cease, of course. Indeed it appears that electrical stimulation applied at the right site, intensity, and duration can cause plastic changes in the brain that correlate with changes in function. Similarly, the wrong site, duration, and intensity may inhibit plastic changes.

23.8 Learned non-use

Learned non-use can occur when a behavior is not performed for a period of time extending into the interval when performance is actually possible physiologically (Taub et al., 1993; Miltner et al., 1999; Liepert et al., 2001). Learned non-use in dysphagia

(a)

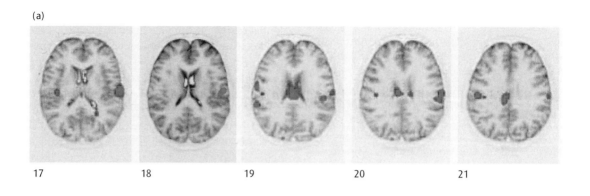

17   18   19   20   21

(b)

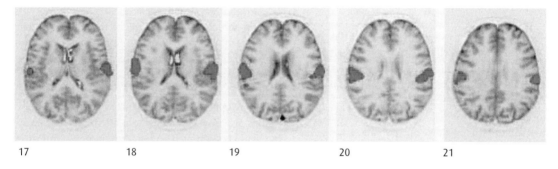

17   18   19   20   21

Figure 23.5. Patterns of activation (a) before and (b) after electrical stimulation in normal swallowers. Activation increased bilaterally (Fraser C. et al., 2002 reprinted with permission).

has not been studied, but it should be. A typical pattern of managing the dysphagic person is tube feeding. Unlike the case of limb paralysis where movement is never performed, in dysphagia even a tube-fed person will continue to swallow saliva unless the dysphagia is profound in which saliva is suctioned or spit into a container. Nonetheless the number of swallows is drastically reduced. As some tube-fed persons are not systematically followed, this reduced rate of swallowing may persist long after some additional swallowing of food and drink is possible. Thus tube feeding presents the researcher with a natural laboratory for studying cortical effects of non-use. A priority would be to determine if a period of tube feeding changes cortical representation of swallowing structures. Next it would be important to test the effects of treatment in cases of learned non-use.

23.9 Negative effects of treatment

The potential negative effects of inappropriately timed or intense treatments especially in relation to severity of neurologic deficit (Kozlowski et al., 1996; Kozlowski and Shallert, 1998; Shallert and Kozlowski, 1998; Shallert et al., 2000) warrants research. It is known that the wrong intensity of electrical stimulation can inhibit cortical functioning. It may well be that such inhibition is a function of lesion size. Smaller lesions may have what Shallert and colleagues (2000) call a "penumbra of vulnerable yet potentially salvageable tissue surrounding the core of the infarct" (p. 159). The wrong treatment intensity and this vulnerable tissue can be further degraded. The tradition in speech–language pathology is to intervene early but possible negative effects of early intervention require further study. Dysphagia clinicians are not used to thinking about harm; that attitude may need to change.

23.10 Alternative explanations of treatment effects

In addition to plasticity, other explanations, especially for immediate effects of treatment can be posited. These include what Moerman and Jonas (2002) call an information effect, more popularly known as a placebo effect. Indeed, as in all treatments, a placebo effect is anticipated in dysphagia management. Another possible explanation, which is probably distinct from the placebo effect, is that patients merely increase attention, concentration, or effort, thereby enhancing performance. The effect is to use more of what might be called the residual support for swallowing. Like the information or placebo effect, this effort effect is to be understood on the way to a fuller appreciation of how rehabilitation changes performance. An issue to be resolved by research is to discover if these influences are different from what are called short-term mechanism of plasticity (Nudo et al., 2000). These authors describe short-term plasticity as "an immediate reorganization in response to altered afferent inputs" (p. 182). The implication is that these short-term changes reflect differences in "synaptic efficacy." Presumably placebo effects and – if they are different – effects resulting from increased attention would be supported by changes in nervous system activity remote from the cortical swallowing centers. Short-term plastic changes are likely to be supported by perilesional changes.

Peripheral and central effects

Huckabee and Cannito (1999) have observed that the relationship among peripheral changes from treatment by which they mean a variety of performance and muscle level changes and central or plastic changes in the nervous system should be investigated. Doubtless these relationships will be complex. A variety of hypotheses can be tested. Early peripheral changes may precede changes in the nervous system. They may follow changes in the central nervous system (Hamdy et al., 1998). They may be associated simultaneously with widely distributed, even bilateral, alterations in brain activity. Late in treatment, the alterations may be more focal involving subcortical regions, perilesional areas, or homologous areas on the brain's side opposite the lesion. These and other permutations, based on underlying pathophysiology of the swallow; locus of damage; and type, intensity, and duration of treatment are yet to be tested. However, a beginning in the understanding of plastic changes with dysphagia treatment has been made.

23.11 Conclusions

Clinicians are convinced most dysphagia management is successful in restoring safe, adequate, pleasurable eating and drinking. The evidence on which this conviction rests is taken from single case and small N studies, however, so the probability of Type II errors is high. Randomized clinical trials will address this shortcoming. In even shorter supply is evidence for experience-dependent plasticity in dysphagia. The early data are promising for electrical stimulation, especially of the pharynx, but are non-existent for all other methods. These data need to be collected. As the science of dysphagia matures, the "why" questions will be more frequently asked. The relationships of peripheral and central changes will be elucidated and ways of maximizing both will be developed. In the interim, clinicians will continue to practice in ways guided by the extant data and their professional experience. Clinical-scientists will continue working to provide a firmer database. Both groups can afford to be confident because the reality of plasticity, even in the damaged adult brain, is now widely recognized.

REFERENCES

Agency for Healthcare Research and Quality (2001). In: *Evidence Report/Technology Assessment: Number 43.* AHRQ Publication #01-E058. Agency for Healthcare Research and Quality, Rockville, MD.

Bosma, J.F., Donner, M.W., Tanaka, E. and Robertson, D. (1986). The anatomy of the pharynx, pertinent to swallowing. *Dysphagia,* **1**, 24.

Carrau, R.T. and Murray, T. (1999). *Comprehensive Management of Swallowing Disorders,* Singular Publishing, San Diego.

Crary, M.A. and Groher, M.E. (2003). *Introduction to Adult Swallowing Disorders,* Butterworth Heinemann, St. Louis.

Filipek, P.A. (2000). The developmental disorders: does plasticity play a role? In: *Cerebral Reorganization of Function After Brain Damage* (eds Levin, H.S. and Grafman, J.), Oxford University Press, Oxford, pp. 165–290.

Fraser, C., Power, M., Hamdy, S., Rothwell, J., Hobday, D., Hollander, I., Tyrell, P., Hobson, A., Williams, S. and Thompson, D. (2002). Driving plasticity in adult human motor cortex is associated with improved motor function after brain injury. *Neuron,* **34**, 831–840.

Fujiu, M. and Logemann, J.A. (1996). Effect of a tongue-holding maneuver on posterior pharyngeal wall movement during deglutition. *Am J Speech-Lang Patholo,* **5**, 23–30.

Fujiu, M., Logemann, J.A. and Pauloski, B.R. (1995). Increased postoperative posterior pharyngeal wall movement in patients with anterior oral cancer; preliminary findings and possible implications for treatment. *Am J Speech-Lang Pathol,* **4**, 24–30.

Hamdy, S., Aziz, Q., Rothwell, J.C., Singh, K.D.C., Barlow, J., Hughes, D.G., Tallis, R.C. and Thompson, D.G. (1996). The cortical topography of human swallowing musculature in health and disease. *Nat Med,* **11**, 1217–1224.

Hamdy, S., Aziz, Q., Rothwell, J.C., Crone, R., Hughes, D.G., Tallis, R.C. and Thompson, D.G. (1997). Explaining oropharyngeal dysphagia after unilateral hemispheric stroke. *Lancet,* **350**, 686–692.

Hamdy, S., Aziz, Q., Rothwell, J.C., Power, M., Singh, K.D.C., Nicholson, D.A., Tallis, R.C. and Thompson, D.G. (1998). Recovery of swallowing after dysphagic stroke relates to functional reorganization in the intact motor cortex. *Gastroenterology,* **115**, 1104–1112.

Hamdy, S., Rothwell, J.C., Brooks, D.J., Bailey, D., Aziz, Q. and Thompson, D.G. (1999). Identification of the cerebral loci processing human swallowing with H2150 PET activation. *J Neurol,* **81**, 1917–1926.

Hirano, K., Takahashi, K., Uyama, R., Yamashita, Y., Yokoyama, M., Michiwaki, Y., Michi, K., Seki, K., Sano, T., Okano, T. and

Groher, M.E. (1999). Objective evaluation of swallow maneuver (show a swallow maneuver) using CT images. *Dysphagia,* **14**, 127 (abstract).

Horner, J., Bouyer, F.G., Alberts, M.J. and Helms, M.J. (1991). Dysphagia following brain-stem stroke: clinical correlates and outcome. *Arch Phys Med Rehab,* **48**, 1170–1173.

Huckabee, M.L. and Cannito, M.P. (1999). Outcomes of swallowing rehabilitation in chronic brainstem dysphagia: a retrospective evaluation. *Dysphagia,* **14**, 93–109.

Huckabee, M.L. and Pelletier, C.A. (1999). *Management of Adult Neurogenic Dysphagia,* Singular Publishing, San Diego.

Kelly, B.N. and Huckabee, M.L. (2003). Cerebral dominance in swallowing neural networks. *New Zeal J Speech-Lang Ther,* **58**, 47–53.

Kozlowski, D.A. and Shallert, T. (1998). Relationship between dendritic pruning and behavioral therapy following sensorimotor cortex lesions. *Behav Brain Res,* **97**, 89–98.

Kozlowski, D.A., James, D.C. and Shallert, T. (1996). Use-dependent exaggeration of neuronal injury following unilateral sensorimotor cortex lesions. *J Neurosci,* **16**, 4776–4786.

Langmore, S.E. (2000). Fiberoptic endoscopic evaluation of swallowing. In: *Evaluation of Dysphagia in Adults: Expanding the Diagnostic Options* (ed. Mills, R.H.), Pro-ed, Austin, pp. 145–178.

Lazzara, G., Lazarus, C.L. and Logemann, J.A. (1986). Impact of thermal stimulation on the triggering of the swallowing reflex. *Dysphagia,* **1**, 73–80.

Liepert, J., Uhde, I., Graf, S., Leidner, O. and Weiller, C. (2001). Motor cortex plasticity during forced-use therapy in stroke patients: a preliminary study. *J Neurol,* **248**, 315–321.

Logemann, J.A. (1997). *Evaluation and Treatment of Swallowing Disorders,* Pro-ed, Austin.

Logemann, J.A., Pauloski, B.R., Rademaker, A.W. and Colangelo, L.A. (1997). Super-supraglottic swallow in irradiated head and neck cancer patients. *Head Neck,* **19**, 535–540.

Mann, G. (2000). *MASA: The Mann Assessment of Swallowing Ability,* Singular Publishing, San Diego.

Martin, R.E. and Sessle, B.J. (1993). The role of the cerebral cortex in swallowing. *Dysphagia,* **8**, 195–202.

Mendelsohn, M.S. and Martin, R.E. (1993). Airway protection during breath-holding. *Ann Otol Rhinol Laryngol,* **102**, 941–944.

Miller, A.J. (1986). Neurophysiological basis of swallowing. *Dysphagia,* **1**, 91–100.

Miller, A.J. (ed.) (1999). *The Neuroscientific Principles of Swallowing and Dysphagia,* Singular Publishing, San Diego.

Miltner, W.H.R., Bauder, H., Sommer, M., Dettmers, C. and Taub, E. (1999). Effects of constraint-induced movement therapy on patients with chronic motor deficits after stroke: a replication. *Stroke,* **30**, 586–592.

Moerman, D.E. and Jonas, W.B. (2002). Deconstructing the placebo effect and finding the meaning response. *Ann Intern Med*, **136**, 471–476.

Nudo, R.J., Barbay, S. and Kleim, J.A. (2000). Role of neuroplasticity in functional recovery after stroke. In: *Cerebral Reorganization of Function After Brain Damage* (eds Levin, H.S. and Grafman, J.), Oxford University Press, Oxford, pp. 168–200.

Power, M., Fraser, C., Hobson, A., Rothwell, J.C., Mistry, S., Nicholson, D.A., Thompson, D.G. and Hamdy, S. (2004). Changes in pharyngeal corticobulbar excitability and swallowing behavior after oral stimulation. *Amer J Physiol: Gastr Liver Physiol*, **286**, G45–G50.

Rosenbek, J.C., Robbins, J., Fishback, B. and Levine, R.L. (1991). Effects of thermal application on dysphagia after stroke. *J Speech Hear Res*, **34**, 1257–1268.

Rosenbek, J.C., Roecker, E.B., Wood, J.L. and Robbins, J. (1996). Thermal application reduces the duration of stage transition in dysphagia after stroke. *Dysphagia*, **11**, 225–233.

Rosenbek, J.C., Robbins, J. and Williford, W.O. (1998). Comparing treatment intensities of tactile-thermal application. *Dysphagia*, **13**, 1–9.

Shaker, R., Easterling, C., Kern, M., Nitschke, T., Massey, B., Daniels, S., Grande, B., Kazandjian, M. and Dikeman, K. (2002). Rehabilitation of swallowing by exercise in tube-fed patients with pharyngeal dysphagia secondary to abnormal UES opening. *Gastroenterology*, **122**, 1314–1321.

Shallert, T. and Kozlowski, D.A. (1998). Brain damage and plasticity: use-related neural growth and overuse-related exaggeration of injury. In: *Cerebrovascular Disease: Pathology, Diagnosis, and Management* (eds Ginsbert, M.D. and Bogousslavsky, J.), Blackwell Science, Cambridge, MA, pp. 611–619.

Shallert, T., Bland, S., Leasure, J.L., Tillerson, J., Gonzales, R., Williams, L., Aronowski, J. and Grotta, J. (2000). Motor rehabilitation, use-related neural events, and reorganization of the brain after injury. In: *Cerebral Reorganization of Function After Brain Injury* (eds Levin, H.S. and Grafman, J.), Oxford University Press, Inc., Oxford, pp. 145–167.

Sharkawi, A.E., Ramig, L., Logemann, J.A., Pauloski, B.R., Rademaker, A.W., Smith, C.H., Pawlas, A., Baum, S. and Wemer, C. (2002). Swallowing and voice effects of lee silverman voice therapy (LSVT): a pilot study. *J Neurol Neurosurg Psychiatr*, **72**, 31–36.

Taub, E., Miller, N.E., Novack, T.A., Cook III, E.W., Fleming, W.C., Nepomuceno, C.S., Connell, J.S. and Crago, J.E. (1993). Technique to improve chronic motor deficit after stroke. *Arch Phys Med Rehab*, **74**, 347–354.

24

Autonomic dysfunction

Brenda S. Mallory

Department of Rehabilitation Medicine, Columbia University College of Physicians & Surgeons, New York, USA

That "humans absolutely require a functionally intact sympathetic nervous system to tolerate the 'non-emergency' behavior of simply standing up" is testimony to the importance of the autonomic nervous system (ANS) and although orthostatic intolerance is the hallmark of sympathetic neurocirculatory failure it is but one manifestation among many of autonomic dysfunction (Goldstein et al., 2002). Clinical manifestations of ANS dysfunction can result from the disordered autonomic control of the cardiovascular, sudomotor, alimentary, urinary, and sexual systems. The etiology of autonomic dysfunction may be primary, such as pure autonomic failure (PAF), secondary, such as that due to cervical spinal cord injury (SCI) or due to drugs and chemical toxins (Mathias, 2003). An understanding of the components of the ANS, their function and their supraspinal, spinal and peripheral organization is essential to appreciate autonomic dysfunction. Additionally, the disturbance of ANS function such as that seen in persons with cervical SCI results not only from the loss of normal supraspinal control of the ANS, but also from changes caused by synaptic reorganization and neuronal plasticity in the damaged spinal cord.

24.1 Anatomy and physiology

The ANS has three peripheral components (the sympathetic, parasympathetic, and enteric nervous systems) and a supraspinal and spinal organization that is essential to its regulation of visceral function and maintenance of internal homeostasis. The control systems of the ANS involve: (1) supraspinal controlling and integrative neuronal centers; (2) supraspinal, spinal, ganglionic, and peripheral interneurons; and (3) afferent neurons (Shields Jr., 1993). Afferent neurons have cell bodies in the dorsal root ganglia or cranial nerve somatic sensory ganglia. The sympathetic and parasympathetic nerves form an efferent pathway comprised of preganglionic and postganglionic neurons (Fig. 24.1). The second-order postganglionic neurons synapse upon smooth and cardiac muscle and also control glandular secretion. *Norepinephrine* (NE) is the main chemical messenger of the sympathetic nervous system and *Acetylcholine* (Ach) is the main messenger of the parasympathetic nervous system. Ach is also the neurotransmitter for all preganglionic axons, both parasympathetic and sympathetic. Thermoregulatory sweating is mediated by sympathetic postganglionic axons that release Ach (Shields Jr., 1993).

Ach receptors are of two types, muscarinic and nicotinic. Preganglionic axons synapse upon nicotinic receptors and postganglionic axons synapse upon muscarinic receptors. There are five identified subtypes of muscarinic receptors (M_1–M_5) involved in peripheral and central cholinergic responses (Table 24.1) (Gainetdinov and Caron, 1999). In mice, cholinergic contraction of smooth muscle is mediated primarily by the M_3 subtype with a small contribution mediated by the M_2 subtype (about 25% and 5% of the cholinergic contractility in the ileum longitudinal muscles and the detrusor muscles, respectively) (Takeuchi et al., 2004). M_2/M_3 knockout mice show virtually no cholinergic contraction of the ileal longitudinal smooth muscles *in vitro* yet maintain coordinated peristalsis suggesting that peristaltic movements can be maintained by local mediators

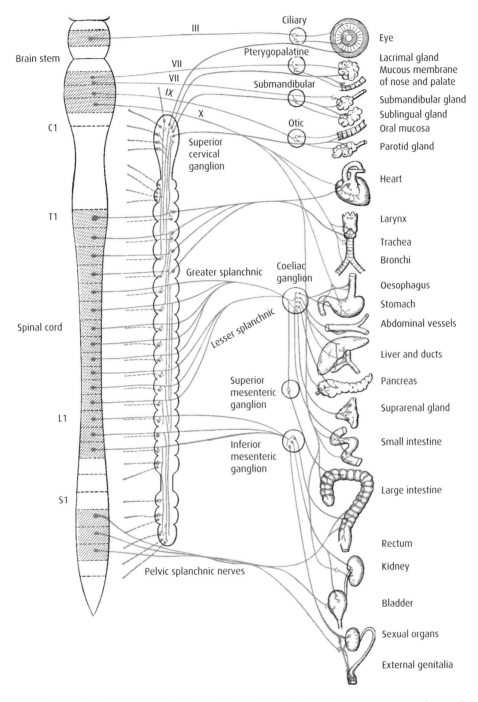

Figure 24.1. The efferent pathways of the ANS. The solid lines indicate parasympathetic and sympathetic pathways and the interrupted lines indicate postganglionic rami to the cranial and spinal nerves (after Meyer and Gottlieb).

Table 24.1. Neurotransmitters in autonomic dysfunction.

Neurotransmitter	Receptor	Function
Acetylcholine	M_1	Salivation
	M_2	Smooth muscle contraction
		Negative myocardial chronotropic and ionotropic effect
	M_3	Smooth muscle contraction
		Salivation
		Pupillary constriction
	M_4	Salivation
	M_5	
Norepinephrine Epinephrine	α_1-AR	Arterial vasoconstriction
		Contracts the smooth muscle of the bladder trigone and urethra
		Facilitates parasympathetic ganglionic transmission
		Contraction of the IUS
		Contraction of the IAS
	α_{1A}-AR	Prostate smooth muscle contraction
	α_{1B}-AR	
	α_{1D}-AR	
	α_2-AR	Arterial and venous vasoconstriction
		Centrally mediated vasodilatation
		Sympathetic postganglionic prejunctional vasodilatation
		Inhibition of parasympathetic ganglionic transmission
		Relaxation of the IAS
	α_{2A}-AR	
	α_{2B}-AR	
	α_{2C}-AR	Increased calcium sensitivity of vascular smooth muscle contraction
	β_1-AR	Coronary and cerebral artery vasodilatation
		Positive myocardial chronotropic and ionotropic effect
		Renin release from juxtaglomerular granular cells
	β_2-AR	Arterial and venous vasodilatation
		NOergic prejunctional release of NO
		Positive myocardial chronotropic and ionotropic effect
		Inhibits detrusor smooth muscle
	β_3-AR	Inhibits detrusor smooth muscle
Arginine vasopressin	V_1	Facilitates sympathetic postganglionic mediated vasoconstriction via presynaptic and postsynaptic mechanisms
	V_2	Synthesis of aquaporin-2 mRNA
Adenosine triphosphate	P_2	Detrusor smooth muscle contraction
Nitric oxide		Vasodilatation
		Urethral smooth muscle relaxation
Angiotensin II	AT_1	Vasoconstriction
	AT_2	Vasodilatation
Serotonin	$5\text{-}HT_{1P}$	Causes submucosal IPANs to initiate peristaltic and secretory reflexes
	$5\text{-}HT_4$	Facilitates release of neurotransmitters from submucosal IPANs

and by motoneurons releasing neurotransmitters other than Ach (Takeuchi et al., 2004). Compared to wild type or M_2 knockout mice, M_3 knockout mice had longer voiding intervals and larger micturition volumes and while atropine inhibited voiding in wild type or M_2 knockout mice, atropine had no effect on any cystometric parameters in M_3 knockout mice suggesting that non-cholinergic mechanisms can compensate for a chronic loss of M_3 receptors (Igawa et al., 2004). M_3 receptors also seem to be the major receptor subtype involved in muscarinic agonist-induced salivation, however muscarinic M_1 and M_4 receptor subtypes may also play a role (Matsui et al., 2000; Bymaster et al., 2003). (The predominant muscarinic receptors regulating body temperature are M_2 receptors, but M_3 receptors may also be involved (Gomeza et al., 1999; Bymaster et al., 2003). Pupillary constriction is likely mediated via M_3 receptors as M_3 knockout mice have dilated pupils (Matsui et al., 2000).

There are also multiple subtypes of adrenoreceptors (AR). α-AR are subdivided into α_1-AR and α_2-AR based on the relative potency of certain alpha agonists and antagonists (Guimaraes and Moura, 2001). α_1-AR are further divided into α_{1A}-, α_{1B}-, and α_{1D}-AR. α_2-AR are further divided into α_{2A}-, α_{2B}-, and α_{2C}-AR. α_1-AR are mostly postsynaptic and excitatory and α_2-AR are usually presynaptic and inhibitory. Presynaptic α_2-AR inhibit the release of NE from sympathetic axons and result in sympathetic inhibition. β-AR are divided into β_1-, β_2-, and β_3- AR. β_2-AR that do not respond to NE can be considered as hormone receptors for circulating adrenaline from the adrenal medulla as they are not functionally innervated by sympathetic nerves (Guimaraes and Moura, 2001). Although there are many exceptions, α-AR are excitatory and β-AR are inhibitory. The classic neurotransmitters, Ach and NE, are not the only neurotransmitters in the ANS. Putative cotransmitters and neuromodulators include dopamine, adenosine triphosphate (ATP) and other nucleotides, angiotensin II, and neuropeptides such as neuropeptide Y (NPY), enkephalin, somatostatin, and vasoactive intestinal peptide (VIP) (Kirstein and Insel, 2004). One function of neuropeptides is to augment the action of the classical transmitter. In the dopamine-β-hydroxylase deficiency syndrome, patients have a congenital absence of the enzyme required for the synthesis of NE and epinephrine (E) and suffer from severe orthostatic hypotension, noradrenergic failure, and ptosis of the eyelids (Garland et al., 2002). These patients have been successfully treated with L-dihydroxyphenylserine (L-DOPS), a prodrug acted upon by endogenous dopa decarboxylase to yield NE (Garland et al., 2002).

Visceral afferents from the trigeminal, facial, glossopharyngeal and vagus nerves terminate topographically in the nucleus tracti solitarii (NTS) (Saper, 2002). Visceral afferents that convey sensations of temperature and nociceptive visceral stimulation, sensations that reach conscious perception, are principally spinal afferents. Most spinal visceral afferents are thought to ascend via the spinothalamic and spinoreticular tracts while some may enter the dorsal columns (Saper, 2002). The rostral NTS is innervated by axons concerned with taste from the anterior two thirds of the tongue followed by the posterior third of the tongue. Fibers from the esophagus terminate in the central NTS subnucleus and fibers from the vagus nerve that innervate more caudal parts of the gastrointestinal (GI) tract end more caudally in the medial part of the NTS (Saper, 2002). Axons from carotid body and aortic arch baroreceptors terminate within the dorsomedial part of the NTS while respiratory chemoreceptors and laryngeal, bronchial, tracheal, and pulmonary mechanoreceptor afferents end in the lateral NTS (Saper, 2002). NTS neurons are under tonic gamma-aminobutyric acid (GABA)ergic inhibition (Mifflin, 2001).

The output of the NTS is to the parabrachial nucleus, which in turns projects to the contralateral ventroposterior parvicellular nucleus (VPpc) of the thalamus. In humans a lesion of the dorsolateral pons that includes the parabrachial nucleus causes an ipsilateral taste deficit while a thalamic lesion causes a contralateral taste deficit (Saper, 2002). The VPpc in turn innervates an insular visceral sensory cortex (Saper, 2002). The relay from the NTS to parabrachial nucleus to VPpc to insular cortex may be the pathway by which cranial nerve visceral afferents reach consciousness .The spinal visceral afferent system converges extensively with the cranial nerve visceral sensory system from the NTS to the insular cortex (Saper, 2002).

24.2 Autonomic dysfunction in blood pressure control

Arterial or high-threshold baroreceptors are located in the carotid sinus and walls of the aortic arch while cardiac or low-threshold baroreceptors are located in the atria and ventricles. Baroreceptor afferent fibers are inhibited by a decrease in arterial blood pressure and excited by a rise in blood pressure. Afferent axons with information from the baroreceptors project through the vagus and glossopharyngeal nerves, with their cell bodies in the petrosal and nodose ganglia, to terminate primarily in the NTS of the medulla (Sun, 1995). There is also evidence that baroreceptor inhibition of sympathetic activity can be exerted at the spinal cord level, suggesting that some fibers conveying baroreceptor afferent information course directly to the spinal cord (Coote and Lewis, 1995).

At resting blood pressure, the predominant effect of baroreceptor afferents is a tonic excitatory input to the NTS (Zhang and Mifflin, 2000; Stauss, 2002). Both *N*-methyl-D-aspartate (NMDA) and non-NMDA excitatory amino acid (EAA) receptor subtypes are involved in the integration of baroreceptor afferent inputs within the NTS (Zhang and Mifflin, 1998). A fall in arterial blood pressure activates three limbs of the baroreceptor response: (1) a reduction of excitatory drive from the NTS to the nucleus ambiguous which increases heart rate by slowing vagal firing, (2) a reduction of excitation on inhibitory interneurons in the caudal ventrolateral medulla that project to neurons in the rostral ventrolateral medulla (RVLM) that in turn excite vasoconstrictor sympathetic preganglionic neurons (SPN) in the intermediolateral (IML) cell column of the thoracic and lumbar spinal cord segments T1–L2 (Shields Jr., 1993), and (3) activation of vasopressin-synthesizing neurons in the hypothalamus (Saper, 2002).

The tonic activity of RVLM neurons on sympathetic vasomotor tone may be due to their intrinsic pacemaker properties or a balance of tonic excitatory and inhibitory synaptic inputs (Sun et al., 1988; Dampney et al., 2003). Although it is uncertain what these specific synaptic inputs are, glutamate in the RVLM is important for the maintenance of arterial pressure (Sved, 2004) and RVLM neurons receive tonic GABAergic inhibition (Dampney et al., 2003). The descending input to SPN involved in regulating resistance vessels is predominantly sympathoexcitatory from the glutamatergic neurons of the RVLM (Amendt et al., 1979; Sun, 1995; Morrison, 2003). There are also sympathoinhibitory descending inputs from GABAergic, glycinergic, and adrenergic neurons onto SPN although it is thought that inhibiting excitatory inputs, such as those from the RVLM, largely produces SPN inhibition (Sun, 1995).

In the cat, about 90% of postganglionic axons in nerves innervating skeletal muscle are vasoconstrictor axons. Preganglionic muscle vasoconstrictor neurons (MVC) are: (1) under powerful inhibitory control of the arterial baroreceptor reflexes; (2) excited by arterial chemoreceptors, trigeminal receptors (e.g. by immersion of the face in water), and a variety of somatic and visceral inputs (e.g. nociceptors and stretch receptors in the urinary bladder); and (3) demonstrate respiratory modulation (Janig and Habler, 2003). Sympathetic vasoconstrictor neurons in prevertebral ganglia are known to receive sensory collateral afferent input, as are segments of the vasculature that also receive autonomic innervation (Gibbins et al., 2003). This indicates that vasomotor neurons may be modulated by peripheral inputs independent of central controllers and afferent inputs may alter vasomotor activity via prejunctional sites on postganglionic sympathetic nerves in addition to their actions at postjunctional sites (i.e. muscle or endothelium) (Coffa and Kotecha, 1999; Gibbins et al., 2003).

Baroreflex failure may develop in patients with surgery, injury or radiation to the neck. Clinical manifestations of baroreflex failure include hypertensive crisis, volatile hypertension, orthostatic tachycardia, and malignant vagotonia (Ketch et al., 2002;

Table 24.2. Treatment of autonomic dysfunction.

Autonomic dysfunction	Treatment
Baroreflex failure	Clonidine
	Benzodiazepines
	Guanadrel
	Guanethidine
Orthostatic hypotension	Support stockings
	Abdominal binder
	Muscle pumping
	Sodium (10 g per day)
	Fluids (2 l per day)
	Water drinking (500 cc in 5 min)
	Fludrocortisone
	Midodrine
	DDAVP
	Erythropoietin
	Bionic baroreflex
Autonomic dysreflexia (AD)	Remove the eliciting cause (usually bladder distension)
	Captopril (25 mg sublingual)
	Nitro paste (2.5 cm of 2% above the SCI)
	Nifedipine (10 mg bite and swallow)
	Intravenous drip of sodium nitroprusside
	Others are hydralazine, mecamylamine, diazoxide, prazosin and clonidine
	Fecal disempaction using 2% lidocaine jelly
	Epidural or spinal anesthesia for labor and delivery
	Terazosin for prophylaxis
Detrusor hyperactivity	Oxybutynin
	Tolterodine
	Baclofen
	Gabapentin
	Intravesicular capsaicin
	Intravesicular resiniferatoxin
	Detrusor botulinum toxin injection
DESD	Isosorbide dinitrate (10 mg sublingual)
	Urethral sphincter botulinum toxin injection
Gastroparesis	Elimination of drugs that reduce gastric motility
	Correction of hyperglycemia
	Dietary changes to increase fluids, decrease intake of fats and fiber and restrict meal size
	Antiemetic agents (phenothiazines and serotonin receptor antagonists)
	Prokinetic agents (metoclopramide, erythromycin, domperidone, and tegaserod)
	Pyloric botulinum toxin injection
	Gastric electric stimulation

Biaggioni, 2003). Treatment of hypertension includes clonidine, benzodiazepines, and agents that inhibit the release or NE from peripheral sympathetic nerve endings such as Guanadrel and guanethidine (Table 24.2) (Ketch et al., 2002). Hypotension has been treated with fludrocortisone while bradycardia may necessitate placement of a pacemaker (Ketch et al., 2002). Orthostatic hypotension is not a prominent symptom of baroreflex failure and Biaggioni suggests that other afferent pathways, such as from the otoliths, compensate for the absent carotid sinus baroreceptors (Biaggioni, 2003). Otolith organs have been shown to have excitatory effects on sympathetic outflow and may maintain blood pressure during postural movements (Ray, 2000).

Multiple system atrophy (MSA) is a disorder of the ANS with functioning efferent postganglionic sympathetic and parasympathetic nerves but with a central autonomic impairment (Parikh et al., 2002). Patients with MSA have severe orthostatic hypotension and supine hypertension. Orthostatic hypotension is defined as a fall in systolic blood pressure (SBP) of more than 20 mmHg or a fall in diastolic blood pressure (DBP) of more than 10 mmHg within 3 min of standing and may be asymptomatic or accompanied by symptoms of cerebral hypoperfusion (1996). Supine plasma NE is near normal in MSA subjects but does not increase appropriately in response to standing up (Parikh et al., 2002). Supine hypertension may be explained by a constant remaining postganglionic sympathetic activity. The supine hypertension has been treated with transdermal nitroglycerin (Shannon et al., 1997). In mild forms of orthostatic hypotension, non-pharmacologic therapy, such as support stockings, abdominal binders, muscle pumping, and increased dietary salt (10 g of sodium per day), and fluid (2 l per day in adults) intake, may be sufficient treatment (Freeman, 2003). Straining activities and exercises that would increase intrathoracic pressure and reduce venous return should be avoided (Freeman, 2003). Water drinking (500 cc in 5 min) causes increased blood pressure in many patients with severe orthostatic hypotension from autonomic failure in MSA and PAF (Shannon et al., 2002). The effect is seen within 5 min of drinking, peaks at about 35 min and last for at least 60 min (Shannon et al., 2002). Primary pharmacologic therapy includes the synthetic mineralocorticoid fludrocortisone and the peripheral selective direct α_1-AR agonist midodrine. Second line agents include desmopressin acetate (DDAVP) and erythropoietin (Freeman, 2003). Recently, a bionic baroreflex system has shown promise in alleviating the effects of

baroreflex failure. Arterial pressure sensors in animals can react to a fall in blood pressure and activate an epidural spinal cord stimulator that can in turn activate spinal sympathetic outflow and increase blood pressure (Yanagiya et al., 2004).

The sympathoexcitatory descending input to SPN is disrupted after a high spinal cord transection and quadriplegic subjects experience an initial drop in systemic arterial pressure (Lehmann et al., 1987; Mathias, 1991). In animal studies, resistances of the muscle and visceral vascular beds are decreased equally (Yardley et al., 1989). Also in animal studies, there is a reduction in sympathetic nerve activity following acute SCI with the exception of the mesenteric and splenic nerves (Qu et al., 1988; Stein and Weaver, 1988). However, the sympathetic nerve activity that remains following SCI in experimental animals becomes less synchronized and may not support vascular tone adequately regardless of the magnitude of SPN discharge. (McCall and Gebber, 1975; Stein et al., 1989). Bravo and coworkers suggest that the decrement in arterial pressure and heart rate immediately after SCI in animals results from Ach release from parasympathetic fibers and the cholinergic stimulation of vasodilating nitric oxide (NO) release from endothelium (Bravo et al., 2001). The acute cardiovascular abnormalities that follow acute cervical SCI in humans (bradycardia, hypotension, supraventricular arrhythmias, and primary cardiac arrest; see Volume II, Chapter 37), resolve spontaneously within 2–6 weeks (Lehmann et al., 1987).

The ability over time of quadriplegic humans to maintain blood pressure in a sitting position improves for reasons that are not clear (Groomes and Huang, 1991). Spinal sympathetic reflexes that include blood pressure elevation in response to bowel or bladder distension or to water drinking can trigger transient increases in blood pressure but are unlikely to play a major role in the maintenance of arterial pressure (Tank et al., 2003). Several studies have shown that vascular resistance in the lower limbs of chronic SCI subjects is higher than in control subjects (Hopman et al., 2002; Kooijman et al., 2003). This may be due to structural changes resulting from venous atrophy and stiffness which would limit venous dispensability and thereby maintain central volume and prevent orthostasis (Wecht et al., 2003). Furthermore, the development of spasticity may contribute to the recovery of arterial pressure owing to increased central venous volume resulting from enhanced venous return and to physical compression on the arterial side of the skeletal muscle beds, which would increase vascular resistance (Osborn et al., 1989).

Animal studies have been unable to attribute the normalization of arterial pressure following spinal cord transection to either (1) increased vascular sensitivity to a constantly low level of sympathetic activity or (2) a steadily increasing level of sympathetic nerve discharge (Osborn et al., 1989). Quadriplegic subjects have been shown to have much lower plasma NE levels in contrast to intact subjects (Mathias et al., 1975; Schmid et al., 1998; 2000; Gao et al., 2002). This is consistent with the finding of reduced sympathetic nerve activity to peroneal muscle nerve fascicles in subjects with spinal cord lesions (Stjernberg et al., 1986). In addition, when quadriplegic subjects change from a lying to a sitting position there is no significant increase in either NE or E (Mathias et al., 1975) which appears to be due to a reduction in NE release and not to a decrease in NE clearance (Krum et al., 1990). Mathias and colleagues (1976) reported an enhanced pressor response to NE in humans with cervical SCI, however their results may not have been due to denervation sensitivity, as suggested, but may have resulted from the absence of baroreceptor mediated sympathoinhibition (Osborn et al., 1989). Arnold and coworkers found a left shift of the dose-response curve for local infusions of NE to reduce dorsal foot vein diameter, suggesting that α-AR responsiveness is increased in quadriplegic persons (Arnold et al., 1995). However, increased α-AR responsiveness in a cutaneous vein may not necessarily indicate that α_1-AR in arteries, which contribute most to systemic vascular tone (Guimaraes and Moura, 2001), are similarly hyperresponsive. Kooijman et al. found that α-AR mediated vascular tone in the lower limbs of subjects with T4–T12 complete chronic SCI was preserved and postulated

that this was related to a spinal sympathetic reflex, local venoarteriolar reflex or α-AR hypersensitivity to circulating catecholamines (Kooijman et al., 2003).

If hypotension following spinal cord transection is principally the result of a decrease in sympathetic activity to vascular beds with relatively weak autoregulatory properties, such as skin and skeletal muscle, normalization of blood pressure following SCI may occur because autoregulatory controllers of blood flow completely dominate within 24 h following spinal cord transection with the result that any remaining sympathetic vasoconstrictor activity is without effect (Osborn et al., 1989). Finally, improvement in blood pressure control in chronic SCI may be due to long-term regulation by renal fluid control (Teasell et al., 2000).

24.3 Renin-angiotensin system and arginine vasopressin

Animal studies have indicated that after lesions of RVLM, arterial pressure is maintained by the renin-angiotensin system and by arginine vasopressin (AVP) (also known as antidiuretic hormone) (Cochrane and Nathan, 1994). The secretion of AVP by the posterior pituitary gland is predominantly controlled by: (1) changes in plasma osmolality, which are sensed by osmoreceptors in the hypothalamus and (2) changes in blood volume and blood pressure relayed from cardiovascular receptors in the carotid sinus and thorax via the glossopharyngeal and vagal cranial nerves to the NTS and thence to the paraventricular and supraoptic nuclei of the hypothalamus (Poole et al., 1987).

In the kidney, circulating AVP activates the V_2 receptors on the luminal tubular membrane and appears to stimulate the synthesis of aquaporin-2 mRNA in addition to regulating the insertion of aquaporin-2 into the luminal membrane of the collecting tubules. Aquaporin-2 causes an increase in water permeability allowing the movement of free water from the collecting duct into the tubular cell (Antunes-Rodrigues et al., 2004).

Renin release is controlled by neural and non-neural stimuli. An increase in efferent renal nerve activity causes renin release via stimulation of postjunctional β-AR on the renin-containing juxtaglomerular granular cells (DiBona and Kopp, 1997). Non-neural stimuli that control renin release are: (1) NaCl sensed at the macula densa; (2) humoral factors with angiotensin II, vasopressin, endothelin, and ATP inhibiting renin release; and (3) the renal vascular baroreceptor mechanism with increases in renal perfusion pressure decreasing renin secretion and with decreases in renal perfusion pressure resulting in increased prostacyclin synthesis and increased renin secretion (Burns et al., 1993). Renin acts on angiotensinogen in the plasma, forming angiotensin, which is converted to angiotensin II, a major vasoconstricting hormone.

Research findings show that quadriplegic persons have increased plasma renin levels and high normal aldosterone levels (Johnson and Park, 1973; Kooner et al., 1988), possibly owing to renin release by the juxtaglomerular cells in response to the decreased renal perfusion that accompanies low arterial pressures (Mathias et al., 1980). Increased release of aldosterone is probably a direct effect of the increased serum renin level (Groomes and Huang, 1991). Hohenbleicher and coworkers studied a 71-year-old woman with PAF and found that a fall in mean arterial pressure (MAP) below 80 mmHg with graded head-up tilt resulted in no signs of sympathetic activity and a distinct rise in plasma renin activity which could be masked by a high salt intake (Hohenbleicher et al., 1997). Animal studies indicate that there is a MAP threshold of about 80–90 mmHg below which there is a pressure-dependent renin release and Hohenbleicher was able to demonstrate that this threshold is also present in humans (Hohenbleicher et al., 1997).

AVP is a potent vasoconstrictor peptide and its vasoconstriction is mediated by the V_1 receptor (Weber et al., 1997). In addition, AVP facilitates sympathetic postganglionic mediated vasoconstriction via presynaptic and postsynaptic mechanisms that are also V_1-receptor mediated (Streefkerk et al., 2003). Quadriplegic subjects, unlike control or paraplegic subjects, have a decline in MAP during progressive head-up tilt which is associated with a marked increase in plasma vasopressin concentration once the MAP is reduced at least 25% (Sved et al., 1985; Ozcan et al., 1991; Wall et al., 1994). Infusion of hypertonic saline causes plasma AVP to rise in both control and quadriplegic subjects; however, at any given level of plasma osmolality, plasma AVP tends to be higher in the quadriplegic subjects than in the control subjects (Kooner et al., 1988). Studies such as these suggest that quadriplegic persons not only have appropriate cardiovascular and osmotic control of AVP secretion, but plasma AVP may increase to levels that are potentially capable of exerting a pressor effect (Wall et al., 1994).

24.4 Autonomic dysreflexia

One manifestation of abnormal cardiovascular control in persons with SCI is autonomic dysreflexia (AD), which is manifested by hypertension, sweating, headache, and bradycardia (Kewalramani, 1980; Braddom and Rocco, 1991; Consortium for spinal cord Medicine, 1997). AD is reported to affect 30–90% of quadriplegic and high paraplegic (above the T6 level) persons in the chronic stage of SCI and 6% of patients in the acute phase (within 1 month) after SCI (Krassioukov et al., 2003). Kirshblum and coworkers found that 70% of subjects with chronic complete SCI above T6 level have an increase in SBP greater than 40 mmHg during their bowel program (Kirshblum et al., 2002). In addition, spinal reflexes activated by bladder distension, pressure sores, or childbirth may initiate AD (Giannantoni et al., 1998). These spinal reflex pathways that contribute little to normal cardiovascular control when they are restrained by supraspinal pathways, may become the dominate regulators of arterial pressure when they control the splanchnic and renal circulation (innervated by sympathetic outflow below T5) (Gao et al., 2002).

Propriospinal pathways link visceral and somatic afferents with SPN in the IML column of the spinal cord, however SCI results in the interruption of spinal sympathetic pathways linking the supraspinal cardiovascular centers with the peripheral sympathetic outflow. The parasympathetic efferent pathways through the vagus nerve, as well as the afferent arc of the baroreceptor reflex through the glossopharyngeal and vagus nerves remain intact after SCI resulting in an increase in vagal efferent activity and a decrease in sympathetic activity above the spinal lesion during AD.

SCI subjects have normal baroreceptor reflex sensitivity at rest (Krum et al., 1992; Legramante et al., 2001; Gao et al., 2002). During AD induced by urinary bladder percussion in C4–T5 spinal cord injured subjects, vagal activation resulted in an initial rapid bradycardia, however the heart rate returned to baseline levels towards the end of a 3 min percussion period presumably due to the counterbalance of generalized sympathetic activation (Gao et al., 2002).

Treatment of AD requires that the eliciting cause be eliminated or that pharmacologic treatment be instituted (Amzallag, 1993; Lee et al., 1995; Comarr and Eltorai, 1997; Naftchi and Richardson, 1997; Karlsson, 1999; Blackmer, 2003). Esmail and coworkers suggests that 25 mg of captopril be administered sublingually as a first line treatment if SBP is at or greater than 150 mmHg (Esmail et al., 2002). The Joint National Committee on Detection, Evaluation and Treatment of High Blood Pressure has discouraged use of immediate release nifedipine (Anton and Townson, 2004).

Several pathophysiological mechanisms responsible for AD have been postulated and include: (1) disinhibition of sensory pathways, (2) disinhibition of the sympathetic systems, (3) altered reflex responses in SPN, (4) re-innervation of SPN by spinal interneurons, and (5) denervation hypersensitivity. It has been shown in animals that noxious afferent stimulation elicits larger increases in heart rate, blood pressure, excitatory renal sympathetic nerve activity, and cardiac sympathetic efferent nerve activity after acute spinal cord transection (Kimura et al., 1995) and increases in blood pressure to visceral distension are greater in chronically than acutely spinally transected rats (Krassioukov et al., 2002). Sympathetically correlated spinal interneurons

are likely involved in spinal networks responsible for activating SPN following SCI (Krassioukov et al., 2002). A larger percentage of sympathetically correlated spinal interneurons are excited by noxious and innocuous cutaneous stimulation in rats with chronic SCI compared to those with acute SCI (Krassioukov et al., 2002). In the rat, spinal cord transection can convert a previously sympathoinhibitory response to a non-noxious stimulus into a sympathoexcitatory response (Giuliani et al., 1988).

Further evidence of spinal cord neuronal plasticity was found by Krassioukov and Weaver who showed that SPN caudal to spinal transection in rats undergo dendritic degeneration and a decrease in soma size within 1 week after transection that is reversed by 1-month post transection (Krassioukov and Weaver, 1996). Krenz and Weaver (1998) found that the time frame of degeneration and recovery of the dendritic arbor of SPN correlated to the time frame for first reduced and them enhanced vasomotor reflexes in the rat.

The incidence of AD after spinal cord transection in mice is reduced by half in Wld^S mice (a mutant that exhibits delayed Wallerian degeneration) compared to its wild type parental strain and supports the hypothesis that the development of AD depends, in part, on synaptic plasticity triggered by signals elaborated by degenerating axons (Jacob et al., 2003). As sprouting of small diameter primary afferent fibers after SCI may be responsible for the development of AD and as most small diameter primary afferent fibers express calcitonin gene-related peptide (CGRP) (Smith et al., 1993), Jacob and coworkers determined the size of the small diameter primary afferent arbor in spinal cord injured and sham-operated mice by measuring the area occupied by CGRP-immunoreactive fibers (Jacob et al., 2001). Although AD was associated with sprouting of CGRP fibers below the level of injury in this mouse model of SCI (Jacob et al., 2001), sprouting of CGRP-immunoreactive afferent fibers after SCI is not mandatory for the development of AD in all strains of mice (Jacob et al., 2003).

Increasing afferent fiber arbor area in the dorsal horn has been associated with the development of

AD in the rat (Krenz and Weaver, 1998; Weaver et al., 2001). The enlarged afferent fiber arbor following SCI in animals has been shown for fibers containing CGRP (Krenz and Weaver, 1998; Weaver et al., 2001) but not for fibers containing substance P (Marsh and Weaver, 2004). Blocking nerve growth factor (NGF) prevents primary afferent sprouting in spinal cord transected rats and decreases the hypertension induced by colon stimulation (Marsh et al., 2002). Blocking NGF also decreases the density of CGRP immunoreaction in the dorsal horn (Christensen and Hulsebosch, 1997).

The EAA, glutamate, may be the neurotransmitter that mediates the viscerosympathetic spinal reflexes involved in generating AD (Maiorov et al., 1997). In a pharmacologic study in rats, Maiorov and coworkers demonstrated that the glutamate receptors NMDA and alpha-amino-3-hydroxy-5-methyl-4-isoxazolepropionic acid (AMPA) contribute to the increase in MAP secondary to colonic distension in rats following acute and chronic spinal cord transection (Maiorov et al., 1997). The proportion of glutamatergic inputs to SPN in spinal cord transected rats (approximately 40%) was found to be less than that in unoperated rats while the GABAergic proportion (60–68%) was increased (Llewellyn-Smith and Weaver, 2001). Overall, the GABAergic input predominated over the glutamatergic input on both cell bodies and dendrites at 14 days post injury (Llewellyn-Smith and Weaver, 2001). Grossman and coworkers found that SCI in a rat model leads to the formation of AMPA receptors with altered subunit composition which may alter the response of neurons in the spinal cord to glutamate and be responsible for the altered functional state seen after chronic SCI (Grossman et al., 1999).

24.5 Autonomic dysfunction in the urinary tract

Micturition requires the coordinated activity of the smooth muscle of the urinary bladder (Detrusor) and urethra along with the striated muscle of the external urethra sphincter (EUS). Complete SCI proximal to the sacral spinal cord results in an upper motor neuron lesion characterized by a hyperreflexic detrusor, whereas injuries involving the sacral cord or cauda equina result in a lower motor neuron lesion characterized by an areflexic detrusor (Kaplan et al., 1991). Detrusor hyperreflexia is defined as involuntary bladder contractions with increased detrusor pressure of at least 60 cm H_2O during the storage phase (Blaivas et al., 1981). In a study of 489 persons with spinal cord lesions due to a variety of causes, all those who had suprasacral spinal cord lesions without evidence of additional sacral spinal cord or cauda equina involvement had either detrusor hyperreflexia or detrusor-external urethral sphincter dyssynergia (DESD) (Kaplan et al., 1991). DESD is the presence of involuntary contractions of the EUS during involuntary detrusor contractions and may be present in as many as 86% of persons with SCI (Blaivas et al., 1981; Wyndaele, 1987).

Activation of the parasympathetic pathways to the detrusor muscle and inhibition of somatic input to the EUS are the essential neuronal events initiating release of urine. Urinary bladder distension activates bladder mechanoreceptors and supplies the sensory input via afferent fibers in the pelvic nerve projecting to the sacral spinal cord needed to facilitate the activation of both supraspinal and spinal mediated micturition reflexes as well as produce the sensation of bladder fullness (Andersson and Sjogren, 1982; Janig and McLachlan, 1986; Yoshimura, 1999). Spinal afferent pathways ascend in the lateral funiculus or the dorsal funiculus of the spinal cord and terminate in the nucleus gracilis and periaqueductal gray (PAG) (De Groat, 1997). It is thought that neurons in the PAG relay information to the pontine micturition center (PMC) to initiate micturition (De Groat, 1997). In cats the PMC corresponds to the nucleus locus coeruleus (Sugaya et al., 2003). The descending pathway of the micturition reflex is in the dorsolateral funiculus, in close proximity to the ascending tracts (Sakakibara et al., 1995). Neurons in the PMC project to: (1) the sacral IML column where they make direct contact with bladder motoneurons and (2) the sacral intermediomedial cell column also known as the dorsal gray commissure where they make contact with GABAergic interneurons that may inhibit EUS motoneurons (Blok and Holstege, 2000).

GABA is the main inhibitory neurotransmitter in the brain and spinal cord. It has been shown that the supraspinal micturition reflex pathway including the PMC is under tonic GABAergic inhibitory control in animals (Mallory et al., 1991; De Groat and Yoshimura, 2001). At the sacral spinal cord level GABA agonists also inhibit sacral parasympathetic preganglionic neurons in animals (De Groat and Yoshimura, 2001). Baclofen, a $GABA_B$ agonist, decreases bladder hyperactivity in patients with spinal cord pathology (Steers et al., 1992). Gabapentin has been found to successfully treat chronic refractory genitourinary pain (Sasaki et al., 2001) and preliminary data suggests that gabapentin may reduce detrusor over activity (Andersson, 2004).

A substantial majority of patients with Parkinson's disease (PD), characterized by dopamine depletion in the striatum (Hornykiewicz and Kish, 1987), have symptoms of bladder hyperactivity characterized by urinary urgency, frequency, and incontinence (Yoshimura et al., 2003). The most common urodynamic finding in PD is detrusor hyperreflexia (Pavlakis et al., 1983; Berger et al., 1987). In 1-methyl-4-phenyl-1, 2,3,6-tetrahydropyridine (MPTP)- induced parkinsonian cynomolgus monkeys, bromocriptine, a centrally acting dopamine D_2-like receptor agonist, was able to reduce the bladder volume micturition threshold by 25% compared to pergolide which decreased the bladder volume micturition threshold by 50% via D_1 receptor activation (Yoshimura et al., 1998). In a rodent model of 6-hydroxydopamine (6-OHDA)-induced parkinsonism, degeneration of dopaminergic neurons in the nigrostriatal pathway resulted in bladder hyperactivity. The hyperactivity was reduced by dopamine receptor agonists acting on D_1/D_5 receptors at a supraspinal site while dopamine receptor agonists acting on D_2/D_4, but not D_3 receptors, had facilitatory effects on the micturition reflex acting predominantly at a lumbosacral spinal site (Yoshimura et al., 2003). The inhibition of micturition produced by activation of central D_1/D_5

receptors in the rodent model of PD may be mediated by activation of the GABAergic system in the basal ganglia (Yoshimura et al., 2003).

Electrical stimulation of the locus coeruleus in cats elicits urinary bladder contraction via a descending NE pathway that activates preganglionic neurons in the IML column of S1–S3 spinal cord segments by means of α_1-AR (Westlund et al., 1982; Yoshimura et al., 1988). The descending limb of the micturition pathway in rats was facilitated by noradrenergic inputs acting on spinal α_{1A}-AR in one study (Yoshiyama and De Groat, 2001), however another study in rats found that intrathecal tamsulosin (an α_{1A}-/α_{1D}-AR antagonist) did not change the frequency or amplitude of isovolumetric bladder contraction whereas naftopidil (an α_{1D}-AR antagonist) decreased the amplitude of bladder contraction (Sugaya et al., 2002). The α_2-AR agonists clonidine and oxymetazoline but not tizanidine cause bladder hyperactivity in male rats possibly by acting at α_2-AR at spinal and supraspinal sites (Kontani et al., 2000).

In cats Aδ-fiber bladder afferents respond to bladder distension while C-fiber bladder afferents respond primarily to noxious stimulation (De Groat and Yoshimura, 2001). Aδ-fiber bladder afferents initiate the supraspinal and spinal micturition reflex while C-fiber afferents, which usually do not respond to bladder distention, may become mechanosensitive after SCI and may trigger micturition and induce bladder hyperreflexia following SCI (Cheng et al., 1999). Most bladder C-fibers carry the vanilloid receptor subtype 1 (VR1) that binds capsaicin. Capsaicin causes an initial excitation of C-fibers followed by a lasting refractory state, termed desensitization (Igawa et al., 2003). In animals, intravesical capsaicin or resiniferatoxin (RTX), a potent analog of capsaicin, can reduce bladder hyperactivity and AD induced by bladder distention (Chancellor and De Groat, 1999; Igawa et al., 2003; Cruz, 2004; Giannantoni et al., 2004). Installation of capsaicin into the urinary bladder of subjects with SCI acutely triggers AD with maximum cardiovascular effects seen 5–10 min after installation followed by a gradual return to baseline within 40 min (Igawa et al.,

2003). After intravesical capsaicin treatment, AD is eliminated for about 3 months (Igawa et al., 2003). Intravesical installation of RTX has been used in SCI humans to treat detrusor hyperreflexia (Kim et al., 2003; Watanabe et al., 2004).

NGF can induce hyperexcitability of C-fiber bladder afferent pathways after spinal cord transection in rats that is reversed by intrathecal NGF antibodies (Seki et al., 2004). DESD in chronic spinalized rats is associated with an increase in NGF levels in the L6 spinal cord that can be neutralized by the application of intrathecal NGF-Ab or subcutaneous capsaicin (which desensitizes C-fiber afferents) (Seki et al., 2004). Increased production of NGF in the bladder and spinal cord may lead to increased transport of NGF to afferent neurons thereby inducing bladder afferent pathway hyperexcitability. Manipulation of NGF level in bladder afferent pathways may effectively treat DESD following SCI in humans (Seki et al., 2004).

Preganglionic parasympathetic neurons in the IML of the sacral cord segments S2–S4 project preganglionic fibers in the pelvic nerve to the pelvic plexus (Andersson and Sjogren, 1982). Parasympathetic postganglionic nerves excite detrusor smooth muscle via release of Ach acting on the M_3 muscarinic receptor subtype in the bladder muscle or by the release of ATP acting on purinergic receptors in the bladder muscle (De Groat and Yoshimura, 2001). The parasympathetic input to the urethral smooth muscle is inhibitory and mediated by NO (Yoshimura, 1999; Mamas et al., 2001). NO donors may be useful in the treatment of DESD. Male spinal cord injured patients with neurogenic detrusor overactivity and DESD were given 10 mg of isosorbide dinitrate sublingually which significantly reduced EUS pressures at rest and during dyssynergic contraction of the urinary bladder while bladder pressures at rest and during contraction as well as the reflex volume remained unchanged (Reitz et al., 2004).

The major current therapies for detrusor over activity, oxybutynin and tolterodine, both display high-affinity antagonism at the M_3 receptor and have more selectivity for the bladder than the salivary glands (Nelson et al., 2004). Oxybutynin patches seem to be associated with fewer incidences of dryness of the mouth, constipation, dizziness, and nausea as compared to oral medications though they may result in skin reactions (Bang et al., 2003). Detrusor injection of 200 U of botulinum-A toxin is effective in the treatment of detrusor over activity that is refractory to anticholinergic agents (Kuo, 2004). Botulinum-A toxin leads to paralysis of the detrusor smooth muscle by preventing the release of Ach from cholinergic nerve endings at the neuromuscular junction (Yokoyama et al., 2002). Botulinum-A toxin injection is also effective in treating DESD seen in patients with multiple sclerosis and SCI when injected either transurethrally or transperineally into the EUS (Leippold et al., 2003). Botulinum-A toxin injections into the EUS have also been used to decrease outlet resistance in patients with an acontractile detrusor in order to effect micturition (Leippold et al., 2003).

SPN that project to the lower urinary tract are found in spinal cord segments T10–L2 in humans (Andersson and Sjogren, 1982). Most preganglionic sympathetic fibers project through the lumbar splanchnic nerves to the inferior mesenteric ganglion (IMG), and a smaller number of preganglionic sympathetic fibers project via the sacral paravertebral chain ganglia into the pelvic nerve to the pelvic plexus (Janig and McLachlan, 1987). The hypogastric nerve (also known as the presacral nerve) is composed of both preganglionic and postganglionic sympathetic fibers that pass from the IMG to the pelvic plexus (Janig and McLachlan, 1987). Most preganglionic sympathetic fibers innervating the pelvic viscera form synapses in the IMG or the pelvic plexus (Janig and McLachlan, 1987). The sympathetic postganglionic neurons release NE which (1) inhibits detrusor smooth muscle via β_2- or β_3-AR, (2) contracts the smooth muscle of the bladder trigone and urethra via α_1-AR, and (3) inhibits (via α_2-AR) or facilitates (via α_1-AR) parasympathetic ganglionic transmission (De Groat, 1997). The β_3-AR is the predominant β receptor in human bladder tissue (Yamaguchi, 2002) and may be a potential target for treatment of detrusor overactivity (Andersson,

2004). In the rat, activation of β_3-AR inhibited spontaneously contracting strips of detrusor muscle suggesting a role in the treatment of urge urinary incontinence (Woods et al., 2001).

Combined degeneration and ongoing regeneration of intrinsic detrusor nerves is found in patients with upper motoneuron neurogenic bladder dysfunction and is independent of dysfunction duration (Haferkamp et al., 2003). Supraspinal neurogenic bladder dysfunction is associated with a higher percentage of admixed normal axons compared to dysfunction caused spinal upper motoneuron deficits (Haferkamp et al., 2003).

The *urethral sphincter* mechanism has internal and external components (McGuire, 1986). The internal urethral sphincter (IUS) is the smooth muscle of the urethra that extends from the bladder outlet through the pelvic floor (McGuire, 1986). The striated muscle of the EUS is composed of the intrinsic EUS found within the urethral wall and the extrinsic EUS composed of the muscles of the pelvic floor and urogenital diaphragm (Elbadawi, 1996). The EUS is the most important active mechanism for maintenance of urinary continence (McGuire, 1986). The urethral sphincter mechanism is tonically active during urine storage and it becomes inactive during normal micturition. Pressure along the urethra during urine storage is highest (about 100–120 cm H_2O in the human) in the mid-urethra (about 3 cm from the bladder neck in the human female and 4–5 cm from the bladder neck in the membranous urethra in the human male) (Brading, 1999). Motoneurons in Onuf's nucleus innervate the EUS via the pudendal nerve, however the EUS may have an autonomic innervation as well (McGuire, 1986). In human adult cadavers, the intrinsic EUS was found to be densely innervated by cholinergic nerves with rare nerves containing NE or NPY (von Heyden et al., 1998). Nerves containing NE, Ach, NPY and galanin innervated the IUS (von Heyden et al., 1998). Activation of α_1-AR elicits contraction in the IUS (Brading, 1999). The α_{1A}-/α_{1D}-AR antagonist tamsulosin has been shown to have minimal blood pressure effects in older individuals while relieving the symptoms of bladder outlet obstruction (Gu et al., 2004).

The guarding or continence reflex prevents urine incontinence when there is a sudden increase in bladder pressure such as may be initiated by a laugh or sneeze (Thor, 2003). The afferent limb of this reflex is via the pelvic nerve to the sacral spinal cord to sphincter motoneurons in Onuf's nucleus. There is a high density of serotonin (5-HT)$_{1A}$ and 5-HT$_2$ receptors in this nucleus (Thor, 2003). The efferent limb of the guarding reflex is via the pudendal nerve to the EUS to facilitate urine storage by stimulating nicotinic cholinergic receptors on the striated muscle fibers and causing muscle contraction (Thor, 2003). The 5-HT/NE-uptake inhibitor duloxetine facilitates sphincter contraction during bladder filling but not during micturition in animals models (Thor, 2003) and has been shown to be safe and effective at 80 mg per day in the treatment of stress urinary incontinence (Van Kerrebroeck, 2004).

The Vocare Bladder System based on the Finetech-Brindley Bladder Controller is Food and Drug Administration (FDA) approved to provide urination or to decrease post void residual urine in patients with complete SCI with intact parasympathetic innervation of the bladder. Extradural electrodes are placed on the S2–S4 nerves via a S1–S3 laminectomy and posterior sacral rhizotomy (S2–S5) is performed through a T11–L2 laminectomy (Creasey et al., 2001). The loss of the posterior roots prevents detrusor hyperreflexia and abolishes reflex defecation, reflex erection in males and reflex vaginal lubrication in females (Steers et al., 2002) and is likely responsible for reduced AD following this procedure (Hohenfellner et al., 2001).

24.6 Autonomic dysfunction in the GI tract

GI tract function is to retain nutrients and eliminate waste. These functions are accomplished by the motility, secretion, and absorption processes of the GI tract, which are regulated via exocrine, endocrine, and neural mechanisms. GI neuronal reflex pathways may be located entirely within the gut or involve the brain and/or spinal cord (Furness and Costa, 1980). The enteric nervous system is extensive and contains as many neurons (10^8) as there are in the spinal cord (Furness and Costa, 1980). Enteric nervous system neurons are not the same as postganglionic parasympathetic neurons and the majority of enteric neurons do not have direct contact with parasympathetic preganglionic axons. The enteric nervous system consists of two ganglionated and several aganglionated plexuses: (1) the submucosal plexus (Meissner's plexus), which innervates the mucosa and regulates secretion; (2) the myenteric plexus (Auerbach's plexus), which innervates the circular and longitudinal smooth muscle layers and regulates motility; and (3) several aganglionated plexuses that supply all layers of the gut (Hansen, 2003).

The enteric nervous system has three types of nerve cells: (1) motoneurons that innervate smooth muscle cells, (2) interneurons that connect different neurons, and (3) intrinsic primary afferent neurons (IPANs). Enteric neurons may contain more than one neurotransmitter and some neurons seem to contain as many as seven putative transmitters (Lundgren, 2002). Ach largely mediates fast excitatory postsynaptic potentials on nicotinic cholinergic receptors while many substances are associated with slow excitatory and inhibitory postsynaptic potentials (Hansen, 2003).

Enteric motoneurons

Enteric motoneurons are further categorized as muscle motoneurons, secretomotor neurons, enteric vasodilator neurons and motoneurons to enteric endocrine cells and enteric motoneurons can be either excitatory or inhibitory. Although over 30 substances have been identified as putative neurotransmitters in the enteric nervous system, the main neurotransmitters of excitatory motoneurons that innervate the longitudinal and circular muscle of the enteric nervous system are Ach, neurokinin A and substance P, while the main neurotransmitters of inhibitory motoneurons are VIP, NO, GABA, NPY, ATP, and carbon monoxide (Goyal and Hirano, 1996; Hansen, 2003). Secretomotor neurons result in water and electrolyte secretion in the small and large intestine, bicarbonate secretion in the duodenum and

gastric acid secretion in the stomach. VIP is known to be a secretagogue in the small intestine (Eklund et al., 1979). The enteric endocrine cells are a highly specialized mucosal cell subpopulation of endodermal origin with regional differences in distribution and hormonal content (Rindi et al., 2004). Changes in the number of enteric endocrine cells has been observed in human gastric mucosa in disorders such as gastritis or impaired acid production suggesting that enteric endocrine cells can adapt to local stimuli (Rindi et al., 2004).

Intrinsic primary afferent neurons

IPANs have cell bodies in the wall of the small intestine and respond to tension, mucosal mechanical distortion and to chemicals on the surface of the mucosa (Clerc and Furness, 2004). These afferents synapse with each other as well as with interneurons and motoneurons of the myenteric plexus (Furness et al., 1998). IPANs are thought to be indirectly excited by intermediate substances such as 5-HT released from the enteric endocrine cells or biologically active compounds, such as cytokines, prostaglandins, and NO released by epithelial cells when exposed to microorganisms (Kagnoff and Eckmann, 1997; Furness et al., 1998; Lundgren, 2002). Submucosal IPANs can initiate peristaltic and secretory reflexes via 5-HT$_{1P}$ receptor activity when stimulated by 5-HT released into the lamina propria by enteric endocrine cells which have microvilli projecting into the lumen of the GI tract and stores of 5-HT in secretion granules at their bases (Gershon, 2004). Mucosal epithelial cells remove and thereby inactivate 5-HT via seratonin reuptake transporter (SERT) (Gershon, 2004). Stimulated submucosal IPANs release Ach and CGRP which actives second-order neurons with nicotinic fast excitatory post synaptic potentials (EPSPs) and/or CGRP mediated slow EPSPs. Release of neurotransmitters from submucosal IPANs is increased by the action of 5-HT on 5-HT$_4$ receptors (Pan and Gershon, 2000). When inflamed, IPANs in the guinea-pig distal colon have been shown to have an increased excitability and have been implicated in the dysmotility of inflammatory bowel diseases (Linden et al., 2003). Tegaserod, a 5-HT$_4$ receptor partial agonist that stimulates GI motility and intestinal secretion, has been shown to be efficacious in treating patients with chronic constipation or irritable bowel syndrome with constipation (Johanson, 2004).

Extrinsic primary afferent neurons

Extrinsic primary afferent neurons have three pathways that connect the gut to the central nervous system (Berthoud et al., 2004). Upper GI afferents have axons in the vagus nerve with cell bodies in the nodose ganglia, colorectal afferents have axons in the pelvic nerve with cell bodies in the sacral dorsal root ganglia and throughout the GI tract afferents have axons in the splanchnic sympathetic nerves with cell bodies in the thoracolumbar dorsal root ganglia (Berthoud et al., 2004). Extrinsic primary afferent neurons have terminal endings in the mucosa, muscle layers including the myenteric plexus or the serosa (Berthoud et al., 2004) and convey sensations of satiety, nausea, and pain to the central nervous system (CNS). Mucosal receptors respond to mechanical stimuli such as gentle stroking of the epithelium, lumenal chemicals, cold or lumenal osmolarity, 5-HT$_{1A}$ and 5-HT$_2$ receptors (Hillsley and Grundy, 1998). This is different than submucosal IPANs, which are stimulated via 5-HT$_{1P}$ and 5-HT$_4$ receptors (Gershon, 2004). Muscle receptors in the gastric, duodenal, and jejunal smooth muscle respond to distension and contraction of the viscus (Andrews, 1986). Serosal receptors are activated by mechanical stimuli. The splanchnic nerves, which convey afferents from the gut to the spinal cord, are thought to mediate painful sensations, although vagus nerve afferents may also be involved in gut nociception (Andrews, 1986; Grundy, 2002). The sensation of hunger is reduced in vagotomized patients, but it is not eliminated, perhaps because the hypothalamus monitors the levels of circulating nutrients (Andrews, 1986).

Extrinsic efferent innervation

Extrinsic efferent innervation of the GI tract occurs through the parasympathetic and sympathetic divisions of the ANS. Preganglionic neurons in the dorsal motor complex of the vagus innervate the GI tract from the esophagus to the distal colon. Mechano- and chemotransmission from the GI tract elicits a number of different vago-vagal reflexes, which consist basically of sensory vagal afferents, second-order integrative neurons of the NTS, and efferent vagal neurons of the dorsal motor nucleus of the vagus (DMV). One vagal efferent pathway from the DMV is cholinergic-muscarinic and induces an increase of GI functions such as motility and acid output and the second is non-adrenergic, non-cholinergic (NANC) and causes a decrease in gastric motility when activated, mainly via release of NO onto gastric smooth muscle (Travagli et al., 2003).

SPN in the mediolateral gray matter of the spinal cord send efferent fibers through the splanchnic nerves to the celiac and superior mesenteric prevertebral ganglia (plexuses). SPN to the colon and pelvic viscera project to the superior mesenteric ganglion (SMG) and IMG via the lumbar splanchnic nerves. The stomach receives sympathetic postganglionic fibers principally from the celiac plexus but also from the left phrenic plexus, bilateral gastric and hepatic plexuses, and the sympathetic trunk. Postganglionic sympathetic efferent nerves emerge from the celiac and SMG to run along mesenteric blood vessels and innervate the small intestine. Postganglionic fibers from the SMG innervate the colon from the cecum to the distal transverse colon. Postganglionic fibers from the IMG project via lumbar colonic nerves that run along the inferior mesenteric artery to innervate the left side of the colon. Postganglionic fibers from the IMG also project via the hypogastric nerves and join the pelvic plexus (also known as the inferior hypogastric plexus) to innervate the distal colon (Janig and McLachlan, 1987). Other sympathetic preganglionic axons enter paravertebral chain ganglia and form synapses with postganglionic neurons there (Kuo et al., 1984).

Some sympathetic postganglionic neurons are visceral vasoconstrictor neurons and innervate vascular smooth muscle while others are motility-regulating (MR) neurons that innervate visceral smooth muscle (Longo et al., 1989). The majority of lumbar sympathetic postganglionic neurons are noradrenergic, but many contain a peptide as well (Lundberg et al., 1982). Sympathetic ganglia receive synaptic input from (1) preganglionic neurons with cell bodies in the spinal cord, (2) primary sensory neurons with cell bodies in the dorsal root ganglia, and (3) neurons arising in visceral intramural ganglia (enteric nervous system). The apparent convergence of multiple synaptic inputs onto individual principal ganglionic neurons suggests that the outflow from these neurons is the result of integration of synaptic information from several sources (Keef and Kreulen, 1990). In the guinea-pig ileum, activation of α_2-AR on interneurons in the myenteric plexus and intrinsic sensory neurons is needed for sympathetic inhibition of intestinal motility (Stebbing et al., 2001).

The actions of the stomach in response to a meal are storage, secretion, mixing, and emptying. Vagal stimulation induces relaxation of the fundus and contraction of the antrum (Read and Houghton, 1989). Mesenteric sympathetic nerve stimulation inhibits contraction in the small intestine (Read and Houghton, 1989). The normal interdigestive state of the GI tract of humans is characterized by cyclical contractions of the smooth muscle layers in the stomach, small intestine or colon that can propagate over large regions of the GI tract. These recurring contractions are called the migrating motor complexes (MMC) or the interdigestive motor complex (IDMC) and are divided into four phases (Spencer et al., 2003). Phase I is the quiescent phase. Phase II has both non-migrating and peristaltic contractions that propagate over short distances. Phase III consists of recurring periods of intense regular motor activity that propagate over long lengths of the bowel. Phase III can be followed by a brief interval of less intense activity called phase IV. MMC-like activity can be recorded *in vitro* (Spencer et al., 2003). The phases of the interdigestive state disappear after a meal and are replaced by the ongoing phasic contractile activity of the fed pattern (Kunze and Furness, 1999).

Phasic contractions of the GI tract occur during intervals between MMC and during the MMC (Spencer et al., 2003). Slow waves are spontaneous myogenic oscillations in membrane potential generated by the interstitial cells of Cajal (Dickens et al., 1999). Ward and coworkers suggests that propagation of slow waves in the canine gastric antrum is facilitated by a voltage-dependent dihydropyridine-resistant Ca^{2+} influx (Ward et al., 2004). However, at least in the mouse, slow waves do not seem necessary for generation of either phasic contractions or the MMC (Spencer et al., 2003). While the MMC are abolished by atropine or hexamethonium, the phasic contractions are not, suggesting that the MMC require enteric nerves and the phasic contractions do not as they are likely myogenic (Spencer et al., 2003). The hormone motilin appears to be related to the MMC (Tack, 1995). Erythromycin has motilin agonist properties and its administration can induce a MMC (Tack, 1995). One case report describes the successful resolution of refractory SCI-induced gastroparesis with erythromycin lactobionate (Clanton Jr. and Bender, 1999). Another prokinetic peptide, Ghrelin, is expressed mainly in the stomach, by neuroendocrine cells in humans, and is secreted into the circulation. Ghrelin increases gastric acid secretion, gastric motility, and gastric emptying. When administered systemically or intracerbroventricularly, Ghrelin stimulates food intake (Spencer et al., 2003).

GI Dysfunction

GI Dysfunction following SCI includes impairment of gastric motility, gastric emptying and intestinal motility. In humans, gastric distension and ileus occur immediately after traumatic spinal cord transection, however, in long-term quadriplegic persons an intact supraspinal sympathetic pathway is not an absolute requirement for initiation and propagation of antral phase III motor activity (Fealey et al., 1984). Chronic quadriplegic subjects continue to have delayed gastric emptying (Fealey et al., 1984; Segal et al., 1995). Chronic paraplegic persons have been reported to have delayed gastric emptying, but this appears to be a non-specific finding related to prolonged immobilization (Rock et al., 1981). Segal and coworkers identified a biphasic pattern of gastric emptying in chronic quadriplegic subjects where the initial (20–30 min) gastric emptying (which resembled the patterns seen in control and paraplegic subjects) was followed by a delayed phase II (Segal et al., 1995).

Gastroparesis or delayed gastric emptying without evidence of mechanical obstruction is a chronic disorder of varying severity and symptoms (Lin et al., 2003). Symptoms include early satiety, nausea, vomiting bloating, and upper abdominal discomfort (Parkman et al., 2004). The gold standard for the diagnosis of gastroparesis is gastric emptying scintigraphy of a solid-phase meal (Parkman et al., 2004). Treatment of gastroparesis includes elimination of drugs that reduce gastric motility (anticholinergics, narcotics, tricyclic antidepressants, and calcium channel blockers), correction of hyperglycemia, and dietary changes to increase fluids, decrease intake of fats and fiber and restrict meal size (Parkman et al., 2004). Medical treatment includes antiemetic agents (phenothiazines and 5-HT receptor antagonists) and prokinetic agents (metoclopramide, erythromycin, domperidone, and tegaserod) (Parkman et al., 2004). Newer treatments for refractory gastroparesis include pyloric botulinum toxin injection and gastric electric stimulation (Lin et al., 2003; Parkman et al., 2004).

Most human individuals after SCI have chronic constipation and the loss of voluntary control of the initiation of defecation (Stone et al., 1990). Normally, fecal material entering the rectum results in relaxation of the internal anal sphincter (IAS) (rectoanal reflex) and contraction of the external anal sphincter (EAS) to prevent incontinence (holding reflex) (Banwell et al., 1993). Stool elimination results from voluntary relaxation of the EAS and the puborectalis muscle (Sun et al., 1995). Sacral parasympathetic spinal reflex activity independent of supraspinal pathways and having afferent and efferent limbs in the pelvic nerve is needed for the initiation of propulsive activity during defecation (De Groat and Krier, 1978). In guinea-pigs, distension of the rectum elicits the rectoanal reflex with cholinergic mediated contraction of the rectum and synergistic nitrergic mediated relaxation of the IAS (Yamanouchi et al., 2002). The rectoanal reflex is inhibited by sympathetic outflow through the lumbar colonic nerves (Yamanouchi et al., 2002). In the opossum, sympathetic suppression of IAS relaxation during the rectoanal reflex is mediated by α_2-AR while sympathetically mediated increased in resting tone of the IAS is mediated by α_1-AR (Yamato and Rattan, 1990). A pontine defecation reflex center has been postulated to exist in dogs and rats as pontine transection at the cerebellar peduncle was able to abolish propulsive contractions of the descending colon and rectum in response to colorectal or gastric distention while preserving small contractions (Nagano et al., 2004).

Compared to individuals without SCI, individuals with supraconal SCI have higher rectal tone and individuals with conal or cauda equina lesions have lower rectal tone (Krogh et al., 2002). IAS relaxation occurs after rectal distension in individuals with SCI above T12 (Sun et al., 1995). Complete sacral posterior rhizotomy does not eliminate the IAS relaxation induced by rectal distention. However, reflex contraction of the EAS in response to either rectal distention or increases intraabdominal pressure is eliminated by sacral posterior rhizotomy indicating that these contractions are mediated by a spinal reflex (Sun et al., 1995). In persons with complete SCI above T12 transit of contents is slowed throughout the large bowel, regardless of the level of the spinal cord lesion (Beuret-Blanquart et al., 1990). Studies have identified (1) prolonged rectosigmoid transit times (Beuret-Blanquart et al., 1990; Krogh et al., 2003); (2) transit delays more marked in the descending colon, sigmoid, and rectum than in the cecum, ascending colon, and transverse colon (Menardo et al., 1987; Leduc et al., 1997); or (3) transit delays involving the entire colon (Keshavarzian et al., 1995). Leduc found an association between shorter colonic transit time in individuals with SCI and successful rectal emptying but was unable to demonstrate an association between changes in colonic transit time and a number of symptoms observed in individuals with SCI including fecal incontinence, abdominal pain, time for bowel care, and quality of life (Leduc et al., 2002).

Colonic motor activity increases when food is ingested into the stomach (Hertz and Newton,

1913). The afferent limb of the gastrocolic reflex can be blocked by intragastric lidocaine, and the increase in distal colonic spike activity can be blocked by anticholinergics or naloxone, indicating participation of cholinergic and opiate receptors. As ablation or section of the spinal cord in the rat does not eliminate the gastrocolic reflex, at least for the distal colon, colonic cyclical organization is not initiated by spinal or supraspinal influences (Du et al., 1987). The local enteric nervous system or the prevertebral ganglionic system, or both, are probably responsible for the cyclical organization of distal colonic motility in rats. However, the gastrocolic reflex in the transverse colon persists in rats after spinal cord transection but not after spinal cord ablation, suggesting that it was organized in the spinal cord (Du et al., 1987). Gastrocolic reflexes have been found in subjects with SCI (Connell et al., 1963; Fajardo et al., 2003) although the absolute level of colonic contractility is reduced compared to controls without SCI (Fajardo et al., 2003). Subjects with SCI had higher activity in the descending colon than in the rectosigmoid while control subjects did not demonstrate this regional difference (Fajardo et al., 2003).

A future treatment option for fecal incontinence or constipation is electrical stimulation. Electrical stimulation to the muscles of the anterior abdominal wall via an abdominal belt has been shown to improve defecatory function in patients with SCI (Korsten et al., 2004). The Vocare Bladder System is FDA approved to aid in bowel evacuation as a secondary intended use. Electrical stimulation via an anal plug has been shown to be effective in treating patients with functional constipation (Chang et al., 2003).

24.7 Thermoregulatory dysfunction

Temperature regulation is controlled by a hierarchy of neuronal structures located throughout the brain and the spinal cord with the hypothalamus at the top coordinating and adjusting the activity of lower level thermoregulatory systems (Satinoff, 1978; Boulant, 2000). Body temperature in homeotherms is maintained within narrow limits of an adjustable reference temperature or set-point determined by the hypothalamus (Hammel et al., 1963; Satinoff, 1978). Within this neutral zone no thermoregulatoy responses are activated (Satinoff, 1978). Animals that have been decerebrated or spinalized or have had the entire hypothalamus removed still demonstrate thermoregulatory responses however these responses are elicited only with a more intense thermal threshold than is normally required suggesting a widened neutral zone (Satinoff, 1978).

Neurons in the anterior hypothalamus preoptic area (POA) have intrinsic temperature sensitivity and drive many thermoregulatory effector mechanisms (McAllen, 2004). Pyrogens alter POA thermoregulation by elevating set-point temperatures (Boulant, 2000). In response to cooling, neurons in the POA elicit shivering and non-shivering thermogenesis, cutaneous vasoconstriction, behavioral responses that conserve body heat and increases in levels of thyroxine, catecholamines, and glucocorticoids whereas POA warming elicits cutaneous vasodilation, sweating, and behavioral responses that enhance heat loss (Boulant, 2000). The median forebrain bundle appears to be an important pathway connecting neurons in the POA to the brainstem and is considered the efferent pathway from the POA to effector areas controlling skin blood flow and shivering (Nagashima et al., 2000).

Nakamura suggests that the POA regulates temperature in response to pyrogenic PGE_2 signals or warming via a descending pathway that activates vesicular glutamate transporter 3 (VGLUT3)-expressing neurons in the medullary raphe and that these thermoregulatory medullary raphe neurons tonically receive GABAergic inhibitory inputs (Takamori et al., 2000; Nakamura et al., 2004). VGLUT3-expressing medullary raphe neurons (which are involved in thermoregulation in rats) have been shown to have direct projections to SPN and SPN are known to express ionotropic glutamate receptors (Nakamura et al., 2004). This evidence suggests that the descending thermoregulatory pathway in the spinal cord is mediated via the neurotransmitter glutamate.

Changes in environmental and body temperatures are detected by thermosensitive neurons in the POA, brainstem, spinal cord, and periphery (Satinoff,

1978; Patapoutian et al., 2003). Thermoreceptors in the POA are activated by local warming or cooling and simultaneously receive thermally related input from warm and cold receptors in the skin conveyed via the lateral spinothalamic tract (Boulant, 2000). Thermosensation is thought to be mediated primarily by a subset of transient receptor potential (TRP) ion channels that are located in or near nerve terminals in the skin and convert thermal information into chemical and electrical signals (Patapoutian et al., 2003). There are several molecularly defined thermosensitive channels: one is a potassium channel, TREK-1, four are members of the TRP vanilloid (TRPV1–4) subset of channels, one is a TRP melastatin (TRPM8) subset channel also known as cold- and menthol-sensitive receptor (CMR1) and one is a TRPA subset channel TRPA1 also known as ankyrin-like with transmembrane domains 1 (ANKTM1) (McKemy et al., 2002; Benham et al., 2003; Story et al., 2003; Bandell et al., 2004). VR1 now called TRPV1 is activated by noxious heat and the vanilloid, capsaicin, however the temperature threshold for TRPV1 can be modulated allowing for a degree of plasticity in its thermoresponsivity (Caterina et al., 1997; Benham et al., 2003). Vanilloid receptor like protein 1 (VRL1) now called TRPV2 is activated by noxious heat >53°C. TRPV3 receptors are activated at temperature thresholds ranging from 23 to 39°C. TRPV4 receptors respond to temperatures around normal body temperature (Patapoutian et al., 2003). The expression of TRPV4 in the hypothalamus and in skin keratinocytes suggests that TRPV4 may participate in peripheral and central heat thermotransduction (Guler et al., 2002). TRPV4 in skin keratinocytes may release a chemical mediator such as ATP in order to trigger surrounding neurons (Guler et al., 2002). TRPM8 receptors are activated by cold (with a threshold about 25°C), as well as by menthol and icilin (McKemy et al., 2002). TRPA1 receptors are activated by cold (with a threshold about 17°C) as well as by a number of chemical agents (cinnamon oil, mustard oil, wintergreen and capsaicin) that are known to evoke nociceptive sensations (Story et al., 2003; Bandell et al., 2004; Green, 2004). The two-pore domain mechano-gated potassium channel TREK-1

is opened gradually and reversibly by heat and is also highly expressed within dorsal root ganglion sensory fibers as well as in the POA which makes this potassium channel an ideal candidate as a physiological thermoreceptor (Maingret et al., 2000).

Body temperature in humans is regulated by behavioral and autonomic mechanisms. Behavioral mechanisms include changing the thermal environment, changing posture, and changing the amount of insulating clothing. Physiological responses to cold stress include vasoconstriction and shivering and non-shivering thermogenesis while the physiological responses to heat stress include sweating and vasoconstriction. Core (T_c) and skin surface (T_{sk}) temperature contribute about equally toward thermal comfort, which is important for behavioral responses, whereas T_c predominates in regulation of the autonomic thermoregulatory responses (Frank et al., 1999).

Impairment of temperature regulation is a recognized hazard for persons with SCI (Schmidt and Chan, 1992). Thermoregulatory dysfunction is most severe for persons with a complete cervical SCI because shivering can only occur above the level of the injury and hypothalamic control of sympathetically mediated vasomotor control and sweating is lost below the level of the lesion (Downey et al., 1967). Non-shivering thermogenesis or chemical thermogenesis secondary to increases in cellular metabolism, although important for some animals, has not been clearly demonstrated in humans although non-shivering thermogenesis may be important for the survival of infants (Cannon and Nedergaard, 2004). Behavioral modification however is an important mechanism for thermoregulation in persons with complete high-level SCIs (Downey et al., 1967).

Cold signals from central and peripheral thermoreceptors induce shivering (an involuntary tremor of skeletal muscles) in order to produce heat. The POA inhibits shivering while the posterior hypothalamus generates excitatory signals for shivering (Nagashima et al., 2000). In paraplegic subjects, peripheral and deep or central temperature receptors sensitive to cold are able to initiate shivering but only above the level of the SCI (Downey et al., 1967). Spinal cord cooling in spinal-transected animals has been shown to elicit shivering indicating that the spinal cord contains the basic mechanisms for this response (Simon, 1974).

Cooling of peripheral or central areas results in a reduction of *skin blood flow* due to vasoconstriction that reduces heat loss and causes a simultaneous increase in flow to central vascular regions (Simon, 1974; Chotani et al., 2000). Cold-induced vasoconstriction results from a reflex increase in sympathetic output and a direct cold-induced augmentation of α_{2C}-AR responsiveness (Chotani et al., 2000). The augmented responsiveness of normally silent α_{2C}-AR is mediated by cold-induced activation of the Rho/Rho kinase pathway, which stimulates the translocation of α_{2C}-AR to the cell surface and increases the calcium sensitivity of vascular smooth muscle contraction (Bailey et al., 2004). Reflex cutaneous vasoconstriction in response to whole-body cooling is mediated by noradrenergic and non-noradrenergic mechanisms, probably via a sympathetic cotransmitter that may be NPY and/or ATP (Stephens et al., 2001a; Charkoudian, 2003). Vasomotor responses below the level of SCI have been variously reported as either absent or present (Cooper et al., 1957; Appenzeller and Schnieden, 1963; Benzinger, 1969; Corbett et al., 1971; Tsai et al., 1980). Tsai and coworkers reported that all vasomotor responses to cooling or warming in the paraplegic lower extremities of men were absent following acute SCI (T5–T11) but by 4 months after injury the ipsilateral local vasomotor responses to warming and cooling in the paraplegic lower extremities returned to normal (Tsai et al., 1980).

When heated, warm receptors in the POA activate efferent pathways for heat loss that result in cutaneous vasodilation via excitatory signals to vasodilative neurons and inhibitory signals to vasoconstrictive neurons in the midbrain (Zhang et al., 1997; Nagashima et al., 2000). Cutaneous blood flow can increase considerably in response to hyperthermia and constitute up to 60% of cardiac output (Charkoudian, 2003). While cutaneous vasoconstriction is tonically active in thermoneutral environments, hyperthermia triggers active cutaneous vasodilation, which dissipates heat (Charkoudian,

2003). A yet unidentified cotransmitter from sympathetic cholinergic nerves mediates active cutaneous vasodilation (Kellogg Jr., et al., 1995). In addition to reflex active cutaneous vasodilation, local cutaneous warming elicits vasodilation via both a fast responding local axon reflex and a more slowly responding vasodilator system that relies on the local production of NO (Minson et al., 2001). CGRP (which is a principal transmitter of neurogenic dilatation of arterioles) or Substance P are the likely substances involved in the initial rapid vasodilation resulting from antidromic release from a subpopulation of C-fiber nociceptive afferents via an axon reflex (Holzer, 1998; Kellogg Jr., et al., 1999; Minson et al., 2001; Stephens et al., 2001b; Warner et al., 2004).

Paraplegic men have been shown to have significant differences in skin blood flow response to hyperthermia when compared to intact control subjects (Freund et al., 1984). Heating insensate skin to 40°C in paraplegic subjects resulted in little or no increases in forearm blood flow (FBF) while the same pattern of heating in spinal cord intact control subjects resulted in vigorous vaso- and sudomotor responses. In addition whole-body heating of paraplegic subjects resulted in sweating above the level of the spinal cord lesion and increases in FBF that was less than that reported for hyperthermic spinal cord intact men. Freund and coworkers suggested that one reason for the attenuated response of FBF to whole-body heating was diminished thermoregulatory effector outflow resulting from the diminished afferent input which, after SCI, could originate only from above the level of the lesion (Freund et al., 1984). Tam and colleagues reached a similar conclusion (Tam et al., 1978). They reported that a person with T6 paraplegia had to achieve a higher core temperature threshold (37.2–37.9°C) to generate sweating and related vasodilatation responses, compared to the core temperature threshold (36.2–37.1°C) of a normal control subject. Since paraplegic persons appear to exhibit markedly attenuated skin blood flow in response to hyperthermia they are limited in their ability to dissipate excess heat (Freund et al., 1984).

In humans, heat dissipation is predominantly due to sweating (Cheshire and Freeman, 2003). Two to four million eccrine sweat glands receive dual innervation by both cholinergic and adrenergic fibers and are stimulated by cholinergic, α-adrenergic, and β-adrenergic agonists; however, cholinergic stimulation provokes the largest response (Quinton, 1983; Cheshire and Freeman, 2003). Spinal lesions are associated with anhidrosis below the level of the lesion and normal evaporative cooling is maintained by increased compensatory sweating from sentient skin (Seckendorf and Randall, 1961; Normell, 1974; Downey et al., 1976; Quinton, 1983). Although AD is often associated with sweating above the level of the spinal cord lesion, reflex sweating also occurs below the level of lesion in SCI during AD (Silver, 2000). There is also evidence for thermal reflex sweating below the level of SCI in humans (Seckendorf and Randall, 1961; Silver et al., 1991). Although sweating (up to 30% of what would be expected in controls) has been observed on the entire cutaneous surface below the level of SCI in response to environmental heating, the amount of sweating was not sufficient to prevent an elevation in body temperature in patients with cervical SCI (Silver et al., 1991). Anhidrosis may be associated with a number of neurologic disorders (including MSA and PAF) and can cause heat intolerance (Cheshire and Freeman, 2003; Thami et al., 2003; Low, 2004).

24.8 Summary

Neuronal components of the ANS in the spinal cord, peripheral ganglia and enteric nervous system are capable of complex integrative functions. When the ANS is deranged, the clinical manifestations are many and various and management will often involve different specialists. The manifestations of autonomic dysfunction following SCI result from the interruption of descending pathways as well as the effects of synaptic reorganization and neuronal plasticity.

REFERENCES

1996. The definition of orthostatic hypotension, pure autonomic failure, and multiple system atrophy. *J Auton Nerv Syst*, **58**(1–2), 123–124.

Amendt, K., Czachurski, J., Dembowsky, K.and Seller, H. (1979). Bulbospinal projections to the intermediolateral cell column: a neuroanatomical study. *J Auton Nerv Syst*, **1**(1), 103–107.

Amzallag, M. (1993). Autonomic hyperreflexia. *Int Anesthesiol Clin*, **31**(1), 87–102.

Andersson, K.E. (2004). New pharmacologic targets for the treatment of the overactive bladder: an update. *Urology*, **63**(3 Suppl. 1), 32–41.

Andersson, K.E. and Sjogren, C. (1982). Aspects on the physiology and pharmacology of the bladder and urethra. *Prog Neurobiol*, **19**(1–2), 71–89.

Andrews, P.L. (1986). Vagal afferent innervation of the gastrointestinal tract. *Prog Brain Res*, **67**, 65–86.

Anton, H.A. and Townson, A. (2004). Drug therapy for autonomic dysreflexia. *CMAJ*, **170**(8), 1210.

Antunes-Rodrigues, J., de Castro, M., Elias, L.L., Valenca, M.M. and McCann, S.M. (2004). Neuroendocrine control of body fluid metabolism. *Physiol Rev*, **84**(1), 169–208.

Appenzeller, O. and Schnieden, H. (1963). Neurogenic pathways concerned in reflex vasodilatation in the hand with especial reference to stimuli affecting the afferent pathway. *Clin Sci*, **25**, 413–421.

Arnold, J.M., Feng, Q.P., Delaney, G.A. and Teasell, R.W. (1995). Autonomic dysreflexia in tetraplegic patients: evidence for alpha-adrenoceptor hyper-responsiveness. *Clin Auton Res*, **5**(5), 267–270.

Bailey, S.R., Eid, A.H., Mitra, S., Flavahan, S. and Flavahan, N.A. (2004). Rho kinase mediates cold-induced constriction of cutaneous arteries: role of alpha2C-adrenoceptor translocation. *Circ Res*, **94**(10), 1367–1374.

Bandell, M., Story, G.M., Hwang, S.W., Viswanath, V., Eid, S.R., Petrus, M.J., Earley, T.J. and Patapoutian, A. (2004). Noxious cold ion channel TRPA1 is activated by pungent compounds and bradykinin. *Neuron*, **41**(6), 849–857.

Bang, L.M., Easthope, S.E. and Perry, C.M. (2003). Transdermal oxybutynin: for overactive bladder. *Drugs Aging*, **20**(11), 857–864.

Banwell, J.G., Creasey, G.H., Aggarwal, A.M. and Mortimer, J.T. (1993). Management of the neurogenic bowel in patients with spinal cord injury. *Urol Clin North Am*, **20**(3), 517–526.

Benham, C.D., Gunthorpe, M.J. and Davis, J.B. (2003). TRPV channels as temperature sensors. *Cell Calcium*, **33**(5–6), 479–487.

Benzinger, T.H. (1969). Heat regulation: homeostasis of central temperature in man. *Physiol Rev*, **49**(4), 671–759.

Berger, Y., Blaivas, J.G., DeLaRocha, E.R. and Salinas, J.M. (1987). Urodynamic findings in Parkinson's disease. *J Urol*, **138**(4), 836–838.

Berthoud, H.R., Blackshaw, L.A., Brookes, S.J. and Grundy, D. (2004). Neuroanatomy of extrinsic afferents supplying the gastrointestinal tract. *Neurogastroenterol Motil*, **16**(**Suppl. 1**), 28–33.

Beuret-Blanquart, F., Weber, J., Gouverneur, J.P., Demangeon, S. and Denis, P. (1990). Colonic transit time and anorectal manometric anomalies in 19 patients with complete transection of the spinal cord. *J Auton Nerv Syst*, **30**(3), 199–207.

Biaggioni, I. (2003). Sympathetic control of the circulation in hypertension: lessons from autonomic disorders. *Curr Opin Nephrol Hypertens*, **12**(2), 175–180.

Blackmer, J. (2003). Rehabilitation medicine: 1. Autonomic dysreflexia. *CMAJ*, **169**(9), 931–935.

Blaivas, J.G., Sinha, H.P., Zayed, A.A. and Labib, K.B. (1981). Detrusor-external sphincter dyssynergia. *J Urol*, **125**(4), 542–544.

Blok, B.F. and Holstege, G. (2000). The pontine micturition center in rat receives direct lumbosacral input. An ultrastructural study. *Neurosci Lett*, **282**(1–2), 29–32.

Boulant, J.A. (2000). Role of the preoptic-anterior hypothalamus in thermoregulation and fever. *Clin Infect Dis*, **31**(**Suppl. 5**), S157–S161.

Braddom, R.L. and Rocco, J.F. (1991). Autonomic dysreflexia. A survey of current treatment. *Am J Phys Med Rehabil*, **70**(5), 234–241.

Brading, A.F. (1999). The physiology of the mammalian urinary outflow tract. *Exp Physiol*, **84**(1), 215–221.

Bravo, G., Rojas-Martinez, R., Larios, F., Hong, E., Castaneda-Hernandez, G., Rojas, G. and Guizar-Sahagun, G. (2001). Mechanisms involved in the cardiovascular alterations immediately after spinal cord injury. *Life Sci*, **68**(13), 1527–1534.

Burns, K.D., Homma, T. and Harris, R.C. (1993). The intrarenal renin-angiotensin system. *Semin Nephrol*, **13**(1), 13–30.

Bymaster, F.P., Carter, P.A., Yamada, M., Gomeza, J., Wess, J., Hamilton, S.E., Nathanson, N.M., McKinzie, D.L. and Felder, C.C. (2003). Role of specific muscarinic receptor subtypes in cholinergic parasympathomimetic responses, in vivo phosphoinositide hydrolysis, and pilocarpine-induced seizure activity. *Eur J Neurosci*, **17**(7), 1403–1410.

Cannon, B. and Nedergaard, J. (2004). Brown adipose tissue: function and physiological significance. *Physiol Rev*, **84**(1), 277–359.

Caterina, M.J., Schumacher, M.A., Tominaga, M., Rosen, T.A., Levine, J.D. and Julius, D. (1997). The capsaicin receptor: a heat-activated ion channel in the pain pathway. *Nature*, **389**(6653), 816–824.

Chancellor, M.B. and De Groat, W.C. (1999). Intravesical capsaicin and resiniferatoxin therapy: spicing up the ways to treat the overactive bladder. *J Urol*, **162**(1), 3–11.

Chang, H.S., Myung, S.J., Yang, S.K., Jung, H.Y., Kim, T.H., Yoon, I.J., Kwon, O.R., Hong, W.S., Kim, J.H. and Min, Y.I. (2003). Effect of electrical stimulation in constipated patients with impaired rectal sensation. *Int J Colorectal Dis*, **18**(5), 433–438.

Charkoudian, N. (2003). Skin blood flow in adult human thermoregulation: how it works, when it does not, and why. *Mayo Clin Proc*, **78**(5), 603–612.

Cheng, C.L., Liu, J.C., Chang, S.Y., Ma, C.P. and De Groat, W.C. (1999). Effect of capsaicin on the micturition reflex in normal and chronic spinal cord-injured cats. *Am J Physiol*, **277**(3 Pt 2), R786–R794.

Cheshire, W.P. and Freeman, R. (2003). Disorders of sweating. *Semin Neurol*, **23**(4), 399–406.

Chotani, M.A., Flavahan, S., Mitra, S., Daunt, D. and Flavahan, N.A. (2000). Silent alpha(2C)-adrenergic receptors enable cold-induced vasoconstriction in cutaneous arteries. *Am J Physiol Heart Circ Physiol*, **278**(4), H1075–H1083.

Christensen, M.D. and Hulsebosch, C.E. (1997). Spinal cord injury and anti-NGF treatment results in changes in CGRP density and distribution in the dorsal horn in the rat. *Exp Neurol*, **147**(2), 463–475.

Clanton Jr., L.J. and Bender, J. (1999). Refractory spinal cord injury induced gastroparesis: resolution with erythromycin lactobionate, a case report. *J Spinal Cord Med*, **22**(4), 236–238.

Clerc, N. and Furness, J.B. (2004). Intrinsic primary afferent neurones of the digestive tract. *Neurogastroenterol Motil*, **16**(**Suppl. 1**), 24–27.

Cochrane, K.L. and Nathan, M.A. (1994). Pressor systems involved in the maintenance of arterial pressure after lesions of the rostral ventrolateral medulla. *J Auton Nerv Syst*, **46**(1–2), 9–18.

Coffa, P.F. and Kotecha, N. (1999). Modulation of sympathetic nerve activity by perivascular sensory nerves in the arterioles of the guinea-pig small intestine. *J Auton Nerv Syst*, **77**(2–3), 125–132.

Comarr, A.E. and Eltorai, I. (1997). Autonomic dysreflexia/hyperreflexia. *J Spinal Cord Med*, **20**(3), 345–354.

Connell, A.M., Frankel, H. and Guttman, L. (1963). The motility of the pelvic colon following complete lesions of the spinal cord. *Paraplegia*, **1**, 98–110.

Consortium for spinal cord Medicine (1997). Acute management of autonomic dysreflexia: adults with spinal cord injury presenting to health-care facilities. *J Spinal Cord Med*, **20**(3), 284–308.

Cooper, K.E., Ferres, H.M. and Guttmann, L. (1957). Vasomotor responses in the foot to raising body temperature in the paraplegic patient. *J Physiol (Lond)*, **136**, 547–555.

Coote, J.H. and Lewis, D.I. (1995). The spinal organisation of the baroreceptor reflex. *Clin Exp Hypertens*, **17(1–2)**, 295–311.

Corbett, J.L., Frankel, H.L. and Harris, P.J. (1971). Cardiovascular reflex responses to cutaneous and visceral stimuli in spinal man. *J Physiol*, **215(2)**, 395–409.

Creasey, G.H., Grill, J.H., Korsten, M., HS, U., Betz, R., Anderson, R. and Walter, J. (2001). An implantable neuroprosthesis for restoring bladder and bowel control to patients with spinal cord injuries: a multicenter trial. *Arch Phys Med Rehabil*, **82(11)**, 1512–1519.

Cruz, F. (2004). Mechanisms involved in new therapies for overactive bladder. *Urology*, **63(3 Suppl. 1)**, 65–73.

Dampney, R.A., Horiuchi, J., Tagawa, T., Fontes, M.A., Potts, P.D. and Polson, J.W. (2003). Medullary and supramedullary mechanisms regulating sympathetic vasomotor tone. *Acta Physiol Scand*, **177(3)**, 209–218.

De Groat, W.C. (1997). A neurologic basis for the overactive bladder. *Urology*, **50(Suppl. 6A)**, 36–52.

De Groat, W.C. and Krier, J. (1978). The sacral parasympathetic reflex pathway regulating colonic motility and defecation in the cat. *J Physiol*, **276**, 481–500.

De Groat, W.C. and Yoshimura, N. (2001). Pharmacology of the lower urinary tract. *Annu Rev Pharmacol Toxicol*, **41**, 691–721.

DiBona, G.F. and Kopp, U.C. (1997). Neural control of renal function. *Physiol Rev*, **77(1)**, 75–197.

Dickens, E.J., Hirst, G.D. and Tomita, T. (1999). Identification of rhythmically active cells in guinea-pig stomach. *J Physiol*, **514(Pt 2)**, 515–531.

Downey, J.A., Chiodi, H.P. and Darling, R.C. (1967). Central temperature regulation in the spinal man. *J Appl Physiol*, **22(1)**, 91–94.

Downey, J.A., Huckaba, C.E., Kelley, P.S., Tam, H.S., Darling, R.C. and Cheh, H.Y. (1976). Sweating responses to central and peripheral heating in spinal man. *J Appl Physiol*, **40(5)**, 701–706.

Du, C., Ferre, J.P. and Ruckebusch, Y. (1987). Spinal cord influences on the colonic myoelectrical activity of fed and fasted rats. *J Physiol*, **383**, 395–404.

Eklund, S., Jodal, M., Lundgren, O. and Sjoqvist, A. (1979). Effects of vasoactive intestinal polypeptide on blood flow, motility and fluid transport in the gastrointestinal tract of the cat. *Acta Physiol Scand*, **105(4)**, 461–468.

Elbadawi, A. (1996). Functional anatomy of the organs of micturition. *Urol Clin North Am*, **23(2)**, 177–210.

Esmail, Z., Shalansky, K.F., Sunderji, R., Anton, H., Chambers, K. and Fish, W. (2002). Evaluation of captopril for the management of hypertension in autonomic dysreflexia: a pilot study. *Arch Phys Med Rehabil*, **83(5)**, 604–608.

Fajardo, N.R., Pasiliao, R.V., Modeste-Duncan, R., Creasey, G., Bauman, W.A. and Korsten, M.A. (2003). Decreased colonic motility in persons with chronic spinal cord injury. *Am J Gastroenterol*, **98(1)**, 128–134.

Fealey, R.D., Szurszewski, J.H., Merritt, J.L. and DiMagno, E.P. (1984). Effect of traumatic spinal cord transection on human upper gastrointestinal motility and gastric emptying. *Gastroenterology*, **87(1)**, 69–75.

Frank, S.M., Raja, S.N., Bulcao, C.F. and Goldstein, D.S. (1999). Relative contribution of core and cutaneous temperatures to thermal comfort and autonomic responses in humans. *J Appl Physiol*, **86(5)**, 1588–1593.

Freeman, R. (2003). Treatment of orthostatic hypotension. *Semin Neurol*, **23(4)**, 435–442.

Freund, P.R., Brengelmann, G.L., Rowell, L.B. and Halar, E. (1984). Attenuated skin blood flow response to hyperthermia in paraplegic men. *J Appl Physiol*, **56(4)**, 1104–1109.

Furness, J.B. and Costa, M. (1980). Types of nerves in the enteric nervous system. *Neuroscience*, **5(1)**, 1–20.

Furness, J.B., Kunze, W.A., Bertrand, P.P., Clerc, N. and Bornstein, J.C. (1998). Intrinsic primary afferent neurons of the intestine. *Prog Neurobiol*, **54(1)**, 1–18.

Gainetdinov, R.R. and Caron, M.G. (1999). Delineating muscarinic receptor functions. *Proc Natl Acad Sci USA*, **96(22)**, 12222–12223.

Gao, S.A., Ambring, A., Lambert, G. and Karlsson, A.K. (2002). Autonomic control of the heart and renal vascular bed during autonomic dysreflexia in high spinal cord injury. *Clin Auton Res*, **12(6)**, 457–464.

Garland, E.M., Hahn, M.K., Ketch, T.P., Keller, N.R., Kim, C.H., Kim, K.S., Biaggioni, I., Shannon, J.R., Blakely, R.D. and Robertson, D. (2002). Genetic basis of clinical catecholamine disorders. *Ann NY Acad Sci*, **971**, 506–514.

Gershon, M.D. (2004). Review article: serotonin receptors and transporters – roles in normal and abnormal gastrointestinal motility. *Aliment Pharmacol Ther*, **20(Suppl. 7)**, 3–14.

Giannantoni, A., Di Stasi, S.M., Scivoletto, G., Mollo, A., Silecchia, A., Fuoco, U. and Vespasiani, G. (1998). Autonomic dysreflexia during urodynamics. *Spinal Cord*, **36(11)**, 756–760.

Giannantoni, A., Di Stasi, S.M., Stephen, R.L., Bini, V., Costantini, E. and Porena, M. (2004). Intravesical resiniferatoxin versus botulinum-A toxin injections for neurogenic detrusor overactivity: a prospective randomized study. *J Urol*, **172(1)**, 240–243.

Gibbins, I.L., Jobling, P. and Morris, J.L. (2003). Functional organization of peripheral vasomotor pathways. *Acta Physiol Scand*, **177(3)**, 237–245.

Giuliani, S., Maggi, C.A. and Meli, A. (1988). Capsaicin-sensitive afferents in the rat urinary bladder activate a spinal sympathetic cardiovascular reflex. *Naunyn Schmiedebergs Arch Pharmacol*, **338**(4), 411–416.

Goldstein, D.S., Robertson, D., Esler, M., Straus, S.E. and Eisenhofer, G. (2002). Dysautonomias: clinical disorders of the autonomic nervous system. *Ann Intern Med*, **137**(9), 753–763.

Gomeza, J., Shannon, H., Kostenis, E., Felder, C., Zhang, L., Brodkin, J., Grinberg, A., Sheng, H. and Wess, J. (1999). Pronounced pharmacologic deficits in M2 muscarinic acetylcholine receptor knockout mice. *Proc Natl Acad Sci USA*, **96**(4), 1692–1697.

Goyal, R.K. and Hirano, I. (1996). The enteric nervous system. *New Engl J Med*, **334**(17), 1106–1115.

Green, B.G. (2004). Temperature perception and nociception. *J Neurobiol*, **61**(1), 13–29.

Groomes, T.E. and Huang, C.T. (1991). Orthostatic hypotension after spinal cord injury: treatment with fludrocortisone and ergotamine. *Arch Phys Med Rehabil*, **72**(1), 56–58.

Grossman, S.D., Wolfe, B.B., Yasuda, R.P. and Wrathall, J.R. (1999). Alterations in AMPA receptor subunit expression after experimental spinal cord contusion injury. *J Neurosci*, **19**(14), 5711–5720.

Grundy, D. (2002). Neuroanatomy of visceral nociception: vagal and splanchnic afferent. *Gut*, **51**(**Suppl. 1**), i2–i5.

Gu, B., Reiter, J.P., Schwinn, D.A., Smith, M.P., Korstanje, C., Thor, K.B. and Dolber, P.C. (2004). Effects of alpha 1-adrenergic receptor subtype selective antagonists on lower urinary tract function in rats with bladder outlet obstruction. *J Urol*, **172**(2), 758–762.

Guimaraes, S. and Moura, D. (2001). Vascular adrenoceptors: an update. *Pharmacol Rev*, **53**(2), 319–356.

Guler, A.D., Lee, H., Iida, T., Shimizu, I., Tominaga, M. and Caterina, M. (2002). Heat-evoked activation of the ion channel, TRPV4. *J Neurosci*, **22**(15), 6408–6414.

Haferkamp, A., Dorsam, J., Resnick, N.M., Yalla, S.V. and Elbadawi, A. (2003). Structural basis of neurogenic bladder dysfunction. III. Intrinsic detrusor innervation. *J Urol*, **169**(2), 555–562.

Hammel, H.T., Jackson, D.C., Stolwijk, J.A., Hardy, J.D. and Stromme, S.B. (1963). Temperature regulation by hypothalamic proportional control with an adjustable set point. *J Appl Physiol*, **18**, 1146–1154.

Hansen, M.B. (2003). The enteric nervous system I: organisation and classification. *Pharmacol Toxicol*, **92**(3), 105–113.

Hertz, A. and Newton, A. (1913). The normal movement of the colon in man. *J Physiol (Lond)*, **47**, 57–65.

Hillsley, K. and Grundy, D. (1998). Sensitivity to 5-hydroxytryptamine in different afferent subpopulations within mesenteric nerves supplying the rat jejunum. *J Physiol*, **509**(**Pt 3**), 717–727.

Hohenbleicher, H., Klosterman, F., Schorr, U., Seyfert, S., Persson, P.B. and Sharma, A.M. (1997). Identification of a renin threshold and its relationship to salt intake in a patient with pure autonomic failure. *Hypertension*, **30**(5), 1068–1071.

Hohenfellner, M., Pannek, J., Botel, U., Dahms, S., Pfitzenmaier, J., Fichtner, J., Hutschenreiter, G. and Thuroff, J.W. (2001). Sacral bladder denervation for treatment of detrusor hyperreflexia and autonomic dysreflexia. *Urology*, **58**(1), 28–32.

Holzer, P. (1998). Neurogenic vasodilatation and plasma leakage in the skin. *Gen Pharmacol*, **30**(1), 5–11.

Hopman, M.T., Groothuis, J.T., Flendrie, M., Gerrits, K.H. and Houtman, S. (2002). Increased vascular resistance in paralyzed legs after spinal cord injury is reversible by training. *J Appl Physiol*, **93**(6), 1966–1972.

Hornykiewicz, O. and Kish, S.J. (1987). Biochemical pathophysiology of Parkinson's disease. *Adv Neurol*, **45**, 19–34.

Igawa, Y., Satoh, T., Mizusawa, H., Seki, S., Kato, H., Ishizuka, O. and Nishizawa, O. (2003). The role of capsaicin-sensitive afferents in autonomic dysreflexia in patients with spinal cord injury. *BJU Int*, **91**(7), 637–641.

Igawa, Y., Zhang, X., Nishizawa, O., Umeda, M., Iwata, A., Taketo, M.M., Manabe, T., Matsui, M. and Andersson, K.E. (2004). Cystometric findings in mice lacking muscarinic M$_2$ or M$_3$ receptors. *J Urol*, **172**(6)(**Pt 1 of 2**), 2460–2464.

Jacob, J.E., Gris, P., Fehlings, M.G., Weaver, L.C. and Brown, A. (2003). Autonomic dysreflexia after spinal cord transection or compression in 129Sv, C57BL, and Wallerian degeneration slow mutant mice. *Exp Neurol*, **183**(1), 136–146.

Jacob, J.E., Pniak, A., Weaver, L.C. and Brown, A. (2001). Autonomic dysreflexia in a mouse model of spinal cord injury. *Neuroscience*, **108**(4), 687–693.

Janig, W. and Habler, H.J. (2003). Neurophysiological analysis of target-related sympathetic pathways—from animal to human: similarities and differences. *Acta Physiol Scand*, **177**(3), 255–274.

Janig, W. and McLachlan, E.M. (1986). Identification of distinct topographical distributions of lumbar sympathetic and sensory neurons projecting to end organs with different functions in the cat. *J Comp Neurol*, **246**(1), 104–112.

Janig, W. and McLachlan, E. M. (1987). Organization of lumbar spinal outflow to distal colon and pelvic organs. *Physiol Rev*, **67**(4), 1332–1404.

Johanson, J.F. (2004). Review article: tegaserod for chronic constipation. *Aliment Pharmacol Ther*, **20**(**Suppl. 7**), 20–24.

Johnson, R.H. and Park, D.M. (1973). Effect of change of posture on blood pressure and plasma renin concentration in men with spinal transections. *Clin Sci*, **44**(6), 539–546.

Kagnoff, M.F. and Eckmann, L. (1997). Epithelial cells as sensors for microbial infection. *J Clin Invest*, **100**(1), 6–10.

Kaplan, S.A., Chancellor, M.B. and Blaivas, J.G. (1991). Bladder and sphincter behavior in patients with spinal cord lesions. *J Urol*, **146**(1), 113–117.

Karlsson, A.K. (1999). Autonomic dysreflexia. *Spinal Cord*, **37**(6), 383–391.

Keef, K.D. and Kreulen, D.L. (1990). Comparison of central versus peripheral nerve pathways to the guinea pig inferior mesenteric ganglion determined electrophysiologically after chronic nerve section. *J Auton Nerv Syst*, **29**(2), 95–112.

Kellogg Jr., D.L., Liu, Y., Kosiba, I.F. and O'Donnell, D. (1999). Role of nitric oxide in the vascular effects of local warming of the skin in humans. *J Appl Physiol*, **86**(4), 1185–1190.

Kellogg Jr., D.L., Pergola, P.E., Piest, K.L., Kosiba, W.A., Crandall, C.G., Grossmann, M. and Johnson, J.M. (1995). Cutaneous active vasodilation in humans is mediated by cholinergic nerve cotransmission. *Circ Res*, **77**(6), 1222–1228.

Keshavarzian, A., Barnes, W.E., Bruninga, K., Nemchausky, B., Mermall, H. and Bushnell, D. (1995). Delayed colonic transit in spinal cord-injured patients measured by indium-111 Amberlite scintigraphy. *Am J Gastroenterol*, **90**(8), 1295–1300.

Ketch, T., Biaggioni, I., Robertson, R. and Robertson, D. (2002). Four faces of baroreflex failure: hypertensive crisis, volatile hypertension, orthostatic tachycardia, and malignant vagotonia. *Circulation*, **105**(21), 2518–2523.

Kewalramani, L.S. (1980). Autonomic dysreflexia in traumatic myelopathy. *Am J Phys Med*, **59**(1), 1–21.

Kim, J.H., Rivas, D.A., Shenot, P.J., Green, B., Kennelly, M., Erickson, J.R., O'Leary, M., Yoshimura, N. and Chancellor, M.B. (2003). Intravesical resiniferatoxin for refractory detrusor hyperreflexia: a multicenter, blinded, randomized, placebo-controlled trial. *J Spinal Cord Med*, **26**(4), 358–363.

Kimura, A., Ohsawa, H., Sato, A. and Sato, Y. (1995). Somatocardiovascular reflexes in anesthetized rats with the central nervous system intact or acutely spinalized at the cervical level. *Neurosci Res*, **22**(3), 297–305.

Kirshblum, S.C., House, J.G. and O'connor, K.C. (2002). Silent autonomic dysreflexia during a routine bowel program in persons with traumatic spinal cord injury: a preliminary study. *Arch Phys Med Rehabil*, **83**(12), 1774–1776.

Kirstein, S.L. and Insel, P.A. (2004). Autonomic nervous system pharmacogenomics: a progress report. *Pharmacol Rev*, **56**(1), 31–52.

Kontani, H., Tsuji, T. and Kimura, S. (2000). Effects of adrenergic alpha2-receptor agonists on urinary bladder contraction in conscious rats. *Jpn J Pharmacol*, **84**(4), 381–390.

Kooijman, M., Rongen, G. A., Smits, P. and Hopman, M.T. (2003). Preserved alpha-adrenergic tone in the leg vascular bed of spinal cord-injured individuals. *Circulation*, **108**(19), 2361–2367.

Kooner, J.S., Frankel, H.L., Mirando, N., Peart, W.S. and Mathias, C.J. (1988). Haemodynamic, hormonal and urinary responses to postural change in tetraplegic and paraplegic man. *Paraplegia*, **26**(4), 233–237.

Korsten, M.A., Fajardo, N.R., Rosman, A.S., Creasey, G.H., Spungen, A.M. and Bauman, W.A. (2004). Difficulty with evacuation after spinal cord injury: colonic motility during sleep and effects of abdominal wall stimulation. *J Rehabil Res Dev*, **41**(1), 95–100.

Krassioukov, A.V., Furlan, J.C. and Fehlings, M.G. (2003). Autonomic dysreflexia in acute spinal cord injury: an under-recognized clinical entity. *J Neurotraum*, **20**(8), 707–716.

Krassioukov, A.V., Johns, D.G. and Schramm, L.P. (2002). Sensitivity of sympathetically correlated spinal interneurons, renal sympathetic nerve activity, and arterial pressure to somatic and visceral stimuli after chronic spinal injury. *J Neurotraum*, **19**(12), 1521–1529.

Krassioukov, A.V. and Weaver, L.C. (1996). Morphological changes in sympathetic preganglionic neurons after spinal cord injury in rats. *Neuroscience*, **70**(1), 211–225.

Krenz, N.R. and Weaver, L.C. (1998). Changes in the morphology of sympathetic preganglionic neurons parallel the development of autonomic dysreflexia after spinal cord injury in rats. *Neurosci Lett*, **243**(1–3), 61–64.

Krogh, K., Mosdal, C., Gregersen, H. and Laurberg, S. (2002). Rectal wall properties in patients with acute and chronic spinal cord lesions. *Dis Colon Rectum*, **45**(5), 641–649.

Krogh, K., Olsen, N., Christensen, P., Madsen, J.L. and Laurberg, S. (2003). Colorectal transport during defecation in patients with lesions of the sacral spinal cord. *Neurogastroenterol Motil*, **15**(1), 25–31.

Krum, H., Brown, D.J., Rowe, P.R., Louis, W.J. and Howes, L.G. (1990). Steady state plasma [3H]-noradrenaline kinetics in quadriplegic chronic spinal cord injury patients. *J Auton Pharmacol*, **10**(4), 221–226.

Krum, H., Louis, W.J., Brown, D.J. and Howes, L.G. (1992). Pressor dose responses and baroreflex sensitivity in quadriplegic spinal cord injury patients. *J Hypertens*, **10**(3), 245–250.

Kunze, W.A. and Furness, J.B. (1999). The enteric nervous system and regulation of intestinal motility. *Annu Rev Physiol*, **61**, 117–142.

Kuo, D.C., Hisamitsu, T. and De Groat, W.C. (1984). A sympathetic projection from sacral paravertebral ganglia to the pelvic nerve and to postganglionic nerves on the surface of the urinary bladder and large intestine of the cat. *J Comp Neurol*, **226**(1), 76–86.

Kuo, H.C. (2004). Urodynamic evidence of effectiveness of botulinum A toxin injection in treatment of detrusor overactivity
refractory to anticholinergic agents. *Urology*, **63**(5), 868–872.

Leduc, B.E., Giasson, M., Favreau-Ethier, M. and Lepage, Y.
(1997). Colonic transit time after spinal cord injury. *J Spinal
Cord Med*, **20**(4), 416–421.

Leduc, B.E., Spacek, E. and Lepage, Y. (2002). Colonic transit
time after spinal cord injury: any clinical significance?
J Spinal Cord Med, **25**(3), 161–166.

Lee, B.Y., Karmakar, M.G., Herz, B.L. and Sturgill, R.A. (1995).
Autonomic dysreflexia revisited. *J Spinal Cord Med*, **18**(2),
75–87.

Legramante, J.M., Raimondi, G., Massaro, M. and Iellamo, F.
(2001). Positive and negative feedback mechanisms in the
neural regulation of cardiovascular function in healthy and
spinal cord-injured humans. *Circulation*, **103**(9), 1250–1255.

Lehmann, K.G., Lane, J.G., Piepmeier, J.M. and Batsford, W.P.
(1987). Cardiovascular abnormalities accompanying acute
spinal cord injury in humans: incidence, time course and
severity. *J Am Coll Cardiol*, **10**(1), 46–52.

Leippold, T., Reitz, A. and Schurch, B. (2003). Botulinum toxin
as a new therapy option for voiding disorders: current state
of the art. *Eur Urol*, **44**(2), 165–174.

Lin, Z., Forster, J., Sarosiek, I. and McCallum, R.W. (2003).
Treatment of gastroparesis with electrical stimulation. *Dig
Dis Sci*, **48**(5), 837–848.

Linden, D.R., Sharkey, K.A. and Mawe, G.M. (2003). Enhanced
excitability of myenteric AH neurones in the inflamed
guinea-pig distal colon. *J Physiol*, **547**(Pt 2), 589–601.

Llewellyn-Smith, I.J. and Weaver, L.C. (2001). Changes in
synaptic inputs to sympathetic preganglionic neurons after
spinal cord injury. *J Comp Neurol*, **435**(2), 226–240.

Longo, W.E., Ballantyne, G.H. and Modlin, I.M. (1989). The
colon, anorectum, and spinal cord patient. A review of the
functional alterations of the denervated hindgut. *Dis Colon
Rectum*, **32**(3), 261–267.

Low, P.A. (2004). Evaluation of sudomotor function. *Clin
Neurophysiol*, **115**(7), 1506–1513.

Lundberg, J.M., Hokfelt, T., Anggard, A., Terenius, L., Elde, R.,
Markey, K., Goldstein, M. and Kimmel, J. (1982).
Organizational principles in the peripheral sympathetic
nervous system: subdivision by coexisting peptides
(somatostatin-, avian pancreatic polypeptide-, and vasoactive intestinal polypeptide-like immunoreactive materials).
Proc Natl Acad Sci USA, **79**(4), 1303–1307.

Lundgren, O. (2002). Enteric nerves and diarrhoea. *Pharmacol
Toxicol*, **90**(3), 109–120.

Maingret, F., Lauritzen, I., Patel, A.J., Heurteaux, C., Reyes, R.,
Lesage, F., Lazdunski, M. and Honore, E. (2000). TREK-1 is a
heat-activated background K(+) channel. *EMBO J*, **19**(11),
2483–2491.

Maiorov, D.N., Krenz, N.R., Krassioukov, A.V. and Weaver, L.C.
(1997). Role of spinal NMDA and AMPA receptors in
episodic hypertension in conscious spinal rats. *Am J
Physiol*, **273**(3 Pt 2), H1266–H1274.

Mallory, B.S., Roppolo, J.R. and De Groat, W.C. (1991).
Pharmacological modulation of the pontine micturition
center. *Brain Res*, **546**(2), 310–320.

Mamas, M.A., Reynard, J.M. and Brading, A.F. (2001).
Augmentation of nitric oxide to treat detrusor-external
sphincter dyssynergia in spinal cord injury. *Lancet*,
357(9272), 1964–1967.

Marsh, D.R. and Weaver, L.C. (2004). Autonomic dysreflexia,
induced by noxious or innocuous stimulation, does not
depend on changes in dorsal horn substance p.
J Neurotraum, **21**(6), 817–828.

Marsh, D.R., Wong, S.T., Meakin, S.O., MacDonald, J.I.,
Hamilton, E.F. and Weaver, L.C. (2002). Neutralizing
intraspinal nerve growth factor with a trkA-IgG fusion
protein blocks the development of autonomic dysreflexia
in a clip-compression model of spinal cord injury.
J Neurotraum, **19**(12), 1531–1541.

Mathias, C.J. (1991). Role of sympathetic efferent nerves in
blood pressure regulation and in hypertension.
Hypertension, **18**(Suppl. 5), III22–III30.

Mathias, C.J. (2003). Autonomic diseases: management.
J Neurol Neurosurg Psychiatr, **74**(Suppl. 3), iii42–iii47.

Mathias, C.J., Christensen, N.J., Corbett, J.L., Frankel, H.L.,
Goodwin, T.J. and Peart, W.S. (1975). Plasma catecholamines, plasma renin activity and plasma aldosterone in
tetraplegic man, horizontal and tilted. *Clin Sci Mol Med*,
49(4), 291–299.

Mathias, C.J., Frankel, H.L., Christensen, N.J. and Spalding, J.M.
(1976). Enhanced pressor response to noradrenaline in
patients with cervical spinal cord transection. *Brain*, **99**(4),
757–770.

Mathias, C.J., Christensen, N.J., Frankel, H.L. and Peart, W.S.
(1980). Renin release during head-up tilt occurs independently of sympathetic nervous activity in tetraplegic man.
Clin Sci (Lond), **59**(4), 251–256.

Matsui, M., Motomura, D., Karasawa, H., Fujikawa, T., Jiang, J.,
Komiya, Y., Takahashi, S. and Taketo, M.M. (2000). Multiple
functional defects in peripheral autonomic organs in mice
lacking muscarinic acetylcholine receptor gene for the M3
subtype. *Proc Natl Acad Sci USA*, **97**(17), 9579–9584.

McAllen, R.M. (2004). Preoptic thermoregulatory mechanisms
in detail. *Am J Physiol Regul Integr Comp Physiol*, **287**(2),
R272–R273.

McCall, R.B. and Gebber, G.L. (1975). Brain stem and spinal synchronization of sympathetic nervous discharge. *Brain Res*, **89**(1), 139–143.

McGuire, E.J. (1986). The innervation and function of the lower urinary tract. *J Neurosurg*, **65**(3), 278–285.

McKemy, D.D., Neuhausser, W.M. and Julius, D. (2002). Identification of a cold receptor reveals a general role for TRP channels in thermosensation. *Nature*, **416**(6876), 52–58.

Menardo, G., Bausano, G., Corazziari, E., Fazio, A., Marangi, A., Genta, V. and Marenco, G. (1987). Large-bowel transit in paraplegic patients. *Dis Colon Rectum*, **30**(12), 924–928.

Mifflin, S.W. (2001). What does the brain know about blood pressure? *News Physiol Sci*, **16**, 266–271.

Minson, C.T., Berry, L.T. and Joyner, M.J. (2001). Nitric oxide and neurally mediated regulation of skin blood flow during local heating. *J Appl Physiol*, **91**(4), 1619–1626.

Morrison, S.F. (2003). Glutamate transmission in the rostral ventrolateral medullary sympathetic premotor pathway. *Cell Mol Neurobiol*, **23**(4–5), 761–772.

Naftchi, N.E. and Richardson, J.S. (1997). Autonomic dysreflexia: pharmacological management of hypertensive crises in spinal cord injured patients. *J Spinal Cord Med*, **20**(3), 355–360.

Nagano, M., Ishimizu, Y., Saitoh, S., Okada, H. and Fukuda, H. (2004). The defecation reflex in rats: fundamental properties and the reflex center. *Auton Neurosci*, **111**(1), 48–56.

Nagashima, K., Nakai, S., Tanaka, M. and Kanosue, K. (2000). Neuronal circuitries involved in thermoregulation. *Auton Neurosci*, **85**(1–3), 18–25.

Nakamura, K., Matsumura, K., Hubschle, T., Nakamura, Y., Hioki, H., Fujiyama, F., Boldogkoi, Z., Konig, M., Thiel, H.J., Gerstberger, R., Kobayashi, S. and Kaneko, T. (2004). Identification of sympathetic premotor neurons in medullary raphe regions mediating fever and other thermoregulatory functions. *J Neurosci*, **24**(23), 5370–5380.

Nelson, C.P., Gupta, P., Napier, C.M., Nahorski, S.R. and Challiss, R.A. (2004). Functional selectivity of muscarinic receptor antagonists for inhibition of M3-mediated phosphoinositide responses in guinea pig urinary bladder and submandibular salivary gland. *J Pharmacol Exp Ther*, **310**(3), 1255–1265.

Normell, L.A. (1974). Distribution of impaired cutaneous vasomotor and sudomotor function in paraplegic man. *Scand J Clin Lab Invest*, **138**, 25–41.

Osborn, J.W., Taylor, R.F. and Schramm, L.P. (1989). Determinants of arterial pressure after chronic spinal transection in rats. *Am J Physiol*, **256**(3 Pt 2), R666–R673.

Ozcan, O., Ulus, I.H., Yurtkuran, M. and Karakaya, M. (1991). Release of vasopressin, cortisol and beta-endorphin in tetraplegic subjects in response to head-up tilt. *Paraplegia*, **29**(2), 120–124.

Pan, H. and Gershon, M.D. (2000). Activation of intrinsic afferent pathways in submucosal ganglia of the guinea pig small intestine. *J Neurosci*, **20**(9), 3295–3309.

Parikh, S.M., Diedrich, A., Biaggioni, I. and Robertson, D. (2002). The nature of the autonomic dysfunction in multiple system atrophy. *J Neurol Sci*, **200**(1–2), 1–10.

Parkman, H.P., Hasler, W.L. and Fisher, R.S. (2004). American Gastroenterological Association technical review on the diagnosis and treatment of gastroparesis. *Gastroenterology*, **127**(5), 1592–1622.

Patapoutian, A., Peier, A.M., Story, G.M. and Viswanath, V. (2003). ThermoTRP channels and beyond: mechanisms of temperature sensation. *Nat Rev Neurosci*, **4**(7), 529–539.

Pavlakis, A.J., Siroky, M.B., Goldstein, I. and Krane, R.J. (1983). Neurourologic findings in Parkinson's disease. *J Urol*, **129**(1), 80–83.

Poole, C.J., Williams, T.D., Lightman, S.L. and Frankel, H.L. (1987). Neuroendocrine control of vasopressin secretion and its effect on blood pressure in subjects with spinal cord transection. *Brain*, **110**(Pt 3), 727–735.

Qu, L., Sherebrin, R. and Weaver, L.C. (1988). Blockade of spinal pathways decreases pre- and postganglionic discharge differentially. *Am J Physiol*, **255**(6 Pt 2), R946–R951.

Quinton, P.M. (1983). Sweating and its disorders. *Annu Rev Med*, **34**, 429–452.

Ray, C.A. (2000). Interaction of the vestibular system and baroreflexes on sympathetic nerve activity in humans. *Am J Physiol Heart Circ Physiol*, **279**(5), H2399–H2404.

Read, N.W. and Houghton, L.A. (1989). Physiology of gastric emptying and pathophysiology of gastroparesis. *Gastroenterol Clin North Am*, **18**(2), 359–373.

Reitz, A., Knapp, P.A., Muntener, M. and Schurch, B. (2004). Oral nitric oxide donors: a new pharmacological approach to detrusor-sphincter dyssynergia in spinal cord injured patients? *Eur Urol*, **45**(4), 516–520.

Rindi, G., Leiter, A.B., Kopin, A.S., Bordi, C. and Solcia, E. (2004). The "normal" endocrine cell of the gut: changing concepts and new evidences. *Ann NY Acad Sci*, **1014**, 1–12.

Rock, E., Malmud, L. and Fisher, R.S. (1981). Motor disorders of the stomach. *Med Clin North Am*, **65**(6), 1269–1289.

Sakakibara, R., Hattori, T., Tojo, M., Yamanishi, T., Yasuda, K. and Hirayama, K. (1995). The location of the paths subserving micturition: studies in patients with cervical myelopathy. *J Auton Nerv Syst*, **55**(3), 165–168.

Saper, C.B. (2002). The central autonomic nervous system: conscious visceral perception and autonomic pattern generation. *Annu Rev Neurosci*, **25**, 433–469.

Sasaki, K., Smith, C.P., Chuang, Y.C., Lee, J.Y., Kim, J.C. and Chancellor, M.B. (2001). Oral gabapentin (neurontin) treatment of refractory genitourinary tract pain. *Tech Urol*, **7**(1), 47–49.

Satinoff, E. (1978). Neural organization and evolution of thermal regulation in mammals. *Science*, **201**(4350), 16–22.

Schmid, A., Halle, M., Stutzle, C., Konig, D., Baumstark, M.W., Storch, M.J., Schmidt-Trucksass, A., Lehmann, M., Berg, A. and Keul, J. (2000). Lipoproteins and free plasma catecholamines in spinal cord injured men with different injury levels. *Clin Physiol*, **20**(4), 304–310.

Schmid, A., Huonker, M., Barturen, J.M., Stahl, F., Schmidt-Trucksass, A., Konig, D., Grathwohl, D., Lehmann, M. and Keul, J. (1998). Catecholamines, heart rate, and oxygen uptake during exercise in persons with spinal cord injury. *J Appl Physiol*, **85**(2), 635–641.

Schmidt, K.D. and Chan, C.W. (1992). Thermoregulation and fever in normal persons and in those with spinal cord injuries. *Mayo Clin Proc*, **67**(5), 469–475.

Seckendorf, R. and Randall, W.C. (1961). Thermal reflex sweating in normal and paraplegic man. *J Appl Physiol*, **16**(5), 796–800.

Segal, J.L., Milne, N. and Brunnemann, S.R. (1995). Gastric emptying is impaired in patients with spinal cord injury. *Am J Gastroenterol*, **90**(3), 466–470.

Seki, S., Sasaki, K., Igawa, Y., Nishizawa, O., Chancellor, M.B., De Groat, W.C. and Yoshimura, N. (2004). Suppression of detrusor-sphincter dyssynergia by immunoneutralization of nerve growth factor in lumbosacral spinal cord in spinal cord injured rats. *J Urol*, **171**(1), 478–482.

Shannon, J., Jordan, J., Costa, F., Robertson, R.M. and Biaggioni, I. (1997). The hypertension of autonomic failure and its treatment. *Hypertension*, **30**(5), 1062–1067.

Shannon, J.R., Diedrich, A., Biaggioni, I., Tank, J., Robertson, R.M., Robertson, D. and Jordan, J. (2002). Water drinking as a treatment for orthostatic syndromes. *Am J Med*, **112**(5), 355–360.

Shields Jr., R.W. (1993). Functional anatomy of the autonomic nervous system. *J Clin Neurophysiol*, **10**(1), 2–13.

Silver, J.R. (2000). Early autonomic dysreflexia. *Spinal Cord*, **38**(4), 229–233.

Silver, J.R., Randall, W.C. and Guttmann, L. (1991). Spinal mediation of thermally induced sweating. *J Neurol Neurosurg Psychiatr*, **54**(4), 297–304.

Simon, E. (1974). Temperature regulation: the spinal cord as a site of extrahypothalamic thermoregulatory functions. *Rev Physiol Biochem Pharmacol*, **71**, 1–76.

Smith, G.D., Seckl, J.R. and Harmar, A.J. (1993). Distribution of neuropeptides in dorsal root ganglia of the rat; substance P,

somatostatin and calcitonin gene-related peptide. *Neurosci Lett*, **153**(1), 5–8.

Spencer, N.J., Sanders, K.M. and Smith, T.K. (2003). Migrating motor complexes do not require electrical slow waves in the mouse small intestine. *J Physiol*, **553**(Pt 3), 881–893.

Stauss, H.M. (2002). Baroreceptor reflex function. *Am J Physiol Regul Integr Comp Physiol*, **283**(2), R284–R286.

Stebbing, M., Johnson, P., Vremec, M. and Bornstein, J. (2001). Role of alpha(2)-adrenoceptors in the sympathetic inhibition of motility reflexes of guinea-pig ileum. *J Physiol*, **534**(Pt 2), 465–478.

Steers, W.D., Meythaler, J.M., Haworth, C., Herrell, D. and Park, T.S. (1992). Effects of acute bolus and chronic continuous intrathecal baclofen on genitourinary dysfunction due to spinal cord pathology. *J Urol*, **148**(6), 1849–1855.

Steers, W.D., Wind, T.C., Jones, E.V. and Edlich, R.F. (2002). Functional electrical stimulation of bladder and bowel in spinal cord injury. *J Long Term Eff Med Implants*, **12**(3), 189–199.

Stein, R.D. and Weaver, L.C. (1988). Multi- and single-fibre mesenteric and renal sympathetic responses to chemical stimulation of intestinal receptors in cats. *J Physiol*, **396**, 155–172.

Stein, R.D., Weaver, L.C. and Yardley, C.P. (1989). Ventrolateral medullary neurones: effects on magnitude and rhythm of discharge of mesenteric and renal nerves in cats. *J Physiol*, **408**, 571–586.

Stephens, D.P., Aoki, K., Kosiba, W.A. and Johnson, J.M. (2001a). Nonnoradrenergic mechanism of reflex cutaneous vasoconstriction in men. *Am J Physiol Heart Circ Physiol*, **280**(4), H1496–H1504.

Stephens, D.P., Charkoudian, N., Benevento, J.M., Johnson, J.M. and Saumet, J.L. (2001b). The influence of topical capsaicin on the local thermal control of skin blood flow in humans. *Am J Physiol Regul Integr Comp Physiol*, **281**(3), R894–R901.

Stjernberg, L., Blumberg, H. and Wallin, B.G. (1986). Sympathetic activity in man after spinal cord injury. Outflow to muscle below the lesion. *Brain*, **109**(Pt 4), 695–715.

Stone, J.M., Nino-Murcia, M., Wolfe, V.A. and Perkash, I. (1990). Chronic gastrointestinal problems in spinal cord injury patients: a prospective analysis. *Am J Gastroenterol*, **85**(9), 1114–1119.

Story, G.M., Peier, A.M., Reeve, A.J., Eid, S.R., Mosbacher, J., Hricik, T.R., Earley, T.J., Hergarden, A.C., Andersson, D.A., Hwang, S.W., McIntyre, P., Jegla, T., Bevan, S. and Patapoutian, A. (2003). ANKTM1, a TRP-like channel expressed in nociceptive neurons, is activated by cold temperatures. *Cell*, **112**(6), 819–829.

Streefkerk, J.O., Pfaffendorf, M. and van Zwieten, P.A. (2003). Vasopressin-induced facilitation of adrenergic responses in the rat mesenteric artery is V1-receptor dependent. *Auton Autacoid Pharmacol*, **23**(1), 35–41.

Sugaya, K., Nishijima, S., Miyazato, M., Ashitomi, K., Hatano, T. and Ogawa, Y. (2002). Effects of intrathecal injection of tamsulosin and naftopidil, alpha-1A and -1D adrenergic receptor antagonists, on bladder activity in rats. *Neurosci Lett*, **328**(1), 74–76.

Sugaya, K., Ogawa, Y., Hatano, T., Nishijima, S., Matsuyama, K. and Mori, S. (2003). Ascending and descending brainstem neuronal activity during cystometry in decerebrate cats. *Neurourol Urodyn*, **22**(4), 343–350.

Sun, M.K. (1995). Central neural organization and control of sympathetic nervous system in mammals. *Prog Neurobiol*, **47**(3), 157–233.

Sun, M.K., Hackett, J.T. and Guyenet, P.G. (1988). Sympathoexcitatory neurons of rostral ventrolateral medulla exhibit pacemaker properties in the presence of a glutamate-receptor antagonist. *Brain Res*, **438**(1–2), 23–40.

Sun, W.M., MacDonagh, R., Forster, D., Thomas, D.G., Smallwood, R. and Read, N.W. (1995). Anorectal function in patients with complete spinal transection before and after sacral posterior rhizotomy. *Gastroenterology*, **108**(4), 990–998.

Sved, A.F. (2004). Tonic glutamatergic drive of RVLM vasomotor neurons? *Am J Physiol Regul Integr Comp Physiol*, **287**(6), R1301–R1303.

Sved, A.F., McDowell, F.H. and Blessing, W.W. (1985). Release of antidiuretic hormone in quadriplegic subjects in response to head-up tilt. *Neurology*, **35**(1), 78–82.

Tack, J. (1995). Georges Brohee Prize 1994. Motilin and the enteric nervous system in the control of interdigestive and postprandial gastric motility. *Acta Gastroenterol Belg*, **58**(1), 21–30.

Takamori, S., Rhee, J.S., Rosenmund, C. and Jahn, R. (2000). Identification of a vesicular glutamate transporter that defines a glutamatergic phenotype in neurons. *Nature*, **407**(6801), 189–194.

Takeuchi, T., Fujinami, K., Goto, H., Fujita, A., Taketo, M.M., Manabe, T., Matsui, M. and Hata, F. (2005). Roles of M2 and M4 muscarinic receptors in regulating acetylcholine release from myenteric neurons of mouse ileum. *J Neurophysiol*, **93**, 2841–2848.

Tam, H.S., Darling, R.C., Cheh, H.Y. and Downey, J.A. (1978). The dead zone of thermoregulation in normal and paraplegic man. *Can J Physiol Pharmacol*, **56**(6), 976–983.

Tank, J., Schroeder, C., Stoffels, M., Diedrich, A., Sharma, A.M., Luft, F.C. and Jordan, J. (2003). Pressor effect of water drinking in tetraplegic patients may be a spinal reflex. *Hypertension*, **41**(6), 1234–1239.

Teasell, R.W., Arnold, J.M., Krassioukov, A. and Delaney, G.A. (2000). Cardiovascular consequences of loss of supraspinal control of the sympathetic nervous system after spinal cord injury. *Arch Phys Med Rehabil*, **81**(4), 506–516.

Thami, G.P., Kaur, S. and Kanwar, A.J. (2003). Acquired idiopathic generalized anhidrosis: a rare cause of heat intolerance. *Clin Exp Dermatol*, **28**(3), 262–264.

Thor, K.B. (2003). Serotonin and norepinephrine involvement in efferent pathways to the urethral rhabdosphincter: implications for treating stress urinary incontinence. *Urology*, **62**(4 **Suppl. 1**), 3–9.

Travagli, R.A., Hermann, G.E., Browning, K.N. and Rogers, R.C. (2003). Musings on the wanderer: what's new in our understanding of vago-vagal reflexes? III. Activity-dependent plasticity in vago-vagal reflexes controlling the stomach. *Am J Physiol Gastrointest Liver Physiol*, **284**(2), G180–G187.

Tsai, S.H., Shih, C.J., Shyy, T.T. and Liu, J.C. (1980). Recovery of vasomotor response in human spinal cord transection. *J Neurosurg*, **52**(6), 808–811.

Van Kerrebroeck, P. (2004). Duloxetine: an innovative approach for treating stress urinary incontinence. *BJU Int*, **94** (**Suppl. 1**), 31–37.

von Heyden, B., Jordan, U. and Hertle, L. (1998). Neurotransmitters in the human urethral sphincter in the absence of voiding dysfunction. *Urol Res*, **26**(5), 299–310.

Wall, B.M., Runyan, K.R., Williams, H.H., Bobal, M.A., Crofton, J.T., Share, L. and Cooke, C.R. (1994). Characteristics of vasopressin release during controlled reduction in arterial pressure. *J Lab Clin Med*, **124**(4), 554–563.

Ward, S.M., Dixon, R.E., DeFaoite, A. and Sanders, K.M. (2004). Voltage dependent calcium entry underlies propagation of slow waves in canine gastric antrum. *J Physiol*, **561**, 393–810.

Warner, D.O., Joyner, M.J. and Charkoudian, N. (2004). Nicotine increases initial blood flow responses to local heating of human non-glabrous skin. *J Physiol*, **559**(Pt 3), 975–984.

Watanabe, T., Yokoyama, T., Sasaki, K., Nozaki, K., Ozawa, H. and Kumon, H. (2004). Intravesical resiniferatoxin for patients with neurogenic detrusor overactivity. *Int J Urol*, **11**(4), 200–205.

Weaver, L.C., Verghese, P., Bruce, J.C., Fehlings, M.G., Krenz, N.R. and Marsh, D.R. (2001). Autonomic dysreflexia and primary afferent sprouting after clip-compression injury of the rat spinal cord. *J Neurotraum*, **18**(10), 1107–1119.

Weber, R., Pechere-Bertschi, A., Hayoz, D., Gerc, V., Brouard, R., Lahmy, J.P., Brunner, H.R. and Burnier, M. (1997). Effects of SR 49059, a new orally active and specific vasopressin V1 receptor antagonist, on vasopressin-induced vasoconstriction in humans. *Hypertension*, **30**(5), 1121–1127.

Wecht, J.M., De Meersman, R.E., Weir, J.P., Spungen, A.M. and Bauman, W.A. (2003). Cardiac homeostasis is independent of calf venous compliance in subjects with paraplegia. *Am J Physiol Heart Circ Physiol*, **284**(6), H2393–H2399.

Westlund, K.N., Bowker, R.M., Ziegler, M.G. and Coulter, J.D. (1982). Descending noradrenergic projections and their spinal terminations. *Prog Brain Res*, **57**, 219–238.

Woods, M., Carson, N., Norton, N.W., Sheldon, J.H. and Argentieri, T.M. (2001). Efficacy of the beta3-adrenergic receptor agonist CL-316243 on experimental bladder hyperreflexia and detrusor instability in the rat. *J Urol*, **166**(3), 1142–1147.

Wyndaele, J.J. (1987). Urethral sphincter dyssynergia in spinal cord injury patients. *Paraplegia*, **25**(1), 10–15.

Yamaguchi, O. (2002). Beta3-adrenoceptors in human detrusor muscle. *Urology*, **59**(5 Suppl. 1), 25–29.

Yamanouchi, M., Shimatani, H., Kadowaki, M., Yoneda, S., Nakagawa, T., Fujii, H. and Takaki, M. (2002). Integrative control of rectoanal reflex in guinea pigs through lumbar colonic nerves. *Am J Physiol Gastrointest Liver Physiol*, **283**(1), G148–G156.

Yamato, S. and Rattan, S. (1990). Role of alpha adrenoceptors in opossum internal anal sphincter. *J Clin Invest*, **86**(2), 424–429.

Yanagiya, Y., Sato, T., Kawada, T., Inagaki, M., Tatewaki, T., Zheng, C., Kamiya, A., Takaki, H., Sugimachi, M. and Sunagawa, K. (2004). Bionic epidural stimulation restores arterial pressure regulation during orthostasis. *J Appl Physiol*, **97**(3), 984–990.

Yardley, C.P., Fitzsimons, C.L. and Weaver, L.C. (1989). Cardiac and peripheral vascular contributions to hypotension in spinal cats. *Am J Physiol*, **257**(5 Pt 2), H1347–H1353.

Yokoyama, T., Kumon, H., Smith, C.P., Somogyi, G.T. and Chancellor, M.B. (2002). Botulinum toxin treatment of urethral and bladder dysfunction. *Acta Med Okayama*, **56**(6), 271–277.

Yoshimura, N. (1999). Bladder afferent pathway and spinal cord injury: possible mechanisms inducing hyperreflexia of the urinary bladder. *Prog Neurobiol*, **57**(6), 583–606.

Yoshimura, N., Kuno, S., Chancellor, M.B., De Groat, W.C. and Seki, S. (2003). Dopaminergic mechanisms underlying bladder hyperactivity in rats with a unilateral 6-hydroxy-dopamine (6-OHDA) lesion of the nigrostriatal pathway. *Br J Pharmacol*, **139**(8), 1425–1432.

Yoshimura, N., Mizuta, E., Yoshida, O. and Kuno, S. (1998). Therapeutic effects of dopamine D1/D2 receptor agonists on detrusor hyperreflexia in 1-methyl-4-phenyl-1,2,3,6-tetrahydropyridine-lesioned parkinsonian cynomolgus monkeys. *J Pharmacol Exp Ther*, **286**(1), 228–233.

Yoshimura, N., Sasa, M., Ohno, Y., Yoshida, O. and Takaori, S. (1988). Contraction of urinary bladder by central norepinephrine originating in the locus coeruleus. *J Urol*, **139**(2), 423–427.

Yoshiyama, M. and De Groat, W.C. (2001). Role of spinal alpha1-adrenoceptor subtypes in the bladder reflex in anesthetized rats. *Am J Physiol Regul Integr Comp Physiol*, **280**(5), R1414–R1419.

Zhang, J. and Mifflin, S.W. (1998). Differential roles for NMDA and non-NMDA receptor subtypes in baroreceptor afferent integration in the nucleus of the solitary tract of the rat. *J Physiol*, **511**(Pt 3), 733–745.

Zhang, J. and Mifflin, S.W. (2000). Subthreshold aortic nerve inputs to neurons in nucleus of the solitary tract. *Am J Physiol Regul Integr Comp Physiol*, **278**(6), R1595–R1604.

Zhang, Y.H., Hosono, T., Yanase-Fujiwara, M., Chen, X.M. and Kanosue, K. (1997). Effect of midbrain stimulations on thermoregulatory vasomotor responses in rats. *J Physiol*, **503**(Pt 1), 177–186.

Abbreviations

5-HT	Serotonin
6-OHDA	6-hydroxydopamine
Ach	Acetylcholine
AD	Autonomic dysreflexia
AMPA	Alpha-amino-3-hydroxy-5-methyl-4-isoxazolepropionic acid
ANS	Autonomic nervous system
AR	Adrenoreceptors
ATP	Adenosine triphosphate
AVP	Arginine vasopressin
CGRP	Calcitonin gene-related peptide
DBP	Diastolic blood pressure
DDAVP	Desmopressin acetate
DESD	Detrusor-external urethral sphincter dyssynergia
DMV	Dorsal motor nucleus of the vagus
E	Epinephrine
EAA	Excitatory amino acid
EAS	External anal sphincter

EPSPs	Excitatory post synaptic potentials	NMDA	*N*-methyl-D-aspartate
EUS	External urethra sphincter	NO	Nitric oxide
FBF	Forearm blood flow	NPY	Neuropeptide Y
GABA	Gamma-aminobutyric acid	NTS	Nucleus tracti solitarii
GI	Gastrointestinal	PAF	Pure autonomic failure
IAS	Internal anal sphincter	PAG	Periaqueductal gray
IDMC	Interdigestive motor complex	PD	Parkinson's disease
IMG	Inferior mesenteric ganglion	PMC	Pontine micturition center
IML	Intermediolateral	POA	Preoptic area
IPANs	Intrinsic primary afferent neurons	RTX	Resiniferatoxin
IUS	Internal urethral sphincter	RVLM	Rostral ventrolateral medulla
M	Muscarinic receptors	SBP	Systolic blood pressure
MAP	Mean arterial pressure	SCI	Spinal cord injury SCI
MMC	Migrating motor complexes	SERT	Seratonin reuptake transporter
MPTP	1-methyl-4-phenyl-1, 2,3,6-tetrahy-dropyridine	SMG	Superior mesenteric ganglion
MR	Motility-regulating	SPN	Sympathetic preganglionic neurons
MSA	Multiple system atrophy	TRP	Transient receptor potential
MVC	Muscle vasoconstrictor neurons	VGLUT3	Vesicular glutamate transporter 3
NANC	Nonadrenergic, noncholinergic	VIP	Vasoactive intestinal peptide
NE	Norepinephrine	VPpc	Ventroposterior parvicellular nucleus
NGF	Nerve growth factor	VR	Vanilloid receptor

Sexual neurorehabilitation

Mindy L. Aisen[1] and Danielle M. Kerkovich[2]

[1]CEO United Cerebral Palsy Research and Educational Foundation and [2]Department of Veterans Affairs, Washington, DC

25.1 Introduction

Sexual dysfunction is a complication of a wide variety of neurologic disorders that include but are not limited to, myelopathies, such as multiple sclerosis (MS) and spinal cord injury (SCI), and central nervous system lesions, such as stroke and traumatic brain injury (TBI). Until recently, society has viewed the addressing of sexual and reproductive activities as taboo, especially when discussing the disabled or the elderly. However, sexuality is a normal physiologic process with profound effects upon quality of life, regardless of physical status, or age (Comfort and Dial, 1991).

Sexuality is the embodiment of sexual and reproductive activities involving complex interactions among biologic, psychologic, and social systems. An individual's perception of their sexuality, as well as society's perception can have an inestimable impact on their self-esteem, and hence their willingness to openly address these issues (Earle, 2001). Such barriers to communication represent a real challenge to practicing clinicians. However, advances in treatment options obligate the clinician providing care to those with neurogenic sexual/reproductive dysfunction to learn to communicate effectively about these issues, provide new therapies and refer patients to the appropriate specialists.

This chapter will provide an introduction to approaches in counseling, an overview of male and female physiology, and a description of common neurologic disorders and their impact on sexuality. Treatment options for those disorders are also reviewed.

25.2 Sexuality counseling for men and women

Having an in-depth understanding of the psychologic and social repercussions that can be a consequence of sexual dysfunction disorders is critical to the rehabilitation process of an individual that suffers from any type of neurologic disorder. Sexuality is an integral part of the human experience. It should be emphasized that it is normal to be interested in engaging and sustaining healthy sexual relationships and to know that other people with impairments have successful, fulfilling sexual experiences. It is also important for clinicians to impart that it is common for neurologically and otherwise impaired individuals to experience feelings of inadequacy and doubt. Such concerns are universal. Therefore, physicians must assert that treatments, whether psychologic, physical, surgical, or medical, are available. Sexual dysfunction is a treatable symptom. Honest communication and open mindedness on behalf of the patient, partner, their support systems, and the physician are essential tools for treatment. These tools are best obtained through proper education and awareness of physical, emotional, psychosocial, intellectual, and spiritual factors affecting sexuality (Goldstein and Brandon, 2004).

Often patients appear ambivalent, refraining from posing any questions or addressing concerns with their healthcare provider. This attitude necessitates clinician-initiation of the discussion by directly asking patients whether they have any concerns about sexual activity or intimate relationships. If no response is given, the clinician may have to broach the subject indirectly or with more gentle prodding allowing the patient time to increase his comfort level. For these reasons, addressing these issues early and throughout any treatment course is important.

Disability often decreases self-esteem resulting in pessimism (anger), anxiety, and depression. These feelings, alone or in combination, can lead to social withdrawal, loss of libido and anxiety over sexual competence further complicated by difficulty retaining a sense of masculinity or femininity (sexuality). However, intimacy issues are not confined to the patient; the partner may also have some sexual trepidation and decreased desire, particularly if he or she is the patient's primary caregiver (Carter et al., 1995; Lechtenberg, 1995; Terra Nova Films, 1995). Therefore, the dogma for many healthcare professionals is that nursing duties be carried out by non-family members whenever possible (Saunders et al., 1997). This helps to ameliorate potential reassignment of the partner's role from lover to a more parental role. The partner may be worried about the patient's inability to consent to sexual activity. Such fears must be allayed by open communication and counseling, but it is important to discern whether any problems or anxieties existed pre-illness, for they are often exacerbated. When required, counseling must be imparted in a sympathetic and non-judgmental manner. The effected individual and the partner must realize that professionals are available to listen and to address their sexual and reproductive concerns. The clinician must explain the origin of difficulties emotionally, functionally, and physiologically. The health care professional is obligated to provide practical suggestions and prescribe interventions including referrals for specialized sexual therapy and subspecialty medical care.

25.3 Essential anatomic and physiologic sexual and reproductive functions

Male anatomy

The prostate gland is a partly muscular and partly glandular male sex gland whose major function is to secrete a slightly alkaline fluid forming part of the seminal fluid. Seminal vesicles, sac-like glands that lie behind the bladder, also release fluid for transport of sperm. The scrotum holds and protects the testicles. Testicles are two small organs that make sperm and testosterone, a hormone important for both primary and secondary sexual characteristics such as muscle development, voice deepening, and body hair. The epididymis is an elongated canal attached to the posterior aspect of the testes. The epididymis stores, matures, and transports spermatozoa into the vas deferens. The vas deferens also stores and transports sperm. The shaft of the penis contains the urethra that drains the bladder and carries sperm out of the body. The glans is the tip of the penis (Fig. 25.1).

The penis' arterial supply is supplied by the internal pudendal arteries, which become the penile arteries. The cavernosal artery, a branch of the penile artery supplies the lacunar spaces through multiple branches. Blood-filled lacunar spaces are important for erection. Venules, located between the erectile tissue, drain the lacunar spaces. Venous return from the penis occurs by way of the deep and superficial dorsal veins of the penis.

Spermatogenesis

Spermatogenesis takes approximately 70 days from the beginning of differentiation of the spermatocyte to the formation of motile sperm (Heller and Clermont, 1963). Transport into the vas deferens via peristaltic movement and intrinsic sperm motility requires an additional 12–21 days (Rowley, 1970).

Spermatogenesis begins with a pulsatile hypothalamic release of gonadotrophin releasing hormone (GnRH) that induces the release of pituitary luteinizing hormone (LH) and follicle stimulating hormone (FSH). LH stimulates Leydig interstitial cells to synthesize and secrete testosterone, which is the primary androgen that controls the functional activity of all male reproductive tract structures. Adequate levels of testosterone are required for spermatogenesis in seminal vesicles, sperm maturation in the epididymis, and the secretory activity

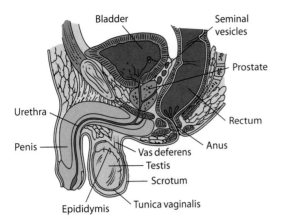

Figure 25.1. Male reproductive tract.

of the prostate and other accessory sex glands (Walsh, 2002). Once spermatogenesis is complete, mature spermatozoa travel through the rete testes and epididymis, where they functionally mature before entering the vas deferens (Walsh, 2002).

Sexual function and erectile physiology

Normal sexual function in men requires sexual desire (libido), erectile, ejaculatory, and orgasmic capacity. Deficits in any of these functions can disrupt normal sexual response as these activities work together to create the hypothalamic messages that traverse the spinal cord at T12–L2 (sympathetic) and S2–S4 (parasympathetic; Rampin, 1997).

In the flaccid state, contraction of the arterial and corporal smooth muscles is mediated by sympathetic alpha-adrenergic receptors. Sexual stimulation results in a decrease in sympathetic input and an increase in parasympathetic activity. Parasympathetic stimulation activates cholinergic receptors of non-adrenergic non-cholinergic (NANC) neurons resulting in the production of nitric oxide (NO), which diffuses into the smooth muscle cells, activates guanylate cyclase, and increases the level of cyclic guanosine monophosphate (GMP) (Rajfer, 1992). Cyclic GMP, in turn, causes an efflux of Ca^{++} from the smooth muscle cells, leading to smooth muscle relaxation. Relaxation of the smooth muscle decreases arterial resistance increasing blood flow to the corpora cavernosa. The

increase in blood volume expands the lacunar spaces resulting in erection. It is the reduction of venous outflow and trapping of blood by fibrous tunicae that maintains the erection (Walsh, 2002).

Sexual intercourse climaxes with ejaculation and the sensory perception of orgasm. Orgasm occurs in conjunction with contraction of smooth muscle of vas deferens, prostate, seminal vesicles, and the buildup of pressure within the proximal urethra. Emission is the propulsion of semen into the posterior urethra by peristaltic contractions of the vas deferens, seminal vesicles, and prostatic smooth muscles. Intermittent relaxation of the sphincter allows semen to enter the bulbous urethra. Ejaculation is a reflex reaction in response to semen entrance into the bulbous urethra (Walsh, 2002).

Detumescence or return of the penis to the flaccid state results when cholinergic receptors are no longer stimulated by parasympathetic input. Increased sympathetic activity results in a decrease in arterial flow, decrease in intracavernosal pressure, and increased venous drainage (Walsh, 2002).

Female anatomy

The female reproductive organs include the vagina, a muscular passage connecting the external genital organs (Fig. 25.2), including the clitoris, to the cervix, or lower part of the uterus. The uterus or womb is a hollow muscular structure. The ovaries are glands that produce hormones and contain tissue sacs where eggs develop (Fig. 25.3). Monthly an egg is released from the ovaries into the fallopian tubes that serve as the conduit between the ovary and the uterus. Fingerlike fimbriae at the opening of the fallopian tubes sweep the egg from the ovary into the fallopian tubes, where fertilization takes place. The fertilized egg then embeds in the uterine wall and fetal growth ensues. If fertilization and implantation do not occur, the menstrual cycle begins again (Townsend, 2001).

Spinal segments T10 to S4 supply the female reproductive organs. Sympathetic efferents from T10 to T11 innervate the ovaries and smooth muscle of the fallopian tubes and uterus, while parasympathetics (S2 to S4) supply the fallopian tubes and vagina.

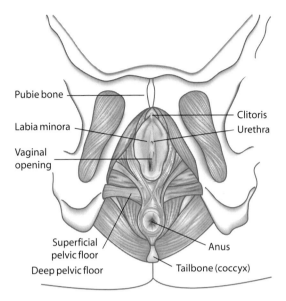

Figure 25.2. External Female Genitalia.

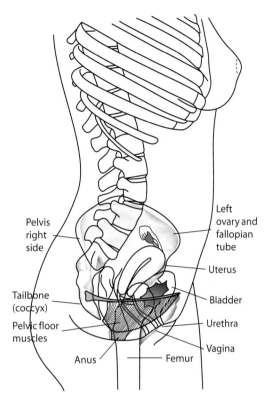

Figure 25.3. Female reproductive system.

Afferent information from the cervix and tubal region is transmitted to T11 to T12 segments through the pelvic nerves (Munarriz, 2002).

Female sexual responses require transmission of somatic, afferent, parasympathetic, and sympathetic signals (Whipple, 1991). Physiologic arousal can be initiated by descending psychic influences, or by tactile stimulation of the clitoris, innervated by afferent fibers of the pudendal nerve (S2–S4). Parasympathetic efferents (S2–S4, responsible for reflex clitoral erection) are activated by descending influences and by afferent sacral synapses. Vaginal lubrication resulting from Bartholin's gland secretions and transudation of fluid across the vaginal wall is parasympathetically mediated (Sipski, 1999).

25.4 Neurologic conditions and sexuality

Myelopathy: SCI and MS

Male sexual function

Loss of one or all three types of erection: psychogenic, reflexogenic, and nocturnal can occur in patients with SCI as a result of trauma (Volume II, Chapter 37) or demyelination (Volume II, Chapter 38). During psychogenic erection, arousal is initiated by audiovisual stimuli or stored fantasy producing sympathetic messages that traverse the spinal cord at T12–L2 and parasympathetic messages at S2–S4. Many patients with sacral SCI retain psychogenic erectile ability even though reflexogenic erection is lost. Psychogenic erections are found more frequently in patients with lower motoneuron lesions below T12 and not in patients with lesions above T9 (Bors and Comarr, 1960; Chapelle, 1980; Master, 2001). Thoracic and cervical cord injuries impair psychogenic erections but do not ablate local spinal reflex pathways involved in erection and ejaculation. Erection and ejaculation are possible. However, decreased rigidity can make penetration difficult or impossible.

In normal males, reflexogenic erection via direct stimulation produces an increase in activity along the ascending tract resulting in sensory perception and stimulation of the cavernous nerves to produce an erection. Reflexogenic erection can be preserved in patients with upper SCI (Walsh, 2002). Many cervical and thoracic cord injured patients have erections after genital stimulation of any kind, including urethral catheterization. Erections are often not sustained adequately for penetration. Impaired ejaculation is common.

Nocturnal erectile activity is often preserved following SCI. However, the level of injury can affect the quality and duration of erection as well as detumescence (Suh, 2003). Ejaculation is a reflex reaction in response to semen entrance into the bulbous urethra. Lesion activity between T12 and L2 impairs or prevents ejaculation. Lumbo-sacral cord lesions can cause erectile dysfunction (ED) by interrupting parasympathetic and somatic pathways, although ejaculation may be preserved (Stewart, 1993). In SCI, the degree of dysfunction is proportional to the severity of injury. After SCI, for patients with stable relationships, the frequency of sexual activity approaches the individual's pre-injury level, but with only 9% reporting intercourse.

Lesions caused by MS may cause impotence or inability to effectively ejaculate. Ninety-one percent of men with MS report a "change" in sexuality; 64% unsatisfactory sexual function, and 47% ED. Sexual libido and orgasmic sensation are commonly altered (Lundberg, 1981). Similar to SCI, the degree of dysfunction depends on the severity and location of the lesion or injury. Similar to SCI from trauma, lower motor lesions prevent vasocongestion, causing weak, or absent reflexive erections, whereas, upper motor neuron lesions in the brainstem and above the lumbar section interfere with psychogenic erections (Dewis and Thornton, 1989). ED is almost always associated with neurogenic bladder dysfunction and pyramidal involvement (DasGupta and Fowler, 2002). Lesions of the lateral horn or connecting pathways in the dorso-lumbar area of the spinal cord, where sympathetic information controlling ejaculation is integrated, can lead to reduced sexual

functioning (DasGupta and Fowler, 2002). MS-related physical changes that indirectly affect sexual activity include fatigue, muscle spasms, muscle weakness, bladder and bowel problems, and distorted body image.

Sexual activity for men with SCI or MS is possible. Again, it is the health care professional's obligation to provide practical suggestions and interventions in a compassionate manner. The chief complaint of men with SCI and MS is ED. Therefore, treatment of male sexual dysfunction has focused on the treatment of ED. For those males who are able to attain reflex erections but not maintain them, the use of a silicon or rubber ring placed at the base of the penis can help maintain an erection. These rings may be used for up to, but no longer than, 30 min due to the risk of ischemia and subsequent complications. If the patient is unable to have an erection, a vacuum suction device may produce an erection which can be maintained using a silicon or rubber ring, as described. Self-administered injections of prostaglandin E1 into the penis can also be used to produce an erection. However, complications may occur, including priapism. Sildenafil citrate (Viagra) has proven effective in cases of both lower and upper motor neuron injury (Derry, 2002). Other male sexual dysfunctions found in SCI and MS patients, such as inorgasmia, impaired libido, and premature ejaculation, have not been well studied (Alexander and Sipski, 1993).

In addition to the inability to ejaculate, males with SCI experience decreases in the quantity and quality of sperm. This decline occurs in the first few weeks post-injury (Sipski and Alexander, 1992). Sperm have a decreased lifespan which may account for decreases in sperm quantity. Morphology can be affected. Malformed sperm cells have a hard time penetrating the egg to achieve fertilization.

Several studies exist examining why sperm quality is poor following SCI. However, no strong leads exist at this time. It is known, however, that an increase in frequency of ejaculation improves sperm quality (Alexander and Sipski, 1993). Secondary effects of SCI that can negatively affect sperm quality include increased scrotal temperature from autonomic dysregulation and frequent urinary tract infections associated with catheterization and medications that affect sperm quantity and/or quality.

Considering the information above, it stands to reason that fertility can be a problem for men with SCI and MS and their partners. For men with little or low-quality sperm, advanced assisted reproductive techniques include intracytoplasmic sperm injection (ICSI) in which a single sperm is injected directly into the cytoplasm of the egg in conjunction with *in vitro* fertilization (IVF). A low-tech approach available for home use and widely used in Europe is electrovibration applied directly to the penis. However, there is a risk of autonomic dysreflexia makes it imperative that patients learn correct electro-vibration techniques in a clinical setting.

Female sexual function

Surveys indicate that up to 76% of women with spinal injury are sexually active, although declines in overall sexual activity do occur. Pre-injury 64% reported sexual intercourse versus 48% post-injury (Sipski, 1995a). Changes in choices of sexual partners are also reported; after injury women more often develop relationships with disabled people and with hospital personnel. Impaired sexual function stems from decreased lubrication, impaired genital sensation, and complications such as urinary infections and autonomic hyper-reflexia. However, SCI women, even those with complete lesions, are able to experience orgasm. Often more time is required, and orgasm is often triggered by stimulation of other arousable body parts (breasts, ear lobes, or lips; Sipski, 1995a).

Women with MS report decreased libido, orgasmic difficulty, severe external dysesthesias, and lack of vaginal lubrication (Lundberg, 1981). The majority (72%) report a change in sexual function, and 39% an unsatisfactory sex life (Lundberg, 1981). Similar to their male counterparts, women with MS experience sexual impairment directly related to the location and severity of lesions. Spinal cord lesions interfere with the transmission of arousal signals. Lower motor neurons alter vasocongestion leading to reduced clitoral swelling and lubrication. Symptoms often develop abruptly, and are often associated with

bowel and bladder dysfunction. Women with complete SCI and upper motor neuron injuries affecting the sacral spinal segments or MS lesions in these areas will maintain the capacity for reflex lubrication while losing the capacity for psychogenic lubrication (Sipski, 1995b). Alternative stimulation techniques and vaginal lubricants are recommended.

Hypersensitivity or dysesthetic pain can be difficult to treat. Results using pharmacologic agents; anticonvulsants and topical anesthetics are disappointing. Anecdotal reports suggest that tricyclic antidepressants may ameliorate some of these symptoms. Some reports also suggest that venlafaxine HCl (effexor), an antidepressant affecting both serotonin and norepinephrine levels, reduce pain associated with dysparunea (Grothe et al., 2004).

Decreased lubrication can be alleviated by the application of water-soluble lubricating jelly (not Vaseline®). Local synapses in sacral and lumbar cord lead to the orgasm reflex, with rhythmic involuntary contraction of uterine and perineal musculature, mediated by pelvic (branch of the hypogastric, L2–L4) and pudendal nerves. Not only the genital region is involved in sexual response, but virtually the entire body as women experience myotonia and venous vasocongestion throughout the trunk, particularly in the breasts and chest wall (Masters and Johnson, 1966).

Menstrual cycle, fertility, and pregnancy in SCI

For premenopausal women with acute SCI, the stress of injury can interrupt the menstrual cycle for 1 year or more (Durkan, 1968; Jefferey, 1997). Fluctuations in estrogen and progesterone levels related to ovulation can affect electrolyte balance and may influence symptoms, such as tone, bladder, and bowel function in SCI. Menstruation then begins again, and fertility returns. SCI does not contraindicate pregnancy. However, the risk of certain SCI-related problems, such as urinary tract infections and pressure ulcers, may increase with pregnancy.

Pregnant women with SCI are susceptible to complications of pregnancy, such as fluid retention, skin breakdown, phlebitis, and constipation. As the uterus expands, the mechanical effects can compromise breathing in tetraplegic women with chest wall weakness, and can aggravate neurogenic bladder symptoms. Although uterine contractions occur, abdominal muscle weakness can limit the woman's ability to "push" during late labor. Autonomic hyperreflexia can be associated with uterine contraction in women with high thoracic or cervical spinal disease. This is a potentially life threatening complication which requires the presence of an anesthesiologist to control sudden surges in blood pressure. In addition, a woman with SCI may not sense the usual indicators of labor, which raise the possibility of an unattended preterm delivery. This suggests that surveillance be maintained as the pregnancy advances, perhaps by hospitalization or by the use of a home uterine contraction monitor. Surgical intervention is frequently required (McCluer, 1991). Post-partum complications include hemodynamic instability and continued autonomic hyperactivity (provoked by uterine contraction and surgical wounds).

Menstrual cycle, fertility, and pregnancy in MS
Hormonal fluctuations of the menstrual cycle can change neurologic symptoms. A rise in core temperature following ovulation may produce an increase in MS symptoms (similar to the "hot bath" test). Increases in neuropathic pain, spasticity, and fatigue have also been reported (Jefferey, 1997).

Similar to those with SCI, pregnant women with MS need close monitoring of the disease and of fetal well-being. More frequent prenatal visits are often needed. There is no established treatment that alters the course of MS however; medications commonly used in the treatment of MS can be used during pregnancy including steroids and anti-inflammatory drugs.

Delivery of the baby may be more difficult in women with MS. While labor itself is not affected, the muscles and nerves needed for pushing can be affected. Women in labor with MS may not have pelvic sensation, and may not feel pain with contractions. This may also make it difficult for them to tell when labor begins, thus making forceps and vacuum-assisted deliveries more likely.

During pregnancy, the MS relapse rate decreases slightly in the first trimester and drops further in the second and third (Jefferey, 1997). Though serum estrogen concentrations fluctuate similarly, no causal relationship has yet been established. Relapse rates after pregnancy increase two- to fourfold, however, no long-term effects on the course of MS have been established (Weinschenker, 1982).

Inappropriate sexual thoughts or behavior have been reported in patients with MS. However, instances are rare and usually present on a background of persistent cognitive impairment or psychiatric dysfunction (Joffe, 1987).

Other central nervous system lesions: TBI and stroke

TBI can result in a variety of specific injuries, each altering a different aspect of the patient's neurologic functioning or behavior (Volume II, Chapter 33). The behavioral consequences of brain damage are the primary source of sexual dysfunction in these patients. Damage to basal frontal or limbic structures, for example, can lead to hypersexuality and disinhibited or inappropriate sexual behavior (Blumer and Benson, 1975; Miller, 1986).

Focal cortical contusions can be primary or secondary to injury, with such frontal or temporal injuries causing inattention, emotional blunting, and a disinterest beyond immediate physical needs (Seliger, 1997). Injury to frontal lobes often results in a neglect of and disregard for social mores leading to emotional or sexual inappropriateness. Brain injuries can also cause distractibility, which is damaging to romantic atmosphere. Individual counseling is important; however, equally as important is advising the patient to focus on the activity. However, patients with profound intellectual impairment may not be able to retain information presented during counseling or grasp the concept of sexual inappropriateness. In these instances, counseling directed at partners, friends, and family is often more effective.

Behavioral consequences of brain injury from stroke (Volume II, Chapter 36) are often similar to TBI, dependent on the location of injury. Damage to basal frontal or limbic structures may cause hyper-sexuality or inappropriate behavior. A significant decline in libido after stroke in both sexes has been reported (Monga, 1986). During the post-stroke period, a decrease in men's ability to achieve erection and ejaculate, and women's ability to have vaginal lubrication and orgasm has been reported. Patient's concerns over weakness, spasticity, and the effect of sexual activity on blood pressure or even causing another stroke may discourage some from sexual encounters. These fears can best be allayed with patient education and reassurance.

Geriatrics

Male sexuality and aging

In addition to pathologies described, accompaniments to normal aging, such as vascular disease or hypertension, can contribute to male sexual dysfunction in the geriatric population. As in SCI and MS, the chief sexual complaint of older men is ED. With increased age, males require increased time, and stimulation to achieve an erection, decreased sensation of impending ejaculation, and decreased ejaculatory volume, followed by rapid detumescence after intercourse (Barclay, 1997).

ED in older men is primarily caused by vascular or neurologic factors (Broderick, 1989). Vascular disease results in ED by two mechanisms, arterial insufficiency and venous leakage. Obstruction from atherosclerotic arterial occlusive disease decreases the perfusion pressure and arterial flow to the lacunar spaces. Additionally, relative penile hypoxia can result in replacement of trabecular smooth muscle with connective tissue resulting in impaired cavernosal expandability. Veno-occlusive dysfunction or venous leakage is characterized by excessive outflow through the subtunical venules, which prevents the development of high pressure within the corpora cavernosa. Risk factors for vascular ED include smoking, hyperlipidemia, hypertension, and diabetes mellitus.

Neurologic disease is the second most common cause of ED in older men. Diabetes mellitus, stroke, and Parkinson's disease can cause autonomic dysfunction that results in impaired vasodilation and erectile failure. Myocardial infarctions and other cardiac conditions, chronic obstructed pulmonary disease, peripheral neuropathy, and a variety of other systemic conditions normally associated with aging, along with the fatigue they cause, can generate physical and psychologic concerns about sexual encounters that can be allayed by a knowledgeable physician. In contrast to ED, libido varies to a modest degree with advancing age. In an ambulatory geriatric population, 53% reported intact libido (Mulligan, 2003).

Female sexuality and aging

Hormonal changes in post-menopausal females can lead to decreased libido, anorgasmia, or dyspareunia (Morley and Kaiser, 1989). High levels of depression have been reported in the female geriatric population. It is not known whether depression is a primary cause or secondary consequence of decreased libido, however, psychotherapy has been shown to be effective. Antidepressants may also be prescribed. Physicians should work with their patients to determine appropriate medications and dosages that support sexual functioning. Dyspareunia can occur with or without depression. Diminished estrogen can result in vaginal thinning and decreased lubrication. Although estrogen replacement therapy can result in maturation of the vaginal epithelium, the optimal form of administration, dosage regimen for improving symptoms and possible risks to the geriatric population have not been well studied.

25.5 Medications and sexual dysfunction

Medications can impair sexual functioning. Estimates show that up to 25% of male medical outpatients have drug-induced ED. Antihypertensives can interfere neurogenically, as in centrally acting sympatholytics, or vascularly, such as angiotensin converting enzyme inhibitors and calcium channel blockers (Prisant, 1994). Diuretics can cause increased zinc excretion leading to decreased testosterone levels (Kinlaw, 1983). Dopamine has been found to exert a stimulatory effect on sexual behavior, while serotonin has an inhibitory effect (Deamer and Thompson, 1991). Thus, selective serotonin re-uptake inhibitor antidepressants may cause impotence and anorgasmia (Rakel, 2004; Saunders, 1997), and other serotonergic antidepressants can cause priapism (Smith and Levitte, 1993; Rand, 1998). Fluoxetine can cause anorgasmia or delayed orgasm (Walker, 1993), while tricyclic antidepressants may cause erectile difficulties (Seliger, 1997). Alpha-adrenergic blockers may interfere with sexual arousal and perfor-mance. Major tranquilizers cause sexual dysfunction, particularly decreased libido (Burks, 1997). Other psychotropic and centrally active drugs can impair sexual function through their sedative actions. These include phenothiazines, butyrophenones, sedatives, and anxiolytics. The anticholinergic and sympatholytic effects of psychoactive drugs can also impair sexual function (Barclay, 1997).

25.6 Secondary complications of neurologic illness and their treatment

In addition to primary effects of neurologic dysfunction and medication side effects, secondary complications of neurologic illness can also impede a patient's sexual activity. Several low-tech options are available. For example, decreasing fluid intake a few hours before intimacy and removing a catheter or taping it to the thigh can minimize the effects of bowel or bladder dysfunction. If a patient is easily fatigued, he could plan ahead for sex by conserving energy or napping. Early morning sex or caffeinated drinks could also help (Burks, 1997). Pain syndromes or spasticity can be helped by medication. Increased genital sensitivity can be treated with topical anesthetics or by molding a bag of frozen peas over the genital area (Burks, 1997). Patients with decreased genital sensitivity should explore other sensual areas, enhance sexual atmosphere, or use shared fantasy and masturbation. Emphasis must be transferred from sex to sexuality and the panorama of enjoyable opportunities it makes possible. For each of these complications, attempting new sexual positions to discover which are the most

comfortable and pleasurable can enhance intimate encounters. Though many patients complain that the time and effort involved in such preparations removes any mystique and spontaneity, patients should instead look upon these measures as opportunities for foreplay (Saunders, 1997).

REFERENCES

Alexander, C.J. and Sipski, M.L. (1993). *Sexuality Reborn: Sexuality Following Spinal Cord Injury*, Videotape. Kessler Institute for Rehabilitation, West Orange, NJ.

Barclay, L. (1997). The geriatric population. In: *Sexual and Reproductive Neurorehabilitation* (ed. Aisen, M.), Humana Press, Totowa, NJ, pp. 219–232.

Blumer, D. and Benson, D.F. (1975). Personality changes with frontal and temporal lobe lesions. In: *Psychiatric Aspects of Neurological Disease* (eds Blumer, D. and Benson, D.F.), Grune and Stratton, New York, pp. 151–170.

Bors, E. and Comarr, A.E. (1960). Neurological disturbances of sexual function with special reference to 529 patients with spinal cord injury. *Urol Surv*, **110**, 191–221.

Broderick, J.P. (1989). Incidence rates in the eighties: the end of the decline in stroke? *Stroke*, **20**, 577.

Burks, J. (1997). Sexual dysfunction in multiple sclerosis. In: *Sexual and Reproductive Neurorehabilitation* (ed. Aisen, M.), Humana Press, Totowa, NJ, pp. 169–196.

Carter, J.M., Flaaten, L. and Hero, C. (1995). *Sex after Stroke*. American Heart Association, Dallas, TX.

Chapelle, P.A. (1980). Penile erection following complete spinal cord injury in man. *Br J Urol*, **52**, 216–219.

Comfort, A. and Dial, L.K. (1991). Sexuality and aging. An overview. *Clin Geriatr Med*, **7**, 1–7.

DasGupta, R. and Fowler, C.J. (2002). Sexual and urological dysfunction in multiple sclerosis: better understanding and improved therapies. *Curr Opin Neurol*, **15**, 271–278.

Deamer, R.I. and Thompson, J.F. (1991). The role of medications in geriatric sexual function. *Clin Geriatr Med*, **7**, 95–111.

Derry, F. (2002). Efficacy and safety of sildenafil citrate (Viagra) in men with *in* and spinal cord injury: a review. *Urology*, **60**, 49–57.

Dewis, M.E. and Thornton, N.G. (1989). Sexual dysfunction in multiple sclerosis. *J Neurosci Nurs*, **21**, 175–179.

Durkan, J.P. (1968). Menstruation after high spinal cord transection. *Am J Obstet Gynecol*, **100**, 521–524.

Earle, S. (2001). Disability, facilitated sex and the role of the nurse. *J Adv Nurs*, **3**, 433–440.

Goldstein, A. and Brandon, M. (2004). *Reclaiming Desire: 4 Keys to Finding Your Lost Libido*, Rodale Press, Emmaus, PA.

Grothe, D.R., Scheckner, B. and Albano, D. (2004). Treatment of pain syndromes with venlafaxine. *Pharmacotherapy*, **5**, 621–629.

Heller, C.G. and Clermont, Y. (1963). Spermatogenesis in man: an estimate of its duration. *Science*, **140**, 184–186.

Jefferey, D. (1997). The menstrual cycle in chronic neurologic disease. The role of the menstrual cycle in chronic disorders of the nervous system. In: *Sexual and Reproductive Neurorehabilitation* (ed. Aisen, M.), Humana Press, Totowa, NJ, pp. 65–72.

Joffe, R.T. (1987). Personal and family history of affective disorder and multiple sclerosis. *J Affect Disord*, **12**, 63–65.

Kinlaw, W.B. (1983). Abnormal zinc metabolism in type II diabetes mellitus. *Am J Med*, **75**, 273–277.

Lechtenberg, R. (1995). *Multiple Sclerosis Fact Book*, F.A. Davis Company, Philadelphia, PA.

Lundberg, P.O. (1981). Sexual dysfunction in female patients with multiple sclerosis. *Int Rehabil Med*, **3**, 32–34.

Master, V.A. (2001). Ejaculatory physiology and dysfunction. *Urol Clin North Am*, **28**, 363–375.

Masters, W. and Johnson, V. (1966). *Human Sexual Response*, Little, Brown and Co., Boston.

McCluer, S. (1991). Reproductive aspects of spinal cord injury in females. In: *Sexual Rehabilitation of the Spinal-Cord-Injured Patient* (ed. Leyson, J.F.J.), Humana Press, NJ, pp. 181–196.

Miller, B.L. (1986). Hypersexuality or altered sexual preference following brain injury. *J Neurol Neurosur Psy*, **49**, 867–873.

Monga, T. (1986). Sexual dysfunction in stroke patients. *Arch Phys Med Rehabil*, **67**, 19–22.

Morley, J.E. and Kaiser, F.E. (1989). Sexual function with advancing age. *Med Clin North Am*, **73**, 1483–1495.

Mulligan, T. (2003). Disorders of male sexual function. *Clin Geriatr Med*, **19**, 473–481.

Munarriz, M. (2002). Biology of female sexual function. *Urol Clin North Am*, **29**, 685–693.

Prisant, L.M. (1994). Sexual dysfunction with anti-hypertensive drugs. *Arch Intern Med*, **154**, 730–736.

Rajfer, J. (1992). Nitric oxide as a mediator of relaxation of the corpus cavernosum in response to nonadrenergic, noncholinergic neurotransmission. *New Engl J Med*, **326**, 90–94.

Rakel, R.E. (2004). *Textbook of Family Practice*, 6th edn, W.B. Saunders Company, Philadelphia, PA.

Rampin, O. (1997). Spinal control of penile erection. *World J Urol*, **15**, 2–13.

Rand, E.H. (1998). Priapism in a patient taking sertaline. *J Clin Psychiat*, **59**, 538.

Rowley, M.J. (1970). Duration of transit of spermatozoa through the human male ductular system. *Fertil Steril*, **21**, 390–396.

Saunders, A. (1997). Principles of sexuality counseling. In: *Sexual and Reproductive Neurorehabilitation* (ed. Aisen, M.), Humana Press, Totowa, NJ, pp. 73–92.

Seliger, G. (1997). Traumatic brain injury. In: *Sexual and Reproductive Neurorehabilitation* (ed. Aisen, M.), Humana Press, Totowa, NJ, pp. 207–218.

Singer, C. (1995). Sexual dysfunction. *Handbook of Autonomic Nervous System Dysfunction* (ed. Korczyn, A.), Marcel Dekker, New York, pp. 381–391.

Sipski, M.L. (1995a). Physiological parameters associated with psychogenic sexual arousal in women with complete spinal cord injuries. *Arch Phys Med Rehabil*, **76**, 811–818.

Sipski, M.L. (1995b). Orgasm in women with spinal cord injuries: a laboratory-based assessment. *Arch Phys Med Rehabil*, **76**, 1097–1102.

Sipski, M.L. (1999). Sexual response in women with spinal cord injuries: implications for our understanding of the abled-bodied. *J Sex Marital Therap*, **25**, 11–22.

Sipski, M.L. and Alexander, C.J. (1992). Sexual function and dysfunction after spinal cord injury. In: *Physical Medicine and Rehabilitation Clinics of North America*, W. B. Saunders Company, Philadelphia, pp. 811–828.

Smith, D.M. and Levitte, S.S. (1993). Association of fluoxetine and return of potency in three elderly men. *J Clin Psych*, **54**, 317–319.

Stewart, J.D. (1993). Autonomic regulation of sexual function. In: *Clinical Autonomic Disorders* (ed. Low, P.), Little, Brown and Co, Boston, pp. 117–123.

Suh, D.D. (2003). Nocturnal penile tumescence and effects of complete spinal cord injury: possible physiologic mechanisms. *Urology*, **61**, 184–189.

Terra Nova Films. (1995). *A Thousand Tomorrows*, Terra Nova Films, Chicago, IL.

Townsend. (2001). *Sabiston Textbook of Surgery*, W.B. Saunders Company, Philadelphia.

Walker, P.W., Cole, J.O., Gardner, E.A., Hughes, A.R. Johnston, J.A., Batey, S.R., Lineberry, C.G. (1993). Improvement in fluoxetine-associated sexual dysfunction in patients switched to Bupropion. *J Clin Psychiatry*, **54**, 459–465.

Walsh. (2002). *Campbell's Urolog*, 8th edn, Elsevier.

Weinschenker, B.G. (1982). Decreased levels of helper T cells. A possible cause of immunodeficiency in pregnancy. *New Engl J Med*, **307**, 307–352.

Whipple, B. (1991). Female sexuality. In: *Sexual Rehabilitation of the Spinal Cord Injured Patient* (ed. Leyson, J.F.J.), Humana Press, New Jersey, pp. 19–38.

Cognitive neurorehabilitation

CONTENTS

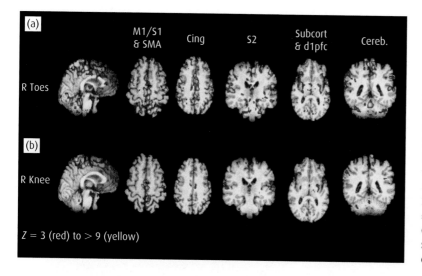

Plate 1 (figure 3.1). Right ankle dorsiflexion and right quadriceps contraction during functional magnetic resonance imaging (fMRI) of a subject with a spinal card injury (SCI) at the conus. R Toes: right toes; R Knee: right knee; SMA: supplementary motor area; Cing: cingulate motor cortex; Subcort: subcortical nodes; Cereb: cerebelum.

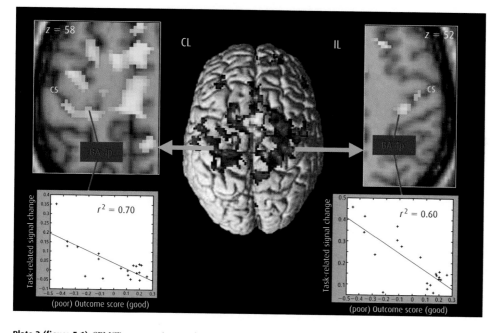

Plate 2 (figure 5.1). SPM{Z} representing voxels in which there is a negative (linear) correlation between task-related BOLD signal and outcome score in a group of 20 chronic stroke patients. Results are surface rendered onto a canonical brain shown from above (left hemisphere on the left). The panels represent the same result displayed on axial slices through a canonical T1-weighted image. The plots represent task-related signal change versus outcome score for the peak voxel in BA 4p contralesional (CL) on the left and ipsilesional (IL) on the right. Each "+" represents one patient. All voxels are significant at $P < 0.05$, corrected for multiple comparisons across whole brain. cs: central sulcus.

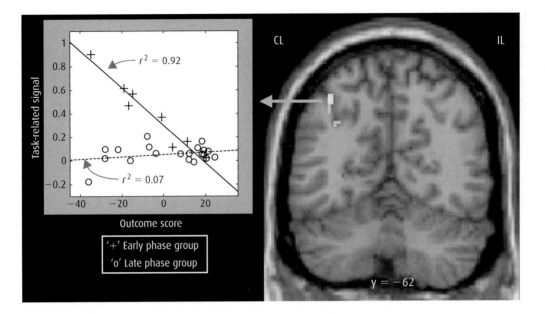

Plate 3 (figure 5.2). A plot of task-related signal change in posterior contralesional (CL) intraparietal sulcus versus outcome/recovery score for a group of early phase patients (10–14 days post stroke) and a group of late phase stroke patients (over 3 months post stroke). The peak voxel in intraparietal sulcus is shown on canonical coronal T_1-weighted brain slice ($P < 0.05$, corrected for multiple comparisons across whole brain).

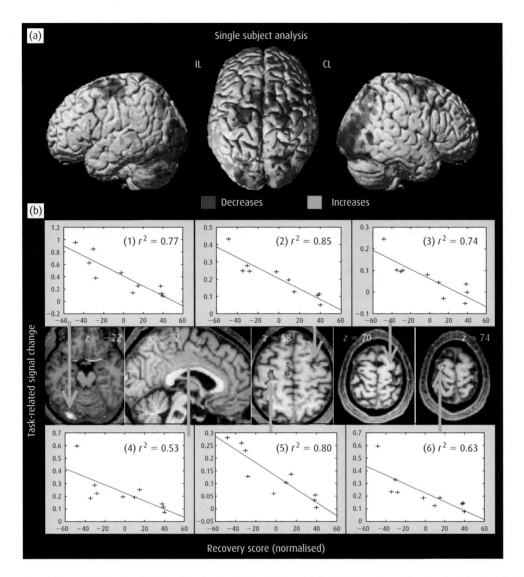

Plate 4 (figure 5.3). Results of single subject longitudinal analysis examining for linear changes in task-related brain activations over sessions as a function of recovery. The patient suffered from a left sided pontine infarct resulting in right hemiparesis. (a) Results are surface rendered onto a canonical brain; red areas represent recovery-related decreases in task-related activation across sessions, and green areas represent the equivalent recovery related increases. All voxels are significant at $P < 0.001$ (uncorrected for multiple comparisons) for display purposes. The brain is shown (from left to right) from the left ipsilesional (IL) side, from above (left hemisphere on the left), and from the right contralesional (CL). (b) Results are displayed on patients own normalised T_1-weighted anatomical images (voxels significant at $P < 0.05$, corrected for multiple comparisons across the whole brain), with corresponding plots of size of effect against overall recovery score (normalised), for selected brain regions. Coordinates of peak voxel in each region are followed by the correlation coefficient and the associated P value: (1) ipsilesional cerebellum ($x = -26, y = -84, z = -22$) ($r^2 = 0.77, P < 0.01$), (2) contralesional (CL) dorsolateral Premotor cortex (PMd) ($x = 38, y = 0, z = 58$) ($r^2 = 0.85, P < 0.01$), (3) CL M1 ($x = 28, y = -14, z = 70$) ($r^2 = 0.74, P < 0.01$), (4) ipsilesional SMA ($x = -2, y = -2, z = 60$) ($r^2 = 0.53, P = 0.02$), (5) ipsilesional M1 ($x = -30, y = -14, z = 58$) ($r^2 = 0.80, P < 0.01$), (6) contralesional (CL) PMd ($x = -18, y = -10, z = 74$) ($r^2 = 0.63, P = 0.01$).

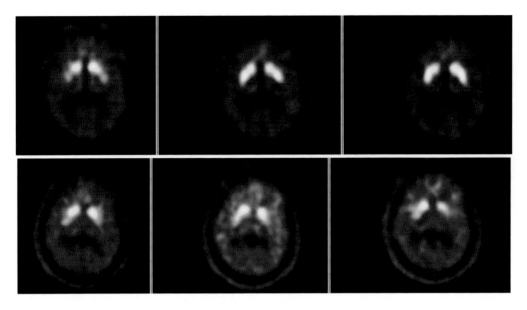

Plate 5 (figure 6.1). Flurodapo–Position emission tomography FD–PET studies in a representative patient receiving bilateral transplantation with 4 donors per side (top panels) and a patient receiving a sham procedure (lower panels). Scans were obtained at baseline (left panels), 1 year (middle panels) and 2 years (right panels). Note the progressive increase in striatal FD uptake in the transplanted patient in comparison to the progressive loss of striatal FD uptake consistent with continued disease progression in the placebo treated patient. Olanow et al. (2003).

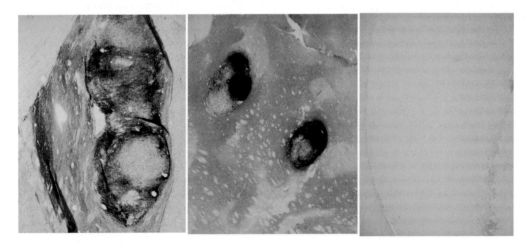

Plate 6 (figure 6.2). Tyrosine hydroxylase (TH)-immunostaining of striatum in patients receiving treatment with bilateral grafts using four donors per side (left panel), one donor per side (middle panel), and a sham placebo procedure (right panel). Note healthy appearing graft deposits and extensive striatal TH innervation with both four and one donors per side. Note also that grafts in the four donor group are larger and have a cylindric appearance whereas in the one donor group they are smaller, more concentric, and more densely packed. Olanow et al. (2003).

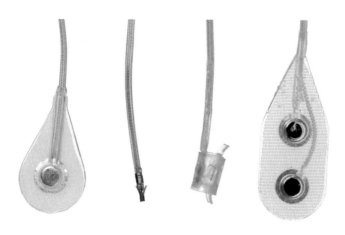

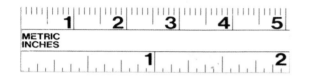

Plate 7 (figure 9.1). Implantable electrodes used in FES applications. The following electrodes are pictured (from left to right): monopolar epimysial, intramuscular, nerve cuff, and bipolar epimysial electrodes.

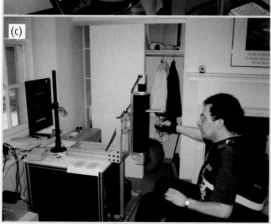

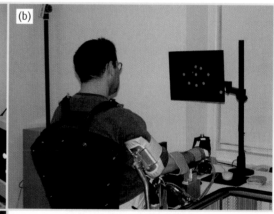

Plate 8 (figure 12.1). Rehabilitation robot modules during clinical trials at the Burke Rehabilitation Hospital (White Plains, NY). (a) and (b) show the shoulder and elbow robot (MIT-MANUS) and the wrist robot, and (c) the anti-gravity spatial module.

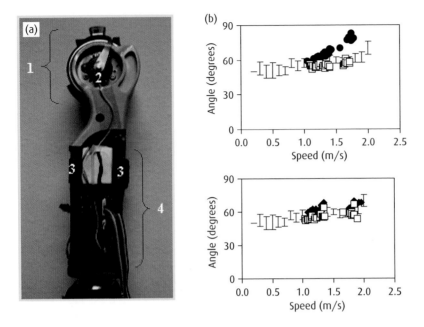

Plate 9 (figure 12.4). An external knee prosthesis for trans-femoral amputees. The damping of the knee joint is modulated to control the movement of the prosthesis throughout each walking cycle. (a) The prosthesis shown on the left comprises magnetorheological (MR) brake (1), potentiometer angle sensor (2), force sensors (3), and battery and electronic board (4). (b) The right plots show the maximum flexion angle during the swing phase versus walking speed. The patient-adaptive knee affords a greater symmetry between affected and unaffected sides.

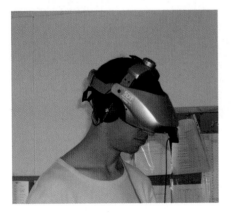

Plate 10 (figure 13.2). Fifth Dimension Technologies (www.5dt.com) Head mounted display (HMD).

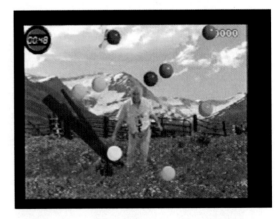

Plate 11 (figure 13.3). VividGroup's Gesture Xtreme-virtual reality (GX-VR) system (www.vividgroup.com) video-capture projection VR system.

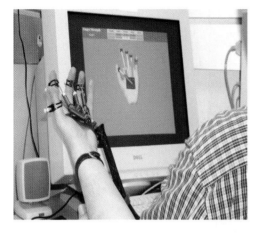

Plate 12 (figure 13.4). Rutgers Master II force-feedback glove.

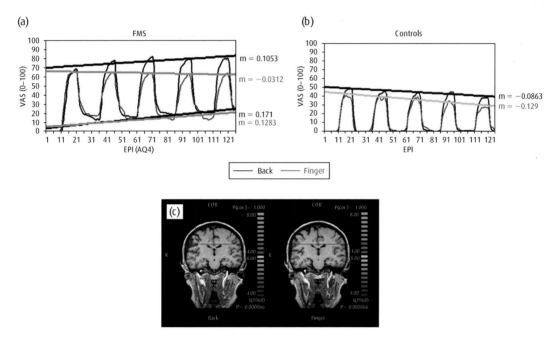

Plate 13 (figure 15.1). The top left panel (a) shows the pain ratings (visual analogue scale (VAS) 0–100) of the fibromyalgia patients to the stimulation of the back (black) or the finger (red). The patients were stimulated in blocks of 20 s with 20-s rest intervals. The top right (b) panel shows the same ratings for the healthy controls. The straight lines show the slope of the ratings. A negative slope indicates a reduction in pain rating and thus habituation and a positive slope indicates sensitization and increased pain ratings. The numbers to the right give the slope. The bottom panel (c) shows the difference in activation between the fibromyalgia patients (FMS) and the healthy controls related to the secondary somatosensory cortex. Note that the FMS patients show more activation both during the back and finger stimulation.

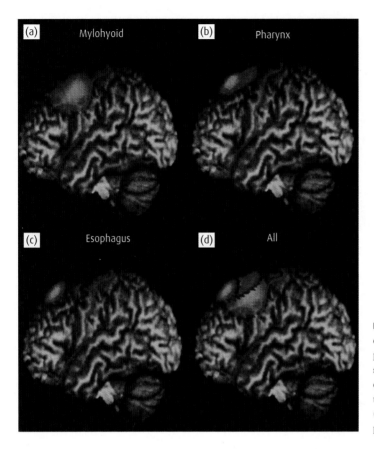

Plate 14 (figure 23.4). Location of regions of cortical control for (a) mylohyoid, (b) pharyngeal, (c) esophageal, and (d) all three states of swallowing in the left hemispheres of normal subjects, as determined by transcranial magnetic stimulation (TMS) (Hamdy et al., 1996, reprinted with permission).

(a)

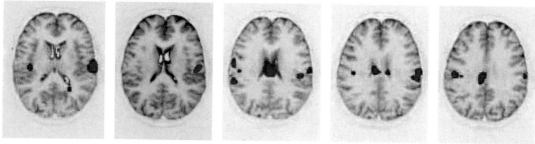

17　　　18　　　19　　　20　　　21

(b)

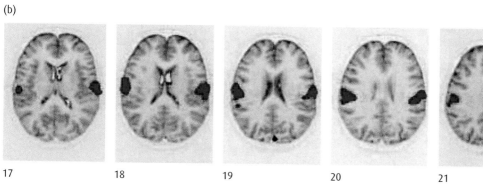

17　　　18　　　19　　　20　　　21

Plate 15 (figure 23.5). Patterns of activation (a) before and (b) after electrical stimulation in normal swallowers. Activation increased bilaterally (Fraser et al., 2002, reprinted with permission).

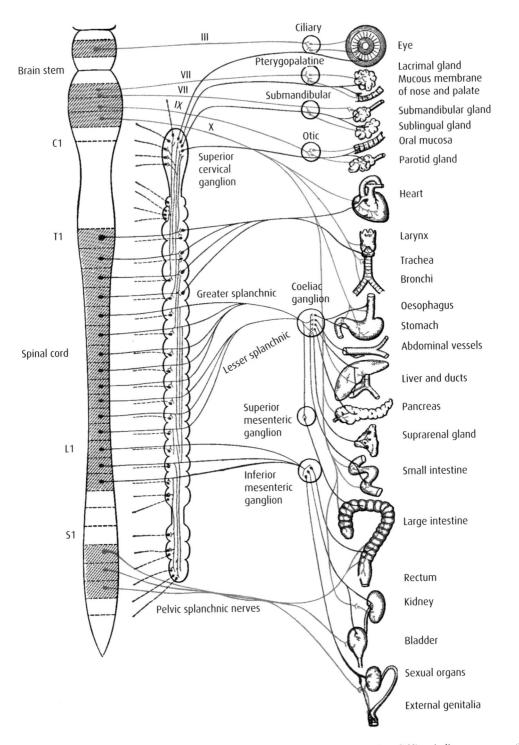

Plate 16 (figure 24.1). The efferent pathways of the automatic nervous system (ANS). The solid lines indicate parasympathetic and sympathetic pathways and the interrupted lines indicate postganglionic rami to the cranial and spinal nerves (after Meyer and Gottlieb).

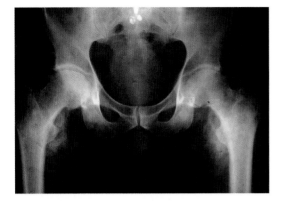

Plate 17 (figure 37.3). Heterotopic ossification surrounding hip joints.

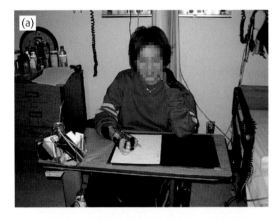

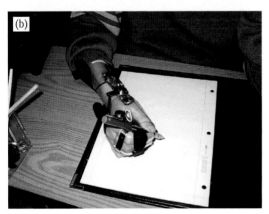

Plate 18 (figure 37.4). (a) Patient with C6 tetraplegia using tenodesis splint for writing and (b) tenodesis splint used to grip pen.

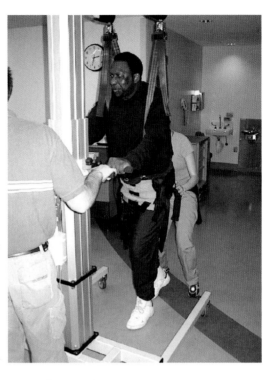

Plate 19 (figure 37.5). Using body weight support system overground.

26

Rehabilitation for aphasia

Stefano F. Cappa

Department of Neuroscience, Vita-Salute University and San Raffaele Scientific Institute, Milano, Italy

Disorders of language, that is, of the ability to express mental contents using words and sentences, and to understand others' mental contents expressed in language, are a frequent consequence of acquired and developmental brain damage and dysfunction. The most common cause of acquired language disorders in adults (aphasia) is cerebrovascular disease, followed by traumatic brain injury (TBI) and tumours. Language disorders are also a prominent clinical feature of several other neurological diseases, such as the dementias. The present overview of aphasia rehabilitation deals only with acquired aphasia due to focal brain damage in adults. However, the impact of language disorders in neurology is more extensive, and the scope of language rehabilitation wider than presented here. The rehabilitation of speech disorders due to motor dysfunction is also not discussed here; the distinction from aphasia is quite clear in the case of the peripheral dysarthrias, but becomes muddled in the case of speech disorders due to cortical damage (anarthria, aphemia, apraxia of speech), which may be associated with aphasia.

26.1 Aphasia: epidemiology and natural history

The available data about the incidence and prevalence of acquired language disorders are limited. The Copenhagen stroke study indicates that aphasia was present in 38% of a series of consecutive patients with acute stroke (Pedersen et al., 1995).

Severe aphasia is a predictor of poor functional outcome in stroke (Paolucci et al., 1996). It has also been shown recently that aphasia is a predictor of increased (doubled) mortality in an 18 months follow-up study (Laska et al., 2004). Much less is known about aphasia associated to closed head injury and other lesions, such as tumours and tumour resections, which involve the language areas of the brain. Language disorders appear to be milder in tumour patients, in comparison with strokes of similar location and extent (Anderson et al., 1990), and complete recovery is more likely in traumatic than in vascular aphasia (Kertesz and McCabe, 1977).

Some degree of recovery can be expected to occur spontaneously in most patients with aphasia due to non-progressive brain diseases. The most important prognostic factors for recovery are severity, lesion size and time post-onset, while age does not appear to play a role independent of other factors, such as co-morbidity (Cappa, 1998).

26.2 Theoretical basis of aphasia rehabilitation

"The relative dearth of effective interventions in neurorehabilitation could be partly attributable to the weak contribution that this field has received from basic sciences such as neuroscience and behavioural psychology" (Taub et al., 2002). A relative lack of communication between basic research and clinical practice has also plagued aphasia research until recently. Some principles explicitly or implicitly underlying the rationale of aphasia rehabilitation are discussed in this section. The endeavour to treat language disorders has a long history, and the approaches are extremely heterogeneous. However, each of them represents the application of a theoretical position about language and the brain, even if not explicitly acknowledged by the proponent of the specific treatment approaches. Most textbook descriptions of aphasia begin with an historical section, which almost invariably includes a discussion of "localizationist" versus holistic approaches. This basic distinction does not relate only to brain organization, but also often implies contrasting ideas about language itself. In a most general way, localizationist approaches emphasize the structural aspects of language. In the traditional associationist approach, the modalities of language use include production, comprehension, repetition, etc., while in more recent, neurolinguistic approaches the emphasis is on the levels of language organization, such as phonology, lexicon and syntax. These "components" of language are associated with distinct specialized neural substrates (areas in older approaches, functional networks in recent times). A corollary of this position is that language is independent of other cognitive functions, both in terms of processing and of neural representation. The holistic approach, on the other hand, emphasizes the unitary nature of language, its relationship with other aspects of cognition, and the distributed nature of its neural substrate. The consequences of one theoretical position versus the other are straightforward. According to a localizationist position, the effect of a brain lesion on the language substrate is the loss of specific function. The ideal aim of treatment is thus restitution through re-learning. If this is not possible, the alternative approach is compensation using intact processing. The holistic approach, on the other hand, emphasizes the possibilities of compensation though procedures such as stimulation, facilitation, etc. At the neural level, the predictions of the former approach are that the effects of rehabilitation depend on recovery of the specialized area or network (if possible), or the "take-over" of the specialized

function by another brain region. On the other hand, the holistic position emphasizes the dynamic re-organization of the brain, in order to compensate for the impaired function (Chapter 5 of Volume II). Several other dichotomies are incompletely overlapping with this distinction. The localizationist approach is focused on the treatment of the impairment level, the holistic on the disability; the former emphasizes the loss of language representation, the latter the blocking of access to linguistic knowledge. At the level of treatment methods, the localizationist approach will be focused on exercises and drills, the holistic approach on "ecological" communication exchange.

Restitution versus compensation

What happens when an aphasic patient recovers, spontaneously or after rehabilitation? Are we observing restitution or compensation? There is long-standing confusion in this respect, due to very loose usage of these terms, and to a defective consideration of the differences between language and communication. It must be emphasized that (some) recovery of communication can be observed in the complete absence of restitution of language structure. There are a number of excellent examples of rehabilitation programmes utilizing this perspective. The most widely known are promoting aphasics communicative effectiveness (PACE) and related "pragmatic" approaches (Davis and Wilcox, 1981). Another example is the "reduced syntax approach" to agrammatism (Springer et al., 2000). At the other end of the spectrum, are the attempts to rebuild specific syntactic structures. An example of this approach is the programme based on the training of syntactically complex sentences, with the aim of obtaining generalization across linguistically related structures, which is enhanced when treatment goes from more complex to less complex constructions (Thompson et al., 2003). Both extremes are considered to be dependent on training; however, in the former approaches what is trained is compensation, or re-organization of communicative strategies, while in the latter it is restitution of syntactic structures.

The contrast between restitution and compensation also has implications for the underlying neurological mechanisms (Goldstein, 1948). We can legitimately speak of restitution if the "damaged substratum" recovers; otherwise, the compensation takes place at the behavioural level, by the mechanisms of adjustment and adaptation. In particular, Goldstein did not believe that true "restitution" could occur through "taking over" by a different substratum. This remains an open question (see below).

Language loss versus language dysfunction

If rehabilitation is based on re-learning, the implication is that brain damage has resulted in the loss of specific language representations. This idea is the basis of efforts to "re-teach" language to the aphasic subject. This has been historically the oldest approach, in which the aphasic patient was considered to be in the condition of an infant or of a foreigner learning an unknown language. The experience gained in fields of special education and second language teaching was thus the natural reference for this kind of treatment, which was widespread in both Europe and the USA. This class of methods, which, with a few exceptions, fell into disrepute for a large part of the twentieth century, has been resurrected by the psycholinguistic approach to aphasia that became prevalent in the 1970s. The detailed and sophisticated analysis of language disorders on the basis of models of normal processing often results in a functional diagnosis, which is based on the definition of the locus of impairment. A possible aim of treatment is then to re-teach the lost representations by means of repetitive exercises. For example, if the disorder affects the phonological lexical forms, it has been shown that treatment results in a selective re-learning of the treated items, with no evidence of generalization to other semantically related words (Miceli et al., 1996). A crucial requirement of this type of programme, which is well suited for homework and computerized treatment with supervision by the rehabilitation specialist, is preserved learning ability. This is an important topic of research, which

has been approached recently with more sophistication than in traditional studies assessing the rote learning abilities of aphasic subjects.

Many treatment approaches, on the other hand, are based on the concept that language is not "lost", but is merely inaccessible under standard conditions. This is the central idea of all programmes based on "stimulation" or "facilitation" of language processing. The origin of this idea can be traced to theoretical concepts introduced into aphasiology by Hughlings Jackson (1932), and in particular to his dynamic conception of behaviour. His fundamental observation that the patient's responses cannot always be predicted led to the recognition of the phenomenon of automatic-voluntary dissociation, which has had a lasting influence on rehabilitation practices. Jackson's distinction between "inferior" and "superior" forms of language use was an integral part of his theory of functional levels of the nervous system. Several approaches to language rehabilitation take this concept as a starting point, and are based on the assumption that it is possible, by means of different techniques, to improve the patient's ability to access the language representations not only automatically, but in a voluntary ("propositional", in Jackson's term) way (for a discussion of this approach, see Basso, 2003). A related proposal, within the Eastern European neurophysiological tradition, is the development of "de-blocking" techniques championed by Weigl and Kreindler (1960). At the empirical level, a crucial issue is whether it is possible to decide if a language representation is lost or inaccessible in a specific patient. This point has been the focus of an interesting proposal by Elizabeth Warrington and her co-workers (Warrington and Cipolotti, 1996) of a set of criteria that define a "storage" as opposed to an "access" disorder. In the case of word comprehension, the presence of an effect of the stimulus presentation rate, of the semantic relatedness of the stimulus array, and of word frequency, and the consistency/inconsistency of the responses tend to separate patients into two distinct groups. Dementia patients behave with the "loss" profile, while "access" disorder seems to be typical of vascular aphasia. The differential pattern lends itself to some intriguing neurological speculations (Gotts and Plaut, 2002).

Learning theories

Caramazza and Hillis (1993) summarized the ideal requirements of a theory of rehabilitation: (a) a detailed analysis of the cognitive conditions pre- and post-therapy; (b) a learning theory; (c) a theory of the therapeutic procedures and (d) a detailed knowledge of the characteristics of the patients and of their brains that may be relevant for the treatment (see Chapter 7 of Volume II). Most treatment approaches incorporate principles of behavioural therapy, such as reinforcement, modelling, etc. Recently, some experimental approaches based on specific learning principles have been applied to aphasia treatment. For example, the theory of "learned non-use" with the correlated proposal of constraint-induced rehabilitation techniques has sound neurobiological foundations (see Chapter 18 of Volume II). In the primate model, deafferentation induces a mobility loss, which can recover if the motility of the intact arm is blocked (see Chapter 14 of Volume I). The approach has been applied to human motor rehabilitation, with interesting results (Sterr et al., 2002). The effect appears to be mediated by cortical re-organization (Liepert et al., 2000). The approach has been extended recently by Pulvermuller et al. (2001) to aphasia rehabilitation. Another approach which has evoked considerable interest is based on the concept of errorless learning (Baddeley, 1992; Fillingham et al., 2003). Fridriksson et al. (2005) report positive effects in the treatment of naming disorders, using a spaced retrieval procedure, an errorless learning method.

An interesting development in the field is the connectionist modelling of rehabilitation. The main focus of this theoretical enterprise is the dynamics of treatment methods, an aspect that is completely absent in the functional information-processing models. Specific examples are the treatment proposals that have been formulated on the basis of Dell's model of lexical retrieval by Nadine Martin and her colleagues (2002), and on the hypotheses on

generalization of treated items, based on Plaut's model of reading (1996).

26.3 Aphasia rehabilitation techniques

Among interventions for acquired cognitive deficits, the rehabilitation of speech and language disorders following brain damage has the longest tradition, dating back to the 19th century (Howard and Hatfield, 1987). A variety of approaches have been applied to the rehabilitation of aphasia. The following summary scheme is based on Basso (2003).

Stimulation and facilitation

The theoretical underpinnings of this approach have been described in the previous section. The main representatives of the school are Schuell, Wepman and Darley (see Basso, 2003). The treatment approach is centred on language comprehension, particularly in the auditory modality, and is tailored for the individual patients on the basis of the severity of impairment, rather than on the specific features of linguistic breakdown.

Behavioural modification

The emphasis of the behavioural approach is on the learning process, and is an application to aphasia treatment of programmed instruction based on operant conditioning. The techniques include shaping and fading, and other principles of behaviour modification. While formal behavioural approaches, such as the one described by Holland (1970), are now seldomly employed, principles of behavioural modification are incorporated in most treatment approaches.

Neo-associationist

The focus on a detailed psycholinguistic and neurological description of the classic aphasic syndromes by the Boston School (Harold Goodglass, Norman Geschwind, Edith Kaplan and others) resulted in the proposal of a number of treatment approaches. These are described in detail in the book by Helm-Eastabrooks and Albert (1991), and include very heterogeneous approaches, such as melodic intonation therapy (MIT) and treatment of aphasic perseveration. What the methods have in common is a structured programme targeted to specific aspects of language impairment, and an emphasis on quantitative evaluation of results.

Neurolinguistic-cognitive

This approach originates from the early attempts to apply linguistic theory to aphasia in the sixties and seventies, flourishing with the development of cognitive neuropsychology. The emphasis is on detailed assessment of language in single cases, and analysis of the pattern of linguistic dysfunction on the basis of a model of normal processing, resulting in a "functional" diagnosis. The implication for rehabilitation remains an open question but it is generally believed that the precise identification of the locus of functional damage should provide the grounds for a rational intervention (Howard and Hatfield, 1987; Hillis, 1993). The usual dichotomy, that is, emphasis on restitution of impaired function or on compensation based on intact processes, applies also to intervention based on cognitive analysis. For example, in the case of reading disorders, a large number of attempts have been based on the "dual route" model. These include training the impaired mechanism (e.g. grapheme-to-phoneme conversion in the case of deep dyslexia (De Partz, 1986) and using the preserved ability to read content words to aid the reading of functors and verbs (Friedman et al., 2002)). The literature reporting specific approaches is now quite extensive. The reader is referred to Basso (2003) and to Hillis (2002), for updated reviews of experimental treatments based on the cognitive neuropsychology of language.

Pragmatic approaches

The pragmatic approach proposes treatment methods that aim at improving the patient's ability to communicate, regardless of the linguistic or non-linguistic strategies. The most widely known programme, PACE (Davis and Wilcox, 1981), incorporates an original attempt to put therapist and patient in a real communicative situation, in which exchange of "real" information is taking place. The influence of the pragmatic approach has been remarkable. Pragmatic principles have been incorporated in many eclectic treatment programmes, especially for severe aphasia.

Table 26.1 summarizes some structured programmes for aphasia rehabilitation.

26.4 Neurobiological foundations of aphasia rehabilitation

The neural mechanisms underlying the spontaneous recuperation of aphasia are incompletely understood. Even less is known about the neural basis of the effects of rehabilitation. The recovery period can be divided into at least three stages, referring to different physiological mechanisms responsible for clinical improvement (Mazzocchi and Vignolo, 1979). These are an early stage (about 2 weeks post-onset), a lesion stage (up to 6 months post-onset) and a chronic stage (after 6 months). During the early period, the likely mechanisms of clinical improvement are the disappearance of cerebral oedema and of intracranial hypertension, the re-absorption of blood, the normalization of haemodynamics in ischaemic penumbra areas, and the resolution of local inflammation. Another crucial mechanism, which is probably at play mostly in the early stage, is the regression of diaschisis (functional suppression) effects in non-injured areas connected to the damaged region (von Monakow, 1914; Feeney and Baron, 1986).

The mechanisms underlying recovery at later stages are a matter of debate. Recovery may be achieved by adopting novel cognitive strategies for performance, which at the neural level implies the recruitment of uninjured cerebral areas. This may represent an effect of the "degeneracy" of neural systems sustaining cognitive functions (Noppeney et al., 2004). True

Table 26.1. Examples of aphasia rehabilitation programmes.

Programme	Reference	Indications	Examples of exercises
Visual action therapy	Helm-Eastabrooks and Albert (1991)	Global aphasia	Matching of objects and pictures; object use; pantomimes
MIT	Helm-Eastabrooks and Albert (1991)	Non-fluent aphasia with moderate comprehension impairment	Humming, unison singing, unison with fading, immediate and delayed repetition
Treatment of aphasic perseveration	Helm-Eastabrooks and Albert (1991)	Any aphasia with perseverations	Inhibition of verbalization, provision of multiple cues
Language oriented treatment	Shewan and Bandur (1986)	All aphasias	Exercises for specific modalities and areas, graded in difficulty
Promoting aphasics' communicative effectiveness	Davis and Wilcox (1985)	Severe aphasia	Description of concealed pictures by therapist and patient using words, gestures, drawings
Mapping therapy	Marshall (1995)	Agrammatic comprehension	Explanation of the thematic grid of verbs; morphological training
BOX	Visch-Brink et al. (1997)	Lexical-semantic impairment	Semantic decisions on word, sentences and texts

recovery of linguistic function has been attributed to the "re-organization" of the cerebral substrate of language processing, with new brain areas taking over the function of damaged regions. The oldest, still influential hypothesis, proposed by Gowers (1895), is that the involvement of homotopic (i.e. homologous) areas of the controlateral hemisphere may have compensatory functions. In alternative, recovery may be due to the recruitment of peri-lesional areas surrounding the lesioned area. In both cases, it is possible that these areas may be part of redundant language networks, which in the intact brain are inhibited by the "primary" language areas (Heiss et al., 2003). This hypothesis is supported by the evidence of right-hemispheric linguistic abilities, especially at the lexical–semantic level, shown by split-brain subjects (Gazzaniga, 1983).

Modern neuroimaging techniques, especially functional magnetic resonance imaging (fMRI), allow testing directly these hypotheses (Chapter 5 of Volume II). Weiller et al. (1995) were the first to report a functional study of aphasia recovery, which supported the capacity of the right hemisphere to take-over for the damaged dominant hemisphere by means of its compensatory linguistic skills. However,

many other studies ascribe a better and long-term recovery to the contribution of preserved areas of the left hemisphere. In particular, follow-up studies with aphasic patients have revealed the existence of a temporal gradient in the enrolment of cerebral re-organization mechanisms after stroke. The initial engagement of non-damaged homologous areas of the right hemisphere is followed over time by their gradual discarding and a concomitant significant increase of activity in left-hemispheric peri-lesional areas. The passage of functional competence from the right to the left is associated with an improvement of linguistic performances (Karbe et al., 1998). Furthermore, Warburton et al. (1999) and Perani et al. (2003) have demonstrated in recovered aphasic patients that even limited salvage of peri-lesional tissue may have a significant impact on recovery. In line with the experimental evidence, some authors have argued that "right-hemispheric recruitment" in functional recovery may simply reflect the reliance on additional cognitive and linguistic resources, which are not required by normal subjects during linguistic processing.

A few studies attempt to evaluate the neural basis of training-induced modifications on language performance. An important role of the right hemisphere is suggested by the study of Musso et al. (1999), who investigated with positron emission tomography (PET) the neural correlates of intensive verbal comprehension training in a group of aphasics. Intensive 2-h language comprehension training on a modified version of the Token Test (De Renzi and Vignolo, 1962) was carried out during the PET inter-scan intervals. Post-training performance on this test was positively correlated with the pattern of regional cerebral blood flow (rCBF) in the right homologues of Wernicke's area and of Broca's area. Another "acute training" study reported right-sided effects. Blasi et al. (2002) found that the learning of a stem-completion task was associated with specific response decrements in the right frontal and occipital cortex, rather than in the left-sided network engaged by normal subjects. Training-induced effects were prevalent in the right hemisphere also in a recent study of "intentional" therapy (Crosson et al., 2005).

Other investigations suggest that the engagement of spared left-hemispheric regions is also crucial in recovery from aphasia. An influential PET study by Belin et al. (1996) involved patients with chronic non-fluent aphasia, who had shown considerable improvement after the introduction of additional rehabilitation training with MIT. Patients who were poor in repeating words with a natural intonation, improved when they used a MIT-like intonation. The pattern of brain activation during single word repetition with natural intonation indicated extensive right-sided involvement. However, during repetition of words with MIT intonation, the right hemisphere was deactivated, and a significant increase was found in the left-frontal areas. The authors argued that the right-sided activation might reflect a "maladaptive" functional re-organization, due to the presence of the left lesion itself, while actual recovery mediated by MIT training might be associated with the re-activation of undamaged left-hemispheric structures. Additional support for this hypothesis comes from a recent study of the effects of repetitive transcranial stimulation to the right hemisphere (Naeser et al., 2005). Interference with right-sided Broca's

area resulted in improved picture naming in three patients with chronic aphasia. Leger et al. (2002) compared the results of fMRI during a naming task pre- and post-rehabilitation in a patient with prominent phonological errors in speech production. The main difference between the two studies was a re-activation of peri-lesional left-hemispheric areas, particularly Broca's region and the supramarginal gyrus, in the post-treatment study. The complex interplay between right- and left-hemispheric activations is shown by a recent study from our laboratory (Vitali et al., 2003). Using event-related fMRI (er-fMRI), we monitored the neural correlates of naming performance in two anomic patients before and after specific language therapy for anomia (phonological cued naming training). A set of pictures that the patients could not name, either spontaneously or after being phonologically cued, was selected for intensive speech therapy. After acquisition of the first er-fMRI session, training was intensively administered on a daily basis by a speech pathologist, until at least 50% correct naming was achieved on the training picture set. Before and after specific speech therapy, an er-fMRI acquisition was performed during which patients had to overtly name the pictures of the experimental set and items of a control set (that patients were able to name prior to admission to our study). In both patients naming was mainly associated with activation in the non-dominant hemisphere before starting speech therapy, while mainly peri-lesional areas of the dominant hemisphere were activated after speech therapy, supporting the role of the peri-lesional areas of the left hemisphere for effective recovery. However, in one of the patients, who had a lesion involving Broca's area, the right homologue was activated, indicating that the right hemisphere may mediate successful naming.

26.5 Efficacy of aphasia rehabilitation

The need to establish the effectiveness of aphasia rehabilitation has stimulated a number of investigations, dating back to the period after the Second

World War, which have been based on a variety of methodologies. A meta-analysis of studies dealing with the effectiveness of language rehabilitation, limited to aphasia as a result of stroke, has been performed by the Cochrane collaboration. The review covers articles up to January 1999 (Greener et al., 2000). The conclusion of the review is that "speech and language therapy treatment for people with aphasia after a stroke has not been shown either to be clearly effective or clearly ineffective within a randomized clinical trial (RCT). Decisions about the management of patients must therefore be based on other forms of evidence. Further research is required to find out if speech and language therapy for aphasic patients is effective. If researchers choose to do a trial, this must be large enough to have adequate statistical power, and be clearly reported." This conclusion is based on a limited number of RCTs, all of which were considered of poor quality (Table 26.2 reports an updated summary of RCTs). Another review by Cicerone et al. (2000) reached a different conclusion, that is, that "cognitive-linguistic therapies" can be considered as standard practice for aphasia after stroke. Similar, positive conclusions for TBI were based on less consistent evidence. The reasons for this discrepancy can be found in the different criteria used in the two reviews. Several studies included by Cicerone et al. were not considered in the Cochrane review because of lack of true randomization or inclusion of patients with traumatic aphasia. Some of the RCTs comparing therapy with unstructured stimulation were based on a very limited number of treatment sessions. A meta-analysis by Bhogal et al. (2003) showed that studies indicating a significant treatment effect provided 8.8 h of therapy per week for 11.2 weeks, while the negative studies provided only approximately 2 h per week for 22.9 weeks. Total length of therapy was significantly inversely correlated with mean change in porch index of communicative abilities (PICA) scores. The number of hours of therapy provided in a week was significantly correlated to greater improvement on the PICA and the Token Test. These results indicate that an intense therapy programme provided over a brief period of time can improve outcomes of

Table 26.2. RCT of aphasia therapy.

	Evidence of superior effectiveness
Specific treatment versus no support	
Lincoln et al. (1984)	−
Wertz et al. (1986)	+
Specific treatment versus support from volunteers	
Meikle et al. (1979)	−
David et al. (1982)	−
Wertz et al. (1986)	−
Leal et al. (1993)	+
Support from volunteers versus no support	
Wertz et al. (1986)	+
Mackay et al. (1988)	+
Specific treatment versus support from professionals	
Hartmann and Landau (1987)	−
Elman and Bernstein-Hillis (1999)	+
Comparison of two specific treatments	
Di Carlo (1980)	−
Wertz et al. (1981)	−
Smith et al. (1981)	+
Kinsey (1986)	−
Prins et al. (1989)	−
Pulvermuller et al. (2001)	+
Doesborgh, S.J. et al. (2004)	−

speech and language therapy for stroke patients with aphasia.

By definition, all evidence derived from studies other than RCTs is not included in the Cochrane review. This resulted in the exclusion of three large studies (Basso et al., 1979; Shewan and Kertesz, 1984; Poeck et al., 1989) indicating significant benefits of treatment. Single-case studies were also not considered in the Cochrane reviews. This is particularly relevant because most of the recent treatment studies based on the cognitive neuropsychological approach make use of the single-case methodology. A review paper by Robey et al. (1999) reports a critical discussion of this approach, concluding that generally large treatment effects are seen in aphasic patients.

Clearly there is a need for large-scale RCTs evaluating well-defined methodologies of intervention.

The main difficulty of this approach lies in the highly heterogeneous nature of aphasia. For example, it is hard to believe that the same standardized aphasia treatment may be effective for both a patient with fluent neologistic jargon and another with agrammatic non-fluent production. Research in neuropsychology has focused on the assessment of specific, theoretically driven treatments on well-defined areas of impairment, usually by means of single-case methodology (e.g. the effect of a linguistically driven intervention compared with simple stimulation on the ability to retrieve lexical items belonging to a defined class). Both approaches represent potentially fruitful avenues for research in this field.

REFERENCES

Anderson, S.W., Damasio, H. and Tranel, D. (1990). Neuropsychological impairments associated with lesions caused by tumor or stroke. *Arch Neurol*, **47**, 397–405.

Baddeley, A.D. (1992). Implicit memory and errorless learning. A link between cognitive theory and neuropsychological rehabilitation? In: *Neuropsychology of Memory* (eds Squire, L.R. Butters, N.), Guilford Press, New York.

Basso, A. (2003). *Aphasia and its Therapy*, Oxford University Press, Oxford.

Basso, A., Capitani, E. and Vignolo, L.A. (1979). Influence of rehabilitation on language skills in aphasic patients. A controlled study. *Arch Neurol*, **36**, 190–196.

Belin, P., Van Eeckhout, P., Zilbovicius, M., Remy, P., François, C., Guillaume, S., Chain, F., Rancurel, G. and Samson, Y. (1996). Recovery from nonfluent aphasia after melodic intonation therapy: a PET study. *Neurology*, **47**, 1504–1511.

Bhogal, S.K., Teasell, R. and Speechley, M. (2003). Intensity of aphasia therapy, impact on recovery. *Stroke*, **34**, 987–993.

Blasi, V., Young, A.C., Tansy, A.P., Petersen, S.E., Snyder, A.Z. and Corbetta, M. (2002). Word retrieval learning modulates right frontal cortex in patients with left frontal damage. *Neuron*, **36**, 159–170.

Cappa, S.F. (1998). Spontaneous recovery from aphasia. In: *Handbook of Neurolinguistics* (eds Stemmer, B. and Withaker, H.), Academic Press, San Diego.

Caramazza, A. and Hillis, A.E. (1993). For a theory of remediation of cognitive deficits. *Neuropsychol Rehabil*, **3**, 217–234.

Cicerone, K.D., Dahlberg, C., Kalmar, K. and Al, E. (2000). Evidence-based cognitive rehabilitation: recommendations for clinical practice. *Arch Phys Med Rehab*, **81**, 1596–1615.

Crosson, B., Moore, A.B., Gopinath, K., White, K.D., Wierenga, C.E., Gaiefsky, M.E., Fabrizio, K.S., Peck, K.K., Soltysik, D., Milsted, C., Briggs, R.W., Conway, T.W. and Gonzalez Rothi, L.J. (2005). Role of the right and left hemispheres in recovery of function during treatment of intention in aphasia. *J Cogn Neurosci*, **17**, 392–406.

David, R., Enderby, P. and Bainton, D. (1982). Treatment of acquired aphasia: speech therapists and volunteers compared. *J Neurol Neurosurg Psychiatr*, **45**, 957–961.

Davis, G. and Wilcox, M. (1985). *Adult Aphasia Rehabilitation: Aapplied Pragmatics*. Windsor, NFER-Nelson.

Davis, G.A. and Wilcox, M.J. (1981). Incorporating parameters of normal conversation in aphasia. In: *Language Intervention Strategies in Adult Aphasia*, William and Wilkins, Baltimore.

De Partz, M.P. (1986). Re-education of a deep dyslexia patient: rationale of the method and results. *Cogn Neuropsychol*, **3**.

De Renzi, E. and Vignolo, L.A. (1962). The Token test: a sensitive test to detect receptive disturbances in aphasia. *Brain*, **85**, 665–678.

Di Carlo, L. (1980). Language recovery in aphasia: effect of systematic filmed programmed instruction. *Arch Phys Med Rehab*, **61**, 41–44.

Doesborgh, S.J., Van De Sandt-Koenderman, M.W., Dippel, D.W., Van Harskamp, F., Koudstaal, P.J. and Visch-Brink, E.G. (2004). Effects of semantic treatment on verbal communication and linguistic processing in aphasia after stroke: a randomized controlled trial. *Stroke*, **35**, 141–146.

Elman, R.J. and Bernstein-Ellis, E. (1999). The efficacy of group communication treatment in adults with chronic aphasia. *J Speech Lang Hear Res*, **42**, 411–419.

Feeney, D.M. and Baron, J.C. (1986). Diaschisis. *Stroke*, **17**, 817–830.

Fillingham, J.K., Hodgson, C., Sage, K. and Ralph, M.A.L. (2003). The application of errorless learning to aphasic disorders: a review of theory and practice. *Neuropsychol Rehabil*, **13**, 337–363.

Fridriksson, J., Holland, A.L., Beeson, P. and Morrow, L. (2005). Spaced retrieval treatment of anomia. *Aphasiology*, **19**, 99–109.

Friedman, R.B., Sample, D.M. and Lott, S.N. (2002). The role of level of representation in the use of paired associate learning for rehabilitation of alexia. *Neuropsychologia*, **40**, 223–234.

Gazzaniga, M.S. (1983). Right hemisphere language following brain bisection. A 20 years perspective. *Am Psychol*, **38**, 525–537.

Goldstein, K. (1948). *Language and Language Disturbances*, Grune and Stratton, New York.

Gotts, S.J. and Plaut, D.C. (2002). The impact of synaptic depression following brain damage: a connectionist account of "access/refractory" and "degraded-store" semantic impairments. *Cogn Affect Behav Neurosci*, **2**, 187–213.

Gowers, W. (1895). *Malattie del Sistema Nervoso*, Vallardi, Milan.

Greener, J., Enderby, P. and Whurr, R. (2000). Speech and language therapy for aphasia following stroke. *The Cochrane Library*, **4**.

Hartmann, J. and Landau, W. (1987). Comparison of formal language therapy with supportive counseling for aphasia due to acute vascular accident. *Arch Neurol*, **44**, 646–649.

Heiss, W.D., Thiel, A., Kessler, J. and Herholz, K. (2003). Disturbance and recovery of language function: correlates in PET activation studies. *Neuroimage*, **20**(**Suppl. 1**), S42–S49.

Helm-Eastabrooks, N. and Albert, M.A. (1991). *Manual of Aphasia Therapy*, Pro-Ed Publishers, Austin, TX.

Hillis, A.E. (1993). The role of models of language processing in rehabilitation of language impairments. *Aphasiology*, **7**, 5–26.

Hillis, A.E.E. (2002). *The Handbook of Adult Language Disorders*, Psychology Press, New York.

Holland, A.L. (1970). Case studies in aphasia rehabilitation using programmed instruction. *J Speech Hear Disord*, **32**, 11–16.

Howard, D. and Hatfield, F.M. (1987). *Aphasia Therapy: Historical and Contemporary Issues*, Lawrence Erlbaum Associates, Hove and London.

Jackson, H.J. (1932). *Selected Writings*, Hodder and Stoughton, London.

Karbe, H., Thiel, A., Weber-Luxenburger, G., Herholz, K., Kessler, J. and Heiss, W.D. (1998). Brain plasticity in post-stroke aphasia: what is the contribution of the right hemisphere? *Brain Lang*, **64**, 215–230.

Kertesz, A. and McCabe, P. (1977). Recovery patterns and prognosis in aphasia. *Brain*, **100**(**Pt 1**), 1–18.

Kinsey, C. (1986). Microcomputer speech therapy for dysphasic adults: a comparison with two conventionally administered tasks. *Br J Disord Commun*, **21**, 125–133.

Laska, A.C., Hellblom, A., Murray, V., Kahan, T. and Von Arbin, M. (2004). Aphasia in acute strike and relation to outcome. *J Int Med*, **249**, 413–422.

Leal, M.G., Farrajota, L., Fonseca, J., Guerriero, M. and Castro-Caldas, A. (1993). The influence of speech therapy on the evolution of stroke aphasia . *J Clin Exp Neuropsychol*, **15**, 399 (Abstract).

Leger, A., Demonet, J.F., Ruff, S., Aithamon, B., Touyeras, B., Puel, M., Boulanouar, K. and Cardebat, D. (2002). Neural substrates of spoken language rehabilitation in an aphasic patient: an fMRI study. *Neuroimage*, **17**, 174–183.

Liepert, J., Bauder, H., Wolfgang, H.R., Miltner, W.H., Taub, E. and Weiller, C. (2000). Treatment-induced cortical reorganization after stroke in humans. *Stroke*, **31**, 1210–1216.

Lincoln, N., Mulley, G.P., Jones, A.C., et al. (1984). Effectiveness of speech therapy for aphasic stroke patients. *Lancet*, 1197–1200.

Mackay, S., Holmes, D.W., Gersumky, A.T. (1988). Methods to assess aphasic stroke patients. *Geriatr Nurs*, **May/June**, 177–179.

Marshall, J. (1995). The mapping hypothesis and aphasia therapy. *Aphasiology*, **9**, 517–539.

Martin, N., Laine, M. and Harley, T.A. (2002). How can connectionist cognitive models of language inform models of language rehabilitation? In: *The Handbook of Adult Language Disorders* (ed. Hillis, A.E.), Psychology Press, New York.

Mazzocchi, F. and Vignolo, L.A. (1979). Localisation of lesions in aphasia: clinical-CT scan correlations in stroke patients. *Cortex*, **15**, 627–654.

Meikle, M., Wechsler, E., Tupper, A., et al. (1979). Comparative trial of volunteer and professional treatments of dysphasia after stroke. *Br Med J*, **2**, 87–89.

Miceli, G., Amitrano, A., Capasso, R. and Caramazza, A. (1996). The treatment of anomia resulting from output lexical damage: analysis of two cases. *Brain Lang*, **52**, 150–174.

Musso, M., Weiller, C., Kiebel, S., Muller, S.P., Bulau, P. and Rijntjes, M. (1999). Training-induced brain plasticity in aphasia. *Brain*, **122**, 1781–1790.

Naeser, M.A., Martin, P.I., Nicholas, M., Baker, E.H., Seekins, H., Kobayashi, M., Theoret, H., Fregni, F., Maria-Tormos, J., Kurland, J., Doron, K.W. and Pascual-Leone, A. (2005). Improved picture naming in chronic aphasia after TMS to part of right Broca's area: an open-protocol study. *Brain Lang*, **93**, 95–105.

Noppeney, U., Friston, K.J. and Price, C.J. (2004). Degenerate neuronal systems sustaining cognitive functions. *J Anat*, **205**, 433–442.

Paolucci, S., Antonucci, G., Gialloreti, L.E., Traballesi, M., Lubich, S., Pratesi, L. and Palombi, L. (1996). Predicting stroke inpatient rehabilitation outcome: the prominent role of neuropsychological disorders. *Eur Neurol*, **36**, 385–390.

Pedersen, P.M., Joergensen, H.S., Nakayama, H., Raaschou, H.O. and Skyhoj Olsen, T. (1995). Aphasia in acute stroke: incidence, determinants and recovery. *Ann Neurol*, **38**, 659–666.

Perani, D., Cappa, S.F., Tettamanti, M., Rosa, M., Scifo, P., Miozzo, A., Basso, A. and Fazio, F. (2003). A fMRI study of word retrieval in aphasia. *Brain Lang*, **85**, 357–368.

Plaut, D. (1996). Relearning after damage to a connectionist network: toward a theory of rehabilitation. *Brain Lang*, **52**, 25–82.

Poeck, K., Huber, W. and Willmes, K. (1989). Outcome of intensive language treatment in aphasia. *J Speech Hear Disord*, **54**, 471–479.

Prins, R.S., Schoonen, R. and Vermuelen, J. (1989). Efficacy of two different types of speech therapy for aphasic patients. *Appl Psycholinguist*, **10**, 85–123.

Pulvermuller, F., Neininger, B., Elbert, T., Mohr, B., Rockstroh, B., Koebbel, P. and Taub, E. (2001). Constraint-induced therapy of chronic aphasia after stroke. *Stroke*, **32**, 1621–1626.

Robey, R.R., Schultz, M.C., Crawford, A.B. and Sinner, C.A. (1999). Single-subject clinical outcome research: designs, data, effect sizes, and analyses. *Aphasiology*, **13**, 445–472.

Shewan, C.M. and Bandur, D.L. (1986). *Treatment of Aphasia: a Language Oriented Approach*. Taylor and Francis, London.

Shewan, C.M. and Kertesz, A. (1984). Effects of speech and language treatment on recovery from aphasia. *Brain Lang*, **23**, 272–299.

Smith, D.S., Goldenberg, E., Ashburn, A., Kinsella, G., Sheikh, K., Brennan, P.J., Meade, T.W., Zutshi, D.W., Perry, J.D. and Reeback, J.S. (1981). Remedial therapy after stroke: a randomised controlled trial. *Br Med J*, **282**, 517–520.

Springer, L., Huber, W., Schlenck, K.-J. and Schlenck, C. (2000). Agrammatism: deficit or compensation? Consequences for aphasia therapy. *Neuropsychol Rehabil Spec Cogn Neuropsychol Lang Rehabil*, **10**, 279–309.

Sterr, A., Elbert, T., Berthold, I., Kolbel, S., Rockstroh, B. and Taub, E. (2002). Longer versus shorter daily constraint-induced movement therapy of chronic hemiparesis: an exploratory study. *Arch Phys Med Rehabil*, **83**, 1374–1377.

Taub, E., Uswatte, G. and Elbert, T. (2002). New treatments in neurorehabilitation founded on basic research. *Nat Rev Neurosci*, **3**, 228–236.

Thompson C.K., Shapiro, L.P., Kiran, S. and Sobecks, J. (2003). The role of syntactic complexity in treatment of sentence deficits in agrammatic aphasia: the complexity account of treatment efficacy (CATE). *J Speech Lang Hear Res*, **46**, 591–607.

Visch-Brink, E.G., Bajema, I.M., and Van de Sandt-Koenderman, M.E. (1997). Lexical-semantic therapy: box. *Aphasiology*, **11**, 1057–1115.

Vitali, P., Tettamanti, M., Abutalebi, J., Danna, M., Ansaldo, A.I., Perani, D., Cappa, S.F. and Joanette, Y. (2003). Recovery from anomia: effects of specific rehabilitation on brain reorganisation: an er-fMRI study in 2 anomic patients. *Brain Lang*, **87**, 126–127.

Von Monakow, C. (1914). *Die Lokalisation in Grosshirn und der Abbau der Funktion durch Kortikale Herde*, Bergmann, Wiesbaden.

Warburton, E., Price, C.J., Swinburn, K. and Wise, R.J. (1999). Mechanisms of recovery from aphasia: evidence from positron emission tomography studies. *J Neurol Neurosurg Psychiatr*, **66**, 155–161.

Warrington, E.K. and Cipolotti, L. (1996). Word comprehension. The distinction between refractory and storage impairments. *Brain*, **119**(Pt 2), 611–625.

Weigl, E. and Kreindler, A. (1960). Contributions to the interpretation of aphasic disorders as manifestations of blocking. Temporary deblocking of speech motor reactions by word-reading in motor aphasia. *Arch Psychiatr Nervenkr Z Gesamte Neurol Psychiatr*, **200**, 306–323.

Weiller, C., Isensee, C., Rijintjes, M., Huber, W., Mueller, S., Bier, D., Dutschka, K., Woods, R.P., Noth, J. and Diener, H.C. (1995). Recovery from Wernicke's aphasia – a PET study. *Ann Neurol*, **37**, 723–732.

Wertz, R., Collins, M.J., Weiss, D., et al. (1981). Veterans administration cooperative study on aphasia: a comparison of individual and group treatment. *J Speech Hear Res*, **24**, 580–594.

Wertz, R., Weiss, W.G., Aten, J.L., et al (1986). Comparison of clinic, home and deferred language treatment. *Arch Neurol*, **43**, 653–658.

Apraxia

Thomas Platz

Charite – Universitätsmeditin Berlin, Abtlg. für neurologische Rehabilitation, Klinik Berlin, Germany

27.1 Historical note

Liepmann assumed that the expression "apraxia" has first been used by Steinthal in the late 19th century denoting that brain-damaged persons sometimes have lost single skills such as handling an instrument (Liepmann, 1920). Liepmann further notes that a disturbance of limb use that is different from paresis and ataxia had repeatedly been reported in the "older" literature (e.g. by Hughlin Jackson). Memorised entities for movements had been entertained by his contemporary colleagues: Wernicke's "movement images" ("Bewegunsgvorstellungen") as memories for kinesthetic perceptions brought about by the execution of repeated movements and their loss called "motor asymbolia" ("motorische asymbolie") by Meynert, Nothnagel's "memorised pictures" ("Erinnerungsbilder") for type and amplitude of movements, and de Buck's "parakinesias" ("parakinésies"); that is, movement alterations that were meant to be caused by an dissociation between movement idea and executed movements. It was, however, Liepmann's contribution to elaborate on the syndrome "apraxia" in a more systematic way. His ideas are still strongly influencing our current clinical classification. Liepmann classified someone as apraxic if she or he executes a requested movement incorrectly or uses an object incorrectly even though he is not or not sufficiently hindered to use her or his limb correctly by paresis or ataxia, and has understood the task – being without comprehension deficit or at least without deficit to comprehend the given task. The apraxic person cannot use (parts of) his body for some purposes at some points in time because learned mechanisms for movements are impaired. He assumed above mechanisms of motor execution and their deficits such as paresis or ataxia mnestic-associative mechanisms: (1) kinetic engrams; (2) extrakinetic temporospatial, mainly visually encoded movement concepts; and (3) the cooperation between these two. He further noted that apraxic behaviour can be observed with body-centred and object-related movements, meaningful and meaningless movements and frequently has to be elicited by examination since the behaviour while actually handling objects can be flawless. He described various error types such as amorphous movements, coarse movement deviations, substitution, perseveration, and lack of movement with perplexity. Liepmann distinguished: (1) motor and (2) ideational apraxia. Motor apraxia can be present either as (1a) limbkinetic apraxia with loss of simple learned movements (kinetic memory) for a body segment leading to clumsy coarse movements or (1b) ideokinetic apraxia with preserved ability to make skilful movements (with preserved memories for simple movements, i.e. limbkinetic engrams), but failure to evoke these for certain body parts on request (verbal command or imitation). Liepmann postulated that the cooperation between mnestic and perceptive optic, tactile, and kinetic components is disturbed in ideokinetic apraxia and more specifically that the movement idea (concept) and the kinetic component for specific body parts are dissociated. Ideational apraxia affects all body parts and is characterised by a deficient movement idea (concept). While movements themselves are skilful they do not match the task, for example a correct movement is performed with the wrong object, or a semantically similar movement is performed. Liepmann further described the left hemisphere dominance for praxis (in right-handed persons) and developed a detailed anatomical disconnection model for paresis, limbkinetic apraxia, ideokinetic apraxia, and ideational apraxia.

27.2 Apraxic syndromes

More recently, the term apraxia has been used in various circumstances, for example apraxia of speech, (ideomotor) prosodic apraxia, apraxia of eyelid opening, tactile apraxia, constructive apraxia, apraxia of gait, and dressing apraxia denoting quite different clinical entities. This chapter, however, will focus on apraxic syndromes that are similar to those described by Liepmann: ideational (conceptual) apraxia, ideomotor apraxia either as ideomotor limb apraxia or buccofacial apraxia, and limbkinetic apraxia.

Patients who have lost the capability to make use of everyday life tools, for example would not know which tool to use for an object or which action to perform with a tool, have been classified as ideational apraxic. Conversely, patients with frontal apraxia would be characterised by action sequence deficits with multi-step actions, that is *schema-type actions* (e.g. "preparing a slice of bread with butter and jam") or *script-type actions* (e.g. "going to the market to shop"), while they know how to use (single) everyday life tools. Patients who have lost the capability to make simpler or more complex limb or face motions according to a model have been classified as limb or buccofacial ideomotor apraxic. The model could be external (e.g. when asked to imitate) or internal (e.g. when verbally asked to perform a conventional symbolic gesture). Limbkinetic apraxia relates to the inability to perform precise, isolated or independent finger and hand movements. It occurs frequently unilaterally, but the deficit is out of proportion of paresis with slow, coarse, and fragmented finger movements, lack of interdigital cooperation, and deranged manipulative behaviour irrespective of the modality of the evoking stimulus (i.e. verbal, visual, tactile).

One might want to ask whether there are clinical reasons to assume that these different apraxic syndromes exist or whether we would rather have to assume one apraxic syndrome with varying severity. A first approach to this question could be to look for dissociations in their prevalence across patient groups.

The mentioned signs of limbkinetic apraxia could be regarded as signs of mild paresis. They can, however, be observed bilaterally during left hemisphere dysfunction in right-handed subjects (and in the left hand during right hemisphere dysfunction) (Heilman et al., 2000) and with preserved cortico-motorneuronal projections as assessed by transcranial magnetic stimulation in a sample of patients with corticobasal degeneration (CBD) (Leiguarda et al., 2003) supporting Liepmann's notion of a deficit that is not equivalent to central paresis.

In patients with lateralised ischaemic brain lesions as well as patients with CBD ideational apraxia has mainly been observed in patients with ideomotor apraxia, while ideomotor apraxia was frequently observed without ideational apraxia (Leiguarda et al., 1994; Heilman et al., 1997). In patients with Alzheimer's disease (AD), however, signs of ideational apraxia are not uncommon in patients without ideomotor apraxia (Ochipa et al., 1992). Nevertheless, ideomotor apraxia does occur in a considerable proportion of patients with moderate to severe AD (Travniczek-Marterer et al., 1993). Ideomotor recognition failure is usually not observed without ideomotor-production failure while the opposite pattern is frequently seen (Leiguarda et al., 1994). Ideomotor facial and limb apraxia as well as ideational apraxia are more frequently observed after left-sided lateralised ischaemic brain lesions, but do occur after right-sided lateralised ischaemic brain lesions (De Renzi et al., 1980; Ochipa et al., 1989; Heilman et al., 1997; Bizzozero et al., 2000; Pedersen et al., 2001). Aside from lateralised brain lesions bilateral ideomotor apraxia has most frequently seen in a cohort of patients with CBD, less frequently with progressive supranuclear palsy (PSP) – some of these patients also exhibited a limbkinetic type of apraxia – and least frequently among patients with Parkinson's disease (PD) (Leiguarda et al., 1997; Pharr et al., 2001). Neither patients with multiple system atrophy (MSA) or neuroleptic-induced Parkinsonism showed ideomotor or limbkinetic apraxia. Ideomotor apraxia occurs also in patients with Huntington's disease (HD) where its occurrence is related to duration of disease, but not to extrapyramidal motor signs (Shelton and Knopman, 1991; Hamilton et al., 2003).

27.3 Cognitive-motor deficits in apraxia

Limbkinetic apraxia could reflect deficient information processing during the preparation and execution of specific movements components such as the object-related grip formation, a capability that has been shown to involve specific parieto-premotor circuits (e.g. human homologues of monkey areas AIP and F5) (Rizzolatti et al., 1988; Binkofski et al., 1999).

Left hemisphere stroke patients with ideomotor apraxia have difficulties to adopt the required configuration of the hand for actions without showing a general decrease of dexterity or slowness of movement (Sunderland and Sluman, 2000). In addition, they have been shown to produce abnormal hand postures responses to known objects while they performed normally in recognising the hand postures appropriate for interacting with novel objects (Buxbaum et al., 2003). Most of these apraxics were impaired in both recognition and production of hand postures for known objects. This evidence points towards the distinction between representation-driven motor behaviour and "online" object-related visuomotor behaviour.

The observation that memory-driven and online (simple) aimed movements were not disproportionally affected in ideomotor apraxic patients leads to the conclusion that only a subset of memory-driven movements is affected; for example, those that are more complex than simple aimed movements (Ietswaart et al., 2001). In as much as delayed motor response involves prefrontal neurons in monkeys (Funahashi et al., 1989) and thus a type of working memory it is conceivable that this type of representation does not necessarily involve a more abstract level of representation than the primary online visuomotor processes would imply. This might be an explanation for the above-mentioned unaffected delayed response performance among apraxic patients (compare Ietswaart et al., 2001).

Ideomotor apraxic patients might be impaired with model-driven behaviour that affords the representation of combinations of positions of body parts and their changes that a more complex than just a simple reaching movement. Documented joint coordination and trajectory deficits during gestures support this view (Platz and Mauritz, 1995; Poizner et al., 1995). It's historically noteworthy that Kimura argued some 25 years ago that limb apraxia involves impairments in making transitions between positions and/or postures in body-centred space (Kimura, 1977).

Indeed, left hemisphere apraxic stroke patients have difficulties to generate hand–head postures combinations (Goldenberg, 1999) both on their own body and at a life-sized wooden mannikin (Goldenberg et al., 1996), and other combinations of positions of body parts regardless of their meaningfulness and in addition have been shown to have impaired working memory for sequences of such positions (Toraldo et al., 2001). A prominent deficit in ideomotor apraxia could be to reproduce or to adopt complex hand configurations (Sunderland and Sluman, 2000). The impairment of working memory performance for sequencing of body positions could, but does not necessarily imply a specific working memory module: it could reflect a problem of encoding body positions or could even be related to inefficient verbal-encoding strategies (Frencham et al., 2003).

A deficit of learned representations of combinations of positions of body parts related to tool use and preserved visual representations of tools and objects might then lead to body-part-as-tool errors with a compensatory use of these tool representations while producing a tool pantomime (Raymer et al., 1997).

Theoretical accounts of ideomotor apraxia would be incomplete without considering the tactile feedback mechanisms: that is, the integration of somatosensation and action. Apraxic patients seem to have problems to evaluate and compare internal (somatosensory) and external (visual) feedback about movements (Sirigu et al., 1999), but are equally more dependent on visual feedback during movements for both their own body and the extrapersonal space (Haaland et al., 1999) pointing to a deficit in the movement-related representation of intrapersonal spatial properties and their relation to extrapersonal space. Most frequently tactile input facilitates normal gesture production among apraxic patients (De Renzi et al., 1982). As suggested by detailed motion analysis this effect is most likely to be incomplete (Poizner et al., 1995). Even non-specific tactile input can markedly facilitate correct tool-use pantomime (Wada et al., 1999) possibly indicating the recruitment of an alternative route of movement control; for example, the evocation of "automatic" motor skills by somatosensory triggers. There have, however, also been case reports where gesture production was specifically impaired by the presence of tactile cues (Heath et al., 2003).

With regard to ideomotor limb apraxia, arm and hand have been shown to be apractic to the same degree as leg and foot (Lehmkuhl et al., 1983).

Conflicting evidence exists whether ideomotor apraxia affects meaningful (transitive or intransitive) and meaningless movements differentially (De Renzi et al., 1980; Roy et al., 1991; Belanger and Duffy, 1996; Schnider et al., 1997; Haaland et al., 2000), and whether ideomotor apraxia is dependent on the mode of elicitation of gestures, that is by verbal command, visual object presentation, tactile object presentation, and imitation of gesture (De Renzi et al., 1982; Roy et al., 1991; Belanger and Duffy, 1996; Schnider et al., 1997). A lack of balanced item difficulties across modalities might have hindered more unequivocal results in these group studies (performance differences across modalities can only be interpreted as modality related when test items have been of comparable difficulty). The mentioned distinctions are, nevertheless, to some degree supported. The analysis of the correlational structure of verbal and non-verbal performance measures among left hemisphere stroke patients with multi-dimensional scaling supported a two-dimensional structure seperating meaningful (transitive) and meaningless movements (Goldenberg et al., 2003). A functional activation study supports the notion of tool use in gestures being an additional feature beyond representation of combinations of positions of body parts: pantomiming tool-use gestures activated the left intraparietal cortex more strongly than meaningless gestures of comparable complexity (Moll et al., 1998). Observation of single subjects lends some support to the notion that apraxia can at times be (relatively) specific to the mode of elicitation of gestures (De Renzi et al., 1982; Merians et al., 1997). This would imply that not only deficient ideomotor praxis processes proper (i.e. model-drive of motor behaviour that affords the representation of combinations of positions of body parts), but also a deficient modality-specific access (i.e. a disconnection syndrome) could account for apraxic behaviour.

Further, the specific constellation of cognitive-motor deficits might vary across patient groups as indicated by (1) the case of a patient with CBD who in contrast to apraxic stroke patients performed more poorly when he had to work with actual tools as compared to gesture imitation (Merians et al., 1999) or (2) CBD patients who performed gestures with imitation worse than to verbal command (Peigneux et al., 2001) while the reverse has been observed with patients with semantic dementia (Hodges et al., 2000), and (3) right hemisphere stroke patients who – in contrast to left hemisphere stroke patients – had more impaired gesture production with imitation than after visual object presentation (Barbieri and De Renzi, 1988) and (4) were more impaired when imitating meaningless gestures involving fingers (internal hand configuration) as compared to hand (external hand position) or foot (Goldenberg and Strauss, 2002), or (5) patients with AD who were more impaired than stroke patients when performing intransitive limb movements (Foundas et al., 1999). (6) the observation of perceptual matching deficits for meaningless actions in both right and left hemisphere stroke patients (Goldenberg and Hagmann, 1999) is another example.

It has been investigated in stroke and control subjects whether movement-related conceptual knowledge could be distinguished in associative knowledge (i.e. *tool–action associations* such as hammer pound and *tool–object associations* such as hammer and nail) and mechanical knowledge (such as knowing the advantage that tools afford) (Heilman et al., 1997). The results of this cross-sectional study with stroke patients did not provide firm evidence in favour of this hypothesis. Similarly, in a cohort study with left and right brain stroke patients, and control subjects pantomime of tool use, the ability to infer function from structure (novel tool selection tasks), and the ability to use familiar objects correctly have all been deficient in the group of left brain stroke patients only (Goldenberg and Hagmann, 1998a). Inability to use familiar objects was only observed among patients with deficits in both pantomime of tool use and the novel tool selection tasks. In a cohort of semantic dementia patients, however, normal performance on the novel tool selection task contrasted with impaired performance with tasks testing semantic knowledge and object use (Hodges et al., 2000). Thus, mechanical knowledge and semantic knowledge might be dissociable processes.

It is further of interest to know whether action-related semantic knowledge can be regarded as a type of category-specific knowledge (system) dissociable from other semantic knowledge. In the mentioned study by Hodges and coworkers (Hodges et al., 2000), action-related semantic knowledge as inferred from object use, and other semantic knowledge showed a moderately high-to-high association rather favouring the notion of a multimodal semantic system than a separate action semantic system. Similar findings have been obtained in patients with AD (Dumont et al., 2000).

A case study of a semantic dementia patient reported poor knowledge on semantic matching and judgement tasks related to tools with in contrast relatively good actual single-object use and using objects in everyday tasks (Buxbaum et al., 1997). This suggests that impaired semantic knowledge for single-objects use does not necessarily imply deficits in using objects. The correct manual use of objects can presumably be based on alternative cognitive-motor processes: that is, semantic knowledge about tool use (ideational component), the ability to infer function from structure (mechanical knowledge), (cortical) representations of movements (combinations of positions of body parts) related to tool use (ideomotor component), and/or "automatic" motor skills for highly familiar motor tasks in a natural context that may be triggered by visual or possibly even more potently by tactile stimuli.

Ideational apraxia as one reason for impaired object use might be defined as a situation where impaired object use is associated with deficient semantic knowledge about tool use. According to the above-mentioned hypothesis impaired object use would most likely be observed when deficient semantic knowledge about tool use (ideational component) would be combined with an inability to infer function from structure (mechanical knowledge), or possibly more importantly an impairment of representations of movements (combinations of positions of body parts) related to tool use (ideomotor component). Any errors in object handling that occur secondary to deficient semantic knowledge related to tool use representations of movements could then not be corrected based on alternative compensatorically used cognitive-motor processes, for example representations of movements (combinations of positions of body parts) related to tool use. Testing ideational apraxia by actual tool use as frequently done clinically would then result in its most frequent observation in ideomotor apraxics.

Action sequencing needs to be distinguished from action production. A sample of nine patients with frontal lobe lesions were given sets of schema-type actions (e.g. "preparing a slice of bread with butter and jam") and sets of script-type actions (e.g. "going to the market to shop") (Zanini et al., 2002). When they had to arrange cards with either pictures or verbal descriptors of action steps, they showed action sequence deficits especially in the middle of an action, but they did not present wrong actions when they where asked to actually perform these actions or to describe them verbally. It is noteworthy that these patients did not suffer from ideational apraxia. Their action-sequencing deficit was not caused by an action representational deficit, that is a deficit of knowledge *per se*, but rather a disorder of control and use of knowledge that has been termed "frontal apraxia" (Cooper, 2002). Such control deficits could be related to deficient action schema retrieval, maintaining the steps of schemata, performance monitoring, inhibition of salient action, or access to semantic knowledge about objects (Forde and Humphreys, 2000). They might indicate a problem in integrating actions with intentions and monitoring operations in working memory. Noteworthy, representations of roughly hierarchically structured routine sequential activity do not necessarily imply that the processing system itself assumes a hierarchical structure; the task structure could well be re-presented in distributed representations the system uses in performing particular tasks (Botvinick and Plaut, 2004). An at least partially reverse pattern of disorder; that is the ability to sequence pictures of activities that cannot be performed correctly, has been shown for patients with ideational apraxia (Rumiati et al., 2001).

It follows that impaired performance on everyday tasks that has been called "action disorganisation syndrome (ADS)" could be caused by either frontal apraxia or ideational apraxia.

While apraxic behaviour has been associated with learned movements there is little and conflicting evidence whether apraxia affects motor learning. In a sample of AD patients with varying severity of ideomotor apraxia motor skill-learning on a rotor pursuit task was not impaired and improvement scores were not related to severity of apraxia (Jacobs et al., 1999) while a former study with hemiparetic apraxic patients showed reduced learning on such as task as compared to hemiparetic non-apraxic patients (Heilman et al., 1975).

27.4 Model of praxis-related processes

Theoretical models that try to account for the different aspects of apraxia have repeatedly been proposed starting with Liepmann (1920) as described above. A more recent and in the scientific community very influential model is the cognitive-neuropsychological model of limb praxis by Rothi and coworkers (1991). It distinguishes among other components between different input modalities: for example, verbal and visual, an action input and output lexicon, an (action)

semantic system, and a non-lexical route between visual analysis and motor response. The model's strengths are the distinction made between action perception and action production, the reference to semantics, and the acknowledgement of different input modalities for the evocation of actions. Accordingly, it has been able to account for many observations of dissociations regarding apraxic deficits.

The cognitive-neuropsychological model of limb praxis by Rothi and coworkers (1991) has, however, shortcomings in that it focuses on ideomotor limb praxis and emphasises meaningful gestures. Some evidence does, but in total the above-mentioned evidence does not necessarily support the distinctions that are made by the model. Apraxic stroke patients have difficulties to generate hand–head postures combinations both on their own body and at a mannikin, and other combinations of positions of body parts frequently regardless of their meaningfulness supporting the notion that a deficient representation of invariant features of intrinsic and extrinsic egocentric coding for movements is a core deficit in ideomotor apraxia rather than a "lexical" deficit for meaningful movements (gestures) and its separation in a perceptual (input lexicon) and action side (output lexicon). Further, the neuroimaging data and evidence from brain-damaged patients (for reference see Section 27.5) favour more complex theoretical models that would more explicitly account for the distinction between "online dynamic" motor control, "automatic" skills, and model-driven motor control, between buccofacial and limb ideomotor apraxia, the more focal brain networks that seem to be involved in gesture production as compared to less focal brain networks likely to be involved in gesture perception, the distinction between ideomotor and ideational apraxia, between semantics and mechanical knowledge, the processes related to action sequencing, and the parallel and in some instances compensatory interplay of these processes for given actions. The model by Rothi and coworkers cannot easily account for these distinctions.

An alternative frame to describe the cognitive-motor deficits of limbkinetic, ideomotor, and ideational apraxia (as well as frontal apraxia) is partially

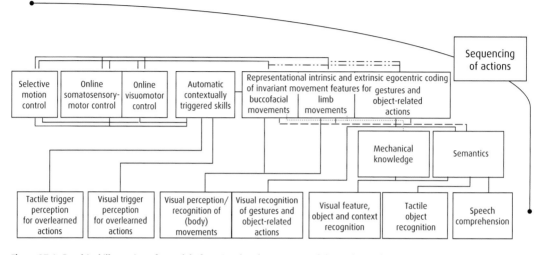

Figure 27.1. Graphical illustration of a model of praxis-related processes and their relationship. The denoted processes are thought to be characterised by the proposition that they can be performed with relative independence under specific circumstances (for explanation see text).

based on the notion of Ungerleider and Mishkin's (1982) dissociation of a ventral "what" and a dorsal "where" visual processing stream and the more recent distinction of two different streams of the dorsal system: the dorso-dorsal and the ventro-dorsal streams (Rizzolatti and Matelli, 2003).

A model of praxis-related processes is illustrated graphically in Fig. 27.1 and will be described in more detail below. Neuroanatomical considerations will be mentioned. The denoted processes are thought to be characterised by the proposition that can be performed with relative independence under specific circumstances. They do, however, neither imply the activity of singular processes (within each box of Fig. 27.1), equally complex processes (across boxes), processes with (comparably) circumscribed brain activations, or processes that are realised by the brain with completely independent network activations (across boxes). Their description as processes that can be relatively independent and their proposed interrelation is meant to promote differential clinical reasoning for apraxic behaviour that is in accordance with the current status of knowledge about both processes related to apraxic behaviour (compare

Section 28.3) and brain activation during human performance (compare Section 28.5).

Selective motion control is viewed as the basic capacity to make fine and precise, isolated, or independent face or limb movements regardless of a specific movement context. Its deficit would frequently be caused by central paresis and thus by the lack of selective innervation. It could, however, indicate limbkinetic apraxia if it was not associated with – or at least out of proportion of – paresis, somatosensory deafferentation, or ataxia. A deficient grasping ability after premotor cortex lesions (human homologue of the monkey's area F5) (Binkofski et al., 1999; Fogassi et al., 2001) could be an example (Fig. 27.2).

A dorso-dorsal action system would perform online, dynamic computations of the positions of body parts with respect to objects ("extrinsic egocentric coding") and of the positions of body parts with respect to one another ("intrinsic egocentric coding") (Buxbaum, 2001; Rizzolatti and Matelli, 2003). Specific partially interdependent processes might be entertained for somatosensorimotor control and visuomotor control. These computations would be necessary for all movements of the body in space.

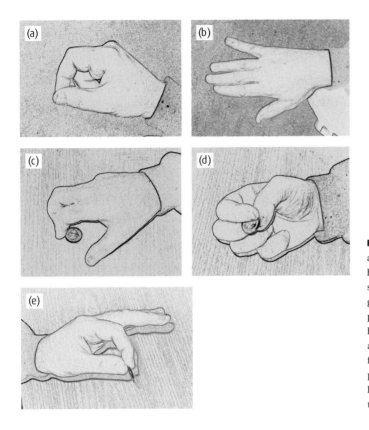

Figure 27.2. Illustration of limbkinetic apraxia for the right hand. This left hemisphere stroke patient had preserved selective innervation to maintain a precision grip (with tactile guidance to reach the position) (a) and to extend his fingers (b) while he had great difficulties to grasp a 2€ coin (c) and could do so only with a deficient grip formation (d). Clinically, he had neither paresis nor somatosensory deficits of his right hand. Further, he had no difficulties to grasp the 2€ coin with his left hand (e).

Movement deficits observed with somatosensory deafferentation (Platz and Mauritz, 1997) or tactile apraxia (Pause et al., 1989) (online somatosensory-motor control) and visuomotor ataxia (Perenin and Vighetto, 1988) (online visuomotor control) would be the clinically observable syndromes when these processes are deficient, typically in patients with superior parietal lobe damage.

There might be instances when visual and tactile environmental cues trigger highly trained and consequently "automatic" skills that do not have to be composed afresh in terms of invariant features of movements of the body in space, but would still be modified during their execution by online dynamic computations adjusting motor behaviour to the specific circumstances. The observed shift from more cortically to more basal ganglia and cerebellar mediated motor control when sequential finger movements (Seitz and Roland, 1992) or a visuomotor sequence (Doyon et al., 1996) have been learned might support the notion of such "automatic skills".

Short-term (imitation of meaningless movements) or long-term (pantomime of meaningful actions) complex movement representations, that is the combination of invariant features of intrinsic and extrinsic egocentric coding for a given movement, become necessary when movements have to be performed outside their typical environmental context. Parieto-frontal networks within the ventro-dorsal stream involving the inferior parietal lobe might be held responsible for these processes. Specific representations might exist for known actions (compare "mirror neurons" (Gallese et al., 1996); coding of unknown movements might be based on their

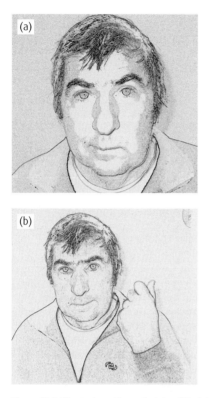

Figure 27.3. Illustration of buccofacial and limb ideomotor apraxic deficits. This left hemisphere stroke patient had been asked to perform movements outside their typical environmental context (i.e. to imitate gestures). He performed an asymmetrical facial movement instead of protruding the tongue when asked to imitate "stick out your tongue" (a). When asked to imitate "brush your teeth" he produced an inadequate positioning of the hand with regard to the mouth (a toothbrush held in his hand would point away from his head and mouth) (b). In both cases this would imply a deficient coding of a typical (invariant) feature of the required gesture. Clinically, he had neither paresis nor somatosensory deficits of his face and left arm.

"visual" features (Rizzolatti and Matelli, 2003). The combined activity of this representational network in the ventro-dorsal action stream (and the ventral stream in some instances) as well as of the dorso-dorsal action stream with its online, dynamic computations of extrinsic and intrinsic egocentric coding would enable the performance of complex movements outside their typical environmental context.

Ideomotor apraxia would reflect the incapacity for this combined activity due to deficient complex movement representations or lack of access to or integration of such representations (Fig. 27.3).

In the case of actual tool use, not only "automatic skills" for this type of tool (when available), representations of object-related actions, that is the combination of invariant features of intrinsic and extrinsic egocentric coding relevant for the use of this type of tool (ventro-dorsal stream), and online, dynamic computations of extrinsic and intrinsic egocentric coding for the specific circumstances (dorso-dorsal stream) would be used, but also semantic knowledge about object use provided by the ventral stream. Ideational apraxia would then result from the incapacity for this even more complex combined activity with (by definition) deficient (action-related) semantic knowledge or lack of access to this knowledge. Based on the conventional clinical testing the diagnosis of ideational apraxia would frequently rest on the observation of impaired actual object use. In this situation, impaired semantic knowledge for tool use might, however, most likely be observable when ideomotor apraxia (i.e. deficient representational intrinsic and extrinsic egocentric coding of invariant movement features) is also present, because this type of representation could mask deficits of semantic knowledge for tool use in the clinical testing situation. Similarly, mechanical knowledge, that is the ability to infer function from structure, might involve processes distinct from semantic knowledge for tool use and could therefore mask such deficits.

Action sequencing needs to be distinguished from performing single actions and can involve more circumscript action sequences, that is schema-type actions (e.g. "preparing a slice of bread with butter and jam"), or more complex action sequences, that is script-type actions (e.g. "going to the market to shop"). In these situations, the integration of actions with intentions and monitoring operations in working memory have to be performed in addition to processes relevant for single actions. Such control processes could involve action schema retrieval, maintaining the steps of schemata, performance monitoring, inhibition of salient action, or access to semantic knowledge about objects. "Frontal apraxia", that is the incapacity to perform action sequencing, would results from the incapacity to perform these processes. With respect to action sequencing, the graphical illustration in Fig. 27.1 merely denotes that action sequencing can involve all processes related to single actions, but involves additional processes that would have to be represented at a different "dimension" of organisation.

The model has been developed based on the currently available knowledge regarding apraxia. Its validation would warrant further testing. Noteworthy, a more recent independent reference states a multi-dimensional scaling of correlations between tests in left hemisphere stroke patients where some of the processes described were separated in a two-dimensional space (Goldenberg, 2003).

27.5 Neuroanatomy of apraxia

The brain's right and left hemisphere, and specific cortical and subcortical brain areas seem to be involved in functional brain networks that contribute to different aspects of praxis.

Various cognitive-motor aspects that are relevant for praxis are represented in different functional brain networks. Investigations of regional cerebral blood flow (rCBF) during the observation of hand actions revealed activation of left frontal (BA45) and temporal areas (BA21) with meaningful hand actions, and of mainly right occipitoparietal pathways related to both "ventral" and "dorsal" streams with meaningless hand actions (Decety et al., 1997). Observing with the intend to recognise activated memory-encoding structures, that is the parahippocampal region, while observation with the intent to imitate activated areas related to the preparation and generation of actions, that is the dorso-lateral prefrontal cortex (DLPFC) and the left pre-supplementary motor area (pre-SMA). Selecting a finger (body schema) rather than a target during aimed movements was related to activity in the anterior intraparietal sulcus extending over the marginal gyrus of the left inferior parietal lobe (de Jong et al., 2001). Selection of finger movements

as compared to repeated motion of the same finger also activates left hemisphere areas (i.e. prefrontal, premotor and intraparietal areas) (Schluter et al., 2001). A functional activation study with body movement observation suggests that body movements are somatotopically represented within the parietal and premotor cortex, mouth actions most ventrally, arm–hand movements at an intermediate position, and foot movements more dorsally (Buccino et al., 2001). Performing and imagery of tool-use gestures as compared to meaningless gestures lead to activations clustering in the left intraparietal cortex (Moll et al., 1998, 2000). The left supramarginal gyrus (SMG) was activated when tool stimuli have been used in various positron emission tomographical (PET) activation studies; the disruption of its activity by transcranial magnetic stimulation impairs the correction of invalid stimulus–response combinations for hand movements (Rushworth et al., 2003). The dorsal inferior parietal lobe has been shown to be specifically activated when objects trigger movements while the ventral inferior parietal lobe was activated by pantomimes whether or not triggered by objects (Rumiati et al., 2004). Activation of the left SMG (BA40) and superior parietal lobule (BA7) have been associated with tool-related gestures while its performance with "body-part-as-object (BPO)" specifically activated the right SMG (Ohgami et al., 2004). Discrimination of hand gestures was associated with activity in the left inferior parietal cortex (BA40) while the discrimination of finger gestures induced a more symmetrical activation and rCBF peaks in the right intraparietal sulcus and in medial visual association areas (BA18/19) (Hermsdörfer et al., 2001).

The distribution of these functional networks is further varying across subjects. The "limbkinetic praxis dominance", "ideomotor praxis dominance", and "language dominance" have been postulated to be associated and most frequently located in the left hemisphere. Subjects with atypical language dominance (right or bilateral), however, exhibit a more bilateral cerebral distribution of both language and praxis function (Meador et al., 1999; Heilman et al., 2000). Case reports and a population-based study support the notion that ideomotor apraxia can occur in right brain damage even among right-handed persons (Raymer et al., 1999; Pedersen et al., 2001).

As suggested by functional neuroimaging studies (see those mentioned above) any hemispheric dominance might be subject to specific cognitive-motor processes that contribute to praxis.

The left hemisphere with frontal areas and especially left parietal areas might frequently be dominant for the representation of invariant features of intrinsic and extrinsic egocentric coding for (complex) movements while the right hemisphere might especially be involved in the generation of finger postures and the visuospatial analysis of complex movements. Intra- and interhemispheric connectivity between brain areas, especially the deep parieto- and occipitofrontal, and anterior callosal fibres are important for the integration of praxis-related brain networks in motor control. Subcortical structures might be especially relevant for highly trained and thus automatic skills, for example skills related to tool use.

These views are supported by observations in brain-damaged persons. In a case study of a patient with an expressive speech disorder and ideomotor apraxia of insidious onset, but preserved gesture recognition a PET scan showed abnormal fludeoxyglucose uptake in the posterior frontal and parietal regions, the left affected more than the right, with a focal metabolic deficit in the left angular gyrus, and bilaterally in the SMA suggesting that these areas are involved in gesture production while gesture recognition networks might be more widely distributed, for example involving right hemisphere areas (Kareken et al., 1998). Similarly, patients with left parietal lobe lesions had a profound deficit when asked to imitate meaningful pantomimed motor acts especially those related to body parts while gesture comprehension was not or only slightly disturbed (Halsband et al., 2001). The performance of patients with premotor cortex lesions, however, was not significantly different from control subjects. Further, patients with CBD and ideomotor apraxia showed superior parietal lobule and SMA hypometabolism as measured with PET (at rest) (Peigneux et al., 2001). Movement-related slow cortical potentials and event-related desynchronisation of alpha (alpha-ERD) and beta (beta-ERD) activity after self-paced voluntary triangular finger movements were studied in 13 stroke patients and 10 age-matched control subjects during movement preparation and actual performance (Platz et al., 2000). The stroke patients suffered from central arm paresis ($n = 8$), somatosensory deficits ($n = 3$), or ideomotor apraxia ($n = 2$). The multimodal electroencephalographical (EEG) analysis suggested impairment-specific changes in the movement-related electrical activity of the brain. Patients with ideomotor apraxia showed more lateralised frontal movement-related slow cortical potentials during both movement preparation and performance, and reduced left parietal beta-ERD during movement preparation. It was concluded that apraxic patients have a relative lack of activity of the mesial frontal motor system and the left parietal cortex. Comparing the areas of overlap of lesion localisation in patients with and without ideomotor limb apraxia revealed that damage to the left middle frontal gyrus (BA46, 9, 8, and 6), and the inferior and superior parietal cortex surrounding the intraparietal sulcus (BA7, 39, and 40) more commonly produce ideomotor limb apraxia than damage to other areas (Haaland et al., 2000). Two patients with ischaemic left mesial brain damage including the SMA showed bilateral ideomotor apraxia for transitive gestures (Watson et al., 1986). In a sample of patients with AD ideomotor apraxia was associated with mild damage of the anterior cingulate cortex (BA24) (Giannakopoulos et al., 1998). In two cohort studies with patients with right and left hemispheric stroke, left brain damage was associated with impaired imitation of meaningless actions, affected imitation of hand and foot gestures more than imitation of finger gestures, and impaired perceptual matching of meaningless hand-to-head actions while right brain damage lead to impaired imitation of finger postures and perceptual matching of meaningless actions (Goldenberg, 1999; Goldenberg and Strauss, 2002).

Previously, it had been shown that small ischaemic brain lesions producing apraxia were mostly frontal and close to the body of the lateral ventricle possibly indicating that lesions of the deep parieto- and occipitofrontal, and anterior callosal fibres can be important in apraxia (Kertesz and Ferro, 1984). Callosal disconnection can result in apraxia of the left hand only (Watson and Heilman, 1983).

To ascertain the role of subcortical structures in praxis, praxis performance has been compared on a variety of tasks in patients with left hemisphere cortical and subcortical lesions (Hanna-Pladdy et al., 2001). The cortical patients presented with deficits in the production of transitive and intransitive gestures-to-verbal command and imitation, as well as impaired gesture discrimination. In contrast, the subcortical group demonstrated mild production–execution deficits for transitive pantomimes, but normal imitation and discrimination.

The notion that apraxia can be due to deep subcortical lesions raises the question as to whether damage to the basal ganglia or thalamus can cause apraxia. Eighty-two such cases of such "deep" apraxias that have been reported in the literature were reviewed (Pramstaller and Marsden, 1996). The main conclusions to be drawn from this meta-analysis are that lesions confined to the basal ganglia (putamen, caudate nucleus, and globus pallidus) rarely, if ever, cause apraxia. Apraxia occurred with deep lesions of the basal ganglia apparently sparing white matter in only eight out of the 82 cases: small lesions confined to the thalamus can sometimes cause apraxia (eight cases).

For buccofacial apraxia a high association with lesions simultaneously in the frontal operculum and the anterior paraventricular white matter has been described (Alexander et al., 1992). Facial apraxia occurs more frequently after left hemisphere damage, but is not infrequently observed among patients with right hemisphere damage (Bizzozero et al., 2000). Accordingly, it seems likely that a distributed neuroanatomical network in both hemispheres is involved in face praxis. Apraxia after unilateral damage might then be accounted for by the proposition that the left and right hemisphere contributions to face praxis do not overlap. Consequently, deficits could not be entirely compensated.

Ideational apraxia from lateralised lesions occurs mainly after left brain damage, but can be observed after right brain damage (Heilman et al., 1997) and has frequently, but not exclusively, been associated with left posterior temporoparietal junction lesions (De Renzi and Lucchelli, 1988). Movement concepts for object use might be represented in either hemisphere as suggested by unimpaired demonstration of object use in either hand (with object in hand) among patients with complete callosotomy (Lausberg et al., 2003). This capacity of either hemisphere, however, might also be related to other control processes supporting actual tool use aside from (action-related) semantic knowledge.

27.6 Clinical testing of apraxia

Signs and symptoms of motor apraxia were described both for ideomotor and ideational apraxia by Poeck who argued that positive signs for apraxia can be observed as "parapraxias", that is typical apraxic performance errors, when certain movement tasks are examined (Poeck, 1986). For ideomotor apraxia, 10 tasks for buccofacial movements and 20 tasks for movements of the upper limb both after verbal command and as imitation tasks with the rated response categories correct execution, or augmentation, fragmentary movement, perseveration, and other types of errors were suggested (Lehmkuhl et al., 1983). For ideational apraxia, the authors suggested 10 sets of five to seven photographs portraying stages of everyday life actions that have to be arranged in the correct order (Lehmkuhl and Poeck, 1981). Group discriminant validity has been demonstrated.

Similarly, De Renzi's group designed a collection of items for both ideomotor and ideational apraxia assessment. With the multiple object test patients are requested to carry out five actions as in everyday life (e.g. preparing a cup of coffee) (De Renzi and Lucchelli, 1988). Perplexity, clumsiness, omission, mislocation, misuse, and sequence errors were specified as error categories. In terms of construct validity, a low correlation with test scores for ideomotor apraxia has been shown in a sample of left brain lesioned patients. For ideomotor apraxia, a movement imitation test with 24 movements including symbolic and non-symbolic, finger and hand positions and sequences (each item ordinally scales from 0 to 3) and a demsonstration-of-use test where the patient has to demonstrate the use of 10 visually presented common objects (without touching them) (each item ordinally scales from 0 to 2) have been designed (De Renzi et al., 1980). Group discriminant validity and a cut-off scores based on performance of healthy subjects have been reported.

The Florida Apraxia Battery (FAB) incorporates a number of tasks that engage different levels of praxis processing: that is, measures of gesture reception (gesture naming, gesture decision, gesture recognition), measures of gesture production (gesture-to-verbal command – the Florida Apraxia Screening Test (FAST), revised (FAST-R), gesture-to-visual tool, gesture-to-tactile tool), praxis imitation (gesture imitation, nonsense praxis imitation), and measures of action semantics (tool selection task) (Rothi et al., 1997). The FAST-R is a 30-item gesture-to-verbal command test including 20 transitive and 10 intransitive pantomimes. Various content errors, temporal errors, and spatial errors related to apraxic performance have been defined. A cut-off score of 15 out of 30 items has been suggested. The Florida Action Recall Test (FLART), developed to assess conceptual apraxia (corresponding to the term ideational apraxia as used in this chapter), consists of 45 line drawings of objects or scenes. The subject must imagine the proper tool to apply to each pictured object or scene and then pantomime its use. Twelve participants with AD (NINCDS-ADRDA criteria) and 21 age- and education-matched controls were tested (Schwartz et al., 2000). Nine AD participants scored below a 2-standard-deviation cut-off on conceptual accuracy, and the three who scored above the cut-off were beyond a 2-standard-deviation cut-off on completion time. The FLART appeared to be a sensitive measure of conceptual apraxia in the early stages of AD.

Roy and coworker suggested a multi-dimensional error notation system with high interrater reliability where gestural performance is evaluated on five performance dimensions: orientation of the hand, action (the movement characteristics of the gesture), the posture of the hand, plane of movement of the hand, and location of the hand in space (Roy et al., 1998). Each dimension is rated with an ordinal scale (0, 1, 2). A composite score reflects overall performance accuracy.

Dobigny-Roman and coworkers (1998) proposed and evaluated more formally and extensively a test of meaningless gesture imitation and studied its relevance in elderly people. The ideomotor apraxia test (IAT) consists of showing 10 gestures, each item is graded from 0 to 3. The IAT was carried out on 55 patients with AD and 26 elderly patients without cognitive impairment. The mean apraxia score was markedly different between the AD group and the normal group. Interrater agreement was excellent (intraclass correlation coefficient = 0.995). Sensitivity and specificity were very good (95% and 88%, respectively). Age and educational level did not influence ideomotor apraxia scores.

Assessment tools for ideomotor apraxia do, however, not necessarily measure the same construct. People with unilateral left hemisphere lesions, diagnosed with apraxia, were compared in their scoring on three tests for ideomotor apraxia and one test for ideational apraxia (Butler, 2002). Correlations between scores of the three ideomotor apraxia tests were low to at the most moderate. In addition, 6 of the 17 apraxic patients scored above cut-off point on one test, but below cut-off point on others. Tests for ideomotor apraxia may therefore identify different people as "apraxic", possibly by eliciting different aspects of apraxia and identifying potential subtypes of the condition. The association between ideomotor test scores and ideational test scores was weak.

Two tests of facial apraxia, assessing upper (eyes and eyebrows; 9 items) and lower (mouth and throat; 29 items) face movements have been proposed (Bizzozero et al., 2000). Individual patients are assessed based on age- and education-adjusted population-based cut-off scores. The tests have very high test–retest reliability (reliability coefficients > 0.90).

Together with Liepelt the author constructed and evaluated a comprehensive test battery for buccofacial and limb ideomotor apraxia as well as ideational apraxia, the Berlin apraxia test (BAXT) (Liepelt and

Platz, 2003). The test assesses (1) separately buccofacial and limb ideomotor apraxia with movements elicited by different command modalities and rated with a complex error notation system; (2) the ability to discriminate observed movements; and (3) tool-use-related semantic knowledge. Item characteristics (objectivity, difficulty, item–test correlation, validity) as well as each subtest's objectivity, reliability (internal consistency, intrarater reliability, test–retest reliability), and validity (criterion, convergent and discriminant, exploratory and confirmatory factorial) have been characterised.

A cross-sectional study with 106 apraxic stroke patients has shown that specifically designed activities of daily living (ADL) observations (van Heugten et al., 1999) can measure disability due to apraxia with more sensitivity than the Barthel ADL index, a conventional functional scale (Donkervoort et al., 2002).

Other approaches to clinical testing of apraxia could be both a detailed kinematic analysis of gestures (Platz and Mauritz, 1995; Hermsdörfer et al., 1996; Merians et al., 1999) and the measurement of response times (Willis et al., 1998). Kinematic analyses revealed motion abnormalities during gesture production with regard to kinematics of movement trajectories such as shape of the trajectory, plane of motion, spatial accuracy of final hand positions, and joint motion. However, apraxic errors from qualitative motion analysis and kinematic abnormalities are not necessarily correlated. With regard to measurement of response time, the time after movement occurs until the gesture movement starts ("pregesture period") has been shown to be prolonged in a group of patients with AD. For both techniques, standardised assessment protocols that fulfil the psychometric affordances of a clinical test would have to be developed and evaluated before their clinical diagnostic use could be recommended.

27.7 Clinical relevance and therapy

Varying prevalence rates for apraxia have been reported. In a hospital-based survey of 100 patients with unilateral left brain damage and 80 patients with unilateral right brain damage, De Renzi and coworkers (1980) documented prevalence rates of 50% and 20%, respectively, for ideomotor limb apraxia. Kertesz and coauthors (1984) found ideomotor apraxia in 83 (54.6%) of 152 patients with a left hemispheric stroke examined within the first month of stroke. Four hundred and ninety-two first left hemisphere stroke patients from 14 rehabilitation centres and 34 nursing homes in the Netherlands who had been referred for occupational therapy had 28% and 37% prevalence rates of apraxia as assessed by clinical judgement (ADL, imitation, object use) (Donkervoort et al., 2000).

Applying two tests of facial apraxia, assessing upper (eyes and eyebrows) and lower (mouth and throat) face movements indicated that 46% and 68% of left hemisphere stroke patients showed apraxia for upper and lower face, respectively (Bizzozero et al., 2000). Further, a substantial proportion of right hemisphere stroke patients also showed facial apraxia (i.e. 44% for upper face and 38% for lower face).

A population-based assessment of the prevalence of buccofacial and limb ideomotor apraxia in 776 unselected acute stroke patients that where assessed within 7 days after stroke documented ideomotor limb apraxia in only 10% in left and 4% in right hemispheric stroke and buccofacial apraxia in only 9% in left and 4% in right hemispheric stroke (Pedersen et al., 2001).

These numbers are astonishingly different and therefore it is difficult to report the "true" prevalence rates. While the former prevalence rates might be overestimated secondary to a selection bias, the latter could be due to detection bias since a simple 3-item test has been used for both buccofacial and ideomotor limb apraxia. The least that can be stated is that apraxia affects a significant proportion of stroke patients.

In addition, it must be noted that spontaneous recovery from ideomotor apraxia occurs over many months after stroke and thus significantly affects prevalence rates (Basso et al., 1987).

In other, spontaneously deteriorating conditions such as AD, CBD, PSP, PD, or HD, limbkinetic apraxia (CBD, PSP), ideomotor apraxia (AD, CBD, PSP,

PD, HD), and ideational apraxia (AD, CBD) can be observed in considerable proportions of patients especially with more advanced disease stages (Shelton and Knopman, 1991; Ochipa et al., 1992; Travniczek-Marterer et al., 1993; Leiguarda et al., 1994, 1997, 2003).

(Ideomotor) apraxia does affect ADL affording arm motor control. This was shown in cohorts of left hemisphere ischaemic stroke patients with ideomotor apraxia when the level of verbal or physical assistance for the initiation, execution, and control that a patient needs to perform activities successfully (Donkervoort et al., 2002), or the degree of caregiver assistance in physical functioning, for example in grooming, bathing, and toileting was rated (Hanna-Pladdy et al., 2003), or when mealtime organisation and adequacy of action components during mealtime were observed (Foundas et al., 1995a).

Ideomotor apraxia does also influence spontaneous conversational gestures (Foundas et al., 1995b) and may negatively affect the use of spontaneous communicative gestures (Borod et al., 1989).

One therapeutic approach could be to teach strategies to compensate for continued apraxic deficits. Using such an approach, improvements have been reported in ADL. In a cohort study with 15 left hemisphere apraxic stroke patients, therapeutic advice has been given for only one of three ADL per week. Reduction of errors for any given activity were only observed in the week when the respective activity has been trained (Goldenberg and Hagmann, 1998b). In another cohort study, 33 left hemisphere apraxic stroke patients who had difficulties to carry out purposeful activities received a 12-week course of strategy training where every 2 weeks one activity was trained with graded therapeutic support with regard to planning, executing, and controlling/correcting this activity (van Heugten et al., 1998). In this study, relatively large therapeutic effects in ADL functioning were observed.

Another more restorative therapeutic approach would be to focus on the primary deficit and to train complex movements and gesture production. Prior casuistic evidence suggested that apraxic errors can be reduced by training, but effects would not generalise to untrained error types or even the same error types in different gestures (Maher and Ochipa, 1997). More recently, however, a randomised controlled trial with 13 ideational and/or ideomotor apraxic left hemisphere stroke patients receiving a more comprehensive complex movement- and gesture-production training programme made up of three sections dedicated to the treatment of complex movements without symbolic value and gestures (with symbolic value) both related and unrelated to the use of objects provided more promising evidence (Smania et al., 2000). Thirty-five experimental sessions, each lasting 50 min, were given. The control group received conventional treatment for aphasia. The patients who received the movement- and gesture-production training programme achieved a significant improvement of performance in both ideational and ideomotor apraxia tests.

Apraxia results not only in relatively coarse apraxic errors: a clinically relatively subtle impairment that can be important for everyday life in hemiparetic subjects is the loss of dexterity of the non-paretic arm and movement deficits when actually handling tools. Persistence of impaired dexterity of the non-paretic arm (Sunderland, 2000) and a reduced accuracy for more demanding aimed movements (Haaland and Harrington, 1994) have been shown to be related to apraxia after left hemisphere stroke. Aiming, tapping, line following, and steadiness have all been shown to be impaired in apraxic patients (Motomura, 1994). Apraxics show various movement deficits when actually using objects, that is improperly coordinated joint motions and irregular trajectories and deviant movement planes that affect performance with everyday life activities (Poizner et al., 1997). In conclusion, it seems that ideomotor apraxia does negatively affect a variety of sensorimotor abilities and skills in everyday life. It is important to note that these deficits occur (also) in the non-paretic arm that many patients have to rely on as a compensatory measure.

In summary, apraxic disorders are prevalent in different neurological patient groups, affect motor competence in everyday life tasks and communication. First promising evidence suggests that apraxia is amenable to both strategy training and restorative training. In current clinical practice, however, its relevance is not widely reflected in a systematic clinical approach to diagnosis of apraxia and consecutive counselling and treatment.

27.8 Conclusions

Apraxic phenomena occur frequently in various neurological conditions. Praxis involves many processes from semantics to "online" dynamic motor control (compare Fig. 27.1). These processes are likely to be differentially impaired in different neurological conditions with their differential neuroanatomical distribution of brain dysfunction and damage since distributed brain networks are involved in various cognitive-perceptual-motor processes related to praxis.

Selective motion control is viewed as the basic capacity to make fine and precise, isolated or independent face or limb movements. Its deficit can indicate limbkinetic apraxia if it is not associated with – or at least out of proportion of – paresis, somatosensory deafferentation, or ataxia. Core deficit in ideomotor apraxia could be deficient short-term (imitation of meaningless movements) or long-term (pantomime of meaningful actions) complex movement representations, that is the combination of invariant features of intrinsic and extrinsic egocentric coding for a given movement, that are most important when movements have to be performed outside their typical environmental context. Ideational apraxia would be defined by a semantic deficit related to action, frontal apraxia by an action-sequencing deficit.

Currently, more detailed neuroscientific knowledge about apraxia and more rigorously developed and validated assessment tools become available. These and the more refined concepts about apraxic disorders can lead to the development and clinical evaluation of specific training concepts that offer restorative or compensatory approaches for patients. First promising evidence suggests that apraxia is amenable to strategy and restorative training.

REFERENCES

Alexander, M.P., Baker, E., Naeser, M.A., Kaplan, E. and Palumbo, C. (1992). Neuropsychological and neuroanatomical dimensions of ideomotor apraxia. *Brain*, **115**, 87–107.

Barbieri, C. and De Renzi, E. (1988). The executive and ideational components of apraxia. *Cortex*, **24**, 535–543.

Basso, A., Capitani, E., Della, S.S., Laiacona, M. and Spinnler, H. (1987). Recovery from ideomotor apraxia. A study on acute stroke patients. *Brain*, **110**, 747–760.

Belanger, S.A. and Duffy, R.J. (1996). The assessment of limb apraxia: an investigation of task effects and their cause. *Brain Cogn*, **32**, 383–404.

Binkofski, F., Buccino, G., Posse, S., Seitz, R.J., Rizzolatti, G. and Freund, H.J. (1999). A fronto-parietal circuit for object manipulation in man: evidence from an fMRI-study. *Eur J Neurosci*, **11**, 3276–3286.

Bizzozero, I., Costato, D., Sala, S.D., Papagno, C., Spinnler, H. and Venneri, A. (2000). Upper and lower face apraxia: role of the right hemisphere. *Brain*, **123**, 2213–2230.

Borod, J.C., Fitzpatrick, P.M., Helm-Estabrooks, N. and Goodglass, H. (1989). The relationship between limb apraxia and the spontaneous use of communicative gesture in aphasia. *Brain Cogn*, **10**, 121–131.

Botvinick, M. and Plaut, D.C. (2004). Doing without schema hierarchies: a recurrent connectionist approach to normal and impaired routine sequential action. *Psychol Rev*, **111**, 395–429.

Buccino, G., Binkofski, F. and Fink, G.R. (2001). Action observation activates premotor and parietal areas in a somatotopic manner: an fMRI study. *Eur J Neurosci*, **13**, 400–404.

Butler, J.A. (2002). How comparable are tests of apraxia? *Clin Rehabil*, **16**, 389–398.

Buxbaum, L.J. (2001). Ideomotor apraxia: a call to action. *Neurocase*, **7**, 445–458.

Buxbaum, L.J., Schwartz, M.F. and Carew, T.G. (1997). The role of semantic memory in object use. *Cogn Neuropsychol*, **14**, 219–254.

Buxbaum, L.J., Sirigu, A., Schwartz, M.F. and Klatzky, R. (2003). Cognitive representations of hand posture in ideomotor apraxia. *Neuropsychologia*, **41**, 1091–1113.

Cooper, R. (2002). Order and disorder in everyday action: the roles of contention scheduling and supervisory attention. *Neurocase*, **8**, 61–79.

Decety, J., Grézes, J., Costes, N., Perani, D., Jeannerod, M., Procyk, E., Grassi, F. and Fazio, F. (1997). Brain activity during observation of actions. *Brain*, **120**, 1763–1777.

de Jong, B.M., van der Graaf, F.H. and Paans, A.M. (2001). Brain activation related to the representations of external space and body scheme in visuomotor control. *Neuroimage*, **14**, 1128–1135.

De Renzi, E. and Lucchelli, F. (1988). Ideational apraxia. *Brain*, **111**, 1173–1185.

De Renzi, E., Motti, F. and Nichelli, P. (1980). Imitating gestures. A quantitative approach to ideomotor apraxia. *Arch Neurol*, **37**, 6–10.

De Renzi, E., Faglioni, P. and Sorgato, P. (1982). Modality-specific and supramodal mechanisms of apraxia. *Brain*, **105**, 301–312.

Dobigny-Roman, N., Dieudonne-Moinet, B., Tortrat, D., Verny, M. and Forette, B. (1998). Ideomotor apraxia test: a new test of imitation of gestures for elderly people. *Eur J Neurol*, **5**, 571–578.

Donkervoort, M., Dekker, J., van den Ende, E., Stehmann-Saris, J.C. and Deelman, B.G. (2000). Prevalence of apraxia among patients with a first left hemisphere stroke in rehabilitation centres and nursing homes. *Clin Rehabil*, **14**, 130–136.

Donkervoort, M., Dekker, J. and Deelman, B.G. (2002). Sensitivity of different ADL measures to apraxia and motor impairments. *Clin Rehabil*, **16**, 299–305.

Doyon, J., Owen, A.M., Petrides, M., Sziklas, V. and Evans, A.C. (1996). Functional anatomy of visuomotor skill learning in human subjects examined with positron emission tomography. *Eur J Neurosci*, **8**, 637–648.

Dumont, C., Ska, B. and Joanette, Y. (2000). Conceptual apraxia and semantic memory deficit in Alzheimer's disease: two sides of the same coin? *J Int Neuropsychol Soc*, **6**, 693–703.

Fogassi, L., Gallese, V., Buccino, G., Craighero, L., Fadiga, L. and Rizzolatti, G. (2001). Cortical mechanism for the visual guidance of hand grasping movements in the monkey: a reversible inactivation study. *Brain*, **124**, 571–586.

Forde, E.M.E. and Humphreys, G.W. (2000). The role of semantic knowledge and working memory in everyday tasks. *Brain Cogn*, **44**, 214–252.

Foundas, A.L., Macauley, B.L., Raymer, A.M., Maher, L.M., Heilman, K.M. and Rothi, L.J. (1995a). Ecological implications of limb apraxia: evidence from mealtime behavior. *J Int Neuropsychol Soc*, **1**, 62–66.

Foundas, A.L., Macauley, B.L., Raymer, A.M., Maher, L.M., Heilman, K.M. and Rothi, L.J. (1995b). Gesture laterality in aphasic and apraxic stroke patients. *Brain Cogn*, **29**, 204–213.

Foundas, A.L., Macauley, B.L., Raymer, A.M., Maher, L.M., Rothi, L.J. and Heilman, K.M. (1999). Ideomotor apraxia in Alzheimer disease and left hemisphere stroke: limb transitive and intransitive movements. *Neuropsychiatr Neuropsychol Behav Neurol*, **12**, 161–166.

Frencham, K.A.R., Fox, A.M. and Maybery, M.T. (2003). The hand movement test as a tool in neuropsychological

assessment: interpretation within a working memory theoretical framework. *J Int Neuropsychol Soc*, **9**, 633–641.

Funahashi, S., Bruce, C.J. and Goldman-Rakic, P.S. (1989). Mnemonic coding of visual space in the monkey's dorsolateral prefrontal cortex. *J Neurophysiol*, **61**, 331–349.

Gallese, V., Fadiga, L., Fogassi, L., Rizzolatti, G. (1996). Action recognition in the premotor Cortex. *Brain*, **119**, 593–609.

Giannakopoulos, P., Duc, M., Gold, G., Hof, P.R., Michel, J.-P. and Bouras, C. (1998). Pathologic correlates of apraxia in Alzheimer disease. *Arch Neurol*, **55**, 689–695.

Goldenberg, G. (1999). Matching and imitation of hand and finger postures in patients with damage in the left or right hemispheres. *Neuropsychologia*, **37**, 559–566.

Goldenberg, G. (2003). Pantomime of object use: a challenge to cerebral localization of cognitive function. *Neuroimage*, **20**(**Suppl. 1**), S101–S106.

Goldenberg, G. and Hagmann, S. (1998a). Tool use and mechanical problem solving in apraxia. *Neuropsychologia*, **36**, 581–589.

Goldenberg, G. and Hagmann, S. (1998b). Therapy of activities of daily living in patients with apraxia. *Neuropsychol Rehabil*, **2**, 123–141.

Goldenberg, G. and Strauss, S. (2002). Hemisphere asymmetries for imitation of novel gestures. *Neurology*, **59**, 893–897.

Goldenberg, G., Hermsdorfer, J. and Spatt, J. (1996). Ideomotor apraxia and cerebral dominance for motor control. *Brain Res Cogn Brain Res*, **3**, 95–100.

Goldenberg, G., Hartmann, K. and Schlott, I. (2003). Defective pantomime of object use in left brain damage: apraxia or asymbolia? *Neuropsychologia*, **41**, 1565–1573.

Haaland, K.Y. and Harrington, D.L. (1994). Limb-sequencing deficits after left but not right hemisphere damage. *Brain Cogn*, **24**, 104–122.

Haaland, K.Y., Harrington, D.L. and Knight, R.T. (1999). Spatial deficits in ideomotor limb apraxia. *Brain*, **122**, 1169–1182.

Haaland, K.Y., Harrington, D.L. and Knight, R.T. (2000). Neural representations of skilled movement. *Brain*, **123**, 2306–2313.

Halsband, U., Schmitt, J., Weyers, M., Binkofski, F., Grützner, G. and Freund, H.-J. (2001). Recognition and imitation of pantomimed motor acts after unilateral parietal and premotor lesions: a perspective on apraxia. *Neuropsychologia*, **39**, 200–216.

Hamilton, J.M., Haaland, K.Y., Adair, J.C. and Brandt, J. (2003). Ideomotor limb apraxia in Huntington's disease: implications for corticostriate involvement. *Neuropsychologia*, **41**, 614–621.

Hanna-Pladdy, B., Heilman, K.M. and Foundas, A.L. (2001). Cortical and subcortical contributions to ideomotor apraxia: analysis of task demands and error types. *Brain*, **124**, 2513–2527.

Hanna-Pladdy, B., Heilman, K.M. and Foundas, A.L. (2003). Ecological implications of ideomotor apraxia: evidence from physical activities of daily living. *Neurology*, **60**, 487–490.

Heath, M., Almeida, Q.J., Roy, E.A., Black, S.E. and Westwood, D. (2003). Selective dysfunction of tool-use: a failure to integrate somatosensation and action. *Neurocase*, **9**, 156–163.

Heilman, K.M., Schwartz, H.D. and Geschwind, N. (1975). Defective motor learning in ideomotor apraxia. *Neurology*, **25**, 1018–1020.

Heilman, K.M., Maher, L.M., Greenwald, M.L. and Rothi, L.J. (1997). Conceptual apraxia from lateralized lesions. *Neurology*, **49**, 457–464.

Heilman, K.M., Meador, K.J. and Loring, D.W. (2000). Hemispheric asymmetries of limb-kinetic apraxia: a loss of deftness. *Neurology*, **55**, 523–526.

Hermsdörfer, J., Mai, N., Spatt, J., Marquardt, C., Veltkamp, R. and Goldenberg, G. (1996). Kinematic analysis of movement imitation in apraxia. *Brain*, **119**, 1575–1586.

Hermsdörfer, J., Goldenberg, G., Wachsmuth, C., Conrad, B., Ceballos-Baumann, A.O., Bartenstein, P., Schwaiger, M. and Boecker, H. (2001). Cortical correlates of gesture processing: clues to the cerebral mechanisms underlying apraxia during the imitation of meaningless gestures. *Neuroimage*, **14**, 149–161.

Hodges, J.R., Bozeat, S., Lambon Ralph, M.A., Patterson, K. and Spatt, J. (2000). The role of conceptual knowledge in object use. Evidence from semantic dementia. *Brain*, **123**, 1913–1925.

Ietswaart, M., Carey, D.P., Della, S.S. and Dijkhuizen, R.S. (2001). Memory-driven movements in limb apraxia: is there evidence for impaired communication between the dorsal and the ventral streams? *Neuropsychologia*, **39**, 950–961.

Jacobs, D.H., Adair, J.C., Williamson, D.J., Na, D.L., Gold, M., Foundas, A.L., Shuren, J.E., Cibula, J.E. and Heilman, K.M. (1999). Apraxia and motor-skill acquisition in Alzheimer's disease are dissociable. *Neuropsychologia*, **37**, 875–880.

Kareken, D.A., Unverzagt, F., Caldemeyer, K., Farlow, M.R. and Hutchins, G.D. (1998). Functional brain imaging in apraxia. *Arch Neurol*, **55**, 107–113.

Kertesz, A. and Ferro, J.M. (1984). Lesion size and location in ideomotor apraxia. *Brain*, **107**, 921–933.

Kertesz, A., Ferro, J.M. and Shewan, C.M. (1984). Apraxia and aphasia: the functional–anatomical basis for their dissociation. *Neurology*, **34**, 40–47.

Kimura, D. (1977). Acquisition of a motor skill after left hemisphere damage. *Brain*, **100**, 275–286.

Lausberg, H., Cruz, R.F., Kita, S., Zaidel, E. and Ptito, A. (2003). Pantomime to visual presentation of objects: left hand dyspraxia in patients with complete callosotomy. *Brain*, **126**, 343–360.

Lehmkuhl, G. and Poeck, K. (1981). A disturbance in the conceptual organization of actions in patients with ideational apraxia. *Cortex*, **17**, 153–158.

Lehmkuhl, G., Poeck, K. and Willmes, K. (1983). Ideomotor apraxia and aphasia: an examination of types and manifestations of apraxic symptoms. *Neuropsychologia*, **21**, 199–212.

Leiguarda, R., Lees, A.J., Merello, M., Starkstein, S. and Marsden, C.D. (1994). The nature of apraxia in corticobasal degeneration. *J Neurol Neurosurg Psychiatr*, **57**, 455–459.

Leiguarda, R.C., Pramstaller, P.P., Merello, M., Starkstein, S., Lees, A.J. and Marsden, C.D. (1997). Apraxia in Parkinson's disease, progressive supranuclear palsy, multiple system atrophy and neuroleptic-induced Parkinsonism. *Brain*, **120(Pt 1)**, 75–90.

Leiguarda, R.C., Merello, M., Nouzeilles, M.I., Balej, J., Rivero, A. and Nogues, M. (2003). Limb-kinetic apraxia in corticobasal degeneration: clinical and kinematic features. *Mov Disord*, **18**, 49–59.

Liepelt, I. and Platz, T. (2003). Reliability and validity of the Berlin apraxia test. *Joint Meeting of the International Neuropsychological Society (INS) and German Neuropsychological Society (GNP)*, 16–19 July 2003, Berlin. *J Int Neuropsychol Soc*, **9**, 521 (abstract).

Liepmann, H. (1920). Apraxie. In: *Ergebnisse der gesamten Medizin* (ed. Brugsch, T.), Urban & Schwarzenberg, Berlin Wien, pp. 516–543.

Maher, L.M. and Ochipa, C. (1997). Management and treatment of limb apraxia. In: *Apraxia. The Neuropsychology of Action* (eds Rothi, L.J. and Heilman, K.M.), Psychology Press, East Sussex, pp. 75–91.

Meador, K.J., Loring, D.W., Lee, K., Hughes, M., Lee, G., Nichols, M. and Heilman, K.M. (1999). Cerebral lateralization: relationship of language and ideomotor praxis. *Neurology*, **53**, 2028–2031.

Merians, A.S., Clark, M., Poizner, H., Macauley, B., Rothi, L.J. and Heilman, K.M. (1997). Visual-imitative dissociation apraxia. *Neuropsychologia*, **35**, 1483–1490.

Merians, A.S., Clark, M., Poizner, H., Jacobs, D.H., Adair, J.C., Macauley, B., Raymer, A.M., Rothi, L.J. and Heilman, K.M. (1999). Apraxia differs in corticobasal degeneration and left-parietal stroke: a case study. *Brain Cogn*, **29**, 204–213.

Moll, J., Oliveira-Souza, R., Souza-Lima, F. and Andreiuolo, P.A. (1998). Activation of left intraparietal sulcus using a fMRI conceptual praxis paradigm. *Arq Neuropsiquiatr*, **56**, 808–811.

Moll, J., Oliveira-Souza, R., Passman, L.J., Cunha, F.C., Souza-Lima, F. and Andreiuolo, P.A. (2000). Functional MRI correlates of real and imagined tool-use pantomimes. *Neurology*, **54**, 1331–1336.

Motomura, N. (1994). Motor performance in aphasia and ideomotor apraxia. *Percept Motor Skill*, **79**, 719–722.

Ochipa, C., Rothi, L.J. and Heilman, K.M. (1989). Ideational apraxia: a deficit in tool selection and use. *Ann Neurol*, **25**, 190–193.

Ochipa, C., Rothi, L.J. and Heilman, K.M. (1992). Conceptual apraxia in Alzheimer's disease. *Brain*, **115**(**Pt 4**), 1061–1071.

Ohgami, Y., Matsuo, K., Uchida, N. and Nakai, T. (2004). An fMRI study of tool-use gestures: body part as object and pantomime. *Neuroreport*, **15**, 1903–1906.

Pause, W., Kunesch, E., Binkofski, F. and Freund, H.-J. (1989). Sensorimotor disturbances in patients with lesions of the parietal cortex. *Brain*, **112**, 1599–1625.

Pedersen, P.M., Jorgensen, H.S., Kammersgaard, L.P., Nakayama, H., Raaschou, H.O. and Olsen, T.S. (2001). Manual and oral apraxia in acute stroke, frequency and influence on functional outcome. The Copenhagen stroke study. *Am J Phys Med Rehabil*, **80**, 685–692.

Peigneux, P., Salmon, E., Garraux, G., Laureys, S., Willems, S., Dujardin, K., Degueldre, C., Lemaire, C., Luxen, A., Moonen, G., Franck, G., Destee, A. and van der Linden, M. (2001). Neural and cognitive bases of upper limb apraxia in corticobasal degeneration. *Neurology*, **57**, 1259–1268.

Perenin, M.T. and Vighetto, A. (1988). Optic ataxia: a specific disruption in visuomotor mechanisms. *Brain*, **111**, 643–674.

Pharr, V., Uttl, B., Stark, M., Litvan, I., Fantie, B. and Grafman, J. (2001). Comparison of apraxia in corticobasal degeneration and progressive supranuclear palsy. *Neurology*, **56**, 957–963.

Platz, T. and Mauritz, K.H. (1995). Human motor planning, motor programming, and use of new task-relevant information with different apraxic syndromes. *Eur J Neurosci*, **7**, 1536–1547.

Platz, T. and Mauritz, K.H. (1997). Syndrome-specific deficits of performance and effects of practice on arm movements with deafferentation due to posterior thalamic lesion. *Behav Neurol*, **10**, 15–19.

Platz, T., Kim, I.H., Pintschovius, H., Winter, T., Kieselbach, A., Villringer, K., Kurth, R. and Mauritz, K.H. (2000). Multimodal EEG analysis in man suggests impairment-specific changes in movement-related electric brain activity after stroke. *Brain*, **123**(**Pt 12**), 2475–2490.

Poeck, K. (1986). The clinical examination for motor apraxia. *Neuropsychologia*, **24**, 129–134.

Poizner, H., Clark, M., Merians, A.S., Macauley, B., Rothi, L.J.G. and Heilman, K.M. (1995). Joint coordination deficits in limb apraxia. *Brain*, **118**, 227–242.

Poizner, H., Merians, A.S., Clark, M., Rothi, L.J.G. and Heilman, K.M. (1997). Kinematic approaches to the study of apraxic disorders. In: *Apraxia. The Neuropsychology of Action* (eds Rothi, L.J.G. and Heilman, K.M.), Psychology Press, East Sussex, pp. 93–109.

Pramstaller, P.P. and Marsden, C.D. (1996). The basal ganglia and apraxia. *Brain*, **119**(**Pt 1**), 319–340.

Raymer, A.M., Maher, L.M., Foundas, A.L., Heilman, K.M. and Gonzalez Rothi, L.J. (1997). The significance of body part as tool errors in limb apraxia. *Brain Cogn*, **34**, 287–292.

Raymer, A.M., Merians, A.S., Adair, J.C., Schwartz, R.L., Williamson, D.J.G., Rothi, L.J.G., Poizner, H. and Heilman, K.M. (1999). Crossed apraxia: implications for handedness. *Cortex*, **35**, 183–199.

Rizzolatti, G. and Matelli, M. (2003). Two different streams from the dorsal visual system: anatomy and functions. *Exp Brain Res*, **153**, 146–175.

Rizzolatti, G., Camarda, R., Fogassi, L., Gentilucci, M., Luppino, G. and Matelli, M. (1988). Functional organization of area 6 in macaque monkey. II. Area F5 and the control of distal movements. *Exp Brain Res*, **71**, 491–507.

Rothi, L.J., Ochipa, C. and Heilman, K.M. (1991). A cognitive neuropsychological model of limb praxis. *Cogn Neuropsychol*, **8**, 443–458.

Rothi, L.J., Raymer, A.M. and Heilman, K.M. (1997). Limb praxis assessment. In: *Apraxia. The Neuropsychology of Action* (eds Rothi, L.J. and Heilman, K.M.), Psychology Press, East Sussex, pp. 61–74.

Roy, E.A., Square-Storer, P. and Hogg, S. (1991). Analysis of task demands in apraxia. *Int J Neurosci*, **56**, 177–186.

Roy, E.A., Black, S.E., Blair, N. and Dimeck, P.T. (1998). Analyses of deficits in gestural pantomime. *J Clin Exp Neuropsychol*, **20**, 628–643.

Rumiati, R.I., Zanini, S., Vorano, L. and Shallice, T. (2001). A form of ideational apraxia as a selective deficit of contention scheduling. *Cogn Neuropsychol*, **18**, 617–642.

Rumiati, R.I., Weiss, P.H., Shallice, T., Ottoboni, G., Noth, J., Zilles, K. and Fink, G.R. (2004). Neural basis of pantomiming the use of visually presented objects. *Neuroimage*, **21**, 1224–1231.

Rushworth, M.F., Johansen-Berg, H., Gobel, S.M. and Devlin, J.T. (2003). The left parietal and premotor cortices: motor attention and selection. *Neuroimage*, **20**(**Suppl. 1**), S89–S100.

Schluter, N.D., Krams, M., Rishworth, M.F.S. and Passingham, R.E. (2001). Cerebral dominance for action in the human brain: the selection of actions. *Neuropsychologia*, **39**, 105–113.

Schnider, A., Hanlon, R.E., Alexander, D.N. and Benson, D.F. (1997). Ideomotor apraxia: behavioral dimensions and neuroanatomical basis. *Brain Lang*, **58**, 125–136.

Schwartz, R.L., Adair, J.C., Raymer, A.M., Williamson, D.J., Crosson, B., Rothi, L.J., Nadeau, S.E. and Heilman, K.M. (2000). Conceptual apraxia in probable Alzheimer's disease as demonstrated by the Florida action recall test. *J Int Neuropsychol Soc*, **6**, 265–270.

Seitz, R.J. and Roland, P.E. (1992). Learning of sequential finger movements in man: a combined kinematic and positron emission tomography (PET) study. *Eur J Neurosci*, **4**, 154–165.

Shelton, P.A. and Knopman, D.S. (1991). Ideomotor apraxia in Huntington's disease. *Arch Neurol*, **48**, 35–41.

Sirigu, A., Da prati, E., Pradat-Diehl, P., Franck, N. and Jeannerod, M. (1999). Perception of self-generated movement following left parietal lesion. *Brain*, **122**, 1867–1874.

Smania, N., Girardi, F., Domenicali, C., Lora, E. and Aglioti, S. (2000). The rehabilitation of limb apraxia: a study in left-brain-damaged patients. *Arch Phys Med Rehabil*, **81**, 379–388.

Sunderland, A. (2000). Recovery of ipsilateral dexterity after stroke. *Stroke*, **31**, 430–433.

Sunderland, A. and Sluman, S.M. (2000). Ideomotor apraxia, visuomotor control and the explicit representation of posture. *Neuropsychologia*, **38**, 923–934.

Toraldo, A., Reverberi, C. and Rumiati, R.I. (2001). Critical dimensions affecting imitation performance of patients with ideomotor apraxia. *Cortex*, **37**, 737–740.

Travniczek-Marterer, A., Danielczyk, W., Simanyi, M. and Fischer, P. (1993). Ideomotor apraxia in Alzheimer's disease. *Acta Neurol Scand*, **88**, 1–4.

Ungerleider, L.G. and Mishkin, M. (1982). Two cortical visual systems. In: *Analysis of Visual Behavior* (eds Ingle, D.J., Goodale, M.A. and Manfield, R.J.W.), MIT Press, Cambridge.

van Heugten, C.M., Dekker, J., Deelman, B.G., et al. (1998). Outcome of strategy training in stroke patients with apraxia: a phase II study. *Clin Rehabil*, **12**, 294–303.

van Heugten, C.M., Dekker, J., Deelman, B.G., Stehmann-Saris, J.C. and Kinebanian, A. (1999). Assessment of disabilities in stroke patients with apraxia: internal consistency and inter-observer reliability. *Occup Ther J Res*, **19**, 55–73.

Wada, Y., Nakagawa, Y., Nishikawa, T., Aso, N., Inokawa, M., Kashiwagi, A., Tanabe, H. and Takeda, M. (1999). Role of somatosensory feedback from tools in realizing movements by patients with ideomotor apraxia. *Eur Neurol*, **41**, 73–78.

Watson, R.T. and Heilman, K.M. (1983). Callosal apraxia. *Brain*, **106(Pt 2)**, 391–403.

Watson, R.T., Fleet, W.S., Gonzalez-Rothi, L. and Heilman, K.M. (1986). Apraxia and the supplementary motor area. *Arch Neurol*, **43**, 787–792.

Willis, L., Behrens, M., Mack, W. and Chui, H. (1998). Ideomotor apraxia in early Alzheimer's disease: time and accuracy measures. *Brain Cogn*, **38**, 220–233.

Zanini, S., Rumiati, R.I. and Shalice, T. (2002). Action sequencing deficit following frontal lobe lesion. *Neurocase*, **8**, 88–99.

Unilateral neglect and anosognosia

Stephanie Clarke and Claire Bindschaedler

Division de neuropsychologie, centre hospitalier universitaire vaudois, Lausanne, Switzerland

28.1 Unilateral neglect

Modular deficit

Unilateral hemineglect is characterised by lack or decrease of attention to stimuli and events on one side of the patient following a contralateral hemispheric lesion. In chronic patients neglect concerns the left hemispace. In extreme cases, patients do not react when they are spoken to from the left side, do not eat food on the left half of their plate, do not shave or make up the left half of their face, or read the left side of their newspaper. Formal testing of hemineglect consists of tests that require cancelling of items on a sheet of paper, copying or drawing of objects, line bisection, dichotic listening or simultaneous tactile stimulation, as well as behavioural and motor assessment (Azouvi et al., 2002, 2003; Perennou et al., 2002).

Hemineglect can affect, sometimes to a varying degree, visual, auditory, somatosensory and motor modalities (Barbieri and De Renzi, 1989).

In the visual modality, hemineglect does not only affect perception but also mental imagery. Bisiach and Luzzatti (1978) described the case of a patient whose hemineglect affected mental images of well-known Milanese landmarks. The perceptual and imagery aspects of visuo-spatial neglect can be affected independently, as demonstrated by the occurrence of selective deficits for extra-personal space, but not for visual images (Anderson, 1993) and a double dissociation between vision and visual imagery (Guariglia et al., 1993; Coslett, 1997). Left visuo-spatial neglect can affect also differently near and far space; selective deficits for one or the other aspect and double dissociations were reported (Guariglia and Antonucci, 1992; Cowey et al., 1994; Beschin and Robertson, 1997). Furthermore, stimuli that are correctly perceived in a type of task may be neglected in another; Marshall and Halligan (1995) described a case of a patient who perceived correctly global forms of figures that were composed of small elements, but on cancellation task this patient crossed only the right half of the small elements.

Auditory neglect, defined as inattention to stimuli within the left hemispace, is mostly diagnosed by left ear extinction in dichotic listening tasks (Heilman and Valenstein, 1972) or by the presence of systematic directional errors to the ipsilesional space in sound localisation tasks (Bisiach et al., 1984; Vallar et al., 1995; Sterzi et al., 1996). Recently two types of auditory neglect have been described, one corresponding to a primarily attentional deficit and the other to distortions of auditory space representations (Bellmann et al., 2001; Clarke and Thiran, 2004).

In the somatosensory modality left sided extinction in a bilateral stimulation paradigm has been interpreted as sign of neglect. The degree of extinction of left hand stimulations was reported to depend in some patients on the position of the hand in respect to the body (Smania and Aglioti, 1995; Aglioti et al., 1999) but not in others (Bartolomeo et al., 2004). Tactile exploration of neglect patients was reported to be reduced within the left hemispace (Haeske-Dewick et al., 1996; Beschin et al., 1997; Karnath and Perenin,

1998), with greater neglect for far space in some patients (Beschin et al., 1996).

Motor neglect is characterised by decreased use of the left side of the body without underlying deficits in strength, reflexes or sensibility (Laplane and Degos, 1983). It can occur in the absence of deficits in purely perceptual neglect tasks (Bottini et al., 1992).

Anatomo-clinical correlations

Anatomo-clinical correlations in cases of left-sided neglect stressed the critical role of right hemispheric lesions (Brain, 1941; McFie et al., 1950) and within this hemisphere, of specific regions (Fig. 28.1). The most common lesion site in left visuo-spatial hemi-neglect involves the inferior parietal lobule (Vallar and Perani, 1986; Fig. 28.1). However visual neglect

can occur also in right frontal lesions (Heilman and Valenstein, 1972) and in particular those of the dorsal aspect of the inferior frontal gyrus (Husain and Kennard, 1996; Fig. 28.1). Hemineglect occurs also in association with subcortical lesions of the thalamus (Watson and Heilman, 1979; Watson et al., 1981), the basal ganglia (Hier et al., 1977; Damasio et al., 1980; Healton et al., 1982) and/or the internal capsula (Ferro and Kertesz, 1984). Several cases of left hemineglect following subcortical lesions were investigated by single positron emission computer tomography (SPECT), demonstrating cortical hypoperfusion (Perani et al., 1987; Bogousslavsky et al., 1988; Weiller et al., 1993). Although left spatial hemineglect is most often discussed in terms of unilateral right lesions, most cases that are referred for clinical evaluation or for rehabilitation may have bilateral

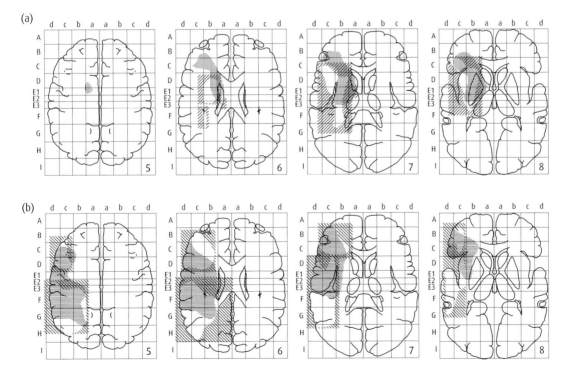

Figure 28.1. Anatomo-clinical correlations of left unilateral neglect. Very different type of right hemispheric lesions can be associated with left unilateral neglect. Top row (a): Example of two cases with subcortical lesions centered on basal ganglia. Bottom row (b): Example of two other cases with mainly parieto-frontal cortical lesions. Adapted from Bellmann et al. (2001).

lesions, as suggested by a recent study (Weintraub et al., 1996). Furthermore it has to be considered that even purely unilateral hemispheric lesions can be accompanied by dysfunction within the intact contralateral hemisphere (Fig. 28.2; Adriani et al., 2003).

Acute stage and beyond

In the acute stage neglect phenomena have been reported after right or left hemispheric lesions. Visual neglect in the contralesional space was found in 83% of right and in 65% of left lesions; hemi-inattention in 70% of right and in 49% of left lesions; tactile extinction in 65% of right and in 35% of left lesions; allaesthesia in 57% of right and in 11% of left lesions; and visual extinction in 23% of right and in 2% of left lesions (Stone et al., 1993).

Several studies described the correlation between the presence of hemineglect beyond the acute stage and poor outcome in terms of independence (Denes et al., 1982; Stone et al., 1992; Buxbaum et al., 2004). Persistent neglect is often associated with large lesions and/or other cognitive deficits (Maguire and Ogden, 2002).

Treatment

Current evidence suggests that neglect rehabilitation is associated with better outcome. In particular, a recent Cochrane review (Bowen et al., 2002) analysed 15 randomised studies and found evidence that cognitive rehabilitation resulted in significant and persisting improvements on impairment level. This study found, however, insufficient evidence to confirm or

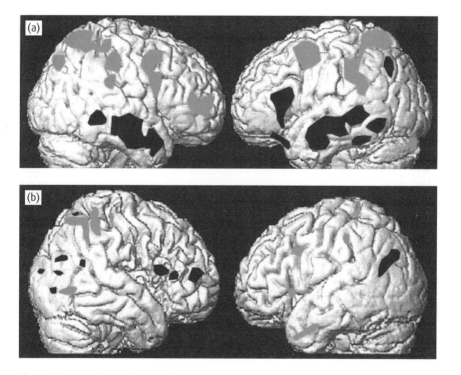

Figure 28.2. Contralateral effects of right unilateral hemispheric lesions. Current evidence suggests that purely right unilateral lesions are associated with dysfunction within the contralateral, intact hemisphere. This is demonstrated here by an activation study of auditory cognitive functions. In normal subjects (a) sound recognition and sound localization activate two distinct cortical networks (in black and grey, respectively), which are both present in either hemisphere. A unilateral right hemispheric lesion disturbs these networks in the damaged but also in the intact, left hemisphere (b) Adapted from Adriani et al. (2003).

exclude an effect at the level of disability or on destination following discharge from hospital. We would like to refer also to other recently published reviews (Robertson and Hawkins, 1999; Robertson, 1999; Diamond, 2001; Pierce and Buxbaum, 2002) and to the guidelines on cognitive rehabilitation published by the European Federation of Neurological Societies (EFNS) Task Force (Cappa et al., 2003)

Many of the current approaches to neglect rehabilitation are based on cognitive models which postulate (i) attentional gradients within each hemispace with differential roles for each hemisphere (Kinsbourne, 1994); (ii) role of spontaneous eye movements in orienting attention (Gainotti, 1994); (iii) multimodal representations sustained by parieto-prefrontal networks (Mesulam, 1981); or (iv) dopaminergic modulation of attention (Gemianini et al., 1998). Several techniques yielded statistically significant improvement measured mostly at the impairment level, more rarely at the disability level. The evidence comes from prospective randomised (Table 28.1) and non-randomised group studies (Table 28.2) as well as single and multiple single case studies.

Restoring attention to the left side

Several techniques aim at improving the attentional imbalance of hemineglect by increasing the attentional load on the left side and retraining visual scanning of the left hemispace.

A combined training of visual scanning, reading, copying and figure description, carried out in daily sessions over 8 weeks, was found to yield statistically significant improvement of neglect symptoms in prospective randomised (Antonucci et al., 1995) and prospective non-randomised studies (Pizzamiglio et al., 1992; Vallar et al., 1997). The success of this training in terms of regression of neglect symptoms is accompanied with increased activation of spared cortical regions of the right hemisphere, as demonstrated in positron emission tomography (PET) activation studies of four patients (Zoccolotti et al., 1992; Pizzamiglio et al., 1998).

Visual scanning training alone was shown to improve significantly neglect in prospective randomised (Weinberg et al., 1977) and multiple single case studies (Gouvier et al., 1987; Wagenaar et al., 1992).

Visual cueing with kinetic stimuli, presented mostly on the left side, was found to bring significant, albeit transient, improvement in three prospective non-randomised studies (Butter et al., 1990; Pizzamiglio et al., 1990; Butter and Kirsch, 1995), and multiple single case study (Karnath, 1996; Kerkoff et al., 1999).

The use of an *alert device*, a buzzer to be turned off by the patients with his left hand, proved useful in a single case study (Robertson et al., 1998b). *Visual cueing* of the left end of items, associated or not with its marking, improved significantly neglect symptoms in a non-randomised study (Lin et al., 1996).

Passive or active movements of the left arm improved neglect significantly in prospective randomised (Kalra et al., 1997; Robertson et al., 2002), prospective non-randomised (Frassinetti et al., 2001) and in single or multiple single case studies (Halligan and Marshall 1989; Robertson et al., 1992; Robertson and North, 1992, 1993; Robertson et al., 1998a; Samuel et al., 2000; Eskes et al., 2003).

Forced use of left visual hemifield or left eye, induced by a patch covering the right eye or (approximately) the right hemifield of both eyes appeared to yield beneficial results in prospective randomised (Beis et al., 1999), prospective non-randomised (Butter and Kirsch, 1992; Walker et al., 1996) and multiple single case studies (Arai et al., 1997).

The use of *visuospatial or verbal instructions* was shown to improve neglect in specific tasks (Ishiai et al., 1990, 1997).

Video feedback, making the patient aware of his deficits, was shown to improve significantly performance on trained tasks in a prospective non-randomised study (Tham and Tegner, 1997) and a multiple single case study (Soderback et al., 1992).

Restoring multisensory representations

Several studies demonstrated that egocentric reference frame of sensory integration is biaised in unilateral neglect (e.g., Bisiach et al., 1984). Applying different stimuli known to influence sensory

Table 28.1. Prospective randomized group studies with statistical analysis, listed in alphabetical order of the first author.

Study	Number of cases	Rehabilitation of neglect	Result
Antonucci et al., 1995	20 neglect cases: 10 with immediate training 10 with delayed training	*Specific training for neglect:* 1. Visual scanning training 2. Reading training 3. Copying of line drawings on a dot matrix 4. Figure description *General cognitive intervention:* Puzzles, chess, card playing, crossword puzzles (done by volunteers) Same specific training as in Pizzamiglio et al., 1990; Pizzamiglio et al., 1992	Statistically significant improvement due to specific training in both groups; no effect of general cognitive intervention
Beis et al., 1999	22 neglect cases: 7, experimental 1 7, experimental 2 8 controls	*Experimental 1*: Right hemifield patches 12 h/day for 3 months *Experimental 2*: Right monocular patch 12 h/day for 3 months *Control*: No patch	Experimental effect was positive, more for experimental 1 than experiemental 2 group
Kalra et al., 1997	47 neglect cases: 24 experimental 23 controls	*Experimental*: Spatiomotor cueing with limb activation *Control*: Conventional therapy	Same baseline; Significantly greater increase in improvement for experimental than control group
Robertson et al., 1990	36 neglect cases: 20 experimental 16 controls	*Experimental*: Scanning training on PC plus combined scanning and attention programme on PC *Control*: Word games, quizzes and logical games on PC	Partial improvement in experimental and control groups; no statistically significant difference in outcome between the two groups
Rossetti et al., 1998 Experiment 2	12 neglect cases: 6 experimental 6 controls	*Experimental*: Pointing with prism goggles deviating by 10 degrees to the right *Control*: Pointing with neutral goggles	Significantly greater improvement with prism than with neutral goggles
Schindler et al., 2002	20 neglect cases: 10 experimental 10 control	*Experimental*: Neck muscle vibration plus visual exploration training *Control*: Visual exploration training	Superior effect of combined treatment: lasting reduction of neglect symptoms and improvement in activities of daily living
Weinberg et al., 1977	57 neglect cases: 25 experimental 32 control	Visual scanning training	Statistically significant improvement in experimental group 1 month after end of training
Wiart et al., 1997 (study 1)	22 neglect cases: 11 experimental 11 controls	*Experiental*: Trunk orientation and scanning 1 h/day plus 2–3 normal rehabilitation sessions per day during 1 month *Control*: 3–4 normal rehabilitation sessions per day during 1 month	Significantly greater improvement in experimental than in control group

Table 28.2. Prospective non-randomised studies with statistical analysis, listed in alphabetical order of the first author.

Study	Number of cases	Rehabilitation of neglect	Result
Bergego et al., 1997	7 neglect cases:	Computer training with moving target versus recreational computing	No statistically signifincant effect of treatment Multiple baseline applied behavioural analysis (ABA)
Butter et al., 1990	18 neglect cases:	1. Dynamic stimuli on left side 2. Static visual stimuli on left side 3. Dynamic visual stimuli in centre	Statistically significant improvement with dynamic stimuli on left side
Butter and Kirsch, 1992	13 neglect cases:	Monocular patching	Neglect improvement in 74% cases
Butter and Kirsch, 1995	24 neglect cases: 11 experimental 13 control	Kinetic visual cues presented on the left side or centrally	Statistically significant increase in detection of left targets; transient effect
Farne et al., 2002	6 neglect cases:	Single prism adaptation session	Statistically significant improvment of several visuo-spatial abilities for 24 h; correlation between presence of after-effects induced by prismatic adaptation and improvement of neglect symptoms
Frassinetti et al., 2001	8 neglect cases:	Complex passive movements with left arm	Statistically significant improvement of neglect in several tests
Frassinetti et al., 2002	13 neglect cases: 7 experimental 6 controls	Prism adaptation applied for 2 weeks	Statistically significant improvement of neglect in several tests with long-term effect
Guarilia et al., 1998	9 cases with right hemispheric damage	Transcutaneous electrical neural stimulation (TENS)	Statistically significant improvement by TENS on left side of neck
Harvey et al., 2003	14 neglect cases: 7 experimental 7 controls	13-day training of picking the rod by the (wrongly) perceived mid-point	Significant and lasting improvement of neglect symptoms
Hommel et al., 1990	9 neglect cases:	Passive stimulations: R/L/both cheek tactile stimulation; Bilateral auditory stimulation: verbal stimulation; music; or white noise	Statistically significant improvement by music or white noise
Ladavas et al., 1994	12 neglect cases:	Overt and covert orienting	Overt and covert orienting equally effective in improving visual extinction and neglect, but not tactile extinction
Kerkoff, 1998	34 cases: 12 experimental with right hemispheric lesion	Visual exploration and visuo-spatial training	Statistically significant improvement in trained tasks

(*Cont.*)

Table 28.2. (cont.)

Study	Number of cases	Rehabilitation of neglect	Result
Lin et al., 1996	2 experimental with left hemispheric lesion 21 normal controls 13 neglect cases:	Line bisection in four conditions: A. No Cue B. Visual Cueing C. Circling digit on left end D. Circling digit on left end and tracing line with finger	B–D decreased neglect: D more than C, which more than B
Robertson et al., 1997	16 neglect cases:	Picking the rod by the (wrongly) perceived mid-point	Transient improvement on line bisection and cancellation tasks
Perennou et al., 2001	36 cases: 6 neglect 8 right lesion (no neglect) 8 left lesion 14 normals	Transcutaneous electric stimulation of neck muscles	Statistically significant improvement of postural stability in neglect patients
Pizzamiglio et al., 1990	53 cases: 33 experimental (neglect) 20 control (10 normal 10 right brain damaged without visual neglect)	Optokinetic stimulation: luminous spots moving in either direction at a speed of 50 cm/s around a luminescent strip on a plexiglass screen	Statistically significant change of performance on line bisection by neglect patients
Pizzamiglio et al., 1992	13 neglect cases:	Visual spatial scanning (searching for numbers in a large visual field) Training of reading and copying Copying of line drawings on a dot matrix Figure description	Stable pretraining baseline Statistically significant decrease of neglect, lasting during 5-months follow-up
Robertson et al., 1995	8 neglect cases:	Sustained attention training in tasks different from outcome measures: – pointing out errors – explain attention – knocking and "attend" by trainer – knocking and "attend" by patient	Statistically significant improvement in unilateral neglect and sustained attention, but not in outcome measures Effect lasted for 24 h–14 days

Study	Cases	Method	Results/Comments
Rode and Perenin, 1994	14 cases: 8 experimental (neglect), 6 control (normal)	– patient raps the table and says "attend" aloud; – patient raps the table and says "attend" subvocally; – patient raps the table mentally and says "attend"	Multiple-baseline-by-function and multiple-baseline-by-subject analysis
Rode et al., 1998b	45 cases: 15 left hemiparetic, 15 right hemiparetic, 15 controls	Vestibular stimulation by irrigation of the left external ear canal with cold water; Vestibular caloric stimulation	In two experiments improvement of mental visual imagery during stimulation; Improvement in cases with right hemispheric lesions
Rorsman et al., 1999	14 neglect cases: 7, experimental 1; 7, experimental 2	Vestibular galvanic stimulation (multiple baseline): Experimental 1: no stimulation – stimulation – no stimulation; Experimental 2: no stimulation – no stimulation – stimulation	Statistically significant improvement on some measures from no stimulation to stimulation
Rossetti et al., 1998	23 cases: 18 experimental, 5 normal controls	Base-left wedge prism goggles with 10 degrees shift of visual field to the right	Midline shift statistically greater in experimental than controls
Tham and Tegner, 1997	14 neglect cases: 7 experimental, 7 control	Video feedback versus conventional feedback	Statistically significant improvement for trained task; no statistically significant difference for not trained tasks
Vallar et al., 1995	3 experiments with 14, 8 and 6 experimental subjects, respectively	Transcutaneous electrical stimulation: of posterior left or right neck	Left-sided stimulation leads to transient neglect improvement, less in severe than in moderate neglect
Vallar et al., 1997	8 neglect cases	Training: 1. Visual spatial scanning 2. Reading and copying 3. Copy of line drawings on a dot matrix 4. Figure description	Statistically significant improvement of neglect; Confirmation of Antunucci et al., 1995; Pizzamiglio et al., 1992
Walker et al., 1996	13 neglect cases	Left versus right eye patching	Increase of neglect after right eye patching, decrease after left eye patching
Webster et al., 2001	40 neglect cases: 20 experimental, 20 controls	Training with computer-assisted programme	Statistically significant improvement in wheel chair mobility

integration in normal subjects, lead to a temporary improvement of this imbalace (see below). Very recent studies demonstrated that applying some of these stimuli over a longer period lead to significant and lasting improvement of neglect.

Vestibular stimulation by cold water infusion into the left outer ear canal showed significant transient effects on different aspects of the unilateral neglect in prospective non-randomised (Rode and Perenin, 1994; Rode et al., 1998b) and single or multiple single case studies (Rubens, 1985; Cappa et al., 1987; Vallar et al., 1990; Geminiani and Bottini, 1992; Vallar et al., 1993; Rode et al., 1998a; Rode et al., 2002).

Galvanic vestibular stimulation improved significantly, albeit transiently, neglect symptoms in a prospective non-randomised study (Rorsman et al., 1999).

Single sessions of *vibration stimulation of neck muscles* on the left side had significantly positive transient effect in multiple single case studies (Karnath et al., 1993; Karnath, 1994, 1995). A recent, partially randomised, study demonstrated that prolonged application of neck muscle vibration, combined with visual exploration training, yields better improvement of neglect symptoms than visual exploration training alone; the effect was still present 2 months later and was accompanied by improvement in activities of daily living (Schindler et al., 2002).

Transcutaneous electrical stimulation of the left-neck muscles has shown significant effects in three prospective non-randomised studies (Vallar et al., 1995; Guariglia et al., 1998; Perennou et al., 2001). However, this same technique yielded little or no effect in another set of patients (multiple single case study; Karnath, 1995).

Changes in *trunk orientation* had significantly positive effects in one prospective randomised (Wiart et al., 1997) and two multiple single case study (Karnath et al., 1993; Schindler and Kerkoff, 1997).

The use of *optical prisms* was first introduced in a paradigm which aimed at moving stimuli into the body-centred ipsilesional space; a 4-week application of rightward prisms in patients with neglect improved the performance in several neglect tests, but not in activities of daily living (Rossi et al., 1990). More recently, the use of prisms was combined with pointing tasks, either ahead or to visually presented locations (Fig. 28.3), called *prism adaptation*. A single session of prim adaptation, using a deviation of 10 degrees to the right, yielded a temporary but statistically significant improvement of neglect symptoms in a prospective randomised study (Rossetti et al., 1998). A group study confirmed such improvement through a session of prism adaptation and demonstrated a correlation between the improvement and the presence of visuo-motor after-effects (Farne et al., 2002). Furthermore, single and multiple single case studies showed parallel improvement in neglect tests and behaviour (Rode et al., 1998a), representational neglect (Rode et al., 2001), haptic neglect (McIntosh et al., 2002), perceptual size judgement (Dijkerman et al., 2003), tactile exctinction (Maravita et al., 2003) and postural imbalance (Tilikete et al., 2001). However, not all neglect patients improve equally through prism adaptation training; a recent single case study reported improvement on standard tests of neglect and on pointing and visual exploration tasks, but not an awareness tasks, such as emotional chimeric faces (Ferber et al., 2003). Furthermore, prism adaptation can affect differently tasks such as straight-ahead pointing and line bisection in different patients (Pisella et al., 2002). It is very likely that different types of neglect respond differently to the prism adaptation treatment (Beversdorf and Heilman,

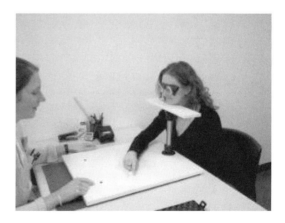

Figure 28.3. Prism adaptation. The use of prisms is combined with pointing tasks, either ahead or to visually presented locations. Adapted from Chesaux (2004).

2003). Daily sessions of prism adaptation over 2 weeks have been shown to yield long-term improvement of neglect symptoms in a prospective non-randomised study (Frassinetti et al., 2002).

Improving non-spatial functions

Neglect was often reported in association with general attentional disability and specific training on the general attentional level was shown to improve neglect symptoms. *Training of sustained attention, increasing of alertness or cueing of spatial attention* were shown to improve significantly neglect in prospective non-randomised studies (Hommel et al., 1990; Ladavas et al., 1994; Robertson et al., 1995; Kerkhoff, 1998). In a recent multiple case study phasic alerting was shown to ameliorate spatial attentional bias in neglect patients (Robertson et al., 1998b).

Proprioceptive feedback and imagery

A certain number of patients with unilateral neglect tend to have a rightward shift in line bisection tasks. A group study demonstrated that the experience of picking the rod by the (wrongly) perceived midpoint can transiently improve performance on neglect tests, such as the bisection and cancellation tasks (Robertson et al., 1997). When neglect patients were exposed for 13 days to the same practise and learned thus to make use of the *proprioceptive feedback*, their

performance improves in a lasting fashion (Harvey et al., 2003).

Specific *training of visual or motor imagery* proved useful in prospective non-randomised (Niermeir, 1998) and single or multiple single case studies (Smania et al., 1997; McCarthy et al., 2002).

Computer training

Computer training yielded mixed results. One prospective randomised (Robertson et al., 1990) and one prospective non-randomised study (Bergego et al., 1997) reported absence of significantly positive effects, while a recent prospective non-randomised study showed statistically significant improvement in wheel chair mobility (Webster et al., 2001). A previous 3-case study (Robertson et al., 1988) found significant improvement in trained skills, but little change in untrained activities.

Dopaminergic treatment

The effect of dopamine agonists on hemispatial neglect was investigated in six studies involving small number of cases (1–7; Table 28.3). Four studies showed improvement of neglect symptoms under bromocriptine, apomorphine, methylphenidate or carbodopa L-dopa therapy (Fleet et al., 1987; Geminiani et al., 1998; Hurford et al., 1998; Mukand et al., 2001), while two obtained a worsening (Grujic et al., 1998; Barrett et al., 1999).

Table 28.3. Dopamine agonist therapy in hemispatial neglect, listed in alphabetical order of the first author.

Study	Number of cases	Treatment	Result
Barrett et al., 1999	1 case	Bromocriptine	Worsening of neglect symptoms
Fleet et al., 1987	2 cases	Bromocriptine	Improvement under therapy, worsening after withdrawal
Geminiani et al., 1998	4 cases	Apomorphine	Transient but significant improvement in perceptual and perceptuomotor functions
Grujic et al., 1998	7 cases	Bromocriptine	Worsening of hemineglect: visual search oriented away from the neglected hemispace
Hurford et al., 1998	1 case	Two trials: Methylphenidate Bromocriptine	Improvement of neglect in both trials
Mukand et al., 2001	4 cases	Carbidopa L-dopa therapy	Improvement in 3 out of 4 cases

28.2 Anosognosia

Deficit of self-awareness

The term anosognosia was introduced in 1914 by Babinski to denote lack of awareness for hemiplegia and qualifies today lack of awareness of impairments such as neglect (Azouvi et al., 2003), cortical blindness (Goldenberg et al., 1995), Wernicke's aphasia (Lebrun, 1987) or executive deficits (Michon et al., 1994). Psychological denial of illness, flattened affect, sensory deficits, neglect or faulty control of action have been proposed as possible mechanisms of anosognosia (for review see e.g., Heilman et al., 1998; Frith et al., 2000).

Anosognosia is relatively frequently found in the acute and postacute stage. Although subsequent recovery or improvement occur in most patients, anosognosia can persist into the chronic stage, even in the absence of general cognitive impairment (Cocchini et al., 2002; Venneri and Shanks, 2004).

Anatomo-clinical correlations

In studies of consecutive patients with unilateral hemispheric lesions, anosognosia was noted more often following right than left lesions, but it did occur after isolated unilateral left lesions (Starkstein et al., 1992; Stone et al., 1992). Lesions associated with anosognosia include temporo-parietal junction, pre- and post-central gyri, thalamus, basal ganglia and the internal capsule (Levine et al., 1991; Starkstein et al., 1992; Ellis and Small, 1997).

Anosognosia of neglect

In cases of right hemispheric lesions, most patients presenting neglect are unaware of their deficit in the initial stage or they tend to underestimate its consequences on everyday life. Anosognosia of neglect tends to be correlated with the severity of neglect and improvement in awareness parallels the recovery from neglect (Azouvi et al., 2003; Buxbaum et al., 2004). However, there appears to be no causal link with hemineglect, since anosognosia was reported in cases without hemineglect (Bisiach et al., 1986) and individual dissociations between the two symptoms can be

observed (Azouvi et al., 2003). Furthermore, recovery from neglect can occur without concomitant improvement of neglect's awareness (Zoccolotti et al., 1992).

Assessment

Quantification of anosognosia for neglect is possible through the use of observational scales such as the Catherine Bergego Scale (Azouvi et al., 2003). Patients are rated by a professional (e.g., an occupational therapist) according to the occurrence of neglect during activities of daily living such as grooming, eating or moving around. They are also asked to rate their behaviour themselves, using the same questionnaire. A difference score between the observer's assessment score and the patient's self-assessment score provides a measure of anosognosia of neglect.

Treatment

Cognitive rehabilitation of neglect anosognosia aims at improving top-down mechanisms by increasing the awareness of neglect symptoms or bottom-up mechanisms by sensory manipulations.

Increasing the awareness of neglect symptoms

Increasing the awareness of neglect symptoms is believed to be a pre-requisite or at least an important step in neglect treatment. This is certainly the case for techniques which aim at improving visual exploration and scanning towards the neglected space and compensating the directional bias towards the ipsilesional side. They require conscious control or compensation of the deficit of unilateral attention.

In most clinical approaches the therapist explains the attentional nature of the deficit and provides then continuous feedback during treatment by drawing the patient's attention towards neglect symptoms such as omissions. Following a cancellation task, he can rotate the sheet of paper by 180° and show the omissions to the patient once they are in the non-neglected hemifield. The therapist can also use auditory cueing (i.e., tapping on the desk on the left side of space) to point out omissions during the task. On reading tasks, when the patients fails to read parts of sentences, the therapist can ask the patient whether what he has just read makes sense and appeal to his judgement to question his performance. In addition to getting feedback from the therapist, the patient should also engage actively in commenting his own performance or in correcting his own production. At the beginning of the treatment, the verbal injunctions for the compensation of the directional bias are given by the therapist and later on by the patient himself. At the end of the treatment, patients should have internalised the verbal instruction to pay particular attention towards the neglected side. This approach leads generally to increased awareness of neglect in parallel to reduction of neglect, since the compensatory strategies are only effective if some degree of insight into the deficit is present. However, awareness of neglect is not necessarily a pre-requisite for recovery from neglect. A patient who sustained a combined training of visual scanning, reading, copying and figure description (as in Pizzamiglio et al., 1990) plus optokinetic stimulation showed good recovery in visual scanning strategies, but remained deeply anosognosic of his visual problems (Zoccolotti et al., 1992).

More formalised feedback can be provided by video-recording. This approach was used in ecological tasks, such as baking (Söderbeack et al., 1992). During the play–replay the therapist made a pause when clear signs of neglect were apparent, asked the patient to comment on irregularities and suggested new strategies, such as to work systematically from left to right, to ensure that everything on the left was seen and to touch the left edge of the oven tray. Better results with video feedback than with conventional feedback have been demonstrated in a subsequent non-randomised study (Tham and Tegner, 1997).

Sensory manipulations

Sensory manipulations such as vestibular stimulation, optokinetic stimulation, electrical transcutenous stimulation or prism adaptation have been shown to yield transient or permanent reduction of extrapersonal and personal neglect as well as improvement of motor performance in neglect patients (see above). Two studies reported additional, albeit transient improvement of anosognosia for hemiplegia following vestibular stimulation (Cappa et al., 1987; Rode et al., 1998 *Cortex*).

28.3 Conclusions

Left unilateral neglect is a modular deficit, which can affect different aspects of visual, auditory, somatosensory and motor processing. The presence of neglect beyond the acute stage is often associated with poor outcome in terms of independence. Current evidence confirms that neglect rehabilitation yields better outcome. Prospective randomised studies demonstrated significant improvement by a range of techniques, including combined training of visual scanning, reading, copying and figure description; trunk orientation plus visual scanning training; neck muscle vibration plus visual exploration training; visual scanning training alone; spatiomotor cueing with limb activation; right hemifield or right eye patching; and prism adaptation training. Additional evidence from non-randomised group and single case studies strongly suggests the efficacy of other cognitive techniques.

The therapy of anosognosia, which often accompanies hemineglect, consists mostly of providing feedback to the patient or is based, in a more experimental fashion, on sensory manipulations.

ACKNOWLEDGEMENTS

We thank Dr. Psych. Anne Bellmann Thiran for her contribution to the review of the literature.

REFERENCES

Adriani, M., Bellmann, A., Meuli, R., Fornari, E., Frischknecht, R., Bindschaedler, C., Rivier, F., Thiran, J-Ph., Maeder, P. and Clarke, S. (2003). Unilateral hemispheric lesions disrupt parallel processing within the contralateral intact hemisphere: an auditory fMRI study. *Neuroimage*, **20**, S66–S74.

Aglioti, S., Smania, N. and Peru, A. (1999). Frames of reference for mapping tactile stimuli in brain-damaged patients. *J Cogn Neurosci*, **11**, 67–79.

Anderson, B. (1993). Spared awareness for the left side of internal visual images in patients with left-sided extrapersonal neglect. *Neurology*, **43**, 213–216.

Antonucci, A., Guariglia, C., Judica, A., Magnotti, L., Paolucci, S., Pizzamiglio, L. and Zoccolotti, P. (1995). Effectivness of neglect rehabilitation in a randomized group study. *J Clin Exp Neuropsychol*, **17**, 383–389.

Arai, T., Ohi, H., Sasaki, H., Hobuto, H. and Tanaka, K. (1997). Hemispatial sunglasses: effect on unilateral spatial neglect. *Arch Phys Med Rehabil*, **78**, 230–232.

Azouvi, P., Samuel, C., Louis-Dreyfus, A., Bernati, T., Bartolomeo, P., Beis, JM., Chokron, S., Leclercq, M., Marchal, F., Martin, Y., de Montety, G., Olivier, S., Perennou, D., Pradat-Diehl, P., Prairial, C., Rode, G., Siéroff, E., Wiart, L. and Rousseaux, M. (2002). Sensitivity of clinical and behavioural tests of spatial neglect after right hemisphere stroke. *J Neurol Neurosurg Psychiatr*, **73**, 160–166.

Azouvi, P., Olivier, S., de Montety, G., Samuel, C., Louis-Dreyfus, A. and Tesio, L. (2003). Behavioural assessment of unilateral neglect: study of the psychometric properties of the catherine bergego scale. *Arch Phys Med Rehabil*, **84**, 51–57.

Barbieri, C. and De Renzi, E. (1989). Patterns of neglect dissociation. *Behav Neurol*, **2**, 13–24.

Barrett, A.M., Crucian, G.P., Schwartz, R.L. and Heilman, K.M. (1999). Adverse effect of dopamine agonist therapy in a patient with motor-inattentional neglect. *Arch Phys Med Rehabil*, **80**, 600–603.

Bartolomeo, P., Perri, R. and Gainotti, G. (2004). The influence of limb crossing on left tactile extinction. *J Neurol Neurosurg Psychiatr*, **75**, 49–55.

Beis, J-M., André, J-M., Baumgarten, A. and Challier, B. (1999). Eye patching in unilateral spatial neglect: efficacy of two methods. *Arch Phys Med Rehabil*, **80**, 71–76.

Bellmann, A., Meuli, R. and Clarke, S. (2001). Two types of auditory neglect. *Brain*, **124**, 676–687.

Bergego, C., Azouvi, P., Deloche, G., Samuel, C., Louis-Dreyfus, A., Kaschel, R. and Willmes, K. (1997). Rehabilitation of unilateral neglect: a controlled multiple-baseline-across-subjects trial using computerised training procedures. *Neuropsychol Rehabil*, **7(4)**, 279–293.

Beschin, N. and Robertson, I.H. (1997). Personal versus extrapersonal neglect: a group study of their dissociation using a reliable clinical test. *Cortex*, **3**, 379–384.

Beschin, N., Cazzani, M., Cubelli, R., Della Sala, S. and Spinazzola, L. (1996). Ignoring left and far: an investigation of tactile neglect. *Neuropsychologia*, **34**, 41–49.

Beschin, N., Cubelli, R., Della Sala, S. and Spinazzola, L. (1997). Left of what? The role of egocentric coordinates in neglect. *J Neurol Neurosurg Psychiatr*, **63**, 483–489.

Beversdorf, D. and Heilman, K.M. (2003). Prism adaptation treatment of neglect. *Neurology*, **60**, 1734–1735.

Bisiach, E. and Luzzatti, C. (1978). Unilateral neglect of representational space. *Cortex*, **14**, 129–133.

Bisiach, E., Cornacchia, L., Sterzi, R. and Vallar, G. (1984). Disorders of perceived auditory lateralization after lesions of the right hemisphere. *Brain*, **107**, 37–52.

Bisiach, E., Vallar, G., Perani, D., Papagno, C. and Berti, A. (1986). Unawareness of disease following lesions of the right hemisphere: anosognosia for hemiplegia and anosognosia for hemianopia. *Neuropsychologia*, **24**, 471–482.

Bottini, G., Sterzi, R. and Vallar, G. (1992). Directional hypokinesia in spatial hemineglect: a case study. *J Neurol Neurosurg Psychiatr*, **55**, 562–565.

Bowen, A., Lincoln, N.B. and Dewey, M. (2002). Cognitive rehabilitation for spatial neglect following stroke. *Cochrane Database Syst Rev*. CD003586.

Brain, W.R. (1941). Visual disorientation with special reference to lesions of the right cerebral hemisphere. *Brain*, **64**, 244–272.

Butter, C.M. and Kirsch, N. (1992). Combined and separate effects of eye patching and visual stimulation on unilateral neglect following stroke. *Arch Phys Med Rehabil*, **73**, 1133–1139.

Butter, C.M. and Kirsch, N. (1995). Effect of lateralized kinetic visual cues on visual search in patients with unilateral spatial neglect. *J Clin Exp Neuropsychol*, **17**, 856–867.

Butter, C.M., Kirsch, N.L. and Reeves, G. (1990). The effect of lateralized dynamic stimuli on unilateral spatial neglect following right hemisphere lesions. *Restor Neurol Neurosci*, **2**, 39–46.

Buxbaum, L.J., Ferraro, M.K., Veramonti, T., Farne, A., Whyte, J., Ladavas, E., Frassinetti, F. and Coslett, H.B. (2004). Hemispatial neglect subtypes, neuroanatomy, and disability. *Neurology*, **62**, 749–756.

Cappa, S., Sterzi, R., Vallar, G. and Bisiach, E. (1987). Remission of hemineglect and anosognosia during vestibular stimulation. *Neuropsychologia*, **25**, 775–782.

Cappa, S.F., Benke, T., Clarke, S., Rossi, B., Stemmer, B. and van Heugten, C.M. (2003). EFNS Guidelines on cognitive rehabilitation: report of an EFNS task force. *Eur J Neurol*, **10**, 11–23.

Chesaux, C. (2004). Effets d'une adaptation prismatique sur les mouvements oculaires chez les patients avec négligence unilatérale. Mémoire de diplôme, FAPSE, Université de Genève.

Clarke, S. and Thiran, A.B. (2004). Auditory neglect: what and where in auditory space. *Cortex*, **40**, 291–300.

Cocchini, G., Beschin, N. and Della Sala, S. (2002). Chronic anosognosia: a case report and theoretical account. *Neuropsychologia*, **40**, 2030–2038.

Coslett, H.B. (1997). Neglect in vision and visual imagery: a double dissociation. *Brain*, **120**, 1163–1171.

Cowey, A., Small, M. and Ellis, S. (1994). Left visuo-spatial neglect can be worse in far than in near space. *Neuropsychologia*, **32**, 1059–1066.

Damasio, A.R., Damasio, H. and Chang Chui, H. (1980). Neglect following damage to frontal lobe or basal ganglia. *Neuropsychologia*, **18**, 123–132.

Denes, G., Semenza, C., Stoppa, E. and Lis, A. (1982). Unilateral spatial neglect and recovery from hemiplegia: a follow-up study. *Brain*, **105**, 543–552.

Diamond, P.T. (2001). Rehabilitative management of post-stroke visuospatial inattention. *Disabil Rehabil*, **23**, 407–412.

Dijkerman, H.C., McIntosh, R.D., Milner, A.D., Rossetti, Y., Tilikete, C. and Roberts, R.C. (2003). Ocular scanning and perceptual size distortion in hemispatial neglect: effects of prism adaptation and sequential stimulus presentation. *Exp Brain Res*, **153**, 220–230.

Ellis, S. and Small, M. (1997). Localization of lesion in denial of hemiplegia after acute stroke. *Stroke*, **28**, 67–71.

Eskes, G.A., Butler, B., McDonald, A., Harrison, E.R. and Phillips, S.J. (2003). Limb activation effects in hemispatial neglect. *Arch Phys Med Rehabil*, **84**, 323–328.

Farnè, A., Rossetti, Y., Toniolo, S. and Làdavas, E. (2002). Ameliorating neglect with prism adaptation: visuo-manual and visuo-verbal measures. *Neuropsychologia*, **40**, 718–729.

Ferber, S., Danckert, J., Joanisse, M., Goltz, H.C. and Goodale, M.A. (2003). Eye movements tell only half the story. *Neurology*, **60**, 1826–1829.

Ferro, J.M. and Kertesz, A. (1984). Posterior internal capsule infarction associated with neglect. *Arch Neurol*, **41**, 422–424.

Fleet, W.S., Valenstein, E., Watson, R.T. and Heilman, K.M. (1987). Dopamin agonist therapy for neglect in humans. *Neurology*, **37**, 1765–1770.

Frassinetti, F., Rossi, M. and Ladavas, E. (2001). Passive limb movements improve visual neglect. *Neuropsychologia*, **39**, 725–733.

Frassinetti, F., Angeli, V., Meneghello, F., Avanzi, S. and Ladavas, E. (2002). Long-lasting amelioration of visuospatial neglect by prism adaptation. *Brain*, **125**, 608–623.

Frith, C.D., Blakemore, S.J. and Wolpert, D.M. (2000). Abnormalities in the awareness and control of action. *Phil Trans Roy Soc London B*, **355**, 1771–1788.

Gainotti, G. (1994). The role of spontaneous eye movements in orienting attention and in unilateral neglect. In: *Unilateral Neglect: Clinical and Experimental Studies* (eds Robertson, E.H., Marshall, J.C.), Lawrence Erlbaum Associates Publishers, Hove, pp. 107–122.

Geminiani, G. and Bottini, G. (1992). Mental representation and temporary recovery from unilateral neglect after vestibular stimulation. *J Neurol Neurosurg Psychiatr*, **55**, 332–333.

Geminiani, G., Bottini, G. and Sterzi, R. (1998). Dopaminergic stimulation in unilateral neglect. *J Neurol Neurosurg Psychiatr*, **65**, 344–347.

Goldenberg, G., Müllbacher, W. and Nowak, A. (1995). Imagery without perception: a case study of anosognosia for cortical blindness. *Neuropsychologia*, **33**, 1373–1382.

Gouvier, W.D., Bua, B.G., Blanton, P.D. and Urey, J.R. (1987). Behavioral changes following visual scanning training: observations of five cases. *Int J Clin Neuropsychol*, **9**, 734–780.

Grujic, Z., Mapstone, M., Gitelman, D.R., Johnson, N., Weintraub, S., Hays, A., Kwasnica, C., Harvey, R. and Mesulam, M.M. (1998). Dopamine agonsts reorient visual exploration away from the neglected hemispace. *Neurology*, **51**, 1395–1398.

Guariglia, C. and Antonucci, G. (1992). Personal and extrapersonal space: a case of neglect dissociation. *Neuropsychologia*, **30**, 1001–1009.

Guariglia, C., Padovani, A., Pantano, P. and Pizzamiglio, L. (1993). Unilateral neglect restricted to visual imagery. *Nature*, **364**, 235–237.

Guariglia, C., Lippolis, G. and Pizzamiglio, L. (1998). Somatosensory stimulation improves imagery disorders in neglect. *Cortex*, **34**, 233–241.

Haeske-Dewick, H.C., Canavan, A.G. and Homberg, V. (1996). Directional hyperattention in tactile neglect within grasping space. *J Clin Exp Neuropsychol*, **18**, 724–732.

Halligan, P.W. and Marshall, J.C. (1989). Perceptual cueing and perceptuo-motor compatibility in visuo-spatial neglect: a single case study. *Cogn Neuropsychol*, **6(4)**, 423–435.

Harvey, M., Hood, B., North, A. and Robertson, I.H. (2003). The effects of visuomotor feedback training on the recovery of hemispatial neglects symptoms: assessment of a 2-week and follow-up intervention. *Neuropsychologia*, **41**, 886–893.

Healton, E.B., Navarro, C., Bressman, S. and Brust, J.C. (1982). Subcortical neglect. *Neurology*, **32**, 776–778.

Heilman, K.M. and Valenstein, E. (1972). Frontal lobe neglect in man. *Neurology*, **22**, 660–664.

Heilman, K.M., Barrett, A.M. and Adair, J.C. (1998). Possible mechanisms of anosognosia: a defect in self-awareness. *Phil Trans Roy Soc London B*, **353**, 1903–1909.

Hier, D.B., Davis, K.R., Richradson, E.P. and Mohr, J.P. (1977). Hypertensive putaminal hemorrhage. *Ann Neurol*, **1**, 152–159.

Hommel, M., Peres, B., Pollack, P., Memin, B., Besson, G., Gaio, J-M. and Perret, J. (1990). Effects of passive tactile and auditory stimuli on left visual neglect. *Arch Neurol*, **47**, 573–576.

Hurford, P., Stringer, A.Y. and Jann, B. (1998). Neuropharmacological treatment of hemineglect: a case report comparing bromocriptine and methylphenidate. *Arch Phys Med Rehabil*, **79**, 346–349.

Husain, M. and Kennard, C. (1996). Visual neglect associated with frontal lobe infarction. *J Neurol*, **243**, 652–657.

Ishiai, S., Sugishita, M., Odajima, N., Yaginuma, M., Gono, S. and Kamaya, T. (1990). Improvement of unilateral spatial neglect with numbering. *Neurology*, **40**, 1395–1398.

Ishiai, S., Seki, I., Koyama, Y. and Izumi, Y. (1997). Disappearance of unilateral spatial neglect following a simple instruction. *J Neurol Neurosurg Psychiatr*, **63**, 23–27.

Kalra, L., Perez, I., Gupta, S. and Wittink, M. (1997). The influence of visual neglect on stroke rehabilitation. *Stroke*, **28**, 1386–1391.

Karnath, H.O. (1994). Subjective body orientation in neglect and the interactive contribution of neck muscle proprioception and vestibular stimulation. *Brain*, **117**, 1001–1012.

Karnath, H.O. (1995). Transcuteneous electrical stimulation and vibration of neck muscles in neglect. *Exp Brain Res*, **105**, 321–324.

Karnath, H.O. (1996). Optokinetic stimulation influences the disturbed perception of body orientation in spatial neglect. *J Neurol Neurosurg Psychiatr*, **60**, 217–220.

Karnath, H.O. and Perenin, M.T. (1998). Tactile exploration of peripersonal space in patients with neglect. *NeuroReport*, **9**, 2273–2277.

Karnath, H.O., Christ, K. and Hartje, W. (1993). Decrease of contralateral neglect by neck muscle vibration and spatial orientation of trunk midline. *Brain*, **116**, 383–396.

Kerkhoff, G. (1998). Rehabilitation of visuospatial cognition and visual exploration in neglect: a cross-over study. *Restor Neurol Neurosci*, **12**, 27–40.

Kerkhoff, G., Schindler, I., Keller, I. and Marquardt, C. (1999). Visual background motion reduces size distortion in spatial neglect. *NeuroReport*, **10**, 319–323.

Kinsbourne, M. (1994). Orientation bias model of unilateral neglect: evidence fro attentional gradients within hemispace. In: *Unilateral Neglect: Clinical and Experimental Studies* (eds Robertson, E.H. and Marshall, J.C.), Lawrence Erlbaum Associates Publishers, Hove, pp. 63–86.

Ladavas, E., Menghini, G. and Umilta, C. (1994). A rehabilitation study of hemispatial neglect. *Cogn Neuropsychol*, **11**, 75–95.

Laplane, D. and Degos, J.D. (1983). Motor neglect. *J Neurol Neurosurg Psychiatr*, **46**, 152–158.

Lebrun, Y. (1987). Anosognosia in aphasics. *Cortex*, **2**, 251–263.

Levine, D.N., Calvanio, R. and Rinn, W.E. (1991). The pathogenesis of anosognosia for hemiplegia. *Neurology*, **41**, 1770–1781.

Lin, K.-C., Cermark, S.A., Kinsbourne, M. and Trombly, C.A. (1996). Effects of left-sided movements on line bisection in unilateral neglect. *J Int Neuropsychol Soc*, **2**, 404–411.

Maguire, A.M. and Ogden, J.A. (2002). MRI brain scan analyses and neuropsychological profiles of nine patients with persisting unilateral neglect. *Neuropsychologia*, **40**, 879–887.

Maravita, A., McNeil, J., Malhotra, P., Greenwood, R., Husain, M. and Driver, J. (2003). Prism adaptation can improve contralesional tactile perception in neglect. *Neurology*, **60**, 1829–1831.

Marshall, J.C. and Halligan, P.W. (1995). Within- and between-task dissociations in visuo-spatial neglect: a case study. *Cortex*, **31**, 367–376.

McCarthy, M., Beaumont, J.G., Thompson, R. and Pringle, H. (2002). The role of imagery in the rehabilitation of neglect in severely disabled brain-injured adults. *Arch Clin Neuropsychol*, **17**, 407–422.

McFie, J., Piercy, M.F. and Zangwill, O.L. (1950). Visual-spatial agnosia associated with lesions of the right cerebral hemisphere. *Brain*, **73**, 167–190.

McIntosh, R.D., Rossetti, Y. and Milner, A.D. (2002). Prism adaptation improves chronic visual and haptic neglect: a single case study. *Cortex*, **38**, 309–320.

Mesulam, M.M. (1981). A cortical network for directed attention and unilateral neglect. *Ann Neurol*, **10**, 309–325.

Michon, A., Deweer, B., Pillon, B., Agid, Y. and Dubois, B. (1994). Relation of anosognosia to frontal lobe dysfunction in Alzheimer's disease. *J Neurol Neurosurg Psychiatr*, **57**, 805–809.

Mukand, J.A., Guilmette, T.J., Allen, D.G., Brown, L.K., Brown, S.L., Tober, K.L. and VanDyck, W.R. (2001). Dopaminergic therapy with carbodopa L-dopa for left neglect after stroke: a case series. *Arch Phys Med Rehabil*, **82**, 1279–1282.

Niermeir, J.P. (1998). The lighthouse strategy: use of a visual imagery technique to treat visual inattention in stroke patients. *Brain Injury*, **12**, 399–406.

Perani, D., Vallar, G., Cappa, S., Messa, C. and Fazio, F. (1987). Aphasia and neglect after subcortical stroke. A clinical/cerebral perfusion correlation study. *Brain*, **110**, 1211–1229.

Perennou, D.A., Leblond, C., Amblard, B., Micallef, J.P., Herisson, C. and Pelissier, J.Y. (2001). Transcuteneous electric nerve stimulation reduces neglect-related postural instability after stroke. *Arch Phys Med Rehabil*, **82**, 440–448.

Perennou, D.A., Amblard, B., Laassel el, M., Benaim, C., Herisson, C. and Pelissier, J. (2002). Understanding the pusher behavior of some stroke patients with spatial deficits: a pilot study. *Arch Phys Med Rehabil*, **83**, 570–575.

Pierce, S.R. and Buxbaum, L.J. (2002). Treatments of unilateral neglect: a review. *Arch Phys Med Rehabil*, **83**, 256–268.

Pisella, L., Rode, G., Farnè, A., Boisson, D. and Rossetti, Y. (2002). Dissociated long lasting improvements of straight-ahead pointing and line bisection tasks in two hemineglect patients. *Neuropsychologia*, **40**, 327–334.

Pizzamiglio, L., Frasca, R., Guariglia, C., Incoccia, C. and Antonucci, G. (1990). Effect of optokinetic stimulation in patients with visual neglect. *Cortex*, **26**, 535–540.

Pizzamiglio, L., Antonucci, G., Judica, A., Montenero, P., Razzano, C. and Zoccolotti, P. (1992). Cognitive rehabilitation og the hemineglect disorder in chronic patients with unilateral right brain damage. *J Clin Exp Neuropsychol*, **14**, 901–923.

Pizzamiglio, L., Perani, D., Cappa, S.F., Vallar, G., Paolucci, S., Grassi, F., Paulesco, E. and Fazio, F. (1998). Recovery of neglect after right hemispheric damage. *Arch Neurol*, **55**, 561–568.

Robertson, I., Gray, J. and McKenzie, S. (1988). Microcomputer-based cognitive rehabilitation of visual neglect: three multiple-baseline single-case studies. *Brain Injury*, **2(2)**, 151–163.

Robertson, I.H. (1999). Cognitive rehabilitation: attention and neglect. *Trend Cogn Sci*, **3**, 385–393.

Robertson, I.H. and North, N. (1992). Spatio-motor cueing in unilateral left neglect: the role of hemispace, hand and motor activation. *Neuropsychologia*, **30**, 553–563.

Robertson, I.H. and North, N. (1993). Active and passive activation of left limbs: influence on visual and sensory neglect. *Neuropsychologia*, **31(3)**, 293–300.

Robertson, I.H. and Hawkins, K. (1999). Limb activation and unilateral neglect. *Neurocase*, **5**, 153–160.

Robertson, I.H., Gray, J., Pentland, B. and Waite, L.J. (1990). Microcomputer-based rehabilitation for unilateral left visual neglect: a randomized contolled trial. *Arch Phys Med Rehabil*, **71**, 663–668.

Robertson, I.H., North, N. and Geggie, C. (1992). Spatiomotor cueing in unilateral left neglect: three case studies of its therapeutic effects. *J Neurol Neurosurg Psychiatr*, **55**, 799–805.

Robertson, I.H., Tegnér, R., Tham, K., Lo, A. and Nimmo-Smith, I. (1995). Sustained attention training for unilateral neglect: theoretical and rehabilitation implications. *J Clin Exp Neuropsychol*, **17(3)**, 416–430.

Robertson, I.H., Nico, D. and Hood, B.M. (1997). Believing what you feel: using proprioceptive feedback to reduce unilateral neglect. *Neuropsychology*, **11**, 53–58.

Robertson, I.H., Hogg, K. and McMillan, T.M. (1998a). Rehabilitation of unilateral neglect: improving function by contralesional limb activation. *Neuropsychol Rehabil*, **8(1)**, 19–29.

Robertson, I.H., Mattingley, J.B., Rorden, C. and Driver, J. (1998b). Phasic alerting of neglect patients overcomes their spatial deficit in visual awareness. *Nature*, **395**, 169–172.

Roberstson, I.H., McMillan, T.M., MacLeod, E., Edgeworth, J. and Brock, D. (2002). Rehabilitation by limb activation training reduces left-sided motor impairment in unilateral neglect patients: a single-blind randomised control trial. *Neuropsychol Rehabil*, **12**, 439–454.

Rode, G. and Perenin, M.T. (1994). Temporary remission of representational hemineglect through vestibular stimulation. *NeuroReport*, **5**, 869–872.

Rode, G., Rossetti, Y., Li, L. and Boisson, D. (1998a). Improvement of mental imagery after prism exposure in neglect: a case study. *Behav Neurol*, **11**, 251–258.

Rode, G., Tiliket, C., Charopain, P. and Boisson, D. (1998b). Postural assymetry reduction by vestibular caloric stimulation in left hemiparetic patients. *Scand J Rehab Med*, **30**, 9–14.

Rode, G., Perenin, M.T., Honoré, J. and Boisson, D. (1998c). Improvement of the motor deficit of neglect patients through vestibular stimulation: evidence for a motor neglect component. *Cortex*, **34**, 253–261.

Rode, G., Rossetti, Y. and Boisson, D. (2001). Prism adaptation improves representational neglect. *Neuropsychologia*, **39**, 1250–1254.

Rode, G., Tilikete, C., Luaute, J., Rossetti, Y., Vighetto, A. and Boisson, D. (2002). Bilateral vestibular stimulation does not improve visual hemineglect. *Neuropsychologia*, **40**, 1104–1106.

Rorsman, I., Magnusson, M. and Johansson, B.B. (1999). Reduction of visuo-spatial neglect with vestibular galvanic stimulation. *Scand J Rehab Med*, **31**, 117–124.

Rossetti, Y., Rode, G., Pisella, L., Farné, A., Li, L., Boisson, D. and Perenin, M.-T. (1998). Prism adaptation to rightward optical deviation rehabilitates left hemispatial neglect. *Nature*, **395**, 166–169.

Rossi, P.W., Kheyfets, S. and Reding, M.J. (1990). Fresnel prisms improve visual perception in stroke patients with homonymous hemianopia or unilateral visual neglect. *Neurology*, **40**, 1597–1599.

Rubens, A.B. (1985). Caloric stimulation and unilateral visual neglect. *Neurology*, **35**, 1019–1024.

Samuel, C., Louis-Dreyfus, A., Kaschel, R., Makiela, E., Troubat, M., Anselmi, N., Cannizzo, V. and Azouvi, P. (2000). Rehabilitation of very severe unilateral neglect by visuo-spatio-motor cueing: two single case studies. *Neuropsychol Rehabil*, **10(4)**, 385–399.

Schindler, I. and Kerkoff, G. (1997). Head and trunk orientation modulate visual neglect. *NeuroReport*, **8**, 2681–2685.

Schindler, I., Kerkhoff, G., Karnath, H.O., Keller, I. and Goldenberg, G. (2002). Neck muscle vibration induces lasting recovery in spatial neglect. *J Neurol Neurosurg Psychiatr*, **73**, 412–419.

Smania, N. and Aglioti, S. (1995). Sensory and spatial components of somaesthetic deficits following right brain damage. *Neurology*, **45**, 1725–1730.

Smania, N., Bazoli, F., Piva, D. and Guidetti, G. (1997). Visuomotor imagery and rehabilitation of neglect. *Arch Phys Med Rehabil*, **78**, 430–436.

Soderback, I., Bengtsson, I., Ginsburg, E. and Ekholm, J. (1992). Video feedback in occupational therapy: its effect in patients with neglect syndrome. *Arch Phys Med Rehabil*, **73**, 1140–1146.

Starkstein, S.E., Fedoroff, J.P., Price, T.R., Leiguarda, R. and Robinson, R.G. (1992). Anosognosia in patients with cerebrovascular lesions: a study of causative factors. *Stroke*, **23**, 1446–1453.

Sterzi, R., Piacentini, S., Polimeni, M., Liverani, F. and Bisiach, E. (1996). Perceptual and premotor components of unilateral auditory neglect. *J Int Neuropsychol Soc*, **2**, 419–425.

Stone, S.P., Patel, P., Greenwood, R.J. and Halligan, P. W. (1992). Measuring visual neglect in acute stroke and predicting its recovery: the visual neglect recovery index. *J Neurol Neurosurg Psychiatr*, **55**, 431–436.

Stone, S.P., Halligan, P.W. and Greenwood, R.J. (1993). The incidence of neglect phenomena and related disorders in patients with an acute right or left hemisphere stroke. *Age Ageing*, **22**, 46–52.

Tham, K. and Tegner, R. (1997). Video feedback in the rehabilitation of patients with unilateral neglect. *Arch Phys Med Rehabil*, **78**, 410–413.

Tilikete, C., Rode, G., Rossetti, Y., Pichon, J., Li, L. and Boisson, D. (2001). Prism adaptation to rightward optical deviation improves postural imbalance in left-hemiparetic patients. *Curr Biol*, **11**, 524–528.

Vallar, G. and Perani, D. (1986). The anatomy of unilateral neglect after right-hemipshere stroke lesions: a clinical/CT-scan correlations study in man. *Neuropsychologia*, **24**, 609–622.

Vallar, G., Sterzi, R., Bottini, G., Cappa, S. and Rusconi, M.L. (1990). Temporary remission of left hemianesthesia after vestibular stimulation: a sensory neglect phenomenon. *Cortex*, **26**, 123–131.

Vallar, G., Bottini, G., Rusconi, M.L. and Sterzi, R. (1993). Exploring somatosensory hemineglect by vestibular stimulation. *Brain*, **116**, 71–86.

Vallar, G., Rusconi, M.L., Barozzi, S., Bernardini, B., Ovadia, D., Papagno, C. and Cesarani, A. (1995). Improvement of left visuo-spatial hemineglect by left-sided transcutaneous electrical stimulation. *Neuropsychologia*, **33**, 73–82.

Vallar, G., Guariglia, C., Magnotti, L. and Pizzamiglio, L. (1997). Dissociation between position sense and visual-spatial components of hemineglect through a specific rehabilitation treatment. *J Clin Exp Neuropsychol*, **19(5)**, 763–771.

Venneri, A. and Shanks, M.F. (2004). Belief and awareness: reflections on a case of persistent anosognosia. *Neuropsychologia*, **42**, 230–238.

Wagenaar, R.C., Van Wieringen, P.C.W., Netelbos, J.B., Meijer, O.G. and Kuik, D.J. (1992). The transfer of scanning training effects in visual inattention after stroke five single-case studies. *Disabil Rehabil*, **14**, 51–60.

Walker, R., Young, A.W. and Lincoln, N.B. (1996). Eye patching and the rehabilitation of visual neglect. *Neuropsychol Rehabil*, **6**, 219–231.

Watson, R.T. and Heilman, K.M. (1979). Thalamic neglect. *Neurology*, **29**, 690–694.

Watson, R.T., Valenstein, E. and Heilman, K.M. (1981). Thalamic neglect: possible role of the medial thalamus and nucleus reticularis in behavior. *Arch Neurol*, **38**, 501–506.

Webster, J.S., McFarland, P.T., Rapport, L.J., Morrill, B., Roades, L.A. and Abadee, P.S. (2001). Computer-assisted training for improving wheelchair mobility in unilateral neglect patients. *Arch Phys Med Rehabil*, **82**, 769–775.

Weiller, C., Willmes, K., Reiche, W., Thron, A., Isensee, C., Buell, U. and Ringelstein, E.B. (1993). The case of aphasia or neglect after striatocapsular infarction. *Brain*, **116**, 1509–1525.

Weinberg, J., Diller, L., Gordon, W.A., Gerstman, L.J., Liebermann, A., Lakin, P., Hodges, G. and Ezrachi, O. (1977). Visual scanning training effect on reading-related tasks in acquired right brain damage. *Arch Phys Med Rehabil*, **58**, 479–486.

Weintraub, S., Daffner, K.R., Ahern, G.L., Price, B.H. and Mesulam, M.M. (1996). Right sided hemispatial neglect and bilateral cerebral lesions. *J Neurol Neurosurg Psychiatr*, **60**, 342–344.

Wiart, L., Bon Saint Côme, A., Debelleix, X., Petit, H., Josph, P.A., Mazaux, J.M. and Barat, M. (1997). Unilateral neglect syndrome rehabilitation by trunk rotation and scanning training. *Arch Phys Med Rehabil*, **78**, 424–429.

Zoccolotti, P., Guariglia, C., Pizzamiglio, L., Judica, A., Razzano, C. and Pantano, P. (1992). Good recovery in visual scanning in a patient with persistent anosognosia. *Int J Neurosci*, **62**, 93–104.

Memory dysfunction

Jonathan Evans

Section of Psychological Medicine, University of Glasgow, Glasgow, UK

29.1 Introduction

It seems likely that in the future memory rehabilitation will be quite different from how it is now. There will be considerably more biologically based restitution-oriented intervention options available to the patient and clinician. However, for the present time, the most effective approaches to memory rehabilitation are those that enable people with memory dysfunction to compensate for their impairment. This can be through the use of learning methods that promote more effective acquisition of knowledge or skills, or through the use of memory aids such as diaries, calendars or electronic devices, which function as cognitive prostheses. In this chapter, following a brief introduction to the different forms of memory, recent studies that provide the basis for future developments in biologically based memory rehabilitation will be reviewed, along with examples of compensatory learning methods, strategies and aids. Figure 29.1 provides a summary list of the approaches to rehabilitation reviewed in this chapter.

29.2 Forms of memory

It is now well established that memory is not a unitary concept or process, at either a psychological or anatomical level. Several different conceptual divisions have been proposed. These include the division between short-term, or working memory (the mental workspace in which information can be held briefly and manipulated) and long-term memory (the long-term repository of knowledge). Within long-term memory, divisions have been made at the level of stimulus material (verbal versus non-verbal), type of information (context-free, factual or semantic information versus information relating to personal experience or episodic information), and accessibility to conscious recollection (declarative/explicit versus non-declarative/implicit memory). Squire (1992, 1998) proposed a taxonomy of memory systems to reflect these conceptual divisions, as illustrated by Christian et al. in Chapter 2 of Volume I. Most memory rehabilitation has been focused on improving, or compensating for, impaired declarative memory. With regard to anatomy, a very wide range of brain structures are involved in remembering processes. Critical to declarative memory functioning are the medial temporal lobes, with their reciprocal connections to areas of the neocortex, which support the acquisition of new episodic and semantic information, and are involved in the recollection of older autobiographical episodic memories (Nadel and Moscovitch, 1997). Medial temporal lobe structures are vulnerable to direct damage or indirect disruption in a variety of neurological conditions (e.g. encephalitis, anoxia, Alzheimer's disease, head injury, anterior communicating artery aneurysm rupture), and might be considered the focus of restorative approaches to memory rehabilitation.

29.3 Restitution-oriented therapies

After brain injury there is usually a period during which cognitive functions impaired by primary and

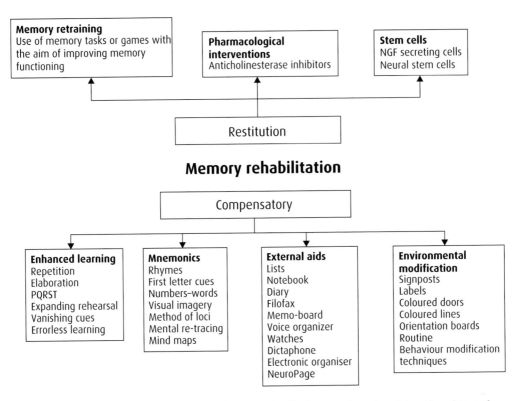

Figure 29.1. Schematic representation of the range of memory rehabilitation strategies reviewed. Apart from the use of pharmacological interventions in the context of DAT, there is little evidence to support use of restitution-based therapies for memory impairment. Compensatory techniques remain the treatments of choice at present. DAT: dementia of the Alzheimer's type.

secondary damage recover. Although the full extent of functional recovery will be affected by many factors, the one thing that appears to have the most significant impact on recovery is the severity of the initial injury, as reflected by measures such as length of coma or period of post-traumatic amnesia (Russell, 1971; Haslam et al., 1994). This suggests that there is a relatively straightforward association between the amount of initial damage and the level of long-term (permanent) impairment. However, the fact that the association is not perfect leads to questions as to what factors may contribute to enhancing recovery of function, despite initially severe injury, and secondly what interventions will weaken that association further. The aim of restitution-oriented therapies for memory impairment (or indeed any impairment) is, in effect, to restore the physical or the functional integrity of

the memory systems of the brain. Recent work investigating the use of neural stem cells as delivery mechanisms for neuroprotective agents or as replacement brain tissue has focused on measuring outcome in terms of improved memory functioning and may be seen as attempts to restore physical integrity. Pharmacological and some memory training interventions might be considered to be attempts to restore functional integrity of memory systems.

Neural stem cell interventions

Two major strands of research into the use of neural stem cells can be identified. In the first, studies have examined the use of cells that are genetically engineered to secrete nerve growth factor (NGF, for detailed discussions of the neurobiology of NGFs see

Chapters 16 and 23 of Volume I). Studies have shown that NGF stimulates functional recovery from cognitive impairments associated with aging (in rats), either when administered as a purified protein or by means of implantation of modified NGF-secreting cells into the medial septum and nucleus basalis magnocellularis (Martinez-Serrano et al., 1996). Philips et al. (2001) looked at the use of NGF-secreting cells after brain injury. In their study, Philips et al. transplanted cells into cortex adjacent to injury sites after experimentally induced brain injury in rats. There was evidence that implantation of these cells resulted in less CA3 hippocampal neuronal cell death and produced improved cognitive and neuromotor functioning compared to a number of control groups. In this case, NGF is thought to function in a neuroprotective manner, effectively rescuing cells that may otherwise have died as a result of the presence of extracellular excitatory amino acids, calcium, free radicals and cytokines in the acute post-injury phase (Philips et al., 2001, p. 770).

However, Virley et al. (1999, p. 2322) note that significant protection against hippocampal cell loss by prospective neuroprotective agents after prolonged ischaemic anoxia has been difficult to demonstrate. When administered very soon after onset of anoxia, cells at risk of death may be rescued, but treatments cannot reverse cell death that has already occurred, so limiting their therapeutic potential. The question arises therefore as to whether lost neurones can be replaced. As Macklis and Kempermann discuss in Chapter 18 of Volume I, until relatively recently it was thought that the adult brain was incapable of generating new neurons or having new neurons added to its structure. However, the last decade of research into neurogenesis has identified specific regions of the brain in which new neurons are generated from neural precursor cells. This has also stimulated work exploring whether new neural cells can be grown from harvested precursor cells and transplanted into lesioned areas. A number of studies (Field et al., 1991; Netto et al., 1993; Hodges et al., 1996, 1997) have shown that transplanting foetal hippocampal cells into a lesioned hippocampus can be effective in producing functional integration into the host brain and

promoting cognitive recovery of memory functioning in rats. Toda et al. (2001) demonstrated improvements in spatial memory in rats transplanted with adult hippocampus-derived neural stem cells. Virley et al. (1999), responding to ethical and practical constraints in using foetal grafts, showed that similar functional recovery of memory functioning could be obtained using cloned neural stem cells (Maudsley hippocampal cell line, clone 36 – MHP36). These cells, derived from mouse hippocampal neuroepithelium, possess the characteristic that they divide at a low temperature, but stop dividing and differentiate into mature brain cells at brain temperature on implantation. Virley et al. (1999) used these cells in common marmosets. Following lesioning of the hippocampus CA1 field and then implantation of stem cells, improvement to control levels was shown on retention and new learning on conditional discrimination tasks. Sinden et al. (2000) note that MHP36 cell grafts are effective in reversing sensory and motor deficits and reducing lesion volume following occlusion of the middle cerebral artery in animal models, though the same cell grafts were unable to reverse motor deficits following nigrostriatal lesions. This work therefore offers considerable promise for the future, with a particular focus on the rehabilitation of memory. However, to date, this work has not been translated into humans with comparable brain damage and this clearly presents a major challenge.

The basal forebrain cholinergic system, which innervates other key structures important for memory (medial temporal lobe, frontal lobe) has also been the target for pharmacological interventions.

Pharmacological interventions

Atrophy of neurones in the basal forebrain cholinergic system is associated with normal ageing and dementia of the Alzheimer's type (DAT), and is thought to underlie associated deficits in memory functioning. This region is also vulnerable to damage following head injury. Several interventions have now been developed that aim to increase levels of available acetylcholine (ACh). The most common method of doing this is through the use of acetylcholinesterase

(AChE) inhibitors such as donepezil, tacrine, rivastigmine and galantamine. Several large-scale clinical trials have demonstrated beneficial effects of these drugs. Whilst the level of improvement above baseline levels of functioning is likely to be modest, it would appear that they reduce the level of cognitive and functional decline in functioning associated with progressive conditions such as Alzheimer's disease (e.g. Rogers et al., 2000; Feldman et al., 2001; Winblad et al., 2001; Wimo et al., 2003; Birks and Harvey, 2003). Although many of the studies do not assess or report impact on memory functioning in detail, it is suggested that measures of verbal rehearsal and verbal episodic memory most consistently respond to manipulation of the cholinergic system (see Simard and van Reekum, 1998; Griffin et al., 2003). Furthermore, positron emission imaging studies (e.g. Kaasinen et al., 2002) have shown that donepezil and rivastigmine reduced levels of AChE, particularly in frontal regions. There are only a small number of studies, many of them case studies, which have examined the effect of AChE inhibitors in the context of non-progressive conditions such as head injury. A recent review by Griffen et al. (2003) found 13 studies of AChE inhibitors or choline precursors after a systematic literature search. Only three of these studies were randomised control trials, with a total of 66 participants. Studies have varied considerably in reported outcomes, but in general there have been reported improvements in performance on memory and attention tasks. Another recent study of donepezil by Morey et al. (2003), with seven people having traumatic brain injury (TBI) with persistent memory disorder at least 1.5 years post-injury reported improvements in performance on a visual recall task (with multiple versions), but there was no improvement on a verbal recall task, nor on a verbal fluency task or on a self-report questionnaire rating of memory functions. In studies such as this without control groups it is clearly necessary to be cautious in interpretation of change. A further small study by Kaye et al. (2003) of four patients with TBI treated with donepezil found no change on tests of memory, but based on patient self-report and observation, Kaye et al. suggested that the overall impression was that, "the patients had improved focus, attention and clarity, with patients commenting that their speed of processing appeared better or they were able to keep multiple ideas in mind simultaneously" (p. 383). This raises the possibility that the compounds are primarily affecting attention and arousal, with a more indirect impact on memory functioning, though this remains to be determined. A related hypothesis was suggested by Beckwith et al. (1999) who concluded that donepezil improved executive functioning, but not memory, based on reported changes on the dementia rating scale.

Another pharmacological intervention, for which there is evidence of efficacy, is the use of drugs that limit the effect of glutamate, the main excitatory neurotransmitter. Enhancement of the excitatory action of this amino acid is thought to play a role in the pathogenesis of Alzheimer's disease and in the damage due to ischaemic stroke (Areosa Sastre, McShane and Sherriff 2005). Memantine is an N-methyl-D-aspartate (NMDA) receptor antagonist and is thought to prevent excitatory amino-acid neurotoxicity without interfering with the physiological actions of glutamate necessary for learning and memory. The Cochrane review of conducted by Areosa Satre et al. (2005) concluded, on the basis of ten published trials that memantine has a positive effect on cognition, mood and behaviour, and the ability to perform activities of daily living in patients with moderate to severe Alzheimer's disease (AD). The effect in mild to moderate AD is unknown. Results for vascular dementia were that there was evidence of improvement in cognition, but not in activities of daily living. Although some work in rat models has suggested that memantine may have a neuroprotective effect after brain injury, reducing neuronal cell loss in hippocampal CA2 and CA3 areas (Rao et al., 2001), there has been little published evidence of efficacy of this approach in humans. In the case of dementia, and potentially in brain injury too, the emphasis is primarily on reducing the deterioration in cognitive functioning that otherwise would occur, rather than enhancing cognitive performance above initial baseline levels.

Herbal remedies, widely marketed as cognitive enhancers, such as *Ginkgo biloba* and *Ginseng* have also been evaluated to a limited extent in both healthy volunteers and people with memory impairment. Results have been somewhat mixed and to a degree, controversial. One systematic review (Diamond et al., 2000) concluded that *Ginkgo* shows promise in treating some of the neurological sequelae of DAT, TBI, stroke, normal cognition and other conditions. However, several recent studies of *Ginkgo* have failed to find significant effects on memory in healthy adults (Solomon et al., 2002; Persson et al., 2003), nor in people with dementia and age-associated memory impairment (van Dongen et al., 2003). Other recent studies have reported some benefits, however (Stough et al., 2001; Mix and Crews 2002), resulting in considerable debate as whether *Ginkgo* will only produce benefits on very selective tests or particular subjects, such as those with poor memory (see Nathan et al., 2003). Very little evidence exists for the impact of *Ginkgo* in the context of memory impairments arising from acquired brain injury.

In summary, it is now standard clinical practice to treat the cognitive impairments associated with DAT with AChE inhibitors. Whether or not the pathophysiology of non-progressive brain injuries such as TBI is similar enough to that of DAT is not clear yet and to date far less evidence exists to suggest that such compounds should routinely be used to treat memory and other cognitive impairments after TBI. A small number of studies suggest that pharmacological interventions are promising, but further well-controlled studies are needed.

Memory training

The idea that memory can be improved through some form of mental exercise or practice at remembering underlies some cognitive retraining approaches to memory rehabilitation. A distinction does have to be drawn between retraining approaches which aim to improve memory through simple practice or exercising memory and those approaches that aim to train memory strategies, which would fall into the category of compensatory approaches. Various computer-based packages are available that enable memory to be exercised, through practice on memory exercises or games. There is, however, little evidence that such

memory training techniques bring about changes in underlying memory processes or impact on everyday remembering. In a systematic review of cognitive training and cognitive rehabilitation for early stage Alzheimer's disease and vascular dementia, Clare et al. (2003) examined the small number of studies of cognitive training interventions. The interventions classified as cognitive training varied somewhat. Some were in fact training in the use of mnemonic strategies though others did examine the impact of memory exercises delivered on a computer. Various methodological limitations were noted and the overall conclusion was that there were no statistically significant results on any measure. They also examined cognitive rehabilitation approaches, which they distinguish from cognitive training in that the focus of cognitive training is on improving cognitive functioning *per se*, whereas in cognitive rehabilitation the emphasis is on improving functioning in the everyday context. Clare et al. conclusions are consistent with earlier comments in relation to the wider brain-injured population from Wilson (1997) and Glisky et al. (1986) who suggested that memory retraining methods cannot be recommended as appropriate clinical practice. Similarly, in a review of cognitive rehabilitation, Robertson (1999) noted that "… in the case of memory rehabilitation, there is as yet no evidence for direct and lasting improvement of memory through restitution-oriented therapies. Hence, compensatory approaches to memory problems appear to be, for the time being at least, the treatment of choice" (p. 704). It should be said though that there have not been many large scale well controlled studies of memory retraining and so to date such conclusions are perhaps based on absence of evidence for an effect, rather than on evidence of absence of an effect. Compensatory strategies are discussed in the next section. Before moving on, however, it is worth noting one further novel form of memory training, though it is a method which has not been properly evaluated to date. Thornton (2000) describes the use of quantitative electroencephalogram (QEEG) biofeedback as a means of improving memory functioning. In this study, QEEG variables associated with memory performance on a range of memory tasks were identified. Subjects with brain injury underwent an EEG study to determine which variables present in controls and correlating with memory performance were deficient. In a training program focused on passage recall, a biofeedback paradigm was used in an attempt to improve QEEG data and also memory performance. Thornton reported on three people with brain injury who showed improvement in passage recall over a series of up to 35 passage recall test trials. Although showing some improvement over time, the study is relatively poorly controlled and therefore it is difficult to draw firm conclusions about the method. The technique has been reported in several other applications (e.g. treating anxiety and post-traumatic stress disorder) and so deserves further evaluation in this client group. The following section, however, deals with the intervention approaches that are the mainstay of current memory rehabilitation.

29.4 Compensatory strategies

Within the category of compensatory strategies, there is a range of possible intervention approaches, some of which have been well evaluated. Four different types of approach can be identified:

1 enhanced learning (making more effective use of residual memory skills),
2 mnemonic strategies,
3 external aids,
4 environmental modification.

Enhanced learning

Complete amnesia is relatively rare and most people with memory impairment retain some residual learning capacity. It is therefore important that this capacity is used to maximum effect. This fact was explicitly recognised in the group intervention described by Berg et al. (1991) in which they provide participants with a set of "memory rules". These include:

- *Attention*: Pay more attention to the information to be remembered. Make sure that you are not distracted by your environment and that you consciously focus on whatever you have to remember.

- *Time*: Spend more time on encoding. Generally the more time you spend on encoding the more you will remember. But spend your time economically – not too long without a pause, but frequently and little by little.
- *Repetition*: Whatever you have to remember will sink in more easily if you repeat it. There are several forms of repetition: simple repetition, spaced repetition (with increasing time intervals) and varied repetition (in several ways and situations).

The spaced repetition or retrieval technique is also known as expanding rehearsal. This technique is derived from a general learning principle that spaced practice is a more effective learning technique than massed practice. The technique involves information being presented and tested for recall immediately, then again after a few seconds interval, then after few minutes and so on gradually increasing the time gap before recall is tested. Evidence suggests that this approach is more effective than the same number of repetitions within a shorter period of time with regular intervals between repetitions. Camp et al. (1996) describe the use of spaced retrieval in training people with mild to moderate Alzheimer's disease to perform prospective memory tasks relevant to their day-to-day life. A spaced retrieval procedure is also the basis of the prospective memory-training program described by Sohlberg et al. (1985) in which people are asked to remember to do something after gradually increasing time intervals.

The vanishing cues and errorless learning techniques were both derived from the marrying of methods from behavioural and cognitive psychology. The vanishing cues technique (Glisky et al., 1986) is essentially a "backward chaining" method, similar to the chaining approaches to teach multi-step tasks (such as dressing) to people with severe learning disability. The main application for the vanishing cues technique has been teaching people with amnesia new knowledge. For example, Glisky et al. demonstrated that people with amnesia could learn new computer-related vocabulary using the technique, which involved presenting the individual with the whole of the information they must learn to begin with, and then gradually withdrawing elements of the to-be-learned information. So, if the individual is learning how to print a document, the sentence, "To make a paper copy of a document, press PRINT" would be presented. Then over successive trials, letters from the word print would be successively removed (i.e. PRIN, PRI, PR, P) until no letters were present. The main theoretical influence on this work is the literature on implicit memory and priming, and in particular the finding that people with amnesia often are able to show word stem completion priming (Warrington and Weiskrantz, 1974). However, one possible limitation of the vanishing cues technique is that the benefit of the technique may only be present when there is at least one letter of the target word left, acting as a perceptual prime.

One hypothesis as to why the vanishing cues technique is effective is that it is less likely that people will make mistakes during the learning process. While learning something new, the person with amnesia who makes a mistake on one occasion (e.g. calling somebody by the wrong name), will forget the error, but in addition may be "primed" to make the same mistake again, so reinforcing the error. The implication of this idea is that if the person with memory impairment can be prevented from making errors during the learning process, then learning ought to be more rapid. Errorless learning techniques have been used for many years to teach new skills to teach people with learning disabilities (Jones and Eayrs, 1992) and more recently this technique has been used with people with acquired neurological impairment. Baddeley and Wilson (1994) published the first study demonstrating that people with amnesia learn better when prevented from making mistakes during the learning process. This was a theoretical study in which a stem completion task was used to teach a list of words. However, since then several single case studies have shown the benefit of errorless learning methods in teaching more practical, everyday information (Wilson et al., 1994; Squires et al., 1996; Hunkin et al., 1998). There has been some investigation of this technique for people with DAT (Clare et al., 1999, 2000, 2001, 2002). For example, Clare et al. (1999) were able to teach a 72-year-old man in the early stages of DAT the names of 11 members of his social club. The intervention incorporated verbal elaboration, vanishing cues and expanding rehearsal. Importantly, the gains generalised from photographs, which were used for training, to real faces and were maintained at follow up 9 months later.

Kessels and DeHaan (2003) conducted a meta-analysis on errorless learning and vanishing cues methods. They identified 27 studies that focused on errorless learning or vanishing cues, but 13 of these included no control condition and so were excluded from the analysis. The result of this analysis was that there was a significant effect size for studies of errorless learning, but not for vanishing cues (though only three studies were included).

For people whose aim is to return to some form of formal education, study techniques such as PQRST and mind maps are useful. They are not specifically designed for people with memory impairments, and have received very little in the way of formal evaluation, though clinical experience suggests they may be useful. Both are mean of enhancing the meaningfulness and memorability of information to be learned. PQRST is an acronym for Preview, Question, Read, State and Test (Robinson, 1970). When faced with information to be learned, the text should be previewed (skim read), and a set of questions identified, the answers to which should be obtained during a more detailed reading of the text. After reading the text, the questions are answered. Finally, knowledge for the whole text is tested. Mind mapping is another means of enhancing the multi-modality encoding of information (Buzan and Buzan, 2000). The technique involves producing a one page visual summary of whatever is being learned, with the use of drawings, coloured text, boxes and arrows to link ideas and information. Mind maps may also be useful in any context where a significant amount of information is required to be retained and used (e.g. preparing for a presentation).

Mnemonics

Mnemonics are memory strategies such as those used by the stage performers who demonstrate "great feats of memory" such as remembering the order of a shuffled pack of cards with only brief exposure to each card. The most commonly used mnemonic technique is a form of the method of loci in which a route around a familiar place or a journey with many specific locations is pre-learned. Each item to be remembered is associated with the locations on the route (using visual imagery). These techniques require a great deal of practice and are best for learning lists. For most people with memory impairment such techniques are difficult to use, or unnecessary and few people use them. In a survey we conducted (Evans et al., 2003) of almost 100 people with memory impairment only one "internal" technique was used frequently, which was "mental retracing". This is the simple idea of retracing your steps in order to remember what you have done, or perhaps where you have left an item that is lost. Given that many people with memory impairments, particularly arising from head injury, may also be impulsive (as a result of frontal lobe deficits), teaching a simple "Stop–Think–Retrace Your Steps" approach can be helpful.

One further mnemonic strategy that can also be helpful, particularly in world full of personal identification number (PIN) codes, is one where numbers are converted to words, such that the number of letters in the words corresponds to the PIN number (i.e. 1424 might be represented by the sentence "I like my bank"). No systematic evaluations of this technique have been undertaken though again clinical experiences suggests that in certain circumstances it can be useful (see Evans, 2003, p. 157).

External aids

The most commonly used strategies for supporting memory are external aids. Evans et al. (2003) found that nearly 70% of people with a memory impairment used a calendar, notebook or diary. External memory aids need to form the core "memory system" for most people with significant memory impairment. Indeed most people without memory impairment use some form of external memory aid. However, for the person with a memory impairment, the process of learning to use such aids is not straightforward and may require

considerable support. Despite this need, Tate (1997) noted that memory rehabilitation is still not often provided for patients with severe disorders of memory. Nevertheless, a number of studies have shown that comprehensive training approaches can lead to effective use of memory journals, even in people with severe amnesia (Sohlberg and Mateer, 1989; Kime et al., 1996; Donaghy and Williams, 1998). Ownsworth and McFarland (1999) demonstrated that a combined "diary and self-instructional training" was more effective than "diary alone" in leading people with brain injury to be more consistent in making diary entries and reporting less memory problems. In this case the self-instructional training participants were taught a set of four strategy cues:

1 What are you going to do?
2 Select a strategy for the task.
3 Try out the strategy.
4 Check how the strategy is working.

These were abbreviated to WSTC. In some senses this strategy could be thought of as a means of compensating for co-existing executive or problem-solving deficits that may lead an individual to fail use a memory even if he or she has one available.

Electronic memory aids offer the major advantage of having the facility to prompt an action using alarms. They also provide a means of combining a number of different memory aid functions (e.g. alarmed reminders, schedule, contact information, to-do list) into one portable tool. However, as Evans et al. (2003) showed, only a small number of people with memory impairment seem to be making use of such tools. It is possible that a range of different factors accounts for this finding, including the cost and perhaps the lack of experience of rehabilitation professionals. One factor that was shown to be important in predicting memory aid use after brain injury in the study group of Evans et al. (2003) and also that of Wilson and Watson (1996) was pre-morbid use of memory aids. Given that use of electronic memory aids is low in the general population, this may be a critical factor. Relevant to this issue is the fact that many of the electronic organisers and palm-top computers can be complex and difficult to learn

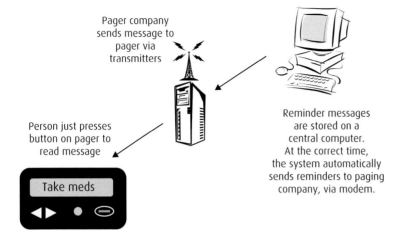

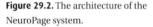

Pager company
sends message to
pager via
transmitters

Person just presses
button on pager to
read message

Take meds

Reminder messages
are stored on a
central computer.
At the correct time,
the system automatically
sends reminders to paging
company, via modem.

Figure 29.2. The architecture of the
NeuroPage system.

for those people without pre-morbid experience. One solution to this problem is to design simpler interfaces for palm-top computers that meet the needs of people with memory and other cognitive impairments. Wright et al. (2001) have shown that it is possible to simplify palm-top computer interfaces for use by people with brain injury. Our group has also developed and undertaken preliminary evaluations of another aid that uses standard Personal Digitial Assistant technology, but with an adapted, simplified user interface (Inglis et al., 2003; Symkoviak et al., 2005). There are some indications that those who are trained to use such aids in a rehabilitation context will continue to use them after discharge (Kim et al., 2000).

One electronic reminding tool that has undergone extensive clinical trials is NeuroPage, a pager-based system designed by Larry Treadgold, the engineer father of a young man who sustained a head injury and Neil Hersh, a neuropsychologist (Hersh and Treadgold, 1994). The architecture of the NeuroPage system is illustrated in Fig. 29.2. The person with the memory impairment wears an ordinary alphanumerical pager. Reminders are entered onto a remote computer and at the correct time, the computer sends the message, via a modem and paging company, to the individual's pager. He or she then simply presses one button to cancel the alert and reads the message. This

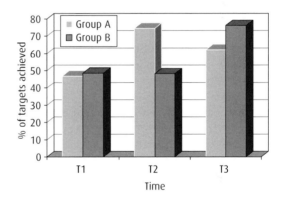

Figure 29.3. Graph illustrating the data from the randomised control trial of NeuroPage. Group A have the pager first at Time 2 (T2) only. Group B has the pager at Time 3 (T3) only.

system has now been evaluated in clinical trials and single case studies, and shown to be very effective (Wilson et al., 1997a, 1999, 2001; Evans et al., 1998). The study by Wilson et al. (2001) was a randomised control trial using a crossover design, in which the impact on everyday tasks was examined in 143 people with memory impairment. The study demonstrated that NeuroPage was effective at increasing functional performance, which is illustrated in Fig. 29.3. What has been found in studies of NeuroPage to date is that for some people performance of a target task is maintained even when NeuroPage is withdrawn as people have reached the point where the task can be carried out without prompting. This suggests that this sort of device could be used on a short-term basis for developing key target behaviours (e.g. remembering to check a to-do list) and then withdrawn. It is important to recognise, of course that generalisation to non-targeted behaviours or new tasks is unlikely to occur in this situation. This system is available on a national basis in the UK and a recent paper (Wilson et al., 2003) described how the system was used by the first 40 people referred to this service. At the present time paging services are beginning to be phased out by many of the current telecommunications companies, in favour of short message (text) services (SMS) for mobile phones. It seems likely that in the near future the paging reminding service will be replaced by a SMS text reminding service, though it would be helpful to have formal evaluation of such a service to ensure that it is as effective for patients as the paging system.

A small number of other electronic reminding devices have also undergone some evaluation. The Voice Organizer (see www.vpti.com) is a hand-held device on which self-dictated reminders are recorded and which are played following a prompt at a time set by the individual. van den Broek et al. (2000) showed that five people with acquired memory impairment showed improvement on two prospective remembering tasks analogous to everyday memory tasks when using the Voice Organizer. Hart et al. (2002) also showed that the Voice Organizer was effective in helping people to remember therapy goals during the course of a rehabilitation programme. Another potential aid is the Timex Data Link watch (www.timex.com) which can provide alarm and text prompts that are programmed on a personal computer (PC) and downloaded to the watch via a universal serial bus (USB) link. Electronic dictaphones can be used to record a number of spoken notes during the day, with the option of transferring information to a diary, electronic organiser, etc. at a later date. Wilson et al. (1997b) also provide a discussion of the development of a comprehensive compensatory memory system, which includes the use of a dictaphone, by one man

(J.C.) who became amnesic following a subarachnoid haemorrhage. Wade and Troy (2001) described the use of a mobile-phone-based system with five people using pre-recorded speech reminders that were sent to the mobile phone. Although showing some promise this system has not been developed further and is not commercially available.

One of the advantages of aids such as the NeuroPage and watches are that they are, in effect, wearable computers. A further development of this sort is Memory Glasses (DeVaul et al., 2003) which provide visual prompts to the wearer via a head-mounted display worn on the subjects glasses. This tool, however, is only in a development stage and has not been evaluated with people with memory impairment.

Dosset boxes, which have multiple sections for storing daily medication doses, can be obtained through pharmacies and are particularly helpful for people who have complicated medication regimes. They can be prepared in advance.

Kapur (1995) and Clare and Wilson (1997) provide good summaries of a range of memory aids. Clare and Wilson's (1997) book also provides a basic introduction to memory problems and how to cope with them for people with memory impairments, their relatives, friends and carers. Gartland (2004) provides a useful discussion of practical considerations for professionals introducing cognitive rehabilitation technology to people with brain injury, emphasing the importance of considering the main purpose of the technology (keeping the focus on what it is that the individual needs the technology for rather than what the technology can do), environmental issues (including amount of support available to the person using the technology outside of the rehabilitation environment) and other factors such as cost.

Environmental modification

For some people, their level of cognitive impairment is so severe that learning to use memory aids or strategies is impossible. For this group, the treatment method of choice is environmental modification. The idea is simply to, as far as possible, reduce the memory demands placed upon the person. The use of signposts, labels or colour coding (e.g. toilet doors always being a particular colour) can aid orientation to the environment. Orientation boards help maintain knowledge of time and place. Reducing clutter and always keeping particular things in particular places (e.g. keys on a key holder) may be helpful. "Smart houses" contain a range of technology that may help people with disabilities including memory impairment live more independently (Wilson and Evans, 2000).

One form of environmental modification is to provide a highly structured environment, involving a great deal of routine. People with severe memory impairment are usually still able to learn routines through repetition. Daily routines provide a way of an individual maintaining a sense of independently completing activities, with minimal demands on memory.

One further area where environmental modification is relevant is in the management of challenging behaviour. Alderman et al. (Alderman and Ward, 1991; Alderman and Burgess, 1994) have discussed the problems of helping people with challenging behaviour to modify their behaviour in the context of a combination of executive and memory impairments. As the severity of learning problems in this client group it is necessary to manipulate environmental contingencies in a very clear and consistent manner. This is often done through the use of token economy reinforcement schedules. However, even here the delay (often several minutes) between behaviour and its contingency (receipt or not of reward) can mean that the memory-impaired individual cannot learn the association between behaviour and its consequence. In this case a further modification has been suggested, using a response cost technique where the client begins with a number of tokens or coins. If he or she exhibits the target inappropriate behaviour he or she has to hand over a set number of coins. Later, the client can exchange coins for a reward item, but only if he or she has sufficient left. The idea here is that the relationship between behaviour and its consequence is much clearer and so more easily learned. Several case studies have demonstrated the value of this approach in helping individuals to reduce the frequency of inappropriate behaviour, and so to participate in other rehabilitation activities.

29.5 Conclusions

The future appears bright as far as the development of restorative treatment techniques is concerned, though many challenges lay ahead before brain repair technology is routinely used as a method of cognitive rehabilitation. For the time being, evidence suggests that compensatory strategies are the treatment of choice for most organic memory disorders. External memory aids remain the most practical, widely used and effective tools. Simple reminding tools such as NeuroPage are proven to improve day-to-day functioning and in some cases reduce the cost of health and social care. Emerging technologies in the form of Internet-ready personal digital assistants and wearable computing platforms may prove useful, extending the range of memory prostheses open to people with impairment. However, the application of learning techniques such as errorless learning methods are, and will continue to be, essential for giving the person with a memory impairment the best chance of acquiring the knowledge and skills required to cope more effectively with day-to-day personal, social and vocational activities.

REFERENCES

Areosa Sastre, A., Sherriff, F. and McShane, R. Memantine for dementia. *The Cochrane Database of Systematic Reviews*, 2005, Issue 3. Art. No.: CD003154. DOI: 10.1002/14651858. CD003154.pub4.

Alderman, N. and Burgess, P. (1994). A comparison of treatment methods for behaviour disorder following herpes simplex encephalitis. *Neuropsychol Rehabil*, **4**, 31–48.

Alderman, N. and Ward, A. (1991). Behavioural treatment of the dysexecutive syndrome: reduction of repetitive speech using response cost and cognitive overlearning. *Neuropsychol Rehabil*, **1**, 65–80.

Baddeley, A.D. and Wilson, B.A. (1994). When implicit learning fails: amnesia and the problem of error elimination. *Neuropsychologia*, **32**, 53–68.

Beckwith, B.E., Bergloff, P., Silvers, N. and Newland, D. (1999). Aricept (Donepezil) improves executive functions, but not memory. *Arch Clin Psychol*, **14**, 45.

Berg, I.J., Koning-Haanstra, M. and Deelman, B.G. (1991). Long term effects of memory rehabilitation: a controlled study. *Neurpsychol Rehabil*, **1**, 91–111.

Birks, J.S. and Harvey, R. (2003). Donepezil for demential due to Alzheimer's disease. In: *Cochrane Review*, The Cochrance Library, Issue 4. John Wiley and Sons, Ltd., Chichester.

Buzan, T. and Buzan, B. (2000). *The Mind Map Book*, BBC Worldwide Ltd., London.

Camp, C.J., Foss, J.W., Stevens, A.B. and O'Hanlon, A.M. (1996). Improving prospective memory task performance in persons with Alzheimer's disease. In: *Prospective Memory: Theory and Applications* (eds Brandimonte, M., Einstein, G.O. and McDaniel, M.A.), Lawrence Erlbaum Associates, Mahwah, New Jersey, pp. 351–367.

Clare, L. and Wilson, B.A. (1997). *Coping with Memory Problems: A Practical Guide for People with Memory Impairments, Their Relatives, Friends and Carers*, Thames Valley Test Company, Bury St Edmunds.

Clare, L, Wilson, B.A., Breen, K. and Hodges, J.R. (1999). Errorless learning of face-name associations in early Alzheimer's disease. *Neurocase*, **5**, 37–46.

Clare, L., Wilson, B.A., Carter, G., Gosses, A., Breen, K. and Hodges, J.R. (2000). Intervening with everyday memory problems in early Alzheimer's disease: an errorless learning approach. *J Clin Exp Neuropsychol*, **22**, 132–146.

Clare, L., Wilson, B.A., Carter, G., Hodges, J.R. and Adams, M. (2001). Long-term maintenance of treatment gains following a cognitive rehabilitation intervention in early dementia of Alzheimer type: a single case study. *Neuropsychol Rehabil*, **11**, 477–494.

Clare, L., Wilson, B.A., Carter, G., Roth, I. and Hodges, J.R. (2002). Relearning of face-name associations in early-stage Alzheimer's disease. *Neuropsychology*, **16**, 538–547.

Clare, L., Woods, R.T., Moniz Cook, E.D., Orrell, M. and Spector, A. (2003). Cognitive rehabilitation and cognitive training for early stage Alzheimer's disease and vascular dementia. In: *Cochrane Review*, The Cochrane Library, Issue 4. John Wiley and Sons, Ltd., Chichester, UK.

DeVaul, R., Pentland, S. and Corey, V.R. (2003). The Memory Glasses: subliminal vs. overt memory support with imperfect information. Paper Presented at: *the 7th IEEE Symposium of Wearable Computers*, October 21–23rd 2003, Crowne Plaza Hotel, White Plains, NY.

Diamond, B.J., Shiflett, S.C., Feiwel, N., Matheis, R.J., Noskin, O., Richards, J.A. and Schoenberger, N.E. (2000). *Ginkgo biloba*

extract: mechanisms and clinical indications. *Arch Phys Med Rehabil*, **81**, 668–678.

Donaghy, S. and Williams, W. (1998). A new protocol for training severely impaired patients in the usage of memory journals. *Brain Injury*, **12**, 1061–1077.

Evans, J.J. (2003). Disorders of memory. In: *Clinical Neuropsychology: A Practical Guide to Assessment and Management for Clinicians* (eds Goldstein, L.H. and McNeil, J.E.), John Wiley and Sons, Ltd., Chichester, UK.

Evans, J.J., Emslie, H. and Wilson, B.A. (1998). External cueing systems in the rehabilitation of executive impairments of action. *J Int Neuropsychol Soc*, **4**, 399–408.

Evans, J.J., Needham, P., Wilson, B.A. and Brentnall, S. (2003). Which memory impaired people make good use of memory aids? Results of a survey of people with acquired brain injury. *J Int Neuropsychol Soc*, **9**, 925–935.

Feldman, H., Gauthier, M.D., Hecker, J., et al. (2001). A 24-week, randomised, double-blind study of donepezil in moderate to severe Alzheimer's disease. *Neurology*, **57**, 613–620.

Field, P.M., Seeley, P.J., Frotscher, M. and Raisman, G. (1991). Selective innervation of embryonic hippocampal transplants by adult host dentate granule cell axons. *Neuroscience*, **41**, 713–727.

Gartland, D. (2004). Considerations in the selection and use of technology with people who have cognitive deficits following acquired brain injury. *Neuropsychol Rehabil*, **14**, 61–75.

Glisky, E.L., Schacter, D.L. and Tulving, E. (1986). Computer learning by memory impaired patients: acquisition and retention of complex knowledge. *Neuropsychologia*, **24**, 313–328.

Griffin, S.L., van Reekum, R. and Masanic, C. (2003). A review of cholinergic agents in the treatment of neurobehavioural deficits following traumatic brain injury. *J Neuropsychiat Clin Neurosc*, **15**, 17–26.

Hart, T., Hawkey, K., Whyte, J. (2002). Use of a portable voice organizer to remember therapy goals in TBI rehabilitation: a within-subjects trial. *J Head Trauma Rehabil*, **17(6)**, 556–570.

Haslam, C., Batchelor, J., Fearnside, M.R., et al. (1994). Post-coma disturbance and post-traumatic amnesia as non-linear predictors of cognitive outcome following severe closed head injury: findings from the Westmead Head Injury Project. *Brain Injury*, **8**, 519–528.

Hersh, N. and Treadgold, L. (1994). NeuroPage: the rehabilitation of memory dysfunction by prosthetic memory and cueing. *Neurorehabilitation*, **4**, 187–197.

Hodges, H., Sowinski, P., Fleming, P., Kershaw, T.R., Sinden, J.D., Meldrum, B.S., et al. (1996). Contrasting effects of fetal CA1 and CA3 hippocampal grafts on deficits in spatial learning and working memory induced by global cerebral ischaemia in rats. *Neuroscience*, **72**, 959–988.

Hodges, H., Nelson, A., Virley, D., Kershaw, T.R. and Sinden, J.D. (1997). Cognitive deficits induced by global cerebral ischaemia: prospects for transplant therapy [Review]. *Pharmacol Biochem Behav*, **56**, 736–780.

Hunkin, N.M., Squires, E.J., Aldrich, F.K. and Parkin, A.J. (1998). Errorless learning and the acquisition of word processing skills. *Neuropsychol Rehabil*, **8**, 433–449.

Inglis, E.A., Szymkowiak, A., Gregor, P., Newell, A.F., Hine, N., Shah, P., Evans, J.J. and Wilson, B.A. (2003). Issues surrounding the user-centred development of a new interactive memory aid. *Universal Access in the Information Society*, **2(3)**, 226–234.

Jones, R.S. and Earys, C.B. (1992). The use of errorless learning procedures in teaching people with a learning disability: a critical review. *Ment Handicap Res*, **5**, 204–212.

Kaasinen, V., Nagren, K., Jarvenpaa, T., Roivainen, A., Yu, M., Oikonen, V., Kurki, T. and Rinne, J.O. (2002). Regional effects of donepezil and rivastigmine on cortical acetylcholinesterase activity in Alzheimer's disease. *J Clin Psychopharmacol*, **22**, 615–620.

Kapur, N. (1995). Memory aids in rehabilitation of memory disordered patients. In: *Handbook of Memory Disorders* (eds Baddeley, A.D., Wilson, B.A. and Watts, F.), John Wiley, Chichester. UK, pp. 533–556.

Kaye, N.S., Townsend III, J.B. and Ivins, R. (2003). An open label trial of donepezil (aricept) in the treatment of persons with mild traumatic brain injury (Letter). *J Neuropsychiat Clin Neurosci*, **15**, 383.

Kessels, R.P.C. and DeHaan, E.H.F. (2003). Implicit learning in memory rehabilitation: a meta analysis on errorless learning and vanishing cues methods. *J Clin Exp Neuropsychol*, **25**, 805–814.

Kim, H.J., Burke, D.T., Dowds, M.M., Boone, K.A. and Park, G.J. (2000). Electronic memory aids for outpatient brain injury: follow up findings. *Brain Injury*, **14**, 187–196.

Kime, S.K., Lamb, D.G. and Wilson, B. A. (1996). Use of a comprehensive programme of external cueing to enhance procedural memory in a patient with dense amnesia. *Brain Injury*, **10**, 17–25.

Martinez-Serrano, A., Fischer, W., Soderstrom, S., Ebendal, T. and Bjorklund, A. (1996). Long-term functional recovery from age-induced spatial memory impairments by nerve growth factor gene transfer to the rat basal forebrain. *Proc Nat Acad Sci USA*, **93**, 6355–6360.

Mix, J.A. and Crews, W.D. (2002). A double blind placebo controlled randomised trial of *Ginkgo biloba* extract Egb761 in a sample of cognitively intact older adults: neuropsychological findings. *Human Psychopharmacol*, **17**, 267–277.

Morey, C.E., Cilo, J.B. and Cusick, C. (2003). The effect of Aricept in persons with persistent memory disorder following traumatic brain injury: a pilot study. *Brain Injury*, 809–815.

Nadel, L. and Moscovitch, M. (1997). Memory consolidation, retrograde amnesia and the hippocampal complex. *Curr Opin Neurobiol*, **7**, 217–227.

Nathan, P.J., Harrison, B.J. and Bartholomeusz, C. (2003). *Ginkgo* and memory. *J Am Med Assoc*, **289**, 546.

Netto, C.A., Hodges, H., Sinden, J.D., LePeillet, E., Kershaw, T., Sowinski, P., et al. (1993). Effects of fetal hippocampal field grafts on ischaemic-induced deficits in spatial navigation in the water maze. *Neuroscience*, **54**, 69–92.

Ownsworth, T.L. and McFarland, K. (1999). Memory remediation in long-term acquired brain injury: two approaches in diary training. *Brain Injury*, **13**, 605–626.

Persson, J., Bringlov, E., Nilsson, L.G. and Nyberg, L. (2003). The memory-enhancing effects of *Ginseng* and *Ginkgo biloba* in healthy volunteers. *Psychopharmacology*, Nov. 25 [ePub ahead of print].

Philips, M.F., Mattiasson, G., Wieloch, T., et al. (2001). Neuroprotective and behavioural efficacy of nerve growth factor-transfected hippocampal progenitor cell transplants after experimental traumatic brain injury. *J Neurosurg*, **94**, 765–774.

Rao, V.L., Dogan, A., Todd, K.G., Bowen, K.K., Dempsey, R.J. (2001). Neuroprotection by memantine, a non-competitive NMDA receptor antagonist after traumatic brain injury in rats. *Brain Res*, **911**, 96–100.

Robertson, I.R. (1999). Setting goals for rehabilitation. *Curr Opin Neurol*, **12**, 703–708.

Robinson, F.B. (1970). *Effective Study*, Harper, New York.

Rogers, S.L., Doody, R.S., Pratt, R.D. and Ieni, J.R. (2000). Long-term efficacy and safety of donepezil in the treatment of Alzheimer's disease: final analysis of a US multicentre open-label study. *Eur Neuropsychopharmacol*, **10**, 195–203.

Russell, W.R. (1971). *The Traumatic Amnesias*, Oxford University Press, London.

Simard, M. and van Reekum, R. (1998). Memory assessment in studies of cognition-enhancing drugs for Alzheimer's disease. *Drugs and Aging*, **14**, 197–230.

Sinden, J.D., Stroemer, P., Grigoryan, G., Patel, S., French, S.J. and Hodges, H. (2000). Functional repair with neural stem cells. *Novartis Found Symp*, **231**, 270–283.

Sohlberg, M.M. and Mateer, K. (1989). *Introduction to Cognitive Rehabilitation: Theory and Practice*, The Guilford Press, New York.

Sohlberg, M.M., Mateer, C.A. and Geyer, S. (1985). *Prospective Memory Screening (PROMS) and Prospective Memory Process Training (PROMPT)*, Association for Neuropsychological Research and Development, Puyallup, WA.

Solomon, P.R., Adams, F., Silver, A., Zimmer, J. and DeVeaux, R. (2002). *Ginkgo* for memory enhancement: a randomized controlled trial. *J Am Med Assoc*, **288**, 835–840.

Squire, L.R. (1992). Declarative and non-declarative memory: multiple brain systems supporting learning and memory. *J Cogne Neurosci*, **4**, 232–243.

Squire, L.R. (1998). Memory systems. *CR Acad Sci Paris Life Sci*, **321**, 153–156.

Squires, E., Hunkin, N.M. and Parkin, A.J. (1996). Memory notebook training in a case of severe amnesia: generalising from paired associate learning to real life. *Neuropsychol Rehabil*, **6**, 55–65.

Stough, C., Clarke, J., Lloyd, J. and Nathan, P.J. (2001). Neuropsychological changes after 30-day *Ginkgo biloba* administration in healthy participants. *Int J europsychopharamcol*, **4**, 131–134.

Szymkowiak, A., Morrison, K., Gregor, P., Shah, P., Evans, J.J. and Wilson, B.A. (2005). A memory aid with remote communication using distributed technology. Person and Ubiquit Comput, **9**, 1–5.

Tate, R.L. (1997). Beyond one-bun, two-shoe: recent advances in the psychological rehabilitation of memory disorders after acquired brain injury. *Brain Injury*, **11**, 907–918.

Thornton, K. (2000). Improvement/rehabilitation of memory functioning with neurotherapy/QEEG biofeedback. *J Head Trauma Rehabil*, **15**, 1285–1296.

Toda, H., Takahashi, J., Iwakami, N., Kimura, T., Hoki, S., Mozumi-Kitamura, K., Ono, S. and Hashimoto, N. (2001). Grafting neural stem cells improved the impaired spatial recogntion in ischemic rats. *Neurosci Lett*, **3136**, 9–12.

van den Broek, M.D., Downes, J., Johnson, Z., Dayus, B. and Hilton, N. (2000). Evaluation of an electronic aid in the neuropsychological rehabilitation of prospective memory deficits. *Brain Injury*, **14**, 455–462.

van Dongen, M., van Rossum, E., Kessels, A., Sielhorst, H. and Knipschild, P. (2003). *Ginkgo* for elderly people with dementia and age-associated memory impairment: a randomised clinical trial. *J Clin Epidemiol*, **56**, 367–376.

Virley, D., Ridley, R.M., Sinden, J.D., Kershaw, T.R., Harland, S., Rashid, T., French, S., Sowinski, P., Gray, J.A., Lantos, P.L. and Hodges, H. (1999). Primary CA1 and conditionally immortal MHP36 cell grafts restore conditional discrimination learning and recall in marmosets after excitotoxic lesions of the hippocampal CA1 field. *Brain*, **122**, 2321–2335.

Wade, T.K. and Troy, J.C. (2001). Mobile phones as a new memory aid: a preliminary investigation using case studies. *Brain Injury*, **15**, 305–320.

Warrington, E.K. and Weiskrantz, L. (1974). The effects of prior learning on subsequent retention in amnesic patients. *Neuropsychologia*, **12**, 419–428.

Wilson, B.A. (1997). Cognitive rehabilitation: how it is and how it should be. *J Int Neuropsychol Soc*, **3**, 487–496.

Wilson, B.A. and Evans, J.J. (2000). Practical management of memory problems. In: *Memory Disorders in Psychiatric Practice* (eds Berrios, G.E. and Hodges, J.R.), Cambridge University Press, Cambridge, pp. 291–310.

Wilson, B.A. and Watson P.C. (1996). A practical framework for understanding compensatory behaviour in people with organic memory impairment. *Memory*, **4**, 465–486.

Wilson, B.A., Baddeley, A.D., Evans, J.J. and Shiel, A. (1994). Errorless learning in the rehbailation of memory impaired people. *Neuropsychol Rehabil*, **4**, 307–326.

Wilson, B.A., Evans, J.J., Emslie, H. and Malinek, V. (1997a). Evaluation of NeuroPage: a new memory aid. *J Neurosurg Neurol Psychiat*, **63**, 113–115.

Wilson, B.A., J.C. and Hughes, E. (1997b). Coping with amnesia: the natural history of a compensatory memory system. *Neuropsychol Rehabil*, **7**, 43–56.

Wilson, B.A., Emslie, H., Quirk, K. and Evans, J.J. (1999). George: learning to live independently with NeuroPage. *Rehabil Psychol*, **44**, 284–296.

Wilson, B.A., Emslie, H., Quirk, K. and Evans, J.J. (2001). Reducing everyday memory and planning problems by means of a paging system: a randomised control crossover study. *J Neurosurg Neurol Psychiat*, **70**, 477–482.

Wilson, B.A., Scott, H., Evans, J.J. and Emslie, H. (2003). Preliminary report of a NeuroPage service within a health care system. *NeuroRehabilitation*, **18**, 3–8.

Wimo, A., Winblad, B., Engedal, K., et al., (2003). An economic evaluation of donepezil in mild to moderate Alzheimer's disease: results of a 1-year, double blind randomised trial. *Dement Geriatr Cognit Disord*, **15**, 44–54.

Winblad, B., Engedal, M.D., Soininen, H., et al. (2001). A 1-year randomised, placebo-controlled study of donepezil in patients with mild to moderate AD. *Neurology*, **57**, 489–495.

Wright, P., Rogers, N., Hall, C., Wilson, B.A., Evans, J.J., Emslie, H. and Bartram, C. (2001). Comparison of pocket-computer memory aids for people with brain injury. *Brain Injury*, **15**, 787–800.

30

Neurorehabilitation of executive function

Mark D'Esposito and Adam Gazzaley

Helen Wills Neuroscience Institute and Department of Psychology,
University of California, Berkeley, CA, USA

The clinical neuropsychological literature includes under the rubric of "executive function" a wide range of cognitive processes such as focused and sustained attention, fluency and flexibility of thought in the generation of solutions to novel problems, and planning and regulating adaptive and goal directed behavior (Luria, 1966; Hecaen and Albert, 1978; Lezak, 1995). As evident by the wide scope of these processes, executive function has been used to capture the highest order of cognitive abilities. Such abilities are sometimes not only difficult to operationally define but difficult to measure, which has led to a large number of clinical and experimental neuropsychologic tests that have been developed as an attempt to tap this range of abilities (Spreen and Strauss, 1991; Lezak, 1995). Evidence from neuropsychologic, electrophysiologic, and functional neuroimaging research supports a critical role of the frontal lobes (specifically the prefrontal cortex) in executive control of goal-directed behavior (Fuster, 1997). The extensive reciprocal frontal lobe connections to virtually all cortical and subcortical structures places the frontal lobes in a unique neuroanatomic position to monitor and manipulate diverse cognitive processes.

Several neurologic disorders can cause predominantly frontal lobe damage, and in patients with these disorders, executive dysfunction is the predominant finding on examination. These disorders include traumatic brain injury, vascular compromise, neoplasms, herpes encephalitis, epilepsy, and neurodegenerative disease. Thus, very different etiologies of frontal lobe damage can produce a common set of behavioral and cognitive findings. Moreover, several of these disorders are quite prevalent (e.g., traumatic brain injury and stroke) highlighting the need to develop therapeutic strategies for compensating or alleviating executive function deficits. Although much progress has been made in remediation of sensorimotor deficits after injury, cognitive therapy remains a challenge, and excluding language function; little progress has been made with effective therapies for improving high-level cognitive abilities such as executive function.

This chapter will begin by describing the cognitive deficits observed in patients with frontal lobe damage, which has resulted in the concept of the "dysexecutive" syndrome. Next, we will review cognitive models of executive dysfunction, which can serve as a foundation for developing potential therapeutic approaches. Finally, we will review current cognitive and pharmacologic approaches towards treating executive function impairments.

30.1 The dysexecutive syndrome

Extensive frontal lobe damage may have little impact on the abilities measured by standardized intelligence tests, or other standard neuropsychologic tests, but this common observation is in marked contrast to the way that these patients perform in unintelligent ways in real life (Shallice and Burgess, 1991). The following is a brief review of the types of cognitive deficits that are observed in patients with frontal lobe damage, which has been called the "dysexecutive syndrome" (Table 30.1).

Inability to initiate, stop, and modify behavior in response to changing stimuli. The inability of patients with frontal lobe damage to alter their behavior in response to changing rules is reflected by poor performance on a commonly administered neuropsychologic measure called the Wisconsin Card Sorting Test (Berg, 1948). During this test, four stimulus cards (one with a red triangle, one with two green stars, one with three yellow crosses, and one with four blue circles) are placed in front of the patient (see Fig. 30.1). The patient is then given a deck of response cards, each card containing from one to four identical figures (stars, triangles, crosses, or circles) in one of four colors. The patient is instructed to place each

response card next to one of the four stimulus cards according to *one* of the stimulus dimensions (i.e., color, form, or number). However, the patient is not told the correct sorting principle, but rather must infer this from the examiner's feedback after each response. After 10 correct sorts by the patient, the examiner changes the sorting principle without warning by saying "incorrect" to previously "correct" trials. Almost invariably, patients with frontal lobe lesions understand what they are supposed to do, and can repeat the rules of the test ("I am supposed to arrange these by color, shape, or number"). Moreover, since four stimulus cards are always visible, patients do not have to remember the sorting principles. However, frontal lobe patients are unable to follow them or use knowledge of incorrect performance based on feedback to alter their behavior (Milner, 1963; Damasio, 1985).

Inability to handle sequential behavior necessary for organization, planning, and problem-solving. Simple daily tasks require many steps. Notably, patients with frontal lobe lesions often do not have difficulty with the individual steps that are necessary to complete a sequential task. For example, these patients can easily perform the basic operations (e.g., adding and subtracting) required to complete complex arithmetic tasks. However, when given more complex problems requiring multiple steps, the patient responds impulsively to an early stimulus

Table 30.1. Clinical features of the dysexecutive syndrome.

- Inability to initiate, stop, and modify behavior in response to changing stimuli.
- Inability to handle sequential behavior necessary for organization, planning, and problem-solving.
- Inability to inhibit responses.
- Perseveration.
- Impaired working memory and strategic aspects of episodic memory.

Wisconsin card sorting test

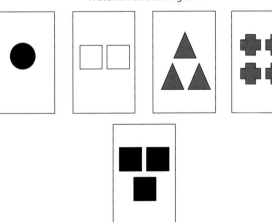

Figure 30.1. During the Wisconsin Card Sorting Task, four stimulus cards (e.g., one with a red circle, one with two yellow squares, one with three green triangles, and one with four blue crosses) are placed in front of the patient (top row, depicted here in shades of grey). The patient is then given a deck of response cards (bottom row), each card containing from one to four identical figures (stars, triangles, crosses, or circles) in one of four colors. The patient is instructed to place each response card next to one of the four stimulus cards according to *one* of the stimulus dimensions (i.e., color, form, or number).

and fails to analyze or execute the component steps required for problem solution (Stuss and Benson, 1984). The following task: "The price of canned peas is two cans for 31 cents. What is the price of one dozen cans?" is almost impossible for patients with frontal lobe damage even though they can perform the direct arithmetic task of multiplying 6 times 31 with ease. Similar errors occur in routine, everyday tasks that require a series of simple steps such as wrapping a present or making a sandwich (Schwartz et al., 1998).

Inability to inhibit responses. The inability to inhibit prepotent responses and filter out distracting information can be revealed with a neuropsychologic test called the Stroop paradigm (Stroop, 1935). This test is based on the observation that it takes less time to read color names (e.g., blue, green, red, and yellow) printed in black type than to read color names printed in a colored ink of a different color (e.g. the word "green" printed in red). This effect is exaggerated in patients with frontal lobe lesions, especially with damage to superior medial regions (Stuss and Benson, 1986), presumably owing to an impaired ability to inhibit the interference created by reading color names printed in an incongruent ink color. A related phenomenon is that frontal patients may display a remarkable tendency to imitate the examiner's gestures and behaviors even when no instruction has been given to do so, and even when this imitation entails considerable personal embarrassment. The mere sight of an object may also elicit the compulsion to use it, although the patient has not been asked to do so and the context is inappropriate, as in a patient who sees a pair of glasses and puts them on, even though he is already wearing his own pair. These symptoms have been called the "environmental dependency syndrome". It has been postulated that the frontal lobes may promote distance from the environment and the parietal lobes foster approach toward one's environment. Therefore, loss of frontal inhibition may result in overactivity of the parietal lobes. Without the frontal lobes our autonomy from our environment would not be possible. A given stimulus would automatically call up a predetermined response regardless of context (Lhermitte, 1986a; Lhermitte et al., 1986b).

Perseveration. This is defined as an abnormal repetition of a specific behavior. It can be observed in patients after frontal lobe damage in a wide range of tasks including motor acts, verbalizations, sorting tests, drawing, or writing. Several different types of perseverative behavior have been described in patients with brain damage such as (1) recurrent perseveration which is the recurrence of a previous response to a subsequent stimulus within the context of an established set, (2) stuck-in-set perseveration which is the inappropriate maintenance of a category or framework of activity, and (3) continuous perseveration which is the abnormal prolongation or continuation without cessation of a current behavior (Sandson and Albert, 1987).

Impaired memory function. Working memory is the short-term storage of information that is not accessible in the environment and the set of processes that keep this information active for later use in behavior (Baddeley, 1986). This system is critically important in cognition, providing a critical physiologic infrastructure for such functions as reasoning, language, comprehension, planning, and spatial processing. Animal and human studies have linked this ability to the prefrontal cortex by demonstrating that frontal lesions impair working memory and normal individuals performing working memory tasks activate prefrontal cortex (Goldman-Rakic, 1987; Fuster, 1997; D'Esposito, 2001). In contrast with this severe working memory impairment, patients with frontal lobe lesions have little impairment on tasks of information storage over longer periods of time. However, frontal patients often appear "forgetful" to family members. This impairment may result from inefficiencies caused by poor attention or poor "executive" function (Shimamura et al., 1991). This type of memory deficit is due to defective retrieval, a function that requires strategy and effort, as opposed to normal storage, a more passive function. There are several other interesting features of these "real-life memory" difficulties. They are defective in recall of temporal order, that is, recalling the context of learned items, even when they can remember these items. For example, a patient instructed to remember words spoken by either a male or a female speaker may later recall or recognize most of the words but cannot correctly identify the speaker. Patients with frontal lobe lesions also do poorly at tasks requiring them to judge the probability that they would recognize the correct answer to a multiple-choice question (e.g., a feeling of knowing), reflecting deficient self-monitoring abilities (Janowsky et al., 1989). In addition, there is a frequent failure at carrying out an intended action, a process know as prospective memory: "remembering to remember" (Fortin et al., 2003). In summary, patients with prefrontal cortical lesions are impaired in the processes involved in planning, organizing, and other strategic aspects of learning and memory that facilitate encoding and retrieval of information.

Together, the range of deficits described above that are observed in patients with frontal lobe damage captures the essence of the dysexecutive syndrome. However, the dysexecutive syndrome cannot be considered unitary given the diverse nature of these deficits. Moreover, any single patient with a frontal lobe lesion may exhibit some of these behavioral deficits and not others. Based on clinical observations, there are two major behavioral/cognitive syndromes (Cummings, 1993) that occur after damage to different regions of the prefrontal cortex (e.g., dorsolateral versus orbitofrontal). These syndromes reflect separable circuits of connections of the prefrontal cortex with subcortical structures. Only damage to the dorsolateral prefrontal cortex causes the most severe impairments in executive dysfunction, as described in this chapter. In contrast, damage to the orbitofrontal cortex, which is intimately connected to the limbic system, spares many cognitive skills but dramatically affects all spheres of social and emotional behavior (Bechara et al., 1998; Stone et al., 1998). The orbitofrontal patient is frequently impulsive, hyperactive, labile, and lacking in proper social skills despite showing reasonable performance on cognitive tasks typically impaired in patients with damage to dorsolateral prefrontal cortex. Careful characterization of the type of deficits observed in patients with frontal lesions has allowed for the development of cognitive models of executive function that will be discussed next.

30.2 Cognitive models of executive function

Two broad cognitive models of executive function exist: those that propose that there is a distinct and dedicated executive control system that directs and monitors the activities of lower level systems in order to guide behavior and those that posit that there is not a dedicated "executive controller" in the brain but rather executive control emerges from the maintenance of task rules and goals. Regardless of the exact nature of the psychologic constructs of models of executive control, proponents of both types of models have reached consensus that these types of processes are likely implemented by the frontal lobes. Each of these cognitive models will be discussed briefly since such models can serve as a foundation for developing therapeutic strategies for treating patients with executive function deficits.

Based on behavioral studies of normal subjects, Baddeley first proposed the existence of a "central executive system" which actively regulates the distribution of limited attentional resources and coordinates information within limited capacity verbal and spatial memory buffers (Baddeley, 1992, 1986). The concept of the central executive system was based on the analogous "supervisory attentional system" introduced by Norman and Shallice (Shallice, 1988) that was proposed to take control over cognitive processing when novel tasks are involved and when existing habits have to be overridden. Thus, in this conceptualization of executive function, there is a dedicated portion of the brain (likely within the frontal lobes) for this set of cognitive operations. However, these models also allow for the possibility that there are many different types of control processes (i.e., updating, shifting, and inhibition) that may have separable neural substrates.

Since these control processes are proposed to have a limited capacity, each additional cognitive operation that a subject performs at one time places increasing demands on this executive control system. For example, two tasks that are performed sequentially will make minimal demands on executive control processes since these tasks can be performed successfully by using separate processing systems. However, two tasks performed concurrently will lead to a decrement in performance, as compared to performance on either task alone, since dual-tasking requires similar processing systems and will make greater demands on executive control processes. This finding from the experimental psychology literature parallels our experience in everyday life – there is clearly a limit to how many tasks one can perform at any one time before performance suffers. Just imagine your ability to fully comprehend and remember what is being told to you while talking on your mobile telephone while driving your car. Importantly, performance on dual-tasks has been shown to be impaired in patients with frontal lobe lesions (Baddeley et al., 1997; McDowell et al., 1997), and activation of the frontal lobes has been demonstrated with functional neuroimaging in healthy young subjects when performing dual tasks (D'Esposito et al., 1995; Szameitat et al., 2002).

Other models of executive function derive from research attempting to understand frontal lobe function and rely on a more unified approach. For example, Fuster (Fuster, 1985, 1997) has proposed that the prefrontal cortex is critically important in tasks that require the temporal integration of information. In proposing his model, Fuster argues explicitly against the interpretation of a homoncular view of executive control writing that "the prefrontal cortex would not superimpose a steering or directing function on the remainder of the nervous system, but rather, by expanding the temporal perspectives of the system, it would allow it to integrate longer, newer, and more complex structures of behavior." Likewise, Cohen and Servan-Schreiber (Cohen and Servan-Schreiber, 1992) propose that frontal lobe damage results in "a degradation in the ability to construct and maintain an internal representation of context, [by which] we mean information held in mind in such a form that it can be used to mediate an appropriate behavioral response." In their model, disordered performance in executive function is seen as a consequence of a change to a single low-level parameter. In this way, two behaviors which appear outwardly different as indexed by poor performance on seemingly different tasks (such as the Stroop paradigm and Wisconsin Card Sorting Test) may have their roots in similar fundamental processes. Other have similar ideas (Kimberg and Farah, 1993), proposing that executive dysfunction is due to a weakening of associations among working memory representations, including mental representations of internal goals, stimuli in the environment, and stored declarative knowledge.

Consideration of these cognitive models may have implications for developing strategies for rehabilitation of executive function. If there are separable executive control processes with independent neural substrates, it may be necessary to develop therapies that target each of these individual component processes independently. Alternatively, executive function emerges from the maintenance of task rules and goals, it is possible that approaches that aim to improve one underlying function may lead to the improvement of other more specific abilities.

30.3 Rehabilitation of executive dysfunction

Intact executive function is essential for most practical skills and impaired executive function is extremely debilitating for both patients and their families. Despite considerable effort by clinicians and researchers to develop rehabilitation strategies for impaired individuals, the path toward effective treatment has been fraught with difficulty and has often yielded disappointing results. Two main approaches, cognitive therapy and pharmacologic intervention, are possible for improving executive function.

Cognitive therapies

It is challenging to develop a standard cognitive therapeutic approach for executive function impairments for several reasons. First, as we have discussed, there are a wide variety of deficits that can result from frontal lobe injury that fit into the rubric of executive disorders (e.g., planning, inhibition, initiation, and self-awareness). Second, there are multiple neurologic conditions that can result in frontal lobe damage (e.g., traumatic brain injury, stroke, and encephalitis). Third, many patients with frontal lobe injury exhibit behavioral deficits such as a lack in self-awareness, poor motivation, or mood disorders that cause a serious impediment to the rehabilitation process. Thus, it is difficult to generalize rehabilitation interventions for such diverse cognitive and behavioral deficits, and such unique patient populations. As a result, many different techniques have been developed, and research studies testing the validity of such techniques are usually presented as case studies describing interventions on individual patients or small series of cases. This leads to uncertainty that these techniques are generalizable.

These limitations as well as different cognitive models of executive function have led to a divergence in the general approach taken by rehabilitation specialists. There are two primary approaches in executive function rehabilitation; a focus on improvement of a real-life function in a particular setting, such as driving skills, or on a specific type of executive deficit as measured in the laboratory, such as selective attention (Mateer, 1999b). The goal of both of these approaches is that the interventions will eventually generalize across settings and skills. The specific rehabilitation strategy then employed, regardless of the general approach, falls within three distinct but overlapping categories: *environmental manipulation*, training of *compensatory techniques,* and *direct interventions* aimed at improving the underlying deficit (Mateer, 1999b). *Environmental manipulation* focuses on factors external to the patient, such as decreasing distracters, simplifying task demands or allowing more time and eliminating the need to do certain tasks. *Compensatory techniques* are devised to allow the patient to accomplish a task in a new manner that minimizes the impaired skills, such as encouraged use of organizers/planners or increasing self-awareness. *Direct interventions* attempt to restore the same skills that are affected by the damage. This is primarily accomplished via repetitive training exercises providing structured practice. The selection of a strategy is usually made on the basis of the type and severity of the deficit, level of self-awareness, and the degree of environmental dependency.

Despite the variety of approaches and strategies, the overall goal is the same–to improve the functioning of individuals in the setting that they live and work by transitioning them from a dependent, externally monitored state to one that is independent and internally monitored. Likewise, the overall organization of a rehabilitation plan is fairly uniform: (1) evaluate the individual's cognitive and behavioral profile, (2) assess the impact on real-life functioning, (3) establish specific, individualized goals, (4) select an intervention strategy, (5) formulate and deliver the plan, and (6) monitor and evaluate the effectiveness of treatment, making adjustments as necessary (Mateer, 1999a, b).

The approach of addressing impairments in specific executive symptoms has been the focus of considerable effort and has utilized many of the strategies described above. A review of the literature reveals that many of the interventions directed at impaired initiation, behavior sequencing, and inhibitory control have employed environmental manipulations and compensatory strategies while those addressing impairments in focused, sustained, selective, alternating, and divided attention, in working memory and prospective memory have often utilized direct interventions (see Table 30.2 for representative examples of published interventions). A comprehensive review of all published reports studying the rehabilitation of executive function is beyond the scope of this chapter. However, it may be helpful to explore several examples of the different rehabilitation options offered by these different strategies.

Environmental manipulations while employing factors external to the patient have no expectations of changing the patient's capacities or abilities. Although it may be an effective strategy for improving function, it places great demands on other individuals and is inflexible . Unlike compensatory strategies and direct interventions, environmental manipulations have not often been investigated in a formal manner, however a recent review outlines available external cueing devices for patients with initiation problems and prospective memory deficits, and offers recommendations for their use, identifies factors important for

Table 30.2. Representative examples of published rehabilitation interventions directed at improving deficits in different executive functions. Interventions directed at impaired initiation, behavior sequencing, and inhibitory control have employed environmental manipulations and compensatory strategies while those addressing impairments in focused, sustained, selective, alternating, and divided attention, in working memory and prospective memory have often utilized direct interventions.

Impaired executive function	Published study	Rehabilitation techniques
Initiation and sequencing of behaviors	Craine, 1982	Training specific behavioral sequences for highly repetitious activities (e.g., grooming dressing). Cues and checklists extensively used.
	Cicerone and Wood, 1987	Self-instructional training procedure (three phases; overt verbalization > overt self-guidance > covert internalized self-monitoring).
	Sohlberg, 1988	Self-analysis cues encouraged awareness of lack of initiation and led to more initiation.
	Gervin, 1991	Paired external cues (song lyrics) with a recorded tempo and melody used to help pacing.
	Burke et al., 1991	Job training by organization of daily tasks to be completed in the same order each day.
	Schwartz et al., 1995	A system of coding errors of action.
Inhibitory control	Alderman and Ward, 1991	Response–cost paradigm: tokens exchanged for rewards and tokens lost for negative behaviors.
Attention and working memory	Sohlberg and Mateer, 1987	APT: auditory and visual tasks to exercise and challenge focused, sustained, selective, alternating, and divided attention.
	Gray et al., 1992	Computerized-attention retraining: reaction time (RT) training, rapid number comparison, digit symbol transfer, alternating Stroop program, and divided attention tasks.
	Sturm et al., 1997	Computerized-adaptive training programs for alertness and selective and divided attention.
	Schmitter-Edgcombe and Beglinger, 2001	Consistent mapping (responding to same class of stimuli) training results in improved automatic attention response.
	Cicerone, 2002	Task treatments derived from working memory experimental procedures; "n-back", random generation, dual-task procedures, and emphasized deliberate use of attention strategies – improved attention, and working memory.
	Brooks et al., 2003	Virtual reality training promotes procedural learning in people with memory impairments.
	Mazer et al., 2003	Visual attention training and visuoperceptial training improve driving performance (*no difference*).
Prospective memory	Sohlberg et al., 1992a, b	Prospective memory training: repetitive sessions designed to increase time after instruction patient remembers to carry out planned action.
	Van den Broek et al., 2000	Electronic memory aid to manage prospective memory errors.
	Tam et al., 2003	Computer software and on-line tele-communication to improve skills.

selecting a particular device, and suggests ways to monitor their efficacy (O'Connell et al., 2003).

An example of the *compensatory technique* is the response–cost procedure developed by Alderman and colleagues (Alderman and Ward, 1991). It is used to treat problems with disinhibition, such as repetitive speech and aggressive behavior. In this paradigm, the patient is given tokens that can be exchanged for a reward, however each time the patient violates a rule set forth by the therapist they lose a token and eventually may drop below a set point to receive the reward. This technique has shown to be successful where as other paradigms such as "time-outs" and positive reinforcement were not (Alderman et al., 1995). Compensatory approaches for impairments in sequencing of actions, as outlined by Schwartz and colleagues (Schwartz, 1995), include a system of coding errors of action, which assists individuals in recognizing errors in omission or order and is transferred to improvements in daily functioning. Compensatory strategies such as these often rely on factors external to the patient, similar to environmental manipulation, but attempt to change the underlying behavior, frequently by attempting to improve self-awareness.

Another type of compensatory approach is substituting an entirely new behavior or skill, such as the use of a memory device. A memory journal training protocol was developed to instruct patients on how to compensate for prospective memory impairments (Donaghy and Williams, 1998). Additionally, technologic advancements are making an impact in this area as a recent survey revealed that 36% of physicians treating traumatic brain injury advocate portable electronic memory devices for their patients (O'Neil-Pirozzi et al., 2004), although cost has been identified as a significant barrier (Hart et al., 2003). New electronic aids are being developed explicity to aid in the rehabilitation of prospective memory impairment (van den Broek et al., 2000).

Strategies employing *direct interventions* probably occupy the largest extent of the executive rehabilitation literature. An example of a frequently used intervention is Attention Process Training (APT) (Sohlberg et al., 1992a, b), although other commercially available programs exist. The rationale is that practice on graded tasks of attention will promote recovery of damaged neural pathways in patients and result in a restoration of attention abilities that can be applied in multiple settings. The goal is to re-train attentional abilities by the completion of a repetitive series of auditory and visual exercises over 1 to 2 months. The tasks proceed in a hierarchic fashion of escalating difficulty, feedback is provided and different types

of attention are addressed: focused, sustained, selective, alternating, and divided. A controlled study of 23 traumatically brain-injured (TBI) patients was designed to evaluate the effectiveness of the APT program (Park et al., 1999). It was found that although there was significant improvement in the TBI group before and after training, there was no difference when compared to the control group.

A recent meta-analysis further evaluated all studies that used such direct intervention techniques, not just the APT. Specifically, it compared the results of studies that only evaluated pre- and post-training performance in patients to those that also incorporated control subjects (Park and Ingles, 2001). Thirty studies with a total of 359 participants met the authors' selection criteria. The analysis revealed that studies that did not use control comparisons revealed large effect sizes while those studies with control comparisons tended to be non-significant, thus suggesting the positive effects of training were the result of practice effects on the tests. This serves to highlight the methodologic significance of establishing controls to assess practice effects when designing studies to evaluate the effectiveness of any intervention. It is important to note, however, that further analysis of individual studies revealed that patients with significant frontal lobe injury were able to learn a variety of specific skills through practice despite the minimal evidence for direct retraining of general attentional processes. This finding was also supported by encouraging results in several studies that have directly focused on the less common approach of specific-skill training, such as the training of activities of daily living (ADLs) (Carter et al., 1983) and driving (Kewman, 1985), suggesting that rehabilitation focused on specific, important skills to the patient might be a powerful rehabilitation approach. Although large-scale studies are beginning to appear, it is clear that further con-trolled studies employing combinations of the two approaches, specific-skill training and process re-training, that also utilize combinations of the three strategies are needed to help direct the practice of executive rehabilitation in patients with frontal lobe damage.

Technologic innovations, such as virtual reality (Brooks and Rose, 2003) and tele-rehabilitation (tele-communication combined with on line software) (Tam et al., 2003) have also started to make its mark on the rehabilitation of cognitive deficits through direct interventions. Although currently applied to memory deficits, these approaches are fertile areas for rehabilitation directed at executive impairments.

Pharmacologic therapies

The function of the cerebral cortex is clearly influenced by the diffuse inputs from brainstem neuromodulatory systems mediated by neurotransmitters such as dopamine, acetylcholine, and serotonin. Based on the anatomic distribution of brainstem dopaminergic projections (see Fig. 30.2), there is a logical basis for proposing a role for dopamine in prefrontal cortical function (for a review, see Arnsten, 1997). The mesocortical and mesolimbic dopaminergic systems originate in the ventral tegmental area of

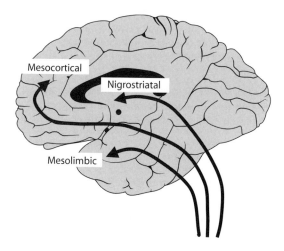

Figure 30.2. Schematic illustration of three brainstem dopaminergic projection systems. The mesocortical and mesolimbic dopaminergic systems originate in the ventral tegmental area of the midbrain and project to prefrontal cortex, anterior cingulate cortex, anterior temporal structures such as the amygdala, hippocampus, and entorhinal cortex and the basal forebrain. The nigrostriatal dopaminergic system originates in the substantia nigra and projects to the striatum.

the midbrain and project to prefrontal cortex, anterior cingulate cortex, anterior temporal structures such as the amygdala, hippocampus, and entorhinal cortex and the basal forebrain (Bannon and Roth, 1983). Also, there is an anterior/posterior gradient in the brain for the concentration of dopamine where it is highest in the prefrontal cortex (Brown et al., 1979).

The functional importance of dopamine to prefrontal function has been demonstrated in several ways. First, in monkeys depletion of dopamine in the prefrontal cortex or pharmacologic blockade of dopamine receptors induces impairment in working memory tasks (Brozoski et al., 1979; Sawaguchi and Goldman-Rakic, 1991). This working memory impairment is as severe as in monkeys with lesion of the prefrontal cortex, and is not observed in monkeys in which other neurotransmitters, such as serotonin or norepinephrine, are depleted. Furthermore, dopaminergic agonists administered to these same monkeys reverses their working memory impairments (Brozoski et al., 1979; Arnsten et al., 1994).

Studying Parkinson's disease (PD) patients "on" and "off" their dopaminergic replacement medication has also made the link between dopamine and prefrontal function. In several studies, PD patients have been found to be impaired on tasks thought to be sensitive to frontal lobe function when they were off their dopaminergic medications (Cooper et al., 1992; Lange et al., 1995; Fournet et al., 1996; Gotham et al., 1988). In one study, the tasks performed poorly by PD patients (the Tower of London, a spatial working memory task, and a test of attentional set-shifting) have also been shown to be specifically impaired in patients with frontal lobe lesions (Lange et al., 1992). This evidence for a specific role of dopamine in prefrontal function is strengthened by the concurrent findings that PD patients perform similarly on and off their medications on long-term memory tasks thought to be sensitive to medial temporal lobe function.

Administration of dopamine receptor agonists to healthy young subjects, which stimulate dopamine receptors in the same way dopamine does, also provides a viable method for examining the role of dopaminergic systems in higher cognitive functions in humans. Healthy young human subjects when given bromocriptine (D-2 receptor agonist) (Luciana et al., 1992; Luciana and Collins, 1997), or pergolide (D-1 and D-2 receptor agonist) (Müller et al., 1998) perform better on working memory tasks when compared to when they are given a placebo. In these studies, the dopaminergic medication had a very specific effect on working memory since it had no effect on other cognitive abilities such as attention or sensorimotor function. Converging on these findings, normal subjects that were administered sulpiride, a D2 receptor antagonist, were impaired on several tasks sensitive to frontal lobe function. Importantly, the impairments could not be accounted for by generalized sedative or motoric influences of the medication (Mehta et al., 1999).

Interestingly, in another study, the effects of bromocriptine on prefrontal function were not the same for all subjects, but interacted with the subject's working memory capacity (Kimberg et al., 1997). Subjects with lower baseline working memory abilities off the drug, tended to demonstrate cognitive improvement on the drug, while those with higher baseline working memory abilities worsened. A similar relationship between dopamine and prefrontal function has been observed in monkeys administered dopaminergic agonist and antagonists. Specifically, a U-shape dose–response curve is observed demonstrating that a specific dosage produces optimal performance on working memory tasks (Arnsten, 1997). This observation suggests that "more" is not "better" but rather there is an optimal level of dopamine concentration that is necessary for optimal function of the prefrontal cortex.

Although these preliminary studies in normal humans are encouraging, there have only been a few studies that have attempted to improve prefrontal deficits in patients. For example, in one such study (McDowell et al., 1998), patients who suffered prefrontal damage from traumatic brain injury were assessed on and off bromocriptine while performing several clinical experimental measures of executive function (e.g., Stroop task, the Wisconsin Card Sorting Task, the trail-making task, dual-task). Significant improvement in performance of traumatic

brain injury patients was observed on bromocriptine, as compared to placebo, on all tasks requiring executive control processes. In contrast, bromocriptine did not improve performance on measures with minimal executive control demands, even if they were cognitively demanding, or other simpler tasks requiring basic attentional, mnemonic, or sensorimotor processes. This pattern of findings provides evidence that the dopaminergic system may specifically modulate executive control processes, and may not be critical for basic mnemonic processes. In another study (Powell et al., 1996), 11 patients with traumatic brain injury or subarachnoid hemorrhage (2 months to 5 years previously) were treated with bromocritpine for a long duration. Bromocriptine treatment was followed by improvement in motivation, which was maintained after withdrawal of the medication in eight of the patients. Finally, in a study of eight patients with vascular or degenerative dementia (Imamura et al., 1998), a 25-day treatment of 10 mg of bromocriptine resulted in reduced perseveration, whereas general attention and overall cognitive function was not affected by the medication.

An important priority for future research should be to further study the effect of dopaminergic drugs on prefrontal function both in healthy young subjects and those with frontal lobe disorders. Based on the studies thus far, dopaminergic pharmacologic intervention may by viable complement to the cognitive therapy in helping to alleviate executive dysfunction.

30.4 Conclusions

Executive function is a concept meant to capture the highest of cognitive abilities. The type of cognitive operations thought to be "executive" in nature allow us to control the enormous number of internal and external representations available to us necessary to guide our behavior in real time, either moment-by-moment or year-by-year. The neural basis of these executive control processes are beginning to mapped out, both on a neuroanatomic and neurochemic level, using sophisticated cognitive neuroscience methodology such as functional magnetic resonance imaging (MRI). Improved understanding of the physiologic basis of executive function will lead to a narrower and more useful view of prefrontal cortical function that will hopefully allow the development of new therapies, both cognitive and pharmacologic, in patients with specific cognitive difficulties from damage to this critical region of the brain.

REFERENCES

Alderman, N., Fry, R.K. and Youngson, H.A. (1995). Improvement of self-monitoring skills, reduction of behavioral disturbance and the dysexecutive syndrome: comparison of response cost and a new programme of self-monitoring training. *Neuropsychol Rehabil*, **5**, 193–221.

Alderman, N. and Ward, A. (1991). Behavioral treatment of the dysexecutive syndrome: reduction of repetitive speech using response–cost and cognitive overlearning. *Neuropsychol Rehabil*, **1**, 65–80.

Arnsten, A. (1997). Catecholamine regulation of the prefrontal cortex. *J Psychopharmacolo*, **11**, 151–162.

Arnsten, K.T., Cai, J.X., Murphy, B.L. and Goldman-Rakic, P.S. (1994). Dopamine D1 receptor mechanisms in the cognitive performance of young adult and aged monkeys. *Psychopharmacology*, **116**, 143–151.

Baddeley, A. (1986). *Working Memory*, Oxford University Press, New York.

Baddeley, A. (1992). Working memory. *Science*, **255**, 556–559.

Baddeley, A., Della Sala, S., Papagano, C. and Spinnler, H. (1997). Dual-task performance in dysexecutive and nondysexecutive patients with a frontal lesion. *Neuropsychology*, **11**, 187–194.

Bannon, M.J. and Roth, R.H. (1983). Pharmacology of mesocortical dopamine neurons. *Pharmacol Rev*, **35**, 53–68.

Bechara, A., Damasio, H., Tranel, D. and Anderson, S.W. (1998). Dissociation of working memory from decision making within the human prefrontal cortex. *J Neurosci*, **18**, 428–437.

Berg, E. (1948). A simple objective test for measuring flexibility in thinking. *J Gen Psycholo*, **39**, 15–22.

Brooks, B.M. and Rose, F.D. (2003). The use of virtual reality in memory rehabilitation: current findings and future directions. *NeuroRehabil*, **18**, 147–157.

Brown, R.M., Crane, A.M. and Goldman, P.S. (1979). Regional distribution of monoamines in the cerebral cortex and subcortical structures of the rhesus monkey: concentrations and in vitro synthesis rates. *Brain Res*, **168**, 133–150.

Brozoski, T.J., Brown, R.M., Rosvold, H.E. and Goldman, P.S. (1979). Cognitive deficit caused by regional depletion of dopamine in prefrontal cortex of rhesus monkey. *Science*, **205**, 929–932.

Burke, W.H., Zencius, A.H., Wesolowski, M.D. and Doubleday, F. (1991). Improving executive function disorders in brain-injured clients. *Brain Inj*, **5**, 241–252.

Carter, L.T., Howard, B.E. and O'Neil, W.A. (1983). Effectiveness of cognitive skill remediation in acute stroke patients. *Am J Occup Ther*, **37**, 320–306.

Cicerone, K.D. (2002). Remediation of "working attention" in mild traumatic brain injury. *Brain Inj*, **16**, 185–195.

Cicerone, K.D. and Wood, J.C. (1987). Planning disorder after closed head injury: a case study. *Arch Phys Med Rehabil*, **68**, 111–115.

Cohen, J.D. and Servan-Schreiber, D. (1992). Context, cortex, and dopamine: a connectionist approach to behavior and biology in schizophrenia. *Psychologic Rev*, **99**, 45–77.

Cooper, J.A., Sagar, H.J., Doherty, M., Jordan, N., Tidswell, P. and Sullivan, E.V. (1992). Different effects of dopaminergic and anticholingergic therapies on cognitive and motor function in Parkinson's disease. *Brain*, **115**, 1701–1725.

Craine, S.F. (1982). In: *Cognitive Rehabilitation: Conceptualization and Intervention* (ed. Trexler, L.E.), Plenum Press, New York.

Cummings, J.L. (1993). Frontal-subcortical circuits and human behavior. *Arch Neurol*, **50**, 873–880.

D'Esposito, M. (2001). In: *Handbook of Functional Neuroimaging of Cognition* (ed. R. Cabeza, A.K.), MIT Press, Cambridge, MA, pp. 293–327.

D'Esposito, M., Detre, J.A., Alsop, D.C., Shin, R.K., Atlas, S. and Grossman, M. (1995). The neural basis of the central executive system of working memory. *Nature*, **378**, 279–281.

Damasio, A., Graff-Radford, N.R., Eslinger, P.J., Damasio, H. and Kassell. N. (1985). Amnesia following basal forebrain lesions. *Arch Neurolo*, **42**, 263–271.

Donaghy, S. and Williams, W. (1998). A new protocol for training severely impaired patients in the usage of memory journals. *Brain Inj*, **12**, 1061–1076.

Fortin, S., Godbout, L. and Braun, C.M. (2003). Cognitive structure of executive deficits in frontally lesioned head trauma patients performing activities of daily living. *Cortex*, **39**, 273–291.

Fournet, N., Moreaud, O., Roulin, J.L., Naegele, B. and Pellat, J. (1996). Working memory in medicated patients with Parkinson's disease: the central executive seems to work. *J Neurol Neurosurg Psychiatr*, **60**, 313–317.

Fuster, J. (1997). *The Prefrontal Cortex: Anatomy, Physiology, and Neuropsychology of the Frontal Lobes*, Raven Press, New York.

Fuster, J.M. (ed.) (1985). *The Prefrontal Cortex and Temporal Integration*, Plenum Press, New York.

Gervin, A.P. (1991). Music therapy compensatory technique using song lyrics during dressing to promote independence in the patient with brain injury. *Music Ther Persp*, **9**, 87–90.

Goldman-Rakic, P.S. (1987). In: *Handbook of Physiology. Section 1. The Nervous System* (eds Plum, F. and Mountcastle, V.), American Physiological Society, Bethesda, Vol 5., (Pt 1), pp. 373–417.

Gotham, A.M., Brown, R.G. and Marsden, C.D. (1988). "'Frontal' cognitive function in patients with Parkinson's disease 'on' and 'off' levodopa. *Brain*, **111**, 299–321.

Gray, M.M., Robertson, I., Pentland, B. and Anderson, S. (1992). Microcomputer-based attentional retraining after brain damage: a randomized controlled trial. *Neuropsychol Rehabil*, **2**, 97–115.

Hart, T., O'Neil-Pirozzi, T. and Morita, C. (2003). Clinician expectations for portable electronic devices as cognitive-behavioural orthoses in traumatic brain injury rehabilitation. *Brain Inj*, **17**, 401–411.

Hecaen, H. and Albert, M.L. (1978). *Human Neuropsychology*, John Wiley & Sons, New York.

Imamura, T., Takanashi, M., Hattori, N., Fujimori, M., Yamashita, H., Ishii, K. and Yamadori, A. (1998). Bromocriptine treatment for perseveration in demented patients. *Alzheimer Dis Assoc Disord*, **12**, 109–113.

Janowsky, J.S., Shimamura, A.P., Kritchevsky, M. and Squire, L.R. (1989). Cognitive impairment following frontal lobe damage and its relevance to human amnesia. *Behav Neurosci*, **103**, 548–560.

Kewman, D.G. (1985). Simulation training of psychomotor skills: teaching the brain-injured to drive. *Rehabil Psychol*, **30**, 11–27.

Kimberg, D. and Farah, M. (1993). A unified account of cognitive impairments following frontal damage: the role of working memory in complex, organized behavior. *J Exp Psychol Learn Memory Cognit*, **122**, 411–428.

Kimberg, D.Y., D'Esposito, M. and Farah, M. (1997). Effects of bromocriptine on human subjects depend on working memory capacity. *NeuroReport*, **8**, 3581–3585.

Lange, K.W., Paul, G.M., Naumann, M. and Gsell, W. (1995). Dopaminergic effects of cognitive performance in patients with Parkinson's disease. *J Neural Trans Suppl*, **46**, 423–432.

Lange, K.W., Robbins, T.W., Marsden, C.D., James, M., Owen, A.M. and Paul, G.M. (1992). L-Dopa withdrawal in Parkinson's disease selectively impairs cognitive performance in tests sensitive to frontal lobe dysfunction. *Psychopharmacology*, **107**, 394–404.

Lezak, M. (1995). *Neuropsychological Assessment*, Oxford University Press, New York.

Lhermitte, F. (1986a). Human autonomy and the frontal lobes. Part II: patient behavior in complex and social situations: the "environmental dependency syndrome". *Ann Neurol*, **19**, 335–343.

Lhermitte, F., Pillon, B. and Serdaru, M. (1986b). Human autonomy and the frontal lobes. Part I: imitation and utilization behavior: a neuropsychological study of 75 patients. *Ann Neurol*, **19**, 326–334.

Luciana, M. and Collins, P.F. (1997). Dopaminergic modulation of working memory for spatial but not object cues in normal humans. *J Cognit Neurosci*, **9**, 330–347.

Luciana, M., Depue, R.A., Arbisi, P. and Leon, A. (1992). Facilitation of working memory in humans by a D2 dopamine receptor agonist. *J Cogniti Neurosci*, **4**, 58–68.

Luria, A.R. (1966). *Higher Cortical Functions in Man*, Basic Books, New York.

Mateer, C.A. (1999a). Executive function disorders: rehabilitation challenges and strategies. *Semin Clin Neuropsychiatr*, **4**, 50–59.

Mateer, C.A. (1999b). In: *Cognitive Neurorehabilitation* (eds Stuss, D., Winocur, G. and Robertson, I.), Cambridge University Press, Cambridge, pp. 314–332.

Mazer, B.L., Sofer, S., Korner-Bitensky, N., Gelinas, I., Hanley, J. and Wood-Dauphinee, S. (2003). Effectiveness of a visual attention retraining program on the driving performance of clients with stroke. *Arch Phys Med Rehabil*, **84**, 541–550.

McDowell, S., Whyte, J. and D'Esposito, M. (1997). Working memory impairments in traumatic brain injury: Evidence from a dual-task paradigm. *Neuropsychologia*, **35**, 1341–1353.

McDowell, S., Whyte, J. and D'Esposito, M. (1998). Differential effect of a dopaminergic agonist on prefrontal function in traumatic brain injury patients. *Brain*, **121**, 1155–1164.

Mehta, M.A., Sahakian, B.J., McKenna, P.J. and Robbins, T.W. (1999). Systemic sulpiride in young adult volunteers simulates the profile of cognitive deficits in Parkinson's disease. *Psychopharmacology (Berl)*, **146**, 162–174.

Milner, B. (1963). Effects of different brain regions on card sorting. *Arch Neurol*, **9**, 90–100.

Müller, U., Pollmann, S. and von Cramon, D.Y. (1998). D1 versus D2-receptor modulation of visuospatial working memory in humans. *J Neuroscience*, **18**, 2720–2728.

O'Connell, M.E., Mateer, C.A. and Kerns, K.A. (2003). Prosthetic systems for addressing problems with initiation: guidelines for selection, training, and measuring efficacy. *Neuro-Rehabilitation*, **18**, 9–20.

O'Neil-Pirozzi, T.M., Kendrick, H., Goldstein, R. and Glenn, M. (2004). Clinician influences on use of portable electronic memory devices in traumatic brain injury rehabilitation. *Brain Inj*, **18**, 179–189.

Park, N.W. and Ingles, J.L. (2001). Effectiveness of attention rehabilitation after an acquired brain injury: a meta-analysis. *Neuropsychology*, **15**, 199–210.

Park, N.W., Moscovitch, M. and Robertson, I.H. (1999). Divided attention impairments after traumatic brain injury. *Neuropsychologia*, **37**, 1119–1133.

Powell, J.H., al-Adawi, S., Morgan, J. and Greenwood, R.J. (1996). Motivational deficits after brain injury: effects of bromocriptine in 11 patients. *J Neurol Neurosurg Psychiatr*, **60**, 416–421.

Sandson, J. and Albert, M.L. (1987). Perseveration in behavioral neurology. *Neurology*, **37**, 1736–1741.

Sawaguchi, T. and Goldman-Rakic, P.S. (1991). D1 dopamine receptors in prefrontal cortex: involvement in working memory. *Science*, **251**, 947–950.

Schmitter-Edgecombe, M. and Beglinger, L. (2001). Acquisition of skilled visual search performance following severe closed-head injury. *J Int Neuropsychol Soc*, **7**, 615–630.

Schwartz, M.F. (1995). Re-examining the role of executive functions in routine action production. *Ann NY Acad Sci*, **769**, 321–335.

Schwartz, M.F., Montgomery, M.W., Buxbaum, L.J., Lee, S.S., Carew, T.G., Coslett, H.B., Ferraro, M., Fitzpatrick-DeSalme, E., Hart, T. and Mayer, N. (1998). Naturalistic action impairment in closed head injury. *Neuropsychology*, **12**, 13–28.

Shallice, T. (1988). *From Neuropsychology to Mental Structure*, Cambridge University Press, Cambridge, England.

Shallice, T. and Burgess, P.W. (1991). Deficits in strategy application following frontal lobe damage in man. *Brain*, **114**, 727–741.

Shimamura, A.P., Janowsky, J.S. and Squire, L.S. (1991). In: *Frontal Lobe Function and Dysfunction* (eds Levin, H., Eisenberg, H. Benton, A.), Oxford University Press, New York.

Sohlberg, M.M. and Mateer, C.A. (1987). Effectiveness of an attention-training program. *J Clin Exp Neuropsychol*, **9**, 117–130.

Sohlberg, M.M., Sprunk, H. and Metzelaar, K. (1988). Efficacy of external cueing system in an individual with severe frontal damage. *Cogn Rehabil*, **6**, 36–40.

Sohlberg, M.M., White, O., Evans, E. and Mateer, C. (1992a). Background and initial case studies into the effects of prospective memory training. *Brain Inj*, **6**, 129–138.

Sohlberg, M.M., White, O., Evans, E. and Mateer, C. (1992b). An investigation of the effects of prospective memory training. *Brain Inj*, **6**, 139–154.

Spreen, O. and Strauss, E. (1991). *A Compendium of Neuropsychological Tests: Administration, Norms, and Commentary*, Oxford University Press, New York.

Stone, V.E., Baron-Cohen, S. and Knight, R.T. (1998). Frontal lobe contributions to theory of mind. *J Cogn Neurosci*, **10**, 640–656.

Stroop, J.R. (1935) Studies of interference in serial verbal reactions. *J Experiment Psychol*, **18**, 643–662.

Sturm, W., Willmes, K., Orgass, B. and Hartje, W. (1997). Do specific attention deficits need specific training. *Neurophysiol Rehabil*, **7**, 81–103.

Stuss, D.T. and Benson, D.F. (1984). Neuropsychological studies of the frontal lobes. *Psychol Bull*, **95**, 3–28.

Stuss, D.T. and Benson, D.F. (1986). *The Frontal Lobes*, Raven Press, New York.

Szameitat, A.J., Schubert, T., Muller, K. and Von Cramon, D.Y. (2002). Localization of executive functions in dual-task performance with fMRI. *J Cogn Neurosci*, **14**, 1184–1199.

Tam, S.F., Man, W.K., Hui-Chan, C.W., Lau, A., Yip, B. and Cheung, W. (2003). Evaluating the efficacy of tele-cognitive rehabilitation for functional performance in three case studies. *Occup Ther Int*, **10**, 20–311.

van den Broek, M.D., Downes, J., Johnson, Z., Dayus, B. and Hilton, N. (2000). Evaluation of an electronic memory aid in the neuropsychological rehabilitation of prospective memory deficits. *Brain Inj*, **14**, 455–462.

Rehabilitation of dementia

Keith M. Robinson[1] and Murray Grossman[2]

[1]*Department of Physical Medicine and Rehabilitation, University of Pennsylvania School of Medicine and*
[2]*Department of Neurology, University of Pennsylvania School of Medicine, Philadelphia, PA, USA*

31.1 There is a neural substrate to support rehabilitation in those with dementia

When the central nervous system is abruptly injured, such as from stroke or traumatic brain injury, the premorbid neural reserve determines how the brain responds spontaneously without explicit therapeutic intervention. This concept also is relevant to those who have neurodegenerative diseases such as dementia, in that even though the neural substrate can be considered in continuous state of decline, the brain spontaneously may attempt to salvage or repair damaged tissue without exposure to treatments. Given exposure to rehabilitative treatments, it has been postulated that the brain will respond at a neural level to support its attempts to salvage/repair damaged tissue and even recover when exposed to these behaviorally based treatments. What remains elusive is when treatments as applied during rehabilitation are either supportive or possibly detrimental to spontaneous neural recovery. Moreover, in the context of dementia, at which point in the disease trajectory that the neural reserve capacity is completely depleted such that even the most passive learning situations are fruitless, is similarly elusive.

The work of Katzman et al. (1989) and Satz (1993) has supported the concept of the determinism of neural repair/recovery by the brain's reserve tissue capacity in their studies of Alzheimer's disease. Reserve capacity has been associated with brain size. Katzman et al. (1989) reported the histopathologic features of a small group of octogenarians who were cognitively intact and healthy. The surprising finding was that these individuals had neuropathological findings consistent with Alzheimer's disease. The

lack of clinicopathological correlation was explained by their relatively large brain sizes indicating a larger neural reserve capacity. Moreover, younger individuals who display an equivalent proportion of cerebral neuropathology and who have small brains may manifest clinical findings of Alzheimer's disease earlier in life, or at least before natural death.

Those factors that determine brain size and neural reserve capacity are speculative. Level of education has received some support from converging data as a determining factor of reserve capacity. For example, there has been reported a higher prevalence of Alzheimer's disease in those who have less education (Zhang et al., 1990; The Canadian Study of Health and Aging 1994). As an indicator of educational level, language has also been studied longitudinally in both younger and older populations: less complex use of language in earlier adulthood predicted the occurrence of Alzheimer's disease in later life (Snowden et al., 1996). Among severity matched patient populations with Alzheimer's disease who have been followed longitudinally, those with higher levels of education die at younger ages, and have more pronounced cerebral perfusion deficits in frontal and parietal lobes during functional imaging of the brain (Stern et al., 1992, 1995; Alexander et al., 1997). These findings suggest that a higher level of education may support maintaining a higher level of cognitive functioning as Alzheimer's disease progresses, in the context of a greater disease burden at the tissue level.

Beyond brain size, neural reserve capacity, and those factors such as education that may contribute to optimizing what one is endowed with genetically, there are additional factors that contribute to cerebral compensation in the context of neural degeneration during dementia. For example, axonal sprouting may maintain partially degenerating neural networks that support cognitive processing. Moreover, alternative neural networks may be developed concurrently or when local sprouting can no longer salvage a degenerating neural network (Stern, 2002). What is unclear is whether behaviorally based rehabilitation interventions can influence these neural mechanisms of tissue salvage/recovery, either positively or negatively.

Functional imaging studies have started to explore the relationships between behaviorally based treatments and tissue responses to these treatments. Backman et al. (1997, 2000) used functional imaging to compare patients with mild Alzheimer's disease and healthy controls during implicit memory tasks such as word stem completion. Alzheimer's disease patients demonstrated increased cerebral perfusion in the occipital association cortex while control subjects demonstrated decreased cerebral perfusion in this area, indicating more efficient cerebral processing with repeated exposure to the stimuli for the healthy control subjects. Clinically, however, the patients with Alzheimer's disease did demonstrate some learning during the implicit memory strategies in these studies. These findings suggest that the patients with Alzheimer's disease may be utilizing the same neural networks as the healthy control subjects during implicit memory processing but with greater inefficiency as reflected by the sustained increase in cerebral perfusion in the occipital association cortex. Sperling et al. (2003) used functional imaging to compare patients with Alzheimer's disease and healthy control subjects during an explicit memory processing task, associative face/name learning. As expected, patients with Alzheimer's disease demonstrated decreased perfusion during task performance in the hippocampal area where explicit memory neural networks are thought to be primarily localized. Moreover, these investigators reported increased activation in novel areas of the brain during task performance including in the medial parietal, posterior cingulate, and superior frontal areas. Clinically, some of the patients with Alzheimer's disease demonstrated learning during associative face/name learning, and it is postulated that alternative

neural networks were being utilized to support explicit learning in these patients. In related studies, Grossman et al. (2003, 2004, Unpublished data, 2004) compared the cerebral perfusion patterns during functional imaging of patients with Alzheimer's disease and healthy control subjects during a semantic memory task that is performed equally well by both groups, specifically, judging "pleasantness" of individual words. A distinct pattern of cerebral perfusion was realized during task performance: patients with Alzheimer's disease demonstrated decreased activation in the posterolateral temporal and inferior parietal areas, and increased perfusion in temporal and frontal areas. Decreased perfusion in the former areas has been associated with Alzheimer's patients' impaired semantic memory. These investigators have hypothesized that patients with Alzheimer's are utilizing alternative neural networks to support semantic memory.

Studies such as these summarized above suggest that neural salvage/repair may occur in those with dementia when there is exposure to behaviorally based cognitive tasks. If the cognitive task is grounded in an implicit learning strategy, there may be cellular efforts to utilize the "usual" neural network to execute the task. In contrast, if the task utilizes an explicit learning strategy, a "bypass" or alternative neural network may be developed to support successful task performance.

31.2 Rehabilitation is relevant for treatment of dementia

Rehabilitation assessments and treatments focus on performance of mundane functions (e.g., eating, dressing, grooming, toileting, bathing, getting out of bed, walking, preparing meals, food shopping, paying bills, etc.) essential to negotiate through everyday life. While these activities are mundane, they can be viewed as cognitively complex for an individual with dementia. Successful performance of these activities is essential for maintaining a sense of control and dignity. Rehabilitation assessments define the specific aspects of functional performance that are impaired and that are preserved, with the intention of developing behaviorally based treatments that restore, enhance, modify or maintain function in everyday life at a level that is realistically and safely optimal for an individual and his/her caregivers, within a living environment that is meaningful.

Control of the rituals necessary to function during the day is defined dynamically by how far the individual with dementia has progressed along the disease trajectory. Loss of function is inevitable as documented by epidemiological studies. Perrault et al. (2002) studied prospectively personal activities of daily living (ADL) of 90 Canadian patients diagnosed with mild dementia: only 17.8% of the group maintained independence in personal ADL over 5 years, or up to 3 months before death if they died within 5 years. Aguero-Torres et al. (2002) observed 223 patients with dementia over a 7-year period in Sweden: at baseline, 31% of the patients had severe functional disability as measured by the Katz ADL scale; after 7 years, 68% of the patients had severe functional disability.

As functional loss occurs, safe and realistic control in everyday life becomes redefined for the individual with dementia. Rehabilitation supports a process of care that dynamically redefines control for the individual and caregivers on their terms. These terms are often influenced by invoking a less negative or more optimistic perception of loss, and a more restrained and focused view of quality of life. Whether or not loss has progressed to the point that learning in the individual with dementia is finite, rehabilitation does not separate the interpersonal and physical environments from the individual during assessments and treatments when redefining control.

Despite loss of cognitive functions, new or alternative ways of participating in everyday life rituals can be developed during rehabilitation. While acknowledging common syndromic and neuropathological features that distinguish different types of dementia (Alzheimer's, frontotemporal, vascular, Parkinsonian, etc.), the clinical presentation among individuals within an identified syndrome is heterogeneous. Thus, individualized assessment of cognition and behavior becomes essential to define their profiles of cognitive and behavioral weaknesses, and strengths.

These individualized diagnostic profiles then become the basis for developing treatment strategies that potentially can be operationalized within an interpersonal and physical environment that may have a varied capacity to support these strategies. The most refined diagnostic and treatment approaches, however, can become meaningless within an environment where caregivers are unavailable, overwhelmed, burned out, disinterested or unable to abandon automatic and counterproductive emotional responses to difficult behaviors.

The assessment and treatment process can involve an array of medical and non-medical specialists including behavioral/cognitive neurologists, rehabilitation medical specialists, cognitive neuroscientists, neuropsychologists, nurses, and traditional rehabilitation therapists such as physical, occupational, speech and language, and recreation therapists. No one specialist monopolizes the process that is viewed as interdisciplinary. Ultimately, treatment strategies are developed and incorporated into everyday life by the individuals with dementia and their caregivers, sometimes in a self-directed manner, or more formally under the guidance of the non-medical rehabilitation specialists mentioned above. Ideally, treatments should occur on-site in the environments where the individuals and caregivers live, work, and play, in that these behaviorally based treatments, when they are effective, may result in successful performance of "hyperspecific" sequences of tasks that utilize cues within idiosyncratic environments (Glisky and Schacter, 1988; Glisky, 1995). For example, learning to use successfully a remote control device to operate a digital cable television with an extensive choice of channels will not necessarily generalize to learning successful use of a mobile cellular telephone, and may not generalize successfully to operate a cable television in someone else's home or in another room in the residential site.

Rehabilitation views inactivity as deleterious for supporting function. "Cognitive inactivity" can be viewed as risk factor for the development of dementia. Higher levels of engagement in cognitive activities during work and leisure time as people grow older can be viewed as a modifiable factor to decrease the risk for developing dementia. Verghese et al. (2003)

Table 31.1. Postulated risk factors for developing Alzheimer's and vascular dementias.

- Older age
- Lower educational level
- Cognitive inactivity
- High dietary intake of lipids especially saturated fats
- Intake of food/water containing aluminium additives
- Low level of physical activity
- Mild cognitive impairment
- Co-morbid chronic conditions that affect neurovascular brain tissue such as diabetes mellitus, cardiovascular and cerebrovascular diseases including hypertension, coronary artery disease and stroke
- Other cardiovascular and cerebrovascular risk factors including smoking, obesity, hyperhomocysteinemia, and hypercholesterolemia and its major transporter, apolipoprotein epilson type 4, associated with the presence of the apolipoproteimemia epsilon gene allele
- Other conditions associated with low cerebral perfusion such as obstructive sleep apnea, heart failure, orthostatic hypotension, and cardiac arrhythmia
- Cognitive impairment associated with a previous condition such as head injury
- Tau protein gene mutations

(Cooper, 2003; DeCarli, 2003; Garcia and Zanibbi, 2004; Grossman, 2003; Haan and Wallace, 2004; Iadecola and Gorelick, 2003; Kotwal et al., 2002; Luchsinger and Mayeux 2004a, b; Messier, 2003; Michikawa, 2003; Miklossy, 2003; Morris, 2003; Poirier, 2003; Refolo and Fillit, 2004; Rocchi et al., 2003; Roman, 2003; Roman et al., 2002; Saykin and Wishart, 2003; Scarmeas and Stern, 2003; Schraen-Maschke et al., 2004; Skoog and Gustafson, 2003; Solfrizzi et al., 2003; Townsend et al., 2002; Verghese et al., 2003; Wakutani et al., 2002; Youssef and Addae, 2002).

prospectively studied over 21 years (median 5.1 years) 469 older people over the age of 75 years old who did not have dementia at the time of baseline assessments: while 121 subjects developed dementia, a higher participation in leisure activities such as reading, playing board games, playing musical instruments, and dancing, was associated with a reduced risk of developing Alzheimer's and vascular dementia, and with reduced rates of decline in memory, independently of other reported risk factors. Common risk factors postulated for the developing dementia are summarized in Table 31.1. Several of these risk factors can be considered modifiable within the context of a rehabilitation philosophy.

31.3 Cognitive/behavioral assessment can be used to predict functional disability and develop treatments in dementia

Neuropsychological studies have demonstrated that the presence of dementia predicts a lower level of functioning. Bennett et al. (2002) prospectively studied 77 Australian patients with vascular dementia using a comprehensive neuropsychological battery. Block design from the Wechsler Adult Intelligence Scale-Revised (WAIS-R) as a probe of executive functioning (visual organization and problem solving) emerged as a significant and independent predictor of decline of ADL over 5.82 years. Digit span forward as a probe of auditory attention, free recall on the 6th trial of the Rey Auditory Verbal Learning Test (RAVLT) as a probe of proactive interference during long-term memory processing, and a behavioral disorder of control (impaired self-monitoring, restlessness, euphoria, disinhibition) emerged as independent and significant predictors of decline in instrumental activities of daily living (IADL) during the same period of time. Boyle et al. (2003) cross-sectionally studied 29 American patients with vascular dementia: subscale score on the attention/initiation/perseveration subscale of the Dementia Rating Scale (DRS) emerged as a specific and significant predictor of IADL performance.

Concurrent review of brain magnetic resonance imaging (MRI) in this study by Boyle and colleagues also demonstrated that a higher volume of subcortical hyperintensities was realized as a significant predictor of lower IADL performance. In a study of patients with Alzheimer's dementia, Glosser et al. (2002) explored the usefulness of visuoperception to predict the performance of IADL in 35 American patients with probable Alzheimer's dementia. A battery of tasks that probed visuoperceptual functions localized in the occipital lobes (shape discrimination), posterior inferotemporal cortical regions (face/object form/written word discrimination), and the dorsolateral parietal lobes (spatial localization) were used in this study: object form discrimination emerged as a significant predictor of performance of visually based IADL such as driving. These studies have utilized quantitative approaches for measuring cognition, and they support that performance on specific cognitive tasks, for example, attentional and executive functioning probes in vascular dementia and visuoperceptual probes in Alzheimer's dementia, can predict functional status. They do not, however, direct us as to how to develop treatments of cognitive impairments in patients with dementia.

Several investigators have proposed that an assessment approach that is more qualitative, ethnographic, and ecologically based, or that observes in detail the strategies that patients utilize to execute tasks that are grounded in "real life" experiences, will inform us better as to how to develop treatments. These methodological approaches primarily have been useful to elucidate specific components of impaired cognitive processing that support the development of models of cognitive operations. These models also can be potentially considered as constructs to guide treatment interventions that are hypothesis-driven, and thus can be offered as models to be tested and further refined during treatment trials. For example, Schwartz et al. (1991, 1995) have developed an assessment approach, the Action Coding System, grounded in the concept of the supervisory attention system (SAS) of Shallice (1988). This has been applied to examining everyday life

functions in patients with dementia. The Action Coding System assumes a hierarchical organization of action from higher order to lower order. At the highest level, the general goal of the action to be performed is defined, for example, eating a bowl of cereal. At an intermediate level, the task is deconstructed into subroutines that are rational sequences of more basic action units, for example, opening the box/pouring the cereal into a bowl, opening the milk/pouring milk into the bowl over the cereal, etc. At the lowest level, the basic action units of the target activity are defined, for example, scooping the cereal with a spoon, bringing the spoon with cereal to the mouth, etc. Basic action units are triggered by "top down" intentional or conscious control by the SAS, and "bottom up" unconscious or automatic motor programs that underpin motor behaviors. The SAS inhibits inappropriate actions triggered by distractions in the environment and reorients the movement sequences to maintain them as rational. Thus, two types of disorders of performing action are defined, those of attentional control and those of automatic mechanisms. Each disorder has a distinct pattern of action errors associated with them. Impairment of attentional control is manifest by object mis-selection, intrusion of irrelevant action, perseverations, and distraction by environmental cues not invested in successful task performance and that induce irrelevant automatic behaviors (utilization behaviors). Impairment of automatic mechanisms is manifest by explicit errors in routine behaviors.

Giovannetti et al. (2002) utilized the Action Coding System and examined awareness of action errors during functional tasks such as making toast and gift wrapping in 54 patients with dementia and 10 control subjects who also participated in a neuropsychological assessment. As expected, the patients with dementia were aware of, and self-corrected, significantly fewer basic action unit errors than the control subjects. Awareness and correction of errors did not correlate significantly with the number of errors committed or with neuropsychological data. Awareness of different types of errors was differentiated for the patients with dementia: there was significantly more awareness of substitution and sequence errors than omissions, perseverations, and utilization behaviors. This study would suggest that those errors that the subjects are aware of are the ones more likely to be remediable with behaviorally based treatment interventions. Feyereisen et al. (1999) utilized the Action Coding System and examined dressing in 25 patients with Alzheimer's dementia. They observed that fastening was the least successful step in the basic action units of the proposed dressing sequence (choosing (62% successful), orienting (60%), putting on (56%), adjusting (59%), fastening (43%)). Successful transitions between basic action units during dressing occurred 60% of the time, and successful execution of the complete sequence occurred 39% of the time. Errors in performing basic action units were associated with donning specific pieces of clothing. For example, the most difficult basic action during donning an undershirt was orienting, whereas for underpants was putting on and adjusting. The most common basic action errors were unsatisfactory execution (e.g., orienting errors such as confusing front and back) in 16 patients, incorrect choice of clothing (e.g. putting on shoes before socks) in 12 subjects and passivity in 11 subjects. Moreover, passivity was the major source of errors during transition between basic action units. Successful transitions and successful performance of basic action units during dressing correlated significantly with dementia severity measured by the mini-mental state examination (MMSE) and the Global Deterioration Scale, and with neurological probes across eight cognitive domains (language, visual attention, visual object recognition, ideomotor praxis, executive functioning, verbal short term memory, visuospatial short term memory, episodic visual, and verbal memory). These findings suggest that the defined processing model for dressing can be tested while strategies for remediating deficient basic action units and deficient transitions between units are introduced in an individualized manner. Thus, the proposed model allows for individualized treatments. Moreover, the basic nature of the remediable errors indicates deficits within the SAS and not with automatic motor

programs. Those patients who display passivity may be more difficult to remediate, and perhaps should not subjected to treatments unless their passivity can be lessened with other treatments such as neuro-modulating medications. Thus, possible treatment strategies include the uses of a variety of attentional and executive strategies to facilitate SAS operations. For example, designing a wardrobe that has a clear and explicit back and front if there are orienting deficits, and that has easy (e.g. velcro) or minimal fastening requirements.

Regardless of the assessment approach that is utilized to support treatment interventions for individuals with dementia, a fundamental factor that may determine a potential therapeutic response is whether the individual has some awareness of the deficits to be remediated, as manifest behaviorally by awareness errors made. One implication here is that those individuals who are anosagnostic should not be subjected to treatments in which they are explicitly made aware of errors they have made, but rather should be exposed to treatments in which their awareness of errors made are minimized. Attempts to make such individuals more aware of their errors may be fruitless, and if they are made more aware of their errors, this may interfere with an increase in self-directed or productive behaviors. Clare et al. (2002a) are exploring this in the context of memory deficits in dementia, and they are developing an assessment tool, the Memory Awareness Rating Scale (MARS), that intends to clarify the demented individual's, as well as the caregiver's, awareness of memory difficulties based on performance during the Rivermead Behavioural Memory Test (RMBT) and during the Rivermead Behavioural Memory Test-Extended Version (RMBT-E). The MARS operationalizes level of awareness by five "discrepancy" scores including between the individual with dementia and the caregiver, and between the predicted performance and actual performances of the demented individual with and without prior experience of the target tasks. This tool will be used to test whether awareness of memory deficits can determine therapeutic response to interventions intended to remediate memory.

31.4 There are models of treatment available to guide rehabilitation of cognitive/behavioral deficits

As a discipline whose treatment interventions have been subjected to rigorous scientific study, rehabilitation is viewed as challenging. Rehabilitation treatments historically have been based on empirical experience that recently is being applied to develop hypotheses and models to be tested during treatment interventions. Before randomized, large group sample size, double blind, controlled clinical trials can be operationalized, scientific investigation in rehabilitation has promoted an array of methodologies (e.g., single case or small group experimental designs, observing subjects at different baselines) that are serving to allow research questions and treatment interventions to become more refined, and to compensate for factors that inevitably confound human performance research. When cognitive/behavioral deficits are the object of behaviorally based treatments, these factors become more complex. For example, distinguishing a treatment effect from spontaneous recovery/decline becomes problematic in individual or group studies in which a sham or "no treatment" group is not included (Wilson, 1993).

Wilson (2002) has argued that cognitive neuropsychology is not lacking models to explain deficits, predict cognitive strengths and weaknesses, and guide behaviorally based treatment that is potentially efficacious. These cognitive neuroscientific models, however, are incomplete when considering rehabilitating patients with cognitive impairments in that they have not encompassed the emotional, social, and behavioral factors that interact with cognitive performance. Moreover, the positively observed outcomes of interventions guided by these models have been often irrelevant to everyday life activities. Wilson, thus, has proposed to merge these "limited" cognitive neuroscientific models with other theoretical lines of investigation and model-building in the areas of learning theory and behavior, neural recovery, emotional, and psychosocial issues, impairment/disability/handicap measurement paradigms, and compensatory behaviors. What results is a multidimensional meta-model of the rehabilitation of cognitive deficits that is just beginning to be operationalized. The components of such a model are summarized in Table 31.2. Some of the applications of this model when treating those with dementia are discussed in this chapter, both above and below. Thus, the models that can guide therapeutic interventions for rehabilitating cognitive deficits in dementia are in early phases of development, and the efficacy and usefulness of these interventions to rehabilitate cognitive/behavioral deficits in dementia are exploratory, at best.

Table 31.2. Components of the rehabilitation model for guiding treatment for those who have cognitive deficits.

- *Diagnostic assessment*: Identifying cognitive strengths and weaknesses using neuropsychological testing
- *Behavioral assessment*: Identifying behaviors that are thought to be manifestations of cognitive difficulties, that interfere with functioning in everyday life, and that are potentially amenable to behavioral management techniques; identifying behaviors that may interfere with learning such as apathy and anosagnosia
- *Functional assessment*: Qualitative or quantitative description of everyday life functioning that postulates explicit relationships among impairment (cognitive deficits), disability or activity participation, and handicap or social role participation
- Prediction of potential for spontaneous recovery, or stabilizing clinical and functional status over the short- and long-term
- Assessment of concurrent emotional and psychosocial issues that can confound recovery and be responsive to treatment such as depression and caregiver stress
- Assessment of compensatory behaviors based on direct observation or inferred from clinical factors such as age, cognitive impairment severity and specificity, and pre-disease patterns of compensation
- Application of errorless learning strategies during behaviorally based interventions aimed to enhance cognitive and physical functioning (Clare and Woods, 2001; Wilson, 2002)

31.5 Individuals who have cognitive impairments can learn

Rehabilitation treatments have emphasized the processes of learning/relearning of skills, for example ADL, mobility, communication, that may be viewed as simple motor tasks, but really are cognitively quite complex for someone with dementia. For example, consider the necessary skills required for autonomous dressing during the rehabilitation of an individual with a diabetes-related lower limb amputation who has concurrent subcortical ischemic small blood vessel disease and a mild frontal-subcortical disconnection syndrome associated with mild neuropsychological deficits in attention, short term memory, executive functions, and working memory. Given the lack of bipedal support, this individual must learn to dress either in a supine or sitting position. This requires learning to use axial trunk control and postural reflexes in a novel way. Moreover, it requires a more calculated degree of anticipatory planning to select clothing in order to have garments within reach for donning in a lying or sitting position. It also involves novel donning behaviors when considering the successful use of an artificial limb. The cognitive resources that this individual must utilize include selective and sustained attention (focusing on the immediate stage in the process of dressing, and maintaining focus to complete this stage); visuoperception (proper orientation of garments between front and back); executive functions (visual organization to select items to be donned in a rational sequence; motor sequencing of the trunk and limbs to move from one stage to the next in a rational sequence); and working memory (realizing where one is in the process so that a stage is not repeated or omitted). Moreover, when novel strategies are introduced that may build upon, but also require modifying previously overlearned or automatic motor activities, responding to the environmental cues that induce these modifications through repeated exposure to the cues, and to the novel strategy through repetition and rehearsal, can ultimately result in changes in the "cognitive motor program" that underpins dressing, such that the new motor sequence for dressing becomes an over-learned or automatic motor skill.

Given the nature of the cognitive deficits of this amputee, it has been argued that those cognitive operations dependent on impaired explicit or conscious control may disallow him/her to dress successfully without the provision of external structure provided by a caregiver to facilitate selection of clothing, and transitioning across the stages of dressing in a logical sequence particularly when a novel item is introduced such as an artificial limb. What may be available are implicit or unconscious, less impaired cognitive operations that support learning to participate successfully in a substantial degree of dressing activities safely and autonomously. Even though this model of intact implicit memory and impaired explicit memory can be useful to understand how individuals with dementia can learn, this model considers only one component of this learning situation, that is, the cognitive resources of the individual. As discussed by Wilson (2002) and Clare and Woods (2001), the affective states of the demented individual and the caregiver creates a more complex context around a learning situation during treatment. Thus, learning theory offers a construct that provides understanding of how an individual with dementia can learn based on the dichotomy of conscious/explicit/declarative memory systems that have a specific cerebral localization (medial temporal lobe-thalamic-basal forebrain, and medial temporal lobe-thalamic-amygdala neural networks) that is disproportionately impaired in dementia, and unconscious/implicit/procedural memory systems that have a more distributed localization that may be relatively spared in the mild and moderate stages of dementia (see Volume I, Chapter 2). Yet, declarative and procedural learning interacts with emotional and psychosocial factors. For example, if this individual or his/her caregiver is anxious or depressed, and if their relationship is difficult, this learning situation in rehabilitation could be counterproductive.

Several implicit memory strategies are being utilized to enhance learning in cognitively impaired individuals, including those with dementia, during rehabilitation. These strategies have included using a structured interpersonal and physical environment to create a sense of familiarity ("environmental cueing") to support more efficient and more frequent performance of productive target tasks, "errorless learning", and operant conditioning. These strategies encompass an array of well recognized behavioral management techniques including shaping, desensitization, chaining, extinction, and reinforcement (Wilson et al., 1994; Alderman, 1996; Son et al., 2002). Errorless learning and operant conditioning have been applied and studied with some rigor during cognitive/behavioral treatment of individuals who have memory and executive functioning deficits.

Errorless learning involves learning without errors or mistakes. To-be-learned information is presented to an individual in a manner to avoid or minimize mistakes and a negative learning experience that occurs during such approaches as trial and error learning and more traditional "Socratic" approaches in which the teacher/therapist discovers what information individuals need to learn by exposing and bringing attention to what their knowledge gaps are. To-be-learned information is provided directly in a manner that avoids guessing. This new information is then collaboratively rehearsed in a manner to avoid a negative experience. Positive feedback is provided when a target task is performed correctly. A neutral response follows erroneous behavior that is then linked to providing essential information and participating in the desired behavior in a nurturing and non-didactic manner. Errorless learning is thought to capitalize on both residually intact explicit and implicit memory systems: the more severe is the dementia, it is assumed the more dependent one is on implicit memory to support learning. It has been applied more often as a strategy for rehabilitation of memory impairments, but it also has also been applied during treatment of deficits in other cognitive domains and in functional motor skills (Wilson, 2002). Baddeley (1992) has argued that errorless learning, when applied within implicit learning situations for individuals with impaired explicit memory, can support behaviorally based learning to be more effective because it provides a constructive strategy to handle errors that can distract or interfere

with learning a target task. While memory-intact individuals have strategies to minimize the effects of making mistakes on their learning, or even "learn from their mistakes", memory-impaired individuals may have these strategies impaired as part of their deficit, and any attention directed toward errors, or when repetition of errors occurs within a given learning situation, these may serve to reinforce errors. Errorless learning provides an externally applied strategy that intends to prevent an experience of making errors that are detrimental to learning as an interference effect.

Wilson et al. (1994) applied errorless learning techniques during a series of small group comparative and single case study experiments that observed whether amnestic patients would learn better under errorless learning conditions than guessing conditions. Errorless learning was observed to be a superior learning strategy during word list learning, face and object naming, and learning to use an electronic memory aid. In another series of experiments, Evans et al. (2000), compared errorless learning, and trial and error learning, across another series of experiments that compared these learning approaches in small samples of memory-impaired subjects. Errorless learning was beneficial only during learning people's names but not during learning a route, learning to program an electronic aid, and face naming.

The differential results of the benefits of errorless learning during this latter set of experiments presented by Evans et al. (2000) was explained by a number of factors: (1) if errorless learning is dependent on relatively available explicit memory systems, those subjects who are "partially amnestic" may benefit more from these strategies than those subjects whose explicit memory systems are more thoroughly obliterated; (2) if errorless learning occurs without available explicit memory systems, but depends on relatively available implicit memory systems, then the differential effect of interference from errors that occurs during different behavioral strategies (e.g., direct demonstration versus chaining) will influence what is learned; that is, different behavioral strategies that are encompassed by errorless learning have a variable ability to minimize the experience of making errors; (3) if other specific elements necessary to learn implicitly, such a making connections to a pre-existing knowledge base and adequate repetition and rehearsal of what one is learning, are not included into the errorless learning strategies, then information acquisition may be limited; (4) the strategies utilized must incorporate during the learning process, techniques that not only support access to, and consolidation of information, but also retrieval of what one is to learn.

Hunkin et al. (1998) have applied errorless learning in the acquisition of word processing skills using commercially available computer software. This study continues a line of investigation initiated by Glisky et al. (Glisky et al., 1986; Glisky and Schacter, 1988; Glisky, 1995) that focuses on procedural learning of skills that one needs to function in the "real world", and can be learned in brain injured individuals who have their explicit memory systems impaired. Procedural learning of one skill, however, may be "hyperspecific", and will usually provide no obvious advantage to support learning of another procedural skill, but may generalize to successful performance of the newly learned skill in different environments. Hunkin et al. (1998) studied a severely memory-impaired individual who had survived a viral encephalitis. The errorless learning strategies utilized in this study of successful learning are summarized in Table 31.3. The labor intensity of such a training program must be appreciated.

When considering another approach to implicit learning, Alderman (1996) has discussed the uses of operant conditioning to treat problematic behaviors usually associated with different frontal lobe syndromes: impulsive/disinhibited/aggressive (orbital frontal), amotivational/abulic (dorsal lateral frontal), poor initiation (medial frontal). While an array of behavioral management techniques has been utilized successfully in rehabilitation to modulate these behaviors to allow more consistent participation in learning situations, what remains challenging is the ability to identify those individuals with difficult behaviors who do not respond well to behavioral modification, or alternatively, who may become inappropriately excluded from rehabilitation. Moreover, treating those who can be threatening or embarrassing to caregivers because of difficult behaviors is challenging. While such factors as anosagnosia, and the presence of a very high frequency of difficult behaviors that overwhelm attempts at behavioral management, can help to identify "behavioral modification non-responders", Alderman (1996) has explored impairment in the "ability to learn itself" as a reason for non-response. For example, for the demented individual who may have few explicit memory systems spared and some implicit memory systems available, is there a point in the disease trajectory associated with more diffuse cerebral involvement, or is there a critical cognitive operation impaired, that indicates that behaviorally based learning cannot occur? Alderman (1996) has explored whether

Table 31.3. An example of an errorless learning strategy to facilitate use of a computer (Hunkin et al., 1998).

1 Customize software menus by removing commands that were not to be learned and that could be distracting

2 Read a sequence of commands aloud from cards

3 Read the commands aloud from cards with commands in the sequence missing, using a multiple choice strategy to select the missing command

4 Read the commands aloud from cards with commands in the sequence missing, searching and selecting the missing command from the computer screen

5 Perform the sequential commands on the computer with direct instruction

6 Execute the commands on the computer without instructions by matching what was executed on the computer with a presented text on paper

7 Steps 5 and 6 in the learning trials are timed and used at outcomes measures

8 Repetition occurs at each step of the learning trials and during each learning session.

neuropsychological factors can be utilized to predict when learning is finite. Specifically, he has explored whether impairments in the central executive of working memory as measured by dual task paradigms could be the critical cognitive operation, that when severely impaired, can undermine responding to behavioral modification techniques. Alderman (1996) compared age and global intelligence matched normal control subjects ($n = 10$) and two groups of non-aphasic brain injured subjects. The brain injured subjects were divided into those who responded ($n = 10$) and those who did not respond ($n = 10$) to behavioral management. When the two groups were compared using neuropsychological probes of the central executive of working memory, the non-responders had a disproportionately and significantly impaired performance during the following secondary tasks with visual tracking as the primary task: digit span reverse, temporal judgement, and conversation. Non-responders performed positively and comparable to responders only when verbal feedback was applied as another secondary task. These findings suggest that impairment in a critical cognitive operation, that is, the central executive of working memory, and not disease severity or more widespread cerebral involvement, better identifies behavioral modification non-responders. Regardless, the non-responders still demonstrated a good performance when positive verbal feedback was provided.

Alderman's (1996) study has several important implications when considering how to create therapeutic contexts for brain injured individuals, including those with dementia, during rehabilitation. The learning environment should minimize internal (e.g., depression, anxiety) and external (e.g., caregiver stress, ambient noise) distractions that could compromise attentional control during target task performance. These distractions can be viewed as factors that will interfere with optimal allocation of attentional resources, that is, the functioning of the central executive of working memory that is a critical and fundamental cognitive operation during learning whether explicit or implicit memory systems are utilized. Non-distracting strategies that

provide positive feedback, such as errorless learning, could be incorporated to optimize the therapeutic interaction. Implicit memory strategies can be linked with strategies that optimize attentional control such as rehearsal and repetition, and managing small bits of to be processed new information.

31.6 Individuals who have dementia can learn

In Chapter 29 Volume II of this text, Evans provides further insights and discussion on the uses of pharmacologic agents and behaviorally based cognitive remediation that have been applied to treat memory-impaired individuals. The use of pharmacologic agents is not discussed below. Many cognitive remediation strategies reviewed below have been developed during treatment of non-demented individuals as discussed briefly above and by Evans (In press) in more depth.

Cognitive remediation in healthy older adults has been viewed as promising for improving performance in the specific cognitive domain that is being treated, and these improvements are generally sustained over time. Ball et al. (2002) reported the results of the Advanced Cognitive Training for Independent and Vital Elderly (ACTIVE) trial, a multi-center, large sample, randomly assigned, group comparative, single blind intervention trial that assessed outcomes prospectively after domain-specific treatments in the areas of verbal episodic memory, verbal reasoning, and visuo-motor speed of processing. Significant improvements in cognitive performance were reported in all three domain-specific treatments groups immediately after treatment, and these improvements were generally sustained over 2 years. In an earlier trial, Neely and Backman (1993) performed verbal memory training in healthy Swedish elders during a small sample, group comparative study that observed performance on word list learning in two treatment groups and a "no treatment" group over 6 months. The treatment in this trial encompassed encoding enhancement strategies such as visual imagery and method of loci, this latter technique encouraging making explicit associations between the to-be-remembered words and familiar places in one's home such that a mental map is formulated. Both treatment groups demonstrated significantly improved word list learning abilities over 6 months. What is implied by these studies is that ongoing cognitive activity, and even "cognitive exercises" may have an important role in retarding cognitive decline and optimizing the neural substrate as one grows older as long as there is a neural reserve that is not "depleted". However, for cognitively impaired individuals, conceptualizing the brain as a "mental muscle" that requires "cognitive exercise" has received little empiric support (Josephsson, 1996; Tate, 1997).

Internally generated, re-organizational, mnemonic strategies aimed to enhance declarative memory such as visual imagery and method of loci have not been viewed as useful for individuals with dementia (Woods, 1994). Backman's (1992) review of memory training in dementia (AD) is somewhat more positive regarding explicit memory retraining strategies. One line of investigation reviewed by Backman, and performed by his investigative group, includes those studies that have demonstrated improved declarative memory in AD patients when supported by compensatory strategies at both encoding when the to-be-remembered information is presented, and at retrieval when the to-be-remembered information is to be recalled. Participation in relevant motor activity during semantic elaboration at encoding and retrieval of target information has been demonstrated to facilitate declarative memory processing in AD patients, as well as in healthy elderly people. However, the higher the degree of "attentional effortfulness" of the encoding/retrieval strategies, the less useful for enhancing memory in AD patients, but not necessarily in healthy elderly people.

Schacter et al. (1985) have viewed those internally generated strategies that facilitate encoding during memory processing, as too effortful cognitively to be useful for brain injured individuals in their everyday lives. These investigators (1985) and others (Camp and Stevens 1990; Lekeu et al., 2002) have studied

less effortful memory retraining strategies such as "spaced retrieval" or "retrieval practice". The theoretical rationale that underpins spaced retrieval is that the initial retrieval of to-be-remembered information will facilitate subsequently successful recall of this information over time during the typical long-term declarative memory processing. Spaced retrieval does not require effortful organizational or elaborative strategies that the mnemonic encoding strategies utilize, but it does impose some order on the retrieval process by systematic variation of the time interval for retrieval to occur after initial exposure to the to-be-remembered information. Camp and Stevens (1990) reported a successful application of spaced retrieval in several patients with dementia utilizing uncomplicated stimuli (name-face associations) and short initial retrieval intervals (<20 seconds). They also utilized an implicit learning strategy of shaping, that is, shortening or lengthening the retrieval strategy within memory training sessions depending on each patient's failed or successful "on line" performance in an effort to optimize correct face-name associations. The retrieval intervals were ultimately extended up to several minutes and then up to 1 week. These latter trials of spaced retrieval had some relevance to everyday life of the studied patients in that the trials occurred within the context of structured activities at an adult day program, and the to-be-learned face-name associations included improving the use of the names of the staff members of the adult day program. An intrinsic element of spaced retrieval that may underpin its effectiveness, as well as the effectiveness of other successful memory retraining strategies, is repetition and rehearsal. Repetition supports reinforcement of correct responses during cognitive remediation within a rather limited repertoire of stimuli and in a somewhat limited manner, while rehearsal offers reinforcement of correct responses using a broader variety of stimuli and training techniques in an effort to generalize the use of the newly learned information in varied contexts. The amount of repetition and rehearsal during cognitive remediation for individuals with dementia will likely need to be greater for a successful outcome to occur (Woods, 1994).

Backman (1992) has articulated several cognitive/behavioral factors that make cognitive remediation challenging in individuals with dementia: poor insight; poor ability to internalize effortful strategies such as mnemonics; a high degree of labor intensity to implement; and little evidence of longer-term benefits. When considering these challenges, Josephsson (1996) has proposed a model of cognitive remediation in individuals with dementia that utilizes preserved functions (implicit memory, automatic motor skills) and that is interactive depending heavily on caregivers to create a structured interpersonal and physical environment. Within this model, several studies that have focused on "skills training" have been executed. Zanetti et al. (2001) explored "procedural memory stimulation", that is, the use of previous experience without conscious recognition, to treat individuals with Alzheimer's dementia. This study focused on "fine tuning" basic ADL and IADL skills within "ecologically relevant" environments (e.g., kitchen, bathroom, etc.). Single blinded timed comparison of performances of successful task execution before and after treatment (4 months later) demonstrated a significant decline (79 seconds) in timed performance for the treatment group and a non-significant increase (34 seconds) in timed performance for the matched control group across all functional tasks. In another functionally based study, Tappan (1994) randomly assigned 63 subjects with a variety of dementias into three matched treatment groups: one-on-one functional skills training; general group stimulation in therapeutic recreation; no treatment. Outcome measures demonstrated no significant improvements in functional status among the groups after the 20 weeks intervention phase, however only the functional skills training group demonstrated significant improvements in their abilities to be more self-directed in ADL performance.

In another "skills training" study, Rossler et al. (2002) compared five AD patients and five age matched depressed patients who were exposed to a training intervention that involved 30 minute one-on-one waltz-lessons daily over a 12 day period. Outcome measurement was based on blinded prospective assessment of deconstructed and overall dancing skills utilizing measures of "implicit learning skills" (rhythm, expression, smoothness, creativity, and use of space) and a measure of "explicit learning skills" (number of learned steps). Significant and disproportionate improvements over time only in implicitly learned skills were observed for the AD subjects in comparison to the depressed controls. In another study, Cott et al. (2002) applied a dual task paradigm (walking and talking) to observe its effects on communication, ambulation and overall functional status in a small group, comparative 16 weeks intervention trial in which AD nursing home residents were randomized to one of four subgroups: walk and talk in pairs, a walk and talk group, a talk-only group, no intervention. Outcome measurement included formal measures of communication, ambulation endurance, and functional status. The significant findings reported in this study were limited to the between group comparisons: the talk-only and the no treatments groups had significant improvement in communication over time, and no groups demonstrated improvements in ambulation endurance or functional status over time. Moreover, the walk and talk group demonstrated a significant decrease in function when comparing baseline and post-intervention status. These findings dispute a small exploratory literature that has observed the positive influence of exercise on cognition in dementia (e.g., see Etnier et al., 1997), and suggest that the application of such a dual task paradigm in a group context with relatively open-ended interactional structure may be deleterious for AD patients.

Other investigators have explored how the immediate context of learning can influence information acquisition during memory retraining in individuals with AD. Hutton et al. (1996) have explored the application of performance-based learning that is subject-driven rather than provider/experimenter-driven (e.g., external cueing) or based on verbal instructions. These investigators have continued a line of work performed and summarized above by Backman (1992) in which relevant motor activity is implemented at both encoding and retrieval of information to enhance memory. These investigators performed a series of experiments that compared three subject-driven encoding and retrieval "enact-ment" strategies with traditional experimenter-driven verbally based encoding and retrieval strategies in small samples of AD subjects and healthy control subjects. The three enactment strategies involved actual performance of each action during sequential stimuli exposure (encod-ing), and variable retrieval techniques defined the retrieval conditions as either verbal, actual motoric, and mimed/simulated motoric. Overall, the three enactment strategies each compared superiorly to the verbally based learning strategy during action sequence recall of both logical and random action sequences for both the AD and control subjects. Moreover, further within-group analyses that com-pared the three different retrieval strategies revealed that both AD and control subjects had significantly better action sequence memory recall performance when motoric retrieval was applied than when mimed or verbal retrieval was utilized. Other obser-vations made during these experiments performed by Hutton et al. (1996) included that the AD subjects learned the action sequences optimally when the presentation of the stimuli occurred in a logical and orderly manner rather than randomly. The more organized learning conditions had a more detailed, deconstructed, and structured logical, temporal sequences. Removing the highly organized struc-ture of the action sequences significantly decreased the action sequence recall for the AD subjects only, but not for the control subjects.

In related learning trials that were directed toward understanding better how the context of learning can influence how individuals with AD learn, Dick et al. (1996, 2000, 2003) examined the influence of contextual interference as operationalized through a variability of practice paradigm during motor learning of an underhand tossing task of a bean bag in subjects with AD. In the initial series of experi-ments, the practice conditions during learning of an underhand tossing task were systematically varied. Essentially, the more structured and less randomly applied the practice conditions, the better the learn-ing and the better the generalization of the learned task in other contexts (e.g., tossing bean bags of

different weights at different targets, horseshoe tossing). The pattern of motor learning in the AD subjects was distinctly different from motor learn-ing in healthy elderly people. AD subjects demon-strated successful motor learning only when practice conditions were consistent, uncomplicated, and highly structured, while healthy elderly demonstrated motor learning, as well as generalized what they learned, during variable practice conditions. These investigators suggested that the difficulty with motor learning/generalization among those with AD was related to difficulty with encoding and storing infor-mation necessary to establish a motor schema or program.

Dick et al. (2000) proposed that in order to facili-tate formation of a motor program and generaliza-tion of its successful execution to related tasks, both contextual and task/motor program conditions need systematically to be manipulated during the learning process. They performed a 10 weeks inter-vention study of AD and matched control subjects during which five practice conditions and three motor program variations (underhand toss, over-hand toss, sidearm toss) were compared within and between the groups. Within each group, subjects were assigned to five training subgroups that included a no treatment group. Significant improve-ment in performance for AD subjects was observed only under the constant practice condition. For the control subjects, significant improvements in underhand and overhand tossing performance were observed across three of the four training condi-tions, and for sidearm tossing, across all four train-ing conditions. Analyses of the ability to generalize overhand and underhand tossing abilities to related tasks (beanbag tossing with a heavier stimulus, horseshoe tossing) realized that the AD subjects only demonstrated significantly improved ability during performance of the more closely related task for underhand tossing with a heavier stimulus under the constant practice condition when com-pared to no training. A different observation for the control subjects was made during comparable analy-ses in that significant improvements in the more closely related underhand and overhand tossing tasks occurred during all different training condi- tion, specifically variable-combined practice in which the most diverse range of options of types of throws, force/speed of throwing and target dis- tances were offered. What can be inferred from this series of experiments by Dick et al. (1996, 2000, 2003) is that individuals with AD have better motor learning and generalization when the learning con- ditions are the least dependent on neural structures that support explicit or declarative learning. There is a distinctly different pattern of learning among non- demented elderly subjects in whom more complex and attentionally demanding and less structured conditions seem optimal to support motor program formation as well as flexibility in their generaliza- tion across related skills.

In a parallel series of experiments, Dick et al. (2001, 2003) observed the influence of visual feed- back on fine motor performance, specifically rotary pursuit learning, in individuals with AD. Rotary pur- suit learning is a task that has been characterized as distinguishing AD dementia patients from other dementia patients, in that AD patients' perform- ances are usually comparable to the performances of non-demented individuals on this task. In these experiments, the ongoing dependence of fine motor control on sensory feedback, or sensory motor inte- gration, was explored by systematic variation of visual feedback during rotary pursuit learning. It is thought that during the early phases of motor learn- ing, visual feedback is essential for motor program formation. As the motor program becomes more automatic during continued practice, there is less dependence on visual feedback and more depend- ence on proprioceptive feedback for successful task execution. In a series of small group, comparative, rotary pursuit learning trials, matched AD and con- trol subjects demonstrated relatively comparable accuracy of performance under conditions in which no visual restrictions occurred, regardless of manip- ulation of conditions that varied task difficulty. However, the mean performance time to complete the trials was significantly longer for the AD group. Under conditions in which visual restrictions were imposed, accuracy of learning performance for the

AD group was significantly worse at the begin- ning and at the end of repetitive training trials with the performance gap between the AD and control groups more pronounced at the end of training, regardless of variability of task difficulty. Moreover, under restricted visual conditions, AD subjects' per- formance did not improve after a finite number of practice trials while control subjects' performance did. What can be inferred from this series of experi- ments is that during fine motor learning, AD sub- jects were less able to shift their dependence on sensory feedback from visual to proprioceptive with ongoing practice, during motor program formation. The fact that AD subjects had to compromise speed for accuracy under both visually unrestricted and restricted conditions may further indicate their lim- ited ability to shift to other sensory systems and utilize limited attentional resources to support improved task performance.

This line of investigation by Dick and colleagues summarized above offers some guiding principles for functional skills training for individuals with AD: (1) the context of learning must be structured but uncomplicated, emphasizing consistency during successive practice trials; (2) learning accuracy is dependent on pacing during practice; (3) repetition beyond a finite number of practice trials may not improve performance; (4) limited generalization to performance of related tasks is not well understood; (5) automatic motor program formation may be dependent more exclusively on ongoing visual feed- back over time.

During implicit learning trials, Clare et al. (1999, 2000, 2002b) promote that errorless learning may be essential for any successful treatment of cognitive deficits in patients with dementia, regardless of effortfulness or attentional demands of cognitive processing. Clare et al. (1999, 2001) applied errorless learning strategies to enhance proper name recall in an individual with mild AD using face-name associ- ations. The intervention was ecologically valid/ meaningful in that it focused on proper name recall of members of the social club to which this individual belonged. Face-name associations were enhanced using several approaches: a mnemonic strategy grounded in verbal elaboration, enhancing access to learned names using errorless learning, and applying expanded rehearsal to reinforce learned associations. Over 10 weeks of training, significant improvement in accuracy of proper name identification was observed from 20% at baseline to 100% after the intervention. These improvements were maintained 9 months after the intervention phase, during which time daily practice was implemented. Once daily practice was stopped at 9 months, naming accuracy declined, but not significantly, to 80% at 1 year and 71% at 2 years. As long as daily practice was occurring, there was excellent generalization of correct use of proper names from the intervention phase when photographs were used, to direct and meaningful interpersonal interactions. Clare et al. (2000) extended their application of errorless learning during a multiple single-case design intervention trial of 6 subjects with mild AD aimed to enhance memory in everyday life situations, such as recalling the names of people who the subjects interacted with regularly, recalling the names of famous people, and recalling personal information and the day, these aiming to reduce repetitive questioning to caregivers about this information. The interventions utilized included using face-name associations to enhance proper name recall, and teaching the subjects procedurally to use external aids such as a diary, a calendar, a memory board, and an electronic pager to facilitate recall of personal information and the day. Significant improvements in name recall at the end of the intervention phase and over 6 months was reported: expanded rehearsal was reported to be a more successful strategy than using vanishing cues when coupled with verbal elaboration under errorless learning conditions to enhance proper name recall. Generalization for using proper names during interpersonal interactions was inconsistent. Moreover, inconsistent decreases in repetitive questioning about personal information and the day after being trained to use the external aids were reported over 6 months. Successful use of the external aids to reduce repetitive questioning was dependent on caregivers who reinforced their uses with daily practice. The integrity of the relationships between subjects and caregivers influenced whether practice using the external aid occurred or not. Clare et al. (2002c) continued this line of investigation in a small sample group study of AD subjects during another intervention trial aimed to enhance face-name associations in which they observed the influence of confounding factors such as affective state, awareness of memory difficulties, dementia severity and caregiver stress on ability to learn. Significant improvements in naming accuracy and ability to generalize were reported after the intervention phase and up to 6 months later, even though daily practice stopped 1 month after the intervention phase. Significant correlations were demonstrated between post-intervention naming accuracy and awareness of memory difficulties as well as dementia severity, but not for affective state or caregiver stress. An interesting between subgroup comparison in this study was performed between five subjects who were taking acetylcholinesterase-inhibiting medications and five subjects never exposed to these medications: this subgroup comparison revealed no significant differences in post-intervention naming accuracy, global cognitive status, memory, and awareness of memory difficulties.

31.7 Caregivers must be involved in the rehabilitation of cognitive/behavioral deficits of individuals who have dementia

Caregivers define the interpersonal and physical environment around the individual with dementia. Caregivers' abilities to create meaningful environments depends on an array of factors including their own intellectual and cognitive functions (e.g., does an elderly spouse also have dementia?), the nature and quality of their relationships with the individual with dementia (is there a long history of emotional tension between spouses? is the homemaker/home health aid underpaid and working several jobs?), and their own abilities to be receptive about applying novel strategies (is there caregiver burn-out?) that aim toward enhancing/maintaining optimal function and minimizing difficult and problematic behaviors. Two basic tenets of behavioral management that must be applied in an effort to optimize the functioning of the individual with dementia are: (1) create a highly structured schedule of activities during the daily life of the demented individual that is predictable, consistent and balanced, with controlled distractions, to prevent over-stimulation, and time-out, to allow rest breaks; (2) reward desired, positive, productive behaviors displayed by the individual with dementia using communication skills that represent reinforcement (positive verbal and non-verbal feedback such as verbal praise, smiling and touching); respond to undesired, negative and counterproductive behaviors by a neutral response, and then attempt to redirect the individual away from the possible stimuli that are triggering difficult behaviors.

Before these tenets can be realistically applied, an effort should be made to define why difficult behaviors are occurring. Most problematic behaviors are thought to be precipitated by intrapersonal (e.g., pain, hunger, anxiety, depression, paranoia, fear) and/or environmental (e.g., sensory overload, perceived threat) "triggers" that induce them. Once these behaviors are initiated, factors that either reinforce them to continue or escalate must further be considered. For example, is a distracting environment challenging the individual's limited attentional resources, disallowing him/her to focus on the task at hand, and sustain participation in this task to completion? Other important questions that should be raised: Is the demented individual non-insightful about his/her undesirable behaviors and its influence on others? Is inappropriate behavior positively reinforced by others who provide too much attention to it, usually in an effort to be disciplinary? Are sensory and perceptual systems so impaired that most environmental feedback is being processed too slowly and/or in a disorganized manner (McGlynn, 1990; Yody et al., 2000)? The literature on the application of behavior management in neurological rehabilitation describes an array of individual cases who have displayed the most severe forms of socially inappropriate and problematic

behaviors (e.g., verbal or physical aggression, hypersexuality, poor insight/self-monitoring, verbal perseveration, abulia/apathy, wandering) and who have been successfully managed with individualized treatment strategies that are initially extremely labor intensive, and over time, must be consistently applied with lesser degrees of labor intensity. What is incompletely explored in this literature is how realistically and usefully transferable these strategies are into the residential environments of individuals with dementia and their caregivers (McGlynn, 1990; Yody et al., 2000).

Slone and Gleason (1999) have articulated a model of behavioral management of problematic behaviors associated with dementia. This model defines 10 categories of assessment and intervention to consider: (1) comfort needs (hunger, thirst, feeling of warm/cold, constipation, incontinence, need to toilet, pain); (2) mood (depression, anxiety); (3) assaultiveness (anger, verbal/physical abuse, resistance to care); (4) patient's perception of problem; (5) activity pattern; (6) triggers; (7) pattern of escalation; (8) premorbid personality traits; (9) caregiver interaction style (10) level of cognitive functioning. Assessment is best served by a multidisciplinary effort, including the hands-on caregivers, to cross-validate intrapersonal and environmental triggers and patterns of escalation, and to define the other categories articulated within this model. The successful behavioral strategies that various caregivers are using to achieve desired behaviors should be defined and then applied consistently across this network of caregivers. This requires communication among caregivers, and willingness for caregivers to modify longstanding counterproductive patterns of interaction with the individual who has dementia. This latter suggestion can be particularly challenging for a spouse and adult children.

When considering the physical environment of individuals with dementia, behavioral agitation during the performance of functional activities such as bathing by caregivers has received limited study. Dunn et al. (2002) compared traditional bed bathing with a modified bed bath technique, "thermal bathing", in a small group, cross-over, comparative study of subjects with dementia. Agitated behaviors significantly were less observed during the thermal bath than the traditional bed bath. The essence of the thermal bath was preventing the wash cloth from cooling, thus disallowing a cold, tactile, noxious stimuli, and eliminating physical tactile overstimulation during the rinsing and drying phases by utilizing a special cleansing solution that did not require rinsing and drying.

When considering the interpersonal environment of the individual with dementia, several studies have observed interventions that are aimed at teaching caregiver skills to manage difficult behaviors and cognitive deficits. Gerdner et al. (2002) observed the impact of "progressively lowered stress threshold intervention" in a group comparative study of family caregiver–Alzheimer dementia patient dyads. The progressively lowered stress threshold intervention is a nursing intervention that promotes that six categories of stressors adversely affect behavior in individuals with neurodegenerative diseases: fatigue, changes in routine/environment/caregivier, internal/external demands that exceed functional abilities, multiple and competing stimuli, physical status. Modifying the interpersonal and physical environment in which the individual lives can serve to reduce the magnitude of these stressors. In this study, family caregivers-patients dyads were randomized either to the intervention group in which caregivers were taught explicit interpersonal and environmental strategies to operationalize stress reduction within the home environment, or to a control group in which usual care and unstructured social contact was provided. The most interesting finding of this intervention trial was that positive outcomes varied as to whether the family caregiver was a spouse or not. For example, difficult behaviors became less frequent in the intervention group only among non-spousal subgroup of family caregivers. However, functional status of the demented individuals improved in the intervention group only among spousal caregivers.

When considering non-family caregiver, Looman et al. (2002) have presented qualitative data based on in-depth interviews with 136 nursing assistants that describes the influence of family behaviors on their abilities to provide personal care for individuals with dementia. Five categories of family behaviors positively influenced nursing assistants' care: expression of thanks/appreciation by family members; successful relationship formation with family members; demonstration of trust/respect by family members; demonstration by family members an understanding about their job burden; demonstration of caring for their relative. In another study of nursing assistants, Hoerster et al. (2001) performed an interventional study that observed four nursing assistant-demented subject dyads during their conversational interactions using a multiple baseline prospective design. The intervention in this study involved training the nursing assistants to utilize personalized memory books to participate in meaningful discourse during, and appropriate pragmatics of, conversation. Such an intervention is akin to reminiscence therapy that has been qualitatively described to be therapeutic in the nursing literature but has received little rigorous investigation. The observations made when comparing baseline and post-treatment time periods included: all four subjects improved their abilities to initiate meaningful conversational discourse, sustain the topic of conversation, decrease ambiguity of content during conversations, and take turns during conversations, using the memory book; all four nursing assistants utilized facilitative behaviors less as their training proceeded in association with these improvements in conversational discourse and pragmatics among the demented subjects.

Spector et al. (2001) reassessed the applications of reality orientation as a "milieu" therapy that has had historical importance in creating therapeutic environments for demented individuals, particularly those who live in institutional environments. Their critical and extensive review of the literature identified only one rigorously performed single blind, randomized controlled trial that reported meaningful improvements in cognition and behavior after a reality orientation intervention (Breuil et al., 1994). These investigators then designed a pilot intervention based on reality orientation's most successful applications in a largely descriptive literature.

The intervention identified several principles to be applied therapeutically: sensory stimulation; identifying the psychological difficulties of everyday life limitations and acknowledging the emotional lives of those with dementia; enhancing cognitive skills using implicit learning strategies such as familiarity and intuition; reciprocal understanding of capabilities and vulnerabilities between those with dementia and their caregivers. A 15 session program was applied in four phases that prospectively focused on multisensory stimulation, remembering the past (reminiscence), naming of familiar people such as caregivers and family members, and practical IADL performance such as using money and finding one's way around their physical environment in a self-directed manner. A small group comparative trial compared subjects/caregivers who were randomly assigned to the intervention and "usual care"/control groups. Improvements that approached significance were observed for the intervention group for global cognition and affective state, and for more strongly decreasing depression than anxiety, but not for improving social communication or reducing caregiver stress.

Suhr et al. (1999) investigated the use of procedural training of "progressive muscle relaxation" (sequential tension and relaxation of various muscle groups) in comparison to visual imagery techniques, to treat behavioral disturbances in individuals with Alzheimer's dementia during a small group comparative trial. The caregivers (usually spouses) were actively involved in the 2 months training process during weekly sessions in a manner of learning external cueing to facilitate each strategy. The findings of this study demonstrated that while neither treatment intervention affected dementia severity, and both treatment interventions reduced anxiety, progressive muscle relaxation significantly was more effective than visual imagery over 2 months for reducing difficult behaviors. Curiously, progressive muscle relaxation, but not visual imagery, was associated with significant improvements in visual memory and verbal fluency/word retrieval at the end of the 2 months treatment trial. The caregivers in this study seemed to engage their "coaching" roles willingly and positively, and negative interpersonal interactions between subjects and caregivers were not reported.

Clare et al. (2002c) explored the influence of participating in cognitive remediation (memory retraining) on the affective states of 65 middle-aged and elderly memory-impaired individuals (mostly with dementias), and on concurrent strain of their family caregivers. A fundamental issue observed here is whether participation by the caregiver in an explicitly therapeutic role adds to the stress of the caregiver ("one more thing to do") that then, may translate into increased anxiety/depression of the patient. After 6 months of individualized treatments, the memory-impaired individuals were less anxious and less depressed, while the caregivers were more depressed and had more strain, but not to significant levels. Qualitative individual analyzes demonstrated that heterogeneous patterns of evolution of mood changes and caregiver strain explained their non-significant results. In a related study, Quayhagen and Quayhagen (2001) examined 56 dementia patient-caregiver dyads during two group comparative experiments in which dyads were randomized to either "active" treatment or "passive" treatment groups. Cognitive remediation interventions were directed at improving memory, word retrieval and problem solving over 3 months in the active treatment group. While cognitive measures significantly improved in the active treatment group, no significant changes in the quality of marital interaction were observed. This latter observation was supplemented by qualitative data in which 71% of the caregivers in the active treatment group reported that they had enhanced communication and interaction with their demented spouses.

As extreme examples of dementia-associated problematic behaviors, aggression, at one end of the spectrum, and apathy, at the other end, have received limited investigation when considering behavioral management by caregivers. Both behaviors have been reported more commonly associated with higher dementia severity, and both occur in over 90% of individuals with dementia during progression of disease. Aggression has been reported as not a persistent behavior during disease progression, while apathy is more persistent once it appears. This may reflect that aggression may be relatively more responsive to neuromodulating medications (neuroleptics, anticonvulsants) than apathy (psychostimulants). Both behaviors are more consistently associated with frontotemporal dementias. Teaching caregivers behavioral management strategies to manage these behaviors has been considered supplemental to pharmacologic management, or when these agents are contraindicated or not tolerated. When behavioral management has been implemented to treat aggression and apathy, improved functional status of the individual has been reported (Landes et al., 2001; Brodaty and Low, 2003).

31.8 Conclusions

1 There is exploratory evidence from functional imaging studies of the brain that there is an adequate cerebral substrate at the tissue level in individuals with mild to moderate severity of dementia to support behaviorally based learning during rehabilitation.

2 Functional loss occurs as dementia progresses.

3 Cognitive assessments using neuropsychological tests are useful to predict functional disability in individuals with dementia, however they are not useful for developing behaviorally based treatments.

4 Ecologically based cognitive assessments are more useful for developing behaviorally based treatments, but they are highly labor intensive.

5 Cognitive neuroscientific models that can guide behaviorally based treatment of dementia during rehabilitation are in the early phases of development.

6 Learning theory that has organized memory and learning processes into declarative/explicit learning and procedural/implicit learning is a useful model to be applied during cognitive remediation in dementia.

7 Several learning strategies have demonstrated a promising influence on maintaining or enhancing functional abilities in dementia including spaced retrieval, task-specific procedural/motor learning within minimally attentionally demanding learning contexts, and motor enactment during memory encoding and retrieval within low attentionally demanding learning contexts. These learning strategies demonstrate limited generalization to functional tasks beyond the target task to be learned, and they have not been adequately studied over longer periods of time, that is, beyond the immediate post-intervention phase of application.

8 Errorless learning should be viewed as a fundamental treatment approach during the rehabilitation of those with dementia regardless of the "attentional effortfulness" of the applied learning strategy.

9 Rigorous study of rehabilitation interventions that are mediated by caregivers is needed, however exploratory studies are demonstrating that caregivers training can improve the functional status of those with dementia, as well as their interpersonal environments.

REFERENCES

Aguero-Torres, H., Qiu, C., Wimblad, B. and Fratiglioni, L. (2002). Dementing disorders in the elderly: evolution of the disease severity over 7 years. *Alz Dis Assoc Disord*, **16**, 221–227.

Alderman, N. (1996). Central executive deficit and response to operant conditioning methods. *Neuropsychol Rehabil*, **6**, 161–186.

Alexander, G.E., Furey, M., Grady, C.L., Pietrini, P., Mentis, M.J. and Schapiro, M.B. (1997). Association of premorbid function with cerebral metabolism in Alzheimer's disease: implication for the reserve hypothesis. *Am J Psychiatr*, **154**, 165–172.

Backman, L. (1992). Memory training and memory improvement in Alzheimer's disease: rules and exceptions. *Acta Neurol Scand*, **139(Suppl.)**, 84–89.

Backman, L., Almkvist, O., Andersson, J.L.R., Nordberg, A., Winblad, B., Reineck, R. and Langstrom, B. (1997). Brain activation in younger and older adults during implicit and explicit retrieval. *J Cogn Neurosci*, **9**, 378–391.

Backman, L., Almkvist, O., Nyberg, L. and Andersson, J.L.R. (2000). Functional changes in brain activity during priming in Alzheimer's disease. *J Cogn Neurosci*, **12**, 134–141.

Baddeley, A.D. (1992). Implicit memory and errorless learning: a link between cognitive theory and neuropsychological rehabilitation? In: *Neuropsychology of Memory* (ed. Squire L.R. and Butters, N.), 2nd edn. The Guildford Press, New York, pp. 309–314.

Ball, K., Berch, D.B., Helmers, K.F., Jobe, J.B., Leveck, M.D., Marsiske, M., Morris, J.N., Rebok, G.W., Smith, D.M., Tennstedt, S.L., Unverzagt, F.W. and Willis, S.L., for the ACTIVE Study Group. (2002). Effects of cognitive training interventions with older adults. *J Am Med Assoc*, **288**, 2271–2281.

Bennett, H., Corbett, A.J., Gaden, S., Grayson, D.A., Kril, J.J. and Broe, A. (2002). Subcortical vascular disease and functional decline: a 6-year predictor study. *J Am Geriat Soc*, **50**, 1969–1977.

Boyle, P.A., Paul, R., Moser, D., Zawacki, T., Gordon, N. and Cohen, R. (2003). Cognitive and neurologic predictors of functional impairment in vascular dementia. *Am J Geriatr Psychiatr*, **11**, 103–106.

Breuil, V., Rotrou, J.D., Forette, F., Tortrat, D., Gananasia-Ganem, A., Frambourt, A., Moulin, F. and Boller, F. (1994). Cognitive stimulation of patients with dementia: preliminary results. *Int J Geriatr Psychiatr*, **9**, 211–217.

Brodaty, H. and Low, L.-F. (2003). Agression in the elderly. *J Clin Psychiatr*, **64**(**Suppl. 4**), 36–43.

Camp, C.J. and Stevens, A.B. (1990). Spaced retrieval: a memory intervention for dementia of the Alzheimer's type (DAT). *Clin Gerontol*, **10**, 651–658.

Clare, L. and Woods, B. (2001). Editorial: a role for cognitive rehabilitation in dementia care. *Neuropsychol Rehabil*, **11**, 193–196.

Clare, L., Wilson, B.A., Breen, K. and Hodges, J.R. (1999). Errorless learning of face-name associations in early Alzheimer's disease. *Neurocase*, **5**, 37–46.

Clare, L., Wilson, B.A., Carter, G., Breen, K., Gosses, A. and Hodges, J.R. (2000). Intervening with everyday memory problems in dementia of Alzheimer's type: an errorless learning approach. *J Clin Exp Neuropsychol*, **22**, 32–146.

Clare, L., Wilson, B.A., Carter, G., Hodges, J.R. and Adams, M. (2001). Long-term maintenance of treatment gains following a cognitive rehabilitation intervention in early dementia of Alzheimer type: a single case study. *Neuropsychol Rehabil*, **11**, 477–494.

Clare, L., Wilson, B.A., Carter, G., Roth, I. and Hodges, J.R. (2002a). Assessing awareness in early-stage Alzheimer's disease: development and piloting of the Memory Awareness Rating Scale. *Neuropsychol Rehabil*, **12**, 341–362.

Clare, L., Wilson, B.A., Carter, G., Roth, I. and Hodges, J.R. (2002b). Relearning face-name associations in early Alzheimer's disease. *Neuropsychology*, **16**, 538–547.

Clare, L., Wilson, B.A., Carter, G., Breen, K., Berrios, G.E. and Hodges, J.R. (2002c). Depression and anxiety in memory clinic attenders and their carers: implication for evaluating the effectiveness of cognitive rehabilitation interventions. *Int J Geriatr Psychiatr*, **17**, 962–967.

Cooper, J.L., (2003). Dietary lipids in the aetiology of Alzheimer's disease: implication for therapy. *Drug Aging*, **20**, 399–418.

Cott, C.A., Dawson, P., Sidani, S. and Wells, D. (2002). The effects of a walking/talking program on communication, ambulation, and functional status in residents with Alzheimer disease. *Alz Dis Assoc Disord*, **16**, 81–87.

DeCarli, C. (2003). The role of cerebrovascular diasease in dementia. *Neurologist*, **9**, 123–136.

Dick, M.B., Shankle, R.W., Beth, R.E., Dick-Muehlke, C., Cotman, C.W. and Kean, M.L. (1996). Acquisition and long term retention of a gross motor skill in Alzheimer's disease patients under constant and varied practice conditions. *J Gerontol: Psychol Sci*, **51**, 103–111.

Dick, M.B., Andel, R., Hseih, S., Bricker, J., Davis, D.S. and Dick-Muehlke, C. (2000). Contextual interference and motor skill learning in Alzheimer's disease. *Aging Neuropsychol Cogn*, **7**, 273–287.

Dick, M.B., Andel, R., Bricker, J., Gorospe, J.B., Hsieh, S. and Dick-Muehlke, C. (2001). Dependence on visual feedback during motor skill learning in Alzheimer's disease. *Aging Neuropsychol Cogn*, **8**, 120–136.

Dick, M.B., Hsieh, S., Bricker, J. and Dick-Muehlke, C. (2003). Facilitation acquisition and transfer of a continuous motor task in healthy older adults and patients with Alzheimer's disease. *Neuropsychology*, **17**, 202–212.

Dunn, J.C., Thiru-Chelvan, B. and Beck, C.H. (2002). Bathing. Pleasure or pain? *J Gerontol Nurs*, **28**, 6–13.

Etnier, J.L., Salazar, W., Landers, D.M., Petruzello, S.J., Han, M. and Nowell, P. (1997). The influence of physical fitness and exercise upon cognitive functioning: a meta-analysis. *J Sport Exerc Psychol*, **19**, 249–277.

Evans, J. (In press). Memory dysfunction …

Evans, J.J., Wilson, B.A., Schuri, U., Andrade, J., Baddeley, A., Bruna, O., Canavan, T., Della Sala, S., Green, R., Laaksonen, R., Lorenzi, L. and Taussik, I. (2000). A comparison of "errorless" and "trial-and-error" learning methods for teaching individuals with acquired memory deficits. *Neuropsychol Rehabil*, **10**, 67–101.

Feyereisen, P., Gendron M. and Seron, X. (1999). Disorders of everyday actions in subjects suffering from senile dementia of Alzheimer's type: an analysis of dressing performance. *Neuropsychol Rehabil*, **9**, 169–188.

Garcia, A. and Zanibbi, K. (2004). Homocysteine and cognitive function in elderly people. *Can Med Assoc J*, **171**, 897–904.

Gerdner, L.A., Buckwalter, K.C. and Reed, D. (2002). Impact of a psychoeducational intervention on caregiver responses to behavioral problems. *Nurs Res*, **51**, 363–374.

Giovannetti, T., Libon, D.J. and Hart, T. (2002). Awareness of naturalistic errors in dementia. *J Int Neuropsychol Soc*, **8**, 633–644.

Glisky, E.L. (1995). Acquisition and transfer of word prosessing skills by an amnestic patient. *Neuropsychol Rehabil*, **5**, 299–318.

Glisky, E.L. and Schacter, D.L. (1988). Acquisition of domain specific knowledge in patients with organic memory disorders. *J Learn Disabil*, **21**, 333–339, 351.

Glisky, E.L., Schacter, D.L. and Tulving, E. (1986). Learning and retention of computer related vocabulary in memory impaired patients: methods of vanishing cues. *J Clin Exp Psychol*, **8**, 292–312.

Glosser, G., Gallo, J., Duda, N., de Vries, J.J., Clark, C.M. and Grossman, M. (2002). Visual perceptual functions predict instrumental activities of daily living in patients with dementia. *Neuropsychiat Neuropsychol Behav Neurol*, **15**, 198–206.

Grossman, H. (2003). Does diabetes protect or provoke Alzheimer's disease? Insights in the pathobiology and future treatment of Alzheimer's disease. *CNS Spectr*, **8**, 815–823.

Grossman, M., Koenig, P., Glosser, G., DeVita, C., Moore, P., Rhee, J., Detre, J., Alsop, D. and Gee, J.C. (2003). Neural basis for semantic memory difficulty in Alzheimer's disease: an fMRI study. *Brain*, **126**, 292–311.

Grossman, M., Koenig, P., DeVita, C., Glosser, G., Moore, P., Gee, J.C., Detre, J. and Alsop, D. (2004). Neural basis for verb processing in Alzheimer's disease: an fMRI study. *Neuropsychology*, **17**, 658–674.

Haan, M.N. and Wallace, R. (2004). Can dementia be prevented? Brain aging in a population-based context. *Annu Rev Publ Health*, **25**, 1–14.

Hoerster, L., Hickey, E.M. and Bourgeois, M.S. (2001). Effects of memory aids on conversations between nursing home residents with dementia and nursing assistants. *Neuropsychol Rehabil*, **11**, 399–427.

Hunkin, N.M., Squires, E.J., Aldrich, F.K. and Parkin, A.J. (1998). Errorless learning and the acquisition of word processing skills. *Neuropsychol Rehabil*, **8**, 433–449.

Hutton, S., Sheppard, L., Rusted, J.M. and Rattner, H.H. (1996). Structuring the acquisition and retrieval environment to facilitate learning in individuals with dementia of the Alzheimer type. *Memory*, **4**, 113–130.

Iadecola, C. and Gorelick, P.B. (2003). Converging pathogenic mechanisms in vascular and neurodegenerative dementia. *Stroke*, **34**, 335–337.

Josephsson, S. (1996). Supporting everyday activities in dementia. *Int Psychogeriatr*, **8**(**Suppl.**), 141–144.

Katzman, R., Aromsom, M., Fuld, P., Kawas, C., Brown, T., Morganstern, H., Fishman, W., Gidez, L., Eder, H. and Ooi, W.L. (1989). Development of dementing illnesses in an 80 year old volunteer cohort. *Ann Neurol*, **25**, 317–324.

Kotwal, G.J., Lahiri, D.K. and Hicks, R. (2002). Potential intervention by vaccinia virus complement control protein ... of the signals contributing to the progression of central nervous system injury to Alzheimer's disease. *Ann NY Acad Sci*, **973**, 317–322.

Landes, A.M., Sperry, S.D., Strauss, M.E. and Geldmacher, D.S. (2001). Apathy in Alzheimer's disease. *J Am Geriatr Soc*, **49**, 1700–1707.

Lekeu, F., Wojtasik, V., Van der Linden, M. and Salmon, E. (2002). Training early Alzheimer's patients to use a mobile phone. *Acta Neurol Belg*, **102**, 114–121.

Looman, W.J., Noelker, L.S., Schur, D., Whitlatch, C.J. and Ejaz, F.K. (2002). Impact of family members on nurse assistants: what helps, what hurts. *Am J Alz Dis Relat Disord*, **17**, 350–356.

Luchsinger, J.A. and Mayeux, R. (2004a). Dietary factors and Alzheimer's disease. *Lancet Neurol*, **3**, 579–587.

Luchsinger, J.A. and Mayeux, R. (2004b). Cardiovascular risk factors and Alzheimer's disease. *Curr Arterioscler Rep*, **6**, 261–266.

McGlynn, S. (1990). Behavioral approaches to neuropsychological rehabilitation. *Psychol Bull*, **108**, 420–441.

Messier, C. (2003). Daibetes, Alzheimer's disease and apolipoprotein genotype. *Exp Gerontol*, **38**, 941–946.

Michikawa, M. (2003). Cholesterol paradox: is high total or low HDL cholesterol level a risk for Alzheimer's disease? *J Neurosci Res*, **72**, 141–146.

Miklossy, J. (2003). Cerebral hypoperfusion induces cortical watershed microinfarct which may further aggravate cognitive decline in Alzheimer's disease. *Neurol Res*, **25**, 605–610.

Morris, M.S. (2003). Homocysteine and Alzheimer's disease. *Lancet Neurol*, **2**, 425–428.

Neely, A.S. and Backman, L. (1993). Maintenance of gains following multifactorial and unifactorial memory training in late adulthood. *Educ Gerontol*, **19**, 105–117.

Perrault, A., Wolfson, C., Egan, M., Rockwood, K. and Hogan, D.B. (2002). Prognostic factors for functional independence in older adults with mild dementia: results from the Canadian study of health and aging. *Alz Dis Assoc Disord*, **16**, 239–247.

Poirier, J. (2003). Apolipoprotein E and cholesterol metabolism in the pathogenesis and treatment of Alzheimer's disease. *Trend Mol Med*, **9**, 94–101.

Quayhagen, M.P. and Quayhagen, M. (2001). Testing of a cognitive intervention for dementia caregiver dyads. *Neuropsychol Rehabil*, **11**, 319–332.

Refolo, L.M. and Fillit, H.M. (2004). Apolipoprotein E4 as a target for developing new therapeutics for Alzheimer's disease. *J Mol Neurosci*, **23**, 151–155.

Rocchi, A., Pellegrini, S., Siciliano, G. and Murri, L. (2003). Causative and susceptibility genes for Alzheimer's disease: a review. *Brain Res Bull*, **61**, 1–24.

Roman, G.C. (2003). Vascular dementia: distinguishing characteristics, treatment, and prevention. *J Am Geriatr Soc*, **51**(**Suppl. 5**), S296-S304.

Roman, G.C., Erkinjuntti, T., Wallin, A., Pantoni, L. and Chui, H.C. (2002). Subcortical ischaemic vascular dementia. *Lancet Neurol*, **1**, 426–436.

Rossler, A., Seifritz, E., Krauchi, K., Spoerl, D., Brokuslaus, I., Proserpi, S.-M., Gendre, A., Savaskan, E. and Hofmann, M. (2002). Skill learning in patients with moderate Alzheimer's disease: a prospective pilot study of waltz-lessons. *Int J Geriatr Psychiatr*, **17**, 1155–1156.

Satz, P. (1993). Brain reserve capacity and symptom onset after brain injury: a formulation and review of evidence for threshold theory. *Neuropsychology*, **7**, 273–295.

Saykin, A.J. and Wishart, H.A. (2003). Mild cognitive impairment: conceptual issues and structural and functional brain correlates. *Semin Clin Neuropsy*, **8**, 12–30.

Scarmeas, N. and Stern, Y. (2003). Cognitive reserve and lifestyle. *J Clin Exp Neuropsychol*, **25**, 625–633.

Schacter, D.L., Rich, S.A. and Stampp, M.S. (1985). Remediation of memory disorders: experimental evaluation of the spaced-retrieval technique. *J Clin Exp Neuropsychol*, **7**, 79–96.

Schraen-Maschke, S., Dhaenens, C.M., Delacourte, A. and Sablonniere, B. (2004). Microtubule-associated protein tau gene: a risk factor in human neurodegenerative diseases. *Neurobiol Dis*, **15**, 449–460.

Schwartz, M.F., Reed, E.S., Montgomery, M., Palmer, C. and Mayer, N.H. (1991). The quantitative description of action disorganization after brain damage: a case study. *Cogn Neuropsychol*, **8**, 381–414.

Schwartz, M.F., Montgomery, M., Fitzpatrick-DeSalme, E.J., Ochipa, C., Coslett, H.B. and Mayer, N.H. (1995). Analysis of a disorder of everyday action. *Cogn Neuropsychol*, **12**, 86–92.

Shallice, T. (1988). *From Neuropsychology to Mental Structure*, Cambridge University Press, Cambridge, UK and New York.

Skoog, I. and Gustafson, D. (2003). Hypertension, hypertensive-clustering factors and Alzheimer's disease. *Neurol Res*, **25**, 675–680.

Slone, D.G. and Gleason, C.E. (1999). Behavior management planning for problem behaviors in dementia: a practical model. *Prof Psychol: Res Prac*, **30**, 27–36.

Snowden, D.A., Kemper, S.J., Mortimer, J.A., Greiner, L.H., Wekstein, D.R. and Markesbery, W.R. (1996). Linguistic ability in early life and cognitive function and Alzheimer's disease in late life. Findings from the nun study. *J Am Med Assoc*, **275**, 528–532.

Solfrizzi, V., Panza, F. and Capurso, A. (2003). The role of diet in cognitive decline. *J Neural Transm*, **110**, 95–110.

Son, G.R., Therrien, B. and Whall, A. (2002). Implicit memory and familiarity among elders with dementia. *J Nurs Scholarship*, **34**, 263–267.

Spector, A., Orrell, M., Davies, S. and Woods, B. (2001). Can reality orientation be rehabilitated? Development and piloting of an evidence-based programme of cognition-based therapies for people with dementia. *Neuropsychol Rehabil*, **11**, 377–397.

Sperling, R.A., Bates, J.F., Chua, E.F., Cocchiarella, A.J., Rentz, D.M., Rosen, B.R., Schacter, D.L. and Albert, M.S. (2003). fMRI studies of associative encoding in young and elderly controls and mild Alzheimer's disease. *J Neurol Neurosurg Psychiatr*, **74**, 44–50.

Stern, Y. (2002). What is cognitive reserve? Theory and research application of the reserve concept. *J Int Neuropsychol Soc*, **8**, 448–460.

Stern, Y., Alexander, G.E., Prohovnik, I. and Mayeux, R. (1992). Inverse relationship between education and parietotemporal perfusion deficit in Alzheimer's disease. *Ann Neurol*, **32**, 371–375.

Stern, Y., Tang, M.-X., Denaro, J. and Mayeux, R. (1995). Increased risk of mortality in Alzheimer's disease patients with more advanced educational and occupational attainment. *Ann Neurol*, **37**, 590–595.

Suhr, J., Anderson, S. and Tranel, D. (1999). Progressive muscle relaxation in the management of behavioural disturbances in Alzheimer's disease. *Neuropsychol Rehabil*, **9**, 31–44.

Tappan, R.M. (1994). The effect of skill training on functional abilities of nursing home residents with dementia. *Res Nurs Health*, **17**, 159–165.

Tate, R.L. (1997). Beyond one-bun, two-shoe: recent advances in the psychological rehabilitation of memory disorders after acquired brain injury. *Brain Injury*, **11**, 907–918.

The Canadian Study of Health and Aging. (1994). Risk factors for Alzheimer's disease in Canada. *Neurology*, **44**, 2073–2080.

Townsend, K.P., Obregon, D., Quadros, A., Patel, N., Volmar, C., Paris, D. and Mullen, M. (2002). Proinflammatory and vasoactive effects of Abeta in the cerebrovasculature. *Ann NY Acad Sci*, **977**, 65–76.

Verghese, J., Lipton, R.B., Katz, M.J., Hall, C.B., Derby, C.A., Kulansky, G., Ambrose, A.F., Sliwinski, M. and Buschke, H. (2003). Leisure activities and the risk of dementia in the elderly. *New Engl J Med*, **348**, 2508–2516.

Wakutani, Y., Kowa, H., Kusumi, M., Yamagata, K., Wada-Isoe, K., Adachi, Y., Takeshima, T., Urakami, K. and Nakashima, K. (2002). Genetic analysis of vascular factors in Alzheimer's disease. *Ann NY Acad Sci*, **977**, 232–238.

Wilson, B.A. (1993). Editorial: how do we know that rehabilitation works? *Neuropsychol Rehabil*, **3**, 1–4.

Wilson, B.A. (2002). Towards a comprehensive model of cognitive rehabilitation. *Neuropsychol Rehabil*, **12**, 97–110.

Wilson, B.A., Baddeley, A., Evans, J. and Shiel, A. (1994). Errorless learning in the rehabilitation of memory impaired people. *Neuropsychol Rehabil*, **4**, 307–326.

Woods, B. (1994). Management of memory impairment in older people with dementia. *Int Rev Psychiatr*, **6**, 153–161.

Yody, B.B., Schaub, C., Conway, J., Peters, S., Strauss, D. and Helsinger, S. (2000). Applied behavior management and acquired brain injury: approaches and assessment. *J Head Trauma Rehabil*, **15**, 1041–1060.

Youssef, F.F. and Addae, J.I. (2002). Learning may provide neuroprotection against dementia. *W Indian Med J*, **51**, 143–147.

Zanetti, O., Zanieri, G., DiGiovanni, G., DeVreese, L.P., Pezzina, A., Metitieri, T. and Trabucchi, M. (2001). Effectiveness of procedural memory stimulation in mild Alzheimer's disease: a controlled study. *Neuropsychol Rehabil*, **11**, 263–272.

Zhang, M., Levy, P., Klauber, M.R. and Liu, W.T. (1990). The prevalence of dementia and Alzheimer's disease in Shanghai, China: impact of age, gender, and education. *Ann Neurol*, **27**, 428–437.

Disease-specific neurorehabilitation systems

Contents

32

The organization of neurorehabilitation services: the rehabilitation team and the economics of neurorehabilitation

Richard D. Zorowitz

Associate Professor, Physical Medicine and Rehabilitation; Medical Director, Piersol Rehabilitation Unit; Director, Stroke Rehabilitation, University of Pennsylvania Health System, Philadelphia, PA, USA

The Concise Medical Dictionary (Oxford University Press, 2000 edition) defines "rehabilitation" as:

1 (in *physical medicine*) the treatment of an ill, injured, or disabled patient with the aim of restoring normal health and function or to prevent the disability from getting worse;
2 any means for restoring the independence of a patient after diseases or injury, including employment retraining.

With its emphasis on plasticity and repair of the nervous system, the *Textbook of Neural Repair and Rehabilitation* is predicated on this broad definition rather than the more restricted one assumed traditionally by physical medicine and rehabilitation; that is, "development of a person to the fullest physical, psychologic, social, vocational, avocational, and educational potential, consistent with his or her physiologic or anatomic impairment and environmental limitations (DeLisa, 1993)." Nevertheless, because rehabilitation does not presume perfect restoration of anatomical connections, implicit in the concept of rehabilitation is a holistic, comprehensive, and transdisciplinary team approach, which includes patient education in primary and secondary prevention of disease processes. Thus patients and caregivers are integral parts of the rehabilitation team.

32.1 The World Health Organization model of rehabilitation

Restoring patients' overall functioning in their social environment requires development of complex outcomes measures and the vocabulary to support them. The World Health Organization (WHO) International Classification of Functioning, Disability, and Health (ICF) provides a foundation for discussing the tenets of traditional rehabilitation and its social context (World Health Organization, 2001) but is limited as a descriptive tool for the broader view of neurorehabilitation, which incorporates plasticity and repair of the nervous system. It is described briefly here because it helps to define the outcomes for disease-specific systems of rehabilitation, and has become the basis for much clinical rehabilitation research. The ICF provides a standard language and framework for the description of *health* (the medical conditions themselves) and *health-related states* (such as education and labor). In ICF, *functioning* is an umbrella term encompassing all body functions, activities, and participation. *Disability* is an umbrella term for impairments, activity limitations, or participation restrictions. ICF defines *health domains* that are described from the perspective of the body, the individual, and society, in two basic lists: (1) body functions and structures and (2) activities and participation. ICF also lists environmental factors that interact with all these constructs. *Impairments* are problems in body function or structure, for example deafness or degeneration of the cochlear hair cells. (The failure to define structural abnormalities separately from their functional consequences reflects an under-emphasis on the medical and reparative aspects of rehabilitation.) *Activity* is the execution of a task or action by an individual. *Participation* is involvement in a life situation. The purpose of rehabilitation is to reduce, minimize, and mitigate impairments, activity limitations, and participation restrictions as much as possible.

Environmental factors make up the physical, social, and attitudinal environment in which people live and conduct their lives, and may influence a functional outcome or return to community. ICF takes these factors into account. Changes in *physical environment* may reflect a multitude of natural or human-made products or systems of products, equipment and technology in an individual's immediate environment that are gathered, created, produced or manufactured. *Assistive products and technology* are defined as any product, instrument, equipment or technology adapted or specially designed for improving the functioning of a disabled person (Table 32.1). *Natural and human-made changes to environment* may include changes in physical geography, population, plants and animals, climate, natural events, human-caused events, light, time-related changes, sound, vibration, and air quality. *Social* environments may include people or animals that provide practical physical or emotional support, nurturing, protection, assistance, and relationships to other persons, in their home, place of work, school, or at play or in other aspects of their daily activities. In this classification, only the amount of physical and emotional support the person or animal provides is included. The attitudes of the person or people that are providing the support are excluded.

Social environments extend beyond individual people or animals. Public, private, or voluntary services that provide benefits, and structured programs and operations in various sectors of society designed to meet the needs of individuals may influence

Table 32.1. Examples of products and technology.

- Products or substances for personal consumption
- Products and technology for:
  - personal use in daily living
  - personal indoor and outdoor mobility and transportation
  - communication
  - education
  - employment
  - culture, recreation and sport
  - practice of religion and spirituality
  - land development
- Design, construction and building products and technology of buildings for:
  - public use
  - private use

Table 32.2. Examples of services, systems, and policies.

Services, systems and policies for the production of consumer goods

Architecture and construction services, systems and policies

Open space planning services, systems and policies

Housing services, systems and policies

Utilities services, systems and policies

Communication services, systems and policies

Transportation services, systems and policies

Civil protection services, systems and policies

Legal services, systems and policies

Associations and organizational services, systems and policies

Media services, systems and policies

Economic services, systems and policies

Social security services, systems and policies

General social support services, systems and policies

Health services, systems and policies

Education and training services, systems and policies

Labor and employment services, systems and policies

Political services, systems and policies

neurorehabilitation outcomes. Policies of governments or other authorities govern and regulate the systems that organize, control and monitor services, structured programs and operations in various sectors of society. Examples of services, systems, and policies are listed in Table 32.2.

Attitudes are observable consequences of customs, practices, ideologies, values, norms, factual beliefs, and religious beliefs. Individual or societal attitudes

Table 32.3. Examples of attitudes.

- Individual attitudes of:
  - immediate family members
  - extended family members
  - friends
  - acquaintances, peers, colleagues, neighbours and community members
  - people in positions of authority
  - people in subordinate positions
  - personal care providers and personal assistants
  - strangers
  - health professionals
  - health-related professionals
- Societal attitudes
- Social norms, practices, and ideologies

about a person's trustworthiness and value as a human being may motivate positive or negative (e.g., stigmatizing, stereotyping, marginalizing, neglecting) practices. The attitudes classified are those of people external to the person whose situation is being described, and not those of the person themselves. The individual attitudes, categorized according to kinds of relationships, are listed in Table 32.3. Values and beliefs are not considered separately from attitudes but are assumed to be the driving forces behind the attitudes.

32.2 Team models of neurorehabilitation

Although the "team" approach is the cornerstone of neurorehabilitation, no research has broken down the "black box" of the process. Nevertheless, medical teams appear to produce more cost-effective and efficient rehabilitation than the more fragmentary, physician-dominated models and began to replace them before World War II (Brown, 1982). After the war, increasing medical knowledge resulted in the need for teams to manage more complex patient populations. In the early 1970s, the team concept was re-evaluated, with emphasis on understanding the group dynamics and cost-effectiveness of the team approach (Halstead, 1976). Unfortunately, there is little evidence to substantiate the importance of the health care team.

The traditional *medical model* reflects a clear chain of responsibility that begins with the attending physician. Any needs identified by a consultant or allied health professional must be approved by the attending physician. If multiple consultations are required, all information must pass through the attending physician, even though there may be duplication or omission of services. Coordination of patient care therefore may be slower and less efficient.

The *multidisciplinary model* provides a means for professionals from different disciplines to meet and coordinate actions on a regular basis. The team remains controlled by an attending physician. The patient may not be a part of the decision-making team. Although communication between the attending physician and allied health professionals may be effective, communication between the disciplines remains limited. Services provided to the patient still may be duplicated, fragmented, or omitted. The lack of discussion results in a lack of effective use of each member's expertise. Once again, functional outcomes may not be optimal.

The *interdisciplinary model* greatly improves upon the multidisciplinary model. The team member works within his or her own sphere of expertise but acts in coordination with other team members and patients to set and coordinate functional goals. Team conferences are used to report functional progress, make decisions as a group, and develop an optimal patient care plan. The patient becomes the center of the team and plays a significant role in goal setting required for transition back to the community. The team is not necessarily led by a physician but can be led by any team member. There can be more exchanges of ideas that might alter the types of therapy given to the patient. Disadvantages to the interdisciplinary model include increased time in completing team conferences; the need for extensive training in the team process; the need for commitments and personality traits in team members that allow some ceding of control so that the team process drives patient care; and the need for the neurorehabilitation physician to be comfortable permitting team decision-making in an era of medical–legal challenges to patient care.

The 1990s brought forth the concept of the *transdisciplinary* team. The transdisciplinary team not only encourages communication across health professionals, but also encourages cross-treatment among disciplines. The concept is based upon the premise that team members who have a better understanding of the expertise and functions of other team members can work more efficiently and effectively. Cross-training allows better patient evaluations, setting of goals, and treatments. Team conferences can be more functionally oriented rather than discipline oriented. Although certain health professionals may take the lead on certain aspects of function (e.g., physical therapy on mobility), in cases of discrepancies, other health professionals may provide input that results in discussion and resolution of problems. While the advantages and disadvantages are similar to those of interdisciplinary teams, the transdisciplinary team breaks down the barriers of therapeutic intervention such that all members have an opportunity to work on all aspects of function to a certain extent with their patients. The additional time and practice will allow patients to have potentially better outcomes in a shorter period of time. Despite the a priori rationales for transdisciplinary team organization, there are as yet no controlled clinical trials to indicate that one type of team approach is better than another, or that the team approach is better than the physician-dominated model. What has been documented is that intensity of rehabilitation correlates with better outcome (see Section Effectiveness of neurorehabilitation below).

32.3 Members of the neurorehabilitation team

The makeup of the rehabilitation team and the requirements for qualification vary from one country to another, although in most cases, the basic principles are similar. The information below is based on the USA experience.

Team dynamics

Neurorehabilitation requires the interactions of many health professionals who provide the diversity of services required by patients with disabilities (Spencer, 1969; Nevlud, 1990; Keith, 1991). Patient needs range from treatment of the acute medical condition that resulted in physical impairments, activity limitations, or participation restrictions, to restorative therapies based on invoking neuroplasticity and repair, to management of chronic medical comorbidities that complicate the course of rehabilitation. Each team member is not only responsible for contributing to each patient's care using his own expertise, but also monitoring issues that can be used by other health professionals to facilitate the treatment plan and optimize functional outcomes. Each discipline is represented by a web site of its umbrella organization. Much of the information presented in this section has been compiled from these web sites.

Physician

The neurorehabilitation physician usually coordinates the rehabilitation team and manages medical conditions related to the rehabilitation etiologic condition and comorbidities. The physician may be a *physiatrist* (fizz ee at' trist), a physician specializing in physical medicine and rehabilitation. The specialty focuses on the restoration of function to people with problems ranging from simple physical mobility issues to those with complex cognitive involvement. Physiatrists may provide rehabilitation care to patients with a variety of neurologic conditions, or may specialize in specific conditions such as stroke, traumatic brain injuries, or spinal cord injuries. Other physicians, such as neurologists and internists, also may practice as neurorehabilitation physicians. In the USA, they usually complete a neurorehabilitation fellowship of at least 1 year without obtaining board certification in physical medicine and rehabilitation.

Rehabilitation nurse (www.rehabnurse.org)

In the USA, a registered nurse with at least 2 years of practice in rehabilitation nursing can earn distinction as a Certified Rehabilitation Registered Nurse (CRRN) by successfully completing an examination that validates expertise. They base their practice on rehabilitation and restoration principles by managing complex medical issues, collaborating with other specialists, providing ongoing patient and caregiver education, and establishing plans of care to maintain optimal wellness. Rehabilitation nurses take a holistic approach to meeting patients' medical, vocational, educational, environmental, and spiritual needs by applying principles taught by other health professionals. They also apply their own expertise in medical issues including bowel, bladder, and skin management. Rehabilitation nurses act not only as inpatient caregivers but also as coordinators, collaborators, counselors, and case managers in both the inpatient and outpatient environments.

Physical therapist (www.apta.org)

Physical therapists are the experts in the examination and treatment of neuromuscular problems that affect peoples' abilities to move. Through exercise training and management, physical therapists help to enhance cardiac and pulmonary function. In addition to treating patients with neurologic disorders, physical therapists direct treatment at preventing injury and loss of movement. Physical therapists work in many inpatient and outpatient settings, serve as industrial consultants, and help athletes to prevent and treat musculoskeletal disorders associated with sports and exercise.

Occupational therapist (www.aota.org)

Occupational therapy helps individuals achieve independence in all facets of their lives. It gives people the "skills for the job of living" necessary for independent and satisfying lives. Services that occupational therapists typically provide include:

1 customized treatment programs to improve one's ability to perform daily activities;
2 comprehensive home and job site evaluations with adaptation recommendations;
3 performance skills assessments and treatment;
4 adaptive equipment recommendations and training;
5 education to family members and caregivers.

Although there are overlaps in the functions of physical and occupational therapists, in the USA, occupational therapists are more involved in retraining of hand and arm functions, while physical therapists tend to be more involved in problems of leg and trunk functions.

Speech–language pathologist (www.asha.org)

Speech–language pathologists assess speech and language development, and treat language and speech disorders such as aphasia, speech apraxia, dysarthria, and cognitive-communication impairment. They also treat people with swallowing disorders. In the USA, speech–language pathologists must have masters or doctoral degrees.

Neuropsychologist (www.apa.org)

Psychology is the study of the mind and behavior, and embraces all aspects of the human experience. A neuropsychologist specializes in studying brain–behavior relationships; that is, they attempt to infer damage to specific parts of the brain by observations on the behavioral deficits that follow brain injury or disease. Neuropsychologists have extensive training in the anatomy, physiology, and pathology of the nervous system. They study brain–behavior relationships under controlled and standardized conditions, using valid and reliable tests that have acceptable levels of sensitivity and specificity in order to identify and treat cognitive and neurobehavioral dysfunction. Tests also allow clinicians to monitor the course of recovery and the patient's potential for return to the community.

Recreational therapist (www.atra-tr.org)

Therapeutic recreation is defined by the United States Department of Labor as a "profession of specialists who utilize activities as a form of treatment for persons who are physically, mentally, or emotionally disabled." Differing from diversional or recreation services, recreational therapy utilizes various activities as a form of active treatment to promote the independent physical, cognitive, emotional, and social functioning of persons disabled as a result of trauma or disease, by enhancing current skills and facilitating the establishment of new skills for daily living and community functioning. In addition, recreational therapists assist the patient in developing or re-developing social skills, discretionary time skills, decision-making skills, coping abilities, self-advocacy, discharge planning for re-integration, and skills to enhance general quality of life. Recreational therapy services offer a diversity of rehabilitation benefits addressing the needs of individuals with a range of disabling conditions (Coyle et al., 1991). In the USA, recreational therapists are standard treatment team members in psychiatric rehabilitation, substance abuse treatment, and physical rehabilitation services. However, because most of these therapies have not been validated in controlled clinical trials, in some countries they are considered "alternative medicine" and are not reimbursable by health insurance.

Many recreational activities and milieus may promote wellness and social reintegration among neurologically impaired persons. Several specialized therapist classes have been recognized in different countries. In the USA, these include the following: *horticultural therapists* (www.ahta.org), *music therapist* (www.musictherapy.org), *dance therapist* (www.adta.org), *art therapist* (www.arttherapy.org), and *animal-assisted therapist* (www.deltasociety.org). Animals may promote nurturing and bonding, and accept patients without respect to physical features or impairments of the patient (Cole and Gawlinski, 1995). At a minimum, the presence of an animal can be entertaining and facilitate socialization (Richeson, 2003). The result of a visit by an animal is mental stimulation and physical contact, which may improve cardiovascular function by reducing blood pressure and pulse (Jorgenson, 1997).

Social worker (www.naswdc.org)

Professional social workers assist individuals to restore or enhance their capacity for social functioning, while creating societal conditions favorable to their goals. In the neurorehabilitation environment,

social workers help people overcome the effects of poverty, discrimination, abuse, addiction, physical illness, divorce, loss, unemployment, educational problems, disability, and mental illness. They help prevent crises and counsel individuals, families, and communities to cope more effectively with the stresses of everyday life. Social workers identify resources that allow patients with disabilities to remain in the community. If patients cannot live in the community, the social worker helps them apply for medical and financial assistance, as well as identifying short-term and extended-care facilities.

Case manager (www.acmaweb.org)

In the USA, the neurorehabilitation case manager is a registered nurse who is certified as a case manager and specializes in occupational injuries. She has knowledge of workers' compensation law and experience in medical case management of work-related injuries, including spinal cord and traumatic brain injuries. The neurorehabilitation case manager facilitates the medical aspect of the workers' compensation claim by meeting with the injured worker, employer, insurance adjuster, physician, and other medical providers. She advocates for the appropriate medical treatment at the appropriate time, and coordinates referrals to specialty physicians, second opinions, physical and occupational therapy, functional capacity evaluations, and work hardening programs. A rehabilitation plan is synthesized and implemented to maximize functional recovery from the injury and attempt return to the community and the work force as appropriate.

Certified rehabilitation counselor (www.crccertification.org)

Rehabilitation counseling is a systematic process that assists patients with physical, mental, developmental, cognitive, and emotional disabilities in the community to maximize their vocational and avocational living goals in the most integrated setting possible. This involves: assessment and appraisal; diagnosis and treatment planning; vocational counseling;

facilitating adjustments to the medical and psychosocial impact of disability; case management, referral, and service coordination; program evaluation and research; interventions to remove environmental, employment, and attitudinal barriers; consultation services among multiple parties and regulatory systems; job analysis, job development, and placement services, including assistance with employment and job accommodations; and consultation about and access to rehabilitation technology. *Similar functions are performed by Certified Disability Management Specialists* (www.cdms.org).

Vocational therapist/counselor

Under the 1983 C159 Vocational Rehabilitation and Employment (Disabled Persons) Convention, each of the ratifying 73 countries have agreed to ensure the "equality of opportunity and treatment to all categories of disabled persons, in both rural and urban areas, for employment and integration into the community" (International Labour Office, 1983). The purpose of vocational rehabilitation is to enable a disabled person to secure, retain, and advance in suitable employment; formulate, implement, and periodically review a national policy on vocational rehabilitation and employment of disabled people; promote employment opportunities for disabled people in the open labor market; promote cooperation and coordination between the public and private bodies engaged in vocational rehabilitation; and evaluate vocational guidance, training, placement, employment, and other related services to enable disabled persons to secure, retain and advance in employment.

In the USA, special grant programs help individuals with physical or mental disabilities to obtain employment and to provide supports such as counseling, medical and psychologic services, job training, and other individualized services.

Prosthetist/orthotist (www.abcop.org)

An orthotist makes and fits braces and splints (orthoses) for patients who need added support for body parts that have been weakened by injury, disease, or disorders of the nerves, muscles, or bones. They work under a physician's orders to adapt purchased braces or create custom-designed braces. Orthotics are often named for the body part(s) they cross, such as AFO (ankle–foot orthosis) or KAFO (knee–ankle–foot orthosis). Orthotics such as Halo braces (a brace that surrounds the head and is held in place with small screws in the skull) or TLSO (thoracolumbar spinal orthosis) may be used to stabilize portions of the spine and prevent further damage to the spinal cord after injury.

A prosthetist makes and fits artificial limbs (prostheses) for patients with disabilities. This includes artificial legs and arms for patients who have had amputations due to conditions such as cancer, diabetes, or injury. While prosthetics are not usually utilized in patients with neurologic conditions, amputation may be a comorbid condition in patients with neurologic impairment.

32.4 Other professionals

Many other professionals may comprise the neurorehabilitation team. A neurologist or neurosurgeon may consult on the patient to treat the disorder causing neurologic disability. The patient may require other medical or surgical specialists to monitor new or comorbid conditions throughout the course of rehabilitation. Psychiatric care may be necessary to manage neuropsychiatric consequences of brain injury.

Podiatrist (www.apma.org)

Many neurorehabilitation patients experience foot health problems during their rehabilitation. Patients with diabetes, peripheral vascular disease, or peripheral neuropathies are prone to disorders of the foot due to poor sensation or circulation. Poor foot care may result in infections or pressure sores which, if not treated promptly, could result in amputation of a toe or portion of the limb.

Dentist (www.ada.org)

By providing routine care for teeth or dentures, dentists assist neurologically disabled patients to improve mastication and swallowing function. Infections or abscesses may need treatment. Less commonly, prosthetics such as palatal lifts may be necessary to close the soft palate and permit more normal swallowing function.

Audiologist (www.asha.org)

Audiology is the study of hearing, hearing disorders, and habilitation/rehabilitation for individuals who have hearing loss. It encompasses the study of how the hearing mechanism works; the assessment of hearing; hearing and listening disorders; and the rehabilitation of individuals who have hearing loss. Audiologists test and diagnose hearing and balance disorders in infants, children, and adults; work with patients who require auditory training and speech reading; select, fit, and dispense hearing aids and assistive devices; and educate patients consumers and professionals on the prevention of hearing loss.

32.5 Effectiveness of neurorehabilitation

Before patients are admitted to a neurorehabilitation program, several factors are considered. First, a preliminary review of the patient's condition and comorbidities using the medical record determines whether the patient is likely to benefit significantly from a specific type of rehabilitation program. Second, the psychosocial status must be reviewed to identify appropriate support systems, including family members or caregivers who can provide supervision or assistance, or financial resources to purchase assistance for the patient. Third, the home layout must be delineated for barriers, such as stairs to the front door and in the home, and for the presence of bedroom and bathroom facilities on the entry floor. These influence the goals that the patient must attain in order to return home. Fourth, the premorbid functional status must be determined to establish functional goals that

enable the patient to return home. These are compared with the current, or pre-rehabilitation, functional status to determine the likelihood that the patient will attain the functional goals necessary to return home and the estimated length of stay required to attain those goals. Finally, the means of paying for the services (third-party payer or private payment) must be identified to establish qualification for the level of care desired and the durable medical equipment to be used at home, and to facilitate payment for prescription medications that will be needed following discharge. Rehabilitation needs and appropriate levels of rehabilitation care are illustrated in Fig. 32.1.

The best guideline to apply to a patient requiring neurorehabilitation is to provide the environment with the most intense therapy that the patient can tolerate. The model of stroke rehabilitation best illustrates this concept. Randomized clinical studies of patients who began intensive stroke rehabilitation from 1 week (Sivenius et al., 1985; Kwakkel et al., 1999; Fang et al., 2003) to more than 1 year after stroke onset (Wade et al., 1992; Logan et al., 1997; Green et al., 2002) showed significant functional improvements in

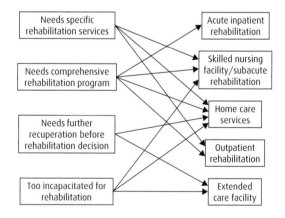

Figure 32.1. Phases of rehabilitation. Decisions about what type of rehabilitation environment is most useful are made on the basis of what patients need, what they are capable of tolerating medically and psychologically, and what their health system will pay for. The latter is generally determined in each country based on cost–benefit analysis.

mobility and activities of daily living when compared to cohorts of stroke survivors receiving less intense rehabilitation. When compared with conventional or less intensive care, stroke rehabilitation in an inpatient rehabilitation facility (IRF) with coordinated, transdisciplinary care significantly reduced the statistical risk of death or institutionalization, or death or dependency, independent of age, sex, or stroke severity (Kramer et al., 1997; Stroke Unit Trialists' Collaboration, 2004). For every 100 patients receiving organized inpatient multidisciplinary rehabilitation, an extra five stroke survivors returned to independent home life (Langhorne and Duncan, 2001). Five years after their events, stroke survivors who were treated in dedicated stroke units (combined acute and rehabilitation) scored higher in energy, physical mobility, emotional reactions, social isolation, and sleep (Indredavik et al., 1998). Even 10 years after their strokes, survivors in combined acute and rehabilitation stroke units were more likely to be alive, had a significantly better functional state, and were more likely to be living at home (Indradavik et al., 1999). Compliance with guidelines such as patient and family education, performance of baseline assessments, family involvement in rehabilitation, monitoring of patient progress, management of impairments, and multidisciplinary evaluation, were most often associated with higher patient satisfaction (Reker et al., 2002). However, in the inpatient rehabilitation environment, there does not appear to be a specific therapy that significantly improves discharge outcomes (Dickstein et al., 1986; Lord and Hall, 1986; Basmajian et al., 1987; Moseley et al., 2004).

There is evidence that intensity of therapy in environments other than inpatient rehabilitation facilities may improve outcomes. In subacute rehabilitation facilities, after controlling for other variables, functional gains were weakly correlated with therapy intensity and rehabilitation duration (Chen et al., 2002). In a meta-analysis of randomized controlled trials comparing stroke survivors with conventional home care and those with early discharge and rehabilitation support in the community setting, hospital stays were reduced by up to 9 days with no significant increase in death, death and institutionalization, or

death and dependency at follow up (Early Supported Discharge Trialists, 2004). Among community-based stroke survivors within 1 year of stroke, seven of every 100 stroke survivors receiving therapy-based rehabilitation services were spared a poor outcome as a result of increasing their personal ADL scores (Outpatient Service Trialists, 2004). In a meta-analysis of seven randomized controlled trials of day hospitals, it was not possible to prove that day hospital rehabilitation was effective for stroke survivors (Dekker et al., 1998).

Correlating functional improvements with neuroanatomic changes, however, has been a bigger challenge. As early as the late 19th century, deafferentation experiments on animals demonstrated "no obvious change in the condition..." up to and over 3 months after the procedure was performed (Mott and Sherrington, 1895). Early in the 20th century, researchers noted that monkeys could use their arms and legs 14 days after decortication (Ogden and Franz, 1917). From such research (c.f., Chapters 8 and 14 of Volume I), the principle that plastic changes in the brain could occur with intensive therapy was suggested, leading to the concept of constraint-induced movement therapy (Taub et al., 1978) (Chapter 18 of Volume II). In 1981, Bach-y-Rita suggested the "unmasking of neural pathways and synapses not normally used but called upon when the dominant system fails" as a result of an excitability that captures the effects of the remaining neurologic input (Bach-y-Rita, 1981).

We now have a better understanding of plastic changes in the central nervous system during rehabilitation (Chapter 15 of Volume I). Once the cerebral cortex could be viewed as functionally and structurally dynamic, researchers learned that behavioral experiences may induce long-term plasticity that are accompanied by changes in dendritic and synaptic structure, as well as the regulation of cortical neurotransmitter systems (Nudo et al., 2001). Even in stroke survivors with aphasia, intensive therapy appeared to produce significant, pronounced improvements on several standard clinical tests, and self-ratings, as well as blinded-observer ratings of patients' communicative effectiveness in everyday life (Pulvermuller et al.,

2001), that were associated with homologous right-hemispheric activation on functional MRI scans (Thulborn et al., 1999) (Chapter 26 of Volume II). Using transcranial magnetic stimulation in stroke survivors undergoing constraint-induced movement therapy, cortical mapping demonstrated that the representation of the affected hand increased significantly until it was nearly identical in size with that of the unaffected hand (Liepert et al., 2000) (Chapter 18 of Volume II). In a randomized trial of task-oriented arm training using passive movement as an activation paradigm, positron emission tomography (PET) scans demonstrated induction of reorganization in bilateral sensory, motor systems, including inferior parietal cortex, premotor cortex, and contralateral sensorimotor cortex (Nelles et al., 2001). While researchers noted that intensive therapy produces functional changes, the mechanisms of change and thresholds required to cause these changes still are not delineated (Chapter 8 of Volume I).

32.6 Economics of neurorehabilitation

An IRF (Department of Health and Human Services, 2001) can be a unit within a general hospital or can be a separate hospital. In the USA, an IRF must meet the following criteria:

- Have in effect a pre-admission screening procedure under which each prospective patient's condition and medical history are reviewed to determine whether the patient is likely to benefit significantly from an intensive inpatient hospital program or assessment.
- Ensure that patients receive close medical supervision and furnish rehabilitation nursing, physical therapy, and occupational therapy, plus, as needed, speech therapy, social or psychologic services, and orthotic and prosthetic services, through the use of qualified personnel.
- Have a director of rehabilitation who meets the criteria specified in the regulations.
- Have a plan of treatment for each inpatient that is established, reviewed, and revised as

needed by a physician in consultation with other professional personnel who provide services to the patient.
- Use a coordinated multidisciplinary team approach in the rehabilitation of each inpatient in the manner specified in the regulations.

IRFs must be fully equipped, staffed, and capable of providing hospital inpatient rehabilitation care; must have written admission criteria that are applied uniformly to both Medicare and non-Medicare patients; have admission and discharge records that are separately identified from those of the hospital in which it is located; have policies specifying that necessary clinical information is transferred to the unit when a patient of the hospital is transferred to the unit; meet applicable state licensure laws; have utilization review standards applicable for the type of care offered in the unit; have beds physically separate from (i.e., not co-mingled with) other beds within a hospital; be serviced by the same fiscal intermediary as the hospital; and be treated as a separate cost center for cost finding and apportionment purposes.

While Medicare guidelines may be the definitive criteria for admission and continued stay in an IRF, they are not the only guidelines used in the healthcare industry. Guidelines such as InterQual (www.interqual.com, McKesson Health Care Solutions LLC) and Milliman Care Guidelines (www.milliman.com, Milliman) are proprietary standards that various health maintenance organizations or preferred provider organizations may use in their pre-certification determinations. Although they cannot be published here, clinicians should be familiar with these and other standards within their own countries, so that they may advocate for potential patients who might benefit from neurorehabilitation services provided in an IRF. For example, in the United Kingdom, Quality Requirement 4 states that "people with long-term neurologic conditions who would benefit from rehabilitation are to receive timely, ongoing, high-quality rehabilitation services in hospital or other specialist settings to meet their continuing and changing needs. When ready, they receive the help they need to return home for ongoing community rehabilitation and support..." (United Kingdom Department of Health, 2005). Many other countries have similarly detailed regulations governing the administration and reimbursement criteria for rehabilitation.

REFERENCES

Bach-y-Rita, P. (1981). Central nervous system lesions: sprouting and unmasking in rehabilitation. *Arch Phys Med Rehabil*, **62**, 413–417.

Basmajian, J.V., Gowland, C.A., Finlayson, A.J., Hall, A.L., Swanson, L.R., Stratford, P.W., Trotter, J.E. and Brandstater, M.E. (1987). Stroke treatment: comparison of integrated behavior-physical therapy vs. traditional physical therapy programs. *Arch Phys Med Rehabil*, **68**, 267–272.

Brown, T.M. (1982). An historical view of health care. In: *Responsibility in Health Care* (ed. Agich, G.J.), D. Reidell, Boston, MA, pp. 3–21.

Chen, C.C., Heinemann, A.W., Granger, C.V. and Linn, R.T. (2002). Functional gains and therapy intensity during subacute rehabilitation: a study of 20 facilities. *Arch Phys Med Rehabil*, **83**(**11**), 1514–1523.

Cole, K.M. and Gawlinski, A. (1995). Animal-assisted therapy in the intensive care unit. A staff nurse's dream comes true. *Nurs Clin North Am*, **30**(**3**), 529–537.

Coyle, C.P., Kinney, W.B., Riley, B. and Shank, J.W. (1991). *Benefits of Therapeutic Recreation: A Consensus View*, Idyll Arbor, Inc., Ravensdale, WA.

Dekker, R., Drost, E.A., Groothoff, J.W., Arendzen, J.H., van Gijn, J.C. and Eisma, W.H. (1998). Effects of day-hospital rehabilitation in stroke patients: a review of randomized clinical trials. *Scand J Rehabil Med*, **30**(**2**), 87–94.

DeLisa, J.A., Martin, G.M. and Currie, D.M. (1993). Rehabilitation medicine: past, present, and future. In: *Rehabilitation Medicine: Principles and Practice*, (ed. Delisa, J.A), 2nd edn., J.B. Lippincott, Philadelphia, PA, p. 3.

Department of Health and Human Services, Centers for Medicare & Medicaid Services (2001). 42 CFR Parts 412 and 413. Medicare program; prospective payment system for inpatient rehabilitation facilities; final rule. *Federal Regist*, **66**(**152**), 41315–41364. Department of Health and Human Services, Baltimore, MD.

Dickstein, R., Hocherman, S., Pillar, T. and Shaham, R. (1986). Stroke rehabilitation: three exercise therapy approaches. *Phys Ther*, **66**(**8**), 1233–1238.

Early Supported Discharge Trialists (2004). Services for reducing duration of hospital care for acute stroke patients (Cochrane review). In: *The Cochrane Library*, Issue 3, John Wiley & Sons, Ltd., Chichester, UK.

Fang, Y., Chen, X., Lin, J., Huang, R. and Zeng, J. (2003). A study on additional early physiotherapy after stroke and factors affecting functional recovery. *Clin Rehabil*, **17**, 608–617.

Green, J., Forster, A., Bogle, S. and Young, J. (2002). *Lancet*, **359**, 199–203.

Halstead, L.S. (1976). Team care in chronic illness: a critical review of the literature of the past 25 years. *Arch Phys Med Rehabil*, **57**(**11**), 507–511.

Indredavik, B., Bakke, F., Slordahl, S.A., Rokseth, R. and Haheim, L.L. (1998). Stroke unit treatment improves long-term quality of life: a randomized controlled trial. *Stroke*, **29**(**5**), 895–899.

Indredavik, B., Bakke, F., Slordahl, S.A., Rokseth, R. and Haheim, L.L. (1999). Stroke unit treatment. 10-year follow-up. *Stroke*, **30**(**8**), 1524–1527.

International Labour Office (1983). *C159 Vocational Rehabilitation and Employment (Disabled Persons) Convention*. Accessed on April 1, 2005: http://www.ilo.org/ public/english/employment/skills/recomm/instr/c_159.htm#Part%20 I.%20Definition%20and%20Scope.

Jorgenson, J. (1997). Therapeutic use of companion animals in health care. *Image J Nurs Scholarship*, **29**(**3**), 249–254.

Keith, R.A. (1991). The comprehensive treatment team in rehabilitation. *Arch Phys Med Rehabil*, **72**, 269–274.

Kramer, A.M., Steiner, J.F., Schlenker, R.E., Eilertsen, T.B., Hrincevich, C.A., Tropea, D.A., Ahmad, L.A. and Eckhoff, D.G. (1997). Outcomes and costs after hip fracture and stroke. A comparison of rehabilitation settings. *J Amer Med Assoc*, **277**(**5**), 396–404.

Kwakkel, G., Wagenaar, R.C., Twisk, J.W.R., Lankhorst, G.J. and Koetsier, J.C. (1999). Intensity of arm and leg training after primary middle cerebral artery stroke: a randomized trial. *Lancet*, **354**, 191–196.

Langhorne, P. and Duncan, P. (2001). Does the organization of postacute stroke care really matter? *Stroke*, **32**(**1**), 268–274.

Liepert, J., Bauder, H., Miltner, W.H.R., Taub, E. and Weiller C. (2000). Treatment-induced cortical reorganization after stroke in humans. *Stroke*, **31**, 1210–1216.

Logan, P.A., Ahern, J., Gladman, J.R. and Lincoln, N.B. (1997). *Clin Rehabil*, **11**(**2**), 107–113.

Lord, J.P. and Hall, K. (1986). Neuromuscular reeducation vs. traditional programs for stroke rehabilitation. *Arch Phys Med Rehabil*, **67**, 88–91.

Moseley, A.M., Stark, A., Cameron, I.D. and Pollock, A. (2004). Treadmill training and body weight support for walking after stroke (Cochrane review). In: *The Cochrane Library*, Issue 3, John Wiley & Sons, Ltd., Chichester, UK.

Mott, F.W. and Sherrington, C.S. (1895). Experiments upon the influences of sensory nerves upon movement and nutrition of the limbs. Preliminary communication. *Proc Roy Soc London Ser B*, **57**, 481–488.

Nelles, G., Jentzen, W., Jueptner, M., Muller, S. and Diener, H.C. (2001). Arm training induced brain plasticity in stroke studied with serial positron emission tomography. *Neuroimaging*, **13(6 Pt 1)**, 1146–1154.

Nevlud, G.N. (1990). The team approach: current trends and issues in rehabilitation. *Texas J Audiol Speech Pathol*, **16**, 21–23.

Nudo, R.J., Plautz, E.J. and Frost, S.B. (2001). Role of adaptive plasticity in recovery of function after damage to motor cortex. *Muscle Nerve*, **24(8)**, 1000–1019.

Ogden, R. and Franz, S.I. (1917). On cerebral motor control: the recovery from experimentally produced hemiplegia. *Psychobiology*, **1**, 33–80.

Outpatient Service Trialists (2004). Therapy-based rehabilitation services for stroke patients at home (Cochrane review). In: *The Cochrane Library*, Issue 3, John Wiley & Sons, Ltd., Chichester, UK.

Pulvermuller, F., Neininger, B., Elbert, T., Mohr, B., Rockstroh, B., Koebbel, P. and Taub, E. (2001). Constraint-induced therapy of chronic aphasia after stroke. *Stroke*, **32(7)**, 1621–1626.

Reker, D.M., Duncan, P.W., Horner, R.D., Hoenig, H., Samsa, G.P., Hamilton, B.B. and Dudley, T.K. (2002). Postacute stroke guideline compliance is associated with greater patient satisfaction. *Arch Phys Med Rehabil*, **83(6)**, 750–756.

Richeson, N.E. (2003). Effects of animal-assisted therapy on agitated behaviors and social interactions of older adults with dementia. *Am J Alzheimer's Dis Other Dement*, **18(6)**, 353–358.

Sivenius, J., Pyorala, K., Heinonen, O.P., Salonen, J.T. and Riekkinen, P. (1985). The significance of intensity of rehabilitation of stroke. A controlled trial. *Stroke*, **16**, 928–931.

Spencer, W.A. (1969). Changes in methods and relationships necessary within rehabilitation. *Arch Phys Med Rehabil*, **50**, 566–580.

Stroke Unit Trialists' Collaboration (2004). Organised inpatient (stroke unit) care for stroke (Cochrane review). In: *The Cochrane Library*, Issue 3, John Wiley & Sons, Ltd., Chichester, UK.

Taub, E., Williams, M., Barro, G. and Steiner S.S. (1978). Comparison of the performance of deafferented and intact monkeys on continuous and fixed ration schedules of reinforcement. *Exp Neurol*, **58(1)**, 1–13.

Thulborn, K.R., Carpenter, P.A. and Just, M.A. (1999). Plasticity of language-related brain function during recovery from stroke. *Stroke*, **30(4)**, 749–754.

United Kingdom Department of Health (2005). *Quality Requirement 4: Early and Specialist Rehabilitation*. Accessed on April 1, 2005: http://www.dh.gov.uk/PolicyAndGuidance/HealthAndSocialCareTopics/LongTermConditions/BestPractice/EarlySpecialistRehabilitation/fs/en.

Wade, D.T., Collen, F.M., Robb, G.F. and Warlow, C.P. (1992). *Br Med J*, **308(6827)**, 609–613.

World Health Organization (2001). *International Classificastion of Functioning, Disability, and Health (ICF)*. World Health Organization, Geneva, Switzerland. Avlailable at: http://www3.who.int/icf/onlinebrowser/icf.cfm

Traumatic brain injury

Michael P. Barnes

*Department of Neurological Rehabilitation, Hunters Moor Regional
Neurological Rehabilitation Centre, Newcastle upon Tyne, UK*

33.1 Introduction

It is regrettable that rehabilitation services for people with traumatic brain injury (TBI) are non-existent in many countries and sparse and fragmented in others. Some countries have developed high quality post-acute rehabilitation facilities, particularly the USA, Canada, Australia, New Zealand and many parts of Western Europe. However, even in these countries there is little coordinated community-based support after discharge from the post-acute facility. There is an urgent need for the development of more comprehensive rehabilitation facilities which will support the individual, and the family, from injury to death.

This chapter will highlight the problems encountered after TBI and suggest clinical strategies and treatment methods by which many of these problems can be alleviated. It is important that this chapter is not read in isolation but is cross-referenced with other chapters in this textbook that are of relevance to the rehabilitation of people with TBI. In particular, the reader's attention is drawn to Volume I, Chapter 14 by Nudo and colleagues on Plasticity After Brain Lesions.

Many of the difficulties encountered by people after TBI are also covered in the chapters of this volume which concentrate on rehabilitation by symptoms and in particular Chapter 28, Neglect and Anosognosia; Chapter 29, Memory Dysfunction; and Chapter 30, Neurorehabilitation of Executive Function. The present chapter will not cover the rehabilitation of the comatose patient, as this is discussed in Chapter 22 of this volume.

33.2 Epidemiology

The reported incidence of TBI varies widely. The NIH Consensus Development Statement (1998) quoted an annual rate of 100 per 100,000 population per annum in the USA. This paper further estimated that there are around 52,000 annual deaths from TBI. This compares to the number of people requiring hospitalisation in the UK following brain injury of around 275 per 100,000 annually. Obviously the majority of these people have a mild brain injury and will make a reasonably quick recovery. However, a significant number have moderate to severe injuries and are at significant risk of longer-term disability. In the UK it is estimated that around 25 per 100,000 people per year are admitted to hospital with a moderate to severe brain injury. Around 10–20% of these people are likely to have a long-term severe disability or remain in prolonged coma. About 65–80% will eventually have a good physical (but not necessarily cognitive or psycho-social) recovery (McLellan et al., 1998; Royal College of Physicians and British Society of Rehabilitation Medicine, 2003; Table 33.1).

The estimates of prevalence vary even more widely. The NIH Consensus Development Statement (1998) estimated prevalence between 2.5 and 6.5 million individuals living with the consequences of TBI in the USA. This compares to the suggested prevalence in the UK of approximately one per 1000 population (Medical Disability Society, 1988). This compares reasonably well with the estimate in the Canadian population of approximately 0.6 per 1000 adults (Moscato et al., 1994).

Table 33.1. Definitions of injury severity.

Mild head injury	Glasgow Coma Score 13–14/coma of less than 15 min
Moderate head injury	Coma of 15 min to 6 h/Glasgow Coma Score 8–12/PTA less than 24 h
Severe head injury	Glasgow Coma Score 7 or less/coma of greater than 6 h/post-traumatic amnesia of 24 h or more

Medical Disability Society (1988). PTA: post-traumatic amnesia.

There is a well-described peak of incidence of TBI between the ages of 15 and 24 years and, in this age group; there is a strong male preponderance in the order of two or three males to every female. There is an additional small peak under the age of 5 years and then a much later rise in incidence in the elderly population.

Approximately half of the injuries are the result of road traffic accidents. However, there is encouraging, albeit modest, decline in the incidence TBI following the introduction, in many countries, of legislation regarding the use of safety belts, airbags and child car seats as well as regulations covering speed limits, road design and traffic control (Munro et al., 1995). There has also been a reduction of avoidable deaths following the introduction of alcohol limits in road users.

The second most frequent cause of TBI, particularly among the elderly population, is falls. Regrettably there is also an increasing incidence of head injury following violence and assault. In the USA violence-related brain injury now accounts for around 20% of all head injuries, broadly divided between firearm and non-firearm assaults. Sports and recreational related injuries only account for a relatively small minority of TBI and greater regulatory control of sports in order to prevent such injuries is to be welcomed.

Alcohol plays a significant part in the majority of TBI, particularly in road traffic accidents but also in falls and violence.

Thus, TBI is a major public health concern and has very significant financial implications for health systems and the economy as a whole. There is a scarcity of research into risk factors and there are large gaps in our knowledge of appropriate prevention strategies.

33.3 Predictors of long-term outcome

It would be very useful if, in the acute stages following TBI, there could be some robust predictor of eventual outcome. This may help to focus on an appropriate rehabilitation strategy and enable accurate information to be imparted to the patient's family. Regrettably there are still no markers that can make such predictions with any useful degree of accuracy. There are, of course, some generalisations that can be made. It is generally true that the worse the extent of the original brain injury, the worse the eventual outcome. There is a crude correlation between outcome and depth of coma (as judged by the Glasgow Coma Score), the duration of coma and the extent of brain damage as judged by computed tomography (CT) or magnetic resonance imaging (MRI) scanning (Signorini et al., 1999). There is also a similar relationship between duration of post-traumatic amnesia (PTA) (McMillan et al., 1996). A PTA, for example, of more than 2 weeks predicts significant neuropsychological deficit in the long term (Vanzomeren and Vandenburg, 1985) and a coma duration of more than 20 days also predicts lack of independence in the community (Pazzaglia et al., 1975). There is some recent evidence that the Injury Severity Score is able to predict rehabilitative potential (Toschlog et al., 2003). However, there is no scoring system that can be thoroughly relied upon to offer such predictions, as any given individual patient may still be the exception that proves the rule. There are certainly some other pointers towards rehabilitation outcome. It is generally accepted that elderly patients have a poorer outcome both in terms of mortality and morbidity (Cifu et al., 1996; Susman et al., 2002). There is evidence that pre-injury socio-economic status as well as educational history can also predict outcome but once again such broad variables are of little assistance in planning appropriate rehabilitation for a given individual. It may be, in the future, that more accurate neuroradiological and neurophysiological investigations may be useful tools to predict recovery but at the present time this is not the case (Garnett et al., 2001).

33.4 Outcome measures

It is axiomatical that a rehabilitation process must include the use of validated outcome measures. All rehabilitation needs to involve an appropriate client-centred, goal setting process and outcome measures are clearly necessary in order to monitor those goals and determine when they have been met. It is also important, in a busy clinical setting, for such measures to be simple and easy to administer, and widely understood not only by the health professionals involved but by the family and, if possible, by the patient. Clearly any outcome measures should have been through a proper validation and reliability analysis. There is much debate in the literature about appropriate outcome measures that should be used to monitor progress after TBI. There is clearly no single measure that should be used in all circumstances. The measure applied will vary according to the time after injury (post-acute measures, community measures, etc.), the main problems to be measured (e.g. nursing measures, cognitive measures, behavioural measures, etc.) and the time course over which the measure is to be employed. A given individual is likely to have, and indeed probably should have, a number of measures used for monitoring over the whole course of a comprehensive rehabilitation programme. Whilst many of the scales debated in the literature are objective it should not be forgotten that the individual's, and their families', subjective opinion must be taken into account. Rigid adherence to an outcome measure as the sole source of goal monitoring is usually inappropriate.

The standard measure of coma is the Glasgow Coma Scale (Teasdale and Jennett, 1974; Teasdale et al., 1978, 1979). This is reproduced as Table 33.2. However, this scale, whilst an essential and useful tool in an acute setting, obviously has limited use in the context of rehabilitation. There is a crude correlation between the level of coma and rehabilitation

Table 33.2. Glasgow Coma Scale.

Item: Response	Score	Details
Eye opening		
None	1	Even to pain (supra-orbital pressure)
To pain	2	Pain from sternum/limb/ supra-orbital ridge
To speech	3	Non-specific response, not necessarily to command
Spontaneous	4	Eyes open, not necessarily aware
Motor response		
None	1	To any pain; limbs remain flaccid
Extension	2	"Decerebrate"; shoulder adducted and internally rotated, forearm pronated
Abnormal flexion	3	"Decorticate"; shoulder flexes/adducts
Withdrawal	4	Arm withdraws from pain, shoulder abducts
Localises pain	5	Arm attempts to remove supra-orbital/chest pressure
Obeys commands	6	Follows simple commands
Verbal response		
None	1	As stated
Incomprehensible	2	Moans/groans; no words
Inappropriate	3	Intelligible, no sustained sentences
Confused	4	Responds with conversation, but confused
Oriented	5	Aware of time, place, person

Teasdale and Jennett (1974); Teasdale et al. (1978, 1979).

outcome but the use of the scale is not of much practical significance to the rehabilitation team. Other short, global, multi-dimensional measures have some use in determining crude outcome. The best known is the five-point Glasgow Outcome Scale (Jennett and Bond, 1975). However, this, and similar, rating scales are by no means sensitive enough to record more subtle change in function over time. More sensitive measures are needed. Probably the most widely used is the 18-item functional independence measure (FIM; *Guide for the Uniformed Data System for Medical Rehabilitation*, 1993). The FIM has been through many validity and reliability studies. It is well recognised and well known but it does suffer from ceiling effects and the original version paid insufficient attention to cognitive and psycho-social information. The latter problems have been addressed by development of the related functional assessment measure (FAM; Hall et al., 1996). The other widely used measure is the Barthel index (Mahoney and Barthel, 1965), which also suffers from ceiling effects. These two measures are particularly designed for use in the post-acute setting. More subtle and longer-term changes in the community setting will need other measures. Some of the commonest are the Craig Handicap, Assessment and Reporting Technique (CHART; Whiteneck et al., 1992), the 15-item Community Integration Questionnaire (CIQ; Willer et al., 1994) and the Newcastle Independence Assessment Form – Research (NIAF-R; Semlyen et al., 1996, 1997).

Such broad measures are useful for monitoring longer-term strategical goals but individual disability measures may also need to be used in parallel. The team may wish to monitor, for example, memory function, depression, behavioural disturbance and a whole variety of other potential shorter-term sub-goals. Such a "basket" of measures should be picked with care by the team (Turner-Stokes, 2002) in order to ensure that scarce rehabilitation time is not simply taken up by the recording of progress, to the detriment of actual delivery of therapy!

33.5 Rehabilitation service models

Rehabilitation programmes come in many shapes and sizes. There is no universally accepted model and indeed it would be inappropriate to suggest that one single model of service is preferable to any other. Services will clearly need to be designed according to local need, resources, geography, personnel availability and a host of other considerations. Services for urban areas are likely to be very different from services in rural communities. Services in developing countries will need to be designed differently, and much more cheaply, than services in "westernised" nations. However, in general terms, rehabilitation

should be seen as a continuum from acute injury to full community reintegration. There are three main stages: post-acute rehabilitation; transition to community and longer-term community support.

Post-acute rehabilitation

It is not the purpose of this chapter to describe the immediate post-acute care of individuals following TBI. There are a number of guidelines produced in recent years that offer advice on the immediate triage, assessment, investigation and early management of head injury (European Brain Injury Consortium, 1997; Society of British Neurological Surgeons, 1998; Royal College of Surgeons of England, 1999; National Institute for Clinical Excellence, 2003). However, it is clear from the literature that rehabilitation should start as early as possible. There can be little doubt that avoidable complications can occur in the early days after injury and the immediate involvement of a rehabilitation team, even in the acute neurosurgical setting, may help to prevent such difficulties. Early studies (e.g. Rusk et al., 1966) document an unacceptable range of complications such as pressure sores, joint contractures, frozen shoulders, urinary and respiratory difficulties – all of which should have been preventable by proper care and rehabilitation. There have been some studies that demonstrated the benefits of early rehabilitation. One of the earliest, and still one of the most convincing, is the study by Cope and Hall in 1982. They studied outcome at 2 years in people transferred early or late post-injury (before or after 35 days). The two groups were matched for severity of injury and depth of coma. The early-transferred group spent less time on the rehabilitation unit, and obviously less time on the acute ward, with the same functional outcome as the later-transferred group. Other studies have generally confirmed that whilst early transfer does not necessarily produce better outcomes in the long term it certainly produces better outcomes, and earlier discharge and thus reduced costs, in the short term (Cowen et al., 1995; High et al., 1996). Thus, the evidence, albeit somewhat sparse, is that individuals should be transferred to a multidisciplinary rehabilitation unit as soon as possible after the acute event. Some authors have tried to produce guidelines on the number of beds and different types of staff required for such a unit but such suggestions are fraught with difficulties as the requirements will clearly change from place to place and certainly from country to country. The need for post-acute rehabilitation will also, to a great extent, depend on the nature and extent of transitional rehabilitation facilities and community back up. Whilst the precise disposition and make-up of the team will involve some local decisions the literature is clear that such a team must work in a multidisciplinary, or preferably an interdisciplinary, fashion. Multidisciplinary teams are made up of a group of professionals who work alongside one another whereas interdisciplinary teams take a more integrated approach where the team as a whole works towards a single set of agreed goals and often undertakes joint sessions with the patient (Mandy, 1996). Some would suggest that transdisciplinary teams are more appropriate where the role of individual disciplines is extended and the team as a whole adopts an overall problem-solving approach so that the interventions frequently cross traditional discipline boundaries (Jackson and Davies, 1995). Behavioural units often need to adopt this approach. The Royal College of Physicians and British Society of Rehabilitation Medicine (2003) in the UK have recently produced national clinical guidelines which set out some basic standards for the provision of specialist neurological rehabilitation services for people with acquired brain injury. In particular such teams should compromise the following:

- A coordinated interdisciplinary team from all relevant clinical disciplines.
- Staff with specialist expertise in the management of brain injury.
- Educational programmes for staff, patients and carers.
- Agreed protocols for common problems, such as management of spasticity, epilepsy, depression, etc.

These guidelines suggest minimum staffing provisions for such services. They also suggest minimum guidelines for the necessary teamwork and communication,

such as the use of a single interdisciplinary patient record system and that a designated member of the team (a keyworker) should be responsible for overseeing and coordinating the patient's programme and acting as a point of communication between the team and the patient/family.

There is now some evidence that this broad interdisciplinary approach produces benefit for the head injured person over and above benefits that may accrue from single discipline and less coordinated rehabilitation programme. Semlyen et al. (1998) prospectively compared outcome at 2 years in two groups of patients discharged from a neurosurgical unit. Some were discharged to a specialist rehabilitation unit and the others to a local district hospital for non-specialist and often uni-disciplinary rehabilitation. Despite the fact that the specialist rehabilitation group had a higher proportion of more serious injuries the 2-year functional outcome was similar in both groups. The specialist rehabilitation group had improved faster and effectively "caught up" with the other group by the time of discharge (usually by 1 year) and such improvements continued over a longer timescale. It is also worth noting that in this study carer distress decreased over time in the specialist rehabilitation group but increased over time in the other group.

There is further evidence of efficacy in the context of specific situations, such as the management of behavioural disturbance (vide infra). There is also evidence of the efficacy of individual techniques, such as the various interventions for spasticity management, memory disturbance, depression, etc. (vide infra).

Some authors have attempted to analyse the effect of intensity of therapy upon outcome in a post-acute rehabilitation setting. Shiel et al. (2001) investigated the effect of an increased intensity of rehabilitation therapy on the rate of which independence was regained, as well as the duration of hospital admission. This was a two centre prospective controlled study with a random allocation to the different intensity groups. Individuals receiving more intensive therapy made more rapid progress and were discharged home sooner. A similar result was obtained in a randomised single blind controlled trial in the

North of England (Slade et al., 2002). The experimental group were timetabled to receive 67% more therapy in any given week than the control group. The patients in the experimental group showed a significant, 14 day, reduction of length of stay. In a different cultural context Zhu et al. (2001) compared, in a randomised assessor-blind trial, two groups of patients after TBI receiving different intensities of rehabilitation treatment – 2 h/day versus 4 h/day. The interim results, in 36 cases, showed there was a trend for more patients in the more intensive therapy group to achieve full FIM scores and a good outcome on the Glasgow Outcome Scale at 2 and 3 months although at 6 months the control group appeared to be catching up in terms of a similar outcome. The studies all seem to show the same trend that more intensive therapy input can lead to a quicker improvement, and thus an earlier discharge, but probably does not carry a significant longer-term benefit. More recently this work has been confirmed in another study by Cifu et al. (2003). Their findings support the assertion that increased therapy intensity, particularly physical and psychological therapies, enhances functional outcome. It is regrettable that in many centres around the world achieving more than 1 or 2 h therapy per day is impossible due to limitations on staffing numbers. A study by Spivack et al. in 1992, for example, recommended 5–6 h of treatment per day which is entirely unachievable in most countries around the world (Spivack et al., 1992).

However, research in TBI rehabilitation is very difficult to conduct and "adequate sample sizes and appropriate comparison groups are difficult to achieve in a clinical rehabilitation environment. Therefore, the fact that most research to date has not been rigorous must not be interpreted to imply that rehabilitation programmes are not effective" (NIH Consensus Development Statement, 1998).

Transition into community

Once an individual has begun to plateau in terms of recovery after TBI then discharge back into the community will need to be planned. This is a difficult time both for the patient and family and there is much evidence that family stress significantly increases after discharge from hospital (Acorn, 1993; Allen et al., 1994). The individual him/herself may often need specific skills training in order to assist with community reintegration. This can include learning independent living skills, such as cooking and shopping and community transport, as well as social and interpersonal skills. Although such programmes can be provided in a post-acute rehabilitation setting an alternative model is provision of such skills training in a "step-down" or transitional rehabilitation unit. These may provide daytime rehabilitation whilst the person lives at home or are sometimes residential facilities. Attendance can clearly vary according to both post-acute and community facilities but individuals would normally stay several months undergoing a phased reintroduction into the community. Regrettably, although such an idea seems to have commonsense merit, there is little evidence regarding effectiveness (Boake, 1990).

Two studies are worth mentioning. The first is by Cope et al. (1991a, 1991b). Individuals were admitted to a residential, non-hospital, facility around 15 months from injury – although there was a significant range from 15 days to 13 years. The study confirmed a positive effect on residential work status and number of attendant care hours. Even making allowance for spontaneous change a positive effect was still found. However, the obvious criticism of the study is that it is single blind and there is no control group. Nevertheless the reduction in care costs amounted to around 41,000 US dollars per annum for patients initially in the severe category. In another two studies (Johnston, 1991; Johnston and Lewis, 1991) 82 people from nine community re-entry facilities were investigated. Most had had a TBI. Comparison between admission and one-year follow-up (rather unsatisfactorily by telephone) showed a reduction in institutional care (from 45% to 7%), a reduction in supervision and positive effects on work status. However, once again there was no control group and it was a rather heterogeneous case mix of individuals and, although the results look impressive, only limited conclusions can be drawn.

Community-based programmes and longer-term support

Only a small minority of people after TBI will be able to access any form of transitional brain injury rehabilitation facility. Indeed many, on a global basis, will not access post-acute rehabilitation facilities and will be discharged from the acute care ward straight back home. Thus, for many people there is a need for active community rehabilitation. Even for those who have been through a post-acute rehabilitation facility and/or a community reintegration facility there is nearly always a need for some form of continuing support. Support is required in order to avoid the emergence of any unnecessary longer-term complications (either physical, psychological, emotional or behavioural) or to provide ongoing advice and assistance on family, social and work life. Ongoing support for the family and carers may also be required. There is now quite good quality evidence of the efficacy of community rehabilitation programmes in the context of stroke. There are, for example, a number of early discharge community teams. These teams accept responsibility for ongoing community rehabilitation of people after stroke, and thus enable the individual to be discharged earlier from acute hospital than would otherwise be the case (Rodgers et al., 1997). Anderson et al. (2002) reviewed seven published trials involving over 1000 patients and demonstrated that early hospital discharge with community rehabilitation support reduced the total length of stay by 13 days without any clinical detrimental effect. These are stroke-based studies and there have been no similar studies in the context of TBI. However, there is no real reason why similar principles should not apply, but there does seem to be a dearth of early discharge brain injury rehabilitation teams. However, there are a few published examples of community-based rehabilitation teams that provide longer-term support. In one of the few evaluative studies, Powell et al. (2002) evaluated multidisciplinary community-based outreach rehabilitation. They found that the community team participants were significantly more likely to show gains on a number of relevant outcome measures than the control group. A similar result in an outpatient rehabilitation programme has recently been reported by Goranson et al. (2003).

Regrettably there is a paucity of such services. In one study in South East England (McMillan and Ledder, 2001) showed that there were fewer than 1.5 community team professionals for every 4000–5000 neurologically disabled people. A total of 35 community teams were identified serving over 14 million population but many teams were more generic and focussed on people with physical disability rather than specifically on TBI. These teams had seen less than 3% of the disabled TBI survivors in their geographical area.

Individuals with TBI can have a complex range of problems requiring input from a variety of different services. An individual can, for example, continue to need input from physiotherapy, occupational therapy, speech and language therapy, clinical neuropsychology and medical disciplines. In addition to such health professionals, they may often need support and advice from other professionals such as social workers, vocational counsellors and lawyers. There is a clear need for proper cooperation and coordination between such professionals. Case management is a system that has gradually been introduced in recent years in order to provide a system for such coordination. Although the role of the case manager varies widely the basic task is not only to coordinate the input of services but also to help the individual identify unmet needs and try to provide for such needs through the maze of statutory and voluntary services. The model has been extensively developed in the USA for head injured people. In some cases the case management role can develop into an advocacy role on behalf of the individual. Some case managers may even hold a budget for the individual and buy-in relevant services on their behalf. There are a number of training courses and professional qualifications for brain injury case managers. There are now a few published studies evaluating the effectiveness of case management after TBI. One study from London, UK, compared individuals randomised prospectively to case management and followed for 2 years (Greenwood et al., 1994). Although contact with rehabilitation was increased in the case management group there was no functional or vocational benefit or reduction in carer distress, compared to controls. Although there have been a few other studies the conclusions are still rather unclear. At a simple and non-scientific level it seems eminently sensible for a complex array of services to be properly coordinated by a case management but it is so far unproven whether such coordination actually translates into functional benefit for the individual. Further studies are awaited. However, lack of evidence should not be taken as lack of efficacy or as an excuse not to supply longer-term community rehabilitation services in a consistent and coordinated fashion.

Many individuals who suffer a TBI are young adults and many will want to find gainful employment. Regrettably the unemployment rate is very high after TBI. Unemployment can clearly have further negative effects on self-esteem, community status, financial standing and relationships within the family, and amongst friends. Many studies confirm the poor rate of return to work after severe head injury. In the seminal study by Brooks et al. (1987a) employment rate fell from 86% pre-injury to 29% post-injury in 98 severely head injury people. They found, not surprisingly, the persisting behavioural, personality and cognitive problems had a significant negative effect on employment. Return to work was less affected by physical disability. Younger people and those with higher prior educational status or who had already been in employment at the time of the injury stood a greater chance of returning to work.

There is evidence that appropriate advice and active vocational rehabilitation can have a positive effect on return to work rates. Some of the most successful schemes have been published in the USA by Wehman et al. (1990). These schemes involve the use of "job coaches" and in the context of "supported employment programmes".

Individuals after brain injury also find difficulty in sustaining a job. Studies have shown that in those who return to work only about 30–50% retain their jobs and most lose their jobs within the first 6 months. Wehman et al. (1990) suggested that stability at work could be achieved if the client could maintain a job for around 20 weeks and after 40 weeks little further active intervention is required.

Consideration for work potential and return to work should be an integral part of the rehabilitation programme.

33.6 Specific rehabilitation

Many of the other chapters in this book will discuss rehabilitation of specific difficulties that may arise after TBI. It is not the purpose of this chapter to discuss in any detail all the different symptoms that can arise after such injuries. However, it is appropriate to discuss some of the more important topics that can specifically follow TBI so that problems that may arise can be seen in an overall context. This section will discuss problems under the following four headings:

1 physical,
2 cognitive and intellectual,
3 behavioural,
4 emotional and personality problems.

Physical

In the early few weeks after injuries physical therapies will normally be directed towards the prevention of complications. In particular, muscle contractures should be avoided by the use of passive stretching, perhaps combined with splinting, casting and botulinum toxin therapy. Physiotherapy input is essential in these early stages to ensure proper positioning in bed or chair and prescription of proper seating systems. The latter will also help to reduce the risk of pressure sores, which are still unfortunately too common in acute wards. Maintaining adequate nutritional input can also be a problem in the short term. Incidence varies but in a large recent study the overall incidence of dysphagia was reported as 5.3% (at least in the paediatric head injury population) with an incidence of 68% for severe TBI, 15% for moderate TBI and only 1% for mild brain injury (Morgan et al., 2003). If oral intake is not desirable because of confusion and risk of inhalation then nasogastric feeding is a short-term possibility. However, if such feeding is needed for more than a few days then there are risks of nasal or pharyngeal ulceration. Confused and cognitively impaired people frequently remove their nasogastric tubes and re-intubation can be upsetting, cause trauma and is costly in terms of nursing time. The tube can become blocked or displaced and overall nasogastric feeding is to be avoided, except to overcome short-term nutritional requirements (Park et al., 1992; Norton et al., 1996). The enteral feeding route of choice is percutaneous endoscopic gastrostomy (PEG). This procedure is better tolerated, there is less risk of blocking or dislodging of tubes and overall PEG tubes seem more acceptable to patients in terms of being more comfortable, less obtrusive and much less likely to interfere with rehabilitation treatments. The tubes can be positioned under radiological guidance or endoscopic guidance or by direct surgical gastrostomy. However, the latter has the highest complication rate. Radiological placement is probably associated with a higher rate of successful tube placements and a lower rate of complications (Wallman et al., 1995). Dietetical advice is necessary to ensure a balanced calorific intake, particularly in the post-acute phase when nutritional requirements can be significantly increased.

Urinary incontinence is commonly present in the post-acute phase after severe TBI (Chua et al., 2003). Although pads can be worn it is essential to keep the skin dry to prevent pressure sores. Catheterisation is acceptable in the short term before a more thorough assessment of bladder function can take place.

Attention needs to be paid to a number of other potential physical problems in the post-acute phase. Deep venous thrombosis (DVT) is a risk during immobilisation. Appropriate preventative measures need to be taken (Bower et al., 1991). Heterotopic ossification (HO) is a possibility after TBI although it is more common after traumatic spinal cord injury. The incidence of HO after head injury is probably around 10–20% of those with severe injuries and up to 80% in people who are unconscious for more than a month (Sazbon et al., 1981). The onset is usually 1–4 months after injury although it can occur later. Early clinical signs include decreased range of movement, acute leg swelling, fever and pain. In unconscious or cognitively impaired people biochemical markers need to be monitored, particularly including persistent elevation of bony alkaline phosphatase (Kim et al., 1990). Treatment is controversial but, in addition to simple range of motion exercises, many centres would now use intravenous Etidronate and consider surgical resection (Banovak and Gonzales, 1997; McAuliffe and Wolfson, 1997).

Post-traumatic epilepsy is obviously a risk after TBI. There are well published tables giving percentages of risk according to severity of injury, presence of depressed skull fracture, presence or absence of epilepsy in the first week after injury or the presence of intracranial haemorrhage requiring surgery. Other risks include PTA greater than 24 h (Jennett, 1975; Annagers et al., 1998). Many centres would initiate prophylactic anticonvulsants, particularly in the high-risk categories.

Cognitive and intellectual

The challenge of the rehabilitation of TBI is to cope not only with the physical consequences but also with the cognitive and intellectual, behavioural and emotional consequences. There are a wide range of cognitive and intellectual impairments that can follow brain injury. Memory function is often the most profoundly affected and has the most significant impact on daily function. Other difficulties include problem solving, attention, perception, neglect, multitasking, new learning and language functions. The assessment and remediation of these difficulties are outlined in other chapters of this book. This chapter simply needs to state that a neuropsychologist is vital part of any brain injury rehabilitation team. It would normally be the neuropsychologist who makes the assessment of the complex range of neuropsychological deficits and should be the main source of advice to other team members regarding appropriate remediation of these problems. There is now evidence, mainly from single case design methodologies, that demonstrate improvement in function, particularly memory and attention, following various rehabilitation strategies (Wilson and Evans, 1996; Robertson et al., 1998). Strategies should clearly not only be directed towards improvement of impairment but also towards the maximisation of intact functions. The development of such strategies need not be complex. The use of a simple "bleeper" to remind individuals of particular tasks is an example of a simple idea with useful functional application (Wilson et al., 1999). The educational involvement of family and carers is also vital in the application of a cognitive rehabilitation strategy. Particularly in the latter stages of rehabilitation, it is often the family and carers that need to help with the many hours of prompting, guidance and supervision of the brain injured person.

Behavioural

Behavioural problems, particularly physical and verbal aggression, can be significant barriers to rehabilitation. Many rehabilitation units in the UK will not admit individuals with moderate or severe behavioural disturbance to a post-acute rehabilitation facility. Whilst this is understandable, given the disruption that such individuals can cause, the paucity of neurobehavioural rehabilitation facilities means that many individuals simply do not receive adequate, or any, rehabilitation. Agitation, confusion and restlessness in the recovery phases after acute brain injury are remarkably common but fortunately such phases are often short and the behaviour reasonably easily contained. A recent Cochrane review demonstrated that the most effective drug for the management of agitation and aggression is a beta-blocker whereas the evidence, surprisingly, for carbamazepine and valpropate was lacking. In such circumstances brief pharmacological management may be necessary although, in general terms, should be avoided (Fleminger et al., 2003). It is only a small minority of people that go on to develop longer term, severe behavioural problems (Greenwood and McMillan, 1993). However, there is now considerable literature demonstrating that a number of different cognitive and behavioural management techniques can be effective in improving difficult behaviour, which in turn can have a positive effect on independent living and reduce dependence on carers. The classic work of Eames and Wood (1985) has been followed by a number of other studies showing the effectiveness of various behavioural techniques (e.g. Alderman and Knight, 1997; Wood and McMillan, 2001). Appropriate behavioural management programmes have been shown to assist people, not only in the post-acute phase, but even some years after injury – both in a residential setting and in a community setting. Although it is generally accepted that severe behavioural disturbance needs a specialist, and often residential, unit there are studies that show that a behavioural modification approach can be introduced successfully into a non-specialised setting (McMillan et al., 1990; Watson et al., 2001). Appropriate resourcing for long-term treatment programmes can be a problem and many such programmes, at least in the UK, are now only funded through legal settlements.

Emotional and personality problems

Many relatives state that the head injured person has undergone a "personality change". This is an unsatisfactory term and it is better to delineate more exactly the parameters of personality that appear to have changed. Some, such as increased forgetfulness or problems with short temper, may be amenable to rehabilitation. Others may not be treatable but assessment and explanation of the problems may assist understanding. There are many changes that may occur following brain injury, including problems with:

- memory,
- judgement,
- planning,
- drive,
- initiation,
- egocentricity,
- lack of emotion,
- irritability,
- aggressiveness,
- increased or decreased sexual interest,
- lack of social restraint, etc.

These changes may lead to significant marital and relationship problems, as well as difficulties with community reintegration and return to work. Indeed the more obvious physical problems, such as wheelchair dependency, dysarthria or visual problems, are often coped with by family members more readily than the more subtle "personality" changes. There is ample evidence of the impact of such problems (Brooks et al., 1987b; Dickmen et al., 2003). The situation is often compounded by a lack of awareness of such difficulties in the head injured person. This makes any rehabilitation or coping strategy difficult to plan and execute (Flashman and MacAllister, 2002). Individuals who are aware and retain some insight into their problems are at risk of depression. Depression, and occasionally suicide, is not uncommon following TBI (Klonoff and Lage, 1995; Seel and Kreutzer, 2003). Cognitive and behavioural approaches for the treatment of depression may be difficult in those with cognitive dysfunction and pharmacological management may be needed. Occasionally other psychiatric problems can arise after TBI such as paranoid psychosis, mania, neuroticisms or obsessive–compulsive disorders (Hibbard et al., 1998). Emotionalism can also occur, although more common after stroke, and usually responds to small doses of antidepressants (Brown et al., 1999).

The foregoing sections have not attempted to be a definitive review of all the difficulties that can arise after TBI. Hopefully, the sections have covered the major problems and many, but not yet all, of these difficulties are potentially amenable to appropriate rehabilitation. Whilst there are undoubtedly gaps in the evidence base for the different approaches such gaps are being steadily reduced. Greater collaboration between basic neuroscience and clinical neurorehabilitation should lead to a greater understanding of recovery and coping mechanisms so that TBI rehabilitation can be placed on a firmer footing.

33.7 Mild head injury

Most of this chapter has been devoted to the consequences of severe head injury. The majority of head injuries are, of course, at the milder end of the spectrum. The great majority of people who suffer a mild head injury make a full recovery within a few weeks. Most will not be admitted to hospital and, assuming there is no impairment of consciousness or other neurological damage, discharged direct from casualty. Many will be given a head injury card warning them of the necessity of returning to hospital should there be any later problem, such as confusion or drowsiness or other neurological difficulty. Some countries have now produced clear and evidence-based guidance for the management of mild head injuries and appropriate discharge advice (National Institute for Clinical Excellence, 2003). Whilst it is undoubtedly true that the majority of symptoms after mild head injury clear up after about a month a significant minority are troubled by longer-term symptoms. The proportion varies considerably in the literature, but at least some symptoms persisting at a year seems to occur in about 25% of individuals (Alexander, 1995). The common symptoms tend to be labelled together as the post-concussional syndrome. The labelling is unfortunate as it gives the impression of a coherent entity whereas the syndrome encompasses a wide range of difficulties in different domains, including cognitive, affective and physical problems. The commonest difficulties are: memory disturbance, problems with attention and concentration, irritability, insomnia, anxiety, headaches, fatigability and dizziness. In some people the symptoms are no more than a nuisance whilst in others they have a considerable disruptive effect on home life, work and leisure.

There are now clearly documented studies confirming axonal injury in mild TBI from neurophysiological, neuroradiological and neuropsychological perspectives (Levin et al., 1992). However, it seems likely that whilst persisting problems do have an organic cause there is also a relationship with psychological factors and/or personality type (McMillan and Glucksman, 1987; Newcombe et al., 1994; Karzmark et al., 1995).

It is a major logistic problem to screen individuals after mild head injury. Most countries have no such follow-up procedure and this probably means that a number of people with troublesome symptoms go unsupported. In New Zealand (Wrightson, 1989) one unit asks people with mild brain injury to attend an outpatient clinic a few weeks after the injury. This enables those with continuing symptoms to be seen and further assessment and advice given. The New Zealand team consists of a full-time psychologist, a physician, a psychiatrist and there is access to the occupational therapy department, medical social worker and the Accident Compensation Corporation. The clinic is also supported by the local head injury society. This model has also been recommended by the Medical Disability Society in the UK (Medical Disability Society, 1988). Wade et al. (1997) recently published a study randomly allocating 1156 people attending hospital after head injury of all severity to early follow-up (7–10 days) or to no follow-up. No differences were found in either group in terms of symptom frequency or severity at 6 months. However, further analysis suggested benefit in those with PTA greater than 1 h. A later, and similarly designed, study also showed benefit from contact in the head injury clinic for those with a PTA less than 7 days (Wade et al., 1998). Other studies have tended to confirm this benefit (McMillan, 1997).

33.8 Conclusion

TBI is common. Fortunately most people suffer a minor injury with a good and rapid recovery. However, a significant minority of people, even those with mild injuries, have significant long-term problems. Obviously the problems are worse in more severe injuries. Such people can exhibit a complex range of physical, cognitive, behavioural and emotional problems which pose a significant challenge to the rehabilitation team. However, there is now emerging evidence that provision of interdisciplinary rehabilitation can make a significant difference in terms of functional outcome. The management of many symptoms is now evidence based. Continued developments in neuroscience should steadily lead to a greater understanding of the mechanisms of neural recovery and neural plasticity which hopefully will lead to a firmer basis for the management of people following TBI.

REFERENCES

Acorn, S. (1993). An education/support programme for families of survivors of head injury. *Can J Rehabil*, **7**, 149–151.

Alderman, M. and Knight, A. (1997). The effectiveness of DRL in the management and treatment of severe behaviour disorders following brain injury. *Brain Injury*, **11**, 79–101.

Alexander, M.P. (1995). Mild traumatic brain injury: pathophysiology, natural history and clinical management. *Neurology*, **45**, 1253–1260.

Allen, K., Linn, R., Gutierrez, H. and Willer, B. (1994). Family burden following traumatic brain injury. *Rehabil Psychol*, **39**, 29–48.

Anderson, C., Ni Mhurchu, C., Brown, P.M. and Carter, K. (2002). Stroke rehabilitation services to accelerate hospital discharge and provide home based care: an overview and cost analysis. *Pharmaco Econom*, **20**, 537–552.

Annagers, J.F., Hauser, W.A., Coan, C.P. and Rocca, W.A. (1998). A population based study of seizures after traumatic brain injury. *New Engl J Med*, **378**, 20–24.

Banovak, K. and Gonzales, F. (1997). Evaluation and management of heterotopic ossification in patients with spinal cord injury. *Spinal Cord*, **35**, 158–162.

Boake, C. (1990). Transitional living centres and head injury rehabilitation. In: *Community Integration Following Traumatic Brain Injury* (eds Kreutzer, J.S. and Wehman, P.), Edward Arnold, Sevenoaks, pp. 115–124.

Bower, A., Voth, E., Henze, T. and Pringe, H.W. (1991). Early heparin therapy in patients with spontaneous intracerebral haemorrhage. *J Neurol Neurosurg Psychiatr*, **54**, 466–467.

Brooks, D.N., Campsie, L., Symmington, C., et al. (1987a). The effects of severe head injury on patients and relatives within seven years of injury. *J Head Trauma Rehabil*, **2**, 1–13.

Brooks, D.N., McKinlay, W.W., Symmington, C., et al. (1987b). Return to work within the first seven years of severe head injury. *Brain Injury*, **1**, 5–19.

Brown, K.W., Sloan, R. and Pentland, B. (1999). Fluoxetine as a treatment for post-stroke emotionalism. *Acta Psychiatr Scand*, **98**, 455–458.

Chua, K., Chuo, A. and Cong, K.H. (2003). Urinary incontinence after traumatic brain injury: incidence, outcomes and correlates. *Brain Injury*, **17**, 469–478.

Cifu, D., Kreutzer, J.S. and Marwitz, J.H. (1996). Functional outcomes of older adults with traumatic brain injury: a prospective multi-centre analysis. *Arch Phys Med Rehabil*, **77**, 883–888.

Cifu, D.X., Kreutzer, J.S., Kolakowsky-Hayner, S.A., et al. (2003). The relationship between therapy intensity and rehabilitative outcomes after traumatic brain injury: a multicenter analysis. *Arch Phys Med Rehabil*, **84**, 1441–1448.

Cope, D.N. and Hall, K.M. (1982). Head injury rehabilitation: benefits of early intervention. *Arch Phys Med Rehabil*, **63**, 433–437.

Cope, D.N., Cole, J.R., Hall, K.M. and Barkan, H. (1991a). Brain injury: analysis of outcome in a post-acute rehabilitation system. Part 1. General analysis. *Brain Injury*, **5**, 111–125.

Cope, D.N., Cole, J.R., Hall, K.M. and Barkan, H. (1991b). Brain injury: analysis of outcome in a post-acute rehabilitation system. Part 2. Sub-analysis. *Brain Injury*, **5**, 127–139.

Cowen, T.D., Meythaler, J.M., De vico, M.J., et al. (1995). Influence of early variables in traumatic brain injury on functional independence measure scores in rehabilitation, length of stay and charges. *Arch Phys Med Rehabil*, **76**, 797–803.

Dickmen, S.S., Machamer, J.E., Powell, J.M. and Temkin, N.R. (2003). Outcome 3–5 years after moderate to severe traumatic brain injury. *Arch Phys Med Rehabil*, **84**, 1449–1457.

Eames, P. and Wood, R. (1985). Rehabilitation after severe brain injury: a follow-up study of a behaviour modification approach. *J Neurol Neurosurg Psychiatr*, **48**, 616–619.

European Brain Injury Consortium (1997). Guidelines for the management of severe head injury in adults. *Acta Neurochir*, **139**, 286–294.

Flashman, L.A. and MacAllister, T.W. (2002). Lack of awareness and its impact in traumatic brain injury. *Neurorehabilitation*, **17**, 285–296.

Fleminger, S., Greenwood, R.J. and Oliver, D.L. (2003). Pharmaological management for agitation and aggression in people with acquired brain injury. *Cochrane Database Syst Rev*, **1**, CD003299.

Garnett, M.R., Cadoux-Hudson, T.A. and Styles, P. (2001). How useful is magnetic resonance imaging in predicting severity and outcome in traumatic brain injury? *Curr Opin Neurol*, **14**, 753–757.

Goranson, T.E., Graves, R.E., Allison, D. and Lafreniere, R. (2003). Community integration following multidisciplinary rehabilitation for traumatic brain injury. *Brain Injury*, **17**, 759–774.

Greenwood, R.J. and McMillan, T.M. (1993). Models of rehabilitation programmes for the brain injured adult. 1. Current service provision. *Clin Rehabil*, **7**, 248–255.

Greenwood, R.J., McMillan, T.M., Brooks, D.N., et al. (1994). The effects of case management after severe head injury. *Br Med J*, **308**, 1199–1205.

Guide for the Uniformed Data System for Medical Rehabilitation (Adult FIM) (1993). Version 4.0. State University of New York and Buffalo, Buffalo, NY.

Hall, K., Mann, N., High, W., et al. (1996). Functional measures after traumatic brain injury: ceiling effects of the FIM, FIM+ FAM, DRS and CIQ. *J Head Trauma Rehabil*, **11**, 27–39.

Hibbard, M.R., Uysal, S., Kepler, K., et al. (1998). Axis one psychopathology in individuals with traumatic brain injury. *J Head Trauma Rehabil*, **13**, 24–39.

High Jr., W.M., Hall, K.M., Rosenthal, M., et al. (1996). Factors affecting hospital length of stay and charges following traumatic brain injury of adults living in the community. *Brain Injury*, **9**, 339–353.

Jackson, A.F. and Davies, M. (1995). A transdiciplinary approach to brain injury rehabilitation. *Br J Ther Rehabil*, **2**, 65–70.

Jennett, B. (1975). *Epilepsy after Non-Missile Head Injuries*, 2nd edn., Heinemann, London.

Jennett, B. and Bond, M. (1975). Assessment of outcome after severe brain damage: a practical scale. *Lancet*, **1**, 480–484.

Johnston, M.V. (1991). Outcomes of community re-entry programme for brain injury survivors. Part II. Further investigations. *Brain Injury*, **5**, 155–168.

Johnston, M.V. and Lewis, F.D. (1991). Outcomes of community re-entry programmes for brain injury survivors. Part 1. Independent living and productive activities. *Brain Injury*, **5**, 141–154.

Karzmark, T., Hall, K. and Englander, J. (1995). Late onset post-concussional symptoms after mild brain injury: the role of pre-morbid, injury related, environmental and personality factors. *Brain Injury*, **59**, 21–26.

Kim, S.W., Charter, R.A., Chia, C.J., et al. (1990). Serum alkaline phosphatase and inorganic phosphorous values in spinal cord injured patients with heterotopic ossification. *Paraplegia*, **28**, 441–447.

Klonoff, P.S. and Lage, G.A. (1995). Suicide in patients with chronic brain injury: risk and prevention. *J Head Trauma Rehabil*, **10**, 16–24.

Levin, H.S., Williams, D.H. and Eisenberg, H.M. (1992). Serial MRI and neurobehavioural findings after mild to moderate closed head injury. *J Neurol Neurosurg Psychiatr*, **55**, 255–262.

Mahoney, F.I. and Barthel, D.W. (1965). Functional assessment. The Barthel index. *Maryland Med J*, **14**, 61–65.

Mandy, B. (1996). Interdisciplinary rather than multidisciplinary or generic practice. *Br J Ther Rehabil*, **3**, 110–112.

McAuliffe, J.A. and Wolfson, A.H. (1997). Early excision of heterotopic ossification above the elbow followed by radiation therapy. *J Bone Joint Surg (America)*, **79**, 749–755.

McLellan, D.L., Barnes, M.P., Eames, P., Iannotti, F., et al. (1998). *Rehabilitation After Traumatic Brain Injury*, British Society of Rehabilitation Medicine, London.

McMillan, T.M. (1997). Minor head injury. *Curr Opin Neurol*, **10**, 479–483.

McMillan, T.M. and Glucksman, E.E. (1987). The neuropsychology of moderate head injury. *J Neurol Neurosurg Psychiatr*, **5**, 393–397.

McMillan, T.M. and Ledder, H.A. (2001). Survey of services provided by community neurorehabilitation teams in South East England. *Clin Rehabil*, **15**, 582–588.

McMillan, T.M., Papadopoulos, H., Cornall, C. and Greenwood, R.J. (1990). Modification of severe behavioural problems following herpes simplex encephalitis. *Brain Injury*, **4**, 399–406.

McMillan, T.M., Jongen, E.L.M.M. and Greenwood, R.J. (1996). Assessment of post-traumatic amnesia after severe closed head injury: retrospective or prospective. *J Neurol Neurosurg Psychiatr*, **60**, 422–427.

Medical Disability Society (1988). *The Management of Traumatic Brain Injury*, The Development Trust of the Young Disabled, London.

Morgan, A., Ward, E., Murdoch, B., et al. (2003). Incidence, characteristics and predictive factors for dysphagia after paediatric traumatic brain injury. *J Head Trauma Rehabil*, **18**, 239–251.

Moscato, B., Trevisan, M. and Willer, B. (1994). The prevalence of traumatic brain injury in co-occurring disabilities in national household survey of adults. *J Neuropsych Clin Neurosci*, **6**, 134–142.

Munro, J., Coleman, P., Nicholl, J., et al. (1995). Can we prevent accident and injury to adolescents? A systematic review of evidence. *Inj Prev*, **1**, 249–255.

National Institute for Clinical Excellence (2003). *Head Injury: Triage, Assessment, Investigation and Early Management of Head Injury in Infants, Children and Adults*, National Institute for Clinical Excellence, London, Guideline 4.

Newcombe, F., Rabbitt, P. and Briggs, M. (1994). Minor head injury: pathophysiological or iatrogenic sequelae. *J Neurol Neurosurg Psychiatr*, **57**, 709–716.

NIH Consensus Development Statement (1998). Rehabilitation of persons with traumatic brain injury. October 26–28; Vol. **16(1)**, 1–41 [online].

Norton, B., Homer-Ward, M., Donnelly, M.T., et al. (1996). A randomised prospective comparison of percutaneous endoscopic gastrostomy and nasogastric tube feeding after acute dysphagic stroke. *Br Med J*, **312**, 13–16.

Park, R.H.R., Allison, M.C., Lang, J., et al. (1992). Randomised comparison of percutaneous endoscopic gastrostomy and nasogastric tube feeding in patients with persistent neurological dysphagia. *Br Med J*, **304**, 1406–1409.

Pazzaglia, P., Frank, G., Frank, F. and Gaist, G. (1975). Clinical course and prognosis of acute post-traumatic coma. *J Neurol Neurosurg Psychiatr*, **38**, 149–154.

Powell, J., Heslin, J. and Greenwood, R. (2002). Community based rehabilitation after severe traumatic brain injury: a randomised controlled trial. *J Neurol Neurosurg Psychiatr*, **72**, 193–202.

Robertson, I.H., Hogg, K. and McMillan, T.M. (1998). Rehabilitation of unilateral neglect: improving function by contralesional limb activation. *Neuropsych Rehabil*, **8**, 19–29.

Rodgers, H., Soutter, J., Kaiser, W., et al. (1997). Early supported hospital discharge following acute stroke: pilot study results. *Clin Rehabil*, **11**, 280–287.

Royal College of Physicians and British Society of Rehabilitation Medicine (2003). *Rehabilitation Following Acquired Brain Injury: National Clinical Guidelines* (ed. Turner-Stokes, L.), RCP and BSRM, London.

Royal College of Surgeons of England (1999). *Report of the Working Party on the Management of Patients with Head Injuries*. Royal College of Surgeons of England, London.

Rusk, H.A., Loman, E.W. and Block, J.M. (1966). Rehabilitation of the patient with head injury. *Clin Neurosurg*, **12**, 312–323.

Sazbon, L., Najenson, T., Tartakovsky, M., et al. (1981). Widespread periarticular new bone formation in long term comatosed patients. *J Bone Joint Surg (America)*, **63**, 120–125.

Seel, R.T. and Kreutzer, J.S. (2003). Depression assessment after traumatic brain injury: an empirically based classification method. *Arch Phys Med Rehabil*, **84**, 1621–1628.

Semlyen, J.K., Hurrell, E., Carter, S. and Barnes, M.P. (1996). The Newcastle Independence Assessment Form (Research): development of an alternative functional measure. *J Neurol Rehabil*, **10**, 251–257.

Semlyen, J.K., Summers, S.J. and Barnes, M.P. (1997). The predictive value of the Newcastle Independence Assessment Form – Research (NIAF-R): further development of an alternative functional measure. *J Neurol Rehabil*, **11**, 213–218.

Semlyen, J.K., Summers, S.J. and Barnes, M.P. (1998). Traumatic brain injury: efficacy of multidisciplinary rehabilitation. *Arch Phys Med Rehabil*, **79**, 678–683.

Shiel, A., Burn, J.P., Henry, D., et al. (2001). The effects of increased rehabilitation therapy after brain injury: results of a prospective controlled trial. *Clin Rehabil*, **15**, 501–514.

Signorini, D.F., Andrews, P.J.D., Jones, P.A., et al. (1999). Predicting survival using simple clinical variables: a case study in traumatic brain injury. *J Neurol Neurosurg Psychiatr*, **66**, 20–25.

Slade, A., Tennant, A. and Chamberlain, M.A. (2002). A randomised controlled trial to determine the effect of intensity of therapy upon length of stay in a neurological rehabilitation setting. *J Rehabil Med*, **34**, 260–266.

Society of British Neurological Surgeons (1998). Guidelines for the initial management of head injuries: recommendations from the Society of British Neurological Surgeons. *Br J Neurosurg*, **14**, 349–352.

Spivack, G., Spettell, C.M., Ellis, D.W. and Ross, S.E. (1992). Effects of intensity of treatment and length of stay on rehabilitation outcomes. *Brain Injury*, **6**, 419–434.

Susman, M., Dirusso, S.M., Sullivan, T., et al. (2002). Traumatic brain injury in the elderly: increased mortality and worse functional outcome at discharge despite lower injury severity. *J Trauma*, **53**, 219–223.

Teasdale, G. and Jennett, B. (1974). Assessment of coma and impaired consciousness. A practical scale. *Lancet*, **2**, 81–83.

Teasdale, G., Knill-Jones, R. and van der Sande, J. (1978). Observer variability in assessing impaired consciousness and coma. *J Neurol Neursurg Psychiatr*, **41**, 603–610.

Teasdale, G., Murray, G., Parker, L. and Jennett, B. (1979). Adding up the Glasgow Coma Scale. *Acta Neurochir*, **27**, 13–16.

Toschlog, E.A., Macelligot, J., Sagraves, S.G., et al. (2003). The relationship of Injury Severity Score and Glasgow Coma Score to rehabilitative potential in patients suffering from traumatic brain injury. *Am Surgeon*, **69**, 491–497.

Turner-Stokes, L. (2002). Standardised outcome assessment in brain injury rehabilitation for young adults. *Disabil Rehabil*, **24**, 383–389.

Vanzomeren, A.H. and Vandenburg, W. (1985). Residual complaints of patients two years after severe head injury. *J Neurol Neurosurg Psychiatr*, **48**, 21–28.

Wade, D., Crawford, S., Wenden, S.J., et al. (1997). Does routine follow-up after head injury help? A randomised controlled trial. *J Neurol Neurosurg Psychiatr*, **62**, 478–484.

Wade, D.T., King, N.S., Wenden, S.J., et al. (1998). Routine follow-up after head injury: a second randomised controlled trial. *J Neurol Neurosurg Psychiatr*, **65**, 177–183.

Wallman, B., D'Agostino, H.B., Walus-Wigle, J.R., et al. (1995). Radiological, endoscopic and surgical gastrostomy: an institutional evaluation and meta-analysis of the literature. *Radiology*, **197**, 699–704.

Watson, C., Rutterford, N.A., Shortland, D., et al. (2001). Reduction of chronic aggressive behaviour 10 years after brain injury. *Brain Injury*, **15**, 1003–1015.

Wehman, P.H., Kreutzer, J.S. and West, M.D. (1990). Return to work for persons with TBI: a supported employment approach. *Arch Phys Med Rehabil*, **71**, 1047–1052.

Whiteneck, G.G., Charlifue, S.W., Gerhart, K.A., et al. (1992). Quantifying handicap: a new measure of long term rehabilitation outcome. *Arch Phys Med Rehabil*, **73**, 519–526.

Willer, B., Offenbacher, K.J. and Coad, M.L. (1994). The community integration questionnaire. A comparative examination. *Am J Phys Med Rehabil*, **73**, 103–111.

Wilson, B.A. and Evans, J.J. (1996). Error free learning in the rehabilitation of individuals with memory impairments. *J Head Trauma Rehabil*, **11**, 54–64.

Wilson, B.A., Evans, J.J., Emslie, H. and Maliaek, V. (1999). Evaluation of NeuroPage: a new memory aid. *J Neurol Neurosurg Psychiatr*, **63**, 113–115.

Wood, R. and McMillan, T.M. (2001). *Neurobehavioural Disability and Social Handicap Following Traumatic Brain Injury*, Psychology Press, Sussex.

Wrightson, P. (1989). Management of disability and rehabilitation services after mild head injury. In: *Mild Head Injury* (eds Levin, H.S., Eisenberg, H.M. and Benton, A.L.), Oxford University Press, New York, pp. 245–256.

Zhu, X.L., Poon, W.S., Chan, C.H. and Chan, S.H. (2001). Does intensive rehabilitation improve the functional outcome of patients with traumatic brain injury? Interim results of a randomised controlled trial. *Br J Neurosurg*, **15**, 464–473.

34

Neurorehabilitation in epilepsy

Andres M. Kanner[1] and Antoaneta Balabanov[2]

[1]Professor of Neurological Sciences, Rush Medical College; Director, Laboratory of Electroencephalography and Video-EEG-Telemetry; Associate Director, Section of Epilepsy and Clinical Neurophysiology and Rush Epilepsy Center and [2]Assistant Professor of Neurological Sciences, Rush Medical College; Associate Attending in Neurological Sciences, Rush University Medical Center, Chicago, IL, USA

34.1 Introduction: is rehabilitation necessary in epilepsy?

We usually do not associate rehabilitation with patients with epilepsy (PWE). Epileptic seizures consist of recurrent episodes during which there is a transient loss of awareness of their surroundings, a display of purposeless behavior or a generalized convulsion; unless the seizure activity evolves into status epilepticus, patients usually recover after a few minutes, though occasionally it may take several hours before their motor, sensory and cognitive functions return to baseline. Yet epilepsy includes cognitive and psychiatric disturbances *in addition to* epileptic seizures. Furthermore, frequent psychosocial obstacles in the form of stigma, discrimination, and plain misinformation about this disease add to the difficulties PWE have to face and in some patients the cognitive and psychiatric disturbances may constitute the principal cause of impairment. For example, a child with an acquired epileptic aphasia of childhood (or Landau–Kleffner syndrome) may have rare clinical seizures that usually respond well to antiepileptic drugs (AED). However, the principal expression of this seizure disorder is a global aphasia and severe behavioral disturbances consisting of motor hyperactivity, impulsive and aggressive behavior (Morrell et al., 1995).

In this article, we review the causes that limit PWE from reaching their full potential academically, professionally and socially, and the potential role of rehabilitation in overcoming these obstacles. Finally, we offer suggestions on how the field of rehabilitation should be incorporated into the evaluation and management of every PWE.

34.2 The impact of epilepsy on the lives of patients

Epilepsy can impose restrictions in the performance of professional activities as a consequence of: (i) the transient cognitive impairment (TCI), (ii) loss of motor control, (iii) loss of sensory input during the actual seizures and (iv) as a consequence of long-term persistent problems with attention, learning and memory processing, which often are subtle and undetected by patients and family until formal testing is performed. The unpredictable timing of seizure occurrence causes patients and their families to limit their social activities, which in turn fosters isolation and interferes with the establishment of long-lasting relations and employment. Endogenous, iatrogenic and reactive psychiatric disorders presenting as anxiety and depressive disorders further interfere with the development of self-confidence in achieving an adequate social adaptation.

In recent years, several health-related quality of life instruments have been developed in the USA and Europe to assess the impact of epilepsy on physical and mental health and social adaptation (Vickrey et al., 1992; Stavem et al., 2000). These studies have shown an improvement in health-related quality of life after successful medical and surgical treatment

(Vickrey et al., 1992). Most studies have used the quality of life in epilepsy (QOLIE) inventory (Vickrey et al., 1992; Meador, 1993). Seizure severity, co-morbid depression, and neurotoxicity consistently have been found to have a negative impact on the quality of life of PWE of different ages. Lower socioeconomic status, need for special education and frequent hospitalizations were also associated with poor quality of life (Devinsky et al., 1990).

While patients with refractory epilepsy tend to score worse on health-related quality of life instruments, even PWE whose seizures are well-controlled display a worse outcome than do age and IQ-matched non-epileptic controls. For example, a population-based Finnish prospective study of 245 children with epilepsy followed over 30 years, showed that they had a more than two-fold increase of early school abandonment and more than three-fold increase in unemployment, failure to marry and to have children (Sillanpaa et al., 1998). These outcomes were unrelated to neuropsychologic function and were not restricted to patients with poorly controlled seizures, but were also observed among adults whose seizures had remitted early in childhood and whose AEDs were discontinued early in the course of their illness. In a prospective, population-based study carried out in Nova Scotia, Camfield et al. (1993) assessed the social outcome after the age of 18 years in 337 children with partial epilepsy and *normal intelligence*. Social isolation was recorded in 16%, financial dependency in 30% and unemployment in 30% of these patients (Camfield and Camfield, 1997). These two studies demonstrate a greater vulnerability of PWE, even in the absence of cognitive impairment or when an optimal seizure control (i.e., seizure freedom and AED discontinued) is achieved. In another study from Finland, approximately 7% of respondents to a questionnaire reported significant dissatisfaction with their life that was associated with a lower income and poor economic status, independent of the degree of control of their epilepsy (Sillanpaa, 1987). In a study carried out in the USA, 65% of PWE considered themselves negatively affected by their disease, including patients with less than one

seizure per year (Schacter et al., 1993). Thus the social adjustment of PWE may not always parallel improvements in seizure control.

Epilepsy has a similar negative impact in children's life and half of children with epilepsy have behavior problems (Hoare and Kerley, 1991; Austin et al., 1992), suffer from social isolation and low-self esteem to a significantly greater degree than children with learning disabilities or other chronic medical disorders (Matthews et al., 1982; Margalit and Heiman, 1983; Austin et al., 1994).

34.3 Common obstacles to "optimal" personal and social development in PWE

The cognitive, psychiatric and psychosocial causes of impaired psychologic, professional and social achievements in PWE can be categorized as seizure related, treatment related or related to environmental/social factors.

Cognitive disturbances in epilepsy

Seizure-related variables

Seizure-related variables relate to the etiology of the seizure disorder, type of epileptic syndrome and seizure, seizure burden, inter-ictal epileptiform discharges and age at seizure onset. However, the relationship between cognitive disturbances and seizure occurrence is not supported by all studies. In a recent review of the literature, a positive relationship between seizure activity and progressive cognitive deterioration was found in 12 of 18 studies; five studies yielded mixed results and two found no association (Dodrill, 2004).

Etiology

Epilepsy caused by infectious encephalitis is more likely associated with severe impairment of more than one cognitive modality than epilepsy caused by a single neurocysticercosis lesion in the temporal lobe. By the same token, children with infantile spasms caused by tuberous sclerosis are at significantly greater risk of developing an autistic disorder than children with idiopathic infantile spasms (Bolton et al., 2002).

Epileptic syndrome

Patients with idiopathic (or primary) generalized epilepsies are more likely to have normal intelligence, whereas patients with partial seizure disorders are more likely to display a variety of cognitive disturbances, depending on the number and location of seizure foci. Thus, seizures of temporal lobe origin tend to be associated with memory problems; if the seizure focus is in the dominant hemisphere, patients are likely to experience word-finding difficulties, while those with bilateral antero-temporal ictal foci are more likely to suffer from episodic memory deficits involving both verbal and visual domains. Patients with frontal lobe epilepsy are likely to display problems with attention span and psychomotor speed.

Seizure burden and density

These relate to the duration of the seizure disorder, seizure frequency and the occurrence of status epilepticus. It is generally accepted that a history of frequent generalized tonic–clonic (GTC) seizures (>100 seizures in lifetime) and status epilepticus are associated with reduced performance on neuropsychologic testing (Dodrill and Wilensky, 1990). In addition, there is evidence of mental dulling, emotional and psychosocial problems, and an inferior general level of functioning in patients who have had a large number of GTC seizures over the course of many years (Dodrill, 2002). The extent to which status epilepticus is a predictor of poorer cognitive outcome in children remains controversial.

Age at onset of epilepsy

Age at onset of epilepsy appears to be a determinant of cognitive and behavioral impairment (O'Leary et al., 1983). Children with onset of seizures before age of 5 years performed significantly worse on IQ tests compared with children whose seizures began later, regardless of whether the seizures were partial or generalized (Aarts et al., 1984).

Inter-ictal epileptiform discharges

Cognitive impairments have been associated with inter-ictal, or subclinical, epileptiform discharges, though the impact on overall cognitive function is limited. Aarts et al. coined the term TCI to reflect this phenomenon (Aarts et al., 1984). Binnie and colleagues demonstrated TCI in 50% of 91 patients during generalized or focal discharges (Binnie, 1987). Right-sided discharges were associated with impairment in visual-spatial tasks, while errors in verbal tasks were demonstrated during left-sided discharges. Error rates increased if the stimulus was presented in the midst of the discharge. The degree of disruption was greater if the epileptiform discharge occurred within 2 s before the stimulus. Similarly, the type of deficit was related to side of discharge in 36% of 69 children (Kateleijn-Nolst Trenite et al., 1990). Because of the multiple variables associated with cognitive disturbances, the increased incidence of learning disabilities and behavioral problems in children with benign focal epilepsies may help establish causality between abundant inter-ictal discharges and cognitive disturbances.

Iatrogenic factors

At high doses, all AEDs can cause cognitive adverse events (CAE). However, some AEDs, cause CAE even at low doses. The degree of cognitive impairment plays a fundamental role in the detection of CAE. While cognitively intact patients are more likely to complain of CAE, certain AEDs can exacerbate the severity of an underlying cognitive disturbance (i.e., speech disturbance).

The cognitive effects of standard and new AED have been evaluated in several randomized, double blind, crossover studies in healthy volunteers (Meador et al., 1991; Meador et al., 1993; Meador et al., 1995). Carbamazepine (CBZ), phenytoin (PHT) and valproic acid (VPA) were associated with comparable CAE of mild severity. In a third of the tests, phenobarbital (PB) yielded more severe cognitive impairment than PHT and VPA. Even AEDs known for their positive psychotropic properties and lack of "reported" CAE, for example, gabapentin (GBP) and lamotrigine (LTG), caused more errors on neuropsychologic testing than non-drug conditions.

AEDs produce similar CAE in children as in adults. PB consistently produced more CAE than did CBZ, PHT and VPA. Despite the appearance of AED tolerance and the absence of detected clinical problems, a child may develop subtle, but significant, changes in intellectual function and behavior (Vining et al., 1987).

Among the newer AEDs, topiramate (TPM)-induced CAE have most concerned neurologists. These CAE include difficulty with word finding, slowing of thought processes and forgetfulness (Martin et al., 1990). Patients are often not aware of these effects, which are most often reported by family members.

Psychiatric disturbances in epilepsy

The prevalence of psychiatric disorders is significantly higher among PWE than the general population (Table 34.1).

Psychiatric disorders in PWE are most frequently inter-ictal (i.e., unrelated temporally to the occurrence of seizures). Isolated and clusters of psychiatric symptoms may also appear from several days to several hours before a seizure (pre-ictal), may be the expression of the seizure (ictal) or may occur within the first 120 h after a seizure (post-ictal).

Table 34.1. Prevalence-rates of psychiatric disorders in epilepsy and the general population.

Disorder	Epilepsy (%)	General population (%)
Depression	11–60	2–4
Anxiety	19–45	2.5–6.5
Psychosis	2–8	0.5–0.7
ADHD	14–35	2–10

Pre-ictal psychiatric symptoms

Dysphoric mood is the most frequently reported pre-ictal psychiatric symptom, appearing several hours to 2–3 days before the seizure. This increases progressively in severity before the seizure and often remits after the ictus (Blanchet and Frommer, 1986). At times, however, symptoms persist into the post-ictal period. In children, the dysphoria is often manifest as irritability, poor frustration tolerance, hyperactivity and aggressive behavior.

Ictal psychiatric symptoms

These symptoms are the clinical expression of a simple partial seizure in which psychiatric symptoms are the sole (or predominant) semiology. In a study of 2000 consecutive PWE, 100 reported ictal psychiatric symptoms. Ictal fear or panic was the most frequently reported symptom, followed by symptoms of depression and pleasurable symptoms (Williams, 1956). It may be difficult to recognize ictal psychiatric symptoms as epileptic phenomena but they are typically brief, stereotypical, occur out of context and are associated with other ictal phenomena. The most frequent symptoms of depression include feelings of anhedonia, guilt and suicidal ideation.

Psychosis can be the primary clinical expression of non-convulsive status epilepticus of simple partial, complex partial or even absence seizure disorders (Trimble, 1991). In the case of simple partial status, the diagnosis may be difficult, as scalp recordings may not detect the ictal pattern (Devinsky et al., 1988).

Post-ictal psychiatric symptoms

These symptoms have long been recognized but rarely studied. Their prevalence has yet to be established. In a recently completed study (Kanner et al., 2004), 100 consecutive patients with refractory partial epilepsy, experienced an average of nine different types of post-ictal symptoms (range: 0–25) within 72 h of the seizure, including three post-ictal cognitive symptoms (range: 0–6) and six post-ictal psychiatric symptoms (range 0–22). To be counted, a symptom had to be experienced after more than 50% of the seizures. Sixty-eight patients reported post-ictal cognitive and psychiatric symptoms, 14 experienced only cognitive and 6 only psychiatric symptoms; 12 reported no post-ictal symptoms. Anxiety and depression were the most frequent post-ictal symptoms (45 and 43 patients, respectively). The duration of post-ictal symptoms ranged from a few minutes to several days, with most symptoms of depression and anxiety having a median duration of 24 h. Thirteen percent reported post-ictal suicidal ideation with a median duration more than 24 h. Clearly, these psychiatric symptoms have an even greater negative impact on the quality of life than the actual seizure.

Post-ictal psychiatric phenomena can mimic a variety of psychiatric disorders, the most severe of which being psychoses. Post-ictal psychosis (PIP) accounts for approximately 25% of psychotic disorders in PWE (Onuma et al., 1995). The PIP reported in the literature have been identified almost exclusively in the course of video electroencephalographic (V-EEG) monitoring. Their prevalence has been estimated at 6% and 10% (Kanner et al., 1996).

Post-ictal psychotic episodes usually have the following characteristics (Logsdail and Toone, 1988; So et al., 1990; Savard et al., 1991; Devinsky et al., 1995; Kanner et al., 1996; Kanemoto et al., 1996):

1 a delay of up to 120 h between their onset and the last seizure;
2 a duration of only a few hours to several weeks;
3 an affect-laden symptomatology including delusions and features of depression or mania;
4 association with increased frequency of secondarily GTC seizures;
5 onset after having seizures for a mean period of more than 10 years;
6 prompt response to low-dose neuroleptic medication or benzodiazepines.

Inter-ictal psychiatric disorders

Depression, anxiety, psychotic and attention deficit disorders are more frequent among PWE than the general population (Costello, 1989; Anthony et al.,

1995; Kessler et al., 1995; Wiegartz et al., 1999; Table 34.1). Inter-ictal depression and anxiety are the most frequent psychiatric co-morbidities in PWE (Mendez et al., 1986; Kanner and Palac, 2000). Two psychiatric disorders have especially great impact on the life of PWE: (i) depression in adults and (ii) attention deficit disorders in children. In community and practice-based studies, the prevalence of depression in PWE ranged from 21–33% (Edeh and Toone, 1987; Jacoby et al., 1996; O'Donoghue et al., 1999), but only 6% of PWE in remission (O'Donoghue et al., 1999). A population-based survey investigated the lifetime prevalence of depression, epilepsy, diabetes, asthma and other chronic medical disorders in 185,000 households (Blum et al., 2002). Among the 2900 PWE, 29% reported having experienced at least one episode of depression. This contrasted with 8.6% prevalence among healthy respondents, 13% among diabetics and 16% among people with asthma.

The relationship between depression and epilepsy may be bi-directional (i.e., patients with depression have a higher risk of suffering from epilepsy). In a population-based, case-control Swedish study of adult patients with newly diagnosed epilepsy, a history of depression *preceding the onset of the seizure disorder* was six times more frequent among PWE than controls (Forsgren and Nystrom, 1990). In a second population-based, case-control study of new onset epilepsy at age 55 years and older, after controlling for the impact on seizures of medical therapies for depression, patients were 3.7 more likely than controls to have a prior history of depression (Hesdorffer et al., 2000). Six centuries ago, Hippocrates had suggested this bi-directional relationship when he wrote: *"melancholics ordinarily become epileptics, and epileptics melancholics: what determines the preference is the direction the malady takes; if it bears upon the body, epilepsy, if upon the intelligence, melancholy"* (Lewis, 1934).

Impact of depression in the quality of life of PWE

The presence of depression is associated with a poor quality of life, independent of the seizure frequency and severity. Among several neuropsychologic variables, mood had the highest correlations with scales of the QOLIE inventory-89 and was the strongest predictor of poor quality of life in regression analyses (Perrine et al., 1995; Lehrner et al., 1999). Mood was the strongest clinical predictor of patients' assessment of their own health status in 125 patients more than 1 year after temporal lobe surgery (Gilliam et al., 1999). In a separate cohort of 194 epilepsy clinic patients, a depressed mood and neurotoxicity to AED were the only variables that correlated significantly with poor self-reported health status (Gilliam, 2002).

Despite its high prevalence in PWE, depression continues to be among the more frequently unrecognized co-morbid disorders (Wiegartz et al., 1999; Kanner et al., 2000). For example, 60% of patients with partial epilepsy had been symptomatic for more than 1 year before any treatment was suggested (Kanner et al., 2000). Only one-third of the 97 patients had been treated within 6 months of their symptoms' onset. The delay was not related to the severity of depression, since the proportion of patients untreated for more than 1 year did not differ between those with major depression and dysthymic disorders.

The reasons for the clinicians' failure to recognize depressive disorders in PWE include:

1. Patients minimize their psychiatric symptoms for fear of being further stigmatized.
2. The clinical manifestations of certain types of depression in epilepsy differ from those in non-epileptic patients and are not recognized by physicians.
3. Clinicians usually do not inquire about psychiatric symptoms.
4. Both patients and clinicians minimize the significance of depressive symptoms, considering them to reflect a "normal adaptation process" to this chronic disease.
5. The concern that antidepressant drugs (AD) may lower the seizure threshold has generated among clinicians a certain reluctance to use psychotropic drugs in PWE.

Depression in epilepsy usually results from multiple causes, including processes endogenous to the epilepsy, genetic predisposition, psychosocial obstacles, effects of AEDs (Table 34.2) and effects of surgical treatment.

Table 34.2. Psychiatric adverse events related to AEDs.

AED	ADHD	Behavior disorders	Mood disorders	Anxiety disorders	Psychosis	Forced normalization
Benzodiazepines	+	+	+	−	+	−
CBZ	−	+	+	−	−	+
Ethosuximide	−	+	+	−	+	+
Felbamate	−	+	+	−	−	+
GBP	−	+	+	−	−	−
LTG	−	+	−	+	+	−
Levetiracetam	+	+	+	−	+	+
Oxcarbazepine	−	−	−	−	−	−
PB/primidone	+	+	+	+	+	+
PHT	−	+	−	−	−	+
Tiagabine	−	+	+	−	−	−
TPM	+	+	+	−	+	+
VPA	−	+	−	−	+	+
Zonisamide	−	+	+	−	−	−

Attention deficit disorder in children with epilepsy

Behavior problems, especially attention-deficit/hyperactivity disorder (ADHD), are common in children with epilepsy. In a population-based study in the Isle of White, behavioral disorders were noted in 29% of children with uncomplicated seizures, and 58% of children with both seizures and additional central nervous system (CNS) dysfunction (Rutter et al., 1970). In a separate population-based study of children with epilepsy, heart disease and a control group, hyperactive behavior was found in 28% of the children with epilepsy versus 13% in children with cardiac disease and 5% in controls (McDermott et al., 1995). Compared to controls the adjusted odds ratio in children with epilepsy was 7.4 for motor hyperactivity. Of 11,160 children ages 6 though 17 obtained from the National Health Interview Survey of 1988, 118 were found to have active seizures ($n = 32$) or to have had seizures in the past ($n = 86$) (Carlton-Ford et al., 1995). Impulsive behavior was identified in 11% of the children with no history of seizures and 39% of the children with current or past epilepsy. There was no statistically significant difference between the active and inactive epilepsy groups.

The reported prevalence of ADHD in children with epilepsy vary depending on patient population and study methodology. In four studies that based diagnosis on the Diagnostic and Statistical Manual (DSM) criteria, the prevalence ranged from 14% to 36%. However, these studies were carried out in hospital-based populations, which tend to present more severe problems. Thus, one study of 109 children with epilepsy revealed the presence of ADHD in 40 (37%) children, with a higher prevalence among the children with intractable generalized seizures (Hempel et al., 1995). A second study found ADHD in 12 of 33 patients with complex partial seizures (Semrud-Clikeman and Wical, 1999), while in a third study, of 96 children with chronic seizures, attentive type ADHD was found in 31 and combined type ADHD in 10 (Dunn, 2001). In studies that did not use the DSM criteria, the reported prevalence of ADHD ranged from 8% to 77% (Dunn, 2001).

In the general population, ADHD, Oppositional Defiant Disorder and Conduct Disorder are consistently more common in boys but the reasons vary (NIH Consensus Statement 1988 Nov 16–18). As in the case of depression, ADHD may be caused by AEDs (Table 34.2), might result from a genetic predisposition, might be associated with the underlying cause of the seizures or other seizure-related variables or may be due to combinations of these factors.

Psychosocial obstacles in epilepsy

Fear and shame about their disease is common among PWE, resulting in "self-perceived stigmatization" and failure of many patients to disclose their condition to family members, friends and employers (Scambler and Hopkins, 1986; Jacoby, 1994). Their concerns are well founded. Approximately 18% of PWE who told their employer about their disorder reported subsequent job problems that impaired their careers (Gil-Nagel and Damberre, 2001). Among 160 patients from a neurology clinic in Australia, 44% reported their career had been limited, 39% thought their schooling had been reduced and 58% complained that their social life was restricted because of epilepsy (Edwards, 1974). Similarly, in a large European questionnaire study, 51% of PWE felt stigmatized, with 18% feeling "highly stigmatized" (Baker et al., 2000).

Stigma can be separated into two types: enacted and felt stigma. The former refers to the negative impression that individuals in society feel about epilepsy, while the latter refers to the negative feeling that patients believe their disease cause in other people (Trostle, 1997). Both types of stigma are interrelated: self-stigma is in part proportional to the negative experiences that PWE have encountered through enacted stigma.

Among 81 patients who participated in a study on patients' concerns of living with epilepsy, the most frequently voiced concerns in order of frequency included: (i) inability to drive (68%), (ii) dependence on others (55%), (iii) limitations at work (50%), (iv) embarrassment (38%), (v) having to take medication

(34%), (vi) the presence of mood changes and stress (31%) and (vii) worries about personal safety (31%) (Gilliam et al., 1997).

34.4 Rehabilitation strategies in the management of PWE

Clearly seizures, cognitive deficits, psychiatric disturbances and psychosocial obstacles can all hinder functioning of PWE, suggesting a need for rehabilitation. Unfortunately, most clinicians limit their management to the control of seizures and do not intervene in the other three areas unless they have become quite severe.

Minimizing cognitive deficits

Cognitive disturbances may interfere in the academic and professional performance of PWE. Optimizing seizure control and avoidance of AED-related adverse events can reduce cognitive disturbances but many patients continue to suffer from cognitive problems related to the seizure disorder and/or the pathology underlying the seizures. For example, children with well-controlled absence seizures may still have short attention spans and a poor academic performance.

All school age children with epilepsy should have a neuropsychologic evaluation to identify problems with attention, memory, learning verbal or visual material and specific learning disabilities. In patients with disturbed verbal or visual processing, it is essential to establish their ability to compensate with alternative modalities. These evaluations must be shared with school counselors and psychologists to tailor remedial help. In children with ADHD, pharmacotherapy with CNS stimulants should be recommended. Unfortunately, clinicians often shun these drugs for fear of worsening seizures. Most adult and pediatric epileptologists agree that these drugs are safe in PWE.

As stated above, even patients with childhood onset seizures that remitted with AEDs, and in whom AEDs were discontinued early during treatment faired worse socially and professionally by early adulthood (Sillanpaa et al., 1990). The causes for this are not known, although overprotectiveness by parents and lower academic and professional expectations may contribute. Thus, an assessment of the family members' attitudes towards the patient's epilepsy should be investigated and the counseling provided to eradicate misconceptions and behaviors that may interfere with the child's ability to develop to his/her full potential.

The above measures also apply to *adults with epilepsy*. Neuropsychologic evaluation may identify cognitive disturbances including problems with attention in patients with primary generalized, frontal lobe and temporal lobe epilepsy, and problems with memory in patients with temporal lobe epilepsy. These memory problems involve primarily the acquisition of memory, mediated by hippocampal structures. CNS stimulants are an option in adults with attention disorders.

There are no drugs known to ameliorate memory deficits in PWE, although a small uncontrolled study that tested the safety and efficacy of donepezil (Aricept) yielded encouraging results (Fisher et al., 2001). To-date, patients must rely on cognitive strategies to compensate for memory problems (see Volume II, Chapter 29).

Patients' seizures often force them to change their type of work because of risks of injury. Vocational counseling and, if necessary, rehabilitation should be available to these patients. However, referral for vocational evaluation should not be limited to patients in need of work change, but to any unemployed patient even if cognitively impaired. Patients who are on disability insurance are allowed to work up to 20 h per week and should be encouraged to do so, not only because of the therapeutic effect of work on their quality of life, but because in patients with refractory epilepsy, work is a strong predictor of work after seizures have been controlled by surgery (see below).

Minimizing psychiatric disturbances

As stated above, the impact of psychiatric co-morbidity on the quality of life of PWE is significant among patients with refractory epilepsy. The presence of depression may actually account for a greater negative impact than the seizures. As with cognitive disturbances, clinicians generally fail to identify and treat co-morbid psychiatric problems until they reach great severity (Wiegartz et al., 1999; Kanner et al., 2000). If psychiatric symptoms result from specific AEDs (see Table 34.2), drug adjustments should be carried out.

Failure of patients to report psychiatric symptoms is another big obstacle, which may result from the misconception on the part of patients and family that "it is part of the epilepsy to feel depressed", or "it is normal to get depressed when you suffer from epilepsy". Furthermore, attempts by health professionals to "destigmatize" epilepsy as a "mental disorder" has resulted in a minimization of the significance of psychiatric symptoms, lest it rekindle the old belief that all epilepsy patients "go crazy".

Identification of psychiatric disturbances before they reach serious proportions requires education of patients and family members as to the type of psychiatric symptoms and disorders that are often associated with a specific type of epilepsy. Thus, patients with primary generalized, frontal and temporal lobe epilepsies must look out for symptoms of impulsive behavior, irritability and poor frustration tolerance, while those with of frontal and temporal lobe partial epilepsy should recognize symptoms of anxiety and depression, both during inter-ictal and peri-ictal periods. In our experience, patients and family members are able to accept and report the presence of psychiatric symptoms when they have a clear understanding of their occurrence.

It is also important to recognize that the psychiatric symptoms can worsen cognitive functions and CAEs. In patients with refractory epilepsy, a history of depression was associated with an increased risk of CAEs related to TPM use (Kanner et al., 2003).

Treatment of psychiatric disturbances may require pharmacotherapy, individual psychotherapy, family therapy or a combination of modalities. Most selective serotonin-reuptake inhibitor antidepressants are safe in epilepsy patients, as are the CNS stimulant drugs. With certain exceptions, antipsychotic drugs can be safely used provided they are started at a low dose and titrated slowly. Fear of seizure exacerbation should not be a reason *not to treat* a psychiatric co-morbid disorder.

Overcoming psychosocial obstacles

Education is the best tool to help patients and their families to overcome psychosocial obstacles caused by epilepsy. Such education must begin on the day of diagnosis and should include an understanding of necessary adjustments to professional and recreational activities and other precautions the patient must take to avert self-injury.

It is helpful to schedule a meeting 3–4 weeks after the diagnosis has been made to discuss the impact of epilepsy on the patient and family members. Such meetings help minimize or even avert over-protective attitudes by parents and spouses, and help maximize the sense of independence by the patient. In adults this is often shattered when driving privileges are revoked. These meetings should focus on the reaction of the family members towards the patient and each other, their fears and concerns about epilepsy and the patient. To minimize family conflicts, parents should be asked about any changes in their level of attention to siblings.

Such meetings should be held regularly during the first 6 months, until the patient and family have accepted the diagnosis and its attendant limitations, and have taken the necessary steps to minimize vocational/professional, academic and social problems. Early referral to support groups is also of great benefit to patients and family.

Patients should understand all available legislation that protects their rights at work and school. The local chapters of the Epilepsy Foundation of America are a great resource for this information. It is important, for example, that parents understand the schools' obligation to provide remedial help or transfer to special classes if the patient needs it. If the public school does not have the necessary facilities, federal law stipulates the obligation of the local school district to pay the costs of private schools in the area that can provide the necessary services.

Education of school-mates, teachers of children with epilepsy or co-workers and supervisors of adults may make a significant difference in the acceptance of PWE at school and work. Our epilepsy program arranges lectures to teachers and school-mates of children with epilepsy about what seizures are and what to do in case of a seizure. Such lectures help eliminate stigma, fears and misconceptions about the disease and minimize the risk of rejection of the child with epilepsy by school-mates and teachers.

Rehabilitation and epilepsy surgery

The role of surgery in the treatment of epilepsy

Seizures remit completely with AED in 70% of PWE (Wiebe et al., 2001). This proportion varies according to epilepsy type. Thus, patients with partial epilepsy have a 50% probability of being seizure free on AEDs, but if its cause is mesial-temporal sclerosis (MTS), only 11–30% of patients will be seizure-free with pharmacotherapy (Engel et al., 2003). Epilepsy surgery became available in a small number of epilepsy centers of North America and Canada in the past 60 years. The last two decades, however, have witnessed a marked increase in the number of epilepsy surgery programs throughout the Americas, Europe, Australia and Asia. The goal of surgical treatment is to remove the epileptogenic area (i.e., the cortical region or neuroanatomic structure responsible for the generation of epileptic seizures). Not all patients with refractory epilepsy are candidates for surgery. The consensus among epilepsy centers is that patients should have:

– Refractory partial epilepsy, defined as persistence of disabling seizures despite monotherapy trials with two or three AEDs at sub-toxic doses (Wiebe et al., 2001).
– A well localized seizure focus.
– An epileptogenic area that can be resected with no or minimal risk.

One would expect that patients meeting the above criteria would be referred for a pre-surgical evaluation within the first 5 years of diagnosis. Yet the mean duration between onset of epilepsy and referral to an epilepsy surgery program is 15–20 years (Burg, 2004). Delay in considering surgery is associated with a prolongation and worsening of cognitive and psychiatric disturbances, and psychosocial problems that eventually will require more complex rehabilitation interventions at the time of the surgery.

Epilepsy surgery can be curative or palliative. The former include resective surgical procedures, of which temporal lobectomies comprise about 75%, frontal lobe resections 15% and resections of occipital and parietal cortices 10%. Palliative surgeries provide a significant reduction in seizure frequency, resulting in improved quality of life. Resection of the corpus callosum is a palliative procedure used in patients with secondary generalized epilepsy (Lennox–Gastaut syndrome) presenting primarily with tonic and atonic seizures.

Remission of seizures after epilepsy surgery depends on: location of the seizure focus; presence of an identifiable lesion on magnetic resonance imaging (MRI) or functional neuroimaging, such as positron emission tomography (PET) or ictal single-photon-emission tomography (SPECT). Thus, 60–70% of patients with temporal lobe epilepsy (TLE) secondary to MTS, cavernous angioma or a benign tumor (e.g., ganglioglioma or dysembrioplastic-neuroepithelioma) are expected to become seizure-free or experience only auras, compared to 40–50% of patients with TLE and a normal MRI, PET or ictal SPECT. In patients with frontal lobe epilepsy, the probability of becoming seizure-free is approximately 60% in the presence of a structural lesion and 30% in its absence (Engel et al., 1993).

The aim of pre-surgical evaluation is to identify the location(s) of the seizure focus (or foci) and the potential risks associated with the surgical procedure. Seizure foci in the dominant hemisphere and in proximity to or involving eloquent cortex are associated with the greatest risks.

In planning post-surgical rehabilitation the following must be evaluated:

– Cognitive and psychiatric risks of the procedure.
– Impact of a seizure-free life on family dynamics.
– Optimal vocational/professional potential of the patient.

This discussion will concentrate on patients undergoing temporal lobectomy, as this is the most frequently performed procedure.

Rehabilitation in temporal lobectomy

Cognitive impairments

Among the temporal lobectomies, most are aimed at the resection of sclerotic mesial-temporal structures, or the resection of a structural lesion that may be located remote from mesial structures. However, even in such cases, resection of mesial structures is often necessary due to involvement of hippocampus (dual pathology) (Morrell, 1991). Accordingly, the most frequent concern in these patients is potential post-surgical memory deficit.

Typically, left-sided (or dominant hemisphere) temporal lobectomies are associated with verbal memory deficits and disturbances in verbal learning, while right-sided lobectomies are associated with visual memory deficits. Deficits that follow a dominant hemisphere temporal lobectomy have been reported in 45–50% of patients (Martin et al., 1998). Those following non-dominant temporal resections are more difficult to document with available tests, and are less often noted. Patients also may be able to compensate for visual memory deficits through verbal means, while the opposite is more difficult. Several factors are associated with memory deficits after a dominant hemisphere temporal lobectomy:

– Persistence of seizures after surgery (Rausch and Crandal, 1982; Novelly et al., 1984; Ojieman and Dodrill, 1985).
– Duration of the seizure disorder and age of onset. Patients with seizure onset before age of 5 years are less likely to display a significant change in verbal memory. Conversely, adult-onset seizures are associated with a higher risk of worsening verbal memory after surgery (Saykin et al., 1989).
– *The extent of the resection.* Patients with *en bloc* left temporal lobe resection showed early and late postoperative memory decline (Rausch and Crandal, 1982).
– *Resection of non-atrophic hippocampus in either hemisphere.* Memory loss appears to be inversely related to the histologic evidence of hippocampal pathology (Herman et al., 1984; Herman et al., 1993; Sass et al., 1994; Kneebone et al., 1995).
– Higher preoperative verbal memory scores on neuropsychologic testing and in dominant hemisphere memory testing during intracarotid sodium amytal test (Chelune et al., 1993) (Wada test) (Kneebone et al., 1995).

Temporal lobectomy can sometimes improve cognitive functions, including verbal and visual-spatial memory. This can result from the cessation of seizure activity and the reduction in dose and number of AEDs. In general, improvements are greatest in functions subserved by the hemisphere contralateral to the resection and are seen in patients who become seizure free after surgery (Seidenberg et al., 1998).

Epilepsy surgery and language functions

The risk of aphasia is about 5.5% in most epilepsy surgery programs following an antero-temporal lobectomy in dominant hemisphere (Popovic et al., 1995).

These usually involve a limited resection of temporal-lateral neocortex (4 cm along superior and middle temporal gyri). Mapping of language cortex with either intra-operative electrical stimulation of with subdural grids is essential in patients with non-lesional TLE in the dominant hemisphere and a normal brain MRI with normal volumetric measurements of mesial-temporal structures. In such patients, temporal resections have to be tailored according to the location and extent of the epileptogenic zone and eloquent cortex.

Yet, despite careful mapping of eloquent cortex, it is not infrequent to find word-finding difficulties that persist of months. The cause of these minor, yet annoying disturbances has been the source of much debate and is yet to establish. One theory attributes these deficits to the resection of a secondary language area located in basal-temporal cortex that is usually resected in antero-temporal lobectomies. For additional discussion of aphasia, see Volume II, Chapter 26.

Psychiatric complications of temporal lobectomies

Temporal lobectomies can be complicated by the emergence of psychiatric complications. This can be divided into three main categories:

1 Mood lability, dysphoric and anxiety symptoms which is noted during the first 6–12 weeks after surgery and tends to remit by the sixth month.
2 De-novo depressive disorders.
3 De-novo psychotic disorders.

Patients with a history of psychiatric disorders preceding the surgical procedure can experience an exacerbation of depressive/anxiety disorders during the months that followed the surgical procedure (Tillwally et al., 2003).

In our experience, the mood lability and dysphoric, and anxiety symptoms seen during the first 12 weeks after surgery are very frequent among patients with a prior history of mood disorder, but patients without a previous psychiatric history are also at risk of developing these symptoms. For example, in a study by Ring et al. half of the patients without preoperative psychopathology developed symptoms of anxiety and depression after surgery and 45% of all patients were noted to have increase emotional lability (Ring et al., 1998). Three months after the surgery the emotional lability and anxiety symptoms had diminished, whereas depressive states tended to persist. Low doses of an SSRI (i.e., sertraline at 50 mg/day or paroxetine at 10–20 mg/day) may be sufficient to result in symptom remission.

A more serious problem is the development of depressive disorders that may range from a dysphoric disorder or may reach the proportion of a major depression that can lead to suicidal attempts and death even several months after surgery, especially among patients with persistent seizures (Blumer et al., 1998). The incidence of post-surgical depression has ranged from 4.5% to 63% among seven patient series, with a mean of 26%. Bruton in 1988 reviewed the incidence of post-surgical depression in 274 patients from the Guy–Maudsley programs in Great Britain. There was a 20-fold increase in the prevalence of depression after surgery, relative to pre-surgical figures (Bruton, 1988). Suicide was found in 2.4% of all patients, accounting for 22% of post-op deaths (Bruton, 1988).

In a case series of 89 consecutive patients who underwent a temporal lobectomy at the Rush Epilepsy Center, 37 patients (41.5%) experienced a post-surgical psychiatric complication, the majority of which consisted of a depressive disorder. Fourteen of these 37 patients experienced a de-novo psychiatric disorder, defined as a first (ever) psychiatric disorder or a new type of psychiatric disorder. Fifteen of these 37 patients (40%) corresponding to 17% of all patients who underwent a temporal lobectomy experienced a chronic psychiatric disorder of severe enough to require several changes of psychotropic medications and a significant negative impact on the patients' recovery. A prior history of depression was a significant predictor of post-surgical depression, presenting as a recurrence of a depressive disorder requiring the restart of antidepressant medication or adjustment of its dose. Post-surgical outcome was not associated with likelihood to experience a post-surgical psychiatric complication.

Psychotic disorders have been reported in 7–10% of patients undergoing a temporal lobectomy, although some of these series included patients with pre-surgical history of psychosis. In our own series, three patients (4%) presented with a de-novo psychotic episode, two of which were brief and psychotropic drugs could be discontinued. The PIP being related to the ictal events, are eliminated if the patients are seizure free after the surgery.

Post-surgical psychogenic non-epileptic events have been reported with surprisingly small incidence rates. In our series five patients (6%) were found to have psychogenic non-epileptic events.

Epilepsy surgery and its effect on psychosocial issues

It is not enough to assume that seizures will remit after a temporal lobectomy and ... everything will be just fine! ... In fact, a successful epilepsy surgery may yield changes in the patient's family dynamics with negative consequences. In addition, patients who could not work or for a variety of reasons did not work prior to surgery are facing for the first time the possibility of gainful employment. Yet, even this obvious (anticipated) consequence of a successful surgery fails to be realized more often than not. Thus, these issues need to be carefully considered during the pre-surgical evaluation to ensure the achievement of all expected psychosocial benefits of a successful temporal lobectomy.

The impact of temporal lobectomy on family relations

The persistence of seizures oblige patients to give up many responsibilities that spouses, parents, siblings or friends assume for years. Many patients look forward to the time when they can take over those responsibilities once seizures remit, but family members are not ready to let go which results in conflict. Thus, it is not rare to see couples break up after epilepsy surgeries. Thus, patients and family members need to have a discussion ahead of time of the expectations of "a life without seizures". Special attention must be paid to the new role the patient will take within the family and the necessary changes that the other family members must make to maximize the patient's full potential.

Temporal lobectomy and employment

Rejoining the work force is one of the most obvious aims following a successful epilepsy surgery among adults that were unemployed because of their seizures. For adults that are already working at the time of surgery, a life without seizures is seen as a possibility to get a job with better pay and greater potential for advancement professionally. In reality, however, a successful surgical procedure is not always followed by a search for gainful work.

The impact of medical therapy and epilepsy surgery on employment was investigated by Vickrey et al. (1996). They found moderate improvement in employment status in both surgical and medical groups with a trend towards a greater degree of improvement in the surgical group. In another study by Sperling et al. (1995), employment was significantly improved after surgery and the degree of improvement strongly correlated with the degree seizure relief. Age of surgery also influenced vocational outcomes with older patients (above age of 40 years) doing worse than young adults. Individuals who were students at the time of the surgery tended to do better in regards to employment.

In a series of 80 consecutive adult patients who underwent a temporal lobectomy at our center, 62 were actively employed and 18 were not. There was a significant association between a history of work before and after surgery ($P < 0.0001$). Twelve of the 18 patients that were not working after surgery had not worked before the surgical procedure, while 54 of the 62 patients working after surgery did so before. In this patient series, seizure-freedom post-surgically was significantly associated with working after surgery (unpublished data).

A review of the literature (Novelly et al., 1984; Sperling et al., 1995; Augustine et al., 1984; Reeves et al., 1997) reveals that the main factor associated with post-surgical employment are:

– reduction of seizures or seizure freedom,
– pre-surgical cognitive ability,
– psychiatric co-morbidity,
– pre-surgical employment,
– improvement in neuropsychologic functions.

As shown by our own data, various studies have confirmed that patients who are employed at the time of the surgery are more likely to continue working after surgery. Lendt et al. (1997) found that not only the pre-surgical employment and good seizure outcome are predictors for pre-surgical employment outcome but also young age at the time of surgery and improvement of general neuropsychologic functioning and especially attention. In another study, Reeves et al. (1997) found that being a student or working full time within a year before the surgery, driving after the surgery and obtaining further education after the surgery are associated with full time work postoperatively. Williams et al. (1994) studied the relationship between preoperative Minnesota multiphasic personality inventory (MMPI) scores and vocational status post-surgically. Patients with higher scores on the MMPI test did better on the working status after the surgery, which was contributed to higher motivation in implementing postoperative goals.

Temporal lobectomy and neurologic complications

The neurologic complications associated with a temporal lobectomy are rare and usually mild, but at times, they can be devastating. The most common neurologic complication after anterior temporal lobe resection consists of an upper homonymous quadrantanopsia contralateral to the operated side, caused by a lesion of Meyer's loop; this complication can occur in up to 70% of the patients (Katz et al., 1989). The visual field defects are usually asymptomatic and can be found only on careful neurologic or neuro-opthalmologic testing. Rarely, a homonymous hemianopsia due to anterior choroidal artery infarcts can be seen, which is also associated with hemiparesis.

Hemiparesis contralateral to the operated side is another complication of temporal lobectomy, and can be seen in up to 3% of the patients (Engel et al., 2003). On the other hand, mild hemiparesis immediately after surgery might be due to the edema during the surgery. This usually resolves by itself or with short course of physical therapy. Hemiparesis, when due to infarction of the anterior choroidal artery may last longer and requires prolonged course of physical therapy and rehabilitation. Cranial nerves palsies occur occasionally after temporal lobectomies. Trochlear nerve palsy might be more common than the oculomotor nerve palsy, but is often underdiagnosed. The cranial nerve palsies are transient, but important, especially when postoperative patient complains of double vision, which is usually attributed to side effects of AED.

Neurorehabilitation interventions in temporal lobectomies

Given the above-cited data, the optimal recovery after temporal lobectomy depends on the seizure outcome and the presence of cognitive impairment, development of de-novo psychiatric symptoms or deterioration of previously existing psychiatric disorders. Therefore, careful preoperative psychosocial, neuropsychologic, vocational and psychiatric assessments should be a mandatory part of the presurgical work up and should be considered as important as the localization of the seizure focus.

More often than not, vocational evaluations and education of the family with respect to expected changes in the patient and other family members are deferred post-surgically, In our opinion, such interventions should be offered as part of the presurgical evaluation.

In case of psychiatric complications appropriate intervention with psychotropic medications and psychotherapeutic counseling should be started as soon as symptoms are identified. Furthermore, patients and family members should be instructed as to the type of psychiatric symptoms that are likely to occur.

In case of memory deficits, there are limited interventions that can be offered. Neuropsychologic training to learn compensatory strategies coupled with vocational consultation can often be of assistance. Finally, in case of more serious neurologic complications, patients may need to be referred for speech, physical and occupational therapy.

It is important that patients be followed closely in the immediate postoperative period and on a regular basis (every 3 months) during the first post-surgical year to ensure an optimal recovery. Thereafter, the patient can be followed every 6–12 months. Finally, close follow up and rehabilitation intervention is extremely important if the patient experiences relapse of seizures regardless of cause or time frame.

34.5 Concluding remarks

Rehabilitation is a necessary component of the over-all management of PWE. When applied appropriately, rehabilitation strategies can avert or minimize the impact of cognitive and psychiatric co-morbidities associated with epilepsy and hence significantly improve the quality of life of these patients. The consideration of rehabilitation strategies should not be restricted PWE that has been refractory to pharmacotherapy or those who undergo epilepsy surgery.

REFERENCES

Aarts, J.H.P., Binnie, C.D., Smit, A.M. and Wilkins, A.J. (1984). Selective cognitive impairment during focal and generalized epileptiform EEG activity. *Brain*, **107**, 293–308.

Anthony, J.C., Eaton, W.W. and Henderson, A.S. (1995). Looking in the future of psychiatric etiology. *Epidemiol Rev*, **17**, 240–242.

Augustine, E., Novelly, R.A., Mattson, R.H., et al. (1984). Occupational adjustment following neurosurgical treatment of epilepsy. *Ann Neurol*, **15**, 68–72.

Austin, J.K., Risinger, M.W. and Beckett, L.A. (1992). Correlates of behavior problems in children with epilepsy. *Epilepsia*, **33(6)**, 1115–1122.

Austin, J.K., Smith, M.S., Risinger, M.W., et al. (1994). Childhood epilepsy and asthma: comparison of quality of life. *Epilepsia*, **35(3)**, 608–615.

Baker, G.A., Brooks, J., Buck, D. and Jacoby, A. (2000). The stigma of epilepsy: a European perspective. *Epilepsia*, **41**, 98–104.

Binnie, C.D. (1987). Seizures, EEG discharges and cognition. In: *Epilepsy, Behavior and Cognitive Function* (eds Trimble, M.R. and Reynolds, E.H.), Wylie, New York, pp. 45–51.

Blanchet, P. and Frommer, G.P. (1986). Mood change preceding epileptic seizures. *J Nerv Ment Dis*, **174**, 471–476.

Blum, D., Reed, M. and Metz, A. (2002). Prevalence of major affective disorders and manic/hypomanic symptoms in persons with epilepsy: a community survey. *Neurology*, (**Suppl. 3**), A-175.

Blumer, D., Wakhlu, S., Davies, K., et al. (1998). Psychiatric outcome of temporal lobectomy for epilepsy: incidence and treatment of psychiatric complications. *Epilepsia*, **39**, 478–486.

Bolton, P.F., Park, R.J., Higgins, J.N., Griffiths, P.D. and Pickles, A. (2002). Neuroepileptic determinants of autism spectrum disorders in tuberous sclerosis complex. *Brain*, **125**, 1247–1255.

Bruton, C.J. (1988). *The Neuropathology of Temporal Lobe Epilepsy*, Oxford University Press, Oxford.

Burg, A.T. (2004). Understanding the delay before the epilepsy surgery: who develops intractable epilepsy and when? *CNS Spectr*, **2**, 136–144.

Camfield, C. and Camfield, P. (1997). Social outcome of children with epilepsy and normal intelligence: long-term follow-up of a population based cohort. In: *Pediatric Epilepsy Syndromes and their Surgical Treatment* (eds Tuxhorn, I., Holthausen, H. and Boenigk, H.), John Libbey, London, pp. 44–47.

Camfield, C.S., Camfield, P.R., Smith, B.M. and et al. (2003). Biological factors as Predictors of Social outcome of epilepsy in intellectually normal children: a population-based study. J Pediatrics; **122**, 869–873.

Carlton-Ford, S., Miller, R., Brown, M., Nealeigh, N. and Jennings, P. (1995). Epilepsy and children's social and psychological adjustment. *J Health Soc Behav*, **36**, 285–301.

Chelune, G.L., Najm, R.I., Luders, H., et al. (1993). Individual change after epilepsy surgery: practice effects and base rate information. *Neuropsychology*, **1**, 41–52.

Costello, E.J. (1989). Developments in child psychiatric epidemiology. *J Am Acad Child Adolescent Psychiatr*, **28**, 836–841.

Devinsky, O., Kelly, K., Porter, R.G. and Theodore, W.H. (1988). Clinical and electroencephalographic features of simple partial seizures. *Neurology*, **43**, 1347–1352.

Devinsky, O., Westbrook, L., Cramer, J., et al. (1990). Risk factors for poor health-related quality of life in adolescents with epilepsy. *Epilepsia*, **40**, 1715–1720.

Devinsky, O., Abrahmson, H., Alper, K., et al. (1995). Postictal psychosis: a case control study of 20 patients and 150 controls. *Epilepsy Res*, **20**, 247–253.

Dodrill, C.B. (2002). Progressive cognitive decline in adolescents and adults with epilepsy. In: Do Seizures Damage the Brain? (eds Sutula, T. and Pitkanen, A.), *Prog Brain Res*, **135**, 399–407.

Dodrill, C.B. (2004). Neuropsychological effects of seizures. *Epilepsy Behav*, **5**, S21–S24.

Dodrill, C.B. and Wilensky, A.J. (1990). Intellectual impairment as an outcome of status epilepticus. *Neurology*, **40** (**Suppl. 2**), S23–S27.

Dunn, D. (2001). Attention deficit disorder in epilepsy. In: *Psychiatric Issues in Epilepsy: A Practical Guide to Diagnosis and Treatment* (eds Ettinger, A. and Kanner, A.M.), Lippincott Williams and Wilkins, Philadelphia, PA.

Edeh, J. and Toone, B. (1987). Relationship between interictal psychopathology and the type of epilepsy. Results of a survey in general practice. *Br J Psychiatr*, **151**, 95–101.

Edwards, V.E. (1974). Social problems confronting a person with epilepsy in modern society. *Proc Aust Assoc Neurol*, **11**, 239–243.

Engel Jr., J., Van Nes, P., Rasmussen, T.B., et al. (1993). Outcome with respect to epileptic seizures. In: *Surgical Treatment for Epilepsies* (ed. Engel Jr., J.), 2nd edn., New York, pp. 609–621.

Engel Jr., J., Wiebe, J., French, J., et al. (2003). Practice Parameter: temporal lobe and localized neocortical resections for epilepsy. *Neurology*, **60**, 538–547.

Fisher, R.S., Bortz, J.J., Blum, D.E., Duncan, B. and Burke, H. (2001). A pilot study of donepezil for memory problems in epilepsy. *Epilepsy Behav*, **2**, 330–334.

Forsgren, L. and Nystrom, L. (1990). An incident case referent study of epileptic seizures in adults. *Epilepsy Res*, **6**, 66–81.

Gilliam, F. (2002). Optimizing health outcomes in active epilepsy. *Neurology*, (**Suppl. 5**), S9–S19.

Gilliam, F., Kuzniecky, R. and Faught, E. (1997). Patient-validated content of epilepsy-specific quality of life measurement. *Epilepsia*, **38**, 233–236.

Gilliam, F., Kuzniecky, R., Meador, K., et al. (1999). Patient-oriented outcome assessment after temporal lobectomy for refractory epilepsy. *Neurology*, **53**(4), 687–694.

Gil-Nagel, A. and Garcia Damberre, P. (2001). The social impact of epilepsy: keeping our patients in the closet. In: *Psychiatric Issues in Epilepsy: A Practical Guide to Diagnosis and Treatment* (eds Ettinger, A. and Kanner, A.M.), Lippincott Williams and Wilkins, Philadelphia, PA, pp. 289–296.

Hempel, A.M., Frost, M.D., Ritter, F.J. and Farnham, S. (1995). Factors influencing the incidence of ADHD in pediatric epilepsy patients. *Epilepsia*, **36**(**Suppl. 4**), 122.

Herman, B.P., Wyler, A.R., Somes, G., et al. (1984). Declarative memory following anterior temporal lobectomy in humans. *Behav Neurosci*, **108**, 310.

Herman, B.P., Wyler, A.R. and Somes, G. (1993). Memory loss following left anterior temporal lobectomy is associated with hippocampal pathology and not extend of hippocampal resection [Abstract]. *J Clin Exp Neurophysiol*, **6**, 350.

Hesdorffer, D.C., Hauser, W.A., Annegers, J.F., et al. (2000). Major depression is a risk factor for seizures in older adults. *Ann Neurol*, **47**, 246–249.

Hoare, P. and Kerley, S. (1991). Psychosocial adjustment of children with chronic epilepsy and their families. *Dev Med Child Neurol*, **33**, 201–215.

Jacoby, A. (1994). Felt versus enacted stigma: a concept revisited. *Soc Sci Med*, **38**, 269–274.

Jacoby, A., Baker, G.A., Steen, N., et al. (1996). The clinical course of epilepsy and its psychosocial correlates: findings from a U.K. Community study. *Epilepsia*, **37**(2), 148–161.

Kanemoto, K., Kawasaki, J. and Kawai, J. (1996). Postictal psychosis: a comparison with acute interictal and chronic psychoses. *Epilepsia*, **37**, 551–556.

Kanner, A.M. and Palac, S. (2000). Depression in epilepsy: a common but often unrecognized comorbid malady. *Epilepsy Behav*, **1**, 37–51.

Kanner, A.M., Stagno, S., Kotagal, P. and Morris, H.H. (1996). Postictal psychiatric events during prolonged video-electroencephalographic monitoring studies. *Arch Neurol*, **53**, 258–263.

Kanner, A.M., Kozak, A.M. and Frey, M. (2000). The use of sertraline in patients with epilepsy: is it safe? *Epilepsy Behav*, **1**, 100–105.

Kanner, A.M., Faught, E., Fix, A., French, J.A., et al. (2003). A past psychiatric history may be a risk factor for topiramate related psychiatric and cognitive adverse events. *Epilepsy Behav*, **4**, 548–552.

Kanner, A.M., Soto, A. and Gross-Kanner, H.R. (2004). Prevalence and clinical characteristics of postictal psychiatric symptoms. *Neurology*, **62**, 708–713.

Kateleijn-Nolst Trenite, D.G.A., Smit, A.M., Velis, D.N., et al. (1990). On-line detection of transient neuropsychological disturbances during EEG discharges in children with epilepsy. *Dev Med Child Neurol*, **32**, 46–50.

Katz, A., Award, I.A., Kong, A.K., et al. (1989). Extent of resection in temporal lobectomy for epilepsy II: memory changes and neurological complications. *Epilepsia*, **30**, 763–771.

Kessler, R.C., McGonagle, K.A., Zhao, S., et al. (1995). Lifetime and 12-month prevalence of DSM-III-R psychiatric disorders in United States. Results from the National Comorbidity Survey. *Arch Gen Psychiatr*, **51**, 8–19.

Kneebone, A.C., Chelune, G.J., Dinner, D., et al. (1995). Use of intracarotid amobarbital procedure to predict material specific memory change fallowing anterior temporal lobectomy. *Epilepsia*, **36**, 857–865.

Lehrner, J., Kalchmayr, R., Serles, R., et al. (1999). Health-related quality of life (HRQOL), activity of daily living (ADL) and depressive mood disorder in temporal lobe epilepsy patients. *Seizure*, **8**(2), 88–92.

Lendth, M., Helmstaedter, C. and Elger, C.E. (1997). Pre- and postoperative socio-economic development of 151 patients with focal epilepsies. *Epilepsia*, **38**, 1330–1337.

Lewis, A. (1934). Melancholia: a historical review. *J Ment Sci*, **80**, 1–42.

Logsdail, S.J. and Toone, B.K. (1988). Postictal psychosis. A clinical and phenomenological description. *Br J Psychiatr*, **152**, 246–252.

Margalit, M. and Heiman, T. (1983). Anxiety and self-dissatisfaction in epileptic children. *Int J Soc Psychiatr*, **29**(3), 220–224.

Martin, R., Kuzniecky, R., Ho, S., et al. (1990). Cognitive effects of topiramate, gabapentin and lamotrigine in healthy young adults. *Neurology*, **52**, 321–327.

Martin, R.C., Sawrie, S.M., Roth, D.L., et al. (1998). Individual memory change after anterior temporal lobectomy: a base rate analysis using registration based outcome methodology. *Epilepsia*, **39**, 1075–1082.

Matthews, W.S., Barabas, G. and Ferrari, M. (1982). Emotional concomitants of childhood epilepsy. *Epilepsia*, **23**, 671–681.

McDermott, S., Mani, S. and Krishnaswami, S. (1995). A population-based analysis of specific behavior problems associated with childhood seizures. *J Epilepsy*, **8**, 110–118.

Meador, K.J. (1993). Research use of the new quality-of-life in epilepsy inventory. *Epilepsia*, **34**(**Suppl. 4**), S34–S38.

Meador, K.J., Loring, D.W., Allen, M.E., et al. (1991). Comparative of carbamazepine and phenytoin in healthy adults. *Neurology*, **41**, 1537–1540.

Meador, K.J., Loring, D.W., Abney, O.L., et al. (1993). Effects of carbamazepine and phenytoin on EEG and memory in healthy adults. *Epilepsia*, **34**, 153–726.

Meador, K.J., Loring, D.W., Moore, E.E., et al. (1995). Comparative cognitive effects of carbamazepine and phenytoin, and valproate in healthy adults. *Neurology*, **45**, 1494–1499.

Mendez, M.F., Cummings, J., Benson, D., et al. (1986). Depression in epilepsy. Significance and phenomenology. *Arch Neurol*, **43**, 766–770.

Morrell, F. (1991). The role of secondary epileptogenis in human epilepsy. *Arch Neurol*, **48**, 1221–1224.

Morrell, F., Whisler, W.W., Smith, M.C., et al. (1995). Landau–Kleffner Syndrome: a treatment with subpial transcortical transections. *Brain*, **118**, 1529–1546.

NIH Consensus Statement (1998). Diagnosis and Treatment of Attention Deficit Hyperactivity Disorder (ADHD). November 16–18, Vol. **16**, pp. 1–37.

Novelly, R.A., Augustine, E.A., Mattson, R.H., et al. (1984). Selective memory improvement and impairment in temporal lobectomy in epilepsy. *Ann Neurol*, **15**, 64–67.

O'leary, D.S., Lovell, M.R., Sackellares, J.C., et al. (1983). Effects of age of onset of partial and generalized seizures on neuropsychological performance in children. *J Nerv Ment Dis*, **171**, 624–629.

O'Donoghue, M.F., Goodridge, D.M., Redhead, K., et al. (1999). Assessing the psychosocial consequences of epilepsy: a community-based study. *Br J Gen Pract*, **49**(**440**), 211–214.

Ojieman, G. and Dodrill, C.B. (1985). Verbal memory deficits after left temporal lobectomy for epilepsy. *J Neurosur*, **62**, 101–107.

Onuma. T., Adachi, N., Ishida, S., et al. (1995). Prevalence and annual incidence of psychosis in patients with epilepsy. *Psychiatr Clin Neurosci*, **49**, 267–268.

Perrine, K., Hermann, B.P., Meador, K.J., et al. (1995). The relationship of neuropsychological functioning to quality of life in epilepsy. *Arch Neurol*, **52**(**10**), 997–1003.

Popovic, E.A., Fabinyi, G.C.A., Brazenor, G.A., et al. (1995). Temporal lobectomy for epilepsy: complications in 200 patients. *J Clin Neurosci*, **2**, 238–244.

Rausch, R. and Crandal, P.H. (1982). Psychological status related to surgical control of temporal lobe seizures. *Epilepsia*, **23**, 191–202.

Reeves, A.L., So, E.L., Evans, R.W., et al. (1997). Factors associated with work outcome after anterior temporal lobectomy for intractable epilepsy. *Epilepsia*, **38**, 689–695.

Ring, H.A., Moriarity, J. and Trimble, M.R. (1998). A prospective study of the early postsurgical psychiatric associations of epilepsy surgery. *J Neurol Neurosurg Psychiatr*, **64**, 601–604.

Rutter, M., Graham, P. and Yule, W.A. (1970). *Neuropsychiatric Study in Childhood*. J.B. Lippincott Co., Philadelphia, PA.

Sass, K.J., Westerveld, M., Bachanan, C.P., et al. (1994). Degree of hippocampal neuron loss determines severity of verbal memory decrease after anteromesiotemporal lobectomy. *Epilepsia*, **35**, 1179–1186.

Savard, G., Andermann, F., Olivier, A., et al. (1991). Postictal psychosis after complex partial seizures: a multiple case study. *Epilepsia*, **32**, 225–231.

Saykin, A.J., Gur, R.C., Sussman, N.M., et al. (1989). Memory before and after temporal lobectomy: effects of laterality and age of onset. *Brain Cong*, **9**, 191–200.

Scambler, G. and Hopkins, A. (1986). Being epileptic: coming to terms with stigma. *Social Health Ill*, **8**, 26–43.

Schacter, S.C., Shafer, P.O. and Murphy, W. (1993). The personal impact of seizures: correlations with seizure frequency, employment, cost of medical care, and satisfaction with physician care. *J Epilepsy*, **6**, 224–227.

Seidenberg, M., Hermann, B., Wyler, A.R., et al. (1998). Neuropsychological outcome following anterior temporal lobectomy in patients with and without the syndrome of mesial temporal epilepsy. *Neuropsychology*, **22**, 303–316.

Semrud-Clikeman, M. and Wical, B. (1999). Components of attention in children with complex partial seizures with and without ADHD. *Epilepsia*, **40**, 211–215.

Sillanpaa, M. (1987). Social adjustment and functioning of chronically ill and impaired children and adolescents. *Acta Paediatr Scand*, **340**(**Suppl.**), S1–S70.

Sillanpaa, M., Jalava, M., Kaleva, D., et al. (1998). Long-term prognosis of seizures with onset in childhood. *New Engl J Med*, **338**(**24**), 1715–1722.

So, N.K., Savard, G., Andermann, F., Olivier, A., et al. (1990). Acute postictal psychosis: a stereo-EEG study. *Epilepsia*, **31**, 188–193.

Sperling, M., Saykin, A., Roberts, F., et al. (1995). Occupational outcome after temporal lobectomy for refractory epilepsy. *Neurology*, **45**, 970–976.

Stavem, K., Bjornaes H. and Lossius, M.I. (2000). Reliability and validity of a Norwegian version of the quality of life in epilepsy inventory (QOLIE-89). *Epilepsia*, **41**, 91–97.

Tillwally, S., Kanner, A.M., Leurgans, S., et al. (2003). Postsurgical psychiatric complications of temporal lobectomy: a study of risk factors. *Neurology*, **60**(**Suppl. 1**), A118.

Trimble, M.R. (1991). *Psychosis of Epilepsy*. Raven Press, New York.

Trostle, J.A. (1997). Social aspects: stigma, beliefs and measurement. In: *Epilepsy: A Comprehensive Textbook* (eds Engel Jr., J., Pedley, T.A.), pp. 2183–2189. Lippincott-Raven, Philadelphia, PA.

Vickrey, B.G., Hays, R.D., Graber, J., et al. (1992). A health related quality of life instrument for patients evaluated for epilepsy surgery. *Med Care*, 299–319.

Vickrey, B.G., Hays, R.D., Rausch, R., et al. (1996). Outcomes in 248 patients who had diagnostic evaluation for epilepsy surgery. *Lancet*, **346**, 1445–1449.

Vining, E.P.G., Mellitis, E.D., Dorsen, M.M., et al. (1987). Psychologic and behavioral effects of antiepileptic drugs in children: a double-blind comparison between phenobarbital and valproic acid. *Pediatrics*, **80**, 64–165.

Wiebe, S., Blume, W.T., Girvin, J.P. and Eliasziw, M. (2001). Effectiveness and efficiency of surgery for temporal-lobe epilepsy. *New Engl J Med*, **345**, 311–318.

Wiegartz, P., Seidenberg, M., Woodard, A., et al. (1999). Co-morbid psychiatric disorder in chronic epilepsy: recognition and etiology of depression. *Neurology*, **53**(**Suppl. 2**), S3–S8.

Williams, D. (1956). The structure of emotions reflected in epileptic experiences. *Brain*, **79**, 29–67.

Williams, K.L., Roth, D.L., Kuzniecky, R., et al. (1994). Psychosocial outcome following temporal lobe surgery. *J Epilepsy*, **7**, 144–151.

Parkinson's disease and other movement disorders

Georg Ebersbach[1], Jörg Wissel[2] and W. Poewe[3]

[1]*Neurologisches Fachkrankenhaus, für Bewegungsstörungen/Parkinson, Beelitz-Heilstätten;* [2]*Neurologische Rehabilitationsklinik, Kliniken Beelitz GmbH, Beelitz-Heilstätten and* [3]*Department of Neurology, Medical University Innsbruck, Innsbruck, Germany*

35.1 Introduction

Parkinson's disease (PD) is one of the most prevalent neurodegenerative diseases and affects between 100 and 200 persons per 100,000 (Schrag, 2002). The prevalence of PD increases with age to affect about 2% of those aged 65 years and above (de Rijk et al., 1997). In addition to idiopathic PD, the term "parkinsonism" is used to label a variety of diseases and syndromes related to different neurodegenerative processes, structural cerebral changes and environmental exposures. Dystonia, although less frequent than PD may also affect up to 700 patients per 100,000 in the population aged above 50 years (Muller et al., 2002). Considering the high prevalence of essential tremor (ET) of 0.4–4% in the overall population (Louis et al., 1998) and the idiopathic restless-legs syndrome affecting some 10% of the population above 65 years (Rothdach et al., 2000) there can be little doubt that movement disorders are among the most prevalent neurologic conditions in the community. In fact medical or surgical therapies are available for most of these but symptomatic efficacy is usually incomplete. This is particularly true for PD and dystonia which will be the focus of this chapter.

35.2 Functional organization of the basal ganglia

The current understanding of basal ganglia dysfunction in PD and other movement disorders is based on the model introduced by Alexander et al. (1986). This model postulates that striatal projections are segregated into discrete loops according to their projection targets. Within these circuits striatal output to the globus pallidus internus (GPi) and substantia nigra pars reticulata (SNr) involves a direct GABAergic (gamma aminobutyric acid) pathway and an indirect pathway via the globus pallidus externus (GPe) and the subthalamic nucleus (STN). The GPi then further projects to thalamocortical relay cells projecting directly to various areas of the cerebral cortex which in turn has excitatory glutamatergic efferents to the striatum (Fig. 35.1(a)). The net result of decreased stimulation of dopamine receptors in the striatum is increased inhibitory output of GPi acting on thalamocortical projections (Fig. 35.1(b)). This model is consistent with the improvement of akinesia after pallidotomy and deep brain stimulation (DBS) of the STN in PD. Yet, since the model fails to account for ameliorace of hyperkinetic disturbances which can be achieved with DBS or ablative surgery in the GPi (Parent and Cicchetti, 1998), it is currently subject to reconsiderations.

35.3 Parkinson's disease

Neurobiology and neurogenetics

PD is characterized neuropathologically by Lewy body type neuronal degeneration in the pars compacta of the substantia nigra resulting in dopamine deficiency in nigrostriatal projection areas. Although

(a)

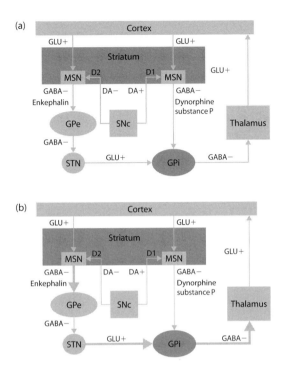

(b)

Figure 35.1. (a) Cortico-striato-thalamocortical motor loops (simplified). Excitatory pathways are marked with "+", inhibitory pathways with "−". Dopaminergic (DA) pathways originating in the substantia nigra pars compacta (SNc) project on striatal medium spiny neurons (MSN). Striatal output to the GPi involves a direct GABAergic pathway and an indirect pathway via the GPe and the STN. Excitatory thalamocortical and corticostriatal projections are glutamatergic (GLU). (b) In PD decreased stimulation of dopamine receptors in the striatum leads to overactivity of the indirect pathway and underactivity of the direct pathway with the net result of increased inhibitory output of GPi acting on thalamocortical projections.

loss of nigral dopaminergic neurons and striatal dopamine deficiency are the pathologic and neurochemical hallmarks of the illness neuropathology is much more widespread. According to a model recently introduced by Braak et al. (2003) the pathologic process starts in the nuclei of the glossopharyngeus and vagal nerve and anterior olfactory nucleus, thereafter pursuing an ascending course involving pontine and midbrain structures and in later stages, limbic and neocortical regions.

PD is still considered a sporadic neurodegenerative disorder and thought to result from a complex interaction between multiple predisposing genes and environmental influences, although these interactions are still poorly understood. However, the number of monogenic forms of PD is steadily increasing with moderate repercussions on the routine diagnostic work-up. The first type of autosomal dominant PD that was recognized (PARK1) is caused by mutations in the gene for alpha-synuclein, one of the principal components of the Lewy body (Polymeropoulos et al., 1997). Autosomal-recessive parkinsonism associated with the parkin mutations is characterized by early onset with dystonia, slow progression and L-dopa responsiveness for prolonged time periods. Pathologic studies in cases with parkin mutations have found depigmentation of substantia nigra and absence of Lewy bodies (Khan et al., 2003; Van De Warrenburg et al., 2001). As parkin–parkinsonism is the most common of the various genetic forms occurring in 40% of patients with early-onset familial parkinsonism but also in a minority of sporadic young-onset patients routine genetic testing for parkin mutations is recommended in subjects with onset of parkinsonism before the age of 30 years.

Clinical features and diagnosis

The classic triad of clinical signs – resting tremor, rigidity and akinesia – asymmetry of symptoms, chronic progressive course and a good to excellent response to levodopa are key features that best differentiate PD from other forms of parkinsonism. In addition to motor signs there is frequent occurrence of vegetative disturbances and neuropsychiatric disorders including depression, dementia and (drug-induced) psychosis. In patients treated with dopaminergic medication drug-induced dyskinesias occur in many cases after a variable interval. Levodopa is clearly more critical in this respect compared to dopamine agonists and may induce peak-dose chorea or dystonic and more stereotyped dyskinesias associated with OFF-phases or threshold levels of levodopa. Clinical features are described in more detail further down in this chapter.

The diagnosis of PD is made on the basis of patient history and clinical signs. Application of validated standards such as UK brain bank criteria (Gibb and Lees, 1988) has led to remarkable accuracy with the clinical diagnosis of idiopathic PD having a positive predictive value of more than 90% for the definite pathologic confirmation (Hughes et al., 2002).

Routine brain imaging does not convey specific structural changes in PD but may help to differentiate idiopathic disease from other causes of parkinsonism. Magnetic resonance imaging (MRI) may show signal abnormalities in the putamen and/or brainstem and cerebellar atrophy in multiple-system atrophy (MSA), midbrain atrophy in progressive supranuclear palsy (PSP) and asymmetric atrophy in corticobasal degeneration (CBD) (Schrag et al., 2000). Furthermore, anatomical imaging can disclose cerebrovascular pathology, calcification of basal ganglia, hydrocephalus or other structural abnormalities which can be associated with parkinsonism.

Functional imaging is sometimes used to confirm clinical classification of parkinsonism. In idiopathic PD positron emission tomography (PET) with [18]Fluoro-dopa and single photon emission computed tomography (SPECT) with ^{123}I-FP-CIT that labels the striatal dopamine transporter show reduced uptake in putamen and to a lesser degree in the caudate nucleus (Morrish et al., 1996). A similar pattern is also found in other parkinsonian syndromes, for example MSA but not in disorders which do not affect the status of nigral dopaminergic neurons (e.g. ET). Studies with ^{123}I-IBZM-SPECT and ^{11}C-raclopride PET that bind to post-synaptic dopamine receptors have reported normal striatal D2 binding in idiopathic PD and reduced binding in other parkinsonian syndromes but sensitivity and specificity of these techniques are limited (Brooks et al., 2002).

The clinical course of idiopathic PD is variable with presence of gait disturbance, old age at onset and occurrence of dementia being reported to be associated with faster rate of progression (Bennett et al., 1996; Jankovic and Kapadia, 2001). In the prelevodopa era Hoehn and Yahr (1967) found severe

Table 35.1. Modified Hoehn and Yahr (1967) staging.

Stage 0	No signs of disease
Stage 1	Unilateral disease
Stage 1.5	Unilateral plus axial involvement
Stage 2	Bilateral disease, without impairment of balance
Stage 2.5	Mild bilateral disease, without recovery on pull test
Stage 3	Mild-to-moderate bilateral disease; some postural instability; physically independent
Stage 4	Severe disability; still able to walk or stand unassisted
Stage 5	Wheelchair bound or bedridden unless aided

disability, corresponding to stages 4 and 5 (Table 35.1) in two-thirds of patients after 5–9 years of disease duration and threefold increased mortality. With the introduction of levodopa progression to advanced stages of disability has slowed, and there is some evidence that life expectancy may now have come near to normal (Muller et al., 2000; Schrag, 2002).

Medical and surgical treatment

Levodopa is the most reliable and effective symptomatic treatment and failure to respond to high doses of levodopa suggests an alternative diagnosis. Yet, long-term therapy with levodopa has its disadvantages since treatment complications reflecting a complex interaction between drug effects and disease progression develop in a majority of patients following sustained treatment. These complications include fluctuations in motor response consisting of predictable ("wearing-OFF") or unpredictable (ON/OFF) loss of effect and drug-induced involuntary movements (dyskinesias). In contrast, treatment with directly acting dopamine agonists is associated with smaller incidence of fluctuations and dyskinesias but is satisfactorily effective only in a minority of patients when given as monotherapy for more than 3–5 years (Rascol et al., 2000; Holloway et al., 2004). Other side-effects of dopaminergic treatment including nausea, orthostatis, edema, somnolence and hallucinosis occur more frequently with dopamine agonists compared to levodopa.

Neurosurgical management of PD has had a renaissance in the last decade mainly driven by a better understanding of basal ganglia circuitries and the introduction of new procedures including functional DBS. Due to its reversibility and adaptability DBS allows to explore new targets and indications at a lower risk compared to ablative stereotactic neurosurgery. The STN and the GPi are the main targets in current neurosurgical PD therapy. DBS of the STN effectively reduces tremor, rigidity and akinesia as well as levodopa-induced dyskinesias and is usually associated with significant reductions in antiparkinsonian drug dose. It seems more effective compared to stimulation of the GPi (Volkmann et al., 2001). Motor symptoms not responding to levodopa in individual patients, which may be the case with imbalance, freezing or dysarthria, are not improved by DBS with the exception of drug-resistant tremor. Furthermore patients with dementia or severe psychosis should not undergo DBS of the STN. Techniques to restore dopaminergic transmission are described in a separate chapter of this book.

Differential diagnosis of parkinsonism

Population-based studies have shown that at least 15% of patients with a diagnosis of PD do not fulfill strict clinical criteria for the disease, and approximately 20% of patients with PD who have already come to medical attention have not been diagnosed (Schrag et al., 2002). In clinical–pathologic studies the most common misdiagnosis relates to other forms of degenerative parkinsonism like PSP, MSA or CBD (Hughes et al., 2002). Clinically based studies have shown that other common errors include ET, drug-induced parkinsonism and vascular parkinsonism (Meara et al., 1999). In addition there is ongoing debate on the distinction between PD with dementia and the so-called dementia with Lewy bodies (DLB).

Essential tremor

ET is a monosymptomatic, in many cases autosomal dominant disorder characterized by an action tremor of the upper extremities (Bain et al., 1994).

Bradykinesia, rigidity and postural instability are not part of the illness but when occurring in the elderly the presence of co-morbid disorder that may interfere with mobility may suggest the diagnosis of PD to the inexperienced clinician. The presence of head tremor, voice tremor and sensitivity to alcohol strongly favor ET (Koller et al., 1994).

Vascular parkinsonism

Vascular parkinsonism, defined as parkinsonism occurring in patients with cerebrovascular disease (Critchley, 1929) has remained a controversial entity. It requires exclusion of Lewy body disease or other neurodegenerative forms of parkinsonism, which may be difficult on clinical grounds alone (Zijlmans et al., 2004). Binswanger's disease or hypertensive subcortical arteriosclerotic encephalopathy is characterized by widespread bilateral deep lacunar white matter infarcts and typically causes a parkinsonian gait disorder with wide-based small stepped gait and freezing ("lower body parkinsonism") (Fitzgerald and Jankovic, 1989). Onset is usually insidious with slow and sometimes stepwise progression while basal ganglia infarcts involving the putamen or putamino-pallido-thalamic outflow or the substantia nigra may give rise to acute onset of contralateral parkinsonism (Zijlmans et al., 2004).

Dementia with Lewy bodies

DLB is currently regarded as the second most common type of degenerative dementia second to Alzheimer's disease (McKeith et al., 2004). According to published consensus criteria it is clinically defined as a progressive dementia syndrome with prominent attentional and visuo-spatial deficits, marked fluctuations in attention and cognition, visual hallucinations and parkinsonism. Although it has been suggested to separate the two conditions based on the onset of dementia relative to parkinsonism and restrict the term PD dementia (PDD) to cases where dementia begins at least 12 months after the motor manifestations of PD (McKeith et al., 1996), it is likely that DLB and PDD are two clinical manifestations within a spectrum of Lewy body diseases (Emre, 2003).

Progressive supranuclear palsy

Also called Steele Richardson Olzewsky syndrome. PSP is a multisystem degeneration which can be easily differentiated from PD when presenting with its typical clinical picture of supranuclear gaze palsy involving predominantly vertical gaze, parkinsonism, pseudobulbar palsy and prominent frontal lobe syndrome. Postural instability and falls not uncommonly occur already in the first year of disease. In the early stages before gaze abnormalities appear or in cases where it does not develop or when a full-blown parkinsonism dominates the clinical picture PSP can be confused with PD (Tolosa et al., 2002). Parkinsonism in PSP rarely improves with dopaminergic treatment. Neuropathologic studies show presence of abundant tau positive neurofibrillary tangles in subcortical and brainstem structures.

Multiple-system atrophy

MSA is a sporadic multisystem degeneration associated with alpha-synuclein deposits in the central nervous system (oligodendrocytic inclusions) but not Lewy bodies or neuritis (Gai et al., 1998). It can present as a predominantly or exclusively cerebellar (olivoponto-cerebellar atrophy) or parkinsonian (striato-nigral degeneration) form associated with variable degrees of autonomic failure. The Parkinson variant of MSA, currently referred to as MSA-p, can be very difficult to differentiate from PD. Only if prominent signs of autonomic failure such as impotence, or postural hypotension develop early in the course of the diseased or a clear cerebellar syndrome is also present can the disorder be reliably diagnosed. Besides dysautonomia other clinical characteristics can help differentiate MSA-p from PD: stridor, rapid course, early instability and falls, stimulus sensitive myoclonus, pyramidal tract signs, severe dysarthria and insufficient or only transient response to L-dopa (Wenning et al., 1995).

Corticobasal degeneration

CBD is a rare tauopathy that shares clinical and biologic features with PSP. CBD can present clinically as an atypical mostly unilateral parkinsonism but also with any of a variety of asymmetrical cortical degeneration syndromes which include primary progressive aphasia, frontal lobe dementia and progressive apraxia. Classically CBD patients present in the sixth decade with slowly progressive unilateral jerky tremulous akinetic rigid and apractic extremity held in a fixed dystonic posture. Alien limb phenomenon develops in approximately 50% of patients and cortical sensory deficits are also common. Motor symptoms rarely respond to levodopa and the disorder progresses relentlessly to become bilateral and produce severe disability in 2–7 years.

Rehabilitative therapy in PD

Attempts to ease motor impairment in PD with physical therapy and other rehabilitative measures date back to the 19th century (Weiner and Singer, 1989). Yet, few controlled clinical trials have actually tested the impact of rehabilitative interventions in PD (Goetz et al., 2002). Clinical practice of rehabilitation in PD thus still relies only partly on scientific evidence and also includes approaches justified by empirical experience, plausibility and intuition.

Rehabilitative therapy in PD intends to provide physical and psychosocial aid that helps to secure quality of life and to reduce the characteristic complications of long-term disease. Rehabilitation cannot halt or reverse the progressive nature of PD but may slow the increase of disability in the course of the chronic disease. Physiotherapy, occupational therapy and speech therapy are the mainstays of rehabilitation in PD which are complemented by spa, music and sport therapy (Ward, 2000). Neuropsychologic interventions have not yet been tried systematically but may have a role in the management of cognitive disturbances in PD. Psychosocial counseling is provided in order to enable patient and caregivers to cope with the evolving disease and may influence mood, social integration and autonomy.

Table 35.2. Motor symptoms which may not respond satisfactorily to dopaminergic medication.

Speech and swallowing disorders
  Hypophonia
  Dysarthria
  Dysprosodia
  Dysphagia
Disequilibrium
  Retropulsion
  Imbalance
  Falls
Complex gait disorders
  Start hesitation
  Turn hesitation
  Freezing
  Festination
Postural disturbances
  Camptocormia ("bent spine")
  Antecollis ("dropped head")

	ON	ON with dyskinesia	OFF	Asleep
06:00–06:30				X
06:30–07:00				X
07:00–07:30			X	
07:30–08:00			X	
08:00–08:30	X			
08:30–09:00	X			
09:00–09:30	X			
09:30–10:00	X			
10:00–10:30	X			
10:30–11:00			X	
11:00–11:30			X	
11:30–12:00			X	

Figure 35.2. Part of an ON/OFF-diary showing response fluctuations in a patient with PD.

Rehabilitative therapy in PD should be aimed at impairments which are not or not sufficiently accessible to pharmacologic treatment. Rigidity, tremor and akinesia are often dramatically reversed by drug effects whereas other symptoms are much less manipulable by medical treatment. Lack of response to dopaminergic drugs predicts (with the exception of drug-resistant tremor) refractoriness to DBS and ablative stereotactic interventions leaving rehabilitative therapy as the sole putatively effective option. Dopa-resistant deficits become increasingly prominent in the late stage of PD (Bonnet et al., 1987) and may cause significant problems even at the onset of disease in atypical Parkinson syndromes such as MSA or PSP. Table 35.2 gives an overview about symptoms which often turn out to be insufficiently influenced by pharmacologic treatment.

Fluctuations of motor performance

An important issue in the rehabilitation of motor symptoms in PD are fluctuations due to pharmacodynamic or circumstantial factors. Response fluctuations including wearing-OFF and ON/OFF-states may dramatically alter motor abilities but also mood and motivation (Witjas et al., 2002). Transitions between ON- and OFF-states frequently occur several times per day often corresponding to the intervals of drug intake (Jankovic, 2002). In general terms, symptoms restricted to the OFF-states are rather a domain of medical treatment including adjustment of medication or deep brain surgery. Rehabilitative strategies should rather concentrate on deficits which persist during ON-states. This implies a thorough clinical observation and analysis of the different motor states in an individual patient prior to the setting of rehabilitative goals. Many patients, when properly instructed, are able to accurately protocol response fluctuations using ON/OFF-diaries (Fig. 35.2) which may help to identify amount, frequency and regularity in the time course of ON- and OFF-phases. Fluctuations are often mild or absent in patients in the early stage of PD, patients with atypical Parkinson syndromes and in patients with extensive co-morbidity (e.g. subcortical arteriosclerotic encephalopathy).

Another type of discontinuous impairment is represented by motor blocks including start and turning hesitation, freezing of gait and speech blockades (Giladi et al., 1992). Motor blocks must be differentiated from fluctuations due to pharma-codynamic responses and are often triggered by circumstantial factors such as narrow pathways, door-steps or stressful situations. Freezing of gait and other motor blocks usually last only seconds and can often be overcome by verbal commands or motor-sensory trick maneuvers. Motor blocks may occur in both, ON- and OFF-states, but can also be confined to OFF- or, very rarely, ON-states in individual patients.

Motor deficits and principles of rehabilitation

A core problem of akinesia in PD is the disturbance of execution of automatized motor routines (Marsden, 1982). Intracerebral recordings in mon-keys have shown that in predictable and easy move-ments phasic internal motor cues from the globus pallidus exert inhibitory action on premovement activity in the supplementary motor cortex facilitat-ing sequential execution of movement components (Brotchie et al., 1991). Due to the impaired genera-tion of internal cues motor control is disrupted and movement requires an increased amount of atten-tional resources. Since both components of motor control, time-keeping and scaling of force can be involved movement execution is hesitant ("akinesia"), slow ("bradykinesia") and performed with reduced amplitude ("hypokinesia"). Changing from one motor program to another (set-shifting) may be dis-turbed and sequencing of repetitive movements may occur with prolonged and/or irregular intervals and reduced and/or irregular amplitudes (Georgiou et al., 1993). External cues may exert disproportion-ate influence on motor performance and can trigger both motor blocks and kinesia paradoxa (Bloem et al., 2004).

Complementary to the increased reliance on external sensory information impaired processing of proprioceptive information, presumably due to disturbed central integration has been described in PD (see Abbruzzese and Berardelli, 2003 for com-prehensive review). In sensorimotor performance deficient proprioceptive integration is reflected by

increased need of visual control of movement (Klockgether and Dichgans, 1994), higher threshold for detecting passively imposed movements (Klockgether et al., 1995), overestimation of actively performed (Moore, 1987) and underestimation of passively imposed (Demirci et al., 1997) movement amplitudes, and reduced precision grip perform-ance (Fellows et al., 1998). In clinical practice dimin-ished awareness for underscaling of amplitude and acceleration of cadence is often evident both for gait and speech. Reduced perception of impaired body posture, in some cases resembling "postural neglect", is a further clinical feature evidencing deficient somatosensory processing.

These alterations of sensorimotor control in PD suggest implementation of specific therapeutic strategies to restore somatosensory perception and to compensate for loss of generation of internal cues. External sensory cues, including acoustic, tac-tile or visual stimuli, are used for the latter purpose and may be provided in order to trigger initiation of movements or to facilitate repetitive and sequential movements. This approach includes delivery of cues by therapists or devices as well as training of patients to employ sensory stimuli or trick maneuvers (Rubinstein et al., 2002).

Physical and occupational therapy

In contrast to the treatment of spasticity which often relies on elaborate and well-defined therapeu-tical concepts, there is no such "school" for the reha-bilitation of motor problems of parkinsonism. Studies focusing on the impact of physical and occupational therapies on PD have tested a variety of exercise programs which are hardly comparable but rather linked by the programmatic effort to improve motor skills by means of a regular training for a prescribed period of time. A recent evidence-based review of interventions to treat PD, produced by a task force commissioned by the Movement Disorder Society (Goetz et al., 2002), identified eight studies on physical and occupational therapy to improve symptomatic control of parkinsonism, dat-ing from 1981 to 1998, which fulfilled predefined minimum quality criteria as follows (Goetz et al., 2002):

• Patients with an established diagnosis of PD.
• Established scales for measuring target symptoms.
• Minimum of 20 patients.
• Minimum of a 4-week treatment period.
• Study report published in English.

Therapeutic interventions in these studies included such diverse approaches as stretching exercises versus active upper body karate training (Palmer et al., 1986), occupational therapy to improve fine motor function (Gauthier et al., 1987), physical therapy aimed at enhancing balance and flexibility in large muscle groups (Comella et al., 1994), exercises of facial muscles (Katsikitis and Pilowsky, 1996), training of spinal flexibility (Schenkman et al., 1998), and other types of passive and active physical therapy (Gibberd et al., 1981; Formisano et al., 1992; Dam et al., 1996). Due to the paucity, diversity and methodologic shortcomings of studies this review as well as a recent Cochrane Review (Deane et al., 2001) concluded that there is insufficient evidence to support or refute the efficacy of physical therapy in PD.

In addition, there is only limited evidence about transfer of motor skills acquired in therapeutical settings to daily motor routines. Gauthier et al. (1987) compared 30 patients which received occupational group therapy twice weekly for 5 weeks with 29 patients who did not receive therapy. Improved motor skills compared to controls in the treatment group was still significant 6 months and, to a lesser degree after 12 months after completion of therapy. In contrast Comella et al. (1994) did not find preservation of motor improvement 6 months after completion of a 4-week training of postural stability and muscle flexibility in spite of sufficient acute response to therapy. The results of Morris et al. (1996) suggest that motor achievements in PD are sometimes confined to the motivational and circumstantial peculiarities of the therapeutical rehabilitative setting. In this study patients with PD were trained to increase step-length by means of sensory cues or mental techniques. Measures of gait that were performed inadvertently off therapy showed that patients reversed to hypokinetic locomotion as soon as attention was withdrawn from the therapeutic goal.

A recent evaluation of a multidisciplinary rehabilitation program including speech and occupational and physiotherapy was presented by Wade et al. (2003) using a randomized crossover design in 94 patients with PD. After a 6-week treatment cycle with weekly interventions significant immediate improvement on disability and quality of life was reported but no effects 18 weeks after termination of the program. It remains to be shown whether more continuous and reiterative protocols are more effective in counteracting the consequences of disease progression.

Behavior modification techniques, cueing and trick maneuvers

Since the publication of Martin's seminal description (1967) numerous behavior modification techniques, using the effect of external cueing like visual lines or metronomes, have been published. One rationale behind implementing cues in the rehabilitation of patients with PD is to substitute defective signaling between basal ganglia and supplementary motor area (SMA). Patients are thus enabled to modify their motor strategies to involve a "closed-loop" performance (Marchese et al., 2000). Another theory is that cues de-automatize motor routines and thus avoid reliance on the disturbed pallidum–thalamus–SMA motor circuit. This should be achieved by means of focused attention or using less overlearned motor strategies, for example marching instead of walking (Morris et al., 1996). Music and mental imaginary incorporated into motor strategies are features that may theoretically activate limbic motor systems (Ito et al., 2000). Azulay et al. (1999) suggested that improvement of gait with floor markers is related to a cerebellar motor pathway. This pathway is activated by optical flow that occurs when visual cues appear to move downward in the visual field during gait. If this dynamic optical flow does not occur, as with stroboscopic lighting, visual cues become ineffective.

Sensory-motor cueing has been used as an isolated trick maneuver or embedded in complex behavioral therapy protocols (Müller et al., 1997). Dam et al., 1996 compared conventional exercises with the same exercises with additional sensory enhancement including performance in front of a mirror, using special colored blocks and other visual cues during the exercises, and listening to audio-cued tapes. In this study patients received therapy for 1 month, then a rest period for 3 months, then a repeat of the therapy with rest, and a third 1-month treatment followed by rest for 3 months. This design corresponds well with routine clinical circumstances where coverage of therapy costs by health insurance is often restricted to intermittent rather than continuous outpatient rehabilitation. Whereas acute effects were similar in both, conventional and cue-enhanced type of therapy, only subjects in the latter group were reported to have continuous improvement of gait and motor scores 1 month after treatment. Another study that compared therapy with and without sensory cues in 20 patients with PD was presented by Marchese et al. (2000). Follow-up (after 6 weeks) only showed persistent improvement in patients who were trained with external cueing.

Special emphasis has been given to the improvement of gait with sensory cueing (see Rubinstein et al., 2002 for comprehensive review). Sensory tricks are used to overcome start hesitation (which has been synonymously termed gait ignition failure) and to maintain steady pacing. Martin (1967) defined various features of visual cues that are critical for their effectiveness. According to Martin visual stimuli need to be on the trajectory and are optimally effective when transverse and contrasting. The best distance between visual cues is about step-length (25–50 cm). Response to one visual cue (e.g. strips attached to the ground) does not predict the response to other visual cues (e.g. inverted walking stick) (Dietz et al., 1990). Cues usually work most dramatic at first presentation and rather lose than gain effectiveness with further use (Stern et al., 1980). Table 35.3 gives examples of different sensorimotor cues than can be incorporated in gait therapy.

Table 35.3. External cues to overcome start hesitation and freezing (examples).

Motor maneuvers
    Shifting of the body
    Walking sidewards or backwards
    Stomping or shaking foot
    Marching
Verbal and auditory stimuli
    Rhythmic commands
    Starting order
    Hand clapping
    Cursing (self-)scolding
    Metronome, music
      RAS (Thaut et al., 1996)
Visual stimuli
    Obstacles
      Balls
      Inverted cane
      Foot of partner
    Markers
      Floor stripes
      Laser-pointer
      Ground structures
Imagined stimuli

Thaut et al. (1996) and McIntosh et al. (1997) suggested rhythmic auditory stimulation (RAS) in order to improve gait velocity. Treatment is based on a home-based training program that require subjects to entrain their walking pace to metronome-pulses embedded into rhythmical instrumental music delivered by audiotapes. Compared to controls receiving no training or training based on internal (self-)pacing patients treated with RAS showed larger gait velocity that was not only attributable to higher cadence (step-rate) but also to improved step-length. The effects of visual cueing on gait have been systematically assessed by Morris et al. (1994) who found immediate performance effects with floor markers which led to normal stride-length. In a later study Morris et al. (1996) reported that training with an attentional strategy, whereby patients were required to concentrate on stride-length produced similar results. Allocation of attention and external encouragement may be critical for the effectiveness of therapy and long-term carry-over of therapeutic progress. Verbal instructions should rather encourage large steps and arm-swing whereas stressing the importance of velocity may result in a faster but abnormal gait pattern (Behrman et al., 1998).

Techniques to improve balance

An important challenge in the rehabilitation of patients with PD is to achieve sufficient equilibrium and to avoid falls. Balance training (Volume II, Chapter 8) is frequently based on exercising on changing support modalities (e.g. with/without manual hold) and surfaces (e.g. foam, moving platforms) (see Fig. 35.3). A recently developed approach (Jöbges et al., 2004) to improve postural stability is based on the repetitive execution of the pull-test maneuver. In this technique patients are tilted backward and sideward by the therapist in order to recover active rebalancing. In a multiple baseline design study

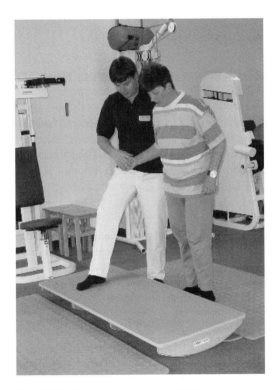

Figure 35.3. Balance training on a swivel platform.

postural responses were significantly improved and gait velocity was faster after a cycle of 14 days of therapy consisting of two 20-min sessions daily. Remarkably, effects were stable for 2 months without additional training.

A further approach to treat disequilibrium is based on exercises strengthening lower limb musculature which have been shown to improve dynamic posturography performance in patients with PD in a small controlled trial (Hirsch et al., 2003). In order to avoid forward falling induced by freezing patients should be advised not to try to overcome their motor block forcefully but to relax first and then calmly reignite locomotion (Bloem et al., 2004).

Besides active exercising, avoidance of risk factors for falls is a complementary element of rehabilitation in patients with PD and disequilibrium including management of orthostasis, surveillance of use of sedative drugs and counseling for environmental and behavioral hazards. If falls cannot be avoided patients should be provided with canes, wheelchairs and protectors for body parts at hazard (hips, knee, head). Some patients with postural problems profit from carrying a backpack with load that is individually adjusted in order to facilitate raising of the trunk and to shift the center of gravity backwards.

Relaxation techniques, spa therapy, diathermy

Although not exclusively classifiable as physiotherapy relaxation techniques are often incorporated into rehabilitative treatment regimes in PD. Progressive muscular relaxation according to Jacobson and other exercises can contribute to ease pain from muscular tension and to improve stress tolerance. The latter may, in some cases, have an effect on motor symptoms which are susceptible to mental strain like tremor and hyperkinesias.

The spectrum of physical therapy is complemented by spa therapy which includes massages, thermal baths and relaxation techniques. Brefel-Courbon et al. (2003) conducted a randomized single-blind study in order to evaluate clinical and economic consequences of spa therapy in 31 patients with PD. Whereas no change was found on the Unified PD rating scale (UPDRS) motor score some aspects of quality of life were improved. Since costs of hospitalization and medication were reduced after spa treatment total health expenditure was found to be decreased with this type of treatment.

Speech therapy

The majority of patients with PD is affected by disorders of speech during some part of their disease which contribute to the communicative restraints imposed by hypomimia, reduced gesturing and immobility. Impairment of speech can manifest with hypophonia, dysarthrophonia and disturbed prosody. Occasionally, analogous to the festination and freezing of gait, there are also severe disorders of speech rhythm and consecutive speech blocks. Shahed and Jankovic (2001) found that, after decades of unremarkable speech, PD can lead to reappearance of stuttering.

Speech therapy is focused on the improvement of communication by exercising articulation, prosody and volume. Another aim is to secure proper swallowing.

Ramig et al. (1996) introduced the "Lee Silverman voice therapy" (LSVT) program that is mainly aimed to increase vocal cord adduction and loudness. This technique has been compared with respiratory exercises in a controlled trial with 35 PD patients. Treatments lasted 1 month during which subjects received 16 sessions. Vocal intensity improved in subjects receiving LSVT and this improvement was still detectable 24 months after cessation of therapy (Ramig et al., 2001). In analogy to the augmentation of strength and amplitude of limb movements that can be achieved with sensory cueing or volitional effort LSVT enables patients to voluntarily mobilize vocal force. The critical issue, as in many rehabilitative approaches in PD, is the carry-over from the artificial setting of therapeutic sessions to everyday communication. In order to allow for this carry-over to occur high-intensity training (including 16

sessions lasting 50–60 min each during 4 weeks) has been recommended for the LSVT technique.

Other techniques, focused more on prosody than volume, have been introduced by Robertson and Thomson (1984) and Johnson and Prang (1990).

Psychosocial counseling

PD is a progressive disorder that affects quality of life and psychosocial situation of both patients and relatives. Evolving motor and mental disturbances, depression and subsequent predicament, and disability require frequent readjustment in coping skills for patients and caregivers. Although relevance of psychosocial problems in PD is reflected by numerous reports only few studies have been undertaken to evaluate the impact of specific psychosocial interventions (Goetz et al., 2002). Ellgring et al. (1993) introduced a comprehensive program based on seminars including coping skills, relaxation techniques, modeling, role-playing and cognitive restructuring. Another approach, based on patient education with personalized written counseling was presented by Montgomery et al. (1994). Due to the lack of sufficient scientific evidence concerning methodology psychosocial interventions often needs to rely on subjective empirical experience. Positive reinforcement of activity, encouragement to be interactive and communicative and noncompetitive exercising of social and motor skills are intuitively recommendable.

35.4 Dystonia

Definition and classification

Dystonia has been defined as a syndrome of sustained muscle contractions, frequently causing twisting and repetitive movements, or abnormal postures (Fahn, 1984). Categorization is complex since the term "dystonia" can be used to describe a symptom, a number of syndromes, or can be the clinical expression of genetic disease. Classifications relating to etiology (Table 35.4), age of onset (before or after 26 years) and distribution of affected body parts are currently used in clinical practice. These classifications are interrelated since, for example, age of onset interacts with the probability of genetic causes (higher in younger subjects) and body distribution (generalized dystonia more likely in childhood onset).

The classes of distribution of dystonia include focal, segmental, multifocal, generalized and hemidystonia. Focal dystonia is restricted to a single body region (neck – torticollis, face – blepharospasm). Segmental dystonia involves contiguous body regions (blepharospasm and oromandibular dystonia – cranial dystonia). Multifocal dystonia comprises at least two separated focal forms (e.g. blepharospasm and writer's cramp). Generalized dystonia includes one lower limb and adjacent pelvic region, and at least one further region, or both legs. In hemidystonia symptoms are restricted to one-half of the body.

Table 35.4. Classification of dystonia.

Primary dystonia (dystonia is the sole clinical sign, some have a genetic basis)
  Autosomal dominant
    Early limb (DYT1, unknown genetic causes)
    Mixed (DYT6, DYT13, others)
    Late focal (DYT7, others)
  Recessive, complex inheritance
  Sporadic
Dystonia-plus syndrome (dystonia plus other features)
  Myoclonus (myoclonus dystonia) DYT11
  Parkinsonism (dopa-responsive dystonia, DYT5, DYT14, DYT12)
Secondary dystonia (identifiable causes)
  For example: anoxia, stroke, toxins, drugs, metabolic disorders
Heredodegenerative diseases
  For example: Wilson's disease, Huntington's disease, etc.
Paroxysmal dystonias
  PKD/PKC, paroxysmal non-kinesiogenic dyskinesia (PNKD)/paroxysmal dystonic choreoathetosis (PDC), paroxysmal exercise-induced dyskinesia/dystonia (PED)

Neurobiology and neurogenetics

Clinical observation and electromyography (EMG) allow to differentiate tonic, phasic, tremulous or myoclonic activity in dystonic muscles (Wissel et al., 2003). There is no abnormality in conventional needle EMG and peripheral and central conduction times (Berardelli et al., 1998). Poly-EMG recordings typically convey co-contraction of antagonistic muscles and overflow phenomenon (involuntary activation of muscles normally not involved in the performance of specific movements) (Wissel et al., 2003). Enhanced excitability of neural reflex circuitries at spinal cord, brainstem and cortical level has been reported by various authors (Tolosa et al., 1988; Rothwell et al., 1983; Deuschl et al., 1995; Kaji et al., 1995; Ikoma et al., 1996). Recently inadequate cortical surround inhibition during performance of voluntary movements has been described by Sohn and Hallett (2004). Basal ganglia dysfunction in idiopathic dystonia has been confirmed by simultaneous EMG and deep brain recordings demonstrating disturbed basal ganglia activation related to dystonic movements (Zhuang et al., 2004).

Idiopathic dystonia includes sporadic and hereditary cases. Presently 14 types of hereditary dystonia have been identified (de Carvalho Aguiar and Ozelius 2002; Klein and Ozelius 2002). DYT1 dystonia is due to a dominant GAG deletion in the gene for torsin A on the long arm of chromosome 9. In a recent study torsin A deposition was found in different midbrain regions considered to be relevant for disturbance of motor control and basal ganglia dysfunction in DYT1 positive dystonia (McNaught et al., 2004).

Secondary dystonia includes cases with brain lesions in the contralateral basal ganglia, mainly in the putamen (Bhathia and Marsden, 1994), intoxications, tardive dystonia following exposure to neuroleptics and post-traumatic forms of dystonia.

Diagnosis and clinical features

In an individual patient, the clinical expression of dystonia depends on the combination of hyperkinetic and hypokinetic patterns. Some patients present tonic abnormal postures with slowness of movements, others phasic hyperkinetic movements with normal tone. Brisk, irregular or pseudorhythmic jerks can be called myoclonus or rapid dystonic movements and many dystonic patients also display tremor. These patterns are not specific to a particular cause of dystonia since identical phenotypes of movement disturbances can be provoked by a variety of familial and secondary forms of dystonia.

Childhood onset or onset in early adulthood with initial limb dystonia is associated with higher risk of progression to multifocal or generalized forms. In contrast, adult-onset and cranio-cervical dystonias seldom progress to multifocal or generalized forms. Most focal dystonias belong to the category of primary dystonia but some clinical features suggest rare secondary forms including abrupt onset, prominent pain from the onset and fixed posture in adult-onset cervical dystonia.

Post-traumatic dystonia, developing after a (usually minor) focal injury may present with typical focal dystonia or fixed dystonia, usually of one limb. The latter pattern is often associated with features of complex regional pain syndrome or features of somatoform disorder or psychogenic dystonia (Schrag et al., 2004).

Paroxysmal kinesiogenic dyskinesias/choreoathetosis (PKD/PKC) is usually due to an autosomal dominant inheritance. The clinical picture consists of brief episodes of involuntary movement, either choreic or dystonic or a mixture of both, usually lasting 30–60 s and mostly affecting the limb(s) on one side of the body. These episodes usually start in childhood and may occur up to dozens of times per day.

Dystonia can be task specific like in case of writer's or musician's cramp, induced by movement (kinesiogenic dystonia) or occur without any specific trigger. The intensity of symptoms can be influenced by physical activation, psychologic stress or sensory tricks (e.g. geste antagonistique in cervical dystonia). Diurnal fluctuations occur in 50% of cases with dopa-responsive dystonia (Segawa et al., 1986).

Initial work-up of dystonia should include MRI and screening for a genetic-, metabolic- or drug-related origin. In cases of young onset absence of dramatic response to levodopa suggestive of dopa-responsive dystonia and clinical/laboratory signs of Wilson's disease (Kayser-Fleischer ring, disturbance of copper metabolism) should be excluded.

Medical and surgical treatment of dystonia

Botulinum toxin injections in dystonic muscles have been shown to be an effective and safe treatment of focal dystonia (Jankovic, 2004). The mechanism of action is a dose dependent, reversible and locally restricted neuromuscular blockade by blocking release of acetylcholine at the motor endplate. Improvement of dystonic symptoms and associated pain typically lasts for 2–4 months. Btx type A (BtxA) is registered in USA (Botox®) and most countries of Europe (Botox®, Dysport® and Xeomin®) for treatment of blepharospasm, and BtxA (USA, Botox®; most countries of Europe Botox®, Dysport® and Xeomin®) and Btx type B (BtxB) (Myo- or Neurobloc®) are registered for cervical dystonia.

Systemic side-effects of BtxA are rare and, like local paresis, dose-related. A change of toxin serotype (from BtxA to BtxB and vice versa) is recommended when secondary non-response to Btx occurs. Sonographic- or EMG-guidance can be useful to ensure precise muscle targeting in difficult locations (Comella et al., 1992; Wissel et al., 2003).

Use of acetylcholine inhibitors (ACI) is the systemic drug treatment of dystonia most consistently reported as beneficial. With the exception of treatment of acute dystonic reactions following exposure to neuroleptics, clinical effects are usually not dramatic. Most open-label reports of anticholinergic therapy of dystonia have used trihexyphenidyl with gradual increase of dosage (Marsden et al., 1984; Gimenez-Roldan et al., 2004). In a controlled double-blind study 30 mg of trihexyphenidyl led to significant improvement of dystonia in about 70% of adult-onset patients (Burke et al., 1986). Whereas children seem to tolerate high doses of trihexyphenidyl use of dosages beyond 15 mg is often limited by side-effects in adults. In cases of non-response or side-effects from acetylcholine-inhibitors (ACI), tetrabenazine (up to150 mg/day) alone or in combination with ACI is recommended. In some patients a triple medication of ACI, tetrabenazine and sulpiride ("Marsden Cocktail") is effective. Third line treatment includes clonazepam, baclofen, levetiracetam or riluzol (Greene et al., 1988). Continuous intrathecal infusion of baclofen can be considered in severe axial or generalized dystonia.

Bilateral DBS of the globus pallidus (Gpi) has been shown to be effective in DYT1 positive generalized dystonia (Coubes et al., 2004; Krauss et al., 2004) and benefit in DYT1 negative primary generalized dystonia is of similar magnitude ranging between 50% and 70% improvement on the Burke–Marsden–Fahn dystonia rating scale (Cif et al., 2003; Yianni et al., 2003). In addition, several case reports have shown effectiveness of DBS in a variety of idiopathic and symptomatic forms of focal and segmental dystonia. Outcome of DBS in dystonia seems to be mainly dependent on the phenotype of dystonia with phasic pattern including mobile dystonia, tremor and myoclonic dystonia being more responsive than fixed dystonic postures (Vercueil et al., 2002). Pallidal stimulation for dystonia requires high energy consumption with frequent replacement of devices. Compared to pallidotomy, DBS for dystonia is associated with less surgical morbidity but much more expensive.

A further surgical treatment option is selective peripheral denervation which may be considered in some cases of torticollis refractory to botulinum toxin (Cohen-Gadol et al., 2003). Ultimately, optimal functional restoration in Parkinson's disease may involve re-establishment of dopaminergic innervation through cell transplantation and gene therapy techniques. Clinical trails have already begun and these are reviewed in Volume I, Chapter 34 and Volume II, Chapter 6.

Rehabilitative treatment of dystonia

Neuromodulation techniques

Leis et al. (1992) showed improvement of cervical dystonia in 50% of patients treated with selective electrical stimulation. Tinazzi et al. (2004) reported high-frequency transcutaneous electrical nerve stimulation (TENS) to be effective in hand dystonia. Modulation of reciprocal inhibition and cortical excitability of forearm flexor and extensor muscles was suggested as the mechanism of action.

Low-frequency repetitive transcranial magnetic stimulation (rTMS) decreases excitability of the cortex stimulated. Application of low-frequency rTMS to contralateral cortical areas involved in dystonia showed temporary relieve of hemidystonia (Lefaucheur et al., 2004) and task-specific dystonia (Murase et al., 2005).

Multidisciplinary rehabilitative treatment of dystonia is time-consuming and should include daily reinforcement in a self-training program (Bleton, 1994; Byl et al., 2002; Zeuner and Hallett, 2003). Physical measures including stretching and local use of massage and warm baths can reduce muscle tonus and alleviate local pain.

Bleton (1994) emphasized physiotherapy and motor retraining programs in patients with cervical dystonia. Exercises should be based on the analysis of abnormal posture and dystonic movements and include repetitive stretching of shortened and reinforcement of weak muscles in a daily training program. Recently a controlled trial evaluating the effects of a standard biofeedback treatment and a physiotherapy program (postural re-education exercises and passive elongation of cervical muscles) reported superiority of physiotherapy (Samania et al., 2003). Evaluation included head realignment, disability and pain 3, 6 and 9 months after the end of the treatments, and showed enduring reduction of disability and pain for up to 3–9 months after treatment.

Evaluation of long-term outcome of treatment approaches in focal hand dystonia in task-specific dystonia in musicians (string instrumentalists) including nerve decompression, traditional physical therapy, retraining, and anticholinergic drugs and botulinum toxin injections or splint devices showed limited benefit with only 38% of the artists being able to maintain their professional careers (Schuele and Lederman, 2004). Byl et al., 2003 reported the effects of a training program for task-specific focal hand dystonia. In this study patients were required to stop performing tasks causing dystonia, to participate in a wellness program (aerobics, postural exercises, stress-free hand use), and to carry out supervised, attended, individualized, repetitive sensorimotor training activities at least once a week for 12 weeks with daily reinforcement at home. Standard tests documented improvements in functional imaging (somatosensory hand representation), target-specific hand control, fine motor skills and sensory discrimination. According to Zeuner and Hallett (2003) learning of braille reading used as a sensory training (30–60 min daily) for 8 weeks improved symptoms in patients with focal hand dystonia.

35.5 Other movement disorders

To date there are, to our knowledge, no randomized clinical trials, comparative group outcome studies or controlled single case studies on the effects of rehabilitation strategies in chorea, myoclonus and tremors. In addition to medical treatment ancillary behavioral modification techniques have been recommended for tic disorders and Tourette syndrome (Jankovic, 2002).

REFERENCES

Abbruzzese, G. and Berardelli, A. (2003). Sensorimotor integration in movement disorders. *Mov Disord*, **18**, 231–240.

Alexander, G.E., DeLong, N.R. and Strick, P.L. (1986). Parallel organization of functional segregated circuits linking basal ganglia and cortex. *Annu Rev Neurosci*, **9**, 351–357.

Azulay, J., Mesure, S., Amblard, B., Blin, O., Sangla, I. and Pouget, J. (1999). Visual control of locomotion in Parkinson's disease. *Brain*, **117**, 1169–1181.

Bain, P.G., Findley, L.J., Thompson, P.D., et al. (1994). A study of hereditary essential tremor. *Brain*, **117**, 805–824.

Behrman, A., Teitelbaum, P. and Cauraugh, J. (1998). Verbal instructional sets to normalize the temporal and spatial gait variables in Parkinson's disease. *J Neurol Neurosurg Psychiatr*, **65**, 580–582.

Bennett, D.A., Beckett, L.A., Murray, A.M., et al. (1996). Prevalence of parkinsonian signs and associated mortality in a community population of older people. *New Engl J Med*, **334**, 71–76.

Berardelli, A., Rothwell, J.C., Hallet, M., Thompson, P.D., Manfredi, M. and Marsden, C.D. (1998). The Pathophysiology of primary dystonia. *Brain*, **121**, 1195–1212.

Bhatia, K.P. and Marsden, C.D. (1994). The behavioural and motor consequences of focal lesions of the basal ganglia in man. *Brain*, **117**, 859–876.

Bleton, J.P. (1994). *Spasmodic Torticollis. Handbook of Rehabilitative Physiotherapy*. Edition Frison-Roche, Paris.

Bloem, B.R., Hausdorff, J.M., Visser, J.E. and Giladi, N. (2004). Falls and freezing of gait in Parkinson's disease: a review of two interconnected, episodic phenomena. *Mov Disord*, **19**, 871–884.

Bonnet, A.M., Loria, Y., Saint-Hilaire, M.H., Lhermitee, F. and Agid, Y. (1987). Does long-term aggravation of Parkinson's disease result from nondopaminergic lesions? *Neurology*, **37**, 1539–1542.

Braak, H., Del Tredici, K., Rub, U., et al. (2003). Staging of brain pathology related to sporadic Parkinson's disease. *Neurobiol Aging*, **24**, 197–211.

Brefel-Courbon, C., Desboeuf, K., Thalamas, C., et al. (2003). Clinical and economic analysis of spa therapy in Parkinson's disease. *Mov Disord*, **18**, 578–584.

Brooks, D.J. (2002). Movement disorders. In: *Functional Imaging in Parkinson's Disease and Movement Disorders* (eds Jankovic, J.J. and Tolosa, E.), 4th edn, Lippincott Williams & Wilkins, Philadelphia, PA, pp. 610–631.

Brotchie, P., Iansek, R. and Horne, M.K. (1991). Motor function of the monkey globus pallidus. 1. Neuronal discharge and parameters of movement. *Brain*, **114**, 1667–1683.

Burke, R.E., Fahn, S. and Marsden, C.D. (1986). Torsion dystonia: a double-blind, prospective trial of high-dosage trihexyphenidyl. *Neurology*, **36**, 160–164.

Byl, N.N., Nagarajan, S.S., Merzenich, M.M., Roberts, T. and McKenzie, A.L. (2002). Correlation of clinical neuromusculoskeletal and central somatosensory performance: variability in controls and patients with severe and mild focal hand dystonia. *Neural Plast*, **9**, 177–203.

Byl, N.N., Nagajaran, S. and McKenzie, A.L. (2003). Effect of sensory discrimination training on structure and function in patients with focal hand dystonia: a case series. *Arch Phys Med Rehabil*, **84**, 1505–1514.

Cif, L., El Fertit, H., Vayssiere, N., et al. (2003). Treatment of dystonic syndromes by chronic electrical stimulation of the internal globus pallidus. *J Neurosurg Sci*, **47**, 52–55.

Cohen-Gadol, A.A., Ahlskog, J.E., Matsumoto, J.Y., Swenson, M.A., McClelland, R.L. and Davis, D.H. (2003). Selective peripheral denervation for the treatment of intractable spasmodic torticollis: experience with 168 patients at the Mayo Clinic. *J Neurosurg*, **98**, 1247–1254.

Comella, C.L., Stebbins, G.T., Brown-Toms, N. and Goetz, C.G. (1994). Physical therapy and Parkinson's disease: a controlled clinical trial. *Neurology*, **44**, 376–378.

Comella, L.C., Buchmann, A.S., Tanner, C.M., Brown-Toms, N.C. and Goetz, C.G. (1992). Botulinum toxin injection for spasmodic torticollis: increased magnitude of benefit with electromyographic assistance. *Neurology*, **42**, 878–882.

Coubes, P., Cif, L., El Fertit, H., Hemm, S., Vayssiere, N., Serrat, S., Picot, M.C., Tuffery, S., et al. (2004). Electrical stimulation of the globus pallidus internus in patients with primary generalized dystonia: long-term results. *J Neurosurg*, **101**, 189–194.

Critchley, M. (1929). Arteriosclerotic parkinsonism. *Brain*, **52**, 23–83.

Dam, M., Tonin, P. and Casson, S. (1996). Effects of conventional and sensory-enhanced physiotherapy on disability of Parkinson's disease patients. *Adv Neurol*, **69**, 551–555.

de Carvalho Aguiar, P.M. and Ozelius, L.J. (2002). Classification and genetics of dystonia. *Lancet Neurol*, **1**, 316–325.

De Rijk, M.C., Tzourio, C., Breteler, M.M., et al. (1997). Prevalence of parkinsonism and Parkinson's disease in Europe: the Euro-Parkinson collaborative study. *J Neurol Neurosurg Psychiatr*, **62**, 10–15.

Deane, K.H., Jones, D., Playford, E.D., Ben Shlomo, Y. and Clarke, C.E. (2001). Physiotherapy for patients with Parkinson's disease (Cochrane Review). *Cochrane Database Syst Rev 3*. CD002817.

Demirci, M., Grill, S., McShane, L. and Hallelett, M. (1997). A mismatch between kinaesthetic and visual perception in Parkinson's disease. *Ann Neurol*, **41**, 781–788.

Deuschl, G., Toro, C., Matsumoto, J. and Hallett, M. (1995). Movement-related cortical potentials in writer's cramp. *Ann Neurol*, **38**, 509–514.

Dietz, M.A., Goetz, C.G. and Stebbins, G.T. (1990). Evaluation of a modified inverted walking stick as a treatment for parkinsonian freezing episodes. *Mov Disord*, **5**, 243–247.

Ellgring, H., Seiler, S., Perleth, B., Frings, W., Gasser, T. and Oertel, W. (1993). Psychosocial aspects of Parkinson's disease. *Neurology*, **43(12 Suppl. 6)**, S41–S44.

Emre, M. (2003). Dementia associated with Parkinson's disease. *Lancet Neurol*, **2**, 229–237.

Fahn, S. (1984). The varied clinical expression of dystonia. *Neurol Clin*, **2**, 541–554.

Fellows, S.J., Noth, J. and Schwarz, M. (1998). Precision grip and Parkinson's disease. *Brain*, **121**, 1771–1784.

Fitzgerald, P.M. and Jankovic, J. (1989). Lower body parkinsonism: evidence for vascular etiology. *Mov Disord*, **4**, 249–260.

Formisano, R., Pratesi, L., Modarelli, F.T., Bonifati, V. and Meco, G. (1992). Rehabilitation and Parkinson's disease. *Scand J Rehabil Med*, **24**, 157–160.

Gai, W.P., Power, J.H., Blumbergs, P.C., et al. (1998). Multiple-system atrophy: a new alpha-synuclein disease? *Lancet*, **352**, 547–548.

Gauthier, L., Dalziel, S. and Gautier, S. (1987). The benefits of group occupational therapy for patients with Parkinson's disease. *Am J Occup Ther*, **41**, 360–365.

Georgiou, N., Iansek, R., Bradshaw, J., Phillips, J., Mattingley, J. and Bradshaw, J. (1993). An evaluation of the role of internal cues in the pathogenesis of parkinsonian hypokinesia. *Brain*, **116**, 1575–1587.

Gibb, W.R. and Lees, A.J. (1988). The relevance of the Lewy body to the pathogenesis of idiopathic Parkinson's disease. *J Neurol Neurosurg Psychiatr*, **51**, 745–752.

Gibberd, F.B., Page, N.G., Spencer, K.M., Kinnear, E. and Hawksworth, J.B. (1981). Controlled trial of physiotherapy and occupational therapy for Parkinson's disease. *Br Med J*, **282**, 1196.

Giladi, N., McMahon, D., Przedborski, S., et al. (1992). Motor blocks in Parkinson's disease. *Neurology*, **42**, 333–339.

Gimenez-Roldan, S., Mateo, D. and Martin, M. (2004). Life-threatening cranial dystonia following trihexyphenidyl withdrawal. *Mov Disord*, **18**, 349–353.

Goetz, C.G., Koller, W.C., Poewe, W., et al. (2002). Management of Parkinson's disease: an evidence-based review. *Mov Disord*, **17(Suppl. 4)**, 156–166.

Greene, P.E., Shale, H. and Fahn, S. (1988). Analysis of open-label trials in torsion dystonia using high dosages of anticholinergics and other drugs. *Mov Disord*, **3**, 46–60.

Hirsch, M.A., Toole, T., Maitland, C.G. and Rider, R.A. (2003). The effects of balance training and high-intensity resistance training on persons with idiopathic Parkinson's disease. *Arch Phys Med Rehabil*, **84(8)**, 1109–1117.

Hoehn, M.M. and Yahr, M.D.P. (1967). Parkinsonism: onset, progression and mortality. *Neurology*, **17**, 427–442.

Holloway, R.G., Shoulson, I., Fahn, S., et al. (2004). Pramipexole vs levodopa as initial treatment for Parkinson disease: a 4-year randomized controlled trial. *Arch Neurol*, **61**, 1044–1053.

Hughes, A.J., Daniel, S.E., Ben-Shlomo, Y. and Lees, A.J. (2002). The accuracy of diagnosis of parkinsonian syndromes in a specialist movement disorder service. *Brain*, **125**, 861–870.

Ikoma, K., Samii, A., Mercuri, B., Wassermann, E.M. and Hallett, M. (1996). Abnormal cortical motor excitability in dystonia. *Neurology*, **46**, 1371–1376.

Ito, N., Hayshi, A., Lin, W., Ohkoshi, N., Watanabe, M. and Shoji, S. (2000). Music therapy in Parkinson's disease: improvement of parkinsonian gait and depression with rhythmic auditory stimulation. In: *Integrated Human Brain Science* (ed. Nakada, N.), Elsevier Science, New York, pp. 435–443.

Jankovic, J. (2002). Tics and Tourette syndrome. In: *Parkinson's Disease and Movement Disorders* (eds Jankovic, J.J. and

Tolosa, E.), 4th edn, Lippincott Williams & Wilkins, Philadelphia, PA, pp. 311–330.

Jankovic, J. (2004). Botulinum toxin in clinical practice. *J Neurol Neurosurg Psychiatr*, **75**, 951–957.

Jankovic, J. and Kapadia, A.S. (2001). Functional decline in Parkinson disease. *Arch Neurol*, **58**, 1611–1615.

Jöbges, M., Heuschkel, G., Pretzel, C., Illhardt, C., Renner, C. and Hummelsheim, H. (2004). Repetitive training of compensatory steps: a therapeutic approach for postural instability in Parkinson's disease. *J Neurol Neurosurg Psychiatr*, **75**, 1682–1687.

Johnson, J.A. and Prang, T.R. (1990). Speech therapy and Parkinson's disease: a review and further data. *Br J Disord Commun*, **25**, 183–194.

Kaji, R., Ikeda, A., Ikeda, T., Kubori, T., Mezaki, T., Kohara, N., Kanda, M., Nagamine, T., Honda, M. and Rothwell, J.C. (1995). Physiological study of cervical dystonia. Task specific abnormality in contingent negative variation. *Brain*, **118**, 511–522.

Katsikitis, M. and Pilowsky, I. (1996). A controlled study of facial mobility treatment in Parkinson's disease. *J Psychosom Res*, **40**, 387–396.

Khan, N.L., Graham, E., Critchley, P., et al. (2003). Parkin disease: a phenotypic study of a large case series. *Brain*, **126**, 1279–1292.

Klein, C. and Ozelius, L.J. (2002). Dystonia: clinical features, genetics, and treatment. *Curr Opin Neurol*, **15**, 491–497.

Klockgether, T. and Dichgans, J. (1994). Visual control of arm movements in Parkinson's disease. *Mov Disord*, **9**, 48–56.

Klockgether, T., Borutta, M., Rapp, H., Spieker, S. and Dichgans, J. (1995). A defect of kinesthesia in Parkinson's disease. *Mov Disord*, **10**, 460–465.

Koller, W.C., Busenbark, K. and Miner, K. (1994). The relationship of essential tremor to other movement disorders: report on 678 patients. Essential Tremor Study Group. *Ann Neurol*, **35**, 717–723.

Krauss, M., Fogel, W., Kloss, M., Rasche, D., Volkmann, J. and Tronnier, V. (2004). Pallidal stimulation for dystonia. *Neurosurgery*, **55**, 1361–1370.

Lefaucheur, J.P., Fenelon, G., Menard-Lefaucheur, I., Wendling, S. and Nguyen, J.P. (2004). Low-frequency repetitive TMS of premotor cortex can reduce painful axial spasms in generalized secondary dystonia: a pilot study of three patients. *Neurophysiol Clin*, **34**, 141–145.

Leis, A.A., Dimitrijevic, M.R., Delapasse, J.S. and Sharkey, P.C. (1992). Modification of cervical dystonia by selective sensory stimulation. *J Neurol Sci*, **110**, 79–89.

Louis, E.D., Ottman, R. and Hauser, W.A. (1998). How common is the most common adult movement disorder? Estimates of the prevalence of essential tremor throughout the world. *Mov Disord*, **13**, 5–10.

Marchese, R., Diverio, M., Zucchi, F., Lentino, C. and Abbruzzese, G. (2000). The role of sensory cues in the rehabilitation of parkinsonian patients: a comparison of two physical therapy protocols. *Mov Disord*, **15**, 879–883.

Marsden, C.D. (1982). The mysterious motor function of the basal ganglia: the Robert Wartenberg Lecture. *Neurology*, **32**, 514–539.

Marsden, C.D., Marion, M.H. and Quinn, N.P. (1984). The treatment of severe dystonia in children and adults. *J Neurol Neurosurg Psychiatr*, **47**, 1166–1173.

Martin, J.P. (1967). *The Basal Ganglia and Posture*, Pitman, London.

McIntosh, G.C., Brown, S.H., Rice, R.R. and Thaut, M.H. (1997). Rhythmic auditory-motor facilitation of gait patterns in patients with Parkinson's disease. *J Neurol Neurosurg Psychiatr*, **62**, 22–26.

McKeith, I., Mintzer, J., Aarsland, D., et al. (2004). Dementia with Lewy bodies. *Lancet Neurol*, **3**, 19–28.

McKeith, I.G., Galasko, D., Kosaka, K., et al. (1996). Consensus guidelines for the clinical and pathologic diagnosis of dementia with Lewy bodies (DLB): report of the consortium on DLB international workshop. *Neurology*, **47**, 1113–1124.

McNaught, K.S., Kapustin, A., Jackson, T., Jengelley, T.A., Jnobaptiste, R., Shashidharan, P., Perl, D.P., Pasik, P. and Olanow, C.W. (2004). Brainstem pathology in DYT1 primary torsion dystonia. *Ann Neurol*, **56**, 540–547.

Meara, J., Bhowmick, B.K. and Hobson, P. (1999). Accuracy of diagnosis in patients with presumed Parkinson's disease. *Age Ageing*, **28**, 99–102.

Montgomery Jr., E.B., Lieberman, A., Singh, G. and Fries, J.F. (1994). Patient education and health promotion can be effective in Parkinson's disease: a randomized controlled trial. PROPATH Advisory Board. *Am J Med*, **97**, 429–435.

Moore, A.P. (1987). Impaired sensorimotor integration in parkinsonism and dyskinesias: a role of corollary discharges? *J Neurol Neurosurg Psychiatr*, **50**, 544–552.

Morris, M.E., Iansek, R., Matyas, T.A. and Summers, J.J. (1994). Ability to modulate walking cadence remains intact in Parkinson's disease. *J Neurol Neurosurg Psychiatr*, **57**, 1532–1534.

Morris, M.E., Iansek, R., Matyas, T.A. and Summers, J.J. (1996). Stride length regulation in Parkinson's disease. Normalisation strategies and underlying mechanisms. *Brain*, **119**, 551–568.

Morrish, P.K., Sawle, G.V. and Brooks, D.J. (1996). Regional changes in [18F]dopa metabolism in the striatum in Parkinson's disease. *Brain*, **119**, 2097–2103.

Muller, J., Wenning, G.K., Jellinger, K., McKee, A., Poewe, W. and Litvan, I. (2000). Progression of Hoehn and Yahr stages in Parkinsonian disorders: a clinicopathologic study. *Neurology*, **55**, 888–891.

Muller, J., Kiechl, S., Wenning, G.K., et al. (2002). The prevalence of primary dystonia in the general community. *Neurology*, **59**, 941–943.

Müller, V., Mohr, B., Rosin, R., Pulvermüller, F., Müller, F. and Birbaumer, N. (1997). Short-term effects of behavioral treatment on movement initiation and postural control in Parkinson's disease: a controlled clinical study. *Mov Disord*, **12**, 306–314.

Murase, N., Rothwell, J.C., Kaji, R., Urushihara, R., Nakamura, K., Murayama, N., Igasaki, T., Sakata-Igasaki, M., Mima, T., Ikeda, A. and Shibasaki, H. (2005). Subthreshold low-frequency repetitive transcranial magnetic stimulation over the premotor cortex modulates writer's cramp. *Brain*, **128**, 104–115.

Palmer, S.S., Mortimer, J.A. and Webster, D.D. (1986). Exercise therapy for Parkinson's disease. *Arch Phys Med Rehabil*, **67**, 741–745.

Parent, A. and Cicchetti, F. (1998). The current model of basal ganglia organization under scrutiny. *Mov Disord*, **13**, 199–202.

Polymeropoulos, M.H., Lavedan, C., Leroy, E., et al. (1997). Mutation in the alpha-synuclein gene identified in families with Parkinson's disease. *Science*, **276**, 2045–2047.

Ramig, L.O., Countryman, S., O'Brien, C., Hoehn, M. and Thompson, L. (1996). Intensive speech treatment for patients with Parkinson's disease: short- and long-term comparison of two techniques. *Neurology*, **47**, 1496–1504.

Ramig, L.O., Sapir, S., Fox, C. and Countryman, S. (2001). Changes in vocal loudness following intensive voice treatment (LSVT) in individuals with Parkinson's disease: a comparison with untreated patients and normal age-matched controls. *Mov Disord*, **16**, 79–83.

Rascol, O., Brooks, D.J., Korczyn, A.D., De Deyn, P.P., Clarke, C.E. and Lang, A.E. (2000). A five-year study of the incidence of dyskinesia in patients with early Parkinson's disease who were treated with ropinirole or levodopa. 056 Study Group. *New Engl J Med*, **342**, 1484–1491.

Robertson, S.J. and Thomson, F. (1984). Speech therapy in Parkinson's disease: a study of the efficacy and long term effects of intensive treatment. *Br J Disord Commun*, **19**, 213–224.

Rothdach, A.J., Trnkwalder, C., Haberstock, J., et al. (2000). Prevalence and risk factors of RLS in an elderly population: the MEMO study. *Neurology*, **54**, 1064–1068.

Rothwell, J.C., Obeso, J.A., Day, B.L. and Marsden, C.D. (1983). Pathophysiology of dystonias. Motor control mechanisms in health and disease. In: *Motor Control Mechanisms in Health and Disease* (ed. Desmedt, J.E.), Raven Press, New York, pp. 851–872.

Rubinstein, T.C., Giladi, N. and Hausdorff, J.M. (2002). The power of cueing to circumvent dopamine deficits: a review of physical therapy treatment of gait disturbances in Parkinson's disease. *Mov Disord*, **17**, 1148–1160.

Samania, N., Corato, E., Tinazzi, M., Montagnana, B., Fiaschi, A. and Aglioti, S.M. (2003). The effect of two different rehabilitation treatments in cervical dystonia: preliminary results in four patients. *Funct Neurol*, **18**, 219–225.

Schenkman, M., Cutson, T.M., Kuchibhatla, M., et al. (1998). Exercise to improve spinal flexibility and function for people with Parkinson's disease: a randomised controlled study. *J Am Geriatr Soc*, **46**, 1207–1221.

Schrag, A. (2002). Epidemiology of movement disorders. In: *Parkinson's Disease and Movement Disorders* (eds Jankovic, J.J. and Tolosa, E.), 4th edn., Lippincott Williams & Wilkins, Philadelphia, PA, pp. 73–89.

Schrag, A., Good, C.D., Miszkiel, K., et al. (2000). Differentiation of atypical parkinsonian syndromes with routine MRI. *Neurology*, **54**, 697–702.

Schrag, A., Ben-Shlomo, Y. and Quinn, N. (2002). How valid is the clinical diagnosis of Parkinson's disease in the community? *J Neurol Neurosurg Psychiatr*, **73**, 529–534.

Schrag, A., Trimble, M., Quinn, N. and Bhatia, K. (2004). The syndrome of fixed dystonia: an evaluation of 103 patients. *Brain*, **127**, 2360–2372.

Schuele, S. and Lederman, R.J. (2004). Long-term outcome of focal dystonia in string instrumentalists. *Mov Disord*, **19**, 43–48.

Segawa, M., Nomura, Y. and Kase, M. (1986). Diurnally fluctuating hereditary progressive dystonia. In: *Extrapyramidal Disorders* (eds Vinken, P.J., Bruyn, G.W. and Klawans, H.L.), Vol. 5, Elsevier, Amsterdam, pp. 529–540.

Shahed, J. and Jankovic, J. (2001). Re-emergence of childhood stuttering in Parkinson's disease: a hypothesis. *Mov Disord*, **16**, 114–118.

Sohn, Y.H. and Hallett, M. (2004). Disturbed surround inhibition in focal hand dystonia. *Ann Neurol*, **56**, 595–599.

Stern, G.M., Lander, C.M. and Lees, A.J. (1980). Akinetic freezing and trick movements in Parkinson's disease. *J Neural Transm* (**Suppl. 16**), 137–141.

Thaut, M.H., McIntosh, G.C., Rice, R.R., Miller, R.A., Rathbun, J. and Brault, J.M. (1996). Rhythmic auditory stimulation in gait training for Parkinson's disease patients. *Mov Disord*, **11**, 193–200.

Tinazzi, M., Zarattini, S., Valeriani, M., Romito, S., Farina, S., Moretto, G., Smania, N., Fiaschi, A. and Abbruzzese, G. (2004). Long-lasting modulation of human motor cortex following prolonged transcutaneous electrical nerve stimulation (TENS) of forearm muscles: evidence of reciprocal inhibition and facilitation. *Exp Brain Res*, **16** [Epub ahead of print].

Tolosa, E., Montserrat, L. and Bayes, A. (1988). Blink reflex studies in focal dystonias: enhanced excitability of brainstem interneurons in cranial dystonia and spasmodic torticollis. *Mov Disord*, **3**, 61–69.

Tolosa, E., Valldeoriola, F. and Pastor, P. (2002) Progressive supranuclear palsy. In: *Parkinson's Disease and Movement Disorders* (eds Jankovic, J.J. and Tolosa, E.), 4th edn, Lippincott Williams & Wilkins, Philadelphia, PA, pp. 73–89.

Van De Warrenburg, B.P., Lammens, M., Luecking, C.B., et al. (2001). Clinical and pathologic abnormalities in a family with parkinsonism and parkin gene mutations. *Neurology*, **56**, 555–557.

Vercueil, L., Krack, P. and Pollak, P. (2002). Results of deep brain stimulation for dystonia: a critical reappraisal. *Mov Disord*, **17(Suppl. 3)**, 89–93.

Volkmann, J., Allert, N., Voges, J., Weiss, P.H., Freund, H.J. and Sturm, V. (2001). Safety and efficacy of pallidal or subthalamic nucleus stimulation in advanced PD. *Neurology*, **56**, 548–551.

Wade, D.T., Gage, H., Owen, C., Trend, P., Grossmith, C. and Kaye, J. (2003). Multidisciplinary rehabilitation for people with Parkinson's disease: a randomised controlled study. *J Neurol Neurosurg Psychiatr*, **74**, 158–162.

Ward, C.D. (2000). Rehabilitation in Parkinson's disease and parkinsonism. In: *Parkinson's Disease and Parkinsonism in the Elderly* (eds Meara, J. and Koller, W.C.), Cambridge University Press, Cambridge, UK, pp. 165–184.

Weiner, W.J. and Singer, C. (1989). Parkinson's disease and non-pharmacological treatment programs. *J Am Geriatr Soc*, **37**, 359–363.

Wenning, G.K., Ben-Shlomo, Y., Maglhaes, M., et al. (1995). Clinical features and natural history of multiple system atrophy: an analysis of 100 cases. *Brain*, **117**, 835–845.

Wissel, J., Müller, J. and Poewe, W. (2003). EMG for identification of dystonic, tremulous and spastic muscles and techniques for guidance of injections. In: *Handbook of Botulinum Toxin Treatment* (eds Moore, P. and Naumann, M.), Blackwell Science, Malden, MA, pp. 76–98.

Witjas, T., Kaphan, E., Azulay, J.P., et al. (2002). *Nonmotor fluctuations in Parkinson's disease: frequent and disabling*. *Neurology*, **59**, 408–413.

Yianni, J., Bain, P., Giladi, N., et al. (2003). Globus pallidus internus deep brain stimulation for dystonic conditions – a prospective audit. *Mov Disord*, **18**, 436–442.

Zeuner, K.E. and Hallett, M. (2003). Sensory training as treatment for focal hand dystonia: a 1-year follow-up. *Mov Disord*, **18**, 1044–1047.

Zhuang, P., Li, Y. and Hallett, M. (2004). Neuronal activity in the basal ganglia and thalamus in patients with dystonia. *Clin Neurophysiol*, **115**, 2542–2557.

Zijlmans, J.C., Daniel, S.E., Hughes, A.J., Revesz, T. and Lees, A.J. (2004). Clinicopathological investigation of vascular parkinsonism, including clinical criteria for diagnosis. *Mov Disord*, **9**, 630–640.

List of abbreviations

CBD	Corticobasal degeneration
DA	Dopamine
DBS	Deep brain stimulation
EMG	Electromyography
ET	Essential tremor
DLB	Dementia with Lewy bodies
GLU	Glutamate
GPe	Globus pallidus externus
GPi	Globus pallidus internus
LSVT	Lee Silverman voice training
MSA	Multiple-system atrophy
PD	Parkinson's disease
PDD	Parkinson's disease dementia
PET	Positron emission tomography
PSP	Progressive supranuclear palsy
RAS	Rhythmic auditory stimulation
SMA	Supplementary motor area
SNr	Substantia nigra pars reticulata
SNc	Substantia nigra pars compacta
SPECT	Single photon emission computed tomography
STN	Subthalamic nucleus
TENS	Transcutaneous electrical nerve stimulation
TMS	Transcranial magnetic stimulation
UPDRS	Unified Parkinson's disease rating scale

36

Neurorehabilitation of the stroke survivor

Richard D. Zorowitz

*Director, Stroke Rehabilitation; Associate Professor of Physical Medicine and Rehabilitation,
University of Pennsylvania, Philadelphia, PA, USA*

Stroke is the third most common cause of death in the Western world, behind heart disease and cancer, and comprises over half of the neurologic admissions to community hospitals. It is a leading cause for placement in nursing homes or extended care facilities (Dombovy et al., 1986). Seven-hundred thousand new or recurrent cases of stroke are reported annually, and there are nearly 5.4 million stroke survivors currently in the USA. The estimated cost of care and earnings lost due to stroke in 2005 totaled $56.8 billion, of which costs due to lost productivity equaled $21.8 billion (American Heart Association, 2005).

Comprehensive rehabilitation may improve the functional abilities of the stroke survivor, despite age and neurologic deficit, and may decrease long-term patient care costs (Feigenson, 1979). Approximately 80% of stroke victims may benefit from inpatient or outpatient stroke rehabilitation (Garraway et al., 1981). Ten percent of patients achieve complete spontaneous recovery within 8–12 weeks, while 10% of patients receive no benefit from any treatment.

The literature suggests that intensive post-stroke rehabilitation significantly improves functional outcomes. One meta-analysis of nine trials involving organized inpatient multi-disciplinary rehabilitation demonstrated significant reductions in death, death or institutionalization, and death or dependency (Langhorne and Duncan, 2001). For every 100 patients receiving organized inpatient multi-disciplinary rehabilitation, an additional five returned home independently. Studies by Indredavik and colleagues demonstrated that patients who were assigned to a specialized stroke service that included rehabilitation services had significantly greater survival rates at 1 year (Indredavik et al., 1991), better quality of life after 5 years (Indredavik et al., 1998), and greater probability of surviving and living at home at 10 years (Indredavik et al., 1999). In a study of medicare recipients in the USA, stroke survivors admitted to inpatient rehabilitation facilities were more likely to return home than those admitted to subacute or traditional nursing homes, despite the higher costs (Kramer et al., 1997). There is an association between the compliance with stroke guidelines and patient satisfaction, even after controlling for functional outcome (Reker et al., 2002). While a small but statistically significant intensity–effect relationship exists between rehabilitation and functional outcomes (Kwakkel et al., 1997), larger, more comprehensive studies are still needed to determine what aspects of rehabilitation are effective and why rehabilitation works.

36.1 Theories of motor recovery

Motor recovery usually occurs in well-described patterns after stroke (Twitchell, 1951). Within 48 h of loss of movement, muscle stretch reflexes become more active on the involved upper and lower extremities in a distal-to-proximal direction. Onset of spasticity ensues thereafter, resulting in resting postures known as *synergy patterns* (Table 36.1). Volitional movement returns in the same patterns, but eventually progresses to isolated movement. Spasticity decreases with increased volitional movement, but muscle stretch reflexes always remain increased despite total recovery. Poor prognostic indicators for motor recovery include: proprioceptive facilitation (tapping) response greater than 9 days; prolonged flaccid period; onset of motion greater than 2–4 weeks; absence of voluntary hand movement greater than 4–6 weeks; and severe proximal spasticity.

Motor recovery occurs despite the presence of brain damage due to the *unmasking of neural pathways and synapses* not normally used for a given function that can be called upon to capture the effects of remaining input and replace the damaged system. First described in the 1980's (Bach-y-rita, 1981a, b), researchers are gaining an understanding of the physiologic mechanisms of motor recovery after stroke (Chapters 8 and 14 of Volume I). Positron emission tomography (PET), functional magnetic resonance imaging (fMRI) (see Chapter 5 of Volume II), and transcranial magnetic stimulation (TMS; Chapter 15 of Volume I) have been helpful in identifying plastic changes in association with improvements in motor function. fMRI has demonstrated extended activation in ipsilateral sensorimotor cortex, ipsilateral premotor and dorsolateral prefrontal cortex, and around the perimeter of the infarcted area during rehabilitation interventions (Cao et al., 1998). Kawamata and colleagues injected basic fibroblast growth factor (bFGF) and demonstrated selective increases in GAP-43 immunoreactivity in intact sensorimotor cortices contralateral to cerebral infarcts, thus providing evidence of axonal sprouting and enhanced recovery of sensorimotor function within the first month after stroke (Kawamata et al., 1997).

Primary representation for movement may expand if spared, and later contract as movements continue to improve (Karni et al., 1995, 1998). Some TMS studies suggest that premotor cortex and the supplementary motor area (SMA) provide bilateral output projections to spinal motor neurons and contribute to movement of the affected hand upon stimulation of the unlesioned cortex (Alagona et al., 2001). PET scans in healthy control subjects and patients with striatocapsular infarcts demonstrated bilateral recruitment of the ventral premotor, supplementary motor, anterior insular, and parietal areas (Weiller et al., 1992). Future carefully-designed protocols will continue to add to the knowledge of post-stroke recovery and may suggest approaches that will maximize functional outcomes.

36.2 Theories of rehabilitation methods

Motor deficits. A number of methods (Table 36.2) are currently used to facilitate movement in affected extremities and teach compensatory techniques to perform activities of daily living (ADL). The most common method involves improving range of motion and strength in the affected extremities as precursors to teaching compensatory strategies in mobility and ADLs.

Some theories involve the facilitation of mass movements. Neurodevelopmental training (NDT)

Table 36.1. Synergy patterns of motor recovery.

Extremity	Pattern	Components
Upper	Flexor	Shoulder flexion, adduction, internal rotation; elbow flexion; wrist flexion; finger flexion
	Extensor	Shoulder, elbow, wrist, finger extension
Lower	Flexor	Hip flexion, adduction; knee flexion; ankle dorsiflexion
	Extensor	Hip, knee extension; ankle plantar flexion

Table 36.2. Techniques of stroke rehabilitation.

Author/type	Theory
Conventional	Range of motion/strengthening Compensatory strategies Mobility/activity of daily Living training
Bobath (NDT)	Suppress synergistic movement Facilitate normal movement
Knott, Voss (PNF)	Suppress normal movement Facilitate defined mass movement
Brunnstrom	Facilitate synergistic movement
Rood	Modify movement with cutaneous sensory stimulation

suggests that abnormal muscle patterns such as associated reactions and mass synergies should be inhibited, and normal patterns should be utilized to facilitate automatic, voluntary movements (Bobath, 1978). Proprioceptive neuromuscular facilitation (PNF) evokes responses through manual stimuli to increase the ease of movement-promoting function (Knott and Voss, 1968). The Brunnstrom theorem enhances specific synergies through use of cutaneous/proprioceptive stimuli and central facilitation, using Twitchell's recovery patterns (Sawner and LaVigne, 1992).

Other theories involve the facilitation of isolated movement. Muscle tone and voluntary motor activity sometimes can be modified using cutaneous sensory stimulation. Biofeedback can be used to modify autonomic function, pain, and motor disturbances, using volitional control and auditory, visual and sensory cues (Brudny et al., 1979; Intiso et al., 1994).

When compared, no one method appears to be more effective than another (Inaba et al., 1978; Dickstein et al., 1986; Lord and Hall, 1986; Basmajian et al., 1987). However, NDT alone may require prolonged periods of time to produce functional results that may be accomplished faster in conjunction with other methods. Biofeedback may not be appropriate if cost, difficulty of application, patient preference, or proprioceptive impairment inhibit its use (Moreland and Thomson, 1994).

Motor learning theory stresses structured practice of goal-oriented tasks with specific feedback patterns for successful transfer and retention of a new skill (Schmidt, 1991). The objective of motor learning is to change motor behavior rather than normalize movement patterns. Activities become new skills and must be taught and performed in different ways constraint-induced movement therapy (CIMT) forces the stroke survivor to increase utilization and incorporation of the affected extremity in ADL's (Kunkel et al., 1999). At the time of printing, a multicenter randomized clinical trial of CIMT is being completed (Winstein et al., 2003; see Chapter 18 of Volume II). In a meta-analysis of 11 trials involving partial weight support treadmill training in stroke survivors, no statistically significant advantage of treadmill training with body weight support was detected, with the exception of walking speed in independent ambulators (Moseley et al., 2005; see Chapter 3 of Volume II). However, exercise therapy specifically targeted at upper or lower extremities induces primary treatment effects on abilities at which the training is specifically aimed (Kwakkel et al., 1999).

More specialized methods of training may be helpful in maximizing functional outcomes. Functional electrical stimulation (FES) (Chapter 9 of Volume II) may be used to increase strength, increase range of motion, decrease edema, and reduce muscle antagonist spasticity and joint contractures in paretic muscles (Sonde et al., 1998; Chae et al., 1998; Francisco et al., 1998). Stroke survivors receiving robot-assisted movement training of the upper extremity (Chapter 12 of Volume II) improved strength and reach, and maintained functional improvements after 6 months (Lum et al., 2002). Repetitive bilateral arm (mirror) training resulted in fMRI activation of contralesional precentral and post-central gyrus, as well as the ipsilesional cerebellum. However, no differences in functional outcome were noted (Luft et al., 2004). In a meta-analysis of 14 trials, acupuncture added no additional effect to stroke rehabilitation on motor recovery, but a small positive effect on disability, possibly due to a true placebo effect and varied study quality, was noted (Sze et al., 2002). Recently, implanted Clonal human (hNT) neurons survived more than 2 years in the human brain without deleterious effects (Nelson et al., 2002; see Chapter 34 of Volume I).

Pharmacologic interventions also may have a role in motor recovery (Chapter 14 of Volume I). Methylphenidate, a mild central nervous system stimulant whose mode of action is not well understood, may decrease depression and improve function in the early stages after stroke (Grade et al., 1998). Too few patients have been studied to determine the effects of amphetamine treatment on recovery from stroke (Martinsson et al., 2005). Fluoxetine may help to facilitate motor recovery independent of its effect as an anti-depressant (Dam et al., 1996). Drugs such as clonidine, prazosin, neuroleptics and other dopamine receptor

antagonists, benzodiazepenes, phenytoin, and phenobarbital actually may impair motor recovery,
although the reasons are not fully understood
(Goldstein, 1995).

Sensory deficits. Sensory deficits (Chapter 6 of
Volume I) most often result from lesions in the ventral nucleus of the thalamus or projections from the
ventral nucleus to the parietal cortex (posterior cerebral artery). Touch, pain, temperature, vibration,
proprioception, or cortical sensory function maybe
involved in any degree or combination. In incomplete sensory deficits, such as partial lesions of the
thalamus, there may be a tendency to recognize all
stimuli as pain, resulting in a *post-stroke central
pain syndrome*. Treatment for sensory deficits
include desensitization to dysesthetic stimuli, transcutaneous nerve stimulation (TENS), visual feedback to compensate for deficits, or medications
such as tricyclic anti-depressants, anti-epileptics,
non-steroidal anti-inflammatory agents, mexile-
tine, or narcotics. Recovery of sensory function
maximizes in 1–2 months in 50–67% of stroke survivors (Van Buskirk and Webster, 1955). See Chapter
16 of Volume II for more details.

36.3 Management of the affected upper extremity

Use of the upper extremity is crucial for performing
ADLs (Chapter 18 of Volume II). Stroke survivors
usually do not place the same degree of importance
on improving upper extremity performance as that
of the lower extremity. Yet, in many cases, teaching
ADLs may be more difficult than teaching ambulation because the affected upper limb is less functional than the affected lower limb. Performance of
ADLs requires visual, cognitive, perceptual, and coordination skills in addition to range of motion, motor
strength, and sensation. Patients can be taught one-
handed techniques to perform feeding, grooming,
dressing, bathing, and writing with the non-
dominant unaffected limb. However, complications
involving the upper extremity may prevent the stroke
survivor from reaching his maximal potential.

Shoulder pain. Up to 72% of stroke survivors will
experience at least one episode of shoulder pain
during the first year of recovery (van Ouwenaller
et al., 1986). Common causes of painful hemiplegic
shoulder include adhesive capsulitis, traction or
compression neuropathy, complex regional pain
syndrome type I (CRPS-I, formerly known as *reflex
sympathetic dystrophy*), shoulder trauma, bursitis,
tendinitis, rotator-cuff tear, and heterotopic ossification. The most common cause of shoulder pain is
impaired passive range of motion, especially external rotation (Bohannon et al., 1986; Zorowitz et al.,
1996). Diagnoses often may be determined from a
physical examination alone, but radiographs, electromyography, bone scans, or MRI may support
clinical findings. Education in an effective self-range
of motion exercise program is responsible for a
decrease in the prevalence of significant shoulder
pain and its complications.

The most serious sequela of shoulder pain is
CRPS-I. The pathogenesis of CRPS-I is not well
understood, but may include activation of nociceptor fibers, subsequent central sensitization of the
pain-signaling system, increased capacity of low-
threshold mechanoreceptors to evoke pain, and
finally activation of nociceptor fibers by the efferent
sympathetic system (Campbell, 1991). Diagnosis is
usually clinical, with metacarpophalangeal (MCP)
tenderness highly predictive (Davis et al., 1977).
However, delayed increased uptake in the wrist or
proximal finger joints on bone scan may support the
diagnosis (Tepperman et al., 1984). Treatment may
include aggressive range of motion of the involved
joint accompanied by the use of non-steroidal agents,
corticosteroids, anti-depressants, TENS, sympathetic
blocks, local injections, or surgical sympathectomy.

Shoulder subluxation. Shoulder subluxation is a
common complication after stroke. The pathogenesis of subluxation is not well understood, but weakness of the supraspinatus muscle has been implicated
as a causative factor (Chaco and Wolf, 1971). The
treatment for ambulatory patients usually includes
shoulder supports. A number of different shoulder
supports should be evaluated for best fit (Zorowitz
et al., 1995). However, some believe that slings do

not prevent or correct shoulder subluxation (Andersen, 1985); do not appreciably affect shoulder range of motion, subluxation, or pain (Hurd et al., 1974); or may reinforce flexor synergy patterns (Bobath, 1978). However, if used, shoulder supports must be easy to don and doff to discourage synergistic patterns and incipient contractures, must permit the affected extremity to function as a postural support, and must not compromise circulation or hamper function.

Treatments for shoulder subluxation, such as FES, have not had positive or negative influences on shoulder pain, but may help to increase passive lateral rotation of the humerus (Price and Pandyan, 2005). Primary wheelchair users may require arm boards, arm troughs, or lapboards to support the extremity with poor recovery. Overhead slings may prevent hand edema, but are usually substituted with foam wedges on the arm board.

Brachial plexus injury. Brachial plexus injuries usually occur as a result of sudden and extreme traction on the affected extremity (Kaplan et al., 1977). Typical signs of brachial plexus injury include atypical functional return, segmental muscle atrophy, finger extensor contracture, and delayed onset of spasticity. Electromyographic demonstration of lower motor neuron abnormalities helps to confirm the diagnosis. Treatment includes gentle range of motion to prevent contracture while traction is avoided, a 45-degree shoulder abduction sling for nighttime positioning, a shoulder support for ambulation to prevent traction neuropathy, and a wheelchair armrest to support the injured arm. As much as 8–12 months may be required for reinnervation to take place.

Spasticity. Spasticity of the affected upper extremity is a common problem in stroke survivors. Treatment usually addresses prevention of deformities, inhibition of tone, maintenance of muscle fiber length, elongation of shortened tissues by prolonged positioning, and reduction of pain (Chapter 17 of Volume II). Conventional wrist–hand orthoses may be fabricated to preserve the balance between extrinsic and intrinsic musculature, provide joint support, and prevent deformities (Smith, 1990). Inhibitory orthoses, such as anti-spasticity splints, decrease

tone by placing a low-intensity, prolonged stretch on appropriate joints (Zislis, 1964; McPherson, 1981; McPherson et al., 1985; Scherling and Johnson, 1989). Serial or dynamic orthotics provide low-intensity prolonged stretch to achieve full range of motion of an affected joint outside a reasonable rehabilitation time frame (Dynamic Solution, 1992).

More aggressive interventions may be used to decrease more diffuse spasticity. Appropriate medications for cerebral spasticity include dantrolene (Katrak et al., 1992), clonidine (Sandford et al., 1992; Yablon and Sipski, 1993), or tizanidine (Roberts et al., 1994; Wallace, 1994; Tizanidine for Spasticity, 1997). Neurolytic agents, such as phenol (Nathan, 1959; Wood, 1978) or denatured alcohol (Herz et al., 1990; Pelissier et al., 1993), may decrease spasticity immediately upon injection, but may cause dysesthesias or edema in the injected limb. Botulinum toxin prevents the release of acetylcholine from the nerve terminal and is better tolerated by most patients (Brashear et al., 2002). Intrathecal baclofen, normally used in patients with traumatic brain or spinal cord injury, can be considered in stroke survivors with severe spasticity (Meythaler et al., 2001). Muscle release or tendon lengthening procedures may be indicated to reverse contractures in conjunction with other interventions (Swanson and Swanson, 1989).

36.4 Management of the affected lower extremity

Ambulation. Probably the most important priority of the stroke survivor is ambulation (Chapter 19 of Volume II). Prerequisites for ambulation include the ability to follow commands; adequate trunk control for sitting and standing; minimal or no contractures of the hip flexor, knee flexor, and ankle plantarflexor muscles; and adequate muscle strength required to stabilize the hip and knee joints. The hip extensor muscles are the most important muscles used in ambulation because of the stability they provide to the hip and knee (Klopsteg and Wilson, 1954).

Gait training begins by teaching transfers to the bed, mat, and wheelchair. The patient must be able to bear weight consistently on the affected extremity. Standing balance must be maximized using visual, proprioceptive, or labyrinthine cues. The patient is taught the most optimal pattern of gait in and out of the parallel bars, and on stairs, ramps, and curbs. Orthoses and assistive devices are used to correct gait deviations, and may decrease energy expenditure during gait when properly use. Ankle–foot orthoses (AFO) stabilize the ankle when dorsiflexor weakness is present, but may help to control excess knee flexion or extension when those muscles are involved as well. Knee–ankle–foot orthoses (KAFO) support the knee when the quadriceps and hamstring muscles cannot provide adequate control across the joint. No energy differential exists between the use of plastic or metal orthoses (Lehmann, 1979).

Wheelchair mobility. Patients who have limited or no ability to ambulate may require wheelchairs for mobility (Chapter 11 of Volume II). Wheelchairs should be prescribed in dimensions which fit the patient most comfortably. The seat should be narrow enough to allow operation of the hand rim with the unaffected arm, and low enough to allow propulsion with the unaffected leg. Removable desk arms and swing-away detachable footrests facilitate the ability to transfer from the wheelchair to other surfaces. One-arm drive wheelchairs are used rarely as most stroke survivors can propel with their unaffected extremities. Lightweight chairs may be issued to patients with cardiac conditions.

36.5 Community re-entry

Driving. Driving may be an important goal for some stroke victims. Occupational therapy administers a pre-driving evaluation, which tests basic cognitive skills needed for driving, such as memory, spatial organization, attention, concentration, and reaction times. Driving skills are tested in a simulator or behind-the-wheel with an instructor. Adaptive aids, such as steering wheel pegs and accelerator extensions, may be incorporated to compensate for motor deficits. Three-fourth of patients with left-hemisphere strokes are able to pass a driving test,

but 50% of patients with right-hemisphere strokes fail driving tests due to cognitive and perceptual deficits (Quigley and DeLisa, 1983).

Vocational Rehabilitation. Approximately 21–33% of stroke survivors under age of 65 years are able to return to work (Weisbroth et al., 1971; Angeleri et al., 1993). Stroke survivors with white-collar jobs are 3.33 times as likely to return to work than those with blue-collar jobs (Saeki et al., 1993). To return to work, patients with left-hemisphere strokes must demonstrate adequate verbal, cognitive, and communication deficits, while patients with right-hemisphere strokes must have adequate ambulation skills, use of left upper extremity, and abstract reasoning skills. Vocational assessments may include neuropsychologic and driving evaluations, work capacity assessments, and on-site evaluations.

36.6 Speech and language disorders

Speech and language disorders may be diagnosed by both formal testing and conversational interaction. Impaired content of speech suggests aphasia or a cognitive-communication impairment. Aphasia is defined as an "acquired impairment of verbal language behavior at the linguistic level," and is characterized by decreased word finding or syntax, word substitutions, and errors in understanding conversational questions or statements (Chapter 26 of Volume II). Aphasias are classified as non-fluent, characterized by slow, telegraphic style of deliver; fluent, characterized by rapid style with paraphasias or neologisms; and global, which involve all modes of speech and may be fluent or non-fluent. The classification of aphasias is listed in Table 36.3.

Cognitive-communication impairment is associated with right-hemisphere dysfunction. It is characterized by decreased concentration, attention, memory, and orientation; confusion; confabulation; concrete or irrelevant thinking; or vague language. Associated functional problems may include unilateral neglect, constructional and dressing apraxias, anosagnosia, and impairments in safety awareness and judgment.

Table 36.3. Classification of aphasias.

Type	Fluent	Comprehension	Repetition
Transcortical motor	(−)	(+)	(+)
Broca	(−)	(+)	(−)
Transcortical mixed	(−)	(−)	(+)
Global	(+ / −)	(−)	(−)
Normal/anomic	(+)	(+)	(+)
Conduction	(+)	(+)	(−)
Transcortical sensory	(+)	(−)	(+)
Wernicke	(+)	(−)	(−)

Impaired acoustic features of speech may indicate an apraxia or dysarthria. Apraxia is defined as a "deficit in willed or planned purposeful movement despite the presence of adequate motor or sensory function, coordination, or comprehension." Apraxias are characterized by inconsistent errors either in programming the positioning of the speech musculature (oral) or in sequencing muscle movements for articulation of volitional speech (verbal).

Dysarthria is defined as "slurred speech." Dysarthric patients present with consistent errors in articulation, decreased normal resonance or phonation, or problems with volume or breath control. The classification of dysarthrias is listed in Table 36.4 (Rosenbek and LaPointe, 1985).

Therapy generally focuses on teaching compensatory strategies and self-correction of errors. Exercises of the oral, lingual, buccal, and laryngeal musculature may increase physiologic support for speech. Facilitation techniques are thought to recruit right-hemisphere areas, which enhance verbal output. Alternative communication techniques and augmentative communication devices may be used as long as apraxia and comprehension deficits do not interfere with their use. Therapy may not be able to restore complex neurologic associations to process language symbols, but may be able to maximize abilities through compensatory strategies (Lincoln et al., 1984). Family education is essential to increase the awareness of the deficits and discuss prognosis. Global aphasia usually has a poor prognosis, while conduction aphasia and anomia often have a complete recovery. Persistent cognitive-communication

Table 36.4. Classification of dysarthrias.

Type	Location	Characteristics
Flaccid	Lower motor neuron	Marked hypernasality
		Breathiness
		Audible inspiration
Spastic	Upper motor neuron	Slow rate
		Low pitch
		Harsh strained-strangled voice
Ataxic	Cerebellum	Excess and equal stress
		Phoneme and interval prolongation
		Dysrhythmia of speech and syllable
		Repetition
		Excess loudness variation
Hypokinetic	Extrapyramidal system	Monopitch
		Monoloudness
		Short rushes of speech
		Inappropriate silences
Hyperkinetic (quick)	Extrapyramidal system	Hypernasality
		Sudden variations in loudness
		Rhythmic phonatory interruptions
		Sudden tic-like grunts, barks, and coprolalia
Hyperkinetic (slow)	Extrapyramidal system	Distinctive deviations unreported

problems may cause an otherwise independent patient to require 24-h supervision. The use of bromocriptine in treating aphasia remains controversial as many of these studies utilize small patient populations (Gupta and Mlcoch, 1992; Gupta et al., 1995; Sabe et al., 1995).

36.7 Common medical complications

Secondary prophylaxis of stroke. Every stroke survivor admitted for rehabilitation must be considered for secondary prophylaxis of stroke. Secondary prophylaxis of hemorrhagic stroke includes control of etiologic factors, such as hypertension. Secondary prevention of stroke is a lifelong endeavor and must include anti-platelet therapy after cerebral ischemia, and warfarin in stroke survivors with atrial fibrillation (Albers et al., 2004). *Carotid endarterectomy* is acceptable for lesions with greater than 60% diameter reduction of distal outflow tract, with or without ulceration, and with or without anti-platelet therapy, irrespective of contralateral artery status, ranging from no disease to occlusion (Biller et al., 1998).

Deep venous thrombosis (DVT). DVT may occur in up to 20–75% of stroke survivors (Turpie, 1997). Clinical signs and symptoms, such as pain, swelling, and warmth of the extremity, are at best marginally diagnostic. Clinical suspicion should be raised in the hemiplegic patient who is not ambulatory and is within 3 months of stroke onset. Non-invasive testing, such as doppler and impedance plethysmography, is a routine part of diagnosis. Patients at risk for DVT should be given thigh–high compression stockings and subcutaneous heparin at regular intervals (Desmukh et al., 1991). Prophylaxis may be discontinued once the patient is ambulating consistently in or out of parallel bars (Bromfield and Reding, 1988).

Pressure sores. Pressure sores result from both extrinsic (pressure, shear forces, friction, moisture) and intrinsic (anemia, contractures, spasticity, diabetes, malnutrition [vitamins B,C,K; zinc], edema, and obesity) etiologies (Nurse and Collins, 1989). Common locations of pressure sores are found in Table 36.5. General measures to prevent pressure sores include adequate nutrition and hydration, as well as proper incontinence care. In bed, appropriate mattresses may distribute pressure, and heel protector boots provide pressure relief to the heel and foot. Patients should maintain a flat position and should be turned regularly. In wheelchairs, patients should be issued appropriate cushions and should be taught techniques of pressure relief.

Bladder dysfunction. A variety of voiding disorders may be observed after stroke (Borrie et al., 1986; see Chapter 24 of Volume II). Reversible causes, such as urinary tract infection, fecal impaction, and

Table 36.5. Locations of pressure sores.

Position	Locations
Supine	Sacrum, heels, occiput, elbow, dorsal thorax, and ear rim
Side-lying	Lateral malleolus, greater trochanter, ribs, shoulder, ear, and lateral knee
Sitting in wheelchair	Ischial tuberosity, sacrum, posterior knee, foot, and shoulder

reduced mobility, should be evaluated and treated (Linsenmeyer and Zorowitz, 1992). Post-void residuals should be measured to assess for urinary retention. Symptoms of urinary incontinence, frequency, and urgency should be noted. Voiding dysfunctions should be characterized by urodynamic studies to determine the appropriate intervention. Toileting every 2–4 h during the day, and fluid restriction after dinner may prevent incontinence in majority of patients (Sogbein and Awad, 1982). External catheters may decrease the incidence of enuresis. Intermittent or indwelling catheterization may be indicated in patients with areflexic bladders.

Bowel dysfunction. Strokes may disinhibit the reflex mechanisms for emptying the bowels (Chapter 24 of Volume II), and sensation or cognitive impairments may prevent control of defecation. Diets should include adequate fluids and fiber. Patients should be toileted after meals to take advantage of the gastrocolic reflex. Stool softeners and bowel stimulants may be prescribed as necessary. Patients who remain incontinent may require suppositories every 1–2 days to prevent incontinence at socially inappropriate times. Persistent bowel incontinence greater than 4 weeks usually is a poor functional predictor.

Dysphagia. Swallowing dysfunction, or dysphagia (Chapter 23 of Volume II), may occur in up to one-third of patients with cortical or brainstem lesions (Veis and Logemann, 1985). Dysphagic patients with hemispheric lesions usually are characterized by contralateral labial and lingual weakness, range of motion, and sensation; delayed pharyngeal swallow; contralateral pharyngeal dysfunction; oral apraxia; auditory comprehension deficits; reduced orientation; perceptual and attention deficits; impulsivity; errors in judgment; and loss of intellectual control over swallowing (Miller and Groher, 1982; Leopold and Kagel, 1983). Patients with brainstem lesions may exhibit reduced strength and range of motion of swallowing muscles; decreased mouth or pharyngeal sensation; absence or delay of pharyngeal swallow; pharyngeal incoordination; unilateral vocal cord paresis; and reduced laryngeal elevation or cricopharyngeal opening (Donner, 1974; Kilman and Goyal, 1976; Hellemans et al., 1981).

Complications of post-stroke dysphagia include malnutrition and aspiration. Malnutrition in stroke survivors is correlated with impaired function, higher stress reactions as measured by urinary cortisol levels, frequency of infection, decubiti, and death (Davalos et al., 1996). Malnourished stroke survivors also had longer lengths of rehabilitation stay (Finestone et al., 1996).

Suspicion of dysphagia should be high in stroke survivors, since only 40% of patients who aspirate may be identified during a bedside evaluation (Splaingard et al., 1988). Presence of aspiration (Alberts et al., 1992) or other types of swallowing disorders (Chen et al., 1990) are not associated with lesion site. However, patients with combined bilateral hemispheric and brainstem lesions were more likely to aspirate than patients with cortical or brainstem lesions alone (Horner et al., 1988). Symptoms associated with aspiration include dysphonia and an impaired gag reflex associated with impaired cough (Linden and Siebens, 1983; Horner and Massey, 1988; Horner et al., 1990; Horner et al., 1991).

Following evaluation by a speech and language pathologist, a videofluorographic swallowing study of liquids, purees, and solids may be undertaken to identify the swallowing disorders and organize a treatment plan. Fiberoptic laryngoscopy may be a useful tool to rule out tracheal aspiration and pharyngeal pooling if they are not observed during laryngoscopy, and the gag reflex is normal (Kaye et al., 1997). Other diagnostic procedures may include ultrasound of the oral musculature (Shawker et al., 1984), scintigraphy to assess gastroesophageal reflux

(Muz et al., 1987), and manometry of the pharynx and esophagus (McConnel et al., 1988).

Treatment of dysphagia includes modification in diet, head positioning, or other compensatory strategies to prevent aspiration. Many stroke survivors will regain normal swallowing function within 2–3 weeks (Gordon et al., 1987). Most patients tolerate a full oral diet by the conclusion of rehabilitation, but some cannot drink thin liquids safely (Gresham, 1990). Although many stroke survivors are fed exclusively by gastrostomy, some patients may be able to tolerate combined oral and gastrostomy feedings. The ability to take even small amounts of food by mouth allows the stroke survivor to practice swallowing and provides some social element when friends and family gather together for a meal.

Depression. Depression occurs in 25–79% of stroke survivors in the acute medical or rehabilitation setting, but less than 5% receive psychotherapeutic or medical intervention (Gordon and Hibbard, 1997). Depression may be related to mourning the loss of function or to the alteration of function of catecholamine-containing neurons. An association between the presence of depression and neuroanatomic location remains controversial. However, depression appears to be more prevalent in stroke survivors 6 months to 2 years post-stroke (Astrom et al., 1993). Diagnosis is usually clinical. Treatment includes psychotherapy and medications. However, no definitive studies support or refute the routine use of pharmacotherapeutic and psychotherapeutic treatments for depression after stroke (Hackett et al., 2005). There also are no definitive studies that support or refute the routine use of pharmacotherapeutic treatments to prevent depression after stroke (Anderson et al., 2005).

Sexual dysfunction. Issues of sexual functioning rarely are addressed with stroke survivors, but are of tremendous importance to many (Chapter 25 of Volume II). Fewer than one-half of all stroke survivors resume unaltered intercourse with their partners (Fugl-Meyer and Jaasko, 1980). Stroke survivors and their partners commonly fear another stroke or increasing blood pressure during intercourse (Monga et al., 1986). Partners report an overall feeling of psychologic change as they assume the role of care-taker for the stroke survivor (Boldrini et al., 1991). Therefore, it is important to discuss sexual issues as openly and honestly as possible. Cardiac limitations should be discussed, and medications should be reviewed. Couples should be encouraged to experiment with sexual techniques and positions, and to communicate their needs and concerns to each other and to the treating physician. The cardiovascular and urologic status of the stroke survivor should be evaluated before any treatment is prescribed. Treatment for erectile dysfunction in males includes intracavernous injection of papaverine, phentolamine, or prostaglandin E1; vacuum tumescence constriction therapy; penile prosthesis; or medications such as transcutaneous nitroglycerin (Sonksen and Biersen-Sorensen, 1992) or levodopa (Yalla et al., 1994). Sildenafil (Viagra®) causes muscle relaxation and blood inflow to the corpus cavernosum by the inhibition of PDE5, but can cause headache, flushing, and dyspepsia. Treatment for impaired vaginal lubrication in females includes artificial lubricants such as saliva, Replens, or K-Y jelly.

36.8 Continuity of care

Rehabilitation care may be a lifelong endeavor. After discharge from the rehabilitation facility, stroke survivors should return to their primary practitioners for routine medical care, but also should be seen periodically by a rehabilitation physician. Blood pressure and weight should be taken, and medications should be reviewed. Progress of mobility and ADL should be reviewed and validated by a family member. Psychosocial issues should be discussed. All equipment should be inspected, and the stroke survivor should be able to demonstrate his home exercise program. A neurologic examination should be performed, including gait with appropriate assistive devices and orthoses (Chapters 10 and 12 of Volume II). Most importantly, time should be allowed for questions. Good communication between the neurorehabilitation physician, the patient, and the family will facilitate optimal care, and provide the patient

with the opportunity to reach his maximal functional potential.

REFERENCES

Alagona, G., Delvaux, V., Gerard, P., DePasqua, V., Pennisi, G., Delwaide, P., Nicolet, F. and de Noordhout, A.M. (2001). Ipsilateral motor responses to focal transcortical magnetic stimulation in healthy and acute stroke patients. *Stroke*, **32**, 1304–1309.

Albers, G.W., Amarenco, P., Easton, J.D., Sacco, R.L. and Teal, P. (2004). Antithrombotic and thrombolytic therapy for ischemic stroke: the Seventh ACCP Conference on Antithrombotic and Thrombolytic Therapy. *Chest*, **126**, 483S–512S.

Alberts, M.J., Horner, J., Gray, L. and Brazer, S.R. (1992). Aspiration after stroke: lesion analysis by brain MRI. *Dysphagia*, **7**, 170–173.

American Heart Association (2005). *Heart and Stroke Statistical Update*, American Heart Association, Inc., Dallas, TX.

Andersen, L.T. (1985). Shoulder pain in hemiplegia. *Am J Occup Ther*, **39**(**1**), 11–19.

Anderson, C.S., Hackett, M.L. and House, A.O. (2005). Interventions for preventing depression after stroke. In: *The Cochrane Library*, Issue 1, 2005. John Wiley & Sons, Ltd., Chichester, UK.

Angeleri, F., Angeleri, V.A., Foschi, N., Giaquinto, S. and Nolfe, G. (1993). The influence of depression, social activity, and family stress on functional outcome after stroke. *Stroke*, **24**, 1478–1483.

Astrom, M., Adolfsson, R. and Asplund, K. (1993). Major depression in stroke patients. A 3-year longitudinal study. *Stroke*, **24**, 976–982.

Bach-y-Rita, P. (1981a). Brain plasticity as a basis of the development of procedures for hemiplegia. *Scand J Rehabil Med*, **13**, 73–83.

Bach-y-Rita, P. (1981b). Central nervous system lesions: sprouting and unmasking in rehabilitation. *Arch Phys Med Rehabil*, **62**, 413–417.

Basmajian, J.V., Gowland, C.A., Finlayson, A.J., Hall, A.L., Swanson, L.R., Stratford, P.W., Trotter, J.E. and Brandstater, M.E. (1987). Stroke treatment: comparison of integrated behavior-physical therapy vs. traditional physical therapy programs. *Arch Phys Med Rehabil*, **68**, 267–272.

Biller, J., Feinberg, W.M., Castaldo, J.E., Whittemore, A.D., Harbaugh, R.E., Dempsey, R.J., Caplan, L.R., Kresowik, T.F., Matchar, D.B., Toole, J.F., Easton, J.D., Adams, H.P., Brass,

L.M., Hobson, R.W., Brott, T.G. and Sternau, L. (1998). Guidelines for carotid endarterectomy. A statement for healthcare professionals from a special writing group of the Stroke Council, American Heart Association. *Circulation*, **97**, 501–509.

Bobath, B. (1978). *Adult Hemiplegia: Evaluation and Treatment*, Spottiswood Ballintype, London.

Bohannon, R.W., Larkin, P.A., Smith, M.B. and Horton, M.G. (1986). Shoulder pain in hemiplegia: statistical relationship with five variables. *Arch Phys Med Rehabil*, **67**, 514.

Boldrini, P., Basagla, N. and Calanca, M.C. (1991). Sexual changes in hemiparetic patients. *Arch Phys Med Rehabil*, **72**, 202–207.

Borrie, M.J., Campbell, A.J., Caradoc-Davies, T.H. and Speers, G.F.S. (1986). Urinary incontinence after stroke: a prospective study. *Age Ageing*, **15**, 177–181.

Brashear, A., Gordon, M.F., Elovic, E., Kassicieh, V.D., Marciniak, C., Do, M., Lee, C.H., Jenkins, S. and Turkel, C., Botox Post-Stroke Spasticity Study Group (2002). Intramuscular injection of botulinum toxin for the treatment of wrist and finger spasticity after a stroke. *New Eng J Med*, **347(6)**, 395–400.

Bromfield, E.B. and Reding, M.B. (1988). Relative risk of deep venous thrombosis or pulmonary embolism post-stroke based upon ambulatory status. *J Neurol Rehabil*, **2(2)**, 51–56.

Brudny, M., Korein, J., Grynbaum, B.B., Belandes, P.V. and Gianutsos, J.G. (1979). Helping hemiparetics to help themselves: sensory feedback therapy. *J Am Med Assoc*, **241(8)**, 814–818.

Campbell, J.M. (1991). Pathogenesis and treatment of peripheral neurogenic pain (paper presentation). *53rd Annual Assembly AAPM&R*, Washington DC, November, 1991.

Cao, Y., D'Olhaberriague, L., Vikingstad, E.M., Levine, S.R. and Welch, K.M. (1998). Pilot study of functional MRI to assess cerebral activation of motor function after poststroke hemiparesis. *Stroke*, **29(1)**, 112–122.

Chaco, J. and Wolf, E. (1971). Subluxation of glenohumeral joint in hemiplegia. *Am J Phys Med*, **50(3)**, 139–143.

Chae, J., Bethoux, F., Bohine, T., Dobos, L., Davis, T. and Friedl, A. (1998). Neuromuscular stimulation for upper extremity motor and functional recovery in acute hemiplegia. *Stroke*, **29(5)**, 975–979.

Chen, M.Y.M., Ott, D.J., Peele, V.N. and Gelfand, D.W. (1990). Oropharynx in patients with cerebrovascular disease: evaluation with videofluoroscopy. *Radiology*, **176**, 641–643.

Dam, M., Tonin, P., De Boni, A., Pizzolato, G., Casson, S., Ermani, M., Freo, U., Piron, L. and Battistin, L. (1996). Effects of fluoxetine and maprotiline on functional recovery in poststroke hemiplegic patients undergoing rehabilitation therapy. *Stroke*, **27(7)**, 1211–1214.

Davalos, A., Ricart, W., Gonzalez-Huix, F., Soler, S., Marrugat, J., Molins, A., Suner, R. and Genis, D. (1996). Effect of malnutrition after acute stroke on clinical outcome. *Stroke*, **27(6)**, 1028–1032.

Davis, S.W., Petrillo, C.R., Eichberg, R.D. and Chu D.S. (1977). Shoulder-hand syndrome in a hemiplegia population: a 5-year retrospective study. *Arch Phys Med Rehabil*, **58**, 353–356.

Desmukh, M., Bisignani, M., Lander, M. and Orchard, T.J. (1991). Deep venous thrombosis in rehabilitating stroke patients: incidence, risk factors, and prophylaxis. *Am J Phys Med Rehabil*, **70(6)**, 313–316.

Dickstein, R., Hocherman, S., Pillar, T. and Shaham, R. (1986). Stroke rehabilitation: three exercise therapy approaches. *Phys Ther*, **66(8)**, 1233–1238.

Dombovy, M.L., Sandok, B.A. and Basford, J.A. (1986). Rehabilitation for stroke: a review. *Stroke*, **17(3)**, 363–369.

Donner, M.W. (1974). Swallowing mechanism and neuromuscular disorders. *Semin Roentgenol*, **9**(4), 273–282.

Feigenson, J.S. (1979). Stroke rehabilitation: effectiveness, benefits, and costs: some practical considerations. *Stroke*, **10(1)**, 1–4.

Finestone, H.M., Greene-Finestone, L.S., Wilson, E.S. and Teasell, R. W. (1996). Prolonged length of stay and reduced functional improvement rate in malnourished stroke rehabilitation patients. *Arch Phys Med Rehabil*, **77(4)**, 340–345.

Francisco, G., Chae, J., Chawla, H., Kirshblum, S., Zorowitz, R., Lewis, G. and Pang, S. (1998). Electromyogram-triggered stimulation for improving the arm function of acute stroke survivors: a randomized pilot study. *Arch Phys Med Rehabil*, **79(5)**, 570–575.

Fugl-Meyer, A.R. and Jaasko, L. (1980). Post-stroke hemiplegia and sexual intercourse. *Scand J Rehabil Med*, **7**, 158–166.

Garraway, W.M., Akhtar, A.J., Smith, D.L. and Smith, M.E. (1981). The triage of stroke rehabilitation. *J Epidemiol Commun Health*, **35**, 39–44.

Goldstein, L.B. (1995). Common drugs may influence motor recovery after stroke. The sygen in acute stroke study investigators. *Neurology*, **45(5)**, 865–871.

Grade, C., Redford, B., Chrostowski, J., Toussaint, L. and Blackwell, B. (1998). Methylphenidate in early poststroke recovery: a double-blind, placebo-controlled study. *Arch Phys Med Rehabil*, **79(9)**, 1047–1050.

Gresham, S.L. (1990). Clinical assessment and management of swallowing difficulties after stroke. *Med J Australia*, **153**, 397–399.

Gupta, S.R. and Mlcoch, A.G. (1992). Bromocriptine treatment of nonfluent aphasia. *Arch Phys Med Rehabil*, **73(4)**, 373–376.

Gupta, S.R., Mlcoch, A.G., Scolaro, C. and Moritz, T. (1995). Bromocriptine treatment of nonfluent aphasia. *Neurology*, **45**(**12**), 2170–2173.

Hackett, M.L., Anderson, C.S. and House, A.O. (2005). Interventions for treating depression after stroke. In: *The Cochrane Library*, Issue 1, 2005. John Wiley & Sons, Ltd., Chichester, UK.

Hellemans, J., Pelemans, W. and Vantrappen, G. (1981). Pharyngoesophageal swallowing disorders and pharyngoesophageal sphincter. *Med Clin North Am*, **65**(**6**), 1149–1171.

Herz, D.A., Looman, J.E., Tiberio, A., Ketterling, K., Kreitsch, R.K., Colwill, J.C. and Grin, O.D. (1990). The management of paralytic spasticity. *Neurosurgery*, **26**, 300–305.

Horner, J. and Massey, E.W. (1988). Silent aspiration following stroke. *Neurology*, **38**, 317–319.

Horner, J., Massey, E.W., Riski, J.E., Lathrop, D.L. and Chase, K.N. (1988). Aspiration following stroke: clinical correlates and outcome. *Neurology*, **38**, 1359–1362.

Horner, J., Massey, E.W. and Brazer, S.R. (1990). Aspiration in bilateral stroke patients. *Neurology*, **40**, 1686–1688.

Horner, J., Buoyner, F.G., Alberts, M.J. and Helms, M.J. (1991). Dysphagia following brain-stem stroke. *Arch Neurol*, **48**(**11**), 1170–1173.

Hurd, M., Farrell, K. and Waylonis, G. (1974). Shoulder sling for hemiplegia: friend or foe? *Arch Phys Med Rehabil*, **55**, 519–522.

Inaba, M., Edberg, E., Montgomery, J. and Gillis, M. (1978). Effectiveness of function training, active exercise, and resistive exercise for patients with hemiplegia. *Phys Ther*, **53**, 28–35.

Indredavik, B., Bakke, F., Solberg, R., Rokseth, R., Haheim, L.L. and Holme, I. (1991). Benefit of a stroke unit: a randomized controlled trial. *Stroke*, **22**(**8**), 1026–1031.

Indredavik, B., Bakke, F., Slordahl, S.A., Rokseth, R. and Haheim, L.L. (1998). Stroke unit treatment improves long-term quality of life: a randomized controlled trial. *Stroke*, **29**(**5**), 895–899.

Indredavik, B., Bakke, F., Slordahl, S.A., Rokseth, R. and Haheim, L.L. (1999). Stroke unit treatment. 10-year follow-up. *Stroke*, **30**(**8**), 1524–1527.

Intiso, D., Santilli, V., Grasso, M.N., Rossi, R. and Caruso, I. (1994). Rehabilitation of walking with electromyographic feedback in foot-drop after stroke. *Stroke*, **25**(**6**), 1189–1192.

Katrak, P.H., Cole, A.M., Poulos, C.J. and McCauley, J.C. (1992). Objective assessment of spasticity, strength, and function with early exhibition of dantrolene sodium after cerebrovascular accident: a randomized double-blind study. *Arch Phys Med Rehabil*, **73**(**1**), 4–9.

Kawamata, T., Dietrich, W.D., Schallert, T., Gotts, J.E., Cocke, R.R., Benowitz, L.I. and Finklestein, S.P. (1997). Intracisternal basic fibroblast growth factor enhances functional recovery and up-regulates the expression of a molecular marker of neuronal sprouting following focal cerebral infarction. *ProcNatl Acad Sci USA*, **94**(**15**), 8179–8184.

Gordon, C., Hewer, R.L. and Wade, D.T. (1987). Dysphagia in acute stroke. *Br Med J Clin Res Educ*, **295**(**6595**), 411–414.

Gordon, W.A. and Hibbard, M.R. (1997). Poststroke depression: an examination of the literature. *Arch Phys Med Rehabil*, **78**(**6**), 658–663.

Kaplan, P.E., Meredith, J., Taft, G. and Betts, H. (1977). Stroke and brachial plexus injury: a difficult problem. *Arch Phys Med Rehabil*, **58**, 415–418.

Karni, A., Meyer, G., Hipolito, C., Jezzard, P., Adams, M. and Underleider, S. (1995). Functional MRI evidence for adult motor cortex plasticity during motor skill learning. *Nature*, **377**, 155–158.

Karni, A., Meyer, G., Hipolito, C., Jezzard, P. and Adams, M. (1998). The acquisition of skilled motor performance. Fast and slow experience-driven changes in primary motor cortex. *Proc Natl Acad Sci USA*, **95**, 861–868.

Kaye, G.M., Zorowitz, R.D. and Baredes, S. (1997). The role of fiberoptic laryngoscopy in evaluating aspiration. *Ann Otol Rhinol Laryngol*, **106**(**6**), 705–709.

Kilman, W.J. and Goyal, R.K. (1976). Disorders of pharyngeal and upper esophageal sphincter motor function. *Arch Int Med*, **136**(**5**), 592–601.

Klopsteg, P.E., Wilson, P.D. (eds) (1954). *Human Limbs and their Substitutes*, McGraw-Hill, New York, NY.

Knott, M. and Voss, D.E. (1968). *Proprioceptive Neuromuscular Facilitation: Patterns and Techniques*, 2nd edn., Harper and Row, Hagerstown, MD.

Kramer, A.M., Steiner, J.F., Schlenker, R.E., Eilertsen, T.B., Hrincevich, C.A., Tropea, D.A., Ahmad, L.A. and Eckhoff, D.G. (1997). Outcomes and costs after hip fracture and stroke. A comparison of rehabilitation settings. *J Am Med Assoc*, **277**(**5**), 396–404.

Kunkel, A., Kopp, B., Muller, G., Villringer, K., Villringer, R., Taub, E. and Flor, H. (1999). *Arch Phys Med Rehabil*, **80**(**6**), 624–628.

Kwakkel, G., Wagenaar, R.C., Koelman, T.W., Lankhorst, G.H. and Koetsier, J.C. (1997). Effects of intensity of rehabilitation after stroke. A research synthesis. *Stroke*, **28**(**8**), 1550–1556.

Kwakkel, G., Wagenaar, R.C., Twisk, J.W., Lankhorst, G.J. and Koetsier, J.C. (1999). Intensity of leg and arm training after primary middle-cerebral-artery stroke: a randomised trial. *Lancet*, **354**(**9174**), 191–196.

Langhorne, P. and Duncan, P. (2001). Does the organization of postacute stroke care really matter? *Stroke*, **32**(**1**), 268–274.

Lehmann, J.F. (1979). Biomechanics of ankle–foot orthoses: prescription and design. *Arch Phys Med Rehabil*, **60**, 200–207.

Leopold, N.A. and Kagel, M.C. (1983). Swallowing, ingestion, and dysphagia: a reappraisal. *Arch Phys Med Rehabil*, **64**, 371–373.

Lincoln, N.B., Milley, G.P., Jones, A.C., McGuirk, E., Lendrem, W. and Mitchell, J.R.A. (1984). Effectiveness of speech therapy for aphasic stroke patients: a randomized controlled trial. *Lancet*, **1**(**8388**), 1197–1200.

Linden, P. and Siebens, A.A. (1983). Dysphagia: predicting laryngeal penetration. *Arch Phys Med Rehabil*, **64**, 281–284.

Linsenmeyer, T.A. and Zorowitz, R.D. (1992). Urodynamic findings of patients with urinary incontinence following cerebrovascular accident. *NeuroRehabilitation*, **2**(**2**), 23–26.

Lord, J.P. and Hall, K. (1986). Neuromuscular reeducation vs. traditional programs for stroke rehabilitation. *Arch Phys Med Rehabil*, **67**, 88–91.

Luft, A.R., Mccombe-Waller, S., Whitall, J., Forrester, L.W., Macko, R., Sorkin, J.D., Schulz, J.B., Goldberg, A.P. and Hanley, D.F. (2004). Repetitive bilateral arm training and motor cortex activation in chronic stroke. A randomized controlled trial. *J Am Med Assoc*, **292**(**15**), 1853–1861.

Lum, P.S., Burgar, C.G., Shor, P.C., Majmundar, M. and van der Loos, M. (2002). Robot-assisted movement training compared with conventional therapy techniques for the rehabilitation of upper-limb motor function after stroke. *Arch Phys Med Rehabil*, **83**(**7**), 952–959.

Martinsson, L., Wahlgren, N.G. and Hårdemark, H.-G. (2005). Amphetamines for improving recovery after stroke. In: *The Cochrane Library*, Issue 1, 2005, John Wiley & Sons, Ltd., Chichester, UK.

McConnel, F.M., Cerenko, D., Hersh, T. and Weil, L.J. (1988). Evaluation of pharyngeal dysphagia with manofluorography. *Dysphagia*, **2**(**4**), 187–195.

McPherson, J.J. (1981). Objective evaluation of a splint designed to reduce hypertonicity. *Am J Occup Ther*, **35**(**3**), 189–194.

McPherson, J.J., Beck, A.H. and Franszczak, N. (1985). Dynamic splint to reduce the passive component of hypertonicity. *Arch Phys Med Rehabil*, **66**, 249–252.

Meythaler, J.M., Guin-Renfroe, S., Brunner, R.C. and Hadley, M.N. (2001). Intrathecal baclofen for spastic hypertonia from stroke. *Stroke*, **32**(**9**), 2099–2109.

Miller, R.M. and Groher, M.E. (1982). The evaluation and management of neuromuscular and mechanical swallowing disorders. *Dysarthria Dysphonia Dysphagia*, **1**, 50–70.

Monga, T.N., Lawson, J.S. and Inglis, J. (1986). Sexual dysfunction in stroke patients. *Arch Phys Med Rehabil*, **67**, 19–22.

Moreland, J. and Thomson, M.A. (1994). Efficacy of electromyographic biofeedback compared with conventional physical therapy for upper-extremity function in patients following stroke: a research overview and meta-analysis. *Phys Ther*, **74**(**6**), 534–543.

Moseley, A.M., Stark, A., Cameron, I.D. and Pollock, A. (2005). Treadmill training and body weight support for walking after stroke (Cochrane Review). In: *The Cochrane Library*, Issue 1, 2005, John Wiley & Sons, Ltd., Chichester, UK.

Muz, J., Mathog, R.H., Miller, P.R., Rosen, R. and Borrero, G. (1987). Detection and quantification of laryngotracheopulmonary aspiration with scintigraphy. *Laryngoscope*, **97**, 1180–1185.

Nathan, P.W. (1959). Intrathecal phenol to relieve spasticity in paraplegia. *Lancet*, **2**, 1099–1102.

Nelson, P.T., Kondziolka, D., Wechsler, L., Goldstein, S., Gebel, J., DeCesare, S., Elder, E.M., Zhang, P.J., Jacobs, A., McGrogan, M., Lee, V.M. and Trojanowski, J.Q. (2002). Clonal human (hNT) neuron grafts for stroke therapy: neuropathology in a patient 27 months after implantation. *Am J Pathol*, **160**(**4**), 1201–1206.

Nurse, B.A. Collins, M.C. (1989). Skin care and decubitus ulcer management in the elderly stroke patient. *PM&R State of the Art Reviews*, **3**(**3**), 549–562.

Pelissier, J., Viel, E., Enjalbert, M., Kotzki, N. and Eledjam, J.J. (1993). Chemical neurolysis using alcohol (alcoholization) in the treatment of spasticity in the hemiplegic. *Cah Anesthesiol*, **41**(**2**), 139–143.

Price, C.I.M. and Pandyan, A.D. (2005). Electrical stimulation for preventing and treating post-stroke shoulder pain (Cochrane Review). In: *The Cochrane Library*, Issue 1, 2005, John Wiley & Sons, Ltd., Chichester, UK.

Quigley, F.L. and DeLisa, J.A. (1983). Assessing the driving potential of cerebral vascular accident patients. *Am J Occup Ther*, **37**(**7**), 474–478.

Reker, D.M., Duncan, P.W., Horner, R.D., Hoenig, H., Samsa, G.P., Hamilton, B.B. and Dudley, T.K. (2002). Postacute stroke guideline compliance is associated with greater patient satisfaction. *Arch Phys Med Rehabil*, **83**(**6**), 750–756.

Roberts, R.C., Part, N.J., Pokorny, R., Muir, C., Leslie, G.C. and Emre, M. (1994). Pharmacokinetics and pharmacodynamics of tizanidine. *Neurology*, **44**(**11 Suppl. 9**), S29–S31.

Rosenbek, J.C. and LaPointe, L.L. (1985). The dysarthrias: description, diagnosis, and treatment. In: *Clinical Management of Neurogenic Communication Disorders* (ed. Johns, D.F.), 2nd edn., Little, Brown, and Company, Boston, MA.

Sabe, L., Salvarezza, F., Garcia Cuerva, A., Leiguarda, R. and Starkstein, S. (1995). A randomized, double-blind, placebo-controlled study of bromocriptine in nonfluent aphasia. *Neurology*, **45**(**12**), 2272–2274.

Saeki, S., Ogata, H., Okubo, T., Takahashi, K. and Hoshuyama, T. (1993). Factors influencing return to work after stroke in Japan. *Stroke*, 24(**8**), 1182–1185.

Sandford, P.R., Spengler, S.E. and Sawasky, K.B. (1992). Clonidine in the treatment of brainstem spasticity. Case report. *Am J Phys Med Rehabil*, 71(**5**), 301–303.

Sawner, K.A. and LaVigne, J.M. (1992). *Brunnstrom's Movement Therapy in Hemiplegia: A Neurophysiological Approach*, 2nd edn., J.B. Lippincott, Philadelphia, PA.

Scherling, E., Johnson, H. (1989). A tone-reducing wrist–hand orthosis. *Am J Occup Ther*, 43(**9**), 609–611.

Schmidt, R.A. (1991). Motor learning principles for physical therapy. In: *Contemporary Management of Motor Control Problems: Proceedings of the II STEP Conference* (ed. Lister, M.J.), Foundation for Physical Therapy, Alexandria VA, pp. 49–63.

Shawker, T.H., Sonies, B.C., Hall, T.E. and Baum, B.F. (1984). Ultrasound analysis of tongue, hyoid, and larynx activity during swallowing. *Invest Radiol*, **19**, 82–86.

Smith, S.A. (1990). Splinting the severely involved hand. *Occup Ther Forum*, December 17, 1990.

Sogbein, S.K. and Awad, S.A. (1982). Behavioural treatment of urinary incontinence in geriatric patients. *Can Med Assoc J*, **127**, 863–864.

Sonde, L., Gip, C., Fernaeus, S.E., Nilsson, C.G. and Viitanen, M. (1998). Stimulation with low-frequency (1.7 Hz) transcutaneous electric nerve stimulation (low tens) increase motor function of the post-stroke paretic arm. *Scand J Rehabil Med*, 36(**2**), 95–99.

Sonksen, J. and Biering-Sorensen, F. (1992). Transcutaneous nitroglycerin in the treatment of erectile dysfunction in spinal cord injured. *Paraplegia*, **30**, 554–557.

Splaingard, M.L., Hutchins, B., Sulton, L.I. and Chadhuri, G. (1988). Aspiration in acute stroke: videofluoroscopy vs. bedside clinical assessment. *Arch Phys Med Rehabil*, **69**, 637–640.

Swanson, A.B. and Swanson, G.D.G. (1989). Evaluation and treatment of the upper extremity in the stroke patient. *Hand Clin North Am*, 5(**1**), 75–96.

Sze, F.K., Wong, E., Or, E.K.H., Lau, J. and Woo, J. (2002). Does acupuncture improve motor recovery after stroke? A meta-analysis of randomized controlled trials. *Stroke*, **33**, 2604–2619.

Tepperman, D.S., Greyson, N.D., Hilbert, L., Jimenez, J. and Williams, J.I. (1984). Reflex sympathetic dystrophy in hemiplegia. *Arch Phys Med Rehabil*, **65**, 442–447.

The Dynamic Slution. (1992). *Dynamic Splinting: Clinical Guidelines*, St. Paul: Empi, Inc.

Tizanidine for Spasticity. (1997). *Med Lett Drugs Ther*, 39(**1004**), 62–63.

Turpie, A.G. (1997). Prophylaxis of venous thromboembolism in stroke patients. *Semin Thromb Hemost*, 23(**2**), 155–157.

Twitchell, T.E. (1951). The restoration of motor function following hemiplegia in man. *Brain*, **74**, 443–480.

Van Buskirk, C. and Webster, D. (1955). Prognostic value of sensory deficits in rehabilitation of hemiplegia. *Neurology*, **5**, 407–411.

Van Ouwenaller, C., Laplace, P.M. and Chantraine, A. (1986). Painful shoulder in hemiplegia. *Arch Phys Med Rehabil*, **67**, 23–26.

Veis, S.L. and Logemann, J.A. (1985). Swallowing disorders in persons with cerebrovascular accident. *Arch Phys Med Rehabil*, 66(**6**), 372–375.

Wallace, J.D. (1994). Summary of the combined clinical analysis of controlled clinical trials with tizanidine. *Neurology*, 11(**Suppl. 9**), S60–S68.

Weiller, C., Chollet, F., Friston, K., Wise, R. and Frackowiak, R. (1992). Functional reorganization of the brain in recovery from striatocapsular infarction in man. *Ann Neurol*, **31**, 463–472.

Weisbroth, S., Esibill, N. and Zuger, R.R. (1971). Factors in the vocational success of hemiplegic patients. *Arch Phys Med Rehabil*, **52**, 441–446.

Winstein, C.J., Miller, J.P., Blanton, S., Taub, E., Uswatte, G., Morris, D., Nichols, D. and Wolf, S. (2003). Methods for a multisite randomized trial to investigate the effect of constraint-induced movement therapy in improving upper extremity function among adults recovering from a cerebrovascular stroke. *NeuroRehabil Neural Repair*, **17**, 137–152.

Wood, K.M. (1978). The use of phenol as a neurolytic agent. *Pain*, **5**, 205–229.

Yablon, S.A. and Sipski, M.L. (1993). Effect of transdermal clonidine on spinal spasticity. *Am J Phys Med Rehabil*, 72(**3**), 154–157.

Yalla, S.V., Vickers, M.A. and Sullivan, M.P. (1994). Sexual dysfunction and spinal cord injury. In: *Impotence: Diagnosis and Management of Erectile Dysfunction* (ed. Bennett, A.H.), W.B. Saunders, Philadelphia, PA, pp. 175–185.

Zislis, J.M. (1964). Splinting of the hand in a spastic hemiplegic patient. *Arch Phys Med Rehabil*, **45**, 41–43.

Zorowitz, R.D., Idank, D., Ikai, T., Hughes, M.B. and Johnston, M.V. (1995). Shoulder subluxation after stroke: a comparison of four supports. *Arch Phys Med Rehabil*, 76(**8**), 763–771.

Zorowitz, R.D., Hughes, M.B., Ikai, T., Idank, D. and Johnston, M.V. (1996). Shoulder subluxation and pain after stroke: correlation or coincidence? *Am J Occup Ther*, 50(**3**), 194–201.

Rehabilitation in spinal cord injury

Diana D. Cardenas and Catherine Warms

Department of Rehabilitation Medicine, University of Washington, Seattle, WA, USA

37.1 Epidemiology of traumatic spinal cord injury

The worldwide incidence of spinal cord injury (SCI) is estimated to be 40 cases per million annually (Sekhon and Fehlings, 2001; National SCI Statistical Center, 2004). In the USA the incidence is approximately 11,000 new cases each year with an additional 4000 cases that do not survive injury long enough to reach a hospital. Prevalence data are less well substantiated due to variability in the severity criteria used to select cases. The estimated number of persons with SCI in the USA is 247,000 (National SCI Statistical Center, 2004).

The National SCI Statistical Center has collected data on approximately 13% of new cases of SCI since 1973. These data (National SCI Statistical Center, 2004) indicate that SCI primarily affects young males (average age at injury is 38 years, 78.2% males). However, with the aging of the USA population, there has been an increase in the proportion of people 60 or more years old at time of injury (4.7% prior to 1980 and 10.9% since 2000). While slightly over half of people with SCI have tetraplegia (56.4%), the proportion of injuries resulting in complete tetraplegia is decreasing and the proportion with incomplete tetraplegia and paraplegia is increasing. Average life expectancy for people with SCI is rising, although actual life expectancy varies with level and completeness of injury as well as age at time of injury. Older people with complete cervical-level injuries have a markedly decreased life expectancy (DeVivo et al., 1993). Motor vehicle crashes are the most common etiology of SCI, accounting for 50.4% since 2000. The most recent data indicate that 11.2% of injuries are attributable

to acts of violence, 23.8% to falls, 9.0% to sports and recreational activities, and 5.6% to other causes. The proportion of injuries due to falls is increasing, while that due to sports is decreasing. Acts of violence were responsible for 13.3% of SCI prior to 1980, increased to 21.8% between 1990 and 1998 and have declined significantly since 2000.

37.2 Initial rehabilitation

The key to rehabilitation of the patient with acute SCI is a strong team approach. The point of transfer is dependent on the medical stability of the patient. The rehabilitation team is typically directed by a rehabilitation physician with other medical and surgical specialists as consultants. The rehabilitation team includes the physicians, nurses, therapists (occupational, physical, speech, respiratory, and recreational), a psychologist, vocational counselor, and usually a case manager.

Neurologic assessment

The neurologic level of injury is determined according to the results of the motor and sensory examination. The level of injury is defined as the caudal most segment with intact motor and sensory innervation. Standard dermatome and myotome references have been established by the American Spinal Injury Association (ASIA) (ASIA and IMSOP, 2000). The injury is classified according to the sensory and motor levels, and by the pattern of injury. The injury is defined as incomplete if there is sparing of sensory or motor function below the neurologic level, including the

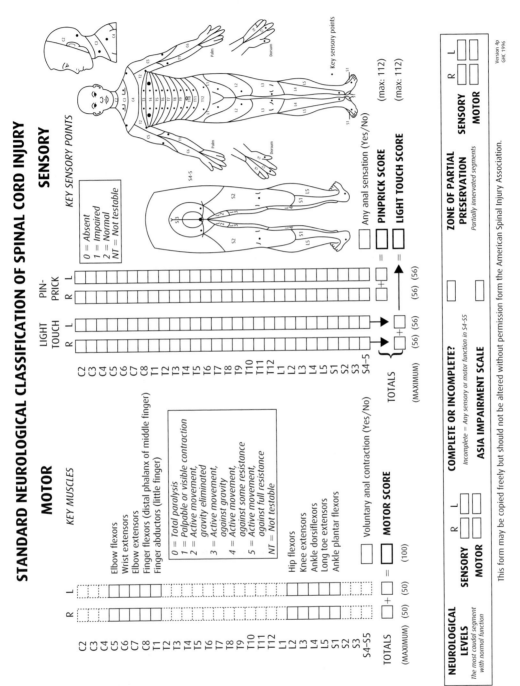

Figure 37.1. Standard Neurological Classification of Spinal Cord Injury, 2000. (Reproduced with permission from the American Spinal Injury Association.)

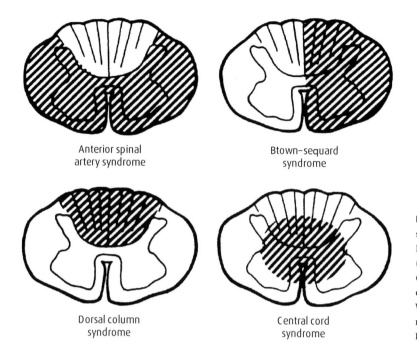

Anterior spinal
artery syndrome

Btown–sequard
syndrome

Dorsal column
syndrome

Central cord
syndrome

Figure 37.2. Incomplete clinical syndromes (original figure from Britell, C.W. and Hammond, M.C. (1994). Spinal cord injury. In: *Chronic Disease and Disability*, eds Hays, R.M., Kraft, G.H., Stolov, W.C., p. 144.). Reproduced and modified with permission from Demos Medical Publishing.

S4/S5 segments. Comprehensive clinical examination and ASIA classification of the SCI individual is important not only for documenting clinical changes, but also for determining functional prognosis. For comprehensive instructions, consult the International Standards for Neurological and Functional Classification of Spinal Cord Injury (ASIA and IMSOP, 2000). Examination and classification is facilitated by the scoring chart (Fig. 37.1). ASIA scoring requires that the key muscle in the myotome have at least grade 3 (antigravity) strength. Intact innervation is presumed if all the segments above have grade 5 strength. Distinct clinical syndromes (Fig. 37.2) can result from SCI.

Central cord syndrome

This involves the central gray matter and the medial white matter, usually due to a cervical hyperextension injury. This results in weaker upper extremities than lower extremities and sacral sensory sparing (Schneider et al., 1954; ASIA and IMSOP, 2000).

Brown–Sequard syndrome occurs from a lesion to half of the spinal cord in the axial plane, resulting in weakness, spasticity and alteration of light touch on one side of the body, with decreased pain and temperature sensation on the opposite side (ASIA and IMSOP, 2000). Causes include gunshot wounds and stabbings (Taylor and Gleave, 1957).

Cauda equina syndrome

This is due to lesions below the conus medullaris, resulting in lower motor neuron (LMN) symptoms, with flaccid lower extremities, bowel and bladder.

Conus medullaris syndrome

Lesions at the level of the conus will usually have a mixture of upper motor neuron (UMN) and LMN characteristics.

Anterior cord syndrome

This usually results from injury to the anterior spinal artery (Ozer and Gibson, 1987), thus causing bilateral weakness, spasticity, and loss of pain/temperature sensation with sparing of vibration, proprioception, and light touch sensations associated with the posterior columns.

Musculoskeletal assessment

Following the period of spinal shock (days to weeks), patients with UMN lesions begin to develop spasticity, usually in an extensor pattern in the legs. Spasticity may be scored by the Ashworth scale (Ashworth, 1964), the modified Ashworth scale (Bohannon and Smith, 1986), the spasm frequency scale (Snow et al., 1990), or by the pendulum test (Nance, 1994) (see Chapter 17 of Volume II).

Musculoskeletal pain after SCI must be distinguished from neuropathic pain caused by neural damage because pharmacologic and non-pharmacologic treatments depend upon the etiology of the pain (see below). SCI individuals are prone to overuse, entrapment neuropathies such as carpal tunnel syndrome or ulnar neuropathies, as well as radiculopathies. These may develop acutely, or after chronic injury, and should be evaluated by electrodiagnostic testing based on clinical presentation.

Pulmonary assessment

Respiratory compromise after SCI is due to impairment of both ventilation and the coughing mechanism. The higher the level of SCI, the more severe are the impairments. Injuries caudal to T12 generally spare pulmonary dysfunction. Since abdominal muscles are supplied by the T6–T12 roots, abdominal and intercostal muscle functions are added with lesions progressively lower between these levels, with improved coughing and expiration. Those with complete lesions at T1–T5 have no abdominal strength and impaired intercostal musculature. At and above the C3 level, diaphragmatic innervation is disrupted, necessitating mechanical ventilation. Initial assessment should evaluate possible trauma-associated injuries such as hemothorax or lung contusions. Concomitant head injury increases the risk of aspiration or the development of neurogenic pulmonary edema. Acute assessment should include

bedside testing of the forced vital capacity (FVC), tidal volume, negative inspiratory pressure for those on mechanical ventilation and arterial blood gases.

Cardiovascular evaluation

Early detection of deep venous thrombosis (DVT), and the associated risk of pulmonary embolism (PE) should be pursued, despite prophylaxis. Assessment for DVT is usually by a venous doppler (duplex scan) and a laboratory D-dimer study may be of value. A ventilation–perfusion scan is usually the preliminary study to rule out PE but pulmonary arteriography or spiral computerized tomography may be more definitive.

Orthostatic hypotension is common immediately after SCI, due to the loss of the sympathetic peripheral vasoconstriction. This must be distinguished from dehydration or low intravascular volume.

Genitourinary evaluation

During the period of spinal shock, the bladder is usually a reflexic, and an indwelling catheter should be placed to allow drainage. Thereafter, assessment of the genitourinary (GU) system is based on whether the injury is a UMN or an LMN (cauda equina) injury, and the presence of detrusor sphincter dysynergia (DSD), the simultaneous contraction of the detrusor muscle and the external urethral sphincter. Baseline GU evaluation during the first weeks post-injury should include renal ultrasound. Urodynamic studies should be done once the bladder is out of spinal shock or by 6 months, whichever comes first (Linsenmeyer and Culkin, 1999). Urodynamic studies assist in determining the functional classification of neurogenic bladder and recommendations for bladder management. Patients with spastic tetraplegia and insufficient hand function (even with splints) may wish to continue with an indwelling foley catheter, since an intermittent catheterization (IC) program (ICP) may make the individual dependent upon an attendant to perform ICP every 4–6h. If condom catheter bladder management is chosen, SCI males with DSD will not be able to adequately drain the bladder without a sphincterotomy. The goals of bladder management are to maintain continence, allow adequate emptying of the bladder, prevent accumulation of post-void residual volumes above 100 ml or maintain IC bladder volumes $\leqslant$500 ml, and enable the individual to be as functionally independent as possible. The bladder management method selected should be acceptable to the patient and fit with the desired lifestyle.

Gastrointestinal evaluation

Immediately post-SCI, paralytic ileus is common, but should resolve within a week as the bowel regains intrinsic activity (Gore et al., 1981). Gastrointestinal bleeding is uncommon, perhaps because of the routine use of ulcer prophylaxis (Cardenas et al., 1995). During the first 3 weeks of hospitalization, the most common gastrointestinal complications are ileus, peptic ulcer, and gastritis (Albert et al., 1991). During the transitional and chronic phases, assessment of neurogenic bowel is similar to that of neurogenic bladder. A scheduled bowel program should be established as soon as possible, and will depend on the type of injury. In the presence of spasticity and a spastic external anal sphincter, an UMN-type of bowel is likely. The UMN bowel program includes judicious use of stool softener and a suppository or mini-enema, followed by digital stimulation of the rectum until the bowels have reflexively evacuated stool. This should be performed daily or every-other-day. Lack of limb spasticity and a flaccid external anal sphincter indicates an LMN-type of bowel. The LMN bowel program includes judicious use of stool-bulking agents and daily or twice-daily manual disimpaction.

Integument evaluation

Neurogenic skin is at significant risk for pressure and shear injury, especially over bony prominences. SCI individuals must immediately be placed on a special mattress that allows equal distribution of pressure, and turned at least every 2 h. The wheelchair must be fitted with a special cushion (see Chapter 11 of Volume II), and the individual's weight

must be shifted every 15 min. The transition of responsibility for maintaining skin integrity and prevention of pressure/shear injury, from caregivers to the patient, is an interdisciplinary rehabilitation team effort. Prevention and comprehensive management of pressure ulcers is described below.

Potential medical and surgical complications

SCI may be complicated by respiratory disorders, DVT and PE, pressure ulcers, autonomic dysreflexia (AD), heterotopic ossification (HO), urinary tract infections (UTIs), renal calculi, gastrointestinal dysfunction, spasticity, and pain. Some of these complications, for example DVT and potentially fatal PE, are much more common during the acute stage after SCI. Others may occur anytime after SCI, for example UTI and pain, and may become lifelong problems. Still other complications, for example AD and spasticity do not occur until after spinal shock subsides.

Respiratory complications

Atelectasis and pneumonia are more common during the first 3 weeks after injury and those with complete injuries are more at risk than those with incomplete injuries. Prevention includes deep breathing exercises, changes in bed position, incentive spirometry, and "quad" coughing for those who do not have adequate abdominal muscle strength. Vigorous pulmonary toilet can decrease the incidence of pulmonary complications. A useful alternative to tracheal suctioning is use of a mechanical in-exsufflator (MI-E). This is a device that provides deep insufflation followed by an immediate decrease in pressure, to create a forced exsufflation. It may be applied via endotracheal or tracheostomy tubes, or via oral–nasal interfaces. MI-E is usually well tolerated, and can be effective in clearing mucous plugs, attenuating atelectasis, and increasing vital capacity. Ventilator weaning after SCI may proceed more slowly than in patients with primary pulmonary disorders, since cervical SCI impairs intercostal and abdominal muscle function.

DVT and PE

The highest risk of DVT is in the first few weeks after injury. The reported incidence of DVT has ranged from 47% to 100% (Myllynen et al., 1985; Merli et al., 1988). DVT prophylaxis should continue for 8–12 weeks depending on risk factors (Green et al., 1997). DVTs should be prevented with compression stockings, sequential-compression devices (SCDs), and either adjusted-dose heparin or low-molecular-weight heparin. The SCD can be discontinued once the patient is wheelchair mobile. Duplex ultrasonography is a useful non-invasive tool for the detection of DVT. Signs and symptoms of PE may be subtle, so the patient with or without DVT must be questioned about chest or shoulder pain or discomfort, cough, or shortness of breath. If any of these are present, the patient must be assessed further.

Pressure ulcers

Pressure ulcers may develop anytime after SCI and are among the costliest complications. Ulcers develop in dependent body areas, usually over bony prominences. Sacral ulcers are the most common during initial hospitalization and ischial ulcers in chronic SCI (Yarkony and Heinemann, 1995). Unrelieved pressure and shear injury are the usual etiologies of skin breakdown, and require patient vigilance and multidisciplinary team assessment and intervention for acute and chronic management. Patients are instructed in weight shifting while in the manual wheelchair, and patients with injuries above the C5 or C6 levels of injury will likely require a power tilting mechanism to relieve pressure. Once a pressure ulcer develops, pressure must be relieved for the wound to heal. This may entail bedrest on a dynamic mattress. In extreme cases with deep ulcers, myocutaneous flap surgery may be required.

Autonomic dysreflexia

The signs and symptoms of AD include an acute elevation of blood pressure associated with headache, sweating above the lesion, nasal congestion, piloerection, and, sometimes, bradycardia. AD may

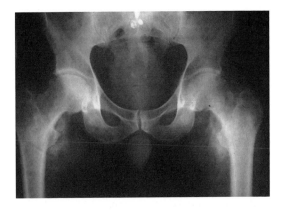

Figure 37.3. Heterotopic ossification surrounding hip joints.

occur in the patient with SCI at or above the T6 level after the period of spinal shock. The most common causative agent is bladder distention followed by bowel distention. But, any noxious stimulus below the level of the lesion may lead to AD. The treatment is directed to removing the stimulus; for example, checking the catheter for kinks if indwelling, or catheterizing the bladder if on IC. Sometimes the blood pressure requires immediate treatment with nitro-paste, nitroglycerin 1/150 sublingually, or an agent, such as hydralazine. *Clinical Practice Guidelines* for detection and treatment of AD have been published by the Consortium for Spinal Cord Medicine (Linsenmeyer et al., 1997).

Heterotopic ossification

This is the abnormal development of bone in the soft tissues surrounding a joint and occurs in 16–53% of patients with SCI (Fig. 37.3) (Finerman and Stover, 1981). The etiology of HO is unknown but is likely related to a combination of immobility and neurogenic and traumatic factors, since it also is seen after traumatic brain injury (TBI), burns, and total hip replacement. HO develops only below the level of the SCI, most commonly at the hips, but also in other locations. A triple-bone scan is helpful diagnostically because it will become abnormal before calcification appears in X-rays (Orzel and Rudd, 1985). Alkaline phosphatase is elevated in HO and falls again when it is treated successfully with disodium etidronate or indomethacin (Stover et al., 1976; Schmidt et al., 1988). In refractory cases surgery and radiation therapy may be necessary.

Spasticity

Spasticity may interfere with function, self-care, or lead to contractures and pain. By 1 year after SCI, 78% of patients and 91% of those with tetraplegia develop spasticity (Maynard et al., 1990). The most basic form of treatment is stretching, but this may provide only very temporary relief of spasms. Several medications are effective (Table 37.1), including baclofen, tizanidine, and sodium dantrolene. Diazepam may provide rapid relief but is addicting and therefore, not a first line drug. Nerve blocks using phenol or botulinum toxin also help. Some patients may not obtain enough relief of spasticity with medications or blocks and benefit from the use of intrathecal baclofen (Nance et al., 1955). The choice of treatment should proceed from the least invasive to the more invasive treatments. Common infections such as UTI may aggravate spasticity and should be treated. Of note antidepressants, particularly the newer selective serotonin reuptake inhibitors (SSRIs), may increase spasticity (Stolp-Smith and Wainberg, 1999).

Urinary tract infections

These are common in patients with SCI during the initial hospitalization and in many persons throughout the remainder of life. The signs and symptoms of UTI may include increased spasticity, cloudy and odorous urine, urinary incontinence, AD, malaise, fever and chills. Patients with complete injuries do not sense dysuria. IC is less likely to lead to recurrent UTIs but only for those who perform self-catheterization, as opposed to having a caregiver perform IC (Cardenas and Mayo, 1987). Indwelling catheters increase the risk of UTIs and are also associated with an increased risk of calculi, epididymitis, fistula formation, and the development of bladder carcinoma (Cardenas and Hooton, 1995).

Chronic pain

This is a common SCI complication. Pain may be sensed both at the level of the injury and below. The incidence of chronic pain has been estimated at 69% (Bonica, 1991). Two major categories of pain are neuropathic and musculoskeletal. Neuropathic pain may be divided into four types: central pain or SCI pain, which occurs below the level of the injury; transitional zone or segmental pain, which occurs at the level of the injury; radicular pain, which may occur at any dermatomal level and is usually unilateral; and visceral pain, which is perceived in the abdomen (Anke et al., 1995; Cardenas et al., 2002a).

Treatment of neuropathic pain in SCI is largely empirical. Drugs that have been used include narcotics, antidepressants, anticonvulsants, and others. Of the antidepressants amitriptyline was not found effective in a recent double-blind, placebo-controlled trial of persons with SCI and chronic pain (Cardenas et al., 2002b). The newer SSRIs do not seem clinically effective for treatment of chronic SCI pain. Gabapentin (Neurontin) has been found beneficial in SCI pain and has a better side effect profile than carbamazepine (Tegretol), an older antiepileptic drug used for chronic neuropathic pain (Levendoglu et al., 2004). Some patients will need to be maintained on narcotics. It is important to establish a strict agreement with the patient regarding dosing because tolerance may develop and the patient may seek more medication. Non-pharmacologic modalities such as acupuncture, relaxation techniques, exercise, and self-hypnosis may be useful for some patients (Warms et al., 2002).

Post-traumatic syringomyelia

The development of a fluid-filled cavity (syrinx) within the spinal cord can be a devastating late complication of SCI. Post-traumatic syringomyelia (PTS) occurs in 1% to 5% of SCI individuals (Rossier et al., 1985; Schurch et al., 1996). The pathogenesis is unclear. The cavity develops at the injury site, followed by enlargement and extension rostrally and caudally. Extension may occur from pressure pulses within the epidural venous system, exacerbated by activities that cause valsalva; for example, coughing, sneezing, straining at stool, exercising. Loss of sensory or motor level or a change in myotatic reflexes should alert the clinician to the possibility of PTS.

Diagnosis is ascertained by neurologic examination followed by magnetic resonance imaging (MRI). A cyst at the level of injury alone is not PTS. There is no definitive correlation between the size of the syrinx and severity of deficit. Once PTS is diagnosed, each patient must be individually considered regarding follow-up and treatment. Surgical treatments include shunts and duraplasty, but they are not always successful.

Cardiovascular complications

The relatively sedentary lifestyle of SCI patients reduces cardiovascular fitness and promotes obesity, glucose intolerance, elevated cholesterol, and low levels of high-density lipoprotein (HDL) (Heldenberg et al., 1981). Cardiac etiologies are second only to pulmonary etiologies as causes of death in chronic SCI (DeVivo et al., 1999). Silent ischemia may occur with higher level of lesions. Hypertension is more prevalent in the SCI population, and is related to increasing age and lesion level.

Endocrine complications

The SCI population has significantly increased risk of developing type II diabetes mellitus secondary to insulin resistance (Duckworth et al., 1980; Bauman and Spungen, 1994), likely due to muscle wasting, adiposity, and relative inactivity.

Antidiuretic hormone (ADH) is secreted in response to hypovolemia and increased serum osmolality (Schmitt and Schroeder, 2003). It is secreted in diurnal surges with highest levels at night, suppressing nocturnal diuresis. In some SCI individuals, the diurnal rhythm may be impaired, and exogenous ADH therapy may be beneficial at night. This is especially important if large nocturnal urine volumes are precluding a successful ICP for bladder management. Patients with dual SCI and brain injury may also develop the syndrome of inappropriate ADH.

Osteoporosis below the level of the lesion develops immediately after SCI, and may result in impaired calcium metabolism. Acutely injured individuals should receive increased fluids to prevent immobilization hypercalcemia, which presents as nausea, abdominal pain, and elevated ionized calcium. Treatment should be initiated with intravenous fluids, but may require biphosphonate medication.

Neurogenic factors affect hypothalamic temperature regulation, and individuals with higher lesion levels may be poikilothermic, at risk for hyperthermia in warm weather, and hypothermia in cool weather.

37.3 Functional outcomes in SCI

The most accurate predictor for recovery from SCI is the standardized physical examination as endorsed by the International Standards for Neurological and Functional Classification of Spinal Cord Injury Patients (ASIA and IMSOP, 2000), that is, the neurologic (motor) level and severity. Other diagnostic tests such as MRI may be helpful. The presence of extensive cord edema and hemorrhage are poor prognostic indicators. The initial strength of a muscle is a significant predictor of achieving functional antigravity strength caudal to any neurologic level of injury. Other factors, such as preservation of sacral pinprick sensation or volitional anal contraction, also portend an improved prognosis. Incomplete injuries have a better prognosis for ambulation and functional outcome than complete injuries. Patient education about recovery mechanisms and prognostic measures is essential to the rehabilitation process because it facilitates planning the course of rehabilitation, equipment needs, discharge disposition, and caregiver support. In addition to the neurologic (motor) level and severity (ASIA impairment scale) of the SCI, other factors affecting functional outcomes include co-morbidities (e.g. TBI), obesity, age, motivation, psychosocial and socioeconomic factors, post-hospitalization setting, access to healthcare, and rehabilitation services after acute rehabilitation. Today's shortened lengths of stay in acute in-patient rehabilitation may also affect functional outcomes. If there is funding, rehabilitation may continue in an outpatient rehabilitation center. It is important to understand the functional outcome predicted by neurologic level, since patients may not achieve these goals by discharge from initial rehabilitation.

Functional improvement occurs faster with incomplete than with complete SCI. For those with incomplete injuries, one-half to two-thirds of the 1-year motor recovery occurs within the first 2 months after injury (Bracken and Holford, 2002). Recovery continues more slowly after 3–6 months (Waters et al., 1994a, b). Recovery of motor function continues past 1 year and has been documented up to 2 years post-injury (Ditunno Jr. et al., 1992) and rarely beyond (McDonald et al., 2002).

SCI with higher ASIA impairment levels have varying degrees of recovery. Research on complete tetraplegia has provided the best predictive data on functional outcomes. Most of this information is regarding muscles at or near the level of injury. Recovery in muscles graded as 1 to 3 – on a 0–5 scale, have a better prognosis than muscles with a muscle grade of zero. For muscles with initial strength of 1–2, 90% achieve antigravity strength (grade 3) by 1 year (Ditunno Jr. et al., 1992). Of those with an initial strength of zero, 64% achieve antigravity strength (grade 3) by 2 years (Ditunno Jr. et al., 1992).

Functional outcome-based guidelines provide estimates of the effect of rehabilitation on functional abilities. This has important implications for the level of care required and for estimating the cost of care for the individual with SCI. The Consortium of Spinal Cord Medicine has developed an outcome-based guideline based on extensive data from research conducted by the National Spinal Cord Injury Statistical Center on the Functional Independence Measure (FIM), expert clinical observation and judgment (Whiteneck et al., 1999).

Outcomes by spinal level

C1–C4 tetraplegia

A patient with a complete lesion at C1–C4 has complete paralysis of trunk, arms and legs, and requires a mechanical ventilator except in the case of C4 tetraplegia. Patients with C1–C2 tetraplegia may be candidates for phrenic nerve stimulation and diaphragmatic pacing. Individuals with C4 tetraplegia may need continuous positive airway pressure (CPAP) or bilevel positive airway pressure (BiPAP) at night to assist with hypoventilation.

The individual with tetraplegia at C1–C4 is dependent for self-care, transfers and bed mobility, but can be independent for drinking fluids with setup of a secured container or sport hydration system and straw approximated to the mouth. Power wheelchair independence including tilting for pressure relief is possible with the use of controls operated by the head, mouth or chin, tongue, voice activation, infrared devices, or breath control. Environmental control units (ECUs), with similar operational inputs as power wheelchairs, increase independence with computer/telephone access, operation of lights, fans, television, doors, security systems, and other home devices. Mouthsticks may be utilized if the individual demonstrates sufficient head control/neck strength. Individuals with C1–C4 tetraplegia are not candidates for independent driving, which requires use of one upper limb to operate a specialized driving system. Although some independence can be achieved via ECUs, a 24-h attendant is required for personal care and homemaking tasks.

C5 tetraplegia

The patient has added at least antigravity (grade 3 on a 0–5 scale) strength in the biceps and also has movement in the deltoid, rhomboids, supraspinatus, infraspinatus, and less than grade 3 movement in wrist extensors. Movements gained include shoulder flexion, extension and abduction, elbow flexion, forearm supination, and weak scapular adduction and abduction. There is paralysis of trunk and legs, absence of elbow extension, pronation, and all hand movement. The patient is unable to perform independent transfers but can operate a power wheelchair, including tilt backs, with appropriately placed controls/switches. Active elbow flexion allows for

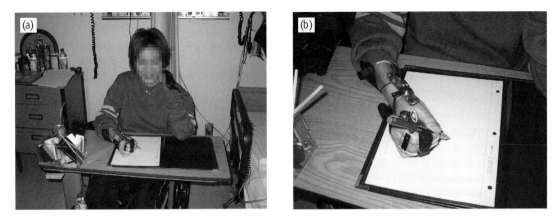

Figure 37.4. (a) Patient with C6 tetraplegia using tenodesis splint for writing and (b) tenodesis splint used to grip pen.

possible independent self-feeding and grooming utilizing splints, overhead slings or mobile arm supports and assistive devices. A ratchet tenodesis splint allows for pinch without wrist extensors. The ratchet mechanism allows external splint activation. C5 is the highest level of tetraplegia that permits driving, given specialized equipment and a wheelchair accessible vehicle. Since most activities will require assistive devices, consideration may be given to tendon transfers for gross hand function once neurologic recovery is considered complete. Individuals will require attendant care daily to assist with self-care and homemaking tasks.

C6 tetraplegia

The individual with C6 tetraplegia has added at least antigravity strength (3/5) in the radial wrist extensors (extensor carpi radialis longus and brevis). Additional muscles partially innervated include supinator, pronator teres, clavicular head of pectoralis major, and latissimus dorsi. Movements gained also include scapular abduction and radial wrist extension. With the addition of wrist extension, tenodesis grasp is possible, which allows the fingers to pinch (Hollar, 1995).

The C6 tetraplegic with at least 3+/5 wrist extension may benefit from a wrist-driven flexor hinge splint (tenodesis splint) to create a three-jaw chuck pinch (Fig. 37.4(a) and (b)). However, there is a tendency for patients to stop using this long term. Therefore, it is sometimes better to allow contractures or muscle shortening to develop in the finger flexors to create a natural tenodesis grasp.

Individuals with C6 tetraplegia can usually achieve independence for feeding, grooming with assistive devices, and use of a tenodesis splint. Upper body dressing independence can be achieved, but some assistance will be required with lower body dressing and a hospital bed may be needed to elevate the head. Modifications to clothing fasteners such as loops, Velcro® closures on shirts, shoes, and pants increase independence. Extensive training is needed for an individual with C6 tetraplegia to achieve independence for transfers. A sliding board and a trapeze over the bed may be necessary. With a tenodesis splint, some men can perform self-catheterization, but may need assistance with clothing and are not able to apply a condom catheter. Women will likely require continued assistance with catheterization. Independent bowel management is not likely, even with assistive devices (digital stimulation, suppository inserter). Independent manual wheelchair propulsion is possible but the wheelchair may require plastic coated rims or knobs. A power wheelchair may be appropriate, especially if the individual is to return to work. Return to driving requires significant evaluation of strength, active range of motion, and functional skills, to determine the most appropriate equipment (seating, steering, hand controls) and van modifications.

At the C6 level, tendon transfers can improve gross hand function. The criteria for tendon transfer include: neurologic recovery is complete and function is maximized, spasticity in the hand is absent or negligible, joints have full range of motion, muscles transferred must be at least 4/5 strength, and the individual must be motivated and committed to extensive post-operative rehabilitation. Tendon transfers of the pronator teres to the flexor digitorum profundus, the brachioradialis to the flexor pollicis longus, and the posterior deltoid to the triceps can provide finger and thumb movement and elbow extension (Waters et al., 1996).

C7–C8 tetraplegia

C7–C8 tetraplegia adds triceps, serratus anterior, pronator quadratus, extensor carpi ulnaris, flexor carpi radialis, flexor digitorum profundus and superficialis, interrossei/lumbricals, and abductor pollicis. Movements gained at C7 include elbow extension of at least grade 3, scapular stabilization, protraction and elevation, ulnar wrist extension, and wrist flexion. At the C8 level, digit flexion and extension, and thumb flexion, extension abduction, and circumduction allow improved hand and finger function.

Individuals with C7 tetraplegia will likely have enough upper extremity motor return to become independent with eating, grooming, dressing, and bathing with appropriate assistive devices and durable medical equipment. Men are likely to achieve independent self-catheterization, but women may still require assistance, especially if leg spasticity is present. Bowel management independence is possible with assistive devices. Independent transfers, weight shifts, pressure reliefs, and manual wheelchair use are feasible with extensive training. Most individuals with C7–C8 SCI have enough shoulder strength to operate a modified van with standard steering wheel and a car with hand controls. A wheelchair-accessible van may be needed if the patient is unable to load/unload their wheelchair independently.

T1–T9 paraplegia

T1–T9 paraplegia adds intrinsic hand muscles. The movements gained at T1 are fully functioning upper limbs. With T2–T9 paraplegia, intercostal and erector spinae muscles are added. Abdominal muscle innervation begins at T6. Independence is achieved in all self-care tasks, including bowel and bladder management and mobility. At lower thoracic levels, standing and ambulation are possible with bracing, but long term these are often abandoned due to very high-energy requirements. There must be adequate tolerance to vertical positioning before ambulation. Standing frame or standing frame/parallel bars and bilateral leg orthoses help achieve vertical tolerance. Bilateral lower-extremity orthoses such as hip–knee–ankle–foot orthoses (HKAFO), reciprocating gait orthosis (RGOs) (T5–T7), knee–ankle–foot orthoses (KAFOs) (T8–T12) with knee locks and ankle–foot orthoses (AFO) with floor reaction modifications may be indicated for individuals with SCI, depending upon completeness and return of function, ambulation goals and personal preference. The "Parastep® system," a functional electrical stimulation (FES) device is an option for ambulation training (see Chapter 9 of Volume II). FES requires the presence of an intact reflex arc, so individuals with LMN lesions are not candidates.

T10–L1 paraplegia

The individual with T10–L1 paraplegia has fully innervated intercostals, external obliques, and rectus abdominus. With L1 paraplegia there is also partial innervation of hip flexors such as iliopsoas. Movements gained include trunk stability and improved potential for ambulation with orthoses. At L1, individuals will likely achieve household ambulation with bilateral KAFOs using a four-point gait with crutches. Independence is achieved in all self-care tasks including bowel and bladder management, and mobility in a wheelchair.

L2–S4/S5 paraplegia

L2–S4/S5 paraplegia leaves fully intact abdominal muscles, most trunk muscles, partially to fully innervated hip flexors, extensors, abductors, knee flexors and extensors, and ankle dorsiflexors and plantar flexors. With L3 paraplegia, quadriceps, and iliopsoas are fully innervated and voluntary knee extension is improved. Ankle dorsiflexion is partially innervated at L4. Ankle plantar flexors are gained at S1. The individual at these levels is fully independent with all self-care and functional mobility. Bowel and bladder management can be performed independently but the methods are dependent upon whether there is a UMN or an LMN lesion. At the L3 level community ambulation using a four-point gait usually requires AFOs with crutches or canes. At this level the individual can usually operate a standard vehicle, sometimes requiring hand controls.

Additional therapeutic considerations

The body weight support system

The body weight support system (BWSS; see below and Chapter 3 of Volume II), used with a treadmill or in combination with parallel bars, may be a good alternative to parallel bars alone for individuals who wish to start ambulation but have questionable proximal leg strength and fear falling. Once they have mastered these techniques, ambulation may progress over ground (Fig. 37.5) and to assistive devices, such as a reciprocating walker, crutches, or canes. Some drawbacks to ambulation that need to be considered and discussed with the individual throughout the process include whether the amount of energy expended is worth the mode of locomotion and whether the strain of additional weight bearing on the arms will lead to overuse syndromes.

Adjustment to SCI

During acute hospitalization and rehabilitation, the injured individual temporarily must depend on

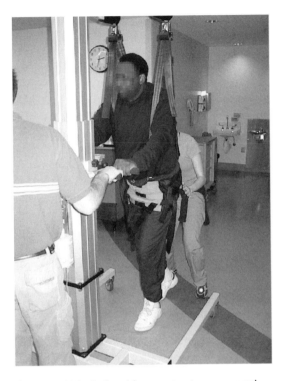

Figure 37.5. Using body weight support system overground.

others, engendering a sense of helplessness and concern about burdening others. Societal norms and healthcare provider beliefs allow for a period of grief and depression after a severe loss and almost impose it on those with SCI. Such "normalization" of depression and grieving can add unintended stress for some patients who may not be experiencing these symptoms (North, 1999).

One model for conceptualizing psychologic adjustment to SCI is the stress appraisal and coping (SAC) model (Fig. 37.6) (Lazarus and Folkman, 1984; Galvin and Godfrey, 2001). This model explains variability in psychologic adjustment as a function of the situation, coping skills and styles, and the individual's stressors and resources. Stress responses are the outcomes of this process and vary from depression, anxiety and distress about physical symptoms to acceptance of disability and satisfaction with life. The SAC model provides a framework for

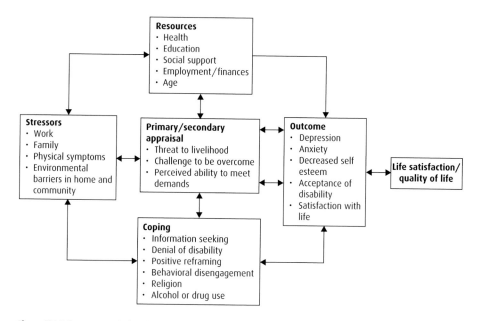

Figure 37.6. Stress appraisal and coping formulation of emotional adjustment to spinal cord injury (original figure Galvin, L.R. and Godfrey, P.D.H. (2001). The impact of coping on emotional adjustment to spinal cord injury: review of the literature and application of a stress appraisal and coping formulation. *Spinal Cord*, **39**(12), 617). Reproduced and modified with permission from Nature Publishing Group.

understanding individual differences in outcomes immediately after SCI and long term.

Appraisal

During rehabilitation and the first year or two after injury, people with SCI tend to compare their current state with their formerly able-bodied selves. Sometimes the need for time to adapt to the changed situation conflicts with the rehabilitation team's need to encourage progress toward independence. With time, a SCI person's appraisal of the situation usually changes. The experience of disability can be a satisfying opportunity for growth and for some, the disability is a way to reinterpret life and regain personal meaning. Since predicting the extent and duration of functional recovery is difficult, the belief in recovery need not be a detriment to the rehabilitation process unless the patient is unwilling to participate in therapies. Sometimes staff express

concerns about "denial" and may believe that forcing an acceptance of "reality" is necessary for adjustment to injury. However, it is important to balance the staff's need for reality with a patient's and family's need for hope, which can be a motivating force to accomplish immediate or short-term goals (Lohne, 2001). Even if the ultimate hope is to "walk out of the hospital" most people with SCI can understand that independence in self-care is a necessary first step.

Stressors

SCI patients experience stress from the hospitalization and disruption in work, home and family roles, and routines. Stress to family members may have a detrimental effect on family health and functioning. Chronic health problems, feelings of frustration, isolation, guilt, and even resentment are reported by family members of newly injured patients (North,

1999). Counseling is required to help family members avoid promoting dependency in the patient through guilt or sympathy, and to support the process of grieving for the family and patient.

Disrupted employment and issues related to returning to work are frequent stressors. While 63% of people admitted to a SCI model system were employed at the time of injury, only 31.7% of people with paraplegia and 26.4% of tetraplegic persons were employed 10 years later (www.spinalcord.uab.edu, 2004). Sometimes SCI necessitates a career change and extensive education and/or re-training. For some people the demands of living with an SCI preclude returning to the workforce. Vocational counseling and social worker assistance during inpatient rehabilitation are important. Planning for transitions to school or vocational training and accessing programs during initial rehabilitation promote long-term adjustment and may decrease stress during the immediate post-discharge period.

Environmental barriers preventing access to home and community may also be a source of stress. Whether or not a given environmental feature will be a barrier depends on the individual's age, mobility, physical strength, and the availability of assistance. It is important to experience such barriers during rehabilitation to promote a sense of mastery and to foster problem-solving abilities. A thorough evaluation of the post-discharge home environment should be done by occupational or physical therapy and an overnight pass before discharge from the hospital is recommended. Gradual re-entry into the community beginning with excursions accompanied by therapeutic recreation staff, transitioning to family escorts and finally independent excursions, will promote confidence and courage.

Resources

An individual's resources for psychologic adjustment include age, level of education, employment/financial resources, and availability of a social support network. Younger individuals generally adjust better than older individuals (Galvin and Godfrey, 2001) perhaps due to fewer commitments to a particular path or lifestyle. Similarly, higher levels of education may contribute to greater flexibility by helping an individual to recognize options rather than focusing on losses. Employment or financial resources that can be maintained after injury offer levels of protection from stresses due to loss of vocation. Finally, more than any other resource, social support is known to moderate the severity of emotional reactions to SCI (Galvin and Godfrey, 2001). Family interactions that foster closeness and participation in more family activities are strongly associated with life satisfaction and positive adjustment (Warren et al., 1996).

Coping skills and styles

Coping skills and strategies are defined by Lazarus and Folkman as "cognitive and behavioral efforts to manage external or internal demands" stemming from a stressful situation. Emotion-focused strategies approach the emotional response to a situation that is perceived to be unchangeable. Emotion-focused coping strategies are often maladaptive in that they attempt to avoid the feelings associated with stressors and include such behaviors as drug and alcohol use, disengagement from the situation, or denial of emotions. Problem-focused strategies, on the other hand, occur in situations where the individual perceives that she/he has some control over the situation and include behaviors aimed at managing the stressful situation. Use of mainly emotion-focused strategies early in rehabilitation predicted poor adjustment up to 2 years post-injury (Galvin and Godfrey, 2001). Poor coping skills are also predictive of depression, anxiety, and perceived stress in long-term SCI (Gerhart et al., 1999). One small study suggested that people using the most problem-focused coping strategies make the greatest improvement over time in their rehabilitation programs (Lou et al., 1997). In a cross-sectional study, people with the best coping skills were most likely to have the highest perceived quality of life (Warren et al., 1996).

The strong correlations between coping skills and adjustment led some researchers and rehabilitation centers to implement programs designed to enhance coping effectiveness early in the rehabilitation process, in order to "immunize" against long-term disruption in mood and poor adjustment. Although there are differing names for such approaches – cognitive behavioral training (CBT), coping effectiveness training (CET), or coping skills education – early evaluations of such approaches show significant reductions in symptoms of depression and anxiety in people experiencing them prior to program participation (Kennedy et al., 2003). Such interventions promote adjustment, restore self-directed behavior, and encourage problem solving.

Outcomes

Severe emotional problems are not as common after SCI as is often believed. Nevertheless it is important for the rehabilitation team to assess frequently for symptoms of developing depression, anxiety, and post-traumatic stress disorder (PTSD). Clinical depression is seen in 23–38% of SCI patients during their initial rehabilitation (Kennedy et al., 2003). This is approximately five times the prevalence in the general population. Higher levels of pain and feeling out of control of one's life predict higher levels of depression (North, 1999). A clinical evaluation for depression should be done if a significant change in behavior is noted or if a consistent pattern of withdrawal, denial, or maladaptive coping is observed. If depression is diagnosed, treatment should be provided including medication and psychotherapy as appropriate.

Anxiety is common in the acute adjustment phase. Factors that contribute to anxiety include sudden changes in body function that may be frightening, lack of control over one's body, environment and life, and lack of mobility that exacerbates fears of being alone or unable to escape a dangerous situation. The hospital environment may contribute to anxiety because of intrusive procedures, lack of privacy, disturbed sleep, and lack of routines. Patients with SCI who are anxious about their situation may benefit from being given control over their schedule, routines, and care. Sleep disturbances should be minimized and psychologic care should

be available on a regular basis. A few patients may benefit from medication for anxiety but most will respond to reassurance, restoration of control, and passage of time.

PTSD consists of intrusive re-experiencing of trauma associated with physiologic arousal and avoidance of situations in which the trauma is re-experienced. In surveys of community-dwelling people with SCI, current prevalence of PTSD is 11% and lifetime prevalence 21–40% (Kennedy and Duff, 2001). PTSD symptoms are often in tandem with other psychologic conditions, especially depression. It is not known whether PTSD results from the trauma (accident or intentional injury), the SCI itself, or a combination of the two. Psychotherapy or medications may be indicated if the patient's symptoms interfere with ability to participate in rehabilitation.

After discharge from the hospital post-rehabilitation, psychosocial adjustment continues in the face of added stressors due to returning to a familiar environment in an unfamiliar body. This immediate post-discharge period and the first few years of living with SCI are known to be periods of high risk for adjustment problems. Suicide risk is higher after SCI than in the general population, with the greatest vulnerability during the first 4 years (Stiens et al., 1997). Risk factors for suicide include previous attempts, age at injury (older age associated with greater risk), alcohol abuse, apathy, shame, weight loss, anger, and destructive behavior. The risk of suicide decreases with time since injury, suggesting that the adjustment process continues for a period of years. Outpatient psychologic support and regular attentive healthcare is extremely important during the immediate post-rehabilitation period.

Despite potential difficulties with adjustment to SCI, over time people with SCI consistently report high levels of satisfaction with life and quality of life, comparable to people without SCI (Post et al., 1998; Putzke et al., 2002). There is a complex relationship among aging, adjustment, and self-reported quality of life. Age is inversely correlated with both psychosocial and functional outcomes, while time since injury is positively correlated with those outcomes. Therefore the effects of chronologic age and time since injury tend to balance each other. For people injured at a younger age, quality of life usually improves with time after SCI, but for people injured at an older age the losses of aging may offset the benefits of experience with SCI.

Health maintenance and lifestyle

Maintaining health after SCI is extremely important since physical symptoms and health problems affect quality of life. Without vigilant self-monitoring, self-care and regular medical follow-up, the number of secondary conditions increases over time. This is true even after controlling for the effects of age and level of injury (Anson and Shepherd, 1996). Surveys of the incidence of secondary conditions among people with long-term SCI found that 95% reported at least one condition, with obesity, pain, spasticity, UTIs, hypotension and pressure sores reported most commonly (Anson and Shepherd, 1996; Noreau et al., 2000). These surveys also found that secondary conditions correlated highly with age and time since injury, frequently led to re-hospitalization, and had a significant impact on social integration.

Alcohol and drug abuse may have preceded SCI in some people. Whether these issues are adequately addressed during rehabilitation depends on the individual's willingness to confront them during this high stress period. After hospital discharge these behaviors commonly return (Young et al., 1995). Beginning or resuming a pattern of using substances as a coping mechanism poses great risks to the ability for self-care, use of good judgment, and choosing to participate in productive activities.

Cigarette smoking may be the most damaging lifestyle behavior for people with SCI. The risks of cardiovascular and respiratory morbidity after SCI are positively associated with age, duration of cigarette use, and the number of cigarettes smoked (Davies and McColl, 2002). Smoking is associated with greater incidence of pressure sores, poor wound-healing, and greater risk of bladder cancer. Exercise and physical activity are important behaviors that may be perceived as difficult or impossible due to the mobility restrictions imposed by the injury. The health benefits of exercise are well known

and may be more important for people with SCI, since many of the secondary conditions associated with SCI are also associated with inactivity. A particular risk of an inactive lifestyle is obesity. Healthcare providers should ask about health behaviors and offer counseling and referrals as needed.

Sexuality

Sexual function after SCI may be changed from pre-injury but the desire to be sexually active and maintain satisfying sexual relationships does not change. The first 6 months after discharge from the hospital are critical for function and realization about sexuality (Fisher et al., 2002). Particular attention to partner issues and relationships is important, since in men with SCI, perceived partner satisfaction, relationship quality, and sexual desire are significant predictors of sexual satisfaction and behavior (Phelps et al., 2001). Every SCI rehabilitation setting should have at least one person who is knowledgeable and comfortable discussing sexuality, and every patient should be offered education and counseling to promote lifelong adjustment.

New and emerging rehabilitation treatments in SCI

Standard SCI rehabilitation

It includes gradual re-mobilization, exercise training, training in activities of daily living and self-care, determination of optimal long-term management of neurogenic bowel and bladder, evaluation for appropriate assistive technologies, extensive education about health self-management and SCI-related complications, and therapies to promote psychologic and social adjustment and return to employment. At present, pharmacologic and cellular therapies specifically targeted to enhance neurologic recovery are limited.

Pharmacotherapy

Currently, the only approved pharmacologic intervention must be administered immediately after injury. Methylprednisolone (MP) was the first treatment shown to improve clinical neurologic recovery in human clinical trials (Bracken et al., 1990, 1997; Bracken and Holford, 1993) when given in high doses (30 mg/kg bolus + 5.4 mg/kg/h over 23–48 h) within 8 h after injury. It is hypothesized to prevent swelling and inflammation and thereby lessen secondary cord injury. MP has been evaluated in five randomized-controlled clinical trials with positive results in three of the five trials and it is currently considered to be the standard of care for acute injury. However, even in the positive trials, improvement in neurologic recovery as compared to controls was minimal, and the rate of infection and sepsis was increased in the group treated with MP. Thus there is controversy about the strength of evidence supporting MP as standard care (Hurlbert, 2001).

Body weight-supported treadmill training

Standard gait training involves strengthening muscles with complete or partial innervation, use of braces or assistive devices and progressive ambulation, beginning on parallel bars and proceeding to indoor or community ambulation. A new rehabilitation technique, body weight-supported treadmill training (BWSTT, a.k.a. "Laufband" therapy; see Chapters 3 and 19 of Volume II), involves partial support of body weight by a harness suspended over a treadmill, unloading paretic limbs by up to 50% (Dobkin et al., 2003a). BWSTT requires therapists to manually assist leg, hip, and trunk control in order to promote repetitive stepping approximating normal gait, a very labor-intensive intervention. BWSTT is believed to enhance recovery of ambulation by providing repetitive sensory input that can strengthen central pattern generator circuitry in the spinal cord (Hulseboch et al., 2000) (see Chapter 13 of Volume I). Several case series and one non-randomized clinical trial with historical controls demonstrated efficacy of BWSTT for improving walking speed, endurance, and head and trunk control (Wernig et al., 1995, 1998; Protas et al., 2001; Barbeau, 2003). However, a large multi-center randomized-controlled trial of 140 patients with recent incomplete SCI (grades B–D) comparing BWSTT with conventional gait training found no significant differences between the two (Barbeau, 2003; Barbeau and Norman, 2003; Dobkin et al., 2003a, b; Kirshblum, 2004). Both modalities enhanced gait parameters, suggesting that any type of intense gait training might enhance locomotor recovery, although the timing and intensity of BWSTT may not have been optimized (see Chapter 3 of Volume II). Due to the labor-intensity of BWSTT, various options for reducing the burden of treatment are being explored including robotic-assistive stepping devices and use of FES. FES may increase sensory input to the central nervous system (CNS) and reduce the requirement for assistance by therapists (Field-Fote, 2000).

Functional electrical stimulation

FES (Chapter 9 of Volume II) of muscles and nerves (FNS) directly bypassing the SCI to produce muscle activation and coordinated movements is another rehabilitative treatment that may be useful for maximizing neural function (Prochazka et al., 2002). The resulting movements can reverse muscle atrophy and may enhance activity-dependent plasticity in the spinal cord (Field-Fote, 2000; Wolpaw and Tennissen, 2001). Specific applications of FES that have been used in the rehabilitation setting include FES to improve upper and lower limb, bladder, and respiratory function.

An implantable neuroprosthesis (freehand) to restore partial motor function in the upper extremity has been approved by the United States Food and Drug Administration for tetraplegic patients after 1 year post-injury (Creasey et al., 2004; Rupp and Gerner, 2004). The system has multiple components that are adapted to the individual and is coupled with an intensive rehabilitation program. Implanting the neuroprosthesis is minimally invasive and allows for removal of the intramuscular electrodes without scarring or residual damage (Mulcahey et al., 2004). Although randomized-controlled trials of this system are not practical, case series (Davis et al., 1998; Taylor et al., 2001, 2002) and a before and after trial with moderate numbers of participants have shown that it is safe, improves grasping and is well accepted by users (Peckham et al., 2001).

Table 37.1. Levels of scientific evidence supporting new treatments. Level I, large randomized trials with clear-cut results; level II, small randomized trials with uncertain results (moderate to high risk of error); level III, non-randomized trials with concurrent or contemporaneous controls; level IV, non-randomized trials with historical controls; level V, case series with no controls.

Rehabilitation treatment	Level of evidence
Body weight supported treadmill training	II (1 negative), IV (1 positive), V (5 positive)
Upper extremity FES (freehand)	IV (1 positive), V (2 positive)
Lower extremity FES gait system (freehand)	V (3 positive)
Bladder stimulation	V (3 positive)
Other FES applications	V (mixed)

FES: functional electrical stimulation.

Short-term use of skin electrodes to stimulate muscle contraction in people with SCI has been done in rehabilitation settings for many years to reverse atrophy and improve strength and cardiovascular fitness. FES-assisted exercise provides substantial cardiovascular fitness benefits over traditional exercise therapy (Glaser, 1991; Gorman, 2003). Examples of these applications include FES ergometry (REGYS, ERGYS) and FES-assisted gait training. The Parastep® is a portable FES unit that is operated by a small microprocessor worn by the patient. A system of surface electrodes placed on gluteal muscles, quadriceps femoris, and the peroneal nerve allows the patient to walk with reciprocal gait using a front-wheeled walker (Kirshblum, 2004). Users of the Parastep® must have a UMN injury (T4–T12) with good upper body strength, functional range of motion at the hip, independence in transfers, and lack of pain sensation in areas where the electrodes provide stimulation. Potential benefits identified in case studies include heart rate increase during training, increased muscle mass and improved ambulation (Winchester et al., 1994; Johnston et al., 2003; Spadone et al., 2003) but the system requires intensive training and usually another person to assist the user, so it is not used often in rehabilitation.

Small before–after trials of electrical stimulation of bladder and bowel using implanted electrodes to promote planned emptying have suggested safety, efficacy (greater bladder filling volumes, fewer UTIs, lower residual volumes, and less incontinence), reduced costs and improved quality of life (Kachourbos and Creasey, 2000; Creasey and Dahlberg, 2001; Creasey et al., 2001). Electroejaculation is commonly used to produce semen for men with SCI and phrenic nerve pacing allows for periods of ventilator-free respiration in high tetraplegics (Creasey et al., 2004).

Although new rehabilitation therapies are continually being developed and evaluated, the evidence supporting the efficacy of each takes much longer to accumulate. Table 37.1 shows the levels of scientific evidence supporting some new treatments, using the standard nomenclature employed in developing clinical guidelines (US Preventive Health Services Task Force, 1996).

Neural repair

Even newer therapies based on cell transplantation (Chapters 18, 25, 28 and 29 of Volume I) and enhancement of axonal regeneration (Chapters 21–24 of Volume I) are primarily in the animal testing stage, although several have been used on human SCI patients in uncontrolled trials and others are in various stages of controlled clinical trials (http://carecure.atinfopop.com/4/OpenTopic?a=frm&s=4754088921&f=8274067031). Since SCI recovery will not be an all or none phenomenon, the good news is that a damaged cord does not need to be completely regenerated in order to provide functional benefits. For example, it has been suggested that fewer than

10% of long-tract axons need to be functional for walking (Blight, 1983; McDonald and Sadowsky, 2002). Most researchers agree that a combination of approaches to neural repair, rather than a single therapy, will be needed and that the choice of therapies will require tailoring to the person and clinical situation. For people with SCI and their families access to information that is current (updated at least annually), accurate and in a format that is understandable is essential. Quality web sites for this purpose include University of Alabama's web site (www.spinalcord.uab.edu), Rutgers University's W.M. Keck Center for Collaborative Neuroscience web site (http://carecure.rutgers.edu/Spinewire/index.html), the Miami Project to Cure Paralysis web site (www.miamiproject.miami.edu), and the University of Washington's Northwest Regional Spinal Cord Injury System web site (http://depts.washington.edu/rehab/sci/). Rehabilitation professionals counseling and teaching these patients and their families should support hope for recovery, education regarding the realities of research progress, advise patience, and encourage active rehabilitation, physical activity in general and active living throughout the process.

REFERENCES

Albert, T.J., Levine, M.J., Balderston, R.A. and Cotler, J.M. (1991). Gastrointestinal complications in spinal cord injury. *Spine*, **16**, S522–S525.

Anke, A.G., Stenehjem, A.E. and Stanghelle, J.K. (1995). Pain and life quality within two years of spinal cord injury. *Paraplegia*, **33**, 555–559.

Anson, C.A. and Shepherd, C. (1996). Incidence of secondary complications in spinal cord injury. *Int J Rehabil Res*, **19**, 55–66.

Ashworth, B. (1964). Preliminary trial of carisoprodol in multiple sclerosis. *Practitioner*, **192**, 540–542.

ASIA and IMSOP. (2000). International standards for neurological classification of spinal cord injury, revised 2000. *Americam Spinal Injury Association and the International Society of Paraplegia*.

Barbeau, H. (2003). Locomotor training in neurorehabilitation: emerging rehabilitation concepts. *Neurorehabil Neural Repair*, **17**, 3–11.

Barbeau, H. and Norman, K.E. (2003). The effect of noradrenergic drugs on the recovery of walking after spinal cord injury. *Spinal Cord*, **41**, 137–143.

Bauman, W.A. and Spungen, A.M. (1994). Disorders of carbohydrate and lipid metabolism in veterans with paraplegia or quadriplegia: a model of premature aging. *Metabolism*, **43**, 749–756.

Blight, A.R. (1983). Axonal physiology of chronic spinal cord injury in the cat: intracellular recording in vitro. *Neuroscience*, **10**, 1471–1486.

Bohannon, R.W. and Smith, M.B. (1986). Interrater reliability of a modified Ashworth scale of muscle spasticity. *Phys Ther*, **67**, 206–207.

Bonica, J.J. (1991). Introduction: semantic, epidemiologic, and educational issues. In: *Pain and Central Nervous System Disease: The Central Pain Syndromes* (ed. Casey, K.L.), Raven Press, New York, pp. 13–291.

Bracken, M. and Holford, T.R. (2002). Neurological and functional status 1 year after acute spinal cord injury. *J Neurosurg*, **96**, 259–266.

Bracken, M.B. and Holford, T.R. (1993). Effects of timing of methylprednisolone or naloxone administration on recovery of segmental and long-tract neurological function in NASCIS 2. *J Neurosurg*, **79**, 500–507.

Bracken, M.B., Shepard, M.J., Collins, W.F., Holford, T.R., Young, W., Baskin, D.S., Eisenberg, H.M., Flamm, E., Leo-Summers, L., Maroon, J., et al. (1990). A randomized, controlled trial of methylprednisolone or naloxone in the treatment of acute spinal-cord injury. Results of the Second National Acute Spinal Cord Injury Study. *New Engl J Med*, **322**, 1405–1411.

Bracken, M.B., Shepard, M.J., Holford, T.R., Leo-Summers, L., Aldrich, E.F., Fazl, M., Fehlings, M., Herr, D.L., Hitchon, P.W., Marshall, L.F., Nockels, R.P., Pascale, V., Perot Jr., P.L., Piepmeier, J., Sonntag, V.K., Wagner, F., Wilberger, J.E., Winn, H.R. and Young, W. (1997). Administration of methylprednisolone for 24 or 48 hours or tirilazad mesylate for 48 hours in the treatment of acute spinal cord injury. Results of the third national acute spinal cord injury randomized controlled trial. National Acute Spinal Cord Injury Study. *J Am Med Assoc*, **277**, 1597–1604.

Cardenas, D.D. and Hooton, T.M. (1995). Urinary tract infection in persons with spinal cord injury. *Arch Phys Med Rehabil*, **75**, 272–280.

Cardenas, D.D. and Mayo, M.E. (1987). Bacteriuria with fever after spinal cord injury. *Arch Phys Med Rehabil*, **68**, 291–293.

Cardenas, D.D., Farrell-Roberts, Sipski, M.L. and Ribner, D. (1995). Management of gastrointestinal, genitourinary, and sexual function. In: *Spinal Cord Injury: Clinical Outcomes from the Model Systems* (eds Stover, S.L., Delisa, J.A. and Whiteneck, G.G.), pp. 120–1441. Aspen, Gaithersburg, MD.

Cardenas, D.D., Turner, J.A., Warms, C.A. and Marshall, H. (2002a). Classification of chronic pain associated with spinal cord injuries. *Arch Phys Med Rehabil*, **83**, 1708–1714.

Cardenas, D.D., Warms, C.A., Turner, J.A., Marshall, H., Brooke, M.M. and Loeser, J.D. (2002b). Efficacy of amitriptyline for relief of pain in spinal cord injury: results of a randomized controlled trial. *Pain*, **96**, 365–373.

Creasey, G.H. and Dahlberg, J.E. (2001). Economic consequences of an implanted neuroprosthesis for bladder and bowel management. *Arch Phys Med Rehabil*, **82**, 1520–1525.

Creasey, G.H., Grill, J.H., Korsten, M.U.H.S., Betz, R., Anderson, R., Walter, J. and Group, I.N.R. (2001). An implantable neuroprosthesis for restoring bladder and bowel control to patients with spinal cord injuries: a multicenter trial. *Arch Phys Med Rehabil*, **82**, 1512–1519.

Creasey, G.H., Ho, C.H., Triolo, R.J., Gater, D.R., DiMarco, A.F., Bogie, K.M. and Keith, M.W. (2004). Clinical applications of electrical stimulation after spinal cord injury. *J Spinal Cord Med*, **27**, 365–375.

Davies, D.S. and McColl, M.A. (2002). Lifestyle risks for three disease outcomes in spinal cord injury. *Clin Rehabil*, **16**, 96–108.

Davis, S.E., Mulcahey, M.J., Smith, B.T. and Betz, R.R. (1998). Self-reported use of an implanted FES hand system by adolescents with tetraplegia. *J Spinal Cord Med*, **21**, 220–226.

DeVivo, M.J., Black, K.J. and Stover, S.L. (1993). Causes of death during the first 12 years after spinal cord injury. *Arch Phys Med Rehabil*, **74**, 248–254.

DeVivo, M.J., Krause, J.S. and Lammertse, D.P. (1999). Recent trends in mortality and causes of death among persons with spinal cord injury. *Arch Phys Med Rehabil*, **8**, 1411–1419.

Ditunno Jr., J.F., Stover, S.K., Freed, M.M. and Ahn, J.H. (1992). Motor recovery of the upper extremities in traumatic quadriplegia: a multicenter study. *Arch Phys Med Rehabil*, **73**, 431–436.

Dobkin, B., Apple, D., Barbeau, H., et al. (2003a). In: *American Congress of Rehabilitation Medicine*. Tucson, AZ.

Dobkin, B.H., Apple, D., Barbeau, H., Basso, M., Behrman, A., Deforge, D., Ditunno, J., Dudley, G., Elashoff, R., Fugate, L., Harkema, S., Saulino, M. and Scott, M. (2003b). Methods for a randomized trial of weight-supported treadmill training versus conventional training for walking during inpatient rehabilitation after incomplete traumatic spinal cord injury. *Neurorehabil Neural Repair*, **17**, 153–167.

Duckworth, W.C., Solomon, S.S., Jallepalli, P., Heckemeyer, C., Finnern, J. and Powers, A. (1980). Glucose intolerance due to insulin resistance in patients with spinal cord injuries. *Diabetes*, **29**, 906–910.

Field-Fote, E.C. (2000). Spinal cord control of movement: implications for locomotor rehabilitation following spinal cord injury. *Phys Ther*, **80**, 477–484.

Finerman, G.A. and Stover, S.L. (1981). Heterotopic ossification following hip replacement or spinal cord injury: two clinical studies with EHDP. *Metab Bone Dis Relat Res*, **3**, 337–342.

Fisher, T.L., Laud, P.W., Byfield, M.G., Brown, T.T., Hayat, M.J. and Fiedler, I.G. (2002). Sexual health after spinal cord injury: a longitudinal study. *Arch Phys Med Rehabil*, **83**, 1043–1051.

Galvin, L.R. and Godfrey, H.P.D. (2001). The impact of coping on emotional adjustment to spinal cord injury (SCI): review of the literature and application of a stress appraisal and coping formulation. *Spinal Cord*, **39**, 615–627.

Gerhart, K.A., Weitzenkamp, D.A., Kennedy, P., Glass, C.A. and Charlifue, S.W. (1999). Correlates of stress in long-term spinal cord injury. *Spinal Cord*, **37**, 183–190.

Glaser, R.M. (1991). Physiology of functional electrical stimulation-induced exercise: basic science perspective. *J Neuro Rehab*, **5**, 49–61.

Gore, R.M., Mintzer, R.A. and Calenoff, L. (1981). Gastrointestinal complications of spinal cord injury. *Spine*, **6**, 538–544.

Gorman, P.H. (2003). Functional electrical stimulation. In: *Spinal Cord Medicine, Principles and Practice* (eds Lin, V.W., Cardenas, D.D., Cutter, N.C., Frost, F.S., Hammond, M.C., Lindblom, L.B., Perkash, I., Waters, R. and Woolsey, R.M.). Demos, New York, NY.

Green, D., Biddle, A.K., Fahey, V., Gardiner, G.A., Hull, R., Lee, M.Y., Merli, G.J., Mossberg, K., Pineo, G., Ragnarsson, K.T., Rosenbloom, D., Simpson, K.N. and Stayer, J.R. (1997). Prevention of thromboembolism in spinal cord injury. *Clinical Practice Guidelines: Consortium for Spinal Cord Medicine and the Paralyzed Veterans of America*, 1–20.

Heldenberg, D., Rubinstein, A., Levtov, O., Werbin, B. and Tamir, I. (1981). Serum lipids and lipoprotein concentrations in young quadriplegic patients. *Atherosclerosis*, **39**, 163–167.

Hollar, L.D. (1995). Occupational therapy for physical dysfunction. In: *Spinal Cord Injury* (ed. Trombly, C.), Williams & Wilkins, Baltimore, MD, pp. 795–8131.

Hulseboch, C.E., Hains, B.C., Waldrep, K. and Young, W. (2000). Bridging the gap: from discovery to clinical trials in spinal cord injury. *J Neurotrauma*, **17**, 1117–1128.

Hurlbert, R.J. (2001). The role of steroids in acute spinal cord injury. An evidence-based analysis. *Spine*, **26**, S39–S46.

Johnston, T.E., Finson, R.L., Smith, B.T., Bonarot, I.D.M., Betz, R.R. and Mulcahey, M.J. (2003). Functional electrical stimulation for augmented walking in adolescents with incomplete spinal cord injury. *J Spinal Cord Med*, **26**, 390–400.

Kachourbos, M.J. and Creasey, G.H. (2000). Health promotion in motion: improving quality of life for persons with neurogenic bladder and bowel using assistive technology. *SCI Nurs*, **17**, 125–129.

Kennedy, P. and Duff, J. (2001). Post traumatic stress disorder and spinal cord injuries. *Spinal Cord*, **39**, 1–10.

Kennedy, P., Duff, J., Evans, M. and Beedie, A. (2003). Coping effectiveness training reduces depression and anxiety following traumatic spinal cord injuries. *Br J Cl Psychol*, **42**, 41–52.

Kirshblum, S. (2004). New rehabilitation interventions in spinal cord injury. *J Spinal Cord Med*, **27**, 342–350.

Lazarus, R. and Folkman, S. (1984). *Stress Appraisal and Coping*. Springer, New York, NY.

Levendoglu, F., Ogun, C.O., Ozerbil, O., Ogun, T.C. and Ugurlu, H. (2004). Gabapentin is a first line drug for the treatment of neuropathic pain in spinal cord injury. *Spine*, **29**, 743–751.

Linsenmeyer, T.A. and Culkin, D. (1999). APS recommendations for the urological evaluation of patients with spinal cord injury. *J Spinal Cord Med*, **22**, 139–142.

Linsenmeyer, T., Biddle, A.K., Cardenas, D., Kuric, J., Mobely, T., Perkash, I., Simpson, K.N. and Zejdlik, C. (1997). Acute management of autonomic dysreflexia: adults with spinal cord injury presenting to health-care facilities. In: *Clinical Practice Guidelines*, Consortium for Spinal Cord Medicine and the Paralyzed Veterans of America, pp. 1–16.

Lohne, V. (2001). Hope in patients with spinal cord injury: A literature review related to nursing. *J Neurosci Nurs*, **33**, 317–325.

Lou, M.F., Dai, Y.T. and Catanzaro, M. (1997). A pilot study to assess the relationships among coping, self-efficacy and functional improvement in men with paraplegia. *Int J Rehabil Res*, **20**, 99–105.

Maynard, F.M., Karunas, R.S. and Waring, W.P. (1990). Epidemiology of spasticity following traumatic spinal cord injury. *Arch Phys Med Rehabil*, **71**, 566–569.

McDonald, J.W. and Sadowsky, C. (2002). Spinal-cord injury. *Lancet*, **359**, 417–425.

McDonald, J.W., Becker, D., Sadowsky, C.L., Jane Sr., J.A., Conturo, T.E. and Schultz, L.M. (2002). Late recovery following spinal cord injury. Case report and review of the literature. *J Neurosurg Spine*, **97**, 252–265.

Merli, G.J., Herbison, G.J. and Ditunno, J.F. (1988). Deep vein thrombosis in acute spinal cord injured patients. *Arch Phys Med Rehabil*, **69**, 661–664.

Mulcahey, M.J., Betz, R.R., Kozin, S.H., Smith, B.T., Hutchinson, D. and Lutz, C. (2004). Implantation of the freehand system during initial rehabilitation using minimally invasive techniques. *Spinal Cord*, **42**, 146–155.

Myllynen, P., Kammonen, M., Rokkanen, P., et al. (1985). DVT and pulmonary embolism in patients with acute spinal cord injury: a comparison with nonparalyzed patients immobilized due to spinal fractures. *J Traum*, **25**, 541–543.

Nance, P., Schryvers, O., Schmidt, B., Dubo, H., Loveridge, B. and Fewer, D. (1955). Intrathecal baclofen therapy for adults with spinal spasticity: therapeutic efficacy and effect on hospital admissions. *Can J Neurol Sci*, **22**, 22–29.

Nance, P.W. (1994). A comparison of clonidine, cyproheptadine and baclofen in spastic spinal cord injured patients. *J Am Paraplegia Soc*, **17**, 150–156.

National SCI Statistical Center (2004). Spinal Cord Injury: facts and figures at a glance. Retrieved October 22, 2004 from University of Alabama at Birmingham, The National SCI Statistical Center website: http://www.spincalcord.uab.edu.

Noreau, L., Proulx, P., Gagnon, L., Drolet, M. and Laramee, M.T. (2000). Secondary impairments after spinal cord injury: a population-based study. *Am J Phys Med Rehabil*, **79**, 526–535.

North, N.T. (1999). The psychological effects of spinal cord injury: a review. *Spinal Cord*, **37**, 671–679.

Orzel, J.A. and Rudd, T.G. (1985). Heterotopic bone formation: clinical, laboratory, and imaging correlation. *J Nucl Med*, **26**, 125–132.

Ozer, M.N. and Gibson, L. (1987). Neurological consultation for persons with spinal cord injury. In: *Physical Medicine and Rehabilitation: State of the Art Reviews* (ed. Redford, J.B.), Hanley and Belfur, Inc., Philadelphia, pp. 3401.

Peckham, P.H., Keith, M.W., Kilgore, K.L., Grill, J.H., Wuolle, K.S., Thrope, G.B., Gorman, P., Hobby, J., Mulcahey, M.J., Carroll, S., Hentz, V.R., Wiegner, A. and Group, I.N.R. (2001). Efficacy of an implanted neuroprosthesis for restoring hand grasp in tetraplegia: a multicenter study. *Arch Phys Med Rehabil*, **82**, 1380–1388.

Phelps, J., Albo, M., Dunn, K. and Joseph, A. (2001). Spinal cord injury and sexuality in married or partnered men: activities, function, needs, and predictors of sexual adjustment. *Arch Sex Behav*, **30**, 591–602.

Post, M.W.M., de Witte, L.P., van Asbeck, F.W.A., van Dijk, A.J. and Schrijvers, J.P. (1998). Predictors of health status and life satisfaction in spinal cord injury. *Arch Phys Med Rehabil*, **83**, 24–30.

Prochazka, A., Mushahwar, V. and Yakovenko, S. (2002). Activation and coordination of spinal motoneuron pools after spinal cord injury. *Prog Brain Res*, **137**, 109–124.

Protas, E.J., Holmes, S.A., Qureshy, H., Johnson, A., Lee, D. and Sherwood, A.M. (2001). Supported treadmill ambulation training after spinal cord injury: a pilot study. *Arch Phys Med Rehabil*, **82**, 825–831.

Putzke, J.D., Richards, J.S., Hicken, B.L. and DeVivo, M.J. (2002). Predictors of life satisfaction: a spinal cord injury cohort study. *Arch Phys Med Rehabil*, **83**, 555–561.

Rossier, A.B., Foo, D., Shillito, J. and Dyro, F.M. (1985). Posttraumatic cervical syringomyelia. Incidence, clinical presentation, electrophysiological studies, syrinx protein and results of conservative and operative treatment. *Brain Res*, **108**, 439–461.

Rupp, R. and Gerner, H.J. (2004). Neuroprosthetics of the upper extremity – clinical application in spinal cord injury and future perspectives. *Biomed Tech (Berl)*, **49**, 93–98.

Schmidt, S.A., Kjaersgaard-Andersen, P., Pedersen, N.W., Kristensen, S.S., Pedersen, P. and Nielsen, J.B. (1988). The use of indomethacin to prevent the formation of heterotopic bone after total hip replacement. A randomized, double-blind clinical trial. *J Bone Joint Surg Am*, **70**, 834–838.

Schmitt, J.K. and Schroeder, D.L. (2003). Endocrine and metabolic consequences of spinal cord injuries. In: *Spinal Cord Medicine, Principles and Practice* (eds Lin, V.W., Cardenas, D.D., Cutter, N.C., Frost, F.S., Hammond, M.C., Lindblom, L.B., Perkash, I., Waters, R. and Woolsey, R.M.), Demos, New York, NY.

Schneider, R.C., Cherry, G. and Pantek, H. (1954). The syndrome of acute central cervical spinal cord injury; with special reference to the mechanisms involved in hyperextension injuries of cervical spine. *J Neurosurg*, **11**, 546–577.

Schurch, B., Wichmann, W. and Rossier, A.B. (1996). Posttraumatic syringomyelia (cystic myelopathy): a prospective study of 449 patients with spinal cord injury. *J Neurol Neurosurg Psychiat*, **60**, 61–67.

Sekhon, L.H.S. and Fehlings, M.G. (2001). Epidemiology, demographics, and pathophysiology of acute spinal cord injury. *Spine*, **26**, S2–S12.

Snow, B.J., Tsui, J.K., Bhatt, M.H., Varelas, M., Hashimoto, S.A. and Calne, D.B. (1990). Treatment of spasticity with botulinum toxin: a double-blind study. *Ann Neurol*, **28**, 512–515.

Spadone, R., Merat, I.G., Bertocchi, E., Mevio, E., Veicsteinas, A., Pedotti, A. and Ferrarin, M. (2003). Energy consumption of locomotion with orthosis versus Parastep®-assisted gait: a single case study. *Spinal Cord*, **41**, 97–104.

Stiens, S.A., Bergman, S.B. and Formal, C.S. (1997). Spinal cord injury rehabilitation: 4. Individual experience, personal adaptation and social perspectives. *Arch Phys Med Rehabil*, **78**, S65–S72.

Stolp-Smith, K.A. and Wainberg, M.C. (1999). Antidepressant exacerbation of spasticity. *Arch Phys Med Rehabil*, **80**, 339–342.

Stover, S.L., Hahn, H.R. and Miller 3rd., J.M. (1976). Disodium etidronate in the prevention of heterotopic ossification following spinal cord injury (preliminary report). *Paraplegia*, **14**, 146–156.

Taylor, R.G. and Gleave, J.R. (1957). Incomplete spinal cord injuries; with Brown–Sequard phenomena. *J Bone Joint Surg Brit*, **39-B**, 438–450.

Taylor, P., Esnouf, J. and Hobby, J. (2001). Pattern of use and user satisfaction of neuro control freehand system. *Spinal Cord*, **39**, 156–160.

Taylor, P., Esnouf, J. and Hobby, J. (2002). The functional impact of the freehand system on tetraplegic hand function. Clinical results. *Spinal Cord*, **40**, 560–566.

US Preventive Health Services Task Force (1996). *Guide to Clinical Preventive Services: An Assessment of the Effectiveness of 169 Interventions*, 2nd edn. Williams and Wilkins, Baltimore.

Warms, C.A., Turner, J.A., Marshall, H.M. and Cardenas, D.D. (2002). Treatments for chronic pain associated with spinal cord injuries: many are tried, few are helpful. *Clin J Pain*, **18**, 154–163.

Warren, L., Wrigley, J.M., Yoels, W.C. and Fine, P.R. (1996). Factors associated with life satisfaction among a sample of persons with neurotrauma. *J Rehab Res Dev*, **33**, 404–408.

Waters, R.L., Adkins, R.H., Yakura, J.S. and Sie, L. (1994a). Motor and sensory recovery following incomplete tetraplegia. *Arch Phys Med Rehabil*, **75**, 67–72.

Waters, R.L., Adkins, R.H., Yakura, J.S. and Sie, L. (1994b). Motor and sensory recovery following incomplete tetraplegia. *Arch Phys Med Rehabil*, **75**, 306–311.

Waters, R.L., Sie, I.H., Gellman, H. and Tognella, M. (1996). Functional hand surgery following tetraplegia. *Arch Phys Med Rehabil*, **77**, 86–94.

Wernig, A., Muller, S., Nanassy, A. and Cagol, E. (1995). Laufband therapy based on "rules of spinal locomotion" is effective in spinal cord injured persons. *Eur J Neurosci*, **7**, 823–829.

Wernig, A., Nanassy, A. and Muller, S. (1998). Maintenance of locomotor abilities following Laufband (treadmill) therapy in para- and tetraplegic persons: follow-up studies. *Spinal Cord*, **36**, 744–749.

Whiteneck, G., Adler, C., Biddle, A.K., Blackburn, S., DeVivo, M.J., Haley, S.M., Hendricks, R.D., Heinemann, A.W., Johnson, K., Marino, R.J., Thomas, H., Waters, R.L. and Yarkony, G.M. (1999). Outcomes following traumatical spinal cord injury: clinical practice guidelines for health-care professionals. In: *Clinical Practice Guidelines*, Consortium for Spinal Cord Medicine and the Paralyzed Veterans of America, pp. 1–291.

Winchester, P., Carollo, J.J. and Habasevich, R. (1994). Physiologic costs of reciprocal gait in FES assisted walking. *Paraplegia*, **32**, 680–686.

Wolpaw, J.R. and Tennissen, A.M. (2001). Activity-dependent spinal cord plasticity in health and disease. *Ann Rev Neurosci*, **24**, 807–843.

Yarkony, G.M. and Heinemann, A.W. (1995). Pressure ulcers. In: *Spinal Cord Injury: Clinical Outcomes from the Model Systems* (eds Delisa, J.A. and Whiteneck, G.G.), Aspen, Gaithersburg, MD, pp. 100–1191.

Young, M.E., Rintala, D.H., Rossi, C.D., Hart, K.A. and Fuhrer, M.J. (1995). Alcohol and marijuana use in a community-based sample of persons with spinal cord injury. *Arch Phys Med Rehabil*, **76**, 525–532.

Multiple sclerosis

Serafin Beer and Jürg Kesselring

Department of Neurology and Neurorehabilitation, Rehabilitation Centre, Valens, Switzerland

38.1 Introduction

Multiple sclerosis (MS) is one of the most common neurological diseases in young adults. Prevalence is especially high in Central and North Europe, North America and Australia with around 100/100,000 inhabitants onset of the disease is mainly in the third and fourth decade of life (Beer and Kesselring, 1994; Hogancamp et al., 1997; Noseworthy et al., 2000; Compston and Coles, 2002). The aetiology is still unknown but a dysregulation of the immune system can be assumed probably initiating the disease process already in childhood in genetically susceptible individuals (Bachmann and Kesselring, 1998; Dyment et al., 2004). Based on this autoimmunity a chronic inflammatory process is set off, allowing immunological active T-cells and monocytes invading the central nervous system (CNS) through a disrupted blood–brain-barrier, thus initiating a cascade of immunological processes (activation of macrophages, microglia, production of immunomediators) and inflammatory reactions which lead to lesions of CNS pathways and finally to glial scaring (Lucchinetti et al., 2000; Noseworthy et al., 2000). The most prominent pathology in MS is demyelination. There is, however, an increasing evidence, that even in an early phase of the disease axonal loss may occur (Trapp et al., 1999; Lucchinetti et al., 2000). Depending on the kind, extent and localisation of such lesions, various functional deficits may occur. Clinically MS runs in two-thirds of the patients a primary relapsing–remitting course, the major number of these cases, however, turning into a secondary progressive course later on. In 20% of MS cases the clinical course is primary chronic progressive (Compston and Coles, 2002).

Symptomatology depends on localisation of lesions in the CNS, although the majority of MS lesions remain asymptomatic. The most common symptoms in relapsing–remitting course are visual disturbances (46%) and sensory disturbances (41%), whereas in primary progressive forms disturbances of gait (88%) and pareses (38%) are most prevalent (Beer and Kesselring, 1988). Other symptoms such as bladder problems and cognitive disturbances develop more commonly later on in the course of the disease and may be more disabling. The consequences of these functional deficits in activities of daily living are very variable: from the patient's view fatigue is one of the most prevalent symptoms with negative impact on activities of daily living, followed by disturbances of balance, pareses and bladder disorders (Kraft et al., 1986).

Diagnosis of MS is based on the clinical or paraclinical demonstration of inflammatory lesions in the CNS disseminated in space and time (Table 38.1). The introduction of magnetic resonance imaging (MRI) in clinical neurology has contributed importantly to early diagnosis in MS, and to improve reliability of diagnosis. MRI makes it possible to demonstrate directly spatial multiplicity as a characteristic of MS intra vitam and to demonstrate the subclinical dynamics of the disease (Miller et al., 1997). Earlier diagnostic criteria by Poser and co-workers

Table 38.1. New diagnostic criteria (McDonald et al., 2001).

Clinical (attacks)	Objective lesions	Additional requirements to make diagnosis
Two or more	Two or more	None: clinical evidence sufficient (additional evidence desirable but must be consistent with MS)
Two or more	One	Dissemination in *space* by MRI *or* positive CSF and two or more MRI lesions consistent with MS *or* further clinical attack involving different site
One	Two or more	Dissemination in *time* by MRI *or* second clinical attack
One (mono-symptomatic)	One	Dissemination in *space* by MRI *or* positive CSF and two more MRI lesions consistent with MS AND
		Dissemination in *time* by MRI *or* second clinical attack
Zero (progression from onset)	One	Positive CSF AND
		Dissemination in *space* by MRI evidence of nine or more T_2 brain lesions *or*
		Two or more cord lesions *or* four to eight brain and one cord lesion *or*
		Positive VEP with four to eight MRI lesions *or*
		Positive VEP with less than four brain lesions plus one cord lesion AND
		Dissemination in time by MRI *or* continued progression for 1 year

VEP: visual-evoked potential.

MRI-findings in MS (McDonald et al., 2001)

At least three of the four following criteria:

- One gadolinium-enhancing lesion or nine T_2-hyperintense lesions
- At least one infratentorial lesion
- At least juxtacortical lesion
- At least three periventricular lesions

MRI evidence of dissemination in time:

- One gadolinium-enhancing lesion in a different site demonstrated in a scan 3 months or more after onset of clinical event
- In absence of gadolinium enhancing lesions at 3 months scan follow-up after additional 3 months showing gadolinium lesion or new T_2 lesion

---

depended on clinical history, examination and evoked potentials as indirect evidence of temporal and spatial multiplicity of the CNS lesions (Poser et al., 1983) complemented by cerebrospinal fluid (CSF) testing as evidence for CNS inflammation. In the new diagnostic criteria proposed by McDonald and co-workers (McDonald et al., 2001), typical MRI findings are accepted as direct evidence for spatial multiplicity and inflammation (gadolinium enhancement) (Table 38.1). Particularly, MRI allows demonstration of new, clinically silent active lesions in serial examinations indicating temporal multiplicity

of inflammatory process. For this reason, diagnosis and therapeutic intervention can be set up earlier. Finally MRI may contribute markedly for discriminating MS from other pathological conditions of the CNS (Kesselring and Miller, 1997). It must be emphasised, however, that, although type and distribution pattern of multifocal lesions (periventricular, corpus callosum, infratentorial) on MRI is very characteristic for MS, it should not be considered as a diagnostic prove on its own: for diagnostic accuracy it is important interpreting MRI findings only in the complete clinical context in order to avoid misapprehensions (McDonald, 1997). The fact, that MS has an early disease onset, a progressive course, and long duration with median survival time of over 40 years after diagnosis, leads to a high prevalence of disabilities with consequences in personal as well as social domains. Fifteen years after diagnosis around 50% of persons with MS use walking aids, 29% need a wheelchair (Weinshenker et al., 1989; Weinshenker, 1994). During the first 10 years of disease 50–80% become unable to work (Rao et al., 1991). This means that the main burden of disease become manifest during the fifth and sixth decade, usually a particularly active life span in social as well as in vocational respect. Thus, socio-economic consequences of MS are substantial: a study on costs for MS in Germany revealed that direct and indirect costs for one person with MS per year are over 65,000 Deutsche Mark (DM) (around 50,000 Euro or US$) (Kiel, 2000). Fifty per cent of direct costs are caused by 17% of the most disabled patients; 6.5% are residing in nursing homes (Carton et al., 1998) (Fig. 38.1).

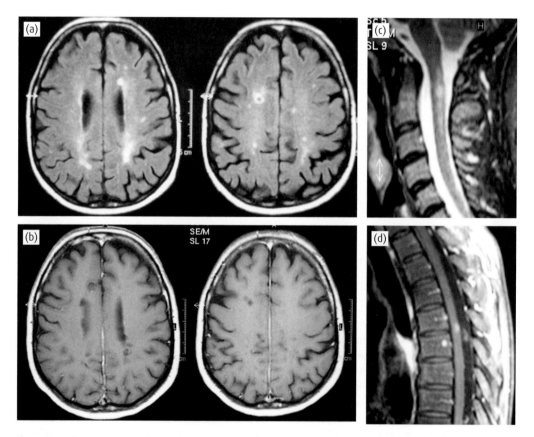

Figure 38.1. *Characteristic MRI-findings in MS.* MRI is helpful in MS diagnosis showing the widespread dissemination in space and pathological diversity of CNS lesions. (a) Hyperintense white matter lesions (FLAIR sequence), typically located in periventricular and juxtacortical regions. (b) T_1-weighted images of the same patient showing some of these lesions to be hypointense ("black holes"), probably reflecting axonal pathology. Spinal lesions are shown in (c) (T_2-weighted, upper cervical spinal cord) and (d) (T_1-weighted with gadolinium, thoracic spinal cord): note gadolinium enhancement indicating active inflammatory process during an acute relapse on thoracic level (d).

38.2 Treatment options

Since the cause of MS is still unknown, effective prevention or cure is not possible. A first evidence for an effective drug treatment for MS derived from a large randomised-controlled study published by Rose and co-workers, showing a benefit of adrenocorticotrophic hormone (ACTH) in treatment of relapses (Rose et al., 1970). Later studies showed that high-dose methylprednisolone is at least as effective as ACTH in this respect (Compston et al., 1987; Milligan et al., 1987). This relapse treatment leads to a reduction of severity and duration of the symptoms with more rapid recovery by restoring blood–brain-barrier leakage and reducing inflammatory oedema (Kesselring et al., 1989). The effect of oral high-dose methylprednisolone is comparable to intravenous treatment, although the latter seems to be better tolerated (Sellebjerg et al., 1998). The steroid treatment itself probably has no effect on the long-term course of the disease.

Immunosuppressive therapies have been tried over decades in MS patients with severe course, mostly with equivocal effect. The introduction of newer, more specific immunomodulating therapies (beta-interferons, glatirameracetate, mitoxantrone and new natalizumab) during the last decade was a breakthrough in the long-term treatment of MS. In large randomised, controlled studies it could be demonstrated for the first time, that frequency of relapses, appearance of new active lesions on MRI and, in part, also clinical progression may be reduced in patients with relapsing–remitting and, to a certain extent, in secondary progressive MS (Multiple-Sklerose-Therapie Konsensus Gruppe (MSTKG), 1999, 2001, 2002; Goodin et al., 2002; Miller et al., 2003). These immunomodulating therapies, however, cannot improve existing deficits, and seems to delay disease progression only by about 1–2 years (The PRISMS Study Group, 2001). Thus, the increase of disability is postponed, but not completely stopped by these treatments.

Although *symptomatic therapies* may reduce consequences of functional deficits, usually they do not eliminate them completely (see Section 38.4.3).

Rehabilitation therefore continues to play an important role in a comprehensive management of MS in order to reduce the consequences of the disease on functional impairment, personal activities and social participation and in order to enable persons to live an independent life with the highest possible quality of life in spite of the disease (Kesselring, 2004). In addition to specific treatment modalities for improving functional deficits, a multidisciplinary approach is necessary to achieve this goal.

38.3 Measuring effectiveness

Evaluation of the effectiveness of rehabilitation measures is particularly difficult in MS for several reasons. One problem is to determine reliably disease activity, course and prognosis. The intra- and inter-individual differences make it very difficult predicting outcome even in patients with the same form of disease (primary relapsing remitting, secondary chronic progressive, primary chronic progressive). Triggering factors for progression and acute relapses are not well understood. Basic pathological processes (inflammation, demyelination, axonal damage) are very heterogeneous and can sometimes be discriminated only with great difficulty by conventional neuroradiology (Miller et al., 1997). Furthermore clinical manifestation of the MS symptomatology may fluctuate due to various factors which may make evaluation of functional capacity more difficult because different functional CNS systems may be affected. One of the most important factors is the so-called Uhthoff's phenomenon, first described by Wilhelm Uhthoff in 1890 in four MS patients with transient loss of vision after physical activities: in thermosensitive patients an increase of body temperature (due to environmental heat or physical activity) may bring on or deteriorate symptoms, which are reversible after cooling down. This temporary clinical deterioration seems to be due to a disruption of central conduction in demyelinated fibres by increased body temperature (Smith and McDonald, 1999; Humm et al., 2004). Due to this phenomenon, performance of MS patients can strongly be influenced by temperature changes (physical activities, temperature of environment).

The impact of pathological changes and functional deficits on activity (disability), participation (handicap) and quality of life may be variable in individual patients. MRI is not very helpful in this respect because there is no close correlation between conventional MRI findings and degree of disability (Miller et al., 1997). Under these circumstances, therefore, it is quite difficult to find a homogenous cohort of patients which satisfies scientific criteria for evaluating effectiveness of a medical intervention. This may be the reason why there are only a limited number of published studies which examine the efficacy of rehabilitation in MS. It is not only of scientific interest to measure outcome with the proper measurements but it also contributes to the evaluation of efficacy of different treatment modalities and to adaptation and development of new therapies. Assessment systems should be related to impairment, disability and handicap, quality of life, goal achievement, coping skills, self-efficacy, and they should be clinically useful, scientifically sound (reliable, valid and responsive), and acceptable (appropriate to sample) (Kesselring, 2004).

38.4 Rehabilitation measures

Therapeutic programmes may vary widely from one rehabilitation clinic to another, but there is a general consensus concerning *personnel and infrastructural requirements* and *essential components* of a rehabilitation programme (Ärztlicher Beirat der Schweizerischen Multiple Sklerose Gesellschaft, 1997; Schneider, 1998; Thompson, 2000; Beer and Kesselring, 2001; Freeman and Thompson, 2003).

Particularly due to the broad spectrum of symptoms and disabilities in MS, a comprehensive assessment of functional disturbances and of personal needs is essential in order to set up an individualised, goal oriented treatment programme (Freeman and Thompson, 2003). The specific therapeutic interventions are only one part of the rehabilitation

programme. Of the same importance are detailed information and instruction of patients and relatives.

The *timing and mode* of rehabilitation treatment in MS patients should be set individually taking into account the degree and impact of disability as personal and environmental factors (Beer, 2003b): in a professionally active patient, who is increasingly limited by the progression of the disease, rehabilitation may be indicated earlier than in a patient, who is able to live independently at home despite his disabilities. The necessity of rehabilitation treatment should be evaluated early in patients, who are at risk loosing important functions, activities or independence. Preservation of functions can be achieved more easily and more reliably than restoration of functions, which have been lost for a longer time. In general patients with more complex functional deficits and disabilities should be admitted for inpatient multidisciplinary rehabilitation treatment, as arrangement of an outpatient multidisciplinary treatment may be quite difficult for logistic reasons. Inpatient rehabilitation should also be considered in patients with increasing disability, who do not respond to outpatient treatment (Feigenson et al., 1981). Even though, best evidence for efficacy of rehabilitation came from studies with patients with chronic progressive MS, there is a growing evidence, that patients with relapsing–remitting course can profit from rehabilitation measures after an acute relapse with incomplete recovery (Craig et al., 2003; Liu et al., 2003).

Realistic goals must be laid down in collaboration with patients and care givers before starting rehabilitation process. In a MS patient, who is unable to walk for a long time, it seems quite unrealistic to aim at walking again: in this patient improvement in other activities of daily living (e.g. independent dressing and undressing, toileting, transfer) is a more appropriate and realistic goal in order to enable the patient to be more independent.

In MS patients with most *severe chronic disabilities* (e.g. bedridden patient) significant improvements of functions and activities usually cannot be expected even by intensive, multidisciplinary rehabilitation. In some of these patients, however, an improvement in some activities, quality of life and a reduction of the need of care can be achieved by a clearly defined, goal-orientated rehabilitation programme. In patients with severe spasticity, multidisciplinary rehabilitation in combination with drug treatment may help improving mobility, thus reducing the risk for secondary complications (pressure sores, contractures a.o.).

Limitations for a comprehensive rehabilitation treatment are severe, irreversible cognitive disturbances, which impede co-operation and learning capabilities. The same is true for patients, who are lacking of motivation, making any improvements quite impossible. Finally severe concomitant diseases may limit training capacity at an appropriate level.

Earlier studies examined mainly small heterogeneous cohorts of MS patients in an open-labelled, non-controlled manner before and after rehabilitative treatment (Feigenson et al., 1981; Greenspun et al., 1987; Aisen et al., 1996; Kidd and Thompson, 1997). In the last decade, however, some randomised-controlled trials have been published on this subject (Freeman et al., 1997; Solari et al., 1999; Wiles et al., 2001; Liu et al., 2003), increasing the evidence of efficacy of rehabilitation measures in MS patients (Table 38.2).

Although a recent study in MS patients suggests that some cortical reorganisation in MS patients (Rocca et al., 2002) occurs, this mechanism of recovery probably plays only a minor role in MS rehabilitation. The main effect is probably rather due to improved compensation, adaptation and reconditioning. Furthermore information and instruction of patients and caregivers, and the use of medical and social resources may contribute to improve coping with disease and disability and thereby improving quality of life of persons with MS and their relatives. The effect of specific therapy modalities can therefore explain only partially the observed long-term effects of inpatient rehabilitation (Freeman et al., 1999).

Multidisciplinary rehabilitation

One of the first trials studying the effect of *multidisciplinary inpatient rehabilitation* in MS patients was published by Feigenson and co-workers in 1981. In a prospective non-controlled study of 20 patients with chronic progressive MS not responding to outpatient treatment, a significant improvement in several disability scores could be seen after an inpatient multidisciplinary rehabilitation programme (duration 53 days) (Feigenson et al., 1981). It was estimated that the yearly costs per patient could be reduced substantially from 25,000 US$ to 19,000 US$ due to lower need for care (Feigenson et al., 1981). Another open-label, non-controlled study by Kidd and co-workers examined the effect of rehabilitation in patients with different patterns of disease: after short inpatient rehabilitation (15 days, $n = 79$) a significant improvement in disability and handicap could be achieved (Kidd and Thompson, 1997). This positive effect was seen also after 3 months. The benefit was more marked in patients with relapsing–remitting disease, a finding assigned to spontaneous recovery from relapses: 19% of these patients had also improved neurologically. Nevertheless, significant improvement could be demonstrated even in progressive forms. These findings were confirmed in a randomised, controlled study by Freeman and co-workers (Freeman et al., 1997): 32 patients, who followed an inpatient multidisciplinary rehabilitation programme over 3 weeks, were compared to a group of MS patients ($n = 34$), who were on a waiting list and came to rehabilitation later. All patients were examined at the beginning of treatment and after 6 weeks: while patients in the control group had a slight deterioration of disability and handicap, patients in the treatment group showed a significant improvement. There were no significant changes in both groups on the functional level measured by Expanded Disability Status Scale (EDSS, see Table 38.3) (Kurtzke, 1983).

A first longitudinal study concerning the duration of the benefit of multidisciplinary inpatient rehabilitation was performed by Francabandera and co-workers: after 3 weeks treatment of MS patients with chronic progressive disease ($n = 67$) there was a significant improvement of disability in the inpatient group compared to outpatient treatment group (Francabandera et al., 1988). This benefit was demonstrable 3 months after treatment, but was no

Table 38.2. Overview of clinical studies on rehabilitation in MS.

	n	Study design	Patient groups	Treatment	Duration	Control	Follow-up	Result
Feigenson et al. 1981	20	Non-controlled, pre/post	Patients failing to respond to outpatient treatment	Inpatient multidisciplinary rehabilitation	53 days	No	After discharge	Significant improvement in different disability scores, substantial decrease of amount of required help and costs of care (interview after 1 year)
Greenspun et al. 1987	28	Retrospective, non-controlled, pre/post	Patients admitted for impatient treatment	Inpatient multidisciplinary rehabilitation	28 days	No	Pre/post, 3 months review	Improvement in different disability scores (CRDS), gains maintained after 3 months
Franchabandera et al. 1988, LaRocca and Kalb 1992	67	Randomised, controlled	Chronic progressive phase	Inpatient multidisciplinary rehabilitation	3 weeks	Outpatient treatment	3, 12 months	Significant improvement of disability (Incapacity Status Scale) at discharge and after 3 months, no differences after 12 months
Kidd et al. 1995	79	Non-controlled, pre/post	Relapsing–remitting, primary/secondary chronic progressive	Inpatient multidisciplinary rehabilitation	15 days	No	3 months	Improvement of disability, handicap, and in EDDS lasting over 3 months
Fuller et al. 1996	45	Randomised, controlled	Patients admitted for inpatient treatment	Inpatient physical therapy	14 days	Waiting list	After discharge	No significant difference in mobility an ADL; reduction of mobility-related distress
Aisen et al. 1996	37	Retrospective, non-controlled, pre/post		Inpatient multidisciplinary rehabilitation	32 days	Steroid treatment only	At discharge (telephone interview after 1–3 years)	Significant improvement in disability (FIM) and FS/EDSS
Freeman et al. 1997	66	Randomised, controlled	Patients in stable progressive phase	Inpatient multidisciplinary rehabilitation	20 days	Waiting list	6 weeks	Significant improvement of disability and handicap (FIM, London, Handicap Scale), no change in EDSS after 6 weeks

(*Cont.*)

Study	N	Design	Patients	Intervention	Treatment duration	Control	Follow-up	Outcome
Di Fabio et al. 1998	46	Randomised, controlled	Patients in progressive phase	Outpatient multidisciplinary rehabilitation	1 year (1 time/week)	Waiting list	1 year	Reduced symptom frequency, reduced fatigue
Freeman et al. 1999	50	Non-controlled, longitudinal	Patients in stable progressive phase	Inpatient multidisciplinary rehabilitation	23 days	No	3, 6, 9, 12 months	Significant improvement of disability and handicap (FIM, London Handicap Scale) after 3 and 6 months, decline of EDSS over study period
Solari et al. 1999	50	Randomised, controlled	Ambulatory patients in stable phase	Inpatient physical therapy	21 days	Home exercise	3, 9, 12 weeks	Significant improvement of disability and mental QoL (FIM, SF-36) after 3/9 weeks, no difference after 12 weeks, no change if EDSS
Wiles et al. 2001	40	Randomised, controlled, crossover	Ambulatory patients in stable phase	Outpatient physical therapy	8 weeks (2 times/week)	No treatment phase	8, 16, 24 weeks	Significant improvement in mobility, balance, gait and reduced falls in treatment groups (Rivermead Mobility Index, balance, VAS) after treatment, no more detectable after 8 weeks
Craig et al. 2003	40	Randomised, controlled	Relapsing–remitting after acute relapse	Outpatient multidisciplinary rehabilitation	Individually	steroid treatment only	1, 3 months	Significant improvement in disability (Guy's Neurological Disability Scale, Barthel Index), motor score (Amende Motor Club Assessment) at 3 months
Patti et al. 2003	111	Randomised, controlled	Primary or secondary chronic progressive	Outpatient multidisciplinary rehabilitation	6 weeks	Home exercise	6, 12 weeks	Significant improvements in disability (FIM), no change in impairment (EDSS)

QoL: quality of life; FS: functional system; VAS: visual analogue scale; SF-36: Short Form (36) Health Survey.

Table 38.3. The EDSS (Kurtzke 1983).

0.0	Normal neurologic examination
1.0	No disability, minimal signs in 1 FS
1.5	No disability, minimal signs in >1 FS
2.0	Minimal disability in 1 FS
2.5	Minimal disability in 2 FS
3.0	Moderate disability in 1 FS, or mild disability in 3–4 FS; fully ambulatory
3.5	Fully ambulatory but with moderate disability in 1 FS and mild disability in 1 or 2 FS; or moderate disability in 2 FS; or mild disability in 5 FS
4.0	Fully ambulatory without aid, up and about 12 h a day despite relatively severe disability; able to walk without aid or rest 500 m
4.5	Fully ambulatory without aid, up and about much of day, able to work a full day, may otherwise have some limitations of full activity or require minimal assistance; relatively severe disability; able to walk without aid or rest 300 m
5.0	Ambulatory without aid or rest 200 m; disability severe enough to impair full daily activities (work a full day without special provisions)
6.0	Intermittent or unilateral constant assistance (cane, crutch or brace) required to walk 100 m with or without resting
6.5	Constant bilateral support (cane, crutch or braces) required to walk 20 m without resting
7.0	Unable to walk beyond 5 m even with aid, essentially restricted to wheelchair, wheels self, transfers alone; active in wheelchair about 12 h a day
7.5	Unable to take more than a few steps, restricted to wheelchair, may need aid to transfer; wheels self, but cannot carry on in standard wheelchair a full day; may require motorised wheelchair
8.0	Essentially restricted to bed, chair or wheelchair, but may be out of bed much of day; retains self-care functions, generally effective use of arms
8.5	Essentially restricted to bed much of day, some effective use of arms, retains some self-care functions
9.0	Confined to bed; can still communicate and eat
9.5	Totally helpless bed patient; unable to communicate effectively or eat/swallow
10.0	Death due to MS

Despite several limitations (non-linear, not sensitive for cognitive dysfunctions, mixing up impairments and disabilities), this is the most widely used scale for assessing clinical progression in MS patients. FS: functional system.

more detectable after 12 month (Francabandera et al., 1988; LaRocca and Kalb, 1992). In a prospective, non-controlled longitudinal study by Freeman and co-workers a group of patients with chronic progressive MS ($n = 50$) were examined regularly every 3 months after a multidisciplinary inpatient rehabilitation treatment of 23 days duration: there was a significant improvement in disability and handicap over 6 months, and in quality of life even over 9 months (Freeman et al., 1999). The findings are even more astonishing as during the same period there was a progressive deterioration on functional level (measured by EDSS) reflecting further progression of the disease process.

DiFabio et al. (1998) studied the influence of an *outpatient multidisciplinary rehabilitation* of MS patients: in a prospective, longitudinal, randomised study significant reduction of frequency of symptoms and in particular of fatigue could be observed in MS patients who had undergone an outpatient therapy programme (physiotherapy, occupational therapy, individual counselling) 1 day/week over 1 year in comparison to a control group. A more recent randomised, controlled trial published by Patti and co-workers (Patti et al., 2003) examined the effect of a short multidisciplinary treatment in MS patients with chronic progressive disease: 58 MS patients randomly assigned to an individualised multidisciplinary outpatient rehabilitation (6 weeks) were compared with a control group (*n* = 53) performing home exercise. After 6 and 12 weeks there was a significant improvement of disability (functional independence measure, FIM) in the treatment group, while impairment level remained unchanged. Thirty-two patients of the treatment group improved by more than 2 FIM steps compared with only 4 in the control group.

Specific therapeutic modalities

Physical therapy aims at improvement of motor functions (as co-ordination, fine-movements), balance and gait and reduction of spasticity by tone modulating exercises. This passive and active training should be complemented by comprehensive instructions and advice to the patients and if necessary to care givers. For better compensation of deficits, adaptation of aids (splints, orthotic device, walking aids, wheelchair) may be necessary in collaboration with an experienced orthopaedic technician. Optimal adaptation to the deficits is an equally important goal as are functional improvements (Steinlin Egli, 1998) (Fig. 38.2).

In a randomised, controlled trial Solari and co-workers examined the effect of *inpatient physical therapy* (duration: 3 weeks, 2 times, 45 min/day) in ambulatory MS patients (*n* = 27) in comparison to a control group (*n* = 23) instructed for a self-training at home (Solari et al., 1999). Significant improvements of disability of mental quality of life were demonstrated

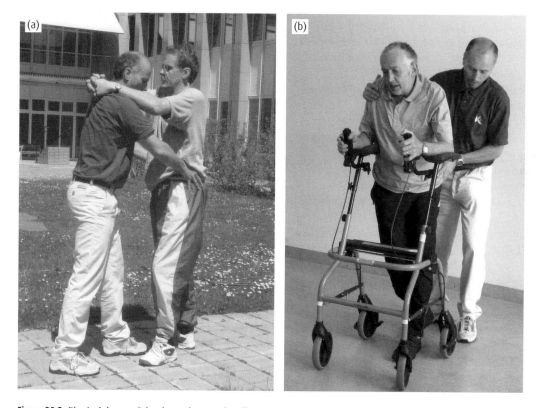

Figure 38.2. *Physical therapy.* It has been shown to be effective in MS patients improving motor functions and mobility. In treating MS patients, the diversity in pathology and clinical course, the wide range of functional deficits and the individual needs must be taken into account adapting programmes individually.

after 3 and 9 weeks, whereas after 12 weeks no significant difference could be demonstrated any more. Both groups remained unchanged on functional level (EDSS). In an earlier controlled study no significant improvement could be demonstrated after inpatient physical therapy during 2 weeks duration (1 time 39 min/day) (Fuller et al., 1996).

Wiles and co-workers studied the effect of an outpatient treatment: in a prospective controlled, crossover trial 40 MS patients were treated in randomised order over 8 weeks on an outpatient basis in a specialised rehabilitation clinic, by a physical therapist at home, or not at all (Wiles et al., 2001). A significant improvement of mobility and disability could be demonstrated during the active treatment periods in comparison to phases without therapy. In addition the frequency of falls could be reduced. Despite the lower costs of therapy for treatment at home, there was no significant difference in outpatient treatment and therapy at home. The effect was of short duration and was no more detectable after 8 weeks (Wiles et al., 2001).

Petajan and co-workers studied in a randomised-controlled trial ($n = 54$) the efficacy of *aerobic training* (3 times/week, 15 weeks): they showed a significant improvement of aerobic capacity and of isometric strength during the observation period in comparison to a control group (Petajan et al., 1996). In addition, transient improvement of psycho-mental factors (anxiety, depression), and of fatigue could be observed. In another study the role of aerobic training during multimodal rehabilitation programmes was analysed (Mostert and Kesselring, 2002): it was shown that by an individually adapted ergometer training at the aerobic threshold (30 min/day during for 4 weeks) the functional capacity could be increased as well as aerobic capacity and level of activity. At the same time an increase on the scores of vitality and social interaction could be demonstrated. Furthermore there was a trend of reduced fatigue. Another important observation in this study was that this individually adapted physical exertion had no negative impact on the clinical symptoms (i.e. triggering Uhthoff's phenomenon) (Mostert and Kesselring, 2002) (Fig. 38.3).

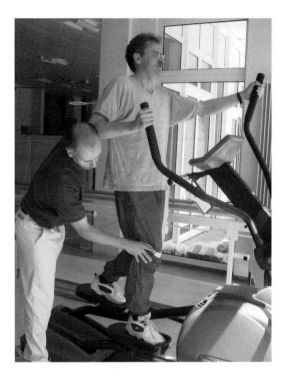

Figure 38.3. *Aerobic training.* As aerobic capacity is reduced in MS patients mainly due to deconditioning, endurance training should be performed at an aerobic level, thus allowing patients to increase general fitness and reduce fatigue symptoms.

Hippotherapy, a riding therapy assisted by a physical therapist, is thought to diminish spasticity by the rhythmic activation of trunk muscles. In addition postural motor control in ataxic patients can be improved (Künzle, 2000) (Fig. 38.4). A similar antispastic effect can be expected by *hydrotherapy*: reduced resistance of movements and of gravity facilitates training of movements in water (Gamper, 1995). Water temperature, however, should not exceed 30°C because of possible deterioration due to Uhthoff's phenomenon (see above). This Uhthoff's phenomenon may be suppressed by cooling therapy. Beenakker et al. showed a reduction of fatigue, improvement of postural stability and muscle strength in 10 heat sensitive MS patients when wearing a cold west with active cooling (7°C, 60 min) in comparison to a

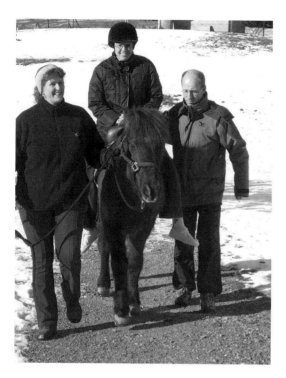

Figure 38.4. *Hippotherapy* (riding). It may be helpful especially in MS patients with spasticity of lower limbs and instability of trunc due to weakness or ataxia.

placebo-cooling suit (Beenakker et al., 2001). In another study it was shown that a cooling bath before training (16°C, 30 min lower body regions) reduced fatigue (White et al., 2000). These functional improvements after cooling are most probably due to partial restoration of central motor conduction capacities in demyelinated fibres (Humm et al., 2004).

For *occupational therapy* (*ergotherapy*) in MS only a few, mainly open-labelled, non-controlled studies are published (Steultjens et al., 2003). In a meta-analysis a positive effect of ergotherapy (tone modulating measures, specific training of manual and practical functions) on muscle function, range of movement and activities of daily living was shown (Baker and Tickle-Degnen, 2001).

As aphasia is rare in MS, specific *logotherapy or speech therapy* is rarely necessary. In patients with dysarthrophonia, however, speech training together with exercises of respiration may help to improve the capacity to articulate. Furthermore, in analogy to stroke patients, training of swallowing with triggering of reflexes, training of the swallowing process and compensatory measures, adaptation of consistency of food and liquids may help to improve the process of swallowing and reduce the risk of aspirations (Bartholome, 1999; Prosiegel et al., 2002). In more severe dysphagia percutaneous endoscopic gastrostomy should be discussed.

In most severely disabled dependent patients in addition to problems with swallowing insufficient respiratory functions and reduced coughing may cause pulmonary infections. In these cases, respiratory *training* may help to improve respiratory functions and cough reflex (Gosselink et al., 2000).

Bladder symptoms are particularly incapacitating in activities of daily living. Urgency is often made worse by motor disabilities which may make it difficult to reach the toilet in due time. Apart from drug therapy, *pelvic floor training* may help to improve bladder symptoms. In a controlled study in 80 MS patients Vahtera et al. could show that pelvic floor training with combined instruction for a home programme led to significant improvements of incontinence, urgency and frequency (Vahtera et al., 1997). Incomplete bladder voiding can be treated by an external bladder stimulator (Queen Square Stimulator), which may lead to a significant reduction of resting urinary volume (Dasgupta et al., 1997; Prasad et al., 2003).

The effect of a *cognitive training* was studied by Plohman and co-workers in 22 MS patients with disturbances of concentration: a significant improvement of attention and a reduction of attention associated problems could be demonstrated after 12 sessions in comparison to a non-specific training (Plohmann et al., 1998). These effects could be demonstrated even several weeks after termination of treatment. In a more recent study the influence of detailed neuropsychological testing with "cognitive intervention" was examined in comparison to the effect of assessment alone: 4 and 8 months after neuropsychological testing there were no significant differences. Therapeutic intervention in this study however consisted only in instructing for a self-training without proper neuropsychological therapy (Lincoln et al., 2002). The group with isolated testing without cognitive intervention declared a reduction of quality of life after 8 months. Therefore isolated neuropsychological evaluation without therapeutic intervention should be avoided.

In a part of the patients with depressive symptoms professional *psychological–psychiatric therapy* may be necessarily supported with drug therapy (Kesselring, 2001).

Group therapies may contribute to enhance motivation, social interaction and participation of patients.

In summary, timing and assignment to a rehabilitation programme should be considered early and should be tailored individually as a part of a comprehensive management of MS patients. As need for support and treatment in MS is changing during the course of disease, it seems reasonable, to set up recommendations based on different disease stages (Freeman et al., 2002). If *functional deficits are lacking or only of minor degree* (EDSS 0–2) the main goal is to maintain or optimise physical and mental fitness. Counselling and instructions for an individual training group (aerobic training, medical training therapy) is a form of prevention without the necessity of specific therapeutic interventions. In *moderate functional impairments* (EDSS 3–5) the goal is improvement or maintenance of motor functions, balance and mobility or reduction of spasticity. The therapeutic programme should include goal-orientated intensive physiotherapy (2–3 times/week) occasionally in combination with other therapeutic modalities (aerobic training, medical training therapy, hippotherapy, hydrotherapy). Patients should be instructed for self-management. If necessary, technical aids should be adapted 3–4 weeks after a first phase of therapy evaluation is performed: if the goals are reached the patient may continue with the instructed home programme. Assessments should be planned after an individually adapted interval. If the goals have not been reached therapy should be continued, if necessary after adapting treatment programme. If goals cannot be reached by outpatient treatment and/or if more complex polysyndromatic functional deficits are present an inpatient multidisciplinary rehabilitation treatment should be considered. In *moderate to severe functional limitations* with use of wheelchairs (EDSS 6–7) the main goal consists in maintenance of wheelchair mobility and highest possible independence as well as in the avoidance of secondary complications. In well instructed and motivated patients a frequency of therapy of 1–2 times/week, accompanied by a medical training therapy for improvement of strength and functions of upper extremities, and tone-reducing measures should be sufficient. In this phase of the disease an optimal adaptation of necessary technical aids is particularly important. Patients should be instructed to perform regularly tone-reducing measures (in particularly standing upright and lying prone). In most *severe functional limitations* when patients are bedridden (EDSS 8–9) the main goals of therapy consist in maintenance of mobility of patients, reduction of caring need and prevention of secondary complication (contractures, pressure sores, respiratory problems). Regular physiotherapy (1 time/week) with tone-reducing exercises should be performed, accompanied by respiratory therapy. In this phase of the disease, comprehensive instruction of relatives and care givers for daily exercises movement, measures for reducing spasticity and for prevention of complications is particularly important. In a favourable course with well-instructed carers regular assessments by an experienced therapist may be sufficient in order to recognise functional deterioration and to adapt the treatment programme if necessary.

Even though, there is a high evidence for some of these treatment programmes, the impact and efficacy of others are based only on lower levels of evidence. In addition, the wide range of disease course and functional deficits and the individual needs must be taken into account. Thus, the recommendations mentioned above should be considered as a framework, which should be adapted to individual patient depending on rehabilitation services available.

Symptomatic therapies

Centrally acting drugs may have a negative influence on the outcome of rehabilitation. Therefore drug therapies in rehabilitation have to be used only very cautiously (Schallert et al., 1986; Goldstein 1995, 1997). In addition to GABA-ergic (gamma aminobutyric acid) effect which may exhibit a negative influence on functional reorganisation, deterioration of cognitive functions and learning capacity may be particularly important. This latter mechanisms seem to be the main reason for negative effects of other drug groups (as neuroleptics, phenytoin, phenobarbital a.o.) on the rehabilitation outcome (Goldstein, 1995; Kowalewski and Kesselring, 2000; Vuadens, 2000). On the other hand, drugs which reduce symptomatology may provide a useful add-on to other rehabilitation measures.

Spasticity often leads to limitations of motor function, range of movement and malpositioning of the joints, often accompanied by pain (see Volume II, Chapter 17). Individual factors as well as type and distribution of spasticity must be taken in consideration when choosing therapeutic options (Beer, 2003a). In generalised tetraspasticity an oral antispastic is used first (baclofen, tizanidine, dantrolene, diazepam). The disadvantage of these medications is the generalised effect lowering muscle tone also in muscle groups with an already reduced tone (e.g. trunk muscles). A major problem may arise in patients with "usefull" spasticity (compensating weakness used for standing, walking), who are at risk loosing important activities reducing spastic muscle tone in weak muscle groups. In patients with combined spasticity and ataxia, medicinal reduction of spasticity may aggravate ataxic movement disorder. Furthermore, side effects such as fatigue and vertigo may occur which reduce physical fitness and co-operation. In patients with severe paraspasticity, who are not responding to oral antispastic treatment, intrathecal baclofen therapy should be considered: in thoroughly selected patients with good response to a test injection, delivery of baclofen intrathecally by an implantated pump has the advantage that required doses are very low (without or with only minimal systemic side effects), timing and amount of baclofen delivery can be controlled precisely, and that the effect is limited predominantly to the lower extremities, limiting risk for negative effects on trunk and upper extremities (Ward, 2002). In regional

spasticity (especially adduction spasticity of the legs) some improvement have been shown by *Botulinum toxin treatment* (Hyman et al., 2000).

As mentioned above, in treatment of spastic syndromes it is important to take into account, that certain patients may profit of spastic increase of muscle tone for standing and walking, and that reduction of spasticity by drugs can lead to dramatic deterioration of mobility. Before treatment, factors triggering or increasing spasticity (as infection, pain, constipation a.o.) should be searched for and, if present, eliminated (Kesselring, 2003).

Neuropsychiatric symptoms are common in MS (Foong and Ron, 2003). Depressive symptoms in particular have a negative influence on functional capacity and quality of life. Modern antidepressive agents (selective serotonin-reuptake inhibitors) may reduce emotional disturbances and thereby support rehabilitation treatment. These medications are also helpful in emotional instability (Kesselring, 2003).

Drug treatment of *ataxia and tremor* is least successful in MS patients. Benzodiazepines (e.g. clonazepam), isoniazid (INH) or ondansetron may relieve symptoms in single cases; the use of such therapies is limited, however, because of intolerable side effects (Kesselring, 2003).

Symptoms of *fatigue*, which are mentioned very frequently and most probably are due to various factors, often reduce physical as well as mental fitness and efficiency in MS patients. In a comparative, double-blind, randomised study ($n = 93$), *amantadine* (2 times, 100 mg daily) over 6 weeks was shown to improve fatigue significantly better than placebo, whereas pemoline did not (Krupp et al., 1995). In clinical practice, however, the effect of amantadine is rather modest, and a recent meta-analysis did criticise the general poor quality of trials lacking investigating the relevance and impact on quality of life. A recently published randomised, double-blind, crossover trial in 36 MS patients, showed a significant improvement of fatigue (Fatigue Severity Scale) during a 3-month treatment with *acetyl L-carnitine* compared with amantadine, concluding that this treatment was superior and better tolerated than amantadine. In a non-randomised, single-blinded, phase 2 study with a titration design during 9 weeks in 72 MS patients fatigue (measured by MS-Fatigue Scale) was improved by *modafinil* (200 mg/d) (Rammohan et al., 2002). Even though treatment was tolerated well, long-term safety and efficacy remains unclear. An alternative could be *methylphenidate*, another drug with central stimulating effects, which however has only shown anecdotal benefit. *Amino-pyridines* (3-4-diaminopyridine, 4-aminopyridine) are thought blocking potassium channels, thus improving central conduction in demyelinated fibres and by this mechanism leading to an improvement of fatigue and of other symptoms (Sheean et al., 1998). In a randomised, double-blind, placebo-controlled, crossover trial in 54 MS patients, 4-aminopyridine (32 mg/d over 6 months) was showed to improve fatigue (Fatigue Severity Scale) in patients with a higher serum levels (>30 ng/l), whereas the whole group and especially patients with lower drug concentrations did not show a significant improvement (Rossini et al., 2001). The treatment was tolerated well in this study; however serious side effects have been described using aminopyridines making safety concerns an important issue of future trials. To support conditioning training nutritional add-ons such as *creatine* (in combination with magnesium) may enhance improvements of physical endurance (Tarnopolsky and Martin, 1999; Tarnopolsky and Beal, 2001): even though for different theoretical reasons, the use of these supplements may be useful during intensive training, there are no clinical trials determining the benefit in rehabilitation of MS patients.

Pain is a frequent problem in MS (see Volume II, Chapter 15). It may be due to central lesions, due to spasticity or malpositioning. The cause should be clarified as far as possible in order to choose most promising therapy options: for example antiepileptic drugs (oxcarbazepin/carbamazepin or gabapentin) in central pain and neuralgia, whereas in pain syndromes due to spasticity treatment of spasticity is of primary importance.

Apart from incontinence, urgency is among the most common bladder symptoms in MS (Volume II, Chapter 24), most often due to a detrusor-hyperactivity. In first choice *tolterodine* is given, an anticholinenergic agent which may improve incontinence and micturition frequency (Abrams et al., 1998). In particularly difficult cases, *intravesical Botulinum toxin injection* into the detrusor muscle may be considered, which seems to be a promising treatment option in patients with hyperactive bladder (Schurch et al., 2000; Leippold et al., 2003).

Sexual dysfunction is frequent in MS patients (Volume II, Chapter 25): in a comparative study, prevalence was much higher in MS patients (73.1%) than in patients with other chronic diseases (39.2%) or healthy controls (12.7%) (Zorzon et al., 1999). The main complaints are anorgasmia/hyporgasmia, decreased vaginal lubrication and reduced libido in women, and impotence or erectile dysfunction, ejaculatory dysfunction and/or orgasmic dysfunction and reduced libido in men (Zorzon et al., 1999). These symptoms may have an important impact on self-esteem and relationship. Even though some of these complaints are due to psychological factors in consequence of the chronic disabling disease, others are due to destruction of central centres important for sexual functioning. Evidence for a somatic dysfunction is given by the fact, that sexual disturbances are correlated with disability, neurological impairment and bladder dysfunction (Zivadinov et al., 1999). Furthermore, MRI data found a correlation with pontine pathology (Zivadinov et al., 2003; Zorzon et al., 2003). Another reason is the use of drugs (as intrathecal baclofen), which can affect erectile function (Denys et al., 1998). Counselling intervention of couples may improve sexual satisfaction (Foley et al., 2001). Drug treatment is mainly limited to erectile dysfunction, which may be treated with oral *sildafinil* (Goldstein et al., 1998; DasGupta and Fowler, 2003). Intracavernous self-injections of vasoactive drugs are another possible treatment (Vidal et al., 1995), which however may be difficult to handle for MS patients with advanced disability.

38.5 Conclusions

MS is a disease affecting young people leading to long-term disability. Although newer immunomodulating drugs may decrease disease progression, and symptomatic treatments are able to alleviate these complaints to a certain extent, there is still an urgent need for rehabilitation in MS patients in order to reduce the consequences of the disease on functional impairment, personal activities and social participation and to enable persons to live an independent life in spite of the disease. Today, there is good evidence, that rehabilitation measures are effective in MS improving disability, handicap and quality of life despite progression of disease. Timing and mode of rehabilitation measures should be selected individually depending on disease phase, functional deficits and personal needs. Rehabilitation measures must be considered early in patients with impending risk for loosing important functions, activities or independence. Patients with progressive disease with complex multisyndromatic deficits or who are not responding to outpatient treatment should be assigned to an inpatient multidisciplinary rehabilitation programme. Multidisciplinary rehabilitation should also be considered in patients with relapsing–remitting MS with insufficient recovery after an acute relapse. Specific therapeutic modalities should be selected based on disease phase and personal needs. Rehabilitation measures should be considered only as a part of a comprehensive, long-term management of this chronic disease. If immunomodulation fails to halt the progression of MS, it may be that therapies aimed at remyelinating demyelinated axons (see Volume I, Chapter 26) and regenerating interrupted axons (see Volume I, Chapter 21–24) can restore anatomical and physiological integrity to the CNS, thereby providing a platform upon which multidisciplinary rehabilitation strategies can be applied.

REFERENCES

Abrams, P., Freeman, R., Anderström, C. and Mattiasson, A. (1998). Tolterodine, a new antimuscarinic agent: as effective but better tolerated than oxibutynin in patients with an overactive bladder. *Brit J Urol*, **81**, 801–810.

Aisen, M.L., Sevilla, D. and Fox, N. (1996). Inpatient rehabilitation for multiple sclerosis. *J Neurol Rehab*, **10**, 43–46.

Ärztlicher Beirat der Schweizerischen Multiple Sklerose Gesellschaft (1997). *Rehabilitation und Multiple Sklerose.* Schweizerische Multiple Sklerose Gesellschaft, SMSG.

Bachmann, S. and Kesselring, J. (1998). Multiple sclerosis and infectious childhood diseases. *Neuroepidemiology*, **17**, 154–160.

Baker, N.A. and Tickle-Degnen, L. (2001). The effectiveness of physical, psychological, and functional interventions in treating clients with multiple sclerosis: a meta-analysis. *Am J Occup Ther*, **55**, 324–331.

Bartholome, G. (1999). Schluckstörungen. In: *NeuroRehabilitation.* (eds Frommelt, P. and Grötzbach, H.), Berlin Wien, Blackwell Wissenschaftsverlag, pp. 107–124.

Beenakker, E.A., Oparina, T.I., Hartgring, A., Teelken, A., Arutjunyan, A.V., et al. (2001). Cooling garment treatment in MS: clinical improvement and decrease in leukocyte NO production. *Neurology*, **57**, 892–894.

Beer, S. (2003a). Medikamentöse Therapien der Spastik bei MS. *ARS Med*, **8**, 383–387.

Beer, S. (2003b). Stationäre Rehabilitation bei Multipler Sklerose. Empfehlungen des Ärztlichen Beirates der Schweizerischen Multiple Sklerose Gesellschaft. *Schweiz Med Forum*, **3**, 1118–1121.

Beer, S. and Kesselring, J. (1988). Die multiple Sklerose im Kanton Bern (CH). Eine epidemiologische Studie. *Fortschr Neurol Psychiat*, **56**, 390–397.

Beer, S. and Kesselring, J. (1994). High prevalence of multiple sclerosis in Switzerland. *Neuroepidemiology*, **13**, 14–18.

Beer, S. and Kesselring, J. (2001). Rehabilitation bei Multipler Sklerose. *Schweiz Med Forum*, **46**, 1143–1146.

Carton, H., Loos, R., Pacolet, J., Versieck, K. and Vlietinck, R. (1998). Utilisation and cost of professional care and assistance according to disability of patients with multiple sclerosis in Flanders (Belgium). *J Neurol Neurosurg Psychiat*, **64**, 444–450.

Compston, A. and Coles, A. (2002). Multiple sclerosis. *Lancet*, **359**, 1221–1231.

Compston, D.A.S., Milligan, N.M., Hughes, P.J., Gibbs, J., McBroom, V., et al. (1987). A double-blind controlled trial of high dose methylprednisolone in patients with multiple sclerosis. 2. Laboratory results. *J Neurol Neurosurg Psychiatr*, **50**, 517–522.

Craig, J., Young, C.A., Ennis, M., Baker, G. and Boggild, M. (2003). A randomised controlled trial comparing rehabilitation against standard therapy in multiple sclerosis patients receiving intravenous steroid treatment. *J Neurol Neurosurg Psychiatr*, **74**, 1225–1230.

Dasgupta, P., Haslam, C., Goodwin, R. and Fowler, C.J. (1997). The 'Queen Square bladder stimulator': a device for assisting emptying of the neurogenic bladder. *Brit J Urol*, **80**, 234–237.

DasGupta, R. and Fowler, C.J. (2003). Bladder, bowel and sexual dysfunction in multiple sclerosis: management strategies. *Drugs*, **63**, 153–166.

Denys, P., Mane, M., Azouvi, P., Chartier-Kastler, E., Thiebaut, J.B., et al. (1998). Side effects of chronic intrathecal baclofen on erection and ejaculation in patients with spinal cord lesions. *Arch Phys Med Rehabil*, **79**, 494–496.

Di Fabio, R.P., Soderberg, J., Choi, T., Hansen, C.R. and Schapiro, R.T. (1998). Extended outpatient rehabilitation: its influence on symptom frequency, fatigue, and functional status for persons with progressive multiple sclerosis. *Arch Phys Med Rehabil*, **79**, 141–146.

Dyment, D.A., Ebers, G.C. and Sadovnick, A.D. (2004). Genetics of multiple sclerosis. *Lancet Neurol*, **3**, 104–110.

Feigenson, J.S., Scheinberg, L., Catalano, M., Polkow, L., Mantegazza, P.M., et al. (1981). The cost-effectiveness of multiple sclerosis rehabilitation: a model. *Neurology*, **31**, 1316–1322.

Foley, F.W., LaRocca, N.G., Sanders, A.S. and Zemon, V. (2001). Rehabilitation of intimacy and sexual dysfunction in couples with multiple sclerosis. *Mult Scler*, **7**, 417–421.

Foong, J. and Ron, M.A. (2003). Neuropsychiatry: cognition and mood disorders. In: *Multiple Sclerosis 2*. (eds McDonald, W.I. and Noseworthy, J.H.), Butterworth-Heinemann, Philadelphia, London, pp. 217–227.

Francabandera, F.L., Holland, N.J., Wiesel-Levison, P. and Scheinberg, L.C. (1988). Multiple sclerosis rehabilitation: inpatient vs. outpatient. *Rehabil Nurs*, **13**, 251–253.

Freeman, J., Ford, H., Mattison, P., Thompson, A., Ridley, J., et al. (2002). Developing MS healthcare standards: evidence-based recommendations for service providers. The Multiple Sclerosis Society of Great Britain and Northern Ireland and the MS Professional Network. *J Neurol* (**Suppl. iv**), iv25–iv29.

Freeman, J.A. and Thompson, A.J. (2003). Rehabilitation in multiple sclerosis. In: *Multiple Sclerosis 2* (eds McDonald, W.I., and Noseworthy, J.H.), Butterworth-Heinemann, Philadelphia, pp. 63–107.

Freeman, J.A., Langdon, D.W., Hobart, J.C. and Thompson, A.J. (1997). The impact of inpatient rehabilitation on progressive multiple sclerosis. *Ann Neurol*, **42**, 236–244.

Freeman, J.A., Langdon, D.W., Hobart, J.C. and Thompson, A.J. (1999). Inpatient rehabilitation in multiple sclerosis: do the benefits carry over into the community? *Neurology*, **52**, 50–56.

Fuller, K.J., Dawson, K. and Wiles, C.M. (1996). Physiotherapy in chronic multiple sclerosis: a controlled trial. *Clin Rehabil*, **10**, 195–204.

Gamper, U.N. (1995). *Wasserspezifische Bewegungstherapie und Training*. Gustav Fischer Verlag, Stuttgart Jena, New York.

Goldstein, I., Lue, T.F., Padma-Nathan, H., Rosen, R.C., Steers, W.D., et al. (1998). Oral sildenafil in the treatment of erectile dysfunction. Sildenafil Study Group. *New Engl J Med*, **338**, 1397–1404.

Goldstein, L.B. (1995). Common drugs may influence motor recovery after stroke. The sygen in acute stroke study investigators. *Neurology*, **45**, 865–871.

Goldstein, L.B. (1997). Influence of common drugs and related factors on stroke outcome. *Curr Opin Neurol*, **10**, 52–57.

Goodin, D.S., Frohman, E.M., Garmany Jr., G.P., Halper, J., Likosky, W.H., et al. (2002). Disease modifying therapies in multiple sclerosis: report of the therapeutics and technology assessment subcommittee of the American Academy of Neurology and the MS Council for Clinical Practice Guidelines. *Neurology*, **58**, 169–178.

Gosselink, R., Kovacs, L., Ketelaer, P., Carton, H. and Decramer, M. (2000). Respiratory muscle weakness and respiratory muscle training in severely disabled multiple sclerosis patients. *Arch Phys Med Rehabil*, **81**, 747–751.

Greenspun, B., Stineman, M. and Agri, R. (1987). Multiple sclerosis and rehabilitation outcome. *Arch Phys Med Rehabil*, **68**, 434–437.

Hogancamp, W.E., Rodriguez, M. and Weinshenker, B.G. (1997). The epidemiology of multiple sclerosis. *Mayo Clin Proc*, **72**, 871–878.

Humm, A., Beer, S., Kool, J., Magistris, M., Kesselring, J. and Rösler, K.M. (2004). Altered central motor conduction time caused by change in body temperature: a quantification of Uhthoff's phenomenon in multiple sclerosis: a magnetic stimulation study. *Clin Neurophysiol*, **115**(**11**), 2493–2501.

Hyman, N., Barnes, M., Bhakta, B., Cozens, A., Bakheit, M., et al. (2000). Botulinum toxin (Dysport) treatment of hip adductor spasticity in multiple sclerosis: a prospective, randomised, double blind, placebo controlled, dose ranging study. *J Neurol Neurosurg Psychiatr*, **68**, 707–712.

Kesselring, J. (2001). Rehabilitation in MS is effective. *Int MS J*, **8**(**2**), 68–71.

Kesselring, J. (2003). Complications of multiple sclerosis: fatigue; spasticity; ataxia; pain; and bowel, bladder, and sexual dysfunktion. In: *Multiple Sclerosis 2* (eds McDonald, W.I. and Noseworthy, J.H.), Butterworth-Heinemann, Philadelphia, London, pp. 217–227.

Kesselring, J. (2004). Neurorehabilitation in multiple sclerosis – what is the evidence-base? *J Neurol*, **251**(**Suppl. 4**), iv25–iv29.

Kesselring, J. and Miller, D. (1997). Differential diagnosis. In: *Magnetic Resonance in Multiple Sclerosis* (eds Miller, D.H., Kesselring, J., McDonald, W.I., Paty, D.W. and Thompson, A.J.),

Cambridge University Press, Cambridge, Melbourne, NY, pp. 63–107.

Kesselring, J., Miller, D.H., MacManus, D.G., Johnson, G., Milligan, N.M., et al. (1989). Quantitative magnetic resonance imaging in multiple sclerosis: the effect of high dose intravenous methylprednisolone. *J Neurol Neurosurg Psychiatr*, **52**, 14–17.

Kidd, D. and Thompson, A.J. (1997). Prospective study of neurorehabilitation in multiple sclerosis. *J Neurol Neurosurg Psychiatr*, **62**, 423–424.

Kiel, G. (2000). Erstmals repräsentative Kostenerhebung für Patienten mit Multiple Sklerose (ed. Rieckmann P. and Würzburg). *Neurol Rehabil*, **6**, 325.

Kowalewski, R. and Kesselring, J. (2000). Pharmakotherapie in der Rehabilitation nach Schlaganfall: Gesichertes und Aussichten. *Neurol Rehabil*, **6**, 1–6.

Kraft, G.H., Freal, J.E. and Coryell, J.K. (1986). Disability, disease duration, and rehabilitation service needs in multiple sclerosis: patient perspectives. *Arch Phys Med Rehabil*, **67**, 164–168.

Krupp, L.B., Coyle, P.K., Doscher, C., Miller, A., Cross, A.H., et al. (1995). Fatigue therapy in multiple sclerosis: results of a double-blind, randomized, parallel trial of amantadine, pemoline, and placebo. *Neurology*, **45**, 1956–1961.

Künzle, U. (2000). *Schweizer Studie über die Wirksamkeit der Hippotherapie-K bei Multiple-Sklerose-Patienten. Hippotherapie.* Springer, Berlin, Heidelberg, New York, Barcelona, Hong Kong, London, Mailand, Paris, Singapore, Tokio, pp. 359–381.

Kurtzke, J.F. (1983). Rating neurological impairment in multiple sclerosis: an expanded disability rating scale (EDSS). *Neurology*, **13**, 1444–1452.

LaRocca, M.G. and Kalb, R.C. (1992). Efficacy of rehabilitation in multiple sclerosis. *J Neurol Rehab*, **6**, 147–155.

Leippold, T., Reitz, A. and Schurch, B. (2003). Botulinum toxin as a new therapy option for voiding disorders: current state of the art. *Eur Urol*, **44**, 165–174.

Lincoln, N.B., Dent, A., Harding, J., Weyman, N., Nicholl, C., et al. (2002). Evaluation of cognitive assessment and cognitive intervention for people with multiple sclerosis. *J Neurol Neurosurg Psychiatr*, **72**, 93–98.

Liu, C., Playford, E.D. and Thompson, A.J. (2003). Does neurorehabilitation have a role in relapsing–remitting multiple sclerosis? *J Neurol*, **250**, 1214–1218.

Lucchinetti, C., Bruck, W., Parisi, J., Scheithauer, B., Rodriguez, M., et al. (2000). Heterogeneity of multiple sclerosis lesions: implications for the pathogenesis of demyelination. *Ann Neurol*, **47**, 707–717.

McDonald, W.I. (1997). The impact of magnetic resonance in multiple sclerosis. In: *Magnetic Resonance in Multiple Sclerosis* (eds Miller, D.H., Kesselring, J., McDonald, W.I., Paty, D.W. and Thompson, A.J.), Cambridge University Press, Cambridge, Melbourne, NY, pp. 63–107.

McDonald, W.I., Compston, A., Edan, G., Goodkin, D., Hartung, H.P., et al. (2001). Recommended diagnostic criteria for multiple sclerosis: guidelines from the international panel on the diagnosis of multiple sclerosis. *Ann Neurol*, **50**, 121–127.

Miller, D.H., Kesselring, J., McDonald, W.I., Paty, D.W. and Thompson, A.J. (1997). *Magnetic Resonance in Multiple Sclerosis.* Cambridge University Press, Cambridge, Melbourne, New York.

Miller, D.H., Khan, O.A., Sheremata, W.A., Blumhardt, L.D., Rice, G.P.A., et al. (2003). A controlled trial of natalizumab for relapsing multiple sclerosis. *New Engl J Med*, **348**, 15–23.

Milligan, N.M., Newcombe, R. and Compston, D.A.S. (1987). A double-blind controlled trial of high dose methylprednisolone in patients with multiple sclerosis: 1. Clinical effects. *J Neurol Neurosurg Psychiatr*, **50**, 511–516.

Mostert, S. and Kesselring, J. (2002). Effects of a short-term exercise training program on aerobic fitness, fatigue, health perception and activity level of subjects with multiple sclerosis. *Mult Scler*, **8**, 161–168.

Multiple-Sklerose-Therapie Konsensus Gruppe (MSTKG) (1999). Immunomodulatorische Stufentherapie der multiplen Sklerose. *Nervenarzt*, **70**, 371–386.

Multiple-Sklerose-Therapie-Konsensus-Gruppe (MSTKG) (2001). Immunomodulatorische Stufentherapie der multiplen Sklerose. Part 1. Ergänzung: Dezember 2000. *Nervenarzt*, **72**, 150–157.

Multiple-Sklerose-Therapie-Konsensus-Gruppe (MSTKG) (2002). Immunomodulatorische Stufentherapie der multiplen Sklerose. Neue Aspekte und praktische Umsetzung, März 2002. *Nervenarzt*, **73**, 556–563.

Noseworthy, J.H., Lucchinetti, C., Rodriguez, M. and Weinshenker, B.G. (2000). Multiple sclerosis. *New Engl J Med*, **343**, 938–952.

Patti, F., Ciancio, M.R., Cacopardo, M., Reggio, E., Fiorilla, T., et al. (2003). Effects of a short outpatient rehabilitation treatment on disability of multiple sclerosis patients – a randomised controlled trial. *J Neurol*, **250**, 861–866.

Petajan, J.H., Gappmaier, E., White, A.T., Spencer, M.K., Mino, L., et al. (1996). Impact of aerobic training on fitness and quality of life in multiple sclerosis. *Ann Neurol*, **39**, 432–441.

Plohmann, A.M., Kappos, L., Ammann, W., Thordai, A., Wittwer, A., et al. (1998). Computer assisted retraining of attentional impairments in patients with multiple sclerosis. *J Neurol Neurosurg Psychiatr*, **64**, 455–462.

Poser, C.M., Paty, D.W., Scheinberg, C.C., McDonald, W.I., Davis, F.A., et al. (1983). New diagnostic criteria for MS: guidelines for research protocols. *Ann Neurol*, **13**, 227–231.

Prasad, R.S., Smith, S.J. and Wright, H. (2003). Lower abdominal pressure versus external bladder stimulation to aid bladder emptying in multiple sclerosis: a randomized controlled study. *Clin Rehabil*, **17**, 42–47.

Prosiegel, M., Heintze, M., Wagner-Sonntag, E., Hannig, C., Wuttge-Hannig, A., et al. (2002). Schluckstörungen bei neurologischen Patienten: Eine prospektive Studie zu Diagnostik, Störungsmustern, Therapie und Outcome. *Nervenarzt*, **73**, 364–370.

Rammohan, K.W., Rosenberg, J.H., Lynn, D.J., Blumenfeld, A.M., Pollak, C.P., et al. (2002). Efficacy and safety of modafinil (Provigil) for the treatment of fatigue in multiple sclerosis: a two centre phase 2 study. *J Neurol Neurosurg Psychiatr*, **72**, 179–183.

Rao, S.M., Leo, G.J., Ellington, L., Nauertz, T., Bernardin, L., et al. (1991). Cognitive dysfunction in multiple sclerosis. II. Impact on employment and social functioning. *Neurology*, **41**, 692–696.

Rocca, M.A., Falini, A., Colombo, B., Scotti, G., Comi, G., et al. (2002). Adaptive functional changes in the cerebral cortex of patients with nondisabling multiple sclerosis correlate with the extent of brain structural damage. *Ann Neurol*, **51**, 330–339.

Rose, A.S., Kuzma, J.W., Kurtzke, J.F., Namerow, N.S., Sibley, W.A., et al. (1970). Cooperative study in the evaluation of therapy in multiple sclerosis: ACTH vs. placebo. Final report. *Neurology*, **20(Suppl.)**, 1–59.

Rossini, P.M., Pasqualetti, P., Pozzilli, C., Grasso, M.G., Millefiorini, E., et al. (2001). Fatigue in progressive multiple sclerosis: results of a randomised, double-blind, placebo-controlled, crossover trial of oral 4-aminopyridine. *Mult Scler*, **7**, 354–358.

Schallert, T., Hernandez, T.D. and Barth, T.M. (1986). Recovery of function after brain damage: severe and chronic disruption by diazepam. *Brain Res*, **379**, 104–111.

Schneider, W. (1998). Rehabilitation Schweiz 1998. *Schweizerische Ärztezeitung*, **79**, 1683–1688.

Schurch, B., Stohrer, M., Kramer, G., Schmid, D.M. and Gaul, G.H.D. (2000). Botulinum-A toxin for treating detrusor hyperreflexia in spinal cord injured patients: a new alternative to anticholinergic drugs? *J Urol*, **164**, 692–697.

Sellebjerg, F., Frederiksen, J.L., Nielsen, P.M. and Olesen, J. (1998). Double-blind, randomized placebo-controlled study of oral, high-dose methylprednisolone in attacks of MS. *Neurology*, **51**, 529–534.

Sheean, G.L., Murray, N.M.F., Rothwell, J.C., Miller, D.H. and Thompson, A.J. (1998). An open-labelled clinical and electrophysiological study of 3,4 diaminopyridine in the treatment of fatigue in multiple sclerosis. *Brain*, **121**, 967–975.

Smith, K.J. and McDonald, W.I. (1999). The pathophysiology of multiple sclerosis: the mechanisms underlying the production of symptoms and the natural history of the disease. *Philos Trans Roy Soc London B Biol Sci*, **354**, 1649–1673.

Solari, A., Filippini, G., Gasco, P., Colla, L., Salmaggi, A., et al. (1999). Physical rehabilitation has a positive effect on disability in multiple sclerosis patients. *Neurology*, **52**, 57–62.

Steinlin Egli, R. (1998). *Physiotherapie bei Multipler Sklerose: Ein funktionelles, bewegungsanalytisches Behandlungskonzept*. Gerog Thieme Verlag, New York, Stuttgart.

Steultjens, E.M., Dekker, J., Bouter, L.M., Cardol, M., Van de Nes, J.C., et al. (2003). Occupational therapy for multiple sclerosis. *Cochrane Database Syst Rev*: CD003608.

Tarnopolsky, M. and Martin, J. (1999). Creatine monohydrate increases strength in patients with neuromuscular disease. *Neurology*, **52**, 854–857.

Tarnopolsky, M.A. and Beal, M.F. (2001). Potential for creatine and other therapies targeting cellular energy dysfunction in neurological disorders. *Ann Neurol*, **49**, 561–574.

The PRISMS Study Group (2001). PRISM-4: long-term efficacy of interferon-B-1a in relapsing MS. *Neurology*, **56**, 1628–1636.

Thompson, A.J. (2000). Multidisciplinary approach. In: *Principles of Treatment in Multiple Sclerosis* (ed. Hawkins, J.S.W.C.P.), Butterworth-Heinemann, Boston, Oxford, pp. 299–315.

Trapp, B.D., Rasohoff, R. and Rudick, R. (1999). Axonal pathology in multiple sclerosis: relationship to neurologic disability. *Neurology*, **12**, 295–302.

Vahtera, T., Haaranen, M., Viramo-Koskela, A.L. and Ruutiainen, J. (1997). Pelvic floor rehabilitation is effective in patients with multiple sclerosis. *Clin Rehabil*, **11**, 211–219.

Vidal, J., Curcoll, L., Roig, T. and Bagunya, J. (1995). Intracavernous pharmacotherapy for management of erectile dysfunction in multiple sclerosis patients. *Rev Neurol*, **23**, 269–271.

Vuadens, P. (2000). Role of drugs in recovery from brain damage. *Rev Med Suisse Romande*, **120**, 717–724.

Ward, A.B. (2002). A summary of spasticity management – a treatment algorithm. *Eur J Neurol*, **9**, 48–52.

Weinshenker, B.G. (1994). Natural history of multiple sclerosis. *Ann Neurol*, **36 (Suppl.)**, S6–S11.

Weinshenker, B.G., Bass, B., Rice, G.P.A., Noseworthy, J., Carriere, W., et al. (1989). The natural history of multiple sclerosis: a geographically based study. I. Clinical course and disability. *Brain*, **112**, 133–146.

White, A.T., Wilson, T.E., Davis, S.L. and Petajan, J.H. (2000). Effect of precooling on physical performance in multiple sclerosis. *Mult Scler*, **6**, 176–180.

Wiles, C.M., Newcombe, R.G., Fuller, K.J., Shaw, S., Furnival-Doran, J., et al. (2001). Controlled randomised crossover trial of the effects of physiotherapy on mobility in chronic multiple sclerosis. *J Neurol Neurosurg Psychiatr*, **70**, 174–179.

Zivadinov, R., Zorzon, M., Bosco, A., Bragadin, L.M., Moretti, R., et al. (1999). Sexual dysfunction in multiple sclerosis. II. Correlation analysis. *Mult Scler*, **5**, 428–431.

Zivadinov, R., Zorzon, M., Locatelli, L., Stival, B., Monti, F., et al. (2003). Sexual dysfunction in multiple sclerosis: a MRI, neurophysiological and urodynamic study. *J Neurol Sci*, **210**, 73–76.

Zorzon, M., Zivadinov, R., Bosco, A., Bragadin, L.M., Moretti, R., et al. (1999). Sexual dysfunction in multiple sclerosis: a case-control study. I. Frequency and comparison of groups. *Mult Scler*, **5**, 418–427.

Zorzon, M., Zivadinov, R., Locatelli, L., Stival, B., Nasuelli, D., et al. (2003). Correlation of sexual dysfunction and brain magnetic resonance imaging in multiple sclerosis. *Mult Scler*, **9**, 108–110.

39

Cerebral palsy and paediatric neurorehabilitation

Peter J. Flett[1] and H. Kerr Graham[2]

[1]Department of Child and Adolescent Development, Neurology and Rehabilitation,
Women's and Children's Hospital, North Adelaide and [2]Royal Children's Hospital, Melbourne, Victoria, Australia

Cerebral palsy (CP) is the most common physical or motor disability affecting children in developed countries, the prevalence being 2.0–2.5 per 1000 live births (Stanley et al., 2000). The prevalence has largely remained constant for decades, with improvements in peri-natal care meaning that more children were saved (including those with disability) and the incidence of very pre-term babies were increased in the 1990s (Stanley et al., 2000). Despite being a common and important clinical problem, there is still lack of precision in the definition of CP (Flett, 2003) or as some prefer "the cerebral palsies" (Miller and Clark, 1998). While the definitions of CP have been refined from time to time, there appears to be general agreement that the condition is characterised by "aberrant control of movement or posture appearing in early life, secondary to central nervous system lesion, damage or dysfunction and not the result of a recognised progressive or degenerative brain disease" (Nelson and Ellenberg, 1978).

There would appear to be at least four features to this heterogenous group of conditions. Firstly, a simple cause–effect relationship is unlikely in most cases. Careful epidemiological and brain-imaging studies suggest that CP frequently has antenatal antecedents, multiple factors and is rarely due to the events of labour and delivery alone. Increasingly, cerebral malformations such as syndromes featuring a neuronal migrational disorder and mitochondrial disorders with or without known chromosomal linkages are being identified. Secondly, CP is the result of a lesion, or lesions, in the immature brain which is non-progressive, that is, it is a static encephalopathy (Mackeith and Polani, 1958). As long as there is a lesion, dysgenesis or injury to the developing motor pathways before the arbitrary cut off of 2 years of age, then it is agreed that the term "CP" may be used. Badawi et al. (1998) have sought to address the problem of standardising the inclusion criteria for selecting people included on CP registers with particular reference to brain dysfunction that must be non-progressive and manifest early in life. Thirdly, as disorders of movement and posture, CP is not unchanging and has a wide variety of musculoskeletal problems and other associated conditions (Flett, 2003). Moreover, Graham (2001) and Graham and Selber, (2003) have argued that the fourth feature to be recognised is the progressive nature of the musculoskeletal pathology, supported by longitudinal studies of gait in children with spastic diplegia. (Bell et al., 2002; Johnson et al., 2002).

Overall, the term "CP", despite its imperfections and lack of precision, was still recently considered by Stanley et al. (2000) to be worth retaining as a blanket description for "non-progressive motor impairment of central origin, recognised in infancy or childhood". CP is the most common diagnostic cause of the upper motor neurone (UMN) syndrome in childhood, a syndrome characterised by positive features (spasticity or dyskinetic, hyper-reflexia, clonus and co-contraction) and negative features (weakness, fatigue, loss of selective motor control (SMC), poor balance, sensory deficits) and aptly described by Gormley (2001), Flett (2003) and also

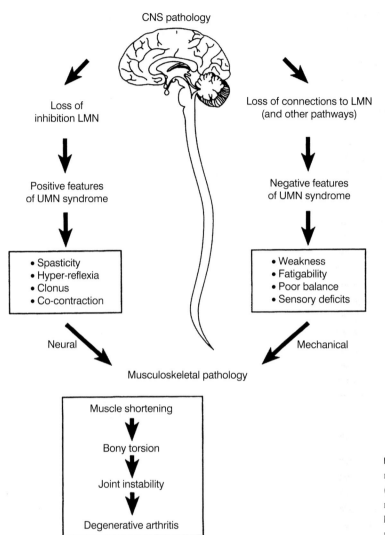

CNS pathology

Loss of
inhibition LMN

Loss of connections to LMN
(and other pathways)

Positive features
of UMN syndrome

Negative features
of UMN syndrome

- Spasticity
- Hyper-reflexia
- Clonus
- Co-contraction

- Weakness
- Fatigability
- Poor balance
- Sensory deficits

Neural

Mechanical

Musculoskeletal pathology

Muscle shortening

Bony torsion

Joint instability

Degenerative arthritis

Figure 39.1. Diagram showing the neuromuscular pathology in CP (Graham and Selber, 2003). CNS: central nervous system; PVL: peri-ventricular leucomalacia; LMN: lower motor neurone.

Graham and Selber (2003; see Fig. 39.1). While the focus has generally been on the positive features especially spasticity for treatment, it is frequently the negative features that have more significant impact on functional prognosis.

For some time now, there has been a search for unambiguous definitions surrounding the topic of spasticity and/or hypertonia in childhood. Moreover, with the advent of effective and specific treatments, it has become essential that definitions and selection criteria are agreed upon and applied as strictly as possible. Sanger et al. (2003) recently defined "spasticity" and "dystonia" and "rigidity" to describe clinical features associated with hypertonia in children. The definitions were designed to allow differentiation of neurological features even when more than one was present simultaneously. While "rigidity" is not a commonly used term in our experience, particular emphasis on "dystonia" is timely due to increasing clinical recognition for practical management purposes. Sanger et al. (2003) defined "dystonia" as a movement disorder in which involuntary sustained or intermittent muscle contractions cause twisting and repetitive movements, abnormal postures, or both. Bressman (1998) described "dystonia" as a "state of sustained muscle contractures producing involuntary fluctuating movements and postures which are often altered by non-specific afferent and emotional stimuli". It is recognised that dystonia will frequently increase with stress and decrease with relaxation or sleep (Lobbozoo et al., 1996). Dystonia may be unilateral, bilateral, focal or generalised.

Better known definitions, historically, of "spasticity" are based on velocity-dependent resistance (Lance, 1980), or on presumed properties of increased sensitivity in the tonic stretch reflex response (Crothers and Paine, 1959). "Spasticity" itself can also be defined as excessive and inappropriate muscular activity occurring in association with the UMN paralysis or syndrome (see Volume II, Chapter 17). In CP, spasticity has both neurophysiological and musculoskeletal components (Gormley, 2001; Flett, 2003).

Thus, there seems to be general consensus on most of the essential elements for the definition of CP, and perhaps also the neuro-physiological features. A modified neurological and practical topographical classification has undergone refinement since Crothers and Paine (1959). They divided patients into the following categories:

1 spastic (pyramidal) CP,
2 dyskinetic (extrapyramidal; see Volume II, Chapter 35) CP,
3 mixed types.

The spastic group has been further subdivided into the topographical distribution or the part of the body that is involved:

- *Hemiplegia*: One side of the body involved, arm and leg; arm often more involved.
- *Diplegia*: Mainly legs involved with some asymmetry expected, arms minimally involved.
- *Quadriplegia*: All four limbs and trunk involved, arms equally or more involved than legs.
- *Triplegia*: Three limbs involved, classically both legs and one arm.

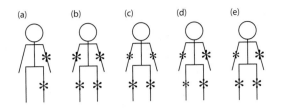

Figure 39.2. Classification of infantile CP according to localisation and ranking of neurological findings (Berweck et al., 2003). (a) hemiplegia (b) quadriplegic (c) diplegic (d) asymmetrical diplegia (e) triplegia.

- *Monoplegia*: Single arm or leg involvement, may be subtle or resolving hemiplegia, rare.
- *Asymmetrical diplegia*: More recently characterised, predominantly one sided but with some involvement of the opposite leg; strong similarities to both hemiplegia and diplegia.

Berweck et al. (2003; Fig. 39.2) have illustrated this recently according to localisation and ranking of neurological findings, based on Michaelis (1999). However, while it is one thing to use such definitions to denote localisation or distribution of neurological involvement, it is another thing to try and rank or grade according to muscle tone or functional impairment. This is of the utmost importance for comparisons of data between centres and CP registers. Further efforts to better define and classify sub-types of CP are necessary for such international comparisons and for research purposes.

Dyskinetic CP embraces dystonia and athetoid variants of the condition, and is commonly associated with spastic or pyramidal tract involvement. Ataxic CP is another uncommon variant, typically mixed spastic/ataxia with unsteadiness of gait in the diplegic distribution. Bulbar CP (Worster–Drought syndrome) primarily affects bulbar functions with minimal limb involvement (Neville, 1997).

39.1 Assessment of spasticity

While traditional clinical evaluation of spasticity will include symptoms and signs together with examination of muscle tone, range of movement (ROM),

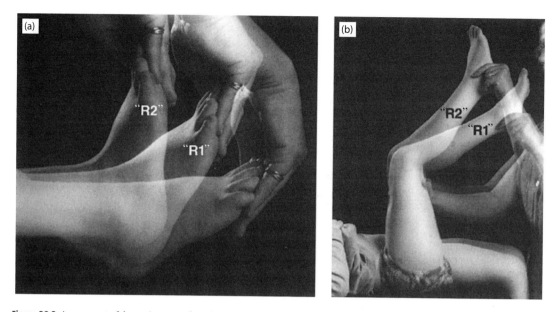

Figure 39.3. Assessment of dynamic range of motion R1 of ankle and knee using modified Tardieu scale. R2 is the slow passive range of motion, while R1 is the point to "catch" in the range of motion during fast movement of the ankle through the full available range of motion. (a) The Tardieu measure is performed at the ankle to test gastrocnemius with the knee extended. (b) The Tardieu measure is performed for the hamstring muscles with the hip flexed to 90° and the opposite hip extended (Boyd and Graham, 1999).

and functional impact, assessment can and should also include validated quantitative and qualitative instruments. The Ashworth and modified Ashworth scales evaluate muscle tone (Ashworth, 1964; Bohannon and Smith, 1987). Damiano et al. (2002a, b) found that instrumented measures, such as an isokinetic dynamometer, tended to have stronger relationships with function than the Ashworth scale. The Tardieu scale (1954), as modified by Boyd et al. (1998) and Boyd (1999) measures the intensity of muscle reaction at specified velocities, thereby producing reproducible measures of spasticity. Figure 39.3 illustrates R1 and R2 measurements, and of clinical relevance is the fact that as R1 approaches R2, spasticity is being replaced by fixed muscle contracture. Morris (2002) concluded that the Tardieu scale appeared to be a more useful clinical measure of spasticity than the Ashworth scales, and that it was a quantitative measure with content validity with promising intra-rater and inter-rater reliability.

Global functional evaluation instruments include the Functional Independent Measure for Children or WeeFIM (Msall et al., 1994) and the Paediatric Evaluation of Disability Inventory or PEDI (Feldman et al., 1990; Haley et al., 1991). Upper extremity functional evaluation scales include the Canadian Occupational Performance Measure or COPM (Pollock et al., 1990), the Melbourne Assessment (Randall 2001) and the Quality of Upper Extremity Skills or QUEST (DeMatteo et al., 1992). For lower extremity function, the Gross Motor Performance Measure or GMPM (Boyce et al., 1995), the Gross Motor Functional Measure or GMFM (Russell et al., 1989) and the Gross Motor Functional Classification System or GMFCS (Palisano et al., 1997; Fig. 39.4) are validated instruments. Health-related quality of life (QOL) instruments include the Child Health Questionnaire or CHQ (Landgraf et al., 1996) and the Paediatric Musculoskeletal-Functional Health Questionnaire or PMFHQ (Daltroy et al., 1998); the Caregiver Questionnaire (Schneider et al., 2001) has

Level I
- Sits unaided, arms free
- Movements in and out of floor sitting and standing without adult assistance
- Free walking (without support/aids)

Level II
- Sits unaided, but some difficulties to hold balance when arms are free; can attain standing from a firm base
- Crawls reciprocally
- Cruises holding onto furniture, walking with support or aids

Level III
- The only attainable free sitting position is "W"-sitting (some assistance may be required)
- Creeping in prone position or crawling (often not reciprocally)
- Attains standing from a firm base; may walks indoors short distances using aids and requiring assistance from caregiver

Level IV
- Requires assistance to attain sitting on the floor, only able to sit with arms propping
- Requires frequently adaptive equipment for sitting and standing
- Moves short distances (indoors) by rolling, creeping or crawling non-reciprocally

Level V
- Unable to hold head and trunk upright when sitting, or up when in prone position
- All motor functions impaired, unable to move along unaided, some mobility may be possible using a power wheel-chair

Figure 39.4. Degree for function disability in spastic motor disorders: levels I–V for 2 and 3 years old according to the GMFCS. The complete classification system encompasses the age groups <2 years, 2 and 3 years, 4 and 5 years and 6–12 years (Palisano et al., 1997).

been modified for CP, is undergoing further testing, and is promising.

Locomotor prognosis

Most functional gains are made in the first decade of life. Nearly all children with spastic hemiplegia walk independently; most of those with spastic diplegia achieve walking by 7 years of age but many require mobility devices and not uncommonly lose their skills and/or endurance towards adulthood. Those with spastic quadriplegia rarely achieve functional walking. In a recent study, Rosenbaum et al. (2002) described motor development in the cerebral palsies as a series of curves of motor development. These curves aid our understanding of gross motor development in children with CP of all degrees of severity. They are also an excellent guide to prognosis, build on earlier work by Badell-Ribera (1985) and Molnar

and Gordon (1976), and have significant implications for our understanding of the potential and limitations of management strategies.

39.2 Management of spasticity

Children with spasticity should be managed in a multi-disciplinary context, and a goal-oriented approach adopted based on clinical findings and the expectations and desires of the family and child. Careful selection to intervene in any muscle tone problem is very important. Some children with CP might depend on, and benefit from, primitive reflex patterns and increased muscle tone for weight bearing, transfers and ambulation (Bower, 2000; Flett, 2003). However, in many other children eliminating spasticity enables them to be more functional (Flett, 2003). Treatment can also be classified as temporary

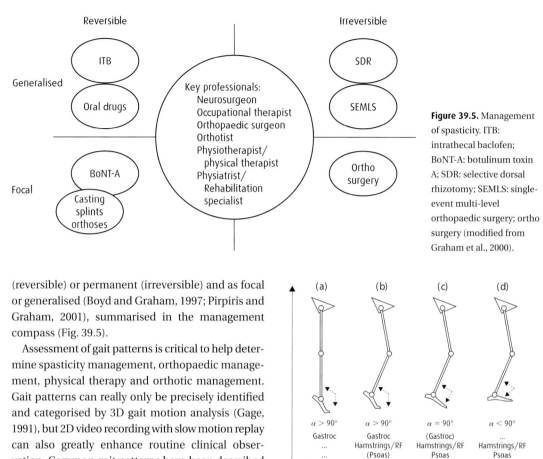

Figure 39.5. Management of spasticity. ITB: intrathecal baclofen; BoNT-A: botulinum toxin A; SDR: selective dorsal rhizotomy; SEMLS: single-event multi-level orthopaedic surgery; ortho surgery (modified from Graham et al., 2000).

(reversible) or permanent (irreversible) and as focal or generalised (Boyd and Graham, 1997; Pirpiris and Graham, 2001), summarised in the management compass (Fig. 39.5).

Assessment of gait patterns is critical to help determine spasticity management, orthopaedic management, physical therapy and orthotic management. Gait patterns can really only be precisely identified and categorised by 3D gait motion analysis (Gage, 1991), but 2D video recording with slow motion replay can also greatly enhance routine clinical observation. Common gait patterns have been described by Rodda and Graham (2001) for spastic diplegia and hemiplegia, and are illustrated in Figs 39.6 and 39.7.

Figure 39.6. Common gait patterns: spastic diplegia. (a) true equinus; (b) jump knee; (c) apparent equinus; (d) crouch gait. Gastroc: gastrocnemius; AFO: ankle–foot orthosis; GRAFO: ground-reaction ankle–foot orthosis; RF: rectus femoris.

39.3 Oral medication

Common indications for such treatment are to reduce as much as possible moderate to severe spasticity, and thereby improve function, facilitate care, delay muscle contractures and improve function (Albright and Neville, 2000). Oral medications act systemically and affect muscles involved to varying degrees of spasticity, including both the target muscles and those for which loss of tone and/or function is undesirable. Unacceptable side effects are common, especially sedation. In general, oral anti-spasticity agents are more likely to be of use to individuals with either generalised spasticity such as in spastic quadriplegia (Flett, 2003) or in combination with other interventions such as botulinum toxin A (BoNT-A) or orthopaedic surgery. Oral medications to treat spasticity in CP require more rigorous scientific evaluation by randomised-controlled trials (RCTs).

Baclofen is a gamma-amino-butyric acid (GABA) agonist agent. Despite being absorbed well, little

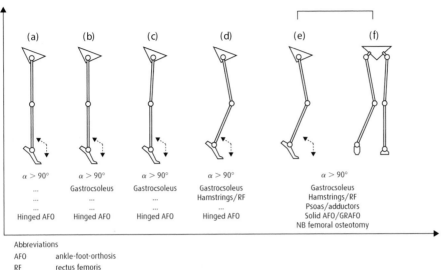

Abbreviations

AFO   ankle-foot-orthosis
RF   rectus femoris
GRAFO ground-reaction-ankle-foot-orthosis

Figure 39.7. Common gait patterns: spastic hemiplegia. (a) Type 1 drop foot; (b) Type 2A true equinus; (c) Type 2B true equinus/recurvatum knee; (d) Type 3 true equinus/jump knee; Type 4 hemiplegia: (e) equinus/jump knee; (f) pelvic rotation, hip flexed adducted, internal rotation. AFO: ankle–foot orthosis; RF: rectus femoris; GRAFO: ground-reaction ankle–foot orthosis.

crosses the blood–brain barrier because of its low liquid solubility. Baclofen is thought to act at the spinal cord level, augmenting deficient GABA release and inhibiting the release of excitatory neuro-transmitters responsible for spasticity. It has no effect on the muscles themselves. Its most common side effect is drowsiness and this factor, coupled with its poor lipid solubility and the blood–brain barrier hurdle, has led to the development of the technology to deliver intrathecal baclofen (ITB). Nevertheless, oral baclofen works well for some children with remarkably good tolerance, it can be useful at night for both relaxation and sedation, and it appears to benefit dystonia as well as spasticity. Combination treatment, such as BoNT-A or orthopaedic surgery, physical therapy and oral baclofen are commonly used in clinical practice with anecdotal benefit, but the results of further scientific studies to prove the extra benefit are awaited. It appears in clinical practice to be best evaluated on an individual trial basis, starting with low doses and gradually increasing to a maximum of 1–2 mg/kg per day (3–4 divided doses).

Dantrolene had been considered to be the drug of choice in spasticity of cerebral origin (Whyte and Robinson, 1990). However, it has been disappointing, and proper studies are now outdated as to its role in childhood (Joynt and Leonard, 1980). The effectiveness of oral baclofen has not been compared with that of dantrolene in rigorously controlled studies (Albright et al., 1995).

Diazepam, a benzodiazepine, is commonly used for short- and long-term spasticity management, including for post-operative muscle spasms. Although it can be quite effective in some cases, unacceptable sedation is usually the cost (Pentoff, 1964). Again, sufficient more recent evidence for clinical effectiveness is lacking.

Tizanidine is a benzothiadozol derivative of clonidine and acts centrally as an alpha-2-adrenergic agent to modulate the release of excitatory neuro-transmitters from afferent terminals and interneurones (Albright and Neville, 2000). It has been extensively studied in adults with spasticity associated with spinal cord injuries and multiple sclerosis (Lapierre et al., 1987; Rice, 1988; Medici et al., 1989). Experience is limited in childhood CP, and as with all oral medications for spasticity, sedation is its most common side effect. For additional discussion of spasticity, see Volume II, Chapter 17.

39.4 Physical therapy, casting, orthoses

Traditional neuro-developmental and physical therapy of CP focussed primarily on striving to rectify abnormal movement patterns and to maintain muscle/joint range for positioning and for daily activity. It also took the view that muscle strengthening exercises in children with CP was neither possible nor desirable because it might increase spasticity (Bower, 2000). However, such approaches failed to address muscle weakness and the negative impact of diminished amounts and intensity of activity on the cardio-respiratory system (Damiano et al., 2002). Muscle strength can be reliably measured in children with CP, and children who participate in strengthening programmes demonstrate increase in muscle power and improvements in function (Damiano and Abel, 1998; Wiley and Damiano, 1998; Dodd et al., 2002). It is probable therefore that the procedural management of spasticity and of surgery could benefit from strength and endurance training before and after treatment to achieve better outcomes. Since repetitive activities have been shown to improve SMC in the normal population, it is assumed that children with CP might also show improvement in SMC with repetitive activity albeit without resolution of other problems associated with CP (Gormley, 2001). McBurney et al. (2003) also undertook a qualitative study which provided further evidence that strength-training programs can be beneficial for young people with CP by increasing strength, reducing activity limitation and promoting participation in leisure activities.

Today, the physiotherapist and occupational therapist are pivotal for developmental and functional assessment, for identifying and selecting muscles and bones for potential medical and surgical interventions and for adjunctive therapy such as serial casting and orthoses. They are also needed for management of posture and seating; for muscle strengthening programs and ROM exercises; and for the "coaching" of parents, carers and teachers about essential and appropriate management activities, including the accessing of equipment.

Despite the wishes of families, convincing evidence that intensive therapy leads to better functional outcomes remains elusive. A RCT of physical therapy in 56 children with CP followed for 18 months compared the outcomes after intensive therapy (defined as 5 h/week) with traditional therapy (1 h/week) to evaluate the effects of pre-determined generalised aims versus specific and measurable goals. They found no statistical change in gross motor function or gross motor performance between the two groups (Bower et al., 2001).

Various types of bracing including twister cables and other similar devices have not been shown to significantly reverse or contain bony torsional deformities in the lower limbs. However, a variable hip abduction orthosis (Standing Walking And Sitting Hip or SWASH Orthosis) in conjunction with BoNT-A may have a role in the prevention of hip displacement, a common deformity in CP that can result in fixed deformity, painful dislocation and loss of function (Boyd et al., 2001).

The judicious combination of physiotherapy, intramuscular injections of BoNT-A plus/minus serial casting, and ankle–foot orthoses are now common clinical practice for the lower limb. Casting mainly acts on muscle length, and systematic trials are awaited to investigate the best way(s) to combine BoNT-A and casting. While the technique and duration of serial casting varies considerably, there is good evidence to show that it is at least equally efficacious to neuromuscular blockade with BoNT-A (Corry, 1998; Flett et al., 1999; Ade-Hall and Moore, 2000).

Subjectively, and according to clinical experience, well selected orthoses may provide stability for functional activity, maintain ROM, contain or delay, or even prevent reoccurrence after other interventions, and facilitate other forms of management.

Morris (2002) undertook a review of lower-limb orthoses used for CP and found that the current levels of evidence to support the efficacy of lower-limb orthoses for children with CP to prevent deformities or improve activities remain low. Morris called for RCTs that balance the differences among individual children between the treatment groups being evaluated. Nevertheless, the key findings from all the studies investigated by Morris were that only orthoses that extend to the knee and have either a rigid ankle, leaf spring, or hinged design with plantar-flexion stop can prevent equinus deformities. Preventing plantar-flexion (or equinus) has been shown to improve walking speed and stride length for the majority of children and thereby improved gait efficiency (Abel et al., 1998; Brunner et al., 1998; Orendurff et al., 1998; Desloovere et al., 1999; Morris, 2002).

39.5 Intrathecal baclofen

Baclofen, a synthetic GABA agonist, is limited by side effects when administered orally. The poor lipid solubility and blood–brain barrier means that the drug only reaches the target tissue in very low concentrations. Using a programmable implanted pump, baclofen can be delivered intrathecally to the target tissue at reasonable dosages, avoiding systemic side effects (Muller, 1992; Kroin et al., 1993). Responsiveness to ITB is confirmed by test injections before insertion of a programmable subcutaneous pump.

ITB has emerged as a powerful and useful technology in the management of severe spasticity, especially where generalised (as in spastic quadriplegia) and where reductions in muscle tone with improvements in comfort and ease of care are possible (Albright et al., 1991; Armstrong et al., 1997; Gerszten et al., 1998). It has also been used in ambulant or semi-ambulant patients, including apparently quite successfully in those with hereditary spastic paraparesis (Boyd et al., 2003), but detailed knowledge of the effects on gait and function are not yet known. Butler and Campbell (2000) reviewed 17 publications and found that a reduction in muscle tone was consistently found; that the body of evidence for significant improvement in function and/or ease of care was still limited or preliminary; and that medical complications were frequent, and sometimes serious, but usually manageable.

Since then, Campbell et al. (2002) has reported on the long-term safety and efficacy of ITB in the management of 21 children with intractable severe spasticity of cerebral origin. Nineteen recipients had spastic quadriplegia and two had spastic diplegia; most with level V on the GMFCS; and most were male. While there was no functional change on GMFM and PEDI, the Ashworth scale showed a marked reduction in spasticity. Most treatment goals were partly achieved; caregivers reported a reduction in oral medication and improvements in comfort, function and ease of care. Caregiver satisfaction was high. Unfortunately, children with GMFCS levels of IV and V experience high rates of adverse events, including death, many of which reflect the underlying severe neurological impairment.

Murphy et al. (2002) reported a consecutive case series of 25 implanted ITB systems, with effective reduction in spasticity but also a high explanation rate of 44% with wound complications as the leading cause.

Bjornson et al. (2003) reported that individual children with spasticity of cerebral origin receiving ITB experienced highly variable and unpredictable consequences in the domains of nutrition, oral motor function, communication and gastrointestinal function. Improvements in these domains of function were found to be important contributors to the QOL for children and families, and deserve close attention.

Albright et al. (2003) reported a prospective multicentre study in 68 patients, of whom 73% were younger than 16 years of age. The conclusions were that ITB provided effective long-term treatment of spasticity of cerebral origin, and its effects did not appear to diminish with time. This therapy was frequently associated with adverse side effects that usually can be alleviated by adjustments in dosage.

A clear advantage with ITB is the potential trade-off between spasticity and weakness that can be managed and programmed according to observations by the physician, physical therapist or occupational therapist and child/family (Flett, 2003). Although effective against spasticity and probably also dystonia (Butler and Campbell, 2000), it does not appear to influence athetosis.

Given that ITB has ongoing costs, including refilling of the pump reservoir every 2–3 months and surgical replacement of the pump every 7–8 years, there will need to be clear and firm guidelines developed for use. There may be some overlap in selection between ITB and selective dorsal rhizotomy (SDR), but upper extremity spasticity might be better treated with ITB than SDR, a trend that could be reinforced by reports of broader functional improvements, such as gait, transfers, self-help skills and communication. It is also likely that there is some overlap in selection between ITB and a combination of BoNT-A with minimally invasive orthopaedic surgery in the moderately affected spastic diplegic child. For example, minimal hip adductor releases without obturator neurectomy plus BoNT-A to medial hamstrings and calves in a young moderately affected child with spastic diplegia could be just as effective, less costly and safe (Flett, 2003). Thus, the ideal candidate for ITB could very well be an older child who is weak, unable to walk and who has had prior orthopaedic procedures (von Koch et al., 2001). The spastic quadriplegic child with well-preserved cognition could be best served by ITB, but so may some of those children with severe cognitive impairment where an alternative to orthopaedic procedures is being sought to facilitate nursing care (Boop et al., 2001).

Long-term prospective randomised trials would more definitely differentiate true functional changes from placebo effects, but would nevertheless be very hard to mask given the marked changes in spasticity (Campbell et al., 2002). Studies rigorously comparing ITB with other treatments such as SDR are needed.

ITB is expensive, invasive and associated with a high incidence of complications, yet in experienced hands and with protocols from the selection phase through to long-term monitoring so as to minimise risks, it would appear that positive functional outcomes can be achieved.

39.6 Selective dorsal rhizotomy

SDR has been used to reduce spasticity and improve function in ambulant children with spastic diplegia (Peacock and Eastman, 1981; Peacock and Arens,

1982; Peacock et al., 1987a, b; Peacock and Stuvedt, 1990) and to ease care of children with spastic quadriplegia (Abbott et al., 1993; McLaughlin et al., 1994; Albright et al., 1995). The rationale for SDR is consistent with neurophysiological evidence that spasticity is the result of decreased inhibition from the UMN corticospinal tracts and inter-neuron inputs (Young, 1994). Regardless of the cause, spasticity is relieved by reducing Ia-mediated excitation by the division of muscle spindle afferent fibres at the level of the posterior rootlets (von Koch et al., 2001).

While there are variations in surgical and electrophysiological techniques, the lumbar spine is usually approached via an en bloc laminoplasty from L1 to S1 and usually 20–40% dorsal rootlets are sectioned. SDR results in an immediate and clinically significant reduction in spasticity, followed by marked improvement in joint ROM and dynamic gait function (Boscarino et al., 1993). While SDR reduces spasticity, it has no effect on SMC, balance or fixed deformities (Boscarino et al., 1993). Postoperatively, an intensive and supervised physical therapy is necessary to ensure maximal outcome (Elk, 1984; Irwin-Carruthers et al., 1995). There are studies reporting that pes planovalgus, hip subluxation and spinal deformities may increase after SDR (Greene et al., 1991; Carroll et al., 1998). The Carroll study actually found that 65% of their patients went onto orthopaedic interventions for contractures and deformity; 37% required subtalar stabilisation for severe planovalgus, and hip subluxation was treated in 25%. Dias and Marty (1992) also reported that subsequent orthopaedic surgical procedures were required in 40–50% patients. However, Heim et al. (1995) found that SDR may prevent the progression of spastic hip displacement.

Long-term follow-up studies have shown that spasticity remained reduced and motor function improved, although orthopaedic procedures were still necessary (Arens et al., 1989; Nishida et al., 1995; Thomas et al., 1997). Similarly, improvements in gait have been reported (Perry et al., 1989; Vaughan et al., 1991; Boscarino et al., 1993; Subramanian et al., 1998; Wright et al., 1998). A child's ability to dorsiflex the foot was found to be a good predictor of independent ambulation after SDR. In children with good motor control prior to SDR, almost normal movement patterns have been observed (Peacock and Staudt 1991). A series by Steinbok et al. (1992) suggested decreased lower extremity spasticity and improved ROM in 50 children with CP after SDR. Improvement in upper-limb function and motor and self-care skills has also been found in children 1 year after SDR (Loewen et al., 1998). In a separate study, however, no improvement in the range of motion of the upper limbs, muscle tone or strength was found (Buckon et al., 1996).

Three randomised-clinical trials of SDR compared with physical therapy without SDR have been published (Steinbok et al., 1997; McLaughlin et al., 1998; Wright et al., 1998). They used single-blind objective measures to evaluate outcomes, appropriate randomisation and study design including the GMFM as the main outcome variable. Although each study reported positive reduction in spasticity, the functional outcomes were not in agreement. One study found no difference in mobility (McLaughlin et al., 1998) while the other two found a statistically significant difference in favour of the group with SDR. There were difficulties in the studies with respect to recruiting patients, pre-operative functional status, electro-physiological monitoring, and percentage of dorsal rootlets cut and the intensity of physical therapy. A meta-analysis by McLaughlin et al. (2002) of these three randomised trials found a reduction in spasticity at the impairment level. However, with regards to function, there was a small but statistically significant advantage to SDR plus physiotherapy compared with physiotherapy alone. The authors also stated that it was disappointing to see only modest improvements in gross motor function despite claims made in uncontrolled studies and despite the time, effort and risk involved. They called for further rigorous studies to evaluate long-term outcomes, both positive and negative.

The best spastic diplegic candidate has been described as being ambulant, having pure spasticity, good SMC and underlying muscle strength, being between the ages of 4 and 8 years, being cognitively intact and with a good social support structure (Gormley, 2001). Others have also said that good

muscle strength to provide support after SDR was important, and aged 3–5 years would be an ideal time (von Koch et al., 2001). It is generally accepted that children selected for SDR should be free of obvious ataxia, athetosis and dystonia (McLaughlin, 2000).

SDR appears to be relatively safe in the short term in experienced hands. Transient post-operative parasthesias are relatively common (McLaughlin et al., 2002). However, a definitive assessment cannot yet be made about long-term effects, especially musculoskeletal effects. Moreover, there does not appear to be any preventative or halting benefits to the progression of such key orthopaedic issues as hip dislocation and scoliosis (Greene et al., 1991; Hodgkinson et al., 1997) and many will still require corrective surgery. Marty et al. (1995) found that during an average 4-year follow-up period on 50 children, that 31 still needed some form of soft tissue orthopaedic surgery procedure. Chicoine et al. (1997) found that the rate of orthopaedic procedures was less if SDR was performed between 2 and 4 years of age than between 5 and 19 years of age, and argued for it to be done as early as possible.

Some children have significant muscle weakness, ataxia, dystonia and/or truncal hypotonia which are "unmasked" by SDR and which limit their post-operative functional improvement (McLaughlin et al., 2002).

There are case reports of back pain and spinal stenosis with neurological loss years after SDR (Gooch and Walker 1996). Boop (2001) stated that laminar replacement may be considered in children undergoing multi-level laminectomy for SDR. They added that further prospective long-term outcome studies are required to determine the incidence of pain, spinal deformity and spinal stenosis following multi-level laminectomy for SDR.

To date, SDR has not been compared prospectively to ITB amongst the more ambulant spastic diplegia group. SDR has been found to be more cost effective than ITB in spastic quadriplegia patients, but the actual efficacy of the two interventions has not been assessed and compared at the same time (Steinbok, 1995).

39.7 The use of BoNT-A

BoNT-A is now established as a definitive therapeutical intervention in the management of childhood spasticity. It acts by short-term chemical denervation of the injected target muscle.

The toxin is one of the most potent bacterial toxins known to humans and is produced by the Gram-positive, anaerobic bacteria *Clostridium botulinum*. There are eight antigenically distinct toxins: A, B, C1, C2, D, E, F and G. While types A, B, E and F are the main toxins affecting humans, BoNT-A is the main one used therapeutically at present.

BoNT-A was first known to act by binding to the neuromuscular junction (Burgen et al., 1949), inhibiting the release of acetylcholine (Ach) from peripheral nerves via a number of steps (Sellin and Thesleff, 1981; Gunderson et al., 1982; Dolly et al., 1984), and producing selective paralysis of muscles. Mechanism of action of botulinum toxins and of the re-establishment of the functional neuromuscular junction after

exposure is illustrated in Figs 39.8 and 39.9. It takes about 3 months for the original nerve endings to be restored while the sprouts are concurrently being eliminated. Thus, BoNT-A is completely reversible pharmacologically and clinically (de Paiva et al., 1999). Other proposed mechanisms to modify the effects of spasticity are increased binding affinity of the toxin to more active (spastic) muscles to decrease true spasticity; and BoNT-A may also decrease peripheral nociception by reducing the release of local nociceptors and reduce perception of pain (Aoki and Guyer, 2001).

BoNT-A can result in atrophy of both the intrafusal muscle fibres (by blocking the gamma motor neurons acting at the muscle spindle) as well as the extrafusal muscle fibres (inhibition of the alpha motor neurones; Rosales et al., 1996). This would suggest that BoNT-A may not only have an effect on the gait of the spastic muscle in CP but also produce change in the muscle spindle, alteration to sensory input and indirect changes in the central nervous system

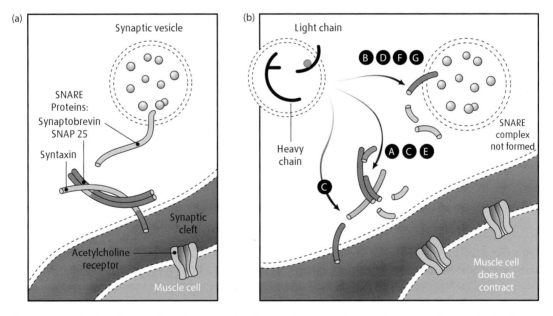

Figure 39.8. Mechanism of action of botulinum toxins: botulinum toxins prevent fusion of the pre-synaptic vesicle by cleaving SNARE proteins (SNAP-25 (synaptosomal-associated protein of 25 kDa), synaptobrevin, and syntaxin). BoNT-A affects SNAP-25. Failure to achieve an effective synaptic fusion complex prevents release of Ach into the synaptic cleft and flaccid muscle paralysis occurs (Koman et al., 2002).

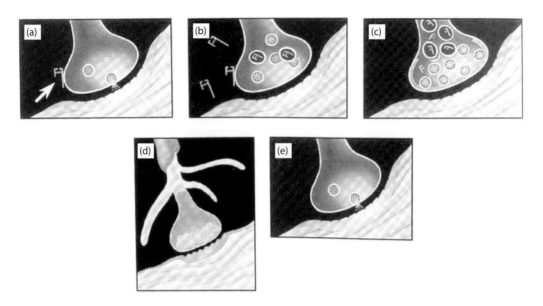

Figure 39.9. Mechanism (five steps) of the re-establishment of the functional neuromuscular junction after exposure to BoNT-A (Aoki, 2001; Koman et al., 2002).

(Giladi, 1997; Aoki and Guyer, 2001; Berardelli, 2002). Inhibition of Ach release may alter the gain of sensory organs leading to changes in the sensory information flowing centrally (Aoki and Guyer, 2001). These data provide preliminary evidence that BoNT-A induced reduction in spindle signals may alter the balance between afferent input and motor output thereby changing cortical excitability (Berardelli, 2002). Moreover, data on brain reorganisation with functional magnetic resonance imaging (functional MRI) support the hypothesis of central brain plasticity in response to peripheral intramuscular injection of BoNT-A (Boyd et al., 2002).

BoNT-A causes a dose dependent, reversible chemical denervation when injected into skeletal muscle. Boyd and Graham (1997) reported that there was considerable evidence to support the use of BoNT-A in the lower limb; they emphasised the importance of an integrated program including physiotherapy, orthoses and orthopaedic surgery. Finally, they developed both an indicative timeline for CP management and also a management algorithm for equinus. Selection factors, injection protocols and recommendations for treatment have been reported (Russman et al., 1997; Graham et al., 2000; Flett, 2003).

The efficacy and the safety of BoNT-A in the management of spasticity in CP has been established in a number of open label, controlled, placebo-controlled/randomised-clinical trials and also two meta-analyses (Cosgrove et al., 1994; Graham et al., 2000; Koman et al., 2000; Boyd and Hays, 2001; Boyd et al., 2001). Comparative studies (Corry et al., 1998; Flett et al., 1999) between BoNT-A and serial fixed casting as clinical best practice in the treatment of dynamic equinus (calf tightness) have shown similar efficacy but BoNT-A was better tolerated, led to a longer period of tone reduction while families emphasised inconvenience with casting (Flett et al., 1999).

Houltram et al. (2001) measured clinical efficacy from two RCTs (Corry et al., 1998; Flett et al., 1999) and demonstrated equivalent efficacy of BoNT-A and serial casting; however, with BoNT-A the effect lasted longer and was clearly the preferred treatment. They further concluded that BoNT-A was not only an effective, safe and acceptable treatment but was associated with only a modest increase in direct medical costs per child per year. Thus, BoNT-A can be considered, according to Houltram et al. (2001), to be a valuable and cost-effective treatment in the conservative management of equinus in children with CP. In Australia, this resulted in full Government subsidy from May 2000.

Common clinical applications in the lower limb include dynamic equinus (Cosgrove et al., 1994; Boyd and Graham, 1997; Koman et al., 2001; Baker et al., 2002), and also adductor spasticity (scissoring) and hamstring spasticity (Corry et al., 1999; Boyd et al., 2001).

A further recent application has been the management of upper-limb spasticity in hemiplegia. Corry (1997) studied the role of BoNT-A in the upper limb in a placebo-controlled trial and concluded that the injections were best suited to those with thumb in palm deformities and marked elbow-flexion spasticity. Fehlings et al. (2000) also found in a randomised, controlled, single-blind trial that BoNT-A injections were effective to improve upper extremity function in children with hemiplegia who had at least modest spasticity. However, electro-myographical guidance was not used. More recently, Hurvitz et al. (2003) found that although BoNT-A reduced tone and increased ROM of the spastic upper extremity, the time course and degree of motor improvement appeared to depend on the complexity of the task.

Pre-operative injection with BoNT-A has been shown to reduce and effectively manage post-operative pain in children with CP undergoing adductor surgery (Barwood et al., 2000).

In general, BoNT-A is a focal or regional intervention, but integrated single-event multi-level treatment (Molenaers et al., 1999; 2001) is now common in clinical practice providing "windows of opportunity" for collateral management strategies such as physical therapy and orthoses to be more effective. Moreover, the same authors found that this integrated approach appears to prolong the duration of BoNT-A treatment, resulting in duration of about 1 year between injections. Assessing for dynamic stiffness or tightness (i.e. neurological) and fixed myostatic contracture (i.e. anatomical) is critical because BoNT-A will not affect the latter. The dynamic component of muscle shortening is usually most evident during walking and other activities, and is largely absent when the child is relaxed. Eames et al. (1999) showed that younger children had a larger dynamic component and also children with diplegia more than hemiplegia. The duration of reduction in spasticity correlated with the dynamic contracture. Again, those with greater amounts of dynamic shortening prior to injection showed a longer response than those who had significant fixed contracture.

BoNT-A is at present manufactured by two companies: Allergan (Botox) and Ipsen (Dysport). They have different dosages and great care must be taken when working out the appropriate dose(s) for the preparation being administered. Single or multiple muscles may be injected per session, and currently, dosage is worked out on a body weight basis: BoNT-A in the range 8–12 units/kg bodyweight of Botox (Allergan) or 20–25 units/kg bodyweight of Dysport (Ipsen). However, some experienced clinicians are already using much larger doses with increased efficacy (Polak et al., 2002). Reconstitution in normal saline is necessary for both preparations, after which there is a shelf life of approximately 4 hr. While accurate localisation of sites in target muscles can be better achieved by electrical stimulation or ultrasound, correct needle positioning can also be confirmed clinically in some lower-limb muscles (e.g. calves) by reciprocal movement of the external end of the needle with passive movements of the joints controlled by that muscle.

Systemic side effects are extremely rare. Care should be taken in children with spastic quadriplegia and dysphagia, and generalised weakness and lethargy have also been attributed to the toxin. However, establishing definite causal relationships in either group is difficult. Neutralising antibodies to BoNT-A are rare in children. Most side effects are gait or function-related, such as excessive weakening or inappropriate target muscles or unrecognised fixed contractures, but the effects are short-lived and/or can be managed other ways. Temporary urinary incontinence or similar symptoms is recognised to occur with hip adductor injections, presumably due to toxin crossing the fascial planes.

Another agent, phenol, has a limited role as a neurolytic agent but can only be used directly for motor nerves such as the obturator nerve for adductor spasticity and the musculocutaneous nerve for elbow flexor spasticity (Gormley, 2001; Pirpiris and Graham, 2001).

39.8 Orthopaedic surgery

Most surgical efforts are directed towards the physical effects of the static neurological damage of CP, but the progressive musculoskeletal pathology has recently been emphasised (Graham, 2001; Graham and Selber, 2003). The stretch of relaxed muscle is considered to be the stimulus for longitudinal growth, and the reduction of this stimulus causes contractures. A normal range of physiological forces must act upon the growth plates and bones, but in CP these forces are commonly disturbed and can lead to hip dysplasia, persistence of neonatal femoral anteversion and scoliosis. The failure of longitudinal growth of skeletal muscle in CP has been aptly called "short muscle disease" (Rang et al., 1986).

The primary aim in the management of spasticity is to prevent the development of fixed contractures. If they occur, correction of fixed musculoskeletal deformities is necessary before the onset of decompensation. Otherwise, once decompensated joint pathology has developed, the surgical options are limited, the rate of complications escalates and the outcome of salvage surgery is frequently indifferent (Graham and Selber, 2003). Coordinated hip surveillance by orthopaedic surgeons and physiotherapists has recently been called for as part of the routine management of children with bilateral CP, following successful prospective clinical, radiological and early surgical intervention (Dobson et al., 2002). The prevalence of hip displacement varies from approximately 1% in spastic hemiplegia, up to 75% in spastic quadriplegia (Dobson et al., 2002). The incidence of hip displacement >30% increases dramatically from GMFCS (Palisano et al., 1997) level I to V (H.K. Graham personal communication). Hip migration percentage can be measured with reasonable

accuracy, thus improving therapy and surgical decision-making (Pountney et al., 2003).

The selection and timing for orthopaedic surgery let alone the variety of procedures available for different ranges of pathology and deformities have produced significant challenges. Graham and Selber (2003) have summarised the most common surgical procedures for spastic hemiplegia, spastic diplegia and spastic quadriplegia, usually preceded by BoNT-A and the use of gait pattern templates and 2D video or instrumented 3D gait analysis (3D GA) in selected cases. It is probable that new anti-spasticity interventions have significantly reduced or delayed the requirements for orthopaedic surgery.

In the lower limb, there has been a definite trend towards delaying surgery until the child's gait has matured in mid to late childhood. At that stage, 3D GA can be employed to help develop the surgical prescription (Gage, 1991; Boyd and Graham, 1997). There has also been a steady trend towards single-event multi-level surgery (SEMLS) (Gage, 1991), in lieu of the "birthday syndrome" where children come in for their annual staged procedure (Rang, 1990; Morton, 1999). However, there is still a need for scientific studies, such as RCTs to prove the efficacy of SEMLS in the various sub-types of CP.

There are good reasons to avoid surgery in some early childhood situations, such as calf lengthening procedures in spastic diplegia (responsible for iatrogenic crouch gait) (Segal et al., 1989), and in hemiparesis (over- or under-lengthening) (Rattey et al., 1993).

Clinical insight into the natural progression of gait and function is important, and 3D GA using computer-based video systems has provided objective confirmation to support the observation that many patients have progressive deterioration of their walking ability in later childhood and adolescence (Johnson et al., 1997).

39.9 Associated medical conditions

Associated and well-recognised disabilities include those of hearing, vision, sensation, epilepsy, communication and cognition. Common general medical issues are growth/nutrition, gastro-oesophageal reflux, oral-motor/swallowing, pulmonary (including aspiration and pneumonia) and salivary control.

39.10 The future

There has been a definite improvement in the attitude and investment of science and clinical practice into the management of children with CP over the last decade especially (Flett, 2003). There is substantial evidence now for better functional and QOL outcomes through our interventions, but we still need to look beyond spasticity and address muscle weakness, SMC and other aspects of CP as well. More work is urgently needed and probably by way of collaborative multi-centre trials. Better understanding of the neurobiology of the brain is an emerging and exciting area of development.

The development and validation of outcome measurement tools for functional ability, societal participation and health-related QOL are also seen as challenges to accomplish and use effectively in management. We need measures that will differentiate real changes from the effect of placebo.

Finally, we should not lose sight of the fact that adults with CP have ongoing problems with locomotion and musculoskeletal status, and might benefit from physical training to remain walking in some cases (Anderson and Mattsson, 2001; see Volume II, Chapter 19). After all, the ability to walk was usually the most significant goal for their parents when they were children (Flett, 2003).

REFERENCES

Abbott, R., Johann-Murphy, M., Shiminski-Maher, T., et al. (1993). Selective dorsal rhizotomy: outcome and complications in treating spastic cerebral palsy. *Neurosurgery*, **33**, 851–857.

Abel, M.F., Juhl, G.A., Vaughan, C.L. and Damiano, D.L. (1998). Gait assessment of fixed ankle–foot orthoses in children with spastic diplegia. *Arch Phys Med Rehabil*, **79**, 126–133.

Ade-Hall, R.A. and Moore, A.P. (2000). *Botulinum Toxin Type A in the Treatment of Lower Limb Spastic Cerebral Palsy,*
Cochrane Database of Systematic Reviews, Issue 3, Cochrane Library (CD 001408). Update Software, Oxford.

Albright, A.L. and Neville, B. (2000). Pharmacological management of spasticity. In: *The Management of Spasticity Associated with the Cerebral Palsies in Children and Adolescents* (eds Neville, B., Albright, A.L.), 1st edn., Churchill Communications. Biddles Ltd, Guildfort, Great Britain. ISBN 09701610 0x, pp. 121–132 (Chapter 9).

Albright, A.L., Cervi, A. and Singetary, J. (1991). Intrathecal baclofen for spasticity in cerebral palsy. *J Am Med Assoc*, **265**, 1418–1422.

Albright, A.L., Barry, M.J., Fasick, M.P. and Janosky, J. (1995). Effects of continuous intrathecal baclofen infusion and selective posterior rhizotomy on upper extremity spasticity. *Pediatr Neurosurg*, **23**, 82–85.

Albright, A.L., Gilmartin, R., Swift, D., Krach, L.E., Ivanhoe, C.B. and McLaughlin, J.F. (2003). Long-term intrathecal baclofen therapy for severe spasticity of cerebral origin. *J Neurosurg*, **98**, 291–295.

Anderson, C. and Mattsson, E. (2001). Adults with cerebral palsy: a survey describing problems, needs, and resources, with special emphasis on locomotion. *Dev Med Child Neurol*, **43**, 76–82.

Aoki, K.R. and Guyer, B. (2001). Botulinum toxin A and other botulinum toxin serotypes: a comparative review of biochemical and pharmacological agents. *Euro J Neurol*, **8(Suppl. 5)**, S21–S29.

Arens, L.J., Peacock, W.J. and Peter, J. (1989). Selective posterior rhizotomy: a long-term follow-up study. *Child Nerv Syst*, **5**, 148–152.

Armstrong, R.W., Steinbok, P., Cochrane, D.D., et al. (1997). Intrathecally administered baclofen for treatment of children with spasticity of cerebral origin. *J Neurosurg*, **87**, 409–414.

Ashworth, B. (1964). Preliminary trial of carisoprodal in multiple sclerosis. *Practitioner*, **192**, 540–542.

Badawi, N., Watson, L., Petterson, B., Blair, E., Slee, J., et al. (1998). What constitutes cerebral palsy? *Dev Med Child Neurol*, **40**, 520–527.

Badell-Ribera, A. (1985). Cerebral palsy: postural-locomotor prognosis in spastic diplegia. *Arch Phys Med Rehabil*, **66**, 614–619.

Baker, R., Jasinski, M., Maciag-Tymecka, I., Michalowska-Mrozek, J., Bonikowski, M., Carr, L., MacLean, J., Lin, J.-P., Lynch, B., Theologis, T., Wendorff, J., Eunson, P. and Cosgrove, A. (2002). Botulinum toxin treatment of spasticity in diplegic cerebral palsy: a randomized, double-blind, placebo-controlled, dose-ranging study. *Dev Med Child Neurol*, **44**, 666–675.

Barwood, S., Baillieu, C., Boyd, R., Brereton, K., Low, J., Nattrass, G. and Graham, H.K. (2000). Analgesic effects of botulinum toxin A: a randomized, placebo-controlled clinical trial. *Dev Med Child Neurol*, **42**, 116–121.

Bell, K.J., Ounpuu, S., DeLuca, P.A., Romness, M.J. (2002). Natural progression of gait in children with cerebral palsy. *J Pediatr Orthop*, **22**, 677–682.

Berardelli, A., Gilio, F. and Currra, A. (2002). Effects of botulinum toxin type A on central nervous system function. In: *Scientific Aspects of Botulinum toxin* (eds Brin, M.F., Jankovic, J. and Hallett, M.), Vol. 16, Lippincott Williams & Wilkins, Philadelphia, PA, pp. 171–177.

Berweck, S., Graham, H.K. and Heinen, F. (2003). Spasticity in children. In: *Handbook of Botulinum Toxin Treatment* (eds Moore, P. and Naumann, M.), 2nd edn. Blackwell Science Ltd., pp. 272–305 (Part 2, Chapter 11).

Bjornson, K.F., McLaughlin, J.F., Loeser, J.D., Nowak-Cooperman, K.M., Russel, M., et al. (2003). Oral motor, communication, and nutritional status of children during intrathecal baclofen therapy: a descriptive pilot study. *Arch Phys Med Rehabil*, **84**, 500–506 (April).

Bohannon, R.W. and Smith, M.B. (1987). Inter-rater reliability of a modified Ashworth scale of muscle spasticity. *Phys Ther*, **67**, 206–207.

Boop, F.A., Woo, R. and Maria, B.L. (2001). Special article: consensus statement on the surgical management of spasticity related to cerebral palsy. *J Child Neurol*, **16**(1), 68–69.

Boscarino, L.F., Ounpuu, S., Davis, R.B., Gage, J.R. and DeLuca, P.A. (1993). Effects of selective dorsal rhizotomy on gait in children with cerebral palsy. *J Pediatr Orthop*, **13**, 174–179.

Bower, E. (2000). Physical management of children and adolescents with spastic cerebral palsy. In: *The Management of Spasticity Associated with the Cerebral Palsies in Children and Adolescents* (eds Neville, B. and Albright, A.L.), Churchill Communications, pp. 63–74 (Chapter 5).

Bower, E., Michell, D., Burnett, M., Campbell, M.J. and McLellan, D.L. (2001). Randomised controlled trial of physiotherapy in 56 children with cerebral palsy followed for 18 months. *Dev Med Child Neurol*, **43**, 4–15.

Boyce, W.F., Gowland, C., Rosenbaum, P.L., Lane, M., Plews, N., et al. (1995). The gross motor performance M: validity and responsiveness of a measure of quality of movement. *Phys Ther*, **75**, 603–613.

Boyd, R. and Graham, H.K. (1997). Botulinum toxin A in the management of children with cerebral palsy: indications and outcome. *Euro J Neurol*, **4**(**Suppl.**), S15–S22.

Boyd, R. and Graham, H.K. (1999). Objective measurement of clinical findings in the use of botulinum toxin type A for the management of children with cerebral palsy. *Euro J Neurol*, **6**(**Suppl. 4**), S23–S35.

Boyd, R.N. and Hays, R.M. (2001). Current evidence for the use of botulinum toxin type A in the management of children with cerebral palsy: a systematic review. *Eur J Neurol*, **8**(**Suppl. 5**), S1–S20.

Boyd, R., Barwood, S., Bailleau, C. and Graham, K. (1998). Validity of a clinical measure of spasticity in children with cerebral palsy in a randomised clinical trial. *Dev Med Child Neurol*, **40**(**Suppl. 1**), 78.

Boyd, R.N., Dobson, F., Parrott, J., Love, S., Oates, J., Larson, A., Burchall, G., Chondros, P., Carlin, J., Nattrass, G. and Graham, H.K. (2001). The effect of botulinum toxin type A and a variable hip abduction orthosis on the gross motor function: a randomized controlled trial. *Eur J Neurol*, **8**(**Suppl. 5**), S109–S119.

Boyd, R., Bach, T., Morris, M., Imms, C., Johnson, L., Graham, H.K., Syngeniotis, A., Johnson, L., Abbott, D.F. and Jackson, G.D. (2002). A randomized trial of botulinum toxin A (BoNT-A) and upper limb training – a functional magnetic resonance imaging and resonant frequency study. *Dev Med Child Neuro*, **44**(**Suppl. 91**), 9.

Boyd, R.N., Selber, P. and Graham, H.K. (2003). Spasticity management in children with cerebral palsy, *Proc Melbourne Gait Course*, **21**, 1–11.

Bressman, S. (1998). Dystonia. *Curr Opin Neurol*, **11**, 363–372.

Brunner, R., Meier, G. and Ruepp, T. (1998). Comparison of a stiff and a spring-type ankle–foot orthosis to improve gait in spastic hemiplegic children. *J Ped Ortho*, **18**, 719–726.

Buckon, C.E., Sienko-Thomas, S., Aiona, M.D. and Piatt, J.H. (1996). Assessment of upper extremity function in children with spastic diplegia before and after selective dorsal rhizotomy. *Dev Med Child Neurol*, **38**, 967–975.

Burgen, A.S.V., Dickens, F. and Zatinan, L.J. (1949). The action of botulinum toxin on the neuromuscular junction. *J Physiol*, **109**, 10–24.

Butler, C. and Campbell, S. (2000). Evidence of the effects of intrathecal baclofen for spastic and dystonic cerebral palsy. *Dev Med Child Neurol*, **42**, 634–645.

Campbell, W.M., Ferrel, A., McLaughlin, J.F., Grant, G.A., Loeser, J.D., et al. (2002). Long-term safety and efficacy of continuous intrathecal baclofen. *Dev Med Child Neurol*, **44**, 660–665.

Carroll, K.L., Moore, K.R. and Stevens, P.M. (1998). Orthopedic procedures after rhizotomy. *J Pediatr Orthop*, **18**, 69–74.

Chicoine, M.R., Park, T.S. and Kaufman, B.A. (1997). Selective dorsal rhizotomy and rates of orthopedic surgery in children with spastic cerebral palsy. *J Neurosurg*, **86**, 34–39.

Corry, I.S., Cosgrove, A.P., Walsh, E.G., McClean, D. and Graham, H.K. (1997). Botulinum toxin A in the hemiplegic upper limb: a double blind trial. *Dev Med Child Neurol*, **39**, 185–193.

Corry, I.S., Cosgrove, A.P., Duffy, C.M., McNeill, S., Taylor, T. and Graham, H. (1998). Botulinum toxin A compared with stretching calves in the treatment of spastic equinus: a randomised prospective trial. *J Pediatr Orthop*, **18**, 304–311.

Corry, I.S., Cosgrove, A.P., Duffy, C.M., Taylor, T.C. and Graham, H.K. (1999). Botulinum toxin A in hamstring spasticity. *Gait Post*, **10**, 206–210.

Cosgrove, A.P., et al. (1994). Botulinum toxin in the management of the lower limb in cerebral palsy. *Dev Med Child Neurol*, **36**, 386–396.

Crothers, B. and Paine, R. (1959). The natural history of cerebral palsy. In: *Classics in Development Medicine* (ed. Mitchell, R.), Vol. 2. JB Lippincott, Philadelphia, PA.

Daltroy, L.H., Liang, M.H., Fossel, A.H. and Goldberg, M.J. (1998). The POSNA pediatric musculoskeletal functional health questionnaire: report on reliability, validity, and sensitivity to change. Pediatric outcomes instrument development group. *Ped Ortho Soc N Am J Pediatr Orthop*, **18**, 561–571.

Damiano, D.L. and Abel, M.F. (1998). Effectiveness of strength training in spastic cerebral palsy. *Gait Post*, **7**, 165–166.

Damiano, D.L., Dodd, K. and Taylor, N.F. (2002a). Should we be testing and training muscle strength in cerebral palsy? *Anno Dev Med Child Neurol*, **44**, 68–72.

Damiano, D.L., Quinlivan, J.M., Owen, B.F., Payne, P., Nelson, K.C. and Abel, M.F. (2002b). What does the Ashworth scale really measure and are instrumented measures more valid and precise? *Dev Med Child Neurol*, **44**, 112–118.

de Paiva, A., Meunier, F.A., Molgo, J., Aoki, K.R. and Dolly, J.O. (1999). Functional repair of motor endplates after botulinum neurotoxin type A poisoning: biphasic switch of synaptic activity between nerve sprouts and their parent terminals. *Proc Natl Acad Sci USA*, **96**, 3200–3205.

DeMatteo, C., Law, M., Russell, D., Pollock, N., Rosenbaum, P. and Walter, S. (1992). *QUEST, Quality of Upper Extremity Skills Test, Co-ordinates Occupational Therapy Services*. West Brunswick, Australia.

Desloovere, K., Huenaerts, C., Molenaers, G., Eyssen, M. and De Cock, P. (1999). *Gait Post*, **10**, 90 (abstract).

Dias, L.S. and Marty, G.R. (1992). Selective posterior rhizotomy. In: *The Diplegic Child. Evaluation and Management* (ed. Sussman, M.D.), American Academy of Orthopaedic Surgeons, Rosemont, IL, pp. 287–294.

Dobson, F., Boyd, R.N., Parrott, J., Nattrass, G.R. and Graham, H.K. (2002). Hip surveillance in children with cerebral palsy. *J Bone Joint Surg*, **84-B(5)**, 720–726.

Dodd, K.J., Taylor, N.F. and Damiano, D.L. (2002). A systematic review of the effectiveness of strength-training programs for people with cerebral palsy. *Arch Phys Med Rehabil*, **83**, 1157–1164.

Dolly, J.O., Black, J., Williams, R.S. and Melling, J. (1984). Acceptors for botulinum toxin reside on the motor nerve terminal and mediate its internalisation. *Nature*, **307**, 457–460.

Eames, N.W.A., Baker, R., Hill, N., Graham, H.K., Taylor, T. and Cosgrove, A.C. (1999). The effect of botulinum toxin A on gastrocnemius length: magnitude and duration of response. *Dev Med Child Neurol*, **41**, 226–232.

Elk, B. (1984). Preoperative assessment and postsurgical occupational therapy for children who have undergone a selective posterior rhizotomy. *S Afr J Occup Ther*, **14**, 45–50.

Fehlings, D., Rang, M., Glazier, J. and Steele. (2000). An evaluation of botulinum-A toxin injections to improve upper extremity function in children with hemiplegic cerebral palsy. *J Ped*, **137(3)**, 331–337.

Feldman, A.B., Haley, S.M. and Coryell, J. (1990). Concurrent and construct validity of the pediatric evaluation of disability inventory. *Phys Ther*, **70**, 602–610.

Flett, P.J. (2003). Review article: Rehabilitation of spasticity and related problems in childhood cerebral palsy. *J Paediatr Child Health*, **39**, 6–14.

Flett, P.J., Stern, L.M., Waddy, H., Connell, T., Seeger, J.D. and Gibson, S.K. (1999). Botulinum toxin A versus fixed cast stretching for dynamic calf tightness in cerebral palsy. *J Paediatr Child Health*, **35**, 71–77.

Gage, J.R. (1991). *Gait Analysis in Cerebral Palsy*. Mackeith Press, London.

Gerszten, P.C., Albright, A.L. and Johnstone, G.F. (1998). Intrathecal baclofen infusion and subsequent orthopaedic surgery in patients with spastic cerebral palsy. *J Neurosurg*, **88**, 1009–1013.

Giladi, N. (1997). The non neuromuscular effects of botulinum toxin injections. *Euro J Neurol*, **2**, 11–16.

Gooch, J.L. and Walker, M.L. (1996). Spinal stenosis after total lumbar laminectomy for selective dorsal rhizotomy. *Pediatr Neurosurg*, **25**, 28–30.

Gormley, M.E. (2001). Treatment of neuromuscular and musculoskeletal problems in cerebral palsy. *Pediatr Rehabil*, **4**, 5–16.

Graham, H.K. (2001). Botulinum toxin type A management of spasticity in the context of orthopaedic surgery for children with spastic cerebral palsy. *Eur J Neurol*, **8(Suppl. 5)**, S30–S39.

Graham, H.K. and Selber, P. (2003). Review article: Musculoskeletal aspects of cerebral palsy. *J Bone Joint Surg (Br)*, **85-B**, 157–166.

Graham, H.K., Aoki, K.R., Autti-Ramo, I., Autti-Ramo, I., Boyd, R., Delgado, M.R., et al. (2000). Recommendations for the use of botulinum toxin type A in the management of cerebral palsy. *Gait Post*, **11**, 67–79.

Greene, W.B., Dietz, F.R., Goldberg, M.J., Gross, R.H., Miller, F. and Sussman, M.D. (1991). Rapid progression of hip subluxation in cerebral palsy after selective posterior rhizotomy. *J Pediatr Orthop*, **11**, 494–497.

Gunderson, C.B.S., Katz, B. and Miledi, R. (1982). The antagonism between botulinum toxin and calcium in motor nerve terminals. *Proc Royal Soc London B*, **216**, 369–376.

Haley, S.M., Ludlow, L.H., Gans, B.M., Faas, R.M. and Inacio, C.A. (1991). Tufts empirical approach to identifying motor performance categories. *Arch Phys Med Rehabil*, **72**, 359–366.

Heim, R.C., Park, T.S., Vogler, G.P., Kaufman, B.A., Noetzel, M.J. and Ortman, M.R. (1995). Changes in hip migration after selective dorsal rhizotomy for spastic quadriplegia in cerebral palsy. *J Neurosurg*, **82**, 567–571.

Hodgkinson, I., Berard, C., Jindrich, M.L., Sindou, M., Martens, P. and Berard, J. (1997). Selective dorsal rhizotomy in children with cerebral palsy. *Stereotact Funct Neurosurg*, **69**, 259–267.

Houltram, J., Noble, I., Boyd, R.N., Corry, I., Flett, P. and Graham, H.K. (2001). Botulinum toxin type A in the management of equinus in children with cerebral palsy: an evidence-based economic evaluation. *Euro J Neurol*, **8** (**Suppl. 5**), 194–202.

Hurvitz, E.A., Conti, G.E. and Brown, S.H. (2003). Changes in movement characteristics of the spastic upper extremity after botulinum toxin injection. *Arch Phys Med Rehabil*, **84**, 444–454.

Irwin-Carruthers, S.H., Davids, L.M., Van Rensburg, C.K., Magasiner, V., Scott, D. (1995). Early physiotherapy in selective posterior rhizotomy. *Physiotherapy*, **41**, 44–49.

Johnson, D.C., Damiano, D.L. and Abel, M.F. (1997). The evolution of gait in childhood and adolescent cerebral palsy. *J Pediatr Orthop*, **17**, 392–396.

Johnson, D.C., Damiano, D.L. and Abel, M.F. (2002). The evolution of gait in childhood and adolescent cerebral palsy. *J Pediatr Orthop*, **22**, 677–682.

Joynt, R.L. and Leonard, J.A. (1980). Dantrolene sodium suspension in the treatment of spastic cerebral palsy. *Dev Med Child Neurol*, **22**, 755–767.

Koman, L.A., Mooney III, J.F., Smith, B.P., Walker, F. and Leon, J.M. (2000). Botulinum toxin type A neuro-muscular blockade in the treatment of lower extremity spasticity in cerebral palsy: a randomized, double-blind, placebo-controlled trial. BOTOX study group. *J Pediatr Orthop*, **20**, 108–115.

Koman, L.A., Brashear, A., Rosenfeld, S., Chambers, H., Russman, B., Rang, M., Root, L., Ferrari, E., Garcia De Yebenes, P.J., Smith, B.P., Turkel, C., Walcott, J.M. and Molloy, P.T. (2001). Botulinum toxin type A neuromuscular blockade in the treatment of equinus foot deformity in cerebral palsy: a multicenter, open-label clinical trial. *Pediatrics*, **108**, 1062–1071.

Koman, L.A., Smith, B.P.S. and Goodman, A. (2002). *Botulinum Toxin Type A in the Management of Cerebral Palsy*. Wake Forest University Press – Scientific Division, Winston-Salem, NC 27157.

Kroin, J.S., Ali, A., York, M. and Penn, R.D. (1993). The distribution of medication along the spinal canal after chronic intrathecal administration. *Neurosurgery*, **33**, 226–230.

Lance, J.W. (1980). Pathophysiology of spasticity and clinical experience with baclofen. In: *Spasticity: Disordered Motor Control* (eds Feldman, R.G., Young, R.R. and Koella, W.P.), Year Book Medical Publishers, Chicago, IL, pp. 185–220.

Landgraf, J.M., Abetz, I. and Ware, J.E. (1996). *The Child Health Questionnaire User's Manual*, 1st edn., The Health Institute, New England Medical Center, Boston, MA.

Lapierre, Y., Bouchard, S., Tansey, C., et al. (1987). Treatment of spasticity with tizanidine in multiple sclerosis. *Can J Neurol Sci*, **14**, 513–517.

Lobbozoo, F., Thon, M.T., Remillard, G., Montplaisir, J.Y. and Lavigne, G.J. (1996). Relationship between sleep, neck muscle activity, and pain in cervical dystonia. *Can J Sci*, **23**, 285–288.

Loewen, P., Steinbok, P., Holsti, L. and MacKay, M. (1998). Upper extremity performance and self-help skill changes in children with spastic cerebral palsy following selective posterior rhizotomy. *Pediatr Neurosurg*, **29**(**4**), 191–198.

Mackeith, R.C. and Polani, P.E. (1958). Cerebral palsy. *Lancet*, **1**, 61.

Marty, G.R., Dias, L.S. and Gaebler-Spira, D. (1995). Selective posterior rhizotomy and soft-tissue procedures for the treatment of cerebral palsy. *J Bone Joint Surg*, **77**, 713–718.

McBurney, H., Taylor, N.F., Dodd, K.J. and Graham, H.K. (2003). A qualitative analysis of the benefits of strength training for young people with cerebral palsy. *Dev Med Child Neurol*, **45**, 658–663.

McLaughlin, J.F., Bjornson, K.F., Astley, S.J., Hays, R.M., Hoffinger, S.A., Armantrout, E.A. and Roberts, T.S. (1994). The role of selective dorsal rhizotomy in cerebral palsy: critical evaluation of a prospective series. *Dev Med Child Neurol*, **36**, 755–769.

McLaughlin, J.F., Bjotson, K.F., Astley, S.J., et al. (1998). Selective dorsal rhizotomy: efficacy and safety in an investigator-masked randomised clinical trial. *Dev Med Child Neurol*, **40**, 220–232.

McLaughlin, J., Bjornson, K., Temkin, N., Steinbok., et al. (2002). Selective dorsal rhizotomy: meta-analysis of three randomised controlled trials. *Dev Med Child Neurol*, **44**, 1–10.

Medici, M., Pebet, M. and Ciblis, D. (1989). A double blind, long-term study of tizanidine (sirdalud) in spasticity due to cerebrovascular lesions. *Curr Med Res Opin*, **11**, 398–407.

Michaelis, R. (1999). Die sogenannten Zerebralparesen. In: *Entwicklungs-neurologie und Neuropediatrie* (eds Michaelis, R. and Niemann, G.W.), Thieme Verlag, Stuttgart, pp. 86–101.

Miller, G. and Clark, G.D. (1998). *The Cerebral Palsies.* Butterworth-Heinemann, Boston.

Molenaers, G., Desloovere, K., Eyssen, M., Decat, J., Jonkers, I. and De Cock, P. (1999). Botulinum toxin type A treatment of cerebral palsy: an integrated approach. *Eur J Neurol*, **6**(**Suppl. 4**), S51–S57.

Molenaers, G., Desloovere, K., DeCat, J., et al. (2001). Single event multilevel botulinum toxin type A treatment and surgery: similarities and differences. *Eur J Neurol*, **8**(**Suppl. 5**), S88–S97.

Molnar, G.E. and Gordon, S.U. (1976). Cerebral palsy: predictive value of selected clinical signs for early prognostication of motor function. *Arch Phys Med Rehabil*, **57**, 153–158.

Morris, C. (2002). A review of the efficacy of lower-limb orthoses used for cerebral palsy. *Dev Med Child Neurol*, **44**, 205–211.

Morton, R. (1999). New surgical interventions for cerebral palsy and the place of gait analysis. *Dev Med Child Neurol*, **41**, 424–428.

Msall, M.E., DiGaudio, K., Rogers, B.T., LaForest, S., Catanzo, N.L., Caampbell, J., Wilczenski, F. and Duffy, L.C. (1994). The functional independence measure for children (Wee FIM). Conceptual basis and pilot use in children with developmental disabilities. *Clin Pediatr*, **33**, 421–430.

Muller, H. (1992). Treatment of severe spasticity: results of a multicentre trial conducted in Germany involving the intrathecal infusion of baclofen in an implantable drug delivery system. *Dev Med Child Neurol*, **34**, 739–745.

Murphy, N.A., Irwin, M.C. and Hoff, C. (2002). Intrathecal baclofen therapy in children with cerebral palsy: efficacy and complications. *Arch Phys Med Rehabil*, **83**(**12**), 1721–1725 (December).

Nelson, K.B. and Ellenberg, J.H. (1978). Epidemiology of cerebral palsy. *Adv Neurol*, **19**, 421–435.

Neville, B.G.R. (1997). The Worster–Drought syndrome: a severe test of paediatric neurodisability services? *Dev Med Child Neurol*, **39**, 782–784.

Nishida, T., Thatcher, S.W. and Marty, G.R. (1995). Selective posterior rhizotomy for children with cerebral palsy – 7-year experience. *Child Nerv Syst*, **11**(**7**), 374–380.

Orendurff, M.S., Chung, J.S. and Dorociak, R.E. (1998). Predictors of stride length barefoot and with ankle foot orthoses in children with cerebral palsy. *Gait Post*, **7**, 148 (abstract).

Palisano, R., Rosenbaum, P., Walter, S., et al. (1997). Development and reliability of a system to classify gross motor function in children with cerebral palsy. *Dev Med Child Neurol*, **39**, 214–223.

Peacock, W.J. and Arens, L.J. (1982). Selective posterior rhizotomy for the relief of spasticity in cerebral palsy. *S Afr Med J*, **62**, 119–124.

Peacock, W.J. and Eastman, R.W. (1981). The neurosurgical management of spasticity. *S Afr Med J*, **60**, 849–850.

Peacock, W.J. and Staudt, L.A. (1991). Functional outcomes following selective posterior rhizotomy in children with cerebral palsy. *J Neurosurg*, **74**, 380–385.

Peacock, W.J. and Stuvedt, L.A. (1990). Spasticity in cerebral palsy and the selective posterior rhizotomy procedure. *J Child Neurol*, **5**, 179–195.

Peacock, W.J., Arens, L.J. and Berman, B. (1987a). Cerebral palsy spasticity. Selective posterior rhizotomy. *Pediatr Neurosci*, **13**, 61–66.

Peacock, W.J., Arens, L.J. and Berman, B. (1987b). An assessment of selective posterior rhizotomy as a procedure for relieving spasticity in cerebral palsy. *Dev Med Child Neurol*, **29**(**Suppl. 155**), 22.

Pentoff, E. (1964). Cerebral palsy: a pharmacological approach. *Clin Pharmacol Ther*, **5**, 947–954.

Perry, J., Adams, J. and Cahan, L.D. (1989). Foot–floor contact patterns following selective dorsal rhizotomy. *Dev Med Neurol*, **31**(**Suppl. 59**), S19 (abstract).

Pirpiris, M. and Graham, H.K. (2001). Management of spasticity in childhood. In: *Upper Motor Neuron Syndrome and Spasticity. Clinical Management and Neurophysiology* (eds Barnes, M.P. and Johnson, G.R.), Cambridge University, Cambridge, pp. 266–305.

Polak, F., Morton, R., Ward, C., Wallace, W.A., Doderlein, L. and Siebel, A. (2002). Double-blind comparison study of two doses of botulinum toxin A injected into calf muscles in children with hemiplegic cerebral palsy. *Dev Med Child Neurol*, **44**, 551–555.

Pollock, N., Baptiste, S., Law, M., McColl, M.A., Opzoomer, A. and Polatajko, H. (1990). Occupational performance measures: a review based on the guidelines for the client-centered practice of occupational therapy. *Can J Occup Ther*, **5**, 77–81.

Pountney, T., Mandy, A. and Gard, P. (2003). Repeatability and limits of agreement in measurement of hip migration percentage in children with bilateral cerebral palsy. *Physiotherapy*, **89**(**5**), 276–281.

Randall, M., Carlin, J.B., Chondros, P. and Reddihough, D. (2001). Reliability of the Melbourne assessment of unilateral upper limb function. *Dev Med Child Neurol*, **43**, 761–776.

Rang, M. (1990). Cerebral palsy. In: *Pediatric Orthopaedics* (eds Morissey, R.T., Lovell, W.W. and Winter, R.B.), 3rd edn., JB Lippincott, Philadelphia, PA, pp. 465–506.

Rang, M., Silver, R. and de la Garza, J. (1986). Cerebral palsy. In: *Pediatric Orthopaedics* (eds Lovell, W.W. and Winter, R.B.), 2nd edn., JB Lippincott, Philadelphia, PA (Chapter 9).

Rattey, T.E., Leahey, L., Hyndman, J., Brown, D.C.S. and Gross, M. (1993). Recurrence after Achilles tendon lengthening in cerebral palsy. *J Pediatr Orthop*, **13**, 185–187.

Rice, G. (1988). Tizanidine vs baclofen in the treatment of spasticity in patients with multiple sclerosis. *Can J Neurol Sci*, **14**, 15–19.

Rodda, J. and Graham, H.K. (2001). Classification of gait patterns in spastic hemiplegia and spastic diplegia: a basis for a management algorithm. *Euro J Neurol*, **8**(**Suppl. 5**), S98–S108.

Rosales, R., Arimura, K., Takenaga, S. and Osame, M. (1996). Extrafusal and intrafusal muscle effects in experimental botulinum toxin A injection. *Muscle Nerve*, **19**, 488–496.

Rosenbaum, P.L., Walter, S.D., Hanna, S.E., et al. (2002). Prognosis for gross motor function in cerebral palsy: creation of motor development curves. *J Am Med Assoc*, **288**, 1357–1363.

Russell, D.J., Rosenbaum, P.L., Cadman, D.T., et al. (1989). The gross motor function measure: a means to evaluate the effects of physical therapy. *Dev Med Child Neurol*, **31**, 341–352.

Russman, B.S., et al. (1997). Cerebral palsy: a rational approach to a treatment protocol, and the role of botulinum toxin in treatment. *Muscle Nerve*, **6**(**Suppl.**), S181–S193.

Sanger, T.D., Delgado, M.R., Gaebler-Spira, D., Hallett, M., Mink, J.W., et al. (2003). Classification and definition of disorders causing hypertonia in childhood. *Pediatrics*, **111**(**1**), e89–e97.

Schneider, J.W., Gurucharri, L.M., Gutierrez, A.L. and Gaebler-Spira, D.J. (2001). Health-related quality of life and functional outcome measures for children with cerebral palsy. *Dev Med Child Neurol*, **43**, 601–608.

Segal, L.S., Thomas, S.E., Mazur, J.M. and Manterer, M. (1989). Calcaneal gait in spastic diplegia after heel cord lengthening: a study with gait analysis. *J Pediatr Orthop*, **9**, 697–701.

Sellin, L.C. and Thesleff, S. (1981). Pre- and post-synaptic actions of botulinum toxin at the rat neuromuscular junction. *J Physiol*, **317**, 487–495.

Stanley, F., Blair, E. and Alberman, E. (2000). Cerebral palsies: epidemiology and causal pathways. In: *Clinics in Developmental Medicine*. Mac-Keith Press, London, p. 151.

Steinbok, P., Daneshvar, H., Evans, D., Kestle, J.R.W. (1995). Cost analysis of continuous intrathecal baclofen versus selective functional posterior rhizotomy in the treatment of spastic quadriplegia associated with cerebral palsy. *Paediatr Neurosurg*, **22**, 255–65.

Steinbok, P., Reiner, A., Beauchamp, R.D., Cochrane, D.D., Keyes, R. (1992). Selective functional posterior rhizotomy for treatment of spastic cerebral palsy in children. *Pediatr Neurosurg*, **18**, 34–42.

Steinbok, P., Reiner, A., Beauchamp, R.D., Armstrong, R.W. and Cochrane, D.D. (1997). A randomised clinical trial to compare selective posterior rhizotomy plus physiotherapy with physiotherapy alone in children with spastic diplegic cerebral palsy. *Dev Med Child Neurol*, **39**, 178–184.

Subramanian, N., Vaughan, C.L., Peter, J.C. and Arens, L.J. (1998). Gait before and 10 years after rhizotomy in children with cerebral palsy spasticity. *J Neuro*, **88**(**6**), 1014–1019.

Tardieu, G., Shentoub, S. and Delarue, R. (1954). A la recherche d'une Technique de mesure de la spasticite. *Rev Neurol*, **91**, 143–144.

Thomas, S.S., Aiona, M.D., Buckon, C.E. and Piatt, J.H. (1997). Does gait continue to improve 2 years after selective dorsal rhizotomy? *J Pediatr Orthop*, **17**, 387–391.

Vaughan, C.L., Berman, B. and Peacock, W.J. (1991). Cerebral palsy and rhizotomy: a 3-year follow-up evaluation with gait analysis. *J Neurosurg*, **74**, 178–184.

von Koch, C.S., Park, T.S., Steinbok, P., Smyth, M. and Peacock, W.J. (2001). Selective posterior rhizotomy and intrathecal baclofen for the treatment of spasticity. *Ped Neurosurg*, **35**, 57–65.

Whyte, J. and Robinson, K. (1990). Pharmacological management. In: *The Practical Management of Spasticity in Children and Adults* (eds Glenn, M.B. and Whyte, J.), Lea and Febiger, Philadelphia, PA, p. 209.

Wiley, M.E. and Damiano, D.L. (1998). Lower extremity strength profiles in spastic cerebral palsy. *Dev Med Child Neurol*, **40**, 100–107.

Wright, F.V., Sheil, E., Drake, J., Wedge, J.H. and Naumann, S. (1998). Evaluation of selective dorsal rhizotomy for the reduction of spasticity in cerebral palsy: a randomized controlled trial. *Dev Med Child Neurol*, **40**, 239–247.

Young, R.R. (1994). Spasticity: a review. *Neurology*, **44**, 512–520.

Neuromuscular rehabilitation: diseases of the motor neuron, peripheral nerve and neuromuscular junction

Hubertus Köller and Hans-Peter Hartung

Department of Neurology, Heinrich-Heine-University, Düsseldorf, Germany

40.1 Introduction

In this chapter, we focus on rehabilitation of patients with diseases of the motor neuron like amyotrophic lateral sclerosis (ALS), spinal muscular atrophy (SMA) and polio and diseases of the peripheral nervous system, especially acute and chronic inflammatory polyneuropathies Guillain–Barré syndrome (GBS) and chronic inflammatory demyelinating polyneuropathy (CIDP) and other neuropathies (Fig. 40.1). Additionally, we include diseases of the neuromuscular junction (myasthenia gravis and Lambert–Eaton myasthenic syndrome (LEMS)). We describe the current knowledge on the pathogenesis, the clinical symptoms, and deficits and current therapy concepts during the acute disease state and for rehabilitation including long-term impairment of activities of daily living.

Quality of life of patients is affected not only by the physical disability as measured in neurologic disability scores but also by spiritual, religious and psychologic factors (Simmons et al., 2000). During the course of the disease ALS patients may accept the disease with its presumed fatal outcome leading to a maintained quality of life despite a deterioration of physical strength (Simmons et al., 2000). The situation seems to be different in myasthenic patients: Although their physical conditions are essentially preserved during most time the knowledge of possible crises with life-threatening muscle weakness and the uncertainty whether or when a crisis may occur severely affects their quality of life

(Padua et al., 2001). There may be also differences in the acceptance of the chronic disease between the patient and their caregivers (Amosun et al., 1995; Mitsumoto and Del Bene, 2000). With disease progression, for example in ALS quality of life of the caregivers may be even more impaired than the quality of life in the patients' self-assessment (Bromberg and Forshew, 2002).

For patients with motor neuron diseases rehabilitation concepts and reports on the course of the disease, the efficacy of therapy to improve muscle strength or to reduce pain, the use of assistive devices for moving or respiration, and the quality of life including the education and working situation are found widely in the literature. Especially survivors of the polio epidemics in the 1940s and 1950s have been followed and data on outcome and results of rehabilitation are available.

Compared to this rich literature, data on rehabilitation, effect of exercise training (White et al., 2004) and long-term outcome of patients suffering from peripheral nerve diseases are rare. While there are a number of studies on the efficacy of acute therapy in GBS and CIDP patients rehabilitation has been rarely studied. This is surprising since the long-term course with only partial recovery and residual deficits in many patients with inflammatory polyneuropathies is common knowledge. However, in the past years multidimensional measures have been introduced to assess quality of life of patients with peripheral neuropathies (Abresch et al., 2001) and neuromuscular diseases (Abresch et al., 1998). These studies

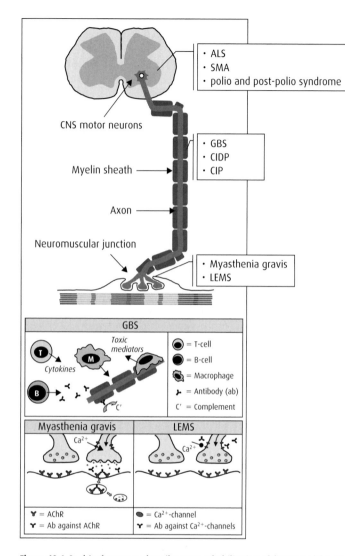

Figure 40.1. In this chapter we describe neurorehabilitation of diseases of the central nervous system motor neurons, peripheral nerves and the neuromuscular junctions. Some important features of the pathogenesis are shown in this cartoon: ALS and SMA as well as polio are diseases of central motor neurons. In GBS and CIDP peripheral nerves are damaged due to an inflammatory process directed against peripheral nerve myelin and axonal epitopes. Myasthenia gravis and LEMS are diseases of the neuromuscular junction mediated by antibodies directed against post-synaptic AChR, myasthenia gravis and presynaptic calcium channels (LEMS), respectively. (Figure by courtesy of Bernd C. Kieseier, Düsseldorf)

show that levels of disability do not predominantly determine the quality of life but lack of information on their disease and services, poor coordination of services, negative attitude and a diminished expectation of their potential are very important. A central issue for maintained quality of life is the level of perceived control and independence (Abresch et al., 1998).

With respect to the costs of medical treatment and support for patients with disabling diseases of the peripheral nervous system, carefully planned and well-conducted studies on the rehabilitation of these diseases are badly needed and probably cost-effective.

40.2 Diseases of the motor neuron: ALS, SMA and poliomyelitis

ALS (motor neuron disease)

Clinical presentation and diagnostic procedures

ALS is characterised by weakness of bulbar, arm and leg muscles attributed to degeneration of upper and lower motor neurons with muscle wasting, fasciculations, extensor plantar responses and clonuses. Diagnosis is definite by the clinical demonstration of a progressive impairment of strength in bulbar arm and leg muscles (Brooks et al., 2000). ALS is the most serious form of motor neuron disease leading to death typically within a few years. Its incidence is 1–2/100,000 and increases with aging (Donaghy, 1999).

ALS results from motor neuron dysfunction and loss of central nervous system motor neurons. While the vast majority of ALS cases are sporadic ones, about 10% are familial and of those, a small proportion results from identified mutations in the gene encoding copper/zinc superoxide dismutase-1 (SOD1). The mechanisms of motor neuron impairment is unknown, however, defective axonal transport, mitochondrial dysfunction and excitotoxicity due to impaired glutamate uptake are implicated mechanisms (Leigh et al., 2003; Bossy-Wetzel et al., 2004). In some sporadic forms, abnormal RNA editing in GluR2 subunits of glutamate receptors leading to an increased calcium entry in the cells is regarded as playing a crucial role in cell toxicity (Kawahara et al., 2004).

Therapy

Therapy consists of riluzole, 100 mg daily, which prolongs the survival of ALS patients by a mean of about 2 months. The efficacy of riluzole was shown in controlled studies, however, the therapeutic effect is only modest (Miller et al., 2002). At present, only riluzole has the approval of the Food and Drug Administration (FDA) for treatment of ALS but other pharmacologic agents are currently under investigation for therapeutic efficacy in ALS patients (Mitchell et al., 2002; Bongioanni et al., 2004). Creatine monohydrate, which seems to be effective in an animal model was ineffective in the therapy of ALS patients in a recently published study (Groeneveld et al., 2003).

Rehabilitation, long-term course of the disease and prognosis

Prognosis is worst in patients with early bulbar or respiratory muscle failure with a median survival of 20 months while patients with an onset other than bulbar or respiratory have a median survival of 29 months (Christensen et al., 1990). Although there are ALS variants associated with dementia (Strong and Rosenfeld, 2003), a large survey on 1118 sporadic ALS patients revealed no decline in mental health status (Norquist et al., 2003).

While therapy of muscle weakness in ALS is of very limited efficacy the control of nutrition, swallowing and, ventilation and the prevention of aspiration and muscle contractions and pain are the most important topics in rehabilitation of ALS patients with a large impact on quality of life and also survival. Recently published studies investigated the rehabilitation care and management of ALS patients in Italy (Chio et al., 1999), North America (Miller et al., 2000), The Netherlands (van den Berg et al., 2003) and in Ireland (Traynor et al., 2003). In the Irish study, the median survival of ALS patients in general neurologic clinics was compared with the survival in multidisciplinary ALS clinics. In the latter, the mean survival was longer especially in bulbar onset patients whose survival was extended by 9.6 months. The reason might at least in part be the close monitoring of bulbar impaired patients by clinicians, specialist nutritionists and speech and swallow therapists. However, there were also some other differences.

The patients were younger in the multidisciplinary ALS clinic and nearly all patients received riluzole in comparison to only 61% in other neurologic clinics in Ireland. The data from the Irish ALS study support a beneficial effect if patients are seen by specialist nutritionists and speech, and swallow therapists who inform the patient about the early use of percutaneous endoscopic gastrostomy (PEG). PEG in ALS patients is safe (Chio et al., 1999) but PEG use by itself showed no survival benefit in the study of Mitsumoto et al. (2003). This negative result may be due to the study design which did not differentiate early or late use of PEG.

Although the use of exercise for ALS patients has been discussed for a very long time (Ashworth et al., 2004), the discussion on its possible beneficial effects is still controversial. Drory and co-workers recently compared muscle strength, spasticity, fatigue, musculoskeletal pain and quality of life in ALS patients with and without a moderate daily exercise program (Drory et al., 2001). Patients with muscle exercise showed significantly less deterioration in muscle strength and spasticity in the first follow-up after 3 months but not in the next after 6 or more months. With respect to the other tested items there was no difference between the two groups. The authors concluded that there is a short-lived positive effect by exercise and they recommend it for ALS patients. With progressive weakness ALS patients often become wheelchair dependent. Wheelchairs should have supports for head, neck, trunk and extremities, and motorized wheelchairs offer otherwise dependent patients a greater sense of partial independence (Trail et al., 2001).

Another important problem of ALS rehabilitation is the control of musculoskeletal pain which was not achieved by an exercise program (Drory et al., 2001) but which has a great impact on the quality of life of patients with progressive neuromuscular diseases (Abresch et al., 2002). Increased pain is associated with diminished levels of general health, vitality, social function, increased fatigue, inability to cope adequately with stress and sleep disturbance. There may be many reasons for pain in ALS patients (e. g. due to muscle weakness and inability to change the

position in advanced stages of the disease). A recently published case report additionally raised the question whether immobilization in an ALS patient may induce a reflex sympathetic dystrophy syndrome with regional pain and autonomic dysfunction (Shibata et al., 2003).

The main goal of therapy and rehabilitation in ALS patients is to maintain quality of life and important issues are enteral feeding, assistive ventilatory device and exercise. Prospective studies are addressing these issues (Mitsumoto and Del Bene, 2000). Patients health-related quality of life decreases with disease expression (Kiebert et al., 2001), however, several studies stated that quality of life is not predominantly determined by the muscle strength and physical function (Simmons et al., 2000; Maillot et al., 2001). Spiritual, religious and psychologic factors play an important role in the determination of quality of life and can obviously not be measured in scores primarily assessing muscle function. It should also be noted that the quality of life of caregivers of ALS patients is also impaired and during the course of the disease scores may even be worse for caregivers than for patients. The latter may reflect a positive process of coping with the disease leading to different expectations in patients (Bromberg and Forshew, 2002). The reduced importance of physical impairment for the quality of life during the course of the disease does not only affect the role and function of ALS caregivers but also of ALS therapists who have to deal with a progressive and fatal disease with the risk to escape or adopt extreme solutions such as euthanasia (Pasetti and Zanini, 2000). Finally in the late stage of disease palliative strategies in multidisciplinary hospices may ease patients' suffering and allow the patient to die with dignity (Carter et al., 1999).

SMA

Clinical presentation and diagnostic procedures

Proximal SMA is a common genetic disorder of the lower motor neuron with high mortality during infancy leading to degeneration of neurons and muscular atrophy. Patients have been classified according to their age of onset and the degree of disability in SMA type I (never able to sit), type II (able to sit but not to walk), type III (able to walk: IIIa onset before 3 years; IIIb onset 3–30 years) and type IV (onset after 30 years) (Zerres et al., 1997). SMA is caused by homozygous deletions or mutations in the survival motor neuron gene 1 (Wirth, 2000) and the severity of the phenotype is partly modulated by the copy number of SMN2 gene.

Prognosis and therapy

The prognosis is very poor especially for SMA type 1 patients who often die within 7–8 months of birth. In the study of Zerres et al. (1997) all SMA type I patients were deceased by age 5 years. Prognosis is better for the other types of SMA with survival rates of more than 75% at an age of 20 years for SMA type II. Life expectancy is not reduced for most IIIb patients and half of type IIIa patients. Nearly 90% of type IIIb are ambulatory at the age of 20 years. At present, there is no approved therapy, however, a small study with riluzole (Russman et al., 2003) and an experimental study with valproic acid in fibroblast cultures (Brichta et al., 2003) open perspectives for SMA treatment.

Rehabilitation of SMA patients

Like in ALS patients, rehabilitation efforts are aimed at maintaining muscle strength, providing assistance of ventilation and nutrition. Unlike ALS patients, SMA patients seem not to suffer from increased musculoskeletal pain leading to an impaired quality of life (Abresch et al., 2002). Since a medical treatment which lessens muscle weakness in SMA patients is not available electrical stimulation of muscles has been used with the aim to improve muscle strength. In a recently published study the effect of low-intensity night-time therapeutic electrical muscle stimulation has been tested. Strength of stimulated muscles was compared to the strength of the same muscles on the contralateral arm in 13 children between 5 and

19 years suffering from SMA (Fehlings et al., 2002). Assessment after 12 months, however, did not show any statistically significant differences between the strength of the treatment and control arm. In advanced stages of muscle weakness patients may develop limb contractures requiring physical therapy such as stretching and positioning, and in some cases even orthopedic surgical management (McDonald, 1998).

Muscle strength (Kroksmark et al., 2001) and forced vital capacity (Steffensen et al., 2002) deteriorate in SMA patients over time and weakness of respiratory muscles causes an increased risk of severe respiratory complications potentially leading to death. Therefore, Koessler et al. (2001) studied the effect of inspiratory muscle training in 9 patients with SMA and 18 patients with Duchennes muscular dystrophy over 2 years. Patients were diagnosed at age 3–5 years and patients older than 10 years were wheelchair dependent. The mean age of all patients was 16.3 years. There was a significant improvement of respiratory muscle function and endurance within 2 years. In SMA patients, ventilatory function is compromised due to weakness of intercostal muscles, paradoxical ventilatory pattern as revealed by kinematic analyses of thoracoabdominal movements during breathing (Lissoni et al., 1998) and mechanically due to progressive scoliosis (Robinson et al., 1995). Breathing may improve upon surgical therapy of the spine and even a significant gain of lung function may be achieved. The ventilatory function of patients may also be bettered with the use of assisted coughing techniques and intermittent positive airway pressure ventilation (Bach and Zhitnikov, 1998). Although impaired ventilatory function is of central importance in treatment and prognosis of SMA patients, there is a great variability in the attitudes and practices of physicians ranging from recommendation of providing "comfort care only" to the recommendation of performing tracheostomy and initiation of mechanical ventilation (Hardart et al., 2002).

SMA patients may also experience difficulties in swallowing and nutrition. Rehabilitation help by specialist nutritionists, and speech and swallow therapists may be necessary similar to the situation in ALS patients (Willig et al., 1994). In rare cases, compared to ALS patients, it might even be necessary to supply the patient with a PEG.

Since unlike ALS, SMA normally starts in early childhood rehabilitation care has also to consider education of the children and the later employment situation. Billard and co-workers showed that children suffering from Duchennes muscular dystrophy have a significantly lower reading age compared to healthy controls which, however, was not the case in SMA children (Billard et al., 1998). Compared to other neuromuscular disorders such as myotonic muscular dystrophy or limb–girdle syndrome SMA patients have a higher educational level and lower levels of unemployment (Fowler et al., 1997).

Poliomyelitis and post-polio syndrome

Clinical presentation

During poliomyelitis epidemics thousands of patients were infected by the poliovirus in many countries throughout the world. During the acute phase of the disease patients suffered from flue-like illness attending by varying degrees of paralysis up to life-threatening respiratory failures. Most patients, however, had only little or no paralysis (Mulder, 1995) prompting the concept of differentiation between "paralytic" and "non-paralytic" polio. Neuronal lesions in brain and spinal cord were also common in autopsies from patients with "non-paralytic" polio (Bruno, 2000) and epidemiologic studies also show late onset weakness in up to 40% of survivors of "non-paralytic" polio. Additionally, pathogenetic studies suggest an ongoing neurodegenerative process in spinal cord motor neurons and in some cases also an ongoing immune activation in spinal fluid (Dalakas, 1995) causing late onset sequelae. This post-polio syndrome is defined by the manifestation of new or increased muscular weakness, fatigue and muscle or joint pain and neuropathic electromyographic changes in patients with a confirmed history of polio (Sunnerhagen and Grimby, 2001; Jubelt 2004).

Long-term prognosis

After introduction of polio vaccination in most countries in the 1950s polio became a rare disease. Prior to vaccination, epidemics occurred and thousands of polio survivors with various degrees of handicap were followed in large surveys in different countries with different health care facilities. Data from the natural course of polio disease were reported from Norway (Schanke et al., 1999; Farbu and Gilhus, 2002; Farbu et al., 2003; Rekand et al., 2003), Sweden (Kling et al., 2002), The Netherlands (Nollet et al., 2003), UK (Pentland et al., 2000), India (Ahuja et al., 1996), Estonia (Rekand et al., 2003), Slovenia (Burger and Marincek, 2000) and Japan (Kumakura et al., 2002). Most of these surveys addressed the question of the incidence and probability of developing post-polio syndrome. The occurrence of a post-polio syndrome was reported to range from about 26% (Farbu et al., 2003) to 55% (Kumakura et al., 2002) of polio survivors. Most studies describe difficulties to move, fatigue, muscular pain, cold intolerance and sleep disturbances as the main problems of patients after polio. Only a minority of patients suffer from respiratory insufficiency. In most patients muscle strength improves during the first one or 2 years after acute polio but disability remains stable afterwards. In the Scottish study, 62% of patients needed inpatient care, 46% received physiotherapy, 29% occupational therapy and 42% required a wheelchair (Pentland et al., 2000). A direct comparison of disability and prognosis of polio patients in the University Hospital in Bergen, Norway, and in Tartu, Estonia, showed differences in the acute phase of polio disability but also in the long-term outcome. The Norwegian patients had more pronounced disability in the acute phase but significantly more Norwegian patients were at gainful work 40 years later (Rekand et al., 2003). The frequency of new symptoms and the use of orthopedic devices, however, did not differ between both populations. The authors concluded that the access to continuous rehabilitation in Norway better enabled the Norwegian polio patients to maintain physical independence and earn their own income.

Rehabilitation of patients with polio and post-polio syndrome

Rehabilitation in polio and post-polio patients is aimed at improving muscle strength, lowering muscle and joint pain, increasing physical independence and quality of life (Jubelt, 2004) not only of the patient but also of the caregiver (Amosun et al., 1995).

Polio patients are handicapped as a consequence of muscle weakness and atrophy after muscle denervation secondary to motor neuron degeneration. As a result, muscle work in polio patients may also be impaired with respect to movement economy. Nollet and co-workers compared muscle power output, oxygen uptake and heart rate in an incremental submaximal cycle ergometry test and found elevated energy costs due to a reduced movement economy in post-polio patients (Nollet et al., 2001). This predisposes polio patients to premature fatigue in sustained activity and raises the question whether exercise training may be helpful or harmful for muscle survival. The latter question was especially addressed in a recently published randomized controlled study which shows that moderate intensity strength training increases muscle strength in polio patients without deleterious effects formerly attributed to overuse (Chan et al., 2003). In this study motor neuron viability was estimated by electrophysiologically measuring motor unit number estimates and surface-detected motor unit action potentials. An earlier study had compared the increase of muscle strength due to a 12-week training program and had found no changes in electromyography or serum creatine kinase (Agre et al., 1997). Spector and co-workers even showed on a cellular level that a supervised progressive resistance strength training increases muscle strength in patients with post-polio muscular atrophy without any histologic signs of muscular damage observed in biopsies taken prior to and after the training period (Spector et al., 1996). Another randomized parallel group study demonstrated the effectiveness of a home exercise program to strengthen hip and knee extensor muscles (Klein et al., 2002). Improvement of leg muscle strength was sufficient to reduce shoulder pain which occurred regularly due to shoulder overuse. The training programs are modified in some studies and training in warm water (Willen et al., 2001) or even warm climate (Strumse et al., 2003) are regarded as especially beneficial for polio patients.

Muscle and joint pain are cardinal symptoms of post-polio syndrome and pain significantly impacts the quality of life of polio patients (Widar and Ahlstrom, 1999). More than 50% of patients experience pain every day mostly during physical activity (Willen and Grimby, 1998). Predictive factors for developing pain are female gender, greater initial motor unit involvement and lower-extremity weakness (Vasiliadis et al., 2002). Although controlled treatment trials for pain in polio patients are lacking some case reports and a report on a small group of patients recommend therapy with gabapentin (Zapp, 1996) or amitriptylin (Trojan and Cashman, 1995).

A number of investigations examined the quality of life of polio survivors in different countries. In a Swedish study (Kling et al., 2002) 57% of polio patients used mobility aids such as cranes or walkers and 21% used wheelchairs. Most patients were independent in eating, daily hygiene or communication while many needed help in mobility-related activities or housework. Similar results were obtained by Thoren-Jonsson and co-workers and others who showed that most polio patients were satisfied with their leisure activities but required assistance in cleaning, shopping and transportation. Many patients try to maintain their independence despite their disabilities (Ahlstrom and Karlsson, 2000; Thoren-Jonsson and Grimby, 2001).

Many former polio patients were working and self-supported. The percentage of former polio patients at gainful work was higher in Norway (71%) than in Estonia (41%) (Rekand et al., 2003). More than 90% of working post-polio patients but only a few patients with a similar impairment due to spinal cord injury experienced increased disability during time at their working place (McNeal et al., 1999). This is in line with the observation that most polio patients reached the same level of education as their siblings but fewer patients were employed full-time at the age of 40 years (Farbu and Gilhus, 2002).

Impairment of pulmonary function in polio patients is related to spinal deformity with scoliosis or kyphosis (Lin et al., 2001) and is most severe during exercise (Weinberg et al., 1999). Only rarely, however, part-time assisted ventilation due to inspiratory muscle weakness is necessary in polio patients. In these cases inspiratory muscle training may help to promote respiratory muscle endurance and improve well-being in patients (Klefbeck et al., 2000). Very rarely polio patients may be so profoundly disabled that they depend on the use of a hands-free environmental control system that activates electric devices by voluntarily induced changes in brain wave signals (Craig et al., 2002; see Volume I, Chapter 33 for discussion of brain-computer interfaces for communication and control).

40.3 Diseases of the peripheral nerve inflammatory and other types of neuropathy

GBS

Clinical presentation and diagnostic procedures

GBS is defined as an acute, largely reversible, idiopathic monophasic demyelinating polyradiculoneuropathy. A misdirected autoimmune response to myelin and/or possibly axolemnal antigens is considered at the root of the disease. In about two-third of patients, the flaccid paralysis is preceded by an infective illness (Govoni and Granieri, 2001). In the classical sensorimotor form of GBS weakness develops acutely within days or subacutely within 2–4 weeks, pareses are symmetrically distributed and reflexes are reduced or abolished. Variants include pure motor forms of GBS, Miller–Fisher form and primary axonal forms of GBS (van der Meche et al., 2001). Diagnosis is based on the clinical presentation, the demonstration of demyelination on electrophysiologic examination and elevation of protein in the cerebrospinal fluid (CSF) (Asbury and Cornblath, 1990). Both, demyelinative changes in nerve conduction studies and elevation

Table 40.1. Current therapy of GBS (according to cochrane reviews).

Therapy	Number of studies/ patients	Result	References (Cochrane reviews)
Corticosteroids	6 studies with 195 patients	No effect	(Hughes and van Der Meche, 2000)
Plasmapheresis	6 studies with 649 patients	Significant efficacy compared to placebo	(Raphael et al., 2002)
IVIG	5 studies with 536 patients	No significant difference compared to plasmapheresis	(Hughes et al., 2004)

of protein contents may be absent during the first week after onset of pareses (Gordon and Wilbourn, 2001).

Therapy during the acute phase

Given the immunopathogenesis of GBS (Kieseier et al., 2004) acute therapy is directed against the immunopathogenic process and includes plasmapheresis and high-dose intravenous immunoglobulin (IVIG, infusion Table 40.1) (Raphael et al., 2002; Hughes et al., 2004). The combination of IVIG and methylprednisolone was not significantly more effective in a recently published Dutch study (van Koningsveld et al., 2004). Recently Hughes and co-workers published recommendations based on evidence by controlled studies for the treatment of GBS and they recommended plasma exchange and IVIG but not corticosteroids and no combination of therapies (Hughes et al., 2003b). Besides, monitoring autonomic function and intensive care management have greatly improved the prognosis of GBS. During rehabilitation significant improvement of function occurred which could be demonstrated by standardized outcome measures (Nicholas et al., 2000).

*Rehabilitation, long-term course
of the disease and prognosis*

While GBS is typically a monophasic disease recurrent episodes of weakness in otherwise typically GBS have been observed (Grand'Maison et al., 1992). These patients have been separated from CIDP patients because of the rapid onset of weakness, the subsequent complete or nearly complete recovery, the high incidence of preceding infections and the normal CSF protein content at the onset of recurrence. In the study of Grand'Maison and co-workers (Grand'Maison et al., 1992) 12 patients suffering from recurrent GBS were reported. The recurrence interval ranged from 2 to 516 months.

In the vast majority of patients, however, GBS is a self-limited disease and the prognosis is favorable for those who survive the acute phase of weakness when mechanical ventilation may be necessary in 25% (Rees et al., 1998) to nearly 40% of patients (Sarada et al., 1994; Melillo et al., 1998). During this stage of the disease the mortality may reach 12% (Govoni and Granieri, 2001). About 20–30% of patients have a mild form of GBS defined as being able to walk unaided at nadir (Van Koningsveld et al., 2000). In different studies, the rate of patients with a complete or nearly complete recovery varied between 62% (Rees et al., 1998) and 88% (Cheng et al., 2000). While the majority of patients recovered well within 1 year, a percentage of about 9% were unable to walk unaided and 4% were still bedridden or ventilated after 1 year (Rees et al., 1998). Compared with mildly affected GBS patients, the prognosis quoad vitam as well as to recover is worse in the group of patients in need of mechanical ventilation at nadir. Fletcher et al. (2000) reported that the 80% of ventilated GBS patients who survived the acute phase may still make a good recovery with 79% regaining independent ambulation. Similar to the findings in a previous study (Ropper, 1986), improvement was still observed beyond 1 year. One patient could only be completely weaned from nocturnal ventilation after 5 years (Fletcher et al., 2000). Interestingly, long-term outcome was not significantly different in ventilated GBS patients between 1976 and 1986, when treatment with IVIG or plasmapheresis

had not been routinely administered, and patients who had fallen ill later and who received standard therapy. Fletcher and co-workers found a good recovery in 60% and 63%, respectively (Fletcher et al., 2000).

The natural course of the disease seems to be similar in children and in adults with an incidence of about 40% of respiratory paralysis in both groups in an Indian study. However, children in this group seem to have a better prognosis with the likelihood to regain independent walking within 1 year being twice as that of adults (Sarada et al., 1994). About 35% of all GBS patients develop long-term disability (Melillo et al., 1998) and 38% of patients had to change their job as a consequence of residua from their disease; 44% had to alter their leisure activities and nearly half of the patients reported an impairment in their psychosocial condition (Bernsen et al., 2002). In a study primarily intended to compare the costs of different treatment regimes data on the efficacy of patient rehabilitation were reported: mildly affected patients who received two plasma exchange therapies resume work after about 100 days whereas patients with severe disease requiring mechanical ventilation were able to work after a mean of 210 days (Esperou et al., 2000). In this study from France, after discharge from the hospital mildly affected patients received 30 sessions of physical therapy within 6 weeks on average whereas severely affected patients additionally received three sessions of physical therapy a week after that 30 initial session in the first 6 weeks. The total health care costs of therapy in hospital and rehabilitation within the first year ranged from 21,000 € in the mildly affected group to more than 60,000 € in more severely affected patients (Esperou et al., 2000). These data are in good accordance with a previously published study by Meythaler et al. (1997). Also in this study the need of mechanical ventilation predicted an extended length of hospitalization in acute care and in rehabilitation as well as the amount of total costs. Unfortunately, these studies do not describe the form of rehabilitation in detail and, to our best knowledge, no studies comparing different rehabilitation concepts or evaluating the efficacy of rehabilitation – similar to the studies on acute therapy – has been published.

CIDP

Clinical presentation and diagnostic procedures

Similar to GBS, CIDP is an inflammatory and demyelinating disease of the peripheral nervous system with a presumed autoimmune origin (Kieseier et al., 2004; Köller et al., 2005). In the pathogenesis of CIDP autoaggressive T-cells, macrophages, soluble factors like cytokines, chemokines, metalloproteinases and adhesion molecules as well as autoantibodies contribute to the inflammation, demyelination and secondary axonal loss in peripheral nerves.

Classical CIDP is clinically defined by the occurrence of symmetrical proximal and distal muscle weakness of subacute onset or progressing for more than 2 months (in contrast to GBS in which disease is maximal within 4 weeks), impaired sensation and absent or reduced tendon reflexes. Demyelination is evidenced by electrophysiologic studies which show reduced motor nerve conduction velocities, partial motor conduction blocks or temporary dispersion, prolonged distal motor latencies or F-wave latencies or histologically in sural nerve biopsies. Inflammation is also mirrored by elevated protein content in CSF analyses (Köller et al., 2005). Several subtypes distinct from classical CIDP have been described and this classification has implications for prognosis and therapy; distal acquired demyelinating symmetrical neuropathy (DADS neuropathy), multifocal motor neuropathy (MMN) and multifocal acquired demyelinating sensory and motor neuropathy (MADSAM or Lewis–Sumner syndrome) (Saperstein et al., 2001).

Therapy during the acute phase

In the acute phase of the disease therapies are directed at blocking the immune process thereby arresting inflammation and demyelination, and preventing secondary axonal degeneration. Standard treatment consists of IVIG (Van Schaik et al., 2002), plasma exchange (Mehndiratta et al., 2004) and corticosteroids (Mehndiratta and Hughes, 2002) whereas the utility of interferons and cytotoxic drugs in CIDP

is presently under investigation but has not yet been confirmed in controlled trials (Hughes et al., 2003a). In open-label studies with small numbers of patients or in case reports, other forms of treatment have been evaluated. Beneficial effects in previously treatment-resistant CIDP patients were reported for the combination of plasmapheresis and IVIG (Walk et al., 2004), mycophenolate mofetil (Gorson et al., 2004), cyclosporin A (Matsuda et al., 2004), etanercept (Chin et al., 2003), cyclophosphamide (Brannagan et al., 2002) and hematopoetic stem cell transplantation (Vermeulen and van Oers 2002). Two recent open-label studies described improvement of patients suffering from IgM antibody-associated demyelinating polyneuropathy under treatment with rituximab, a chimeric humanized monoclonal antibody against CD20 antigen which reduces B lymphocyte counts (Pestronk et al., 2003). However, data based on randomised controlled studies with a sufficient number of patients are not available to allow conclusive treatment recommendations with any of these therapeutic approaches.

Rehabilitation, long-term course of the disease and prognosis

In contrast to the number of treatment studies in the acute phase of CIDP data on the long-term efficacy of treatment have only been rarely reported. Most studies were performed during the first weeks after disease onset or during relapses (Table 40.2). Follow-up data on prognosis and long-term outcome are available mainly from retrospective analyses. During a follow-up period of 4 years Sghirlanzoni et al. (2000) found improvement in nearly 70% of CIDP patients which is in good accordance with the efficacy of therapy in the acute phase (Table 40.2) and in other studies on the long-term course of CIDP (Bouchard et al., 1999). Complete recovery was achieved in 13% of patients (Sghirlanzoni et al., 2000) but mortality is in the same range (Bouchard et al., 1999). CIDP may take a slowly progressive or a relapsing-remitting course with the risk of secondary progressive deterioration. The proportion of patients with a relapsing-remitting course varies in different

Table 40.2. Current therapy of CIDP according to randomized-controlled studies.

Study	Number of patients	Duration	Design	Result	Reference
Plasma exchange versus IVIG in CIDP	15	42 days	Randomized, observer-blinded, cross-over	No significant difference	(Dyck et al., 1994)
Plasma exchange in CIDP	15	28 days	Double blind, sham-controlled cross-over	80% of patients improve upon plasma exchange	(Hahn et al., 1996a)
IVIG in CIDP	30	28 days	Double blind, placebo-controlled, cross-over	63% of patients improve	(Hahn et al., 1996b)
IVIG in CIDP	53	42 days	Double blind, randomized, placebo-controlled	76% of patients improve	(Mendell et al., 2001)
IVIG versus. oral prednisolone in CIDP	32	14 days	Double blind, randomized, cross-over	No significant difference	(Hughes et al., 2001)
Azathioprine in combination with prednisone versus prednisone	30	9 months	Open parallel group randomized	No significant difference	(Dyck et al., 1985)
Interferon-β1a in treatment-resistant CIDP patients	20	28 weeks	Double blind, randomized, placebo controlled, cross-over	No significant benefit of treatment	(Hadden et al., 1999)
IVIG in CIDP-MGUS	22	28	Double blind, randomized, placebo-controlled, cross-over	50% of patients improve within 4 weeks	(Comi et al., 2002)
IVIG in MMN	16	28	Double blind, randomized, placebo-controlled, cross-over	69% of patients improve	(Federico et al., 2000)

studies from 14% (Said, 2002) to 51% (McLeod et al., 1999) and a relapsing-remitting course is predominantly found in younger patients (Hattori et al., 2001). Female gender, young age at onset, relapsing-remitting course and absent evidence of axonal damage on neurophysiologic studies were predictive of a better prognosis (Bouchard et al., 1999; Sghirlanzoni et al., 2000). A number of CIDP patients, however, does not respond to oral immunosuppressive treatment and remains dependent on plasmapheresis (Bromberg et al., 1992). The demonstration of a monoclonal gammopathy was associated with a markedly unfavorable prognosis in some studies (Simmons et al., 1995; Sghirlanzoni et al., 2000) but not invariably (Gorson et al., 1997). Initial presentation with only sensory symptoms, however, did not

carry a better long-term prognosis (van Dijk et al., 1999). In this group of patients weakness developed within 1–6 years in 70% of patients and long-term disability was not different from patients starting with weakness. In the elderly, CIDP is less common and declining with age (Verghese et al., 2001) whereas the percentage of idiopathic axonal neuropathies increase.

Other types of polyneuropathy

Critical illness polyneuropathy

In patients with sepsis and multiple organ failure but also in patients with trauma or burns a polyneuropathy develops in up to 70% of patients and is regarded as a complication of a disease called "systemic inflammatory response syndrome" (SIRS) (Bolton and Young, 2000). Electrophysiologically critical illness polyneuropathy (CIP) is characterized by a reduction of compound muscle and sensory nerve action potential with normal or only slightly reduced nerve conduction velocities and signs of muscle denervation in electromyography. Therapy is directed against SIRS and the prognosis is good in patients surviving the acute phase of the disease. Physiotherapy and rehabilitation should be arranged starting with light exercises to promote muscle strength, to maintain joint mobility and to prevent contractures (Bolton and Young, 2000). IVIG has been tried and seem to be without effect in patients with established CIP (Wijdicks and Fulgham, 1994) but may have some efficacy in preventing the development of CIP (Mohr et al., 1997). In a follow-up study of SIRS survivors Fletcher et al. (2003) reported that most patients clinically recovered completely from CIP in the observation time of 42 month on average. Neurologic examination revealed sensory deficits in 27% of patients, motor weakness in 18% and both sensory and motor impairment in 14% of patients. On electromyographic examination more than 90% showed signs of chronic partial denervation.

Diabetic polyneuropathy

Painful neuropathy is a common complication of poor glycaemic control and may affect 20–30% of diabetes patients (Duby et al., 2004). Diabetic neuropathy presents with distal muscular atrophy and sensory loss, and is characterized in nerve conduction studies by low amplitudes and reduced nerve conduction velocities. Cardiac autonomic neuropathy, gastroparesis and sexual and bladder dysfunction may result from autonomic diabetic neuropathy (Duby et al., 2004). Even in clinically asymptomatic diabetics with normal routine nerve conduction studies double shock stimuli may be able to demonstrate latent neuropathy (Tan and Tan, 2003). Impaired glucose tolerance as determined by oral glucose loading in prediabetic patients is associated with a milder form of neuropathy compared to diabetes patients (Sumner et al., 2003). There is no specific

therapy available for diabetic neuropathy (Arkkila and Gautier, 2003) but improved glycaemic control is shown to slow the progression of neuropathy. Diabetic neuropathy is frequently painful and a number of treatment trials showed efficacy of therapy with various analgetic medications including tramadol (Harati et al., 2000), gabapentin (Backonja and Glanzman, 2003), antidepressants and anticonvulsants (Marchettini et al., 2004). Rehabilitation of patients with diabetic neuropathy additionally faces the problem of neuropathic diabetic foot ulceration with the necessity of pressure reduction, for example by therapeutic footwear (Boulton et al., 2004).

Toxic polyneuropathy

A number of therapeutic agents especially chemotherapeutic medication may cause peripheral neuropathy (Quasthoff and Hartung, 2002; Verstappen et al., 2003). There are some co-medications suggested to reduce the appearance or severity of neuropathy following chemotherapy (Verstappen et al., 2003), however, no specific rehabilitation therapy has been reported. Painful neuropathy will be treated with the same agents as in painful diabetic neuropathy and for patients with poor pain relief upon standard medication spinal cord stimulation may offer an additional therapeutic option (Cata et al., 2004).

40.4 Diseases of the neuromuscular junction: Myasthenia gravis and LEMS

Myasthenia gravis

Clinical presentation and diagnostic procedures

Myasthenia gravis is an acquired autoimmune disease with fluctuating use dependent muscle weakness in most cases due to antibodies against acetylcholine receptors (AChR) (for a recent review see Keesey, 2004). It can occur at any age with an early onset peak between the teens and thirties mainly in women and a late onset peak between the fifties and seventies with a male predominance. The presentation of myasthenia may vary in different patients and affect eye, facial, oropharyngeal, axial and limb muscles whereas tendon reflexes, function of involuntary smooth muscles and skin sensation are intact. The clinical diagnosis of myasthenia is confirmed by serologic assays demonstrating the presence of AChR antibodies and the electrophysiologic demonstration of decremental responses to 2–3 Hz repetitive nerve stimulation in proximal muscles.

Therapy during the acute phase

During the active phase of myasthenia anticholinesterase medication such as pyridostigmine or neostigmine provide relief from myasthenic muscle weakness. In myasthenic crisis plasma exchange is helpful in eliminating antibodies and rapidly improving symptoms. IVIG (typically 0.4 g/kg body weight) may be given as an alternative treatment. Both plasma exchange and IVIG improve patient's muscle strength during crisis and their effect lasts for about 45 days on average. Long-term immunologic treatments encompass immunosuppressive drugs such as prednisone, azathioprine, ciclosporin, mycophenolate mofetil, rituximab and others (Katz and Barohn, 2001; Keesey, 2004). Although the concept of therapeutic thymectomy for non-thymomatous myasthenia gravis is still under debate, in patients with moderate generalized myasthenia thymectomy is recommended by many experts and offers the possibility of a complete symptomfree and drug-free remission (Keesey, 2004).

Rehabilitation, long-term course of the disease and prognosis

The clinical course of myasthenia gravis is highly variable with spontaneous remissions spanning periods of more than 1 year in up to 20%. About half of patients suffering from ocular myasthenia will experience generalized symptoms within 2 years (Sommer et al., 1993; Keesey, 2004). In a retrospective multicenter study 11% of patients had a remission without treatment whereas 77% of patients declined

to maximal muscle weakness within 3 years after onset (Mantegazza et al., 1990). This resembles the three part division of the clinical course of myasthenia gravis known from historic studies: an active stage of 5–7 years with exacerbations, remissions and lability of muscle strength; an inactive stable second stage for about 10 years and burned-out third stage characterized by slow improvement (Simpson and Thomaides, 1987). In a more recent study, Padua et al. (2000) investigated health-related quality of life in patients with myasthenia gravis using self-administered questionnaires and compared the results with scores of physical and mental examination. They found that the Osserman scale and clinical examination findings were significantly related to the patient-oriented measurements in their questionnaires assessing quality of daily life. With disease duration, however, mental composite scores decreased irrespective of the actual physical performance of the patients. The authors concluded from this finding that myasthenia patients suffered from the knowledge of their chronic and potentially dangerous disease even in phases with good compensated muscle strength. For rehabilitation in the acute state but also in long-term management this should be kept in mind and in case of need specific therapy for this aspect should be offered.

LEMS

Clinical presentation and diagnostic procedures

The LEMS is another disease of the neuromuscular junction associated with autoantibodies against P/Q-type voltage-gated calcium channels. It is considered to be autoimmune in nature or a paraneoplastic disorder in association with malignancies most commonly a small cell lung cancer (Sanders, 2003; Newsom-Davis, 2004). Muscle weakness affects predominantly proximal muscle groups. Clinically LEMS can be differentiated from myasthenia gravis by the distribution of weakness, the autonomic symptoms of dry mouth, constipation and erectile dysfunction, and augmentation of muscle strength during exercise. Diagnosis is confirmed by the demonstration of the specific antibody and by the electrophysiologic proof of a significantly increased compound muscle action potential after high-frequency electrical stimulation or after maximal voluntary activation ("incremental response").

Therapy during the acute phase and prognosis

In patients with LEMS associated with a tumor, therapy is aimed at the cancer and patients may improve after successful tumor treatment. Pyridostigmin is not as effective as in myasthenia but most patients improve upon 3,4-diaminopyridine (Sanders, 2003; Newsom-Davis, 2004). In severely affected patients IVIG (Rich et al., 1997) and plasmapheresis in combination with prednisone and azathioprine (Dau and Denys, 1982) is effective. In tumor-associated LEMS the long-term prognosis is mainly determined by the therapeutic efficacy to control the tumor.

REFERENCES

Abresch, R.T., Seyden, N.K. and Wineinger, M.A. (1998). Quality of life. Issues for persons with neuromuscular diseases. *Phys Med Rehabil Clin N Am*, **9**(1), 233–248.

Abresch, R.T., Jensen, M.P. and Carter, G.T. (2001). Health-related quality of life in peripheral neuropathy. *Phys Med Rehabil Clin N Am*, **12**(2), 461–472.

Abresch, R.T., Carter, G.T., Jensen, M.P. and Kilmer, D.D. (2002). Assessment of pain and health-related quality of life in slowly progressive neuromuscular disease. *Am J Hosp Palliat Care*, **19**(1), 39–48.

Agre, J.C., Rodriquez, A.A. and Franke, T.M. (1997). Strength, endurance, and work capacity after muscle strengthening exercise in postpolio subjects. *Arch Phys Med Rehabil*, **78**(7), 681–686.

Ahlstrom, G. and Karlsson, U. (2000). Disability and quality of life in individuals with postpolio syndrome. *Disabil Rehabil*, **22**(9), 416–422.

Ahuja, B., Gupta, V.K. and Tyagi, A. (1996). Paralytic poliomyelitis (1989–1994): report from a sentinel center. *Indian Pediatr*, **33**(9), 739–745.

Amosun, S.L., Ikuesan, B.A. and Oloyede, I.J. (1995). Rehabilitation of the handicapped child–what about the caregiver? *PNG Med J*, **38**(3), 208–214.

Arkkila, P.E. and Gautier, J.F. (2003). Musculoskeletal disorders in diabetes mellitus: an update. *Best Pract Res Clin Rheumatol*, **17**(6), 945–970.

Asbury, A.K. and Cornblath, D.R. (1990). Assessment of current diagnostic criteria for Guillain–Barre syndrome. *Ann Neurol*, **27**(Suppl.), S21–24.

Ashworth, N.L., Satkunam, L.E. and Deforge, D. (2004). Treatment for spasticity in amyotrophic lateral sclerosis/motor neuron disease. *Cochrane Database Syst Rev*, (1), CD004156.

Bach, J.R. and Zhitnikov, S. (1998). The management of neuromuscular ventilatory failure. *Semin Pediatr Neurol*, **5**(2), 92–105.

Backonja, M. and Glanzman, R.L. (2003). Gabapentin dosing for neuropathic pain: evidence from randomized, placebo-controlled clinical trials. *Clin Ther*, **25**(1), 81–104.

Bernsen, R.A., de Jager, A.E., Schmitz, P.I. and van der Meche, F.G. (2002). Long-term impact on work and private life after Guillain–Barre syndrome. *J Neurol Sci*, **201**(1–2), 13–17.

Billard, C., Gillet, P., Barthez, M., Hommet, C. and Bertrand, P. (1998). Reading ability and processing in Duchenne muscular dystrophy and spinal muscular atrophy. *Dev Med Child Neurol*, **40**(1), 12–20.

Bolton, C.F. and Young, G.B. (2000). Critical Illness Polyneuropathy. *Curr Treat Options Neurol*, **2**(6), 489–498.

Bongioanni, P., Reali, C. and Sogos, V. (2004). Ciliary neurotrophic factor (CNTF) for amyotrophic lateral sclerosis/motor neuron disease. *Cochrane Database Syst Rev*, (3), CD004302.

Bossy-Wetzel, E., Schwarzenbacher, R. and Lipton, S.A. (2004). Molecular pathways to neurodegeneration. *Nat Med*, **10**(Suppl.), S2–9.

Bouchard, C., Lacroix, C., Plante, V., Adams, D., Chedru, F., Guglielmi, J.M. and Said, G. (1999). Clinicopathologic findings and prognosis of chronic inflammatory demyelinating polyneuropathy. *Neurology*, **52**(3), 498–503.

Boulton, A.J., Kirsner, R.S. and Vileikyte, L. (2004). Clinical practice. Neuropathic diabetic foot ulcers. *New Engl J Med*, **351**(1), 48–55.

Brannagan III, T.H., Pradhan, A., Heiman-Patterson, T., Winkelman, A.C., Styler, M.J., Topolsky, D.L., Crilley, P.A., Schwartzman, R.J., Brodsky, I. and Gladstone, D.E. (2002). High-dose cyclophosphamide without stem-cell rescue for refractory CIDP. *Neurology*, **58**(12), 1856–1858.

Brichta, L., Hofmann, Y., Hahnen, E., Siebzehnrubl, F.A., Raschke, H., Blumcke, I., Eyupoglu, I.Y. and Wirth, B. (2003). Valproic acid increases the SMN2 protein level: a well-known drug as a potential therapy for spinal muscular atrophy. *Hum Mol Genet*, **12**(**19**), 2481–2489.

Bromberg, M.B. and Forshew, D.A. (2002). Comparison of instruments addressing quality of life in patients with ALS and their caregivers. *Neurology*, **58**(**2**), 320–322.

Bromberg, M.B., Feldman, E.L., Jaradeh, S. and Albers, J.W. (1992). Prognosis in long-term immunosuppressive treatment of refractory chronic inflammatory demyelinating polyradiculoneuropathy. *J Clin Epidemiol*, **45**(**1**), 47–52.

Brooks, B.R., Miller, R.G., Swash, M. and Munsat, T.L. (2000). El Escorial revisited: revised criteria for the diagnosis of amyotrophic lateral sclerosis. *Amyotroph Lateral Scler Other Motor Neuron Disord*, **1**(**5**), 293–299.

Bruno, R.L. (2000). Paralytic vs. nonparalytic polio: distinction without a difference? *Am J Phys Med Rehabil*, **79**(**1**), 4–12.

Burger, H. and Marincek, C. (2000). The influence of post-polio syndrome on independence and life satisfaction. *Disabil Rehabil*, **22**(**7**), 318–322.

Carter, G.T., Bednar-Butler, L.M., Abresch, R.T. and Ugalde, V.O. (1999). Expanding the role of hospice care in amyotrophic lateral sclerosis. *Am J Hosp Palliat Care*, **16**(**6**), 707–710.

Cata, J.P., Cordella, J.V., Burton, A.W., Hassenbusch, S.J., Weng, H.R. and Dougherty, P.M. (2004). Spinal cord stimulation relieves chemotherapy-induced pain: a clinical case report. *J Pain Symptom Manage*, **27**(**1**), 72–78.

Chan, K.M., Amirjani, N., Sumrain, M., Clarke, A. and Strohschein, F.J. (2003). Randomized controlled trial of strength training in post-polio patients. *Muscle Nerve*, **27**(**3**), 332–338.

Cheng, Q., Jiang, G.X., Fredrikson, S., Link, H. and de Pedro-Cuesta, J. (2000). Epidemiological surveillance of Guillain–Barre syndrome in Sweden, 1996–1997. Network members of the Swedish GBS Epidemiology Study Group. *Acta Neurol Scand*, **101**(**2**), 104–110.

Chin, R.L., Sherman, W.H., Sander, H.W., Hays, A.P. and Latov, N. (2003). Etanercept (Enbrel(R)) therapy for chronic inflammatory demyelinating polyneuropathy. *J Neurol Sci*, **210**(**1–2**), 19–21.

Chio, A., Cucatto, A., Calvo, A., Terreni, A.A., Magnani, C. and Schiffer, D. (1999a). Amyotrophic lateral sclerosis among the migrant population to Piemonte, northwestern Italy. *J Neurol*, **246**(**3**), 175–180.

Chio, A., Finocchiaro, E., Meineri, P., Bottacchi, E. and Schiffer, D. (1999b). Safety and factors related to survival after percutaneous endoscopic gastrostomy in ALS. ALS Percutaneous Endoscopic Gastrostomy Study Group. *Neurology*, **53**(**5**), 1123–1125.

Christensen, P.B., Hojer-Pedersen, E. and Jensen, N.B. (1990). Survival of patients with amyotrophic lateral sclerosis in 2 Danish counties. *Neurology*, **40**(**4**), 600–604.

Comi, G., Roveri, L., Swan, A., Willison, H., Bojar, M., Illa, I., Karageorgiou, C., Nobile-Orazio, E., van Den Bergh, P., Swan, T. and Hughes, R. (2002). A randomised controlled trial of intravenous immunoglobulin in IgM paraprotein associated demyelinating neuropathy. *J Neurol*, **249**(**10**), 1370–1377.

Craig, A., Moses, P., Tran, Y., McIsaac, P. and Kirkup, L. (2002). The effectiveness of a hands-free environmental control system for the profoundly disabled. *Arch Phys Med Rehabil*, **83**(**10**), 1455–1458.

Dalakas, M.C. (1995). Pathogenetic mechanisms of post-polio syndrome: morphological, electrophysiological, virological, and immunological correlations. *Ann N Y Acad Sci*, **753**, 167–185.

Dau, P.C. and Denys, E.H. (1982). Plasmapheresis and immunosuppressive drug therapy in the Eaton–Lambert syndrome. *Ann Neurol*, **11**(**6**), 570–575.

Donaghy, M. (1999). Classification and clinical features of motor neurone diseases and motor neuropathies in adults. *J Neurol*, **246**(**5**), 331–333.

Drory, V.E., Goltsman, E., Reznik, J.G., Mosek, A. and Korczyn, A.D. (2001). The value of muscle exercise in patients with amyotrophic lateral sclerosis. *J Neurol Sci*, **191**(**1–2**), 133–137.

Duby, J.J., Campbell, R.K., Setter, S.M., White, J.R. and Rasmussen, K.A. (2004). Diabetic neuropathy: an intensive review. *Am J Health Syst Pharm*, **61**(**2**), 160–173; quiz 175–176.

Dyck, P.J., O'Brien, P., Swanson, C., Low, P. and Daube, J. (1985). Combined azathioprine and prednisone in chronic inflammatory-demyelinating polyneuropathy. *Neurology*, **35**(**8**), 1173–1176.

Dyck, P.J., Litchy, W.J., Kratz, K.M., Suarez, G.A., Low, P.A., Pineda, A.A., Windebank, A.J., Karnes, J.L. and O'Brien, P.C. (1994). A plasma exchange versus immune globulin infusion trial in chronic inflammatory demyelinating polyradiculoneuropathy. *Ann Neurol*, **36**(**6**), 838–845.

Esperou, H., Jars-Guincestre, M.C., Bolgert, F., Raphael, J.C. and Durand-Zaleski, I. (2000). Cost analysis of plasma-exchange therapy for the treatment of Guillain–Barre syndrome. French Cooperative Group on Plasma Exchange in Guillain–Barre Syndrome. *Intens Care Med*, **26**(**8**), 1094–1100.

Farbu, E. and Gilhus, N.E. (2002). Education, occupation, and perception of health amongst previous polio patients compared to their siblings. *Eur J Neurol*, **9**(**3**), 233–241.

Farbu, E., Rekand, T. and Gilhus, N.E. (2003). Post-polio syndrome and total health status in a prospective hospital study. *Eur J Neurol*, **10**(**4**), 407–413.

Federico, P., Zochodne, D.W., Hahn, A.F., Brown, W.F. and Feasby, T.E. (2000). Multifocal motor neuropathy improved by IVIg: randomized, double-blind, placebo-controlled study. *Neurology*, **55**(9), 1256–1262.

Fehlings, D.L., Kirsch, S., McComas, A., Chipman, M. and Campbell, K. (2002). Evaluation of therapeutic electrical stimulation to improve muscle strength and function in children with types II/III spinal muscular atrophy. *Dev Med Child Neurol*, **44**(11), 741–744.

Fletcher, D.D., Lawn, N.D., Wolter, T.D. and Wijdicks, E.F. (2000). Long-term outcome in patients with Guillain–Barre syndrome requiring mechanical ventilation. *Neurology*, **54**(12), 2311–2315.

Fletcher, S.N., Kennedy, D.D., Ghosh, I.R., Misra, V.P., Kiff, K., Coakley, J.H. and Hinds, C.J. (2003). Persistent neuromuscular and neurophysiologic abnormalities in long-term survivors of prolonged critical illness. *Crit Care Med*, **31**(4), 1012–1016.

Fowler Jr., W.M., Abresch, R.T., Koch, T.R., Brewer, M.L., Bowden, R.K. and Wanlass, R.L. (1997). Employment profiles in neuromuscular diseases. *Am J Phys Med Rehabil*, **76**(1), 26–37.

Gordon, P.H. and Wilbourn, A.J. (2001). Early electrodiagnostic findings in Guillain–Barre syndrome. *Arch Neurol*, **58**(6), 913–917.

Gorson, K.C., Allam, G. and Ropper, A.H. (1997). Chronic inflammatory demyelinating polyneuropathy: clinical features and response to treatment in 67 consecutive patients with and without a monoclonal gammopathy. *Neurology*, **48**(2), 321–328.

Gorson, K.C., Amato, A.A. and Ropper, A.H. (2004). Efficacy of mycophenolate mofetil in patients with chronic immune demyelinating polyneuropathy. *Neurology*, **63**(4), 715–717.

Govoni, V. and Granieri, E. (2001). Epidemiology of the Guillain–Barre syndrome. *Curr Opin Neurol*, **14**(5), 605–613.

Grand'Maison, F., Feasby, T.E., Hahn, A.F. and Koopman, W.J. (1992). Recurrent Guillain–Barre syndrome. Clinical and laboratory features. *Brain*, **115**, 1093–1106.

Groeneveld, G.J., Veldink, J.H., van der Tweel, I., Kalmijn, S., Beijer, C., de Visser, M., Wokke, J.H., Franssen, H. and van den Berg, L.H. (2003). A randomized sequential trial of creatine in amyotrophic lateral sclerosis. *Ann Neurol*, **53**(4), 437–445.

Hadden, R.D., Sharrack, B., Bensa, S., Soudain, S.E. and Hughes, R.A. (1999). Randomized trial of interferon beta-1a in chronic inflammatory demyelinating polyradiculoneuropathy. *Neurology*, **53**(1), 57–61.

Hahn, A.F., Bolton, C.F., Pillay, N., Chalk, C., Benstead, T., Bril, V., Shumak, K., Vandervoort, M.K. and Feasby, T.E. (1996a). Plasma-exchange therapy in chronic inflammatory demyelinating polyneuropathy. A double-blind, sham-controlled, cross-over study. *Brain*, **119**, 1055–1066.

Hahn, A.F., Bolton, C.F., Zochodne, D. and Feasby, T.E. (1996b). Intravenous immunoglobulin treatment in chronic inflammatory demyelinating polyneuropathy. A double-blind, placebo-controlled, cross-over study. *Brain*, **119**, 1067–1077.

Harati, Y., Gooch, C., Swenson, M., Edelman, S.V., Greene, D., Raskin, P., Donofrio, P., Cornblath, D., Olson, W.H. and Kamin, M. (2000). Maintenance of the long-term effectiveness of tramadol in treatment of the pain of diabetic neuropathy. *J Diabetes Complicat*, **14**(2), 65–70.

Hardart, M.K., Burns, J.P. and Truog, R.D. (2002). Respiratory support in spinal muscular atrophy type I: a survey of physician practices and attitudes. *Pediatrics*, **110**(2 Pt 1), e24.

Hattori, N., Misu, K., Koike, H., Ichimura, M., Nagamatsu, M., Hirayama, M. and Sobue, G. (2001). Age of onset influences clinical features of chronic inflammatory demyelinating polyneuropathy. *J Neurol Sci*, **184**(1), 57–63.

Hughes, R.A. and van Der Meche, F.G. (2000). Corticosteroids for treating Guillain–Barre syndrome. *Cochrane Database Syst Rev*, (**3**), CD001446.

Hughes, R., Bensa, S., Willison, H., van den Bergh, P., Comi, G., Illa, I., Nobile-Orazio, E., van Doorn, P., Dalakas, M., Bojar, M. and Swan, A. (2001). Randomized controlled trial of intravenous immunoglobulin versus oral prednisolone in chronic inflammatory demyelinating polyradiculoneuropathy. *Ann Neurol*, **50**(2), 195–201.

Hughes, R.A., Swan, A.V. and van Doorn, P.A. (2003a). Cytotoxic drugs and interferons for chronic inflammatory demyelinating polyradiculoneuropathy. *Cochrane Database Syst Rev*, (**1**), CD003280.

Hughes, R.A., Wijdicks, E.F., Barohn, R., Benson, E., Cornblath, D.R., Hahn, A.F., Meythaler, J.M., Miller, R.G., Sladky, J.T. and Stevens, J.C. (2003b). Practice parameter: immunotherapy for Guillain–Barre syndrome: report of the Quality Standards Subcommittee of the American Academy of Neurology. *Neurology*, **61**(6), 736–740.

Hughes, R.A., Raphael, J.C., Swan, A.V. and Doorn, P.A. (2004). Intravenous immunoglobulin for Guillain–Barre syndrome. *Cochrane Database Syst Rev*, (**1**), CD002063.

Jubelt, B. (2004). Post-polio syndrome. *Curr Treat Options Neurol*, **6**(2), 87–93.

Katz, J. and Barohn, R.J. (2001). Update on the evaluation and therapy of autoimmune neuromuscular junction disorders. *Phys Med Rehabil Clin N Am*, **12**(2), 381–397.

Kawahara, Y., Ito, K., Sun, H., Aizawa, H., Kanazawa, I. and Kwak, S. (2004). Glutamate receptors: RNA editing and death of motor neurons. *Nature*, **427**(6977), 801.

Keesey, J.C. (2004). Clinical evaluation and management of myasthenia gravis. *Muscle Nerve*, **29**(4), 484–505.

Kiebert, G.M., Green, C., Murphy, C., Mitchell, J.D., O'Brien, M., Burrell, A. and Leigh, P.N. (2001). Patients' health-related quality of life and utilities associated with different stages of amyotrophic lateral sclerosis. *J Neurol Sci*, **191**(1–2), 87–93.

Kieseier, B.C., Kiefer, R., Gold, R., Hemmer, B., Willison, H.J. and Hartung, H.P. (2004). Advances in understanding and treatment of immune-mediated disorders of the peripheral nervous system. *Muscle Nerve*, **30**(2), 131–156.

Klefbeck, B., Lagerstrand, L. and Mattsson, E. (2000). Inspiratory muscle training in patients with prior polio who use part-time assisted ventilation. *Arch Phys Med Rehabil*, **81**(8), 1065–1071.

Klein, M.G., Whyte, J., Esquenazi, A., Keenan, M.A. and Costello, R. (2002). A comparison of the effects of exercise and lifestyle modification on the resolution of overuse symptoms of the shoulder in polio survivors: a preliminary study. *Arch Phys Med Rehabil*, **83**(5), 708–713.

Kling, C., Persson, A. and Gardulf, A. (2002). The ADL ability and use of technical aids in persons with late effects of polio. *Am J Occup Ther*, **56**(4), 457–461.

Koessler, W., Wanke, T., Winkler, G., Nader, A., Toifl, K., Kurz, H. and Zwick, H. (2001). 2 Years' experience with inspiratory muscle training in patients with neuromuscular disorders. *Chest*, **120**(3), 765–769.

Köller, H., Kieseier, B.C., Jander, S. and Hartung, H.P. (2005). Chronic inflammatory demyelinating polyneuropathy. *New Engl J Med*, **352**(13), 1343–1356.

Kroksmark, A.K., Beckung, E. and Tulinius, M. (2001). Muscle strength and motor function in children and adolescents with spinal muscular atrophy II and III. *Eur J Paediatr Neurol*, **5**(5), 191–198.

Kumakura, N., Takayanagi, M., Hasegawa, T., Ihara, K., Yano, H. and Kimizuka, M. (2002). Self-assessed secondary difficulties among paralytic poliomyelitis and spinal cord injury survivors in Japan. *Arch Phys Med Rehabil*, **83**(9), 1245–1251.

Leigh, P.N., Abrahams, S., Al-Chalabi, A., Ampong, M.A., Goldstein, L.H., Johnson, J., Lyall, R., Moxham, J., Mustfa, N., Rio, A., Shaw, C. and Willey, E. (2003). The management of motor neurone disease. *J Neurol Neurosurg Psychiatr*, **74**(Suppl. 4), iv32–iv47.

Lin, M.C., Liaw, M.Y., Chen, W.J., Cheng, P.T., Wong, A.M. and Chiou, W.K. (2001). Pulmonary function and spinal characteristics: their relationships in persons with idiopathic and post-poliomyelitic scoliosis. *Arch Phys Med Rehabil*, **82**(3), 335–341.

Lissoni, A., Aliverti, A., Tzeng, A.C. and Bach, J.R. (1998). Kinematic analysis of patients with spinal muscular atrophy during spontaneous breathing and mechanical ventilation. *Am J Phys Med Rehabil*, **77**(3), 188–192.

Maillot, F., Laueriere, L., Hazouard, E., Giraudeau, B. and Corcia, P. (2001). Quality of life in ALS is maintained as physical function declines. *Neurology*, **57**(10), 1939.

Mantegazza, R., Beghi, E., Pareyson, D., Antozzi, C., Peluchetti, D., Sghirlanzoni, A., Cosi, V., Lombardi, M., Piccolo, G., Tonali, P., et al. (1990). A multicentre follow-up study of 1152 patients with myasthenia gravis in Italy. *J Neurol*, **237**(6), 339–344.

Marchettini, P., Teloni, L., Formaglio, F. and Lacerenza, M. (2004). Pain in diabetic neuropathy case study: whole patient management. *Eur J Neurol*, **11**(Suppl. 1), 12–21.

Matsuda, M., Hoshi, K., Gono, T., Morita, H. and Ikeda, S. (2004). Cyclosporin A in treatment of refractory patients with chronic inflammatory demyelinating polyradiculoneuropathy. *J Neurol Sci*, **224**(1–2), 29–35.

McDonald, C.M. (1998). Limb contractures in progressive neuromuscular disease and the role of stretching, orthotics, and surgery. *Phys Med Rehabil Clin N Am*, **9**(1), 187–211.

McLeod, J.G., Pollard, J.D., Macaskill, P., Mohamed, A., Spring, P. and Khurana, V. (1999). Prevalence of chronic inflammatory demyelinating polyneuropathy in New South Wales, Australia. *Ann Neurol*, **46**(6), 910–913.

McNeal, D.R., Somerville, N.J. and Wilson, D.J. (1999). Work problems and accommodations reported by persons who are postpolio or have a spinal cord injury. *Assist Technol*, **11**(2), 137–157.

Mehndiratta, M.M. and Hughes, R.A. (2002). Corticosteroids for chronic inflammatory demyelinating polyradiculoneuropathy. *Cochrane Database Syst Rev*, (1), CD002062.

Mehndiratta, M.M., Hughes, R.A. and Agarwal, P. (2004). Plasma exchange for chronic inflammatory demyelinating polyradiculoneuropathy. *Cochrane Database Syst Rev*, (3), CD003906.

Melillo, E.M., Sethi, J.M. and Mohsenin, V. (1998). Guillain–Barre syndrome: rehabilitation outcome and recent developments. *Yale J Biol Med*, **71**(5), 383–389.

Mendell, J.R., Barohn, R.J., Freimer, M.L., Kissel, J.T., King, W., Nagaraja, H.N., Rice, R., Campbell, W.W., Donofrio, P.D., Jackson, C.E., Lewis, R.A., Shy, M., Simpson, D.M., Parry, G.J., Rivner, M.H., Thornton, C.A., Bromberg, M.B., Tandan, R., Harati, Y. and Giuliani, M.J. (2001). Randomized controlled trial of IVIg in untreated chronic inflammatory demyelinating polyradiculoneuropathy. *Neurology*, **56**(4), 445–449.

Meythaler, J.M., DeVivo, M.J. and Braswell, W.C. (1997). Rehabilitation outcomes of patients who have developed Guillain-Barre syndrome. *Am J Phys Med Rehabil*, **76**(5), 411–419.

Miller, R.G., Anderson Jr., F.A., Bradley, W.G., Brooks, B.R., Mitsumoto, H., Munsat, T.L. and Ringel, S.P. (2000). The ALS patient care database: goals, design, and early results. ALS C.A.R.E. Study Group. *Neurology*, **54**(1), 53–57.

Miller, R.G., Mitchell, J.D., Lyon, M. and Moore, D.H. (2002). Riluzole for amyotrophic lateral sclerosis (ALS)/motor neuron disease (MND). *Cochrane Database Syst Rev*, (**2**), CD001447.

Mitchell, J.D., Wokke, J.H. and Borasio, G.D. (2002). Recombinant human insulin-like growth factor I (rhIGF-I) for amyotrophic lateral sclerosis/motor neuron disease. *Cochrane Database Syst Rev*, (**3**), CD002064.

Mitsumoto, H. and Del Bene, M. (2000). Improving the quality of life for people with ALS: the challenge ahead. *Amyotroph Lateral Scler Other Motor Neuron Disord*, **1**(5), 329–336.

Mitsumoto, H., Davidson, M., Moore, D., Gad, N., Brandis, M., Ringel, S., Rosenfeld, J., Shefner, J.M., Strong, M.J., Sufit, R. and Anderson, F.A. (2003). Percutaneous endoscopic gastrostomy (PEG) in patients with ALS and bulbar dysfunction. *Amyotroph Lateral Scler Other Motor Neuron Disord*, **4**(3), 177–185.

Mohr, M., Englisch, L., Roth, A., Burchardi, H. and Zielmann, S. (1997). Effects of early treatment with immunoglobulin on critical illness polyneuropathy following multiple organ failure and gram-negative sepsis. *Intens Care Med*, **23**(11), 1144–1149.

Mulder, D.W. (1995). Clinical observations on acute poliomyelitis. *Ann N Y Acad Sci*, **753**, 1–10.

Newsom-Davis, J. (2004). Lambert–Eaton myasthenic syndrome. *Rev Neurol (Paris)*, **160**(2), 177–180.

Nicholas, R., Playford, E.D. and Thompson, A.J. (2000). A retrospective analysis of outcome in severe Guillain–Barre syndrome following combined neurological and rehabilitation management. *Disabil Rehabil*, **22**(10), 451–455.

Nollet, F., Beelen, A., Sargeant, A.J., de Visser, M., Lankhorst, G.J. and de Jong, B.A. (2001). Submaximal exercise capacity and maximal power output in polio subjects. *Arch Phys Med Rehabil*, **82**(12), 1678–1685.

Nollet, F., Beelen, A., Twisk, J.W., Lankhorst, G.J. and de Visser, M. (2003). Perceived health and physical functioning in post-poliomyelitis syndrome: a 6-year prospective follow-up study. *Arch Phys Med Rehabil*, **84**(7), 1048–1056.

Norquist, J.M., Jenkinson, C., Fitzpatrick, R. and Swash, M. (2003). Factors which predict physical and mental health status in patients with amyotrophic lateral sclerosis over time. *Amyotroph Lateral Scler Other Motor Neuron Disord*, **4**(2), 112–117.

Padua, L., Evoli, A., Aprile, I., Caliandro, P., Mazza, S., Padua, R. and Tonali, P. (2001). Health-related quality of life in patients with myasthenia gravis and the relationship between patient-oriented assessment and conventional measurements. *Neurol Sci*, **22**(5), 363–369.

Pasetti, C. and Zanini, G. (2000). The physician–patient relationship in amyotrophic lateral sclerosis. *Neurol Sci*, **21**(5), 318–323.

Pentland, B., Hellawell, D., Benjamin, J., Prasad, R. and Ainslie, A. (2000). Survey of the late consequences of polio in Edinburgh and the Lothians. *Health Bull (Edinb)*, **58**(4), 267–275.

Pestronk, A., Florence, J., Miller, T., Choksi, R., Al-Lozi, M.T. and Levine, T.D. (2003). Treatment of IgM antibody associated polyneuropathies using rituximab. *J Neurol Neurosurg Psychiatr*, **74**(4), 485–489.

Quasthoff, S. and Hartung, H.P. (2002). Chemotherapy-induced peripheral neuropathy. *J Neurol*, **249**(1), 9–17.

Raphael, J.C., Chevret, S., Hughes, R.A. and Annane, D. (2002). Plasma exchange for Guillain–Barre syndrome. *Cochrane Database Syst Rev*, (**2**), CD001798.

Rees, J.H., Thompson, R.D., Smeeton, N.C. and Hughes, R.A. (1998). Epidemiological study of Guillain–Barre syndrome in south east England. *J Neurol Neurosurg Psychiatr*, **64**(1), 74–77.

Rekand, T., Korv, J., Farbu, E., Roose, M., Gilhus, N.E., Langeland, N. and Aarli, J.A. (2003). Long-term outcome after poliomyelitis in different health and social conditions. *J Epidemiol Commun Health*, **57**(5), 368–372.

Rich, M.M., Teener, J.W. and Bird, S.J. (1997). Treatment of Lambert–Eaton syndrome with intravenous immunoglobulin. *Muscle Nerve*, **20**(5), 614–615.

Robinson, D., Galasko, C.S., Delaney, C., Williamson, J.B. and Barrie, J.L. (1995). Scoliosis and lung function in spinal muscular atrophy. *Eur Spine J*, **4**(5), 268–273.

Ropper, A.H. (1986). Severe acute Guillain–Barre syndrome. *Neurology*, **36**(3), 429–432.

Russman, B.S., Iannaccone, S.T. and Samaha, F.J. (2003). A phase 1 trial of riluzole in spinal muscular atrophy. *Arch Neurol*, **60**(11), 1601–1603.

Said, G. (2002). Chronic inflammatory demyelinative polyneuropathy. *J Neurol*, **249**(3), 245–253.

Sanders, D.B. (2003). Lambert–eaton myasthenic syndrome: diagnosis and treatment. *Ann N Y Acad Sci*, **998**, 500–508.

Saperstein, D.S., Katz, J.S., Amato, A.A. and Barohn, R.J. (2001). Clinical spectrum of chronic acquired demyelinating polyneuropathies. *Muscle Nerve*, **24**(3), 311–324.

Sarada, C., Tharakan, J.K. and Nair, M. (1994). Guillain–Barre syndrome: a prospective clinical study in 25 children and comparison with adults. *Ann Trop Paediatr*, **14**(4), 281–286.

Schanke, A.K., Lobben, B. and Oyhaugen, S. (1999). The Norwegian Polio Study 1994 part II: early experiences of polio and later psychosocial well-being. *Spinal Cord*, **37**(7), 515–521.

Sghirlanzoni, A., Solari, A., Ciano, C., Mariotti, C., Fallica, E. and Pareyson, D. (2000). Chronic inflammatory demyelinating polyradiculoneuropathy: long-term course and treatment of 60 patients. *Neurol Sci*, **21**(**1**), 31–37.

Shibata, M., Abe, K., Jimbo, A., Shimizu, T., Mihara, M., Sadahiro, S., Yoshikawa, H. and Mashimo, T. (2003). Complex regional pain syndrome type I associated with amyotrophic lateral sclerosis. *Clin J Pain*, **19**(**1**), 69–70.

Simmons, Z., Albers, J.W., Bromberg, M.B. and Feldman, E.L. (1995). Long-term follow-up of patients with chronic inflammatory demyelinating polyradiculoneuropathy, without and with monoclonal gammopathy. *Brain*, **118**, 359–368.

Simmons, Z., Bremer, B.A., Robbins, R.A., Walsh, S.M. and Fischer, S. (2000). Quality of life in ALS depends on factors other than strength and physical function. *Neurology*, **55**(**3**), 388–392.

Simpson, J.A. and Thomaides, T. (1987). Treatment of myasthenia gravis: an audit. *Q J Med*, **64**(**244**), 693–704.

Sommer, N., Melms, A., Weller, M. and Dichgans, J. (1993). Ocular myasthenia gravis: a critical review of clinical and pathophysiological aspects. *Doc Ophthalmol*, **84**(**4**), 309–333.

Spector, S.A., Gordon, P.L., Feuerstein, I.M., Sivakumar, K., Hurley, B.F. and Dalakas, M.C. (1996). Strength gains without muscle injury after strength training in patients with post-polio muscular atrophy. *Muscle Nerve*, **19**(**10**), 1282–1290.

Steffensen, B.F., Lyager, S., Werge, B., Rahbek, J. and Mattsson, E. (2002). Physical capacity in non-ambulatory people with Duchenne muscular dystrophy or spinal muscular atrophy: a longitudinal study. *Dev Med Child Neurol*, **44**(**9**), 623–632.

Strong, M. and Rosenfeld, J. (2003). Amyotrophic lateral sclerosis: a review of current concepts. *Amyotroph Lateral Scler Other Motor Neuron Disord*, **4**(**3**), 136–143.

Strumse, Y.A., Stanghelle, J.K., Utne, L., Utne, P. and Svendsby, E.K. (2003). Treatment of patients with postpolio syndrome in a warm climate. *Disabil Rehabil*, **25**(**2**), 77–84.

Sumner, C.J., Sheth, S., Griffin, J.W., Cornblath, D.R. and Polydefkis, M. (2003). The spectrum of neuropathy in diabetes and impaired glucose tolerance. *Neurology*, **60**(**1**), 108–111.

Sunnerhagen, K.S. and Grimby, G. (2001). Muscular effects in late polio. *Acta Physiol Scand*, **171**(**3**), 335–340.

Tan, M. and Tan, U. (2003). Early diagnosis of diabetic neuropathy using double-shock stimulation of peripheral nerves. *Clin Neurophysiol*, **114**(**8**), 1419–1422.

Thoren-Jonsson, A.L. and Grimby, G. (2001). Ability and perceived difficulty in daily activities in people with poliomyelitis sequelae. *J Rehabil Med*, **33**(**1**), 4–11.

Trail, M., Nelson, N., Van, J.N., Appel, S.H. and Lai, E.C. (2001). Wheelchair use by patients with amyotrophic lateral sclerosis: a survey of user characteristics and selection preferences. *Arch Phys Med Rehabil*, **82**(**1**), 98–102.

Traynor, B.J., Alexander, M., Corr, B., Frost, E. and Hardiman, O. (2003). Effect of a multidisciplinary amyotrophic lateral

sclerosis (ALS) clinic on ALS survival: a population based study, 1996–2000. *J Neurol Neurosurg Psychiatr*, **74**(**9**), 1258–1261.

Trojan, D.A. and Cashman, N.R. (1995). Fibromyalgia is common in a postpoliomyelitis clinic. *Arch Neurol*, **52**(**6**), 620–624.

van den Berg, J.P., Kalmijn, S., Lindeman, E., Wokke, J.H. and van den Berg, L.H. (2003). Rehabilitation care for patients with ALS in The Netherlands. *Amyotroph Lateral Scler Other Motor Neuron Disord*, **4**(**3**), 186–190.

van der Meche, F.G., van Doorn, P.A., Meulstee, J. and Jennekens, F.G. (2001). Diagnostic and classification criteria for the Guillain–Barre syndrome. *Eur Neurol*, **45**(**3**), 133–139.

van Dijk, G.W., Notermans, N.C., Franssen, H. and Wokke, J.H. (1999). Development of weakness in patients with chronic inflammatory demyelinating polyneuropathy and only sensory symptoms at presentation: a long-term follow-up study. *J Neurol*, **246**(**12**), 1134–1139.

van Koningsveld, R., van Doorn, P.A., Schmitz, P.I., Ang, C.W. and van der Meche, F.G. (2000). Mild forms of Guillain–Barre syndrome in an epidemiologic survey in The Netherlands. *Neurology*, **54**(**3**), 620–625.

van Koningsveld, R., Schmitz, P.I., Meche, F.G., Visser, L.H., Meulstee, J. and van Doorn, P.A. (2004). Effect of methylprednisolone when added to standard treatment with intravenous immunoglobulin for Guillain–Barre syndrome: randomised trial. *Lancet*, **363**(**9404**), 192–196.

van Schaik, I.N., Winer, J.B. De Haan, R. and Vermeulen, M. (2002). Intravenous immunoglobulin for chronic inflammatory demyelinating polyradiculoneuropathy. *Cochrane Database Syst Rev*, (**2**), CD001797.

Vasiliadis, H.M., Collet, J.P., Shapiro, S., Venturini, A. and Trojan, D.A. (2002). Predictive factors and correlates for pain in postpoliomyelitis syndrome patients. *Arch Phys Med Rehabil*, **83**(**8**), 1109–1115.

Verghese, J., Bieri, P.L., Gellido, C., Schaumburg, H.H. and Herskovitz, S. (2001). Peripheral neuropathy in young–old and old–old patients. *Muscle Nerve*, **24**(**11**), 1476–1481.

Vermeulen, M. and van Oers, M.H. (2002). Successful autologous stem cell transplantation in a patient with chronic inflammatory demyelinating polyneuropathy. *J Neurol Neurosurg Psychiatr*, **72**(**1**), 127–128.

Verstappen, C.C., Heimans, J.J., Hoekman, K. and Postma, T.J. (2003). Neurotoxic complications of chemotherapy in patients with cancer: clinical signs and optimal management. *Drugs*, **63**(**15**), 1549–1563.

Walk, D., Li, L.Y., Parry, G.J. and Day, J.W. (2004). Rapid resolution of quadriplegic CIDP by combined plasmapheresis and IVIg. *Neurology*, **62**(**1**), 155–156.

Weinberg, J., Borg, J., Bevegard, S. and Sinderby, C. (1999). Respiratory response to exercise in postpolio patients with severe inspiratory muscle dysfunction. *Arch Phys Med Rehabil*, **80**(**9**), 1095–1100.

White, C., Pritchard, J. and Turner-Stokes, L. (2004). Exercise for people with peripheral neuropathy. *Cochrane Database Syst Rev*, (**4**), CD003904.

Widar, M. and Ahlstrom, G. (1999). Pain in persons with postpolio. The Swedish version of the multidimensional pain inventory (MPI). *Scand J Caring Sci*, **13**(**1**), 33–40.

Wijdicks, E.F. and Fulgham, J.R. (1994). Failure of high dose intravenous immunoglobulins to alter the clinical course of critical illness polyneuropathy. *Muscle Nerve*, **17**(**12**), 1494–1495.

Willen, C. and Grimby, G. (1998). Pain, physical activity, and disability in individuals with late effects of polio. *Arch Phys Med Rehabil*, **79**(**8**), 915–919.

Willen, C., Sunnerhagen, K.S. and Grimby, G. (2001). Dynamic water exercise in individuals with late poliomyelitis. *Arch Phys Med Rehabil*, **82**(**1**), 66–72.

Willig, T.N., Paulus, J., Lacau Saint Guily, J., Beon, C. and Navarro, J. (1994). Swallowing problems in neuromuscular disorders. *Arch Phys Med Rehabil*, **75**(**11**), 1175–1181.

Wirth, B. (2000). An update of the mutation spectrum of the survival motor neuron gene (SMN1) in autosomal recessive spinal muscular atrophy (SMA). *Hum Mutat*, **15**(**3**), 228–237.

Zapp, J.J. (1996). Post-poliomyelitis pain treated with gabapentin. *Am Fam Physician*, **53**(**8**), 2442, 2445.

Zerres, K., Wirth, B. and Rudnik-Schoneborn, S. (1997). Spinal muscular atrophy–clinical and genetic correlations. *Neuromusc Disord*, **7**(**3**), 202–207.

List of abbreviations

AChR	Acetylcholine receptor
ALS	Amyotrophic lateral sclerosis
CIDP	Chronic inflammatory demyelinating polyneuropathy
CIP	Critical ill polyneuropathy
GBS	Guillain–Barré syndrome
IVIG	Intravenous immunoglobulins
LEMS	Lambert–Eaton myasthenic syndrome
PEG	Percutaneous endoscopic gastrotomy
SIRS	Systemic inflammatory response syndrome
SMA	Spinal muscular atrophy

Muscular dystrophy and other myopathies

James S. Lieberman and Nancy E. Strauss

Department of Rehabilitation Medicine, Columbia University College of Physicians and Surgeons, New York, USA

The Rehabilitation needs of patients with skeletal muscle disease demand a rehabilitation treatment plan that is thoughtful, creative and unique to the needs of the individual patient.

41.1 Definition of myopathy and dystrophy

Although often used interchangeably, it is important to differentiate "myopathy" from "dystrophy". Myopathy refers to any disorder (acquired or congenital/inherited) that can be attributed to pathological, biochemical or electrical changes occurring in muscle fibers or in the interstitial tissue of voluntary musculature, and in which there is no evidence that such changes are due to nervous system dysfunction (Walton and Gardner-Medwin, 1974). The term myopathy (other than the rapidly progressive dystrophies or polymyositis) usually implies a slowly progressive or non-progressive disorder of muscle function. Dystrophy, on the other hand refers to a congenital or inherited disorder of muscle characterized by progressive degeneration of skeletal muscle fibers with weakness and atrophy resulting from a rate of degeneration which outpaces regeneration. The dystrophic process eventually leads to connective tissue replacement of muscle fibers (Harper, 2002). Many of the dystrophies have associated features that are not a result of the muscle weakness. An example of this is Myotonic Dystrophy, which is a systemic disorder affecting multiple organ systems. Dystrophies are genetically transmitted and to date have no known cure. However, research developments continue and rehabilitation intervention resources are vast.

41.2 Classifications of muscle diseases

Various classification systems have been used to categorize the large number of known muscle diseases. Examples of classification systems are by age of onset, inheritance pattern, physiological process, severity, and rate of progression.

A new system of classification was recently proposed (Brooke, 2001). This system is based on proteins or protein abnormalities, each of which is governed by one or several genes, and each is a component mechanism of the muscle "machine". These proteins are grouped according to their role in the contractile mechanism. Muscle diseases with a known protein/molecular defect fall under one of the categories. Conditions for which a gene but not a gene product is identified are listed by chromosome involved.

In rehabilitation, the best way to group myopathic diseases is by functional limitation. However, because there can be a large variability of disease expression within the patient population of each disease, as well as changes in function as the disease progresses, classifying muscle disease in this way is not always practical, and really applies only to rehabilitation. A more useful rehabilitation classification is by functional stage. This classification is (1) ambulatory stage

(2) wheelchair-dependent stage, and (3) stage of prolonged survival (Bach and Lieberman, 1993).

41.3 The rehabilitation approach

Function

Assessing function is a complex, yet essential component in the evaluation of any patient. In order to assess function adequately, the clinician must understand the functional demands of the individual patient relative to their particular lifestyle. The myopathic patient may have a functional disability as a result of decrease in strength and endurance, orthopedic deformity, cardiopulmonary dysfunction and/or cognitive impairment.

Strength and endurance

Muscle strength is decreased in the muscles significantly affected by a muscle disease. Usually, in myopathic disorders, muscle weakness is most pronounced in the proximal musculature. The reverse is true for neuropathies, where weakness is most pronounced in distal musculature (Hilton-Jones and Kissel, 2001; Kitirji, 2002). However, there are distal myopathies and proximal neuropathies. Whether muscle weakness has an effect on function will be dependent on the magnitude of the weakness, distribution of the weakness, and amount of strength required for a functional task.

Endurance limitations resulting from muscle disease depend upon the functional reserve that every individual has for a given activity or task. Determining the amount of endurance required to complete a given task will aid in determining if the endurance limitation is such that task completion is (a) still possible independently; (b) possible but only with more time given to complete it; (c) possible, but only with assistance; or (d) not possible at all. Even if independent task completion is still possible, patients will often choose dependence if it means not using up their functional reserve. Energy conservation becomes essential.

Orthopedic deformity

All muscles do not weaken at the same rate or to the same degree. Therefore, muscle imbalance results from this variability in weakness. Muscle imbalance surrounding a joint causes joint contracture with resulting limitation in passive range of motion that leads to orthopedic deformity. Weakness of muscles that cross more than one joint are more apt to cause contracture. When the lower extremity weight bearing joints of the body are affected by contracture, abnormal body alignment occurs, changing the center of gravity, which can limit or arrest standing and ambulation (Johnson et al., 1992).

Upper extremity functional limitations are primarily due to proximal muscle weakness and contractures are not as prominent as in the lower extremities. Orthopedic deformity of the spine, such as scoliosis, can result in restriction of pulmonary function, impaired sitting balance and cosmetic deformity.

Cardiopulmonary dysfunction

With weakness of muscles of respiration, a restrictive pulmonary pattern on pulmonary function testing develops. This can be further affected by scoliosis when the spinal deformity is in the thoracic region, thus further restricting vital capacity. Limited endurance, fatigue, and poor concentration are among the negative effects of restrictive pulmonary disease. Limited functional reserve can result, leading to further disability. Cardiac involvement is a feature of a number of the myopathies and dystrophies and can ultimately result in cardiomyopathy with conduction abnormalities, heart failure with decreased functional reserve, and ultimately death (Melacini et al., 1996; Hilton-Jones and Kissel, 2001; Meola et al., 2001).

Cognitive dysfunction

Although most myopathic patients have no associated cognitive impairment, it is a feature of a number of muscle diseases (Polakoff et.al., 1998; Hilton-Jones and Kissel, 2001). Cognitive dysfunction has marked deleterious effects on every aspect of the individual's life. Rehabilitation interventions can be very successful in minimizing disability with respect to physical impairment; however, the compensatory techniques for impaired cognition are limited. Therefore, patients with cognitive dysfunction often become severely disabled and handicapped.

In addition, patients with severe physical limitations may have secondary emotional and psychological challenges as a result of their disability. An increased prevalence of depressive disorders in patients with dystrophic disorders has been identified (Fitzpatrick et al., 1986). Learning of the diagnosis of an incurable, hereditary, progressive disease causes feelings of sadness, hope that the diagnosis is wrong and worry about passing it on to future generations (Natterlund et al., 2001). Clinicians must be sensitive to this, utilizing preventive measures, such as support groups, appropriate recreational activities, as well as early detection and proper treatment.

Disease progression

Myopathic disorders may be non-progressive, slowly progressive or rapidly progressive. The rehabilitation program and goals are different for each type of disease.

The Rehabilitation program

The main goals of a rehabilitation program in the myopathic patient are to gain, maintain or restore functional independence. Many methods are used by rehabilitation professionals to score or measure levels of independence (Rosenfeld and Jackson, 2002). Independence can pertain to an activity or task, a form of mobility or overall independence of daily living. The assessment is, therefore, complex in the myopathic patient. For example, a patient with proximal muscle weakness may be an independent, safe ambulator on level surfaces, but be unable to ascend a small curb without assistance. Similarly a patient who may be independent in wheelchair mobility and all aspects of their vocational activities in a wheelchair accessible office, might be unable to transfer from the wheelchair to a toilet independently.

Factors that must be considered when determining whether independence is practical (functional and safe) for a given task or activity include the following:

Safety: For example, a patient with proximal muscle weakness may be independent crossing a street, walking at their maximal speed, but may not be able to cross the street before the light changes due to their maximal speed which is slower than that of a normal individual.

Energy Expenditure: A patient with proximal muscle weakness may be independent ascending a flight of stairs, using bilateral handrails, but may be exhausted when they reach the top. Similarly, a patient with Duchenne's Dystrophy may require such a large energy expenditure to ambulate that they are more functional in a wheelchair.

Architectural Barriers: A patient living in an apartment building may be independent entering their building through a ramped service entrance at the back of their building, far from the elevator, but may or may not be able to independently enter the main entrance of their building because of stairs, and lack of a ramp.

Ability to modify the activity or provide assistance: If an activity is not possible independently because of muscle weakness, decreased endurance, or the use of an assistive device, then the clinician must explore the feasibility of modifying the activity, using an assistive device(s) to aid in performing the activity if the patient does not use one already, modifying the environment, or providing the assistance of another person in order to allow the activity to be successfully completed.

Finally the *monetary cost* of the above options must be considered when determining if they are practical or feasible. Creativity is essential in exploring options, which can aid in assisting patients to achieve, maintain or restore their functional independence. Psychological and self-esteem issues are at the forefront of attempting to avoid dependence (Fardeau-Gautier and Fardeau, 1994).

Providing proper rehabilitation for a patient with a myopathic disorder begins with establishment of the correct diagnosis and the development of a rehabilitation plan. After the rehabilitation plan is developed, it is necessary to inform and educate the patient, their family, their caregivers and their primary care physicians about the correct diagnosis and the proper rehabilitation program.

It is also critical, after the diagnosis is made, that the rehabilitation professionals provide the patient, their family or caregivers and the primary care physician with appropriate education (Galloway et al., 2003) about the specific condition. The patient will ultimately become the expert in their own condition, but until that point is reached, the patient must be educated so that they can gain some control over a condition where they feel they are losing control. In addition, it is necessary to educate school staff, (Kinnealey and Morse, 1979) employers (Fowler et al., 1997) or anyone with a direct relationship with the patient about how the disability may have an effect. The patient's primary physician as well as the rehabilitation team, must be proactive so that they can be helpful in preventing conditions such as cardiopulmonary dysfunction (Muntoni, 2003) in which the patient with a muscle disease may be susceptible. It is recommended that patients with a muscle disease wear Medical Alert identification so that if they are injured and unable to communicate their condition in an emergency situation, the information that they have such a disease is available to the medical personnel caring for the patient in the emergency situation.

With information access advances through computer use and the Internet, patients have a virtually limitless amount of information. The clinician should help them find accurate and appropriate information, instead of inaccurate information, which may be detrimental to the patient. Table 41.1 lists useful websites which are commonly used by both professionals and patients who are acquiring information about muscle diseases in general, and their disease in particular.

Basic Principles in caring for a patient with a muscle disease

1 Most of the muscle diseases have a relatively predictable course with respect to distribution of muscle weakness, progression of weakness,

Table 41.1. Information websites are an excellent resource for patients, families, caregivers and health professionals.

Name of organization	Website address
Muscular Dystrophy Association (MDA)	www.mdausa.org
Facioscapulohumeral Muscular Dystrophy Society, Inc. (FSHD society)	www.fshsociety.org
Myositis Association (TMA)	www.myositis.org
Malignant Hyperthermia Association of the United States	www.mhaus.org
National Organization of Rare Diseases (NORD)	www.rarediseases.org
National Rehabilitation Information Center	www.naric.com
Myasthenia Gravis Foundation of America (MGFA)	www.myasthenia.org
The Amyotrophic Lateral Sclerosis Association (ALSA)	www.alsa.org
Families of Spinal Muscular Atrophy	www.fsma.org
Post-Polio Health International	www.post-polio.org

development of skeletal deformities and impairment of mobility. By being knowledgeable about the disease course, the physician must, to the best of their ability anticipate the next stage of a disease and minimize or prevent complications (Dahlbom et al., 1999).

2 The primary treating physician must make all the appropriate referrals to necessary specialists. Disciplines with expertise applicable to the needs of patients with muscle disease include, but are not limited to, the following: Neurology, Physiatry, Orthopedics, Pulmonology, Cardiology, Nutrition, Genetic Counseling, Social Work, Physical Therapy, Occupational Therapy, Vocational Therapy, Speech Therapy, Respiratory Therapy, Psychology, Recreational Therapy, and Special Education.

3 Once the diagnosis of a muscle disease is established, the physician's responsibility is to ensure that the patient has the highest quality of rehabilitation care available for their condition. Rehabilitation management is at the forefront of the treatment plan.

4 Access and funding become important issues, especially in lifelong disabling conditions. The physician must be aware of what resources are available to each patient and make the proper referrals. Medical insurance companies must be educated to ensure that needed services are covered and are being provided and the physician must be a patient advocate in this situation.

5 Programs such as Early Intervention are excellent for infants and children (newborn to 3 years of age). They provide a wide range of services in the area of therapy when a disabling condition has already been identified. Programs for children from 3–5 years of age include specific school district services available through their Committee on Preschool Special Education. For children 5 years of age and above, there are programs provided by school districts through their Committee on Special Education which ensures that therapy services are provided to minimize any disability that may impact the child's educational experience. The Muscular Dystrophy Association (MDA) is an excellent resource to aid in funding for the diagnosis and treatment of individuals with a neuromuscular disorder. Bach surveyed MDA clinic directors in 220 MDA sponsored clinics. Bach received 167 responses and these responses demonstrate that the clinic directors employed a wide variety of approaches in their patient management (Bach and Chaudhry, 2000).

41.4 Rehabilitation management of patients with a muscle disease

The rehabilitation treatment plan utilizes a goal oriented approach in which objective and subjective measures determine if each goal has been met. Evaluations determining achievement occur at regular intervals so the decision to continue or modify a given rehabilitation plan can be made. The team approach is the basis of all rehabilitation. Team leadership as well as excellent communication between team members is essential to ensure that all members strive for common goals. Table 41.2 lists those

Table 42.2. Individuals who may impact the success of a rehabilitation program.

Patient
Family members
Caregiver/Aide/Personal attendant
Physician(s)*
Physical therapist*
Occupational therapist*
Speech therapist*
Orthotist
Durable medical equipment specialists
Seating specialist
Vocational counselor
Recreational therapist*
Social worker/service coordinator*
Psychologist*
Nurse*
Teacher/Principal/school staff
Employer
Muscular dystrophy association coordinator
Insurance company

The Basic Rehabilitation Team.

professionals who may impact the success of a rehabilitation program for an individual with a muscle disease. Ideally, frequent team meetings are held.

Factors impacting the success of a rehabilitation program

Table 41.3 lists several factors that have direct impact on whether or not a rehabilitation treatment program will be successful. It is imperative that each factor be addressed to ensure that the patient achieves maximum benefit from rehabilitation interventions.

Once the diagnosis is established, the rehabilitation team members are responsible for knowing the disease course and its intrinsic rate of progression, as well as specific disease variability so that the disease effects are anticipated and strategies for achieving reasonable goals can be formulated. For the more rapidly progressive and destructive muscle diseases, success is obviously more limited and goals are altered accordingly. The earlier the program is initiated, the more favorable the outcome, as there are

Table 41.3. Factors impacting the success of a rehabilitation program.

1   Disease course
2   Timing of initiation of rehabilitation program
3   Accessibility of treatment
4   Skill of the staff
5   Motivation of the patient
6   Cooperation of the patient
7   Persistence of the patient and the staff
8   Timing of treatment with respect to the patient's daily
       routine
9   Concurrent medical problems
10   Frequency and duration of the treatment sessions
11   Duration of rehabilitation management
12   Communication between treating clinicians
13   Financial resources available for treatments

still substantial number of trainable muscle fibers (Ansved, 2001).

Ideally the program must be accessible to the patient in a location where the process of transportation will not reduce the positive effects of the treatment. If a patient with a myopathic disorder consumes a significant amount of energy to reach the therapy location, then this will limit the amount of energy remaining for the session itself. Therapy sites to consider include: home-based therapy, hospital-based therapy, school-based therapy and center-based therapy.

The skill of the staff should be such that they are aware of the precautions applicable to this patient population. Avoiding overfatigue, limiting strengthening exercises to the sub-maximal level, being aware of the patterns of musculoskeletal contracture, being aware of bone integrity, and awareness of the patient's cardiopulmonary status, are among the many issues which the therapists must consider when developing their plan of treatment. It is best if the members of the rehabilitation team remain constant so that the entire group will become specialists in the myopathic disorders the group treats.

Patient participation is required for every form of exercise except for passive range of motion and maximally assisted standing. Motivation of the patient,

patient cooperation and patient participation is maximal when reasonably achievable goals, which are important to that patient, are set. Educating the patient on the benefits of exercise and making it pleasurable will help with motivation and inspirational books on physical fitness for the physically challenged may be useful (Simmons, 1986).

The therapy session should occur at a point during the day when it will not interfere with other daily activities and when the patient's endurance is such that they will get maximum benefit.

Concurrent medical problems will impact the patient's ability to exercise and must be adequately addressed. Interruption of the therapy program by intercurrent illness may result in a marked loss of function. Therefore, modifying the program, rather than stopping it, is preferred if at all possible.

The frequency of treatment sessions is determined based on need, availability, and accessibility. Ideally, exercises should be done on a daily basis. Training of family members to assist in a home exercise program and other therapy when therapy is not available is valuable. Most patients can independently participate in exercise with carryover from a prior therapy session. The duration of each session should permit maximal benefit without being excessive in length. The patient should not feel exhausted or experience soreness after therapy.

The physician's written therapy prescriptions should include all essential components including diagnosis, precautions, frequency, duration and goals. Concurrence between the physician and therapists is vital.

Financial resources and medical coverage must be explored so that funding does not become a limiting factor in the success of treatment. The rehabilitation treatment plan usually begins at the time of diagnosis and spans the entire life of the individual.

Goals of any rehabilitation program for a myopathic disease

1 *Preserve Strength and Endurance*: Muscle strength is maintained through frequent contractions, which must produce tension sufficient enough to

exercise the muscle. If tension exerted during exercise is less than 20% of maximal tension, then the muscle loses strength. In our opinion, it imperative that the exercise program in patients with a myopathy must remain sub-maximal although they must exert tension greater than 20% of muscle maximum strength. Lack of physical activity will result in deconditioning of the neuromuscular system, which will have marked deleterious effects in a myopathic patient, whose functional reserve is reduced even at baseline. Disuse atrophy may lead to joint malposition, nerve compression and pain. The best way of preserving strength in a patient with muscle disease is through performance of daily physical activity.

2 *Improve Strength and Endurance*: Sub-maximal exercise programs in patients with muscle disease have been shown to increase strength and endurance (de Lateur and Giaconi, 1979; Hagberg et al., 1980; Bar-Or, 1996; Phillips and Mastaglia, 2000) if properly supervised, avoiding overwork weakness. The positive result of strength increases will carry over to improvement in the patient's mobility, self-care and psychological well being.

3 *Minimize and Prevent Joint Contractures*: Muscle weakness and imbalance result in bony malalignment and contracture. In the myopathic patient, this is more evident in the larger joints of the body, which are needed for weight bearing and the upright posture. Contracture can be the cause of cessation of standing and ambulation, the cause of pain, the cause of skin breakdown, and the cause of cosmetic deformity.

4 *Permit Weight Bearing*: Functional weight bearing is critical to maintaining the muscle disease patient's general health and requires a stable base of support and effective joint alignment. In patients with significant muscle weakness, this goal is often achieved by the use of external supports, such as orthoses, proper footwear (Strauss and Angell, 2001), assistive devices for standing and gait aids.

5 *Prolong Standing/Walking*: The positive effects of standing and upright mobility involve multiple organ systems, such as the genitourinary, digestive, respiratory, cardiac, skeletal, and neuromuscular systems as well as psychological function. A recent study questioned families attending neuromuscular clinics regarding quality of life and found that 89% named activities and health issues related to prolonging ambulation as most important to them (Bothwell et al., 2002). However, the patients (especially in Duchenne's Dystrophy) often prefer to go into a wheelchair because of the high energy costs of ambulation compared to the energy costs of using the wheelchair (Gardner-Medwin, 1979). The opposite view is taken by some experts (Siegal, 1978; Vignos et al., 1996). In our clinics, we attempt to prolong standing and ambulation, as long as it does not impair the patient's safety or require too much use of their energy for their function.

6 *Maximize functional mobility*: To maximize functional mobility, assistive devices and gait aids are used as needed. An understanding of biomechanics is essential to determine which external devices, if any, will assist a patient. For example, a child with Duchenne's muscular dystrophy may be ambulating independently with difficulty. Toe walking, which results from gastrocsoleus contracture, may enable the patient to walk by increasing the knee extension moment and preventing knee collapse. Hyperlordosis, which is compensating for the weak hip extensors, is assisting in keeping the patient upright. Bracing the child and restoring what appears to be proper alignment may actually deprive the patient of compensatory mechanisms and arrest their ambulation. Devices that require upper extremity strength such as crutches, canes and walkers, may not be useful because of weakness of the proximal shoulder girdle region. Mobility aids, such as wheelchairs and scooters, can be liberating and a relief for the patient who is exhausted from walking (Wagner and Katirji, 2002).

7 *Maximize independence for activities of daily living*: When weakness is such that independence in activities of daily living becomes difficult or impossible, creative restructuring of the task with appropriate assistive devices is required.

8 *Minimize the Deleterious Effects of Deconditioning*: Since deconditioning affects multiple organ

systems, the treatment plan must incorporate strategies to minimize its deleterious effects.

41.5 Rehabilitation interventions

The spectrum of rehabilitation interventions for the patient with muscle disease may include exercise and assistive devices.

1 *Exercise*: Exercise is defined as performance of physical exertion for improvement of health or correction of deformity. In the patient with a myopathic disorder, exercises must remain sub-maximal as stressed above.

(a) Strengthening: The effects of strengthening exercises on patients with muscle disease has been well studied. Numerous reports in the literature exist.

A recent study compared published studies of strengthening exercises and endurance training in patients with neuromuscular diseases with respect to age, study design, duration, outcome measures, intervention, and results. The consensus was that supervised sub-maximal resistive exercise programs in selected patients resulted in increased muscle strength without causing overwork weakness, with strength gains in muscles that are not severely dystrophic. In addition moderate intensity aerobic exercises may improve cardiovascular performance (de Lateur and Giaconi, 1979; Wagner and Katirji, 2002). On the other hand high intensity eccentric muscle contractions cause increased serum Creatine Kinase (CK) levels and muscle soreness (Kilmer et al., 2001) and should be used with caution. However, a study of high resistive weight training in patients with slowly progressive or non-progressive muscle disorders revealed a significant increase in muscle performance if the initial muscle strength is greater than 15% of normal (Milner-Brown and Miller, 1988a). Finally, electrical stimulation in combination with voluntary contraction may be a useful modality for strengthening (Milner-Brown and Miller, 1988b; Scott et al., 1990; Zupan et al., 1993).

(b) Range of motion: Range of motion exercises can be passive, active or active assistive in type. Stretching exercises are mandatory for prevention and slowing of contracture progression. Botulium A toxin may have a role in contracture management. For example it was reported that Botulium A Toxin injection into the medial and lateral hamstrings improved a knee contracture in a patient with Duchenne Muscular Dystrophy (von Wendt and Autti-Ramo, 1999). In addition, seating system design should consider range of motion and contracture prevention (Wong and Wade, 1995). Gains in range of motion from the use of orthoses and passive stretching can be lost if it is inconsistent or done in the absence of professional supervision (Seeger et al., 1985).

(c) Balance: Patients with myopathy are consciously aware of their balance as they strive to keep upright and avoid falls. Patients with lower extremity and trunk proximal muscle weakness often use their arm swing while walking to place their arms in a position that will aid the patient in shifting their center of gravity to avoid falling. This is similar to how an acrobat on a tightrope uses a stick. By placing their arms behind them, the patient will pull their center of gravity posteriorly (along with their hyperlordotic posture) to avoid falling forward. Adequate strength, range of motion and alignment are required for balance. Exercises to improve the efficacy and safety of balance are an important part of the exercise regimen.

Standing balance can be challenged by obstructions on the ground, windy weather conditions and carrying items all of which shift the center of gravity and may result in loss of balance. Scanning the ground, practicing balance on uneven terrain and challenging dynamic standing balance are strategies utilized by the therapist.

2) *Assistive devices*: Assistive devices provide external support to aid in the compensation for weak muscles.

(a) Proper footwear: Commonly, a physician will prescribe a pair of shoes, which provides stability, support and alignment only to find that the patient comes to the next appointment wearing a pair of inexpensive, thin, flexible, lightweight shoes. Patients self-select walking shoes to meet their own functional needs, often seeking the following features: (1) Lightweight, (2) Ability to facilitate sensory feedback (thin soled shoes allow more sensory input so the patient can detect subtle changes in terrain in order to correct posture and prevent falling), (3) Desirable coefficient of friction (soles with a higher coefficient of friction provide greater stability but may cause difficulty in advancing the foot; soles with a lower coefficient of friction make it easier to advance the foot, but increase the risk of sliding (Strauss and Angell, 2001).

(b) Orthoses: Chapter 12 of Volume II discusses limb orthotics. In the myopathic patient, the lightest weight orthosis is essential, (Taktak and Bowker, 1995) so that it is not too heavy for the myopathic patient's weak muscles to carry. When a new lower extremity orthosis is introduced, the patient must accommodate to the change in joint position. It is advantageous to try a prefabricated orthosis prior to the fabrication of a custom made orthosis so that a determination of the potential usefulness can be made. Even a perfectly fitting orthosis which provides perfect joint alignment will be abandoned by the patient if it is too heavy, too difficult to don and doff, cosmetically unappealing, or restrictive.

(c) Standing devices: Standing devices are excellent for the pediatric population by allowing interaction at eye level with peers and enjoyment of activities in a standing position while permitting weight bearing. Ankle, knee, hip and trunk support permit their use in patients with marked muscle weakness. Severe equinovarus, or knee and hip flexion contractures may limit or preclude their use. A limitation with adolescents and adults is difficulty in putting the patient in the device as it may take two strong adults to lift a large patient into the standing position.

(d) Gait aids: Canes, crutches and walkers require upper extremity strength sufficient to give support and to allow the patient to advance the device forward. In patients who are able to ambulate safely without a gait aid, the preference is to avoid using it so that they do not become too dependent on the device and subsequently lose their ability to ambulate without it. Patients who are independent on level indoor surfaces may require gait aids solely for outdoor and community ambulation.

(e) Wheelchairs/scooters: Wheelchairs and scooters are devices which can restore independence to patients who are too weak to ambulate safely or comfortably. The term "wheelchair bound" should be avoided as the connotation is negative and confining. Deciding when to order a wheelchair for a patient with muscular dystrophy is difficult as there is no "clear cut time" when it is medically indicated. Our clinic attempts to have the patient ambulate as long as possible so that the negative effects of prolonged sitting, including development of contractures, scoliosis, worsening of restrictive lung disease and deconditioning can be delayed. However, when ambulation becomes unsafe or too energy consumptive, the decision to order a manual versus electric wheelchair must be made. Cessation of walking in progressive diseases should be viewed as a process rather than an endpoint as there is usually transition time when the patient exhibits difficulty walking but does not use the wheelchair full-time. Introducing the concept of a wheelchair early is beneficial in allowing the patient and family more time to adjust (Miller, 1991). Factors to be considered in wheelchair prescription for the patient with a myopathic disease are listed on Table 41.4. Chapter 11 of Volume II discusses wheelchair prescription. Special attention to

Table 41.4. Factors to be considered in determining whether a motorized or a manual wheelchair will suit the patient's needs.

Factors	Manual	Motorized
Weight	Lighter	Heavier
Cost	Less expensive	More expensive
Transport	Easier to transport in car and stairs	More difficult to transport in car and stairs
Maintenance	Easier to maintain and repair	More difficult to maintain and repair
Energy requirement	Requires sufficient upper extremity strength	Requires minimal muscle activity
Exercise achieved with propulsion	Substantial exercise achieved with propulsion	Minimal exercise achieved using controls
Upper extremity overuse injuries developed with repetitive use	Common	Minimal
Cognitive function required for use	Must have adequate visual perception safety awareness	Must have excellent visual perceptual safety awareness
Pressure relief ability	Requires manual position change for pressure relief	Ability to add a tilt in space feature for skin pressure relief

truncal support must be made in this patient population. Children with a rapidly progressive myopathic disorder such as Duchenne's Dystrophy often prefer to go into a wheelchair before their parents are willing to consider this. (See above)

(f) Aids for daily living (ADL) assistive devices: Home adaptive equipment and ADL assistive devices are frequently used. The patient may use the problem-focused coping strategy of devices as well as tricks for better function (Natterlund and Ahlstrom, 1999) to maximize their independence in personal care. Mobile arm supports aid the patient with marked upper extremity weakness in tasks including feeding, driving a motorized wheelchair and performing leisure activities (Yasuda et al., 1986).

41.6 Features of specific disorders

Below is a brief description of selected muscle disorders. A more in-depth description can be found in any of the comprehensive text books dedicated to Neuromuscular Disorders. Rehabilitation strategies are dictated by functional impairment rather than being disease specific (Figure 41.1). There is a large overlap among the rehabilitation of the different disease entities, variability within individuals with the same disease, and variability of impairment throughout the course of each disease.

The dystrophies

Duchenne's muscular dystrophy (Pseudohypertrophic muscular dystrophy)

Duchenne Muscular Dystrophy was the first well characterized dystrophy with historical roots traced back to the 1800's (Tyler, 2003). This X-linked recessive disease is usually identified by age 3 or 4 when gross motor development appears abnormal. Difficulties include problems in running, arising from the floor, climbing stairs and jumping. The characteristic posture of lumbar hyperlordosis, genu recarvatum and toe walking, along with pseudohypertophy of the calf muscles and sometimes the quadriceps and deltoids are characteristic features. With progression of the weakness, the waddling gait becomes inefficient and unsafe, and falls occur frequently. When wheelchair ambulation is chosen (usually at approximately age 12) as a safe form of mobility, contractures begin to progress, especially equinovarus (Figure 41.2), knee flexion, hip flexion, elbow flexion and kyphoscoliosis. Restrictive pulmonary function secondary to weak respiratory muscles is worsened by scoliosis (Figure 41.3).

Although weakness begins primarily in the proximal muscles, it eventually may include all skeletal muscles, but spares extraocular muscles. Associated features

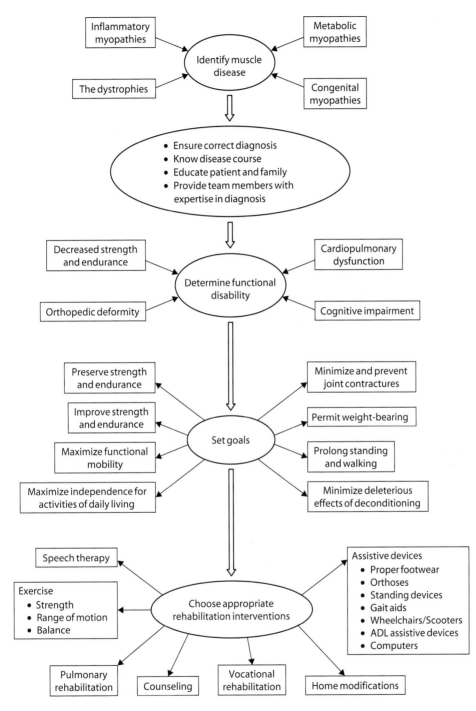

Figure 41.1. Steps in providing appropriate rehabilitation interventions for patients with Muscle Disease.

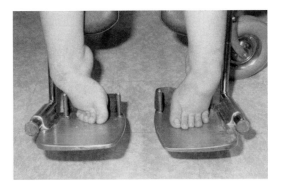

Figure 41.2. An example of equinovarus in a patient with Duchenne's muscular dystrophy.

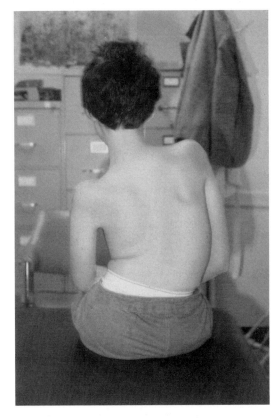

Figure 41.3. An example of scoliosis in a patient with Duchenne's muscular dystrophy.

include an intelligence quotient (IQ) score below the normal population (al-Qudah et al., 1990) and cardiac abnormalities (Oguz et al., 2000; Finsterer and Stollberger, 2003). Lower extremity contracture release

surgery is recommended by some authorities when the ambulatory patient is at risk of losing ambulation due to contractures, but has enough strength and endurance to maintain ambulation with long leg braces if contractures are released. If surgery is performed it is essential to have the patient stand as quickly as possible postoperatively and to limit bedrest. If proper postoperative bracing is not initiated, the contracture will redevelop rapidly. Bracing and surgery are controversial, however and other authorities do not advocate this intervention (see above). Scoliosis surgery is considered and should be performed at a time when pulmonary function tests are favorable enough to tolerate the procedure. Some authorities prefer the use of a body jacket for the scoliosis. The value of non-invasive ventilatory support is clear in reducing the respiratory impairment consequences of inadequate ventilation and secretion clearance (Filart and Bach, 2003). The use of inspiratory and expiratory aids have been shown to prolong survival while decreasing pulmonary morbidity rates (Bach et al., 1997). Mechanical ventilator dependency as an option to extend life requires careful decision making by the patient and their family in concert with their physician (Gilgoff et al., 1989; Miller et al., 1990).

The predictable progressive course of the disease, causing death, secondary to respiratory complications at a young age, usually between age 20 and 25, (Raphael et al., 1994) makes it one of the most studied conditions in which researchers are searching for a cure.

Beckers muscular dystrophy

This X linked recessive dystrophy resembles Duchenne Dystrophy but is more slowly progressive with onset later and survival into mid adult life (McDonald et al., 1995; Ishpekova et al., 1999). Patients are usually walking until approximately age 16 or longer.

Fascioscapulohumeral dystrophy

This slowly progressive autosomal dominant disease mainly affects muscles of the face, shoulders and arms. There is variability with respect to age of onset

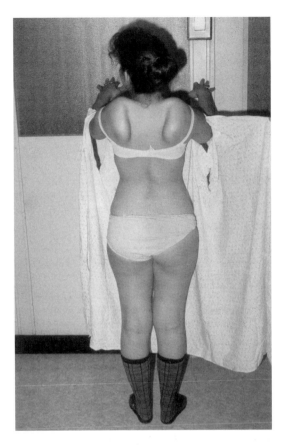

Figure 41.4. An example of shoulder girdle atrophy and scapular winging in a patient with Fascioscapulohumeral dystrophy.

and severity (Kilmer et al., 1995). Distribution of muscle weakness is usually asymmetric and spreads slowly to the hips and lower extremities. The onset of weakness is usually noticed during the end of the first decade and beginning of the second decade with overall progression taking place over several decades with periods of more rapid deterioration. Characteristic physical examination findings parallel the distribution of muscle weakness and include loss of scapular fixation (scapular winging) (Figure 41.4) and inability to abduct the arms. Surgical fixation of the scapula on the thoracic wall may lead to functional improvement; however, potential surgical complications must be considered. (Twyman et al., 1996; Andrews et al., 1998; Mummery et al., 2003). Infantile fascioscapulohumeral dystrophy is usually identified within the first

2 years of life by the inability to smile or fully close the eyes during sleep. Severe progressive weakness causes a typical extreme hyperlordotic gait and usually leads to wheelchair ambulation during childhood. Nerve deafness is a common associated feature.

Emery–Dreifuss disease (Humeroperoneal muscular dystrophy)

This X linked recessive disorder involves slowly progressive wasting and weakness primarily in the scapulohumeraoperoneal distribution with associated contractures of elbows, posterior neck and Achilles tendons. Life threatening cardiac conduction abnormalities occur (Shapiro and Specht, 1991). Triceps and biceps weakness, with relative sparing of the deltoids, and ligamentous thickness are characteristic.

Scapulohumeral dystrophy

This condition, usually an autosomal dominant, presents similarly to fascioscapulohumeral dystrophy but the muscles involved early include those of the peroneal and anterior tibial groups as well as the upper extremity muscles (Brooke, 1986).

Hereditary distal myopathy

Distal muscle weakness, such as one would expect in a neuropathic condition, may, in fact, be secondary to a myopathic condition, and must be differentiated by careful diagnostic workup (Brooke, 1986).

Limb girdle dystrophy/Limb girdle syndrome

A group that share a similar clinical phenotype of progressive weakness of the hips and shoulder girdle, usually with onset in the second or third decade with clinical heterogeneity are characteristic features (McDonald et al., 1995; Bushby, 1999; Mathews and Moore, 2003).

Congenital muscular dystrophy

Manifesting in early life or infancy, it can occur with or without intellectual impairment or major structural brain abnormalities. Those with intellectual impairment or structural brain abnormalities are subdivided into two main entities: Fukuyama congenital myopathic dystrophy and Muscle eye brain syndrome (Tubridy et al., 2001).

The mytotonias

Myotonia, a phenomenon in which there is a delay of relaxation after muscle contraction, is a feature of several disorders. Myotonia can be elicited by voluntary contraction, percussion of muscle, or by electromyography (EMG) needle insertion. Characteristic electromyographic findings include trains of potentials whose amplitude and frequencies wax and wane. The abnormality which occurs at the sarcolemma membrane may have a circuitry abnormality involving other membranes.

Myotonic dystrophy

This autosomal dominant disorder (located on chromosome 19) is a systemic condition with progressive weakness and a primarily distal distribution, but spreading to involve all muscle groups, in adolescence or early childhood. The characteristic appearance is secondary to wasting of the sternocleidomastoid giving a "swan neck appearance," atrophy of the temporalis and masseter muscles, frontal balding, elongated facies, ptosis and general facial weakness. Mental retardation is common. Initially, patients may complain of muscle stiffness, cramping or weakness of the hand and feet. Cataracts, endocrine abnormalities, testicular atrophy and female reproductive abnormalities are features. Smooth muscle abnormalities, with secondary dysfunction of swallowing and pharyngeal musculature, cardiac abnormalities, including arrythmyias and respiratory abnormalities, also occur. When presenting during infancy, hypotonia and facial paralysis are features. Club foot is common. Transmission is from the mother (Brooke, 1986; Pelargonio et al., 2002).

Myotonia congenita (Thompsen's disease)

The common feature is muscle stiffness, especially prominent after resting, but loosening up with exercise. Muscle hypertrophy with well developed musculature is common (Brooke, 1986).

Paramyotonia congenita

Most commonly involving muscles of the face, forearm and hands, this disorder of muscle relaxation is worsened by cold exposure and by exercise (Brooke, 1986).

Inflammatory myopathies

Inflammatory processes due to bacteria, viruses, parasites, tuberculosis and sarcoidosis are among the etiologies of inflammatory muscle disease. Disturbances of the immune system can also be the culprit.

Dermatomyositis/polymyositis are acquired conditions with an acute or subacute course and onset at any age, often beginning with non-specific systemic complaints and may be preceded by infection, drug reaction or immunization. Proximal muscle weakness with frequent involvement of neck flexors and skin rash are characteristic of dermatomyositis. The skin changes can be quite marked, and thickened or atrophic and subcutaneous calcific nodules may be present. Since the rash does not accompany the proximal muscle weakness in polymyositis, it is more difficult to diagnose. Patients may complain of a deep aching in their muscles and muscles may be swollen and tender to palpation. The weakness spreads and can cause significant disability. Cardiac and respiratory involvement may occur. The course is variable. In addition, these disorders may be associated with collagen vascular diseases or with malignancy (Nelson, 1996).

Inclusion Body Myositis causes slowly progressive weakness of the limb girdle musculature as well as associated distal muscle weakness, with onset at any age.

Metabolic myopathies

Metabolic myopathies encompass a diverse group of disorders caused by defects in the biochemical pathways that produce adenosine triphosphate (ATP), the energy currency of the cell (Hirano and DiMauro, 2002). It is essential that the complex pathways of energy production occur reliably in order for muscles to contract properly and react to exercise appropriately. Flaws in the system may result in weakness, fatigue, cramping, myalgias, breakdown of muscle (rhabdomyolysis) or exercise intolerance. Numerous biochemical defects resulting in a wide variety of metabolic myopathies have been identified. Among the disease entities is McArdle's disease (myophosphorylase deficiency) with characteristic muscle cramps, exercise intolerance and myoglobinuria (Nelson, 1996).

Endocrine myopathies may be secondary to hypothyroidism, hyperthyroidism, parathyroid dysfunction, adrenal dysfunction or pituitary dysfunction. Correction of the underlying abnormality usually improves the myopathic symptoms. Nutritional and toxic myopathies add to the etiology of muscle pathology (Nelson, 1996).

The diverse mechanisms of myotoxity are dependent on the specific toxin and can effect muscle tissue directly (focally or generally) or indirectly (secondary toxic effect from subsequent electrolyte imbalance, immunological response or ishchemia) (Amato, 2002). Alcoholic myopathy is one of the most common (Preedy et al., 2001) and can occur either as an acute attack with muscle pain, swelling and weakness, or as a chronic, slowly progressive proximal myopathy.

Congenital myopathies

These relatively non-progressive muscle conditions present as a floppy infant and have a delay in motor milestones. Definitive diagnosis is made by muscle biopsy and the conditions are named according to their histopathological findings. Advances in immunohistochemistry and molecular genetics have led to a more accurate classification and differentiation within this heterogeneous group (Taratuto, 2002). Most congenital myopathies have a large variability in the degree of weakness and a number of individuals that have these disorders are never diagnosed.

Congenital fiber type disproportion

Associated clinical features may include muscle contractures, congenital hip dislocation, high arched palate, Kyphoscoliosis, foot deformities, slim build and short stature. The distribution of weakness is proximal greater than distal, with occasional mild facial weakness. This is most severe in the first 2 years of life and either improve or remain stable (Brooke, 1986).

Central core myopathy

Associated clinical features may include congenital hip dislocation, lordosis (Figure 41.5), kyphoscoliosis, hip deformities, slim build and short stature. The distribution of weakness is diffuse, but primarily proximal, with possible facial and neck muscle involvement. Malignant hyperthermia risk is associated as both conditions have been identified on the same chromosome (Quane et al., 1993).

Nemaline myopathy (Rod body disease)

Associated clinical findings may include a dysmorphic slender face, high arched palate, high arched feet, kyphoscoliosis and jaw malformation. The distribution of weakness is usually diffuse in limbs and trunk and may involve face and bulbar muscles, sparing eye muscles. It may also present later in life in a scapuloperoneal distribution of weakness. A more severe form of the disease involves weakness of respiratory muscles, diaphragm involvement and respiratory failure (Brooke, 1986; Ryan et al., 2001).

Myotubular myopathy (Centronuclear myopathy)

Associated clinical features may be ptosis, extraocular weakness, hip deformities and seizures. Weakness of

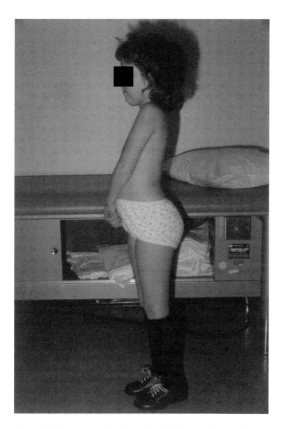

Figure 41.5. An example of hyperlordosis in a patient with a Congenital myopathy.

the facial, extraocular, limb and trunk muscles may be progressive (Brooke, 1986).

41.7 Concerns in the patient with a myopathic disorder

Surgical intervention

The decision to undergo elective surgery in the patient with a myopathic disorder is a difficult one. Thus, the risks and benefits must be carefully weighed. In order to minimize the deleterious effects of deconditioning, bed rest must be limited postoperatively. Proper therapy must be initiated immediately and patient should resume an active lifestyle as quickly as possible. When elective surgery is chosen as the best option for the myopathic patient, it should be done in a Center with muscle disease expertise.

Anesthesia issues

The anesthesiologist must be well aware of the condition of the neuromuscular system, pulmonary function and adverse anesthesia risks prior to determining the mode and type of anesthesia. The risks of malignant hyperthermia as well as other complications must be assessed and adequate precautions must be taken (Lang et al., 1989; Tung et al., 1989; Rittoo and Morris, 1995; Wu et al., 1998; Noordeen et al., 1999; Reid et al., 1999; Kleopa et al., 2000).

Risk versus benefit

Spinal deformity correction

Scoliosis surgery can limit progression of the curve, thus improving sitting balance, and preventing cosmetic deformity (Miller et al., 1991; Bridwell et al., 1999; McCarthy, 1999; Bentley et al., 2001; Berven and Bradford, 2002), and limiting the component of restrictive pulmonary dysfunction, which results from the thoracic rotation and rib cage restriction. In patients who depend on their truncal mobility for reaching or balancing, careful preoperative assessment must include the functional consequences of surgical correction. Orthotic management and seating system customization must also be considered.

Limb deformity correction

When a patient accommodates their balance and center of gravity to a particular deformity, when surgical correction occurs, the rehabilitation team cannot expect the patient to ambulate independently unless they are provided with the proper external support to allow them to learn new compensations. If an ambulatory patient with Duchenne Muscular Dystrophy has advancing lower extremity contractures that are limiting balance and safety, and lower extremity surgery is considered it must be combined with postoperative bracing, gait aids and aggressive physical therapy. Although the deformity can be corrected, the disease cannot; therefore, ambulation remains energy consumptive. The decision to undergo surgery for lower extremity contracture correction may allow ambulation to be prolonged (Bach and McKeon, 1991; Vignos et al., 1996 Forst and Forst, 1999). The overall importance of that to the child and their parents must be considered.

Weight control

Obesity is a growing health concern among today's population and has been studied in the muscular dystrophy population (Edwards et al., 1984; Goldstein et al., 1989; Hankard et al., 1996; Rudnik-Schoneborn et al., 1997; McCrory et al., 1998). In mobility impaired patients, even the slightest weight gain can have significant functional disadvantages. Weight gain, which results from increased caloric intake, decreased energy expenditure, medication side effects (e.g. steroids), edema or pregnancy (approximately 24–28 lbs increase) (Rogers and Matsumura, 1991) may cause the borderline ambulatory patient to cease walking secondary to increased load.

Furthermore, in obesity, pulmonary function changes exacerbate the ventilatory strain associated with exercise. The high metabolic cost of breathing reduces exercise tolerance thus increasing the imbalance between energy availability and expenditure (Hoffman and Gallagher, 2001).

Pregnancy

In addition to the mobility effects of weight gain, when pregnancy is an option in patients with muscle disease, other factors must be considered. (1) Genetic transmission of the disease. (2) Effect of pregnancy on the mother's health. (3) Anesthesia selection during delivery. (4) Mode of delivery. (5) Post-partum health and function of the mother. (6) Perinatal management of the infant. (7) Parenting issues involving strength and endurance. The rehabilitation team, along with the obstetrical team, are often successful in creating solutions to the challenges that arise. However, reports of obstetric complications in women with muscle disease (Nazir et al., 1984; Sun et al., 1985; Gamzu et al.,

2002) suggest that they should all be considered high-risk pregnancies.

When discussing parenting it is necessary to mention that fathers with disability secondary to a myopathic disease must also develop strategies to minimize the physical challenges of childcare. The father's *behavior* has more impact on the relationship between parent and child than does the father's physical *disability* (Buck, 1993).

Effects of deconditioning

The deleterious effects of immobility are discussed in Chapter 21 of Volume II. When muscle tissue is not used, the functional effects are significant. The effects of disuse atrophy must be considered for individual muscle groups as well as for the whole patient. If, for example, a limb is placed in an immobilization device for several hours each day, muscle contraction in the immobilized limb will be limited and weakened and atrophy will occur. The risks and benefits of bracing must be weighed and effects of immobilization must be considered. Night splints used for plantar flexion contracture, hip abduction braces used for hip dysplasia, and the Dennis Browne bar orthosis used for club foot may all be advantageous; however, muscle strength in the related muscle groups should be carefully followed. Isotonic strengthening exercises during times when the brace is off, as well as isometric exercises when the brace is on should be utilized.

Aging with a muscle disease

Normal aging of the neuromuscular system results from quantative as well as qualitive changes in both the peripheral nervous system and muscle itself. *Sarcopenia* refers to age-related changes of reduction in muscle mass reduced muscle strength and alterations in the quality of the remaining muscle tissue. A reduction in the number of functioning motor units with an increase in size of the remaining surviving units suggest cycles of denervation and reinervation from death of motor neurons or peripheral axonal damage (Lexell and Vandervoort, 2002). This cycle occurs in all individuals.

Loss of strength, in addition to other neuromuscular skeletal effects of aging, has negative effects on function (Fiatarone and Evans, 1993), which is especially debilitating in the patient with a myopathic disease. Because of biomechanical abnormalities, degenerative joint disease and overuse, injuries may be more common in patients with myopathic disease. Osteoporosis occurs more rapidly when disuse or decreased muscle force on the bone occurs. It is of utmost importance to listen carefully to our aging patients with muscle disease when they present to the physician with a new complaint. It is too common that their complaint is dismissed as "a symptom of their chronic condition" when it is, in fact, an unrelated symptom which warrants a very complete workup. For example, worsening gait in a patient with a myopathic disease may be from spinal stenosis, hip arthritis, new onset neuropathy or another cause that deserves treatment and can possibly be correctable. Moreover, malignancies of the neurological or skeletal system may present as back pain or weakness and should not be attributed simply to "aging of the patient with a myopathic disease".

41.8 Future research

Recent advances in genome mapping have led to the identification of genes responsible for specific disorders. Progress in the approaches of gene therapy, cell therapy and pharmacological therapy are applied to aid in attacking the problem of treating muscle disease (Chamberlain, 2002; Escolar et al., 2002; Matsuo, 2002; Perkins and Davies, 2002; Skuk et al., 2002).

Gene transfer studies utilizing vectors with dystrophin, utrophin and intergrin recombinant cDNA's continue to be studied and have been shown to prevent the development of muscular dystrophy in transgenic dystrophic mice (Wells and Wells, 2002).

The mechanism of booster genes is being investigated and may eventually lead to therapeutic drugs to provide a boost to degenerating dystrophyic muscle (Engvall and Wewer, 2003).

Myogenic stem cells from bone marrow (Ferrari and Mavilio, 2002) is yet another area with future promise.

Clinical trials using prednisone and other symptomatic pharmacological therapy continues. An important role in pharmacological research is the use of reliable animal models of human disease for preclinical trials to evaluate pharmacological potential (DeLuca et al., 2002).

REFERENCES

al-Qudah, A.A., Kobayashi, J., Chuang, S., Dennis, M. and Ray, P. (1990). Etiology of intellectual impairment in Duchenne muscular dystrophy. *Pediatr Neurol*, **6**, 57–59.

Amato, A. (2002). Endocrine myopathies and toxic myopathies. In: *Neuromuscular Function and Disease: Basic, Clinical, and Electrodiagnostic Aspects* (eds Brown, W.F., Bolton, C.F. and Aminoff, M.J.), Vol. 2, W.B. Saunders, New York, pp. 1399–1427.

Andrews, C.T., Taylor, T.C. and Patterson, V.H. (1998). Scapulo-thoracic arthrodesis for patients with facioscapulohumeral muscular dystrophy. *Neuromuscul Disord*, **8**, 580–584.

Ansved, T. (2001). Muscle training in muscular dystrophies. *Acta Physiol Scand*, **171**, 359–366.

Bach, J.R. and Chaudhry, S.S. (2000). Standards of care in MDA clinics. *Am J Phys Med Rehabil*, **79**, 193–196.

Bach, J.R. and Lieberman, J.S. (1993). Rehabilitation of the patient with disease affecting the motor neuron. In: *Rehabilitation Principles and Practice*, (eds DeLisa, J., Gans, B. Lippincott), 2nd edn, p. 1100.

Bach, J.R. and McKeon, J. (1991). Orthopedic surgery and rehabilitation for the prolongation of brace-free ambulation of patients with Duchenne muscular dystrophy. *Am J Phys Med Rehabil*, **70**, 323–331.

Bach, J.R., Ishikawa, Y. and Kim, H. (1997). Prevention of pulmonary morbidity for patients with Duchenne muscular dystrophy. *Chest*, **112**, 1024–1028.

Bar-Or, O. (1996). Role of exercise in the assessment and management of neuromuscular disease in children. *Med Sci Sport Exer*, **28**, 421–427.

Bentley, G., Haddad, F., Bull, T.M. and Seingry, D. (2001). The treatment of scoliosis in muscular dystrophy using modified Luque and Harrington-Luque instrumentation. *J Bone Joint Surg Br*, **83**, 22–28.

Berven, S. and Bradford, D.S. (2002). Neuromuscular scoliosis: causes of deformity and principles for evaluation and management. *Semin Neurol*, **22**, 167–178.

Bothwell, J.E., Dooley, J.M., Gordon, K.E., MacAuley, A., Camfield, P.R. and MacSween, J. (2002). Duchenne muscular dystrophy–parental perceptions. *Clin Pediatr*, **41**, 105–109.

Bridwell, K.H., Baldus, C., Iffrig, T.M., Lenke, L.G. and Blanke, K. (1999). Process measures and patient/parent evaluation of surgical management of spinal deformities in patients with progressive flaccid neuromuscular scoliosis (Duchenne's muscular dystrophy and spinal muscular atrophy). *Spine*, **24**, 1300–1309.

Brooke, M.H. (1986). *A Clinician's View of Neuromuscular Diseases*, 2nd edn., Williams & Wilkins, Baltimore.

Brooke, M.H. (2001). The classification of muscle diseases. In: *Disorders of Voluntary Muscle* (eds Karpati, G., Hilton-Jones, D. and Griggs, R.C.), 7th edn., Cambridge University Press, Cambridge, pp. 374–384.

Buck, F.M. (1993). Parenting by fathers with physical disabilities. In: *Reproductive Issues for Persons with Physical Disabilities* (eds Haseltine, F.P., Cole, S.S. and Gray, D.B.), Paul H. Brookes, Baltimore, MD, pp. 163–185.

Bushby, K.M. (1999). Making sense of the limb-girdle muscular dystrophies. *Brain*, **122**, 1403–1420.

Chamberlain, J.S. (2002). Gene therapy of muscular dystrophy. *Human Mol Genet*, **11**, 2355–2362.

Dahlbom, K., Ahlstrom, G., Barany, M., Kihlgren, A. and Gunnarsson, L.G. (1999). Muscular dystrophy in adults: a five-year follow-up. *Scand J Rehabil Med*, **31**, 178–184.

de Lateur, B.J. and Giaconi, R.M. (1979). Effects on maximal strength of submaximal exercise in Duchenne's muscular dystrophy. *Am J Phys Med*, **58(1)**, 26–36.

DeLuca, A., Pierno, S. and Liantonio, D.C.C. (2002). Pre-clinical trials in Duchenne dystrophy: what animal models can tell us about potential drug effectiveness. *Neuromuscul Disord*, **12**, S142–S146.

Edwards, R.H., Round, J.M., Jackson, M.J., Griffiths, R.D. and Lilburn, M.F. (1984). Weight reduction in boys with muscular dystrophy. *Dev Med Child Neurol*, **26**, 384–390.

Engvall, E. and Wewer, U.M. (2003). The new frontier in muscular dystrophy research: booster genes. *FASEB J*, **17**, 1579–1584.

Escolar, D.M., Henricson, E.K., Pasquali, L., Gorni, K. and Hoffman, E.P. (2002). Collaborative translational research leading to multicenter clinical trials in Duchenne muscular dystrophy: the Cooperative International Neuromuscular Research Group (CINRG). *Neuromuscul Disord*, **12**, S147–S154.

Fardeau-Gautier, M. and Fardeau, M. (1994). Socioeconomic aspects of neuromuscular disease. In: *Myology* (eds Engel, A.G. and Franzini-Armstrong, C.), 2nd edn., McGraw-Hill, New York, pp. 739–745.

Ferrari, G. and Mavilio, F. (2002). Myogenic stem cells from the bone marrow: a therapeutic alternative for muscular dystrophy? *Neuromuscul Disord*, **12**, S7–S10.

Fiatarone, M.A. and Evans, W.J. (1993). The etiology and reversibility of muscle dysfunction in the aged. *J Gerontol*, **48**, 77–83.

Filart, R.A. and Bach, J.R. (2003). Pulmonary physical medicine interventions for elderly patients with muscular dysfunction. *Clin Geriatr Med*, **19**, 189–204.

Finsterer, J. and Stollberger, C. (2003). The heart in human dystrophinopathies. *Cardiology*, **99**, 1–19.

Fitzpatrick, C., Barry, C. and Garvey, C. (1986). Psychiatric disorder among boys with Duchenne muscular dystrophy. *Dev Med Child Neurol*, **28**, 589–595.

Forst, J. and Forst, R. (1999). Lower limb surgery in Duchenne muscular dystrophy. *Neuromuscul Disord*, **9**, 176–181.

Fowler Jr., W.M., Abresh, R.T., Koch, T.R., Brewer, M.L., Bowden, R.K. and Wanlass, R.L. (1997). Employment profiles in neuromuscular diseases. *Am J Phys Med Rehabil*, **76(1)**, 26–37.

Galloway, G., Murphy, P., Chesson, A.L. and Martinez, K. (2003). MDA and AAEM informational brochures: Can patients read them? *J Neurosci Nurs*, **35**, 171–174.

Gamzu, R., Shenhav, M., Fainaru, O., Almog, B., Kupferminc, M. and Lessing, J.B. (2002). Impact of pregnancy on respiratory capacity in women with muscular dystrophy and kyphoscoliosis. A case report. *J Reprod Med*, **47**, 53–56.

Gardner-Medwin, D. (1979). Controversies about Duchenne muscular dystrophy (2) bracing for ambulation. *Dev Med Child Neurol*, **21**, 659–662.

Gilgoff, I., Prentice, W. and Baydur, A. (1989). Patient and family participation in the management of respiratory failure in Duchenne's muscular dystrophy. *Chest*, **95**, 519–524.

Goldstein, M., Meyer, S. and Freund, H.R. (1989). Effects of overfeeding in children with muscle dystrophies. *J Parenter Enter Nutr*, **13**, 603–607.

Hagberg, J.M., Carroll, J.E. and Brooke, M.H. (1980). Endurance exercise training in a patient with central core disease. *Neurology*, **30**, 1242–1244.

Hankard, R., Gottrand, F., Turck, D., Carpentier, A., Romon, M. and Farriaux, J.P. (1996). Resting energy expenditure and energy substrate utilization in children with Duchenne muscular dystrophy. *Pediatr Res*, **40**, 29–33.

Harper, C.M. (2002). Congenital myopathies and muscular dystrophies. In: *Neuromuscular Function and Disease: Basic, Clinical, and Electrodiagnostic Aspects* (eds Brown, W.F., Bolton, C.F. and Aminoff, M.J.), Vol. 2, W.B. Saunders, New York, pp. 1355–1374.

Hilton-Jones, D. and Kissel, J.T. (2001). The examination and investigation of the patient with muscle disease. In: *Disorders of Voluntary Muscle* (eds Karpati, G., Hilton-Jones, D. and Griggs, R.C.), 7th edn., Cambridge, New York, pp. 349–373.

Hirano, M. and DiMauro, S. (2002). Metabolic myopathies. In: *Advances in Neurology: Neuromuscular Disorders* (eds

Pourmand, R. and Harati, Y.), Vol. 88, Lippincott, Williams, and Wilkins, New York, pp. 217–234.

Hoffman, D.J. and Gallagher, D. (2001). Obesity and weight control. In: *Downey and Darlings' Physiological Basis of Rehabilitation Medicine* (eds Gonzalez, E.G., Myers, S.J., Edelstein, J.E., Lieberman, J.S. and Downey, J.A.), 3rd edn., Butterworth/Heinemann, Boston, pp. 485–505.

Ishpekova, B., Milanov, I., Christova, L.G. and Alexandrov, A.S. (1999). Comparative analysis between Duchenne and Becker types muscular dystrophy. *Electromyogr Clin Neurophysiol*, **39**, 315–318.

Johnson, E.R., Fowler Jr., W.M. and Lieberman, J.S. (1992). Contractures in neuromuscular disease. *Arch Phys Med Rehabil*, **73**(**9**), 807–810.

Katirji, B. (2002). Clinical assessment in neuromuscular disorders. In: *Neuromuscular Disorders in Clinical Practice* (eds Katirji, B., Kaminski, H.J., Preston, D.C., Ruff, R.L. and Shapiro, B.E.), Butterworth Heinemann, Boston, pp. 3–19.

Kilmer, D.D., Abresch, R.T., McCrory, M.A., Carter, G.T., Fowler, W.J., Johnson, E.R. and McDonald, C.M. (1995). Profiles of neuromuscular diseases. Facioscapulohumeral muscular dystrophy. *Am J Phys Med Rehabil*, **74**, S131–S139.

Kilmer, D.D., Aitkens, S.G., Wright, N.C. and McCrory, M.A. (2001). Response to high-intensity eccentric muscle contractions in persons with myopathic disease. *Muscle Nerve*, **24**, 1181–1187.

Kinnealey, M. and Morse, A.B. (1979). Educational mainstreaming of physically handicapped children. *Am J Occup Ther*, **33**, 365–372.

Kleopa, K.A., Rosenberg, H. and Heiman-Patterson, T. (2000). Malignant hyperthermia-like episode in Becker muscular dystrophy. *Anesthesiology*, **93**, 1535–1537.

Lang, S.A., Duncan, P.G. and Dupuis, P.R. (1989). Fatal air embolism in an adolescent with Duchenne muscular dystrophy during Harrington instrumentation. *Anesth Analg*, **69**, 132–134.

Lexell, J. and Vandervoort, A.A. (2002). Age-related changes in the neuromuscular system. In: *Neuromuscular Function and Disease: Basic, Clinical, and Electrodiagnostic Aspects* (eds Brown, W.F., Bolton, C.F. and Aminoff, M.J.), Vol. 1, W.B. Saunders, New York, pp. 591–601.

Matsuo, M. (2002). Duchenne and Becker muscular dystrophy: from gene diagnosis to molecular therapy. *Life*, **53**, 147–152.

Matthews, K.D. and Moore, S.A. (2003). Limb-girdle muscular dystrophy. *Curr Neurol Neurosci Rep*, **3**, 78–85.

McCarthy, R.E. (1999). Management of neuromuscular scoliosis. *Orthop Clin N Am*, **30**, 435–449, viii.

McCrory, M.A., Wright, N.C. and Kilmer, D.D. (1998). Nutritional aspects of neuromuscular diseases. *Phys Med Rehabil Clin N Am*, **9**, 127–143.

McDonald, C.M., Johnson, E.R., Abresch, R.T., Carter, G.T., Fowler, W.J. and Kilmer, D.D. (1995a). Profiles of neuromuscular diseases. Limb-girdle syndromes. *Am J Phys Med Rehabil*, **74**, S117–S130.

McDonald, C.M., Abresch, R.T., Carter, G.T., Fowler, W.J., Johnson, E.R. and Kilmer, D.D. (1995b). Profiles of neuromuscular diseases. Becker's muscular dystrophy. *Am J Phys Med Rehabil*, **74**, S93–S103.

Melacini, P., Vianello, A., Villanova, C., Fanin, M., Miorin, M., Angelini, C. and Dalla Volta, S. (1996). Cardiac and respiratory involvement in advanced stage Duchenne muscular dystrophy. *Neuromuscular Disord*, **6**, 367–376.

Meola, G., Karpati, G. and Griggs, R.C. (2001). The principles of treatment, prevention, and rehabilitation and perspectives on future therapies. In: *Disorders of Voluntary Muscle* (eds Karpati, G., Hilton-Jones, D. and Griggs, R.C.), 7th edn., Cambridge, New York, pp. 739–754.

Miller, J.R. (1991). Family response to Duchenne muscular dystrophy. In: *Muscular Dystrophy and Other Neuromuscular Diseases: Psychosocial Issues* (eds Charash, L.I., Lovelace, R.E., Leach, C.F., Kutscher, A.H., Goldberg, J. and Roye, D.P.J.), Haworth, New York, pp. 31–42.

Miller, J.R., Colbert, A.P. and Osberg, J.S. (1990). Ventilator dependency: decision-making, daily functioning and quality of life for patients with Duchenne muscular dystrophy. *Dev Med Child Neurol*, **32**, 1078–1086.

Miller, R.G., Chalmers, A.C., Dao, H., Filler-Katz, A., Holman, D. and Bost, F. (1991). The effect of spine fusion on respiratory function in Duchenne muscular dystrophy. *Neurology*, **41**, 38–40.

Milner-Brown, H.S. and Miller, R.G. (1988a). Muscle strengthening through high-resistance weight training in patients with neuromuscular disorders. II. *Arch Phys Med Rehabil*, **69**, 14–19.

Milner-Brown, H.S. and Miller, R.G. (1988b). Muscle strengthening through electric stimulation combined with low-resistance weights in patients with neuromuscular disorders. I. *Arch Phys Med Rehabil*, **69**, 20–24.

Mummery, C.J., Copeland, S.A. and Rose, M.R. (2003). Scapular fixation in muscular dystrophy. *Cochrane Database Sys Rev*, **3**.

Muntoni, F. (2003). Cardiac complications of childhood myopathies. *J Child Neurol*, **18**, 191–202.

Natterlund, B. and Ahlstrom, G. (1999). Problem-focused coping and satisfaction with activities of daily living in individuals with muscular dystrophy and postpolio syndrome. *Scand J Caring Sci*, **13**, 26–32.

Natterlund, B., Sjoden, P.O. and Ahlstrom, G. (2001). The illness experience of adult persons with muscular dystrophy. *Disabil Rehabil*, **23**, 788–798.

Nazir, M.A., Dillon, W.P. and McPherson, E.W. (1984). Myotonic dystrophy in pregnancy. Prenatal, neonatal and maternal considerations. *J Reprod Med*, **29**, 168–172.

Nelson, M.R. (1996). Rehabilitation concerns in myopathies. In: *Physical Medicine and Rehabilitation* (eds Bradom, R.L., Buschbacher, R.M., Dumitru, D., Johnson, E.W., Matthews, D. and Sinaki, M.), W.B. Saunders, Philadelphia, PA, pp. 1003–1026.

Noordeen, M.H., Haddad, F.S., Muntoni, F., Gobbi, P., Hollyer, J.S. and Bentley, G. (1999). Blood loss in Duchenne muscular dystrophy: vascular smooth muscle dysfunction? *J Pediatr Orthop, Part B*, **8**, 212–215.

Oguz, D., Olgunturk, R., Tunaoglu, F.S., Gucuyener, K., Kose, G. and Unlu, M. (2000). Evaluation of dysrhythmia in children with muscular dystrophy. *Angiology*, **51**, 925–931.

Pelargonio, G., Dello Russo, A., Sanna, T., De Martino, G. and Bellocci, F. (2002). Myotonic dystrophy and the heart. *Heart*, **88**, 665–670.

Perkins, K.J. and Davies, K.E. (2002). The role of utrophin in the potential therapy of Duchene muscular dystrophy. *Neuromuscul Disord*, **12**, S78–S89.

Phillips, B.A. and Mastaglia, F.L. (2000). Exercise therapy in patients with myopathy. *Curr Opin Neurol*, **13**, 547–552.

Polakoff, R.J., Morton, A.A., Koch, K.D. and Rios, C.M. (1998). The psychosocial and cognitive impact of Duchenne's muscular dystrophy. *Semin Pediatr Neurol*, **5**, 116–123.

Preedy, V.R., Adachi, J., Ueno, Y., Ahmed, S., Mantle, D., Mullatti, N., Rajendram, R. and Peters, T.J. (2001). Alcoholic skeletal muscle myopathy: definitions, features, contribution of neuropathy, impact and diagnosis. *Eur J Neurol*, **8**, 677–687.

Quane, K.A., Healy, J.M.S., Keating, K.E., Manning, B.M., Cauch, F.J., Palmucci, L.M., Doriguzzi, C., Fagerlund, T.H., Berg, K., Ording, H., Bendixen, D., Mortier, W., Linz, U., Muller, C.R. and McCarthy, T.V. (1993). Mutations in the ryanodine receptor gene in central core disease and malignant hyperthermia. *Nat Genet*, **5**, 51–55.

Raphael, J.C., Chevret, S., Chastang, C. and Bouvet, F. (1994). Randomised trial of preventive nasal ventilation in Duchene muscular dystrophy. French multicentre cooperative group on home mechanical ventilation assistance in Duchenne de Boulogne muscular dystrophy. *Lancet*, **343**, 1600–1604.

Reid, J.M. and Appleton, P.J. (1999). A case of ventricular fibrillation in the prone position during back stabilisation surgery in a boy with Duchenne's muscular dystrophy. *Anaesthesia*, **54**, 364–367.

Rittoo, D.B. and Morris, P. (1995). Tracheal occlusion in the prone position in an intubated patient with Duchenne muscular dystrophy. *Anaesthesia*, **50**, 719–721.

Rogers, J. and Matsumura, M. (1991). *Mother-to-be: A Guide to Pregnancy and Birth for Women with Disabilities*, Demos, New York.

Rosenfeld, J. and Jackson, C.E. (2002). Quantitative assessment and outcome measures in neuromuscular disease. In: *Neuromuscular Disorders in Clinical Practice* (eds Katirji, B., Kaminski, H.J., Preston, D.C., Ruff, R.L. and Shapiro, B.E.), Butterworth-Heinemann, Boston, pp. 309–343.

Rudnik-Schoneborn, S., Glauner, B., Rohrig, D. and Zerres, K. (1997). Obstetric aspects in women with facioscapulohumeral muscular dystrophy, limb-girdle muscular dystrophy, and congenital myopathies. *Arch Neurol*, **54**, 888–894.

Ryan, M.M., Schnell, C., Strickland, C.D., Shield, L.K., Morgan, G., Iannaccone, S.T., Laing, N.G., Beggs, A.H. and North, K.N. (2001). Nemaline myopathy: a clinical study of 143 cases. *Ann Neurol*, **50**, 312–320.

Scott, O.M., Hyde, S.A., Vrbova, G. and Dubowitz, V. (1990). Therapeutic possibilities of chronic low frequency electrical stimulation in children with Duchenne muscular dystrophy. *J Neurol Sci*, **95**, 171–182.

Seeger, B.R., Caudrey, D.J. and Little, J.D. (1985). Progression of equinus deformity in Duchenne muscular dystrophy. *Arch Phys Med Rehabil*, **66**, 286–288.

Shapiro, F. and Specht, L. (1991). Orthopedic deformities in Emery–Dreifuss muscular dystrophy. *J Pediatr Orthop*, **11**, 336–340.

Siegel, I.M. (1978). The management of muscular dystrophy: a clinical review. *Muscle Nerve*, 453–460.

Simmons, R. (1986). *Reach for Fitness: A Special Book of Exercises for the Physically Challenged*, Warner, New York.

Skuk, D., Vilquin, J.T. and Tremblay, J.P. (2002). Experimental and therapeutic approaches to muscular dystrophies. *Curr Opin Neurol*, **15**, 563–569.

Strauss, N.E. and Angell, D.K. (2001). Foot conditions related to neuromuscular disorders in adults. In: *Foot and Ankle Rehabilitation* (eds Kim, D.D.J. and Wainapel, S.F.), Vol. 15(3), Hanley and Belfus, Philadelphia, pp. 489–501.

Sun, S. F., Binder, J., Streib, E. and Goodlin, R.C. (1985). Myotonic dystrophy: obstetric and neonatal complications. *South Med J*, **78**, 823–826.

Taktak, D.M. and Bowker, P. (1995). Lightweight, modular knee–ankle–foot orthosis for Duchenne muscular dystrophy: design, development, and evaluation. *Arch Phys Med Rehabil*, **76**, 1156–1162.

Taratuto, A.L. (2002). Congenital myopathies and related disorders. *Curr Opin Neurol*, **15**, 553–561.

Tubridy, N., Fontaine, B. and Eymard, B. (2001). Congenital myopathies and congenital muscular dystrophies. *Curr Opin Neurol*, **14**, 575–582.

Tung, H.C., Chen, Y.J., Su, S.Y. and Chao, C.C. (1989). Epidural anesthesia for major abdominal surgery complicated by muscular dystrophy–a case report. *Ma Tsui Hsueh Tsa Chi Anaesthesiol Sin*, **27**, 75–78.

Twyman, R.S., Harper, G.D. and Edgar, M.A. (1996). Thoracoscapular fusion in facioscapulohumeral dystrophy: clinical review of a new surgical method. *J Shoulder Elb Surg*, **5**, 201–205.

Tyler, K.L. (2003). Origins and early descriptions of "Duchenne muscular dystrophy". *Muscle Nerve*, **28**, 402–422.

Vignos, P.J., Wagner, M.B., Karlinchak, B. and Katirji, B. (1996a) Evaluation of a program for long-term treatment of Duchenne muscular dystrophy. Experience at the University Hospitals of Cleveland. *J Bone Surg Am*, Dec, **78(12)**, 18441–18852.

von Wendt, L.O. and Autti-Ramo, I.S. (1999). Botulinum toxin for amelioration of knee contracture in Duchenne muscular dystrophy. *Euro J Paediatr Neurol*, **3**, 175–176.

Wagner, M.B. and Katirji, B. (2002). Rehabilitation management and care of patients with neuromuscular diseases. In: *Neuromuscular Disorders in Clinical Practice* (eds Katirji, B., Kaminski, H.J., Preston, D.C., Ruff, R.L. and Shapiro, B.E.), Butterworth-Heinemann, Boston, pp. 344–363.

Walton, J.N. and Gardner-Medwin, D. (1974). Progressive muscular dystrophy and myotonic disorders. In: *Disorders of Voluntary Muscle* (ed. Walton, J.), 3rd edn., Churchill-Livingstone, London, pp. 561–613.

Wells, D.J. and Wells, K.E. (2002). Gene transfer studies in animals: what do they really tell us about the prospects for gene therapy in DMD? *Neuromuscular Disord*, **12**, S11–S22.

Wong, C.K. and Wade, C.K. (1995). Reducing iliotibial band contractures in patients with muscular dystrophy using custom dry floatation cushions. *Arch Phys Med Rehabil*, **76**, 695–700.

Wu, C.C., Tseng, C.S., Shen, C.H., Yang, T.C., Chi, K.P. and Ho, Q.M. (1998). Succinylcholine-induced cardiac arrest in unsuspected Becker muscular dystrophy–a case report. *Acta Anaesth Sin*, **36**, 165–168.

Yasuda, Y.L., Bowman, K. and Hsu, J.D. (1986). Mobile arm supports: criteria for successful use in muscle disease patients. *Arch Phys Med Rehabil*, **67**, 253–256.

Zupan, A., Gregoric, M., Valencic, V. and Vandot, S. (1993). Effects of electrical stimulation on muscles of children with Duchenne and Becker muscular dystrophy. *Neuropediatrics*, **24**, 189–192.

Index

Page numbers in **bold** refer to **Volume II** and otherwise to Volume I.

699

Page numbers in **bold** refer to **Volume II** and otherwise to Volume I.

Page numbers in **bold** refer to **Volume II** and otherwise to Volume I.

Page numbers in **bold** refer to **Volume II** and otherwise to Volume I.

Page numbers in **bold** refer to **Volume II** and otherwise to Volume I.

Page numbers in **bold** refer to **Volume II** and otherwise to Volume I.

Page numbers in **bold** refer to **Volume II** and otherwise to Volume I.

Page numbers in **bold** refer to **Volume II** and otherwise to Volume I.

Page numbers in **bold** refer to **Volume II** and otherwise to Volume I.

Page numbers in **bold** refer to **Volume II** and otherwise to Volume I.

Page numbers in **bold** refer to **Volume II** and otherwise to Volume I.